W9-BSN-847

Coronary Care

Coronary Care

Second Edition

Edited by

Gary S. Francis, M.D.
Professor of Medicine, University of Minnesota Medical School; Director, Acute Cardiac Care, University of Minnesota Hospital and Clinic, Minneapolis

Joseph S. Alpert, M.D.
Robert S. and Irene P. Flinn Professor of Medicine, University of Arizona College of Medicine; Head, Department of Medicine, University Medical Center, Tucson

Foreword by
Harold J. C. Swan, M.D., Ph.D.
Professor of Medicine (Emeritus), University of California, Los Angeles, UCLA School of Medicine; Director of Cardiology (Emeritus), Cedars-Sinai Medical Center, Los Angeles

Little, Brown and Company
Boston New York Toronto London

Second Edition

Previous edition titled *Modern Coronary Care* copyright © 1990 by Gary S. Francis and Joseph S. Alpert

Library of Congress Cataloging-in-Publication Data
Coronary care / edited by Gary S. Francis,
Joseph S. Alpert.—2nd ed.
p. cm.
Rev. ed. of: Modern coronary care. c 1990.
Includes bibliographical references and index.
ISBN 0-316-29161-7
1. Myocardial infarction. I. Francis, Gary S., 1943– .
II. Alpert, Joseph S. III. Modern coronary care.
[DNLM: 1. Myocardial Infarction—therapy. 2. Myocardial Infarction—diagnosis. WG 300 C82125 1995]
RC685.I6.M573 1995
616.1′237—dc20
DNLM/DLC
for Library of Congress 95-16985
CIP

Printed in the United States of America
MV-NY

Editorial: Nancy Megley, Richard L. Wilcox
Production Editor: Anne Holm
Copyeditors: Mary Babcock, Anne Miller
Indexer: Betty Hallinger
Production Supervisor/Designer: Cate Rickard
Cover Designer: Cate Rickard

To our parents and teachers, without whom it would never have been started; and to our wives, Margaret and Helle, without whom it would never have been finished

Contents

IV. Mechanical Complications of Acute Myocardial Infarction: Diagnosis and Treatment

V. Miscellaneous Complications of Acute Myocardial Infarction

VI. Special Procedures in Acute Myocardial Infarction

VIII. Post–Myocardial Infarction Considerations

IX. Administrative Decisions in the Coronary Care Unit

Foreword

Rapid changes in our knowledge concerning coronary atherosclerosis and its complications clearly justify a new edition of *Coronary Care.* As our understanding has increased, our management strategies have undergone modification of a greater or lesser degree. In many aspects, a radical shift is taking place, and Drs. Francis and Alpert, together with their contributing authors, have gone to great lengths to see that this is reflected throughout the second edition.

Coronary care is offered to those patients having or suspected of having coronary atherosclerosis and one or more of its thrombotic complications. An appreciation of the vital role of thrombosis in the acute clinical syndromes of unstable angina and acute myocardial infarction is less than two decades old. With total occlusion both myocyte death and intramyocardial collagen disruption occur rapidly. Thus, interventions to prevent occlusion or to restore blood flow are now recognized as the cornerstone of management. Thrombolytic therapy is discussed throughout this second edition, with Chapter 20 specifically addressing unstable angina.

While the "open vessel" theory, addressed in Chapter 27, is reasonable and accepted by all, the timing of that opening is now evidently critical. Late opening may be associated with improved healing and a reduction in the incidence of cardiac arrhythmias. However, the problem of adverse remodeling of large infarcts in many patients remains unsolved. Experimental studies in animals indicate that the current permissible interval between total occlusion and reperfusion of up to 4 hours is far too long. The objective to reduce the time to treatment to a more desirable 90 minutes may be possible for many patients. This requires reconsideration of management in the home (for example, aspirin therapy) and initiation of thrombolytic (and perhaps anticoagulation) therapy by paramedics.

The critical role of disturbed vascular biology in atherogenesis, and in the complications of coronary atherosclerosis, as thoroughly examined in Parts III, IV, and V of this text, is becoming evermore apparent. As the number of related factors and their variable interaction are studied, the designation of this disease as "polygenic, multifactorial" becomes obvious. Platelet function and hemostatic mechanisms exhibit a circadian behavior and can be modified by autonomic triggers. Areas of lipid-rich atheroma proximate to established stenosis with a weakened fibrous cap may provide a powerful thrombogenic effect on flowing blood. A variety of mechanisms are implicated in vascular spasm, plaque rupture, and the natural thrombotic and antithrombotic, coagulative and anticoagulative balances that exist in circulating blood. Recent large-scale clinical trials have, regrettably, focused on the relatively minor advantages of one lytic or anticoagulative agent or combination thereof when compared to another. These trials have deviated attention from the fundamental importance of the time from complete coronary occlusion to the initiation of reperfusion. As Drs. Francis and Alpert discuss throughout *Coronary Care,* clearly a new focus on strategies to facilitate the shortest possible time between symptom onset and drug administration is now necessary. The incidence of chronic heart failure over the past three decades has increased—probably due to patients who have survived larger myocardial infarctions. That we have substituted chronic heart failure for improved hospital mortality is a cause for concern.

The benefits of mechanical revascularization evidenced by older surgical studies are now being confirmed in those patients suitable for prompt direct angioplasty that successfully displaces intravascular thrombus and modifies residual disease of the culprit vessel. These results suggest that a prompt evaluation of coronary anatomy may provide benefit. The management of patients with coronary atherosclerosis following myocardial infarction or unstable angina has been less than satisfactory, and cardiologists must become knowledgeable about diabetes, lipids, and thrombosis. Dependency on dietary intervention to substantially modify abnormal lipid patterns has not been successful—although the resulting benefits of weight loss and modification of high blood pressure are unquestioned. Recent drug studies have demonstrated that significant lipid lowering is accompanied by a marked reduction in clinical events in patients with established coronary artery disease—with or without prior myocardial infarction. Substantial and sustained lipid lowering achieved by the statin class of lipid-lowering drugs points to the probability of major benefit. Chapter 35 combines insightful text with useful tables in its discussion of lipids and lipid-lowering drugs.

New developments concerning coagulation-related risk (fibrinogen, serum iron, platelet adhesiveness, and other factors) are in the forefront of research in this field and will undoubtedly play a significant part in coronary care in the future. These issues, and ongoing consideration of the inflammatory nature of early atherogenesis and the possible relation of a disturbance of endothelial function due to viral infection, offer good reason to believe that a third edition of this excellent text by Drs. Francis and Alpert will be required in the not too distant future.

Harold J. C. Swan

Preface

The last two decades have witnessed remarkable growth in our understanding of acute, unstable ischemic heart disease. A great deal is now known about the pathophysiology of these clinical syndromes. Diagnosis and therapy have also improved quite remarkably. As a result of these advances, morbidity and mortality have declined strikingly. Nevertheless, there is still a great deal of information that needs to be acquired if we are to achieve continuing advances in this arena. Nowhere is this need more challenging than in the patients with acute myocardial infarction. Myocardial reperfusion therapy, angioplasty, and pharmacologic support of patients with acute unstable coronary artery disease are improving constantly. Many uncertainties remain, however. What is clear is that therapy has continued to evolve in the direction of rapid intervention. With changing therapy come new complications, additional costs, and conflicting data. Periodically, it is essential that we pause and review the progress made to date, realizing that the very latest information cannot always be included. It is in this spirit, the contemplative pause, during which information is digested and assimilated, that we present the second edition of *Coronary Care,* a single authoritative source encompassing diagnosis and management of patients with acute coronary syndromes.

The purpose of the first edition of this book was to update physicians and other health care personnel concerning acute coronary care. Contributing authors were asked to provide an up-to-date and balanced review of their topics, realizing that there still was substantial controversy and uncertainty in many areas, such as thrombolytic therapy and emergent angioplasty. Diagnostic and therapeutic options were discussed in detail, with some overlap provided to emphasize varying points of view.

For the second edition, we urged contributors to update their subject area and to refine pathophysiologic, diagnostic, and therapeutic paradigms in light of advances achieved during the 5 years that have passed since the original edition was published. Approaches to the care of patients with acute coronary syndromes will continue to be refined, but our intent is to furnish the reader with the most current data and hypotheses in this era of coronary care.

This text is not intended to be an exhaustive or entirely comprehensive review of the subject matter. For example, electrocardiographic changes present in acute myocardial infarction are not discussed in detail. Myocardial imaging with positron emission tomography (PET) or magnetic resonance imaging (MRI) is mentioned only briefly. In the case of electrocardiography, there are many excellent textbooks available that discuss the subject thoroughly. The imaging techniques of PET and MRI are still evolving, particularly in the context of acute myocardial infarction, and are not used routinely to manage patients with unstable coronary disease. This presentation may change in coming decades and chapter contents will be altered accordingly.

We wish to express our gratitude to the contributing authors who participated in this venture and who provided critical reviews of subject matter related to their areas of expertise. This is truly their book. Nearly all contributors are actively involved in the day-to-day care of patients with acute myocardial infarction, and thus can provide useful and practical guidelines for readers. We are also most grateful to our editors at Little, Brown and Company, without whose tireless efforts this second edition could never have been completed. We are also very grateful to our spouses and families, whose support is essential in any undertaking of this nature. We hope that our readers will find this second edition as useful and comprehensive as the original volume.

G. S. F.
J. S. A.

Contributing Authors

Joseph S. Alpert, M.D. Robert S. and Irene P. Flinn Professor of Medicine, University of Arizona College of Medicine; Head, Department of Medicine, University Medical Center, Tuscon

William F. Armstrong, M.D. Professor of Internal Medicine, University of Michigan Medical School; Director, Echocardiography Laboratory, University of Michigan Medical Center, Ann Arbor, Michigan

Jean T. Barbey, M.D. Assistant Professor of Medicine and Pharmacology, Georgetown University School of Medicine; Director, Cardiac Telemetry and Holter Laboratory, Georgetown Medical Center, Washington

Bradi L. Bartrug, M.S.N. Clinical Associate, School of Nursing, Duke University Medical Center; Cardiology Clinical Nurse Specialist, Department of Heart and Emergency Nursing, Duke University Medical Center, Durham, North Carolina

J. A. Bianco, M.D. Associate Professor of Radiology, University of Wisconsin Medical School; Physician, Department of Nuclear Medicine, University of Wisconsin Clinical Science Center, Madison, Wisconsin

R. Morton Bolman III, M.D. C. Walton and Richard C. Lillehei Professor of Surgery, University of Minnesota Medical School; Chief, Division of Cardiovascular and Thoracic Surgery, University of Minnesota Hospital and Clinic, Minneapolis

Wanda M. Bride, R.N. Head Nurse, Cardiac Care Unit, Duke University Medical Center, Durham, North Carolina

Edward J. Brown, Jr., M.D. Associate Professor of Medicine, Albert Einstein College of Medicine of Yeshiva University; Chief, Cardiology Division, Bronx-Lebanon Hospital Center, New York

Robert P. Byington, Ph.D. Associate Professor of Public Health Sciences, Bowman Gray School of Medicine of Wake Forest University, Winston-Salem, North Carolina

Robert M. Califf, M.D. Associate Professor of Medicine, Duke University School of Medicine, Durham, North Carolina

Kanu Chatterjee, M.B. Professor of Medicine and Lucie Stern Professor of Cardiology, University of California, San Francisco, School of Medicine; Associate Chief, Division of Cardiology, Moffitt-Long Hospital, San Francisco

Lynn. P. Clemow, Ph.D.

Assistant Professor of Medicine, University of Massachusetts Medical School; Clinical Director, Division of Preventive/Behavioral Medicine, University of Massachusetts Medical Center, Worcester, Massachusetts

Jay N. Cohn, M.D.

Professor of Medicine, University of Minnesota Medical School; Head, Cardiovascular Division, University of Minnesota Hospital and Clinic, Minneapolis

James R. Corbett, M.D.

Associate Professor of Radiology, University of Texas Southwestern Medical Center at Dallas, Southwestern Medical School; Director of Nuclear Cardiology, University of Texas Southwestern Medical Center at Dallas

James E. Dalen, M.D.

Dean and Vice Provost for Health Sciences, University of Arizona College of Medicine, Tucson

Charles A. Dennis, M.D.

Chairman, Department of Cardiology, Deborah Heart and Lung Center, Browns Mills, New Jersey

Marcus A. DeWood, M.D.

Director of Research, Spokane Heart Research Foundation, Spokane, Washington

Brooks S. Edwards, M.D.

Professor of Medicine, Mayo Medical School; Consultant, Division of Cardiovascular Diseases, Mayo Clinic, Rochester, Minnesota

Jesse E. Edwards, M.D.

Clinical Professor of Laboratory Medicine and Pathology, University of Minnesota Medical School, Minneapolis; Senior Consultant, Registry of Cardiovascular Pathology, United Hospital, St. Paul, Minnesota

Gordon A. Ewy, M.D.

Professor of Medicine and Chief, Cardiology Division, University of Arizona College of Medicine; Director, Department of Diagnostic Cardiology, University Medical Center, Tucson

Antonio Fernández-Ortiz, M.D., Ph.D.

Assistant Cardiologist, Cardiac Catheterization Laboratory, San Carlos University Hospital, Complutense University, Madrid, Spain

Gary S. Francis, M.D.

Professor of Medicine, University of Minnesota Medical School; Director, Acute Cardiac Care, University of Minnesota Hospital and Clinic, Minneapolis

Curt D. Furberg, M.D., Ph.D.

Professor and Chairman of Public Health Sciences, Bowman Gray School of Medicine of Wake Forest University, Winston-Salem, North Carolina

Valentin Fuster, M.D., Ph.D.

Arthur M. and Hilda A. Master Professor of Medicine and Dean for Academic Affairs, Mount

Sinai School of Medicine of the City University of New York; Director, Cardiovascular Institute, and Vice Chairman, Department of Medicine, Mount Sinai Medical Center, New York

William Ganz, M.D. Professor of Medicine, University of California, Los Angeles, UCLA School of Medicine; Senior Research Scientist, Division of Cardiology, Cedars-Sinai Medical Center, Los Angeles

Otavio C. E. Gebara, M.D. Research Fellow, Harvard Medical School; Research Fellow in Medicine, New England Deaconess Hospital, Boston

Joel M. Gore, M.D. Edward Buchitz Professor of Medicine, University of Massachusetts Medical School; Director, Division of Cardiovascular Medicine, University of Massachusetts Medical Center, Worcester, Massachusetts

Hartmut Henning, M.D. Associate Professor of Medicine, University of British Columbia Faculty of Medicine; Director, Cardiac Care Unit, Vancouver General Hospital, Vancouver, British Columbia

Anne M. Hepner, M.D. Lecturer, Division of Cardiology, University of Michigan Medical School; Staff, Adult Echocardiography Laboratory, University of Michigan Medical Center, Ann Arbor, Michigan

Ik-Kyung Jang, M.D., Ph.D. Assistant Professor of Medicine, Harvard Medical School; Assistant in Medicine, Cardiac Unit, Massachusetts General Hospital, Boston

Martin Juneau, M.D. Assistant Professor of Medicine, Université de Montréal Faculty of Medicine; Chief, Department of Cardiology, Montreal Heart Institute, Montreal

Joel S. Karliner, M.D. Professor of Medicine, University of California, San Francisco, School of Medicine; Chief, Cardiology Section, Veterans Affairs Medical Center, San Francisco

Karl B. Kern, M.D. Associate Professor of Medicine, University of Arizona College of Medicine; Associate Director, Cardiac Catheterization Laboratory, University Medical Center, Tucson

Vibhu R. Kshettry, M.D. Assistant Professor of Cardiovascular and Thoracic Surgery, University of Minnesota Medical School; Director, Circulatory Assist Program, University of Minnesota Hospital and Clinic, Minneapolis

Joseph Loscalzo, M.D., Ph.D.
Distinguished Professor of Cardiovascular Medicine, and Vice Chairman, Department of Medicine, and Director, Whitaker Cardiovascular Institute, Boston University School of Medicine; Chief, Cardiovascular Medicine, Boston University Medical Center Hospital, Boston

Jay W. Mason, M.D.
Professor of Internal Medicine and Chief, Division of Cardiology, University of Utah School of Medicine; Cardiology Staff Physician, Department of Internal Medicine, University of Utah Health Services Center, Salt Lake City

A. Iain McGhie, M.D.
Assistant Professor of Internal Medicine, University of Texas Medical School at Houston; Attending Physician, Department of Internal Medicine/Cardiology, Hermann Hospital, Houston

James E. Muller, M.D.
Associate Professor of Medicine, Harvard Medical School; Chief, Cardiovascular Division, New England Deaconess Hospital, Boston

David R. Murray, M.D.
Assistant Professor of Medicine, University of Texas Medical School at San Antonio; Staff Physician, Division of Cardiology, Audie L. Murphy Memorial Veterans Hospital, San Antonio

Ira S. Ockene, M.D.
Professor of Medicine, University of Massachusetts Medical School, Worcester, Massachusetts

Judith K. Ockene, Ph.D.
Professor of Medicine, University of Massachusetts Medical School; Director, Preventive/Behavioral Medicine, University of Massachusetts Medical Center, Worcester, Massachusetts

Robert A. O'Rourke, M.D.
Professor of Medicine, University of Texas Medical School at San Antonio; Director, Division of Cardiology, University of Texas Health Science Center at San Antonio Teaching Hospitals, San Antonio

Milton Packer, M.D.
Dickinson W. Richards Professor of Medicine, Columbia University College of Physicians and Surgeons; Chief, Division of Circulatory Physiology, and Director, Center for Heart Failure Research, Columbia-Presbyterian Medical Center, New York

John J. Paris, S.J., Ph.D.
Walsh Professor of Bioethics, Boston College; Clinical Professor of Community Health, Tufts University School of Medicine, Boston

Eugene R. Passamani, M.D.
Director, Department of Cardiology, Suburban Hospital, Bethesda, Maryland

Robert W. Peters, M.D.
Professor of Medicine, University of Maryland School of Medicine; Chief, Division of Cardiology, Veterans Affairs Medical Center, Baltimore

Marc A. Pfeffer, M.D., Ph.D.
Associate Professor of Medicine, Harvard Medical School; Physician, Cardiovascular Division, Brigham and Women's Hospital, Boston

Gordon L. Pierpont, M.D., Ph.D.
Associate Professor of Medicine, University of Minnesota Medical School; Medical Director, Coronary Care Unit, Veterans Affairs Medical Center, Minneapolis

Bertram Pitt, M.D.
Professor of Medicine, University of Michigan Medical School; Professor of Medicine, Department of Cardiology, Taubman Medical Center, Ann Arbor, Michigan

Eric N. Prystowsky, M.D.
Consulting Professor of Medicine, Duke University School of Medicine, Durham, North Carolina; Director, Clinical Electrophysiology Laboratory, St. Vincent Hospital, Indianapolis

Peter R. Puleo, M.D.
Attending Cardiologist, Department of Medicine, The Christ Hospital, Cincinnati

David A. Rawling, M.D.
Cardiac Electrophysiologist, The Heart Center of Salt Lake, Salt Lake City

Frank E. Reardon, J.D., M.S.
Partner, Hassan and Reardon Law Offices, Brookline; Chairman, Board of Directors, St. Monica's Nursing Home, Roxbury, Massachusetts

Robert Roberts, M.D.
Professor of Medicine and Cell Biology Baylor College of Medicine; Chief of Cardiology, The Methodist Hospital, Houston

Prediman K. Shah, M.D.
Professor of Medicine, University of California, Los Angeles, UCLA School of Medicine; Shapell and Webb Chair in Cardiology, and Director, In-Patient Cardiology, Cedars-Sinai Medical Center, Los Angeles

John D. Slack, M.D.
Clinical Associate Professor of Medicine, Indiana University School of Medicine; Staff Physician, Department of Cardiology, St. Vincent Hospital, Indianapolis

David H. Spodick, M.D., D.Sc.
Professor of Medicine, University of Massachusetts Medical School; Director, Clinical Cardiology, and Director, Cardiovascular Fellowship Training, St. Vincent Hospital, Worcester, Massachusetts

Borys Surawicz, M.D.
Professor Emeritus of Medicine, Indiana University School of Medicine; Senior Research Associate, Krannert Institute of Cardiology, Indiana University School of Medicine, Indianapolis

Heinrich Taegtmeyer, M.D., D.Phil.
Professor of Internal Medicine, University of Texas Medical School at Houston; Active Staff, Department of Cardiology, Hermann Hospital, Houston

Pierre Théroux, M.D.
Professor of Medicine, Université de Montréal Faculty of Medicine; Director, Coronary Care Unit, Montreal Heart Institute, Montreal

Geoffrey H. Tofler, M.D.
Assistant Professor of Medicine, Harvard Medical School; Cardiologist, New England Deaconess Hospital, Boston

Douglas E. Vaughan, M.D.
Associate Professor of Medicine and Pharmacology, Vanderbilt University School of Medicine; Director, Thrombosis Research, Vanderbilt University Medical Center, Nashville, Tennessee

Galen S. Wagner, M.D.
Associate Professor of Medicine, Duke University School of Medicine, Durham, North Carolina

Ann D. Walling, M.D.
Assistant Professor of Medicine, McGill University Faculty of Medicine; Attending Cardiologist, Sir Mortimer B. Davis–Jewish General Hospital, Montreal

Richard A. Walsh, M.D.
Stonehill Professor of Medicine, University of Cincinnati College of Medicine; Director, Division of Cardiology and Cardiovascular Center, University Hospital, Cincinnati

James T. Willerson, M.D.
Professor and Chairman of Internal Medicine, University of Texas Medical School at Houston; Medical Director, Texas Heart Institute, and Chief, Medical Services, Hermann Hospital, Houston

Andrew A. Wolff, M.D.
Assistant Clinical Professor of Medicine, University of California, San Francisco, School of Medicine; Vice-President, Clinical Research, CV Therapeutics, Palo Alto, California

Raymond L. Woosley, M.D., Ph.D.
Professor of Pharmacology and Medicine and Chairman of Pharmacology, Georgetown University School of Medicine; Member, Medical Staff, Department of Medicine, Georgetown University Hospital, Washington

K. Michael Zabel, M.D.
Fellow in Cardiology, Department of Medicine, Duke University Medical Center, Durham, North Carolina

Doron Zahger, M.D.
Lecturer, Department of Cardiology, Hadassah-Hebrew University; Attending Physician, Department of Cardiology, Hadassah Hospital, Jerusalem

Peter L. Zwerner, M.D.
Assistant Professor of Medicine, University of Massachusetts Medical School, Worcester; Director, Cardiac Catheterization Laboratory, Berkshire Medical Center, Pittsfield, Massachusetts

I.
Pathophysiology and Pathology of Acute Myocardial Infarction

Notice.

The indications and dosages of all drugs in this book have been recommended in the medical literature and conform to the practices of the general medical community. The medications described do not necessarily have specific approval by the Food and Drug Administration for use in the diseases and dosages for which they are recommended. The package insert for each drug should be consulted for use and dosage as approved by the FDA. Because standards for usage change, it is advisable to keep abreast of revised recommendations, particularly those concerning new drugs.

1. Pathophysiology of Acute Myocardial Infarction

Joseph S. Alpert

Nearly 80 years ago two Russian physicians, Obraztsov and Strazhesko, realized that coronary arterial thrombosis led to acute myocardial infarction (AMI) [1]. Shortly thereafter, Herrick made similar observations in the United States [1]. Since these initial descriptions, enormous efforts have been expended to understand the pathophysiology of AMI and its attendant complications. Controversy still surrounds a number of aspects of this pathophysiologic sequence, and our knowledge remains remarkably incomplete. Despite these shortcomings, much has been learned concerning the pathophysiology of AMI, particularly since 1980.

Understanding the pathobiology of AMI is of considerable clinical importance. New therapeutic approaches to this common disease are based on an understanding of its pathophysiology. For example, thrombolytic therapy during the early hours after the onset of infarction is based on the recognition that coronary arterial thrombosis is a central feature of the initial phases of AMI. This chapter reviews the biochemical, ultrastructural, and functional precedents and consequences of AMI.

Atherosclerosis

In most patients with AMI, coronary atherosclerosis is the underlying etiology that eventually leads to infarction. Fatty streaks, the earliest lesions of atherosclerosis, can be found commonly in the coronary arteries of children [2]. With increasing age, fatty streaks evolve into fibromuscular, atherosclerotic plaques. The initial injury to the arterial endothelium that sets in motion the process leading to fatty streaks is apparently mediated by monocytes that adhere to the surface of the coronary arterial endothelium [3]. Platelet adherence, platelet aggregation, and release of smooth muscle and other growth factors cause the embryonic atherosclerotic plaque to increase in size. Adherent monocytes also migrate into the lesion and are transformed into macrophages, which release smooth muscle and fibrous tissue growth factors [2, 3]. The disturbed endothelium is capable of releasing various growth factors as well (Fig. 1-1). The resultant fibrous/smooth muscle plaque demonstrates abnormal transport of lipid from the arterial lumen. Some of this lipid becomes deposited in the plaque, leading to further macrophage infiltration, growth factor release, and smooth muscle fibrous cellular proliferation. Late in this pathophysiologic sequence, necrosis and calcification may develop within the atherosclerotic plaque. A number of possible pathophysiologic events are being considered by various investigators as the first steps in the development of an atherosclerotic plaque. Each of these theories favors a different aspect of the above-mentioned sequence as the primary initiating factor (i.e., platelets, monocytes, lipids). It is possible, however, that all of these sequences are operative at different times and in different individuals, leading to atherosclerotic plaques that are therefore multifactorial in origin.

Myocardial Ischemia

Biochemistry and Electrophysiology

When myocardial oxygen demand exceeds coronary arterial blood flow, myocardial ischemia develops. Cardiac muscle requires large amounts of oxygen and nutrients to function. Indeed, mitochondria, the organelle of oxidative metabolism where adenosine triphosphate (ATP) is generated, make up 25 to 40 percent of the volume of left ventricular

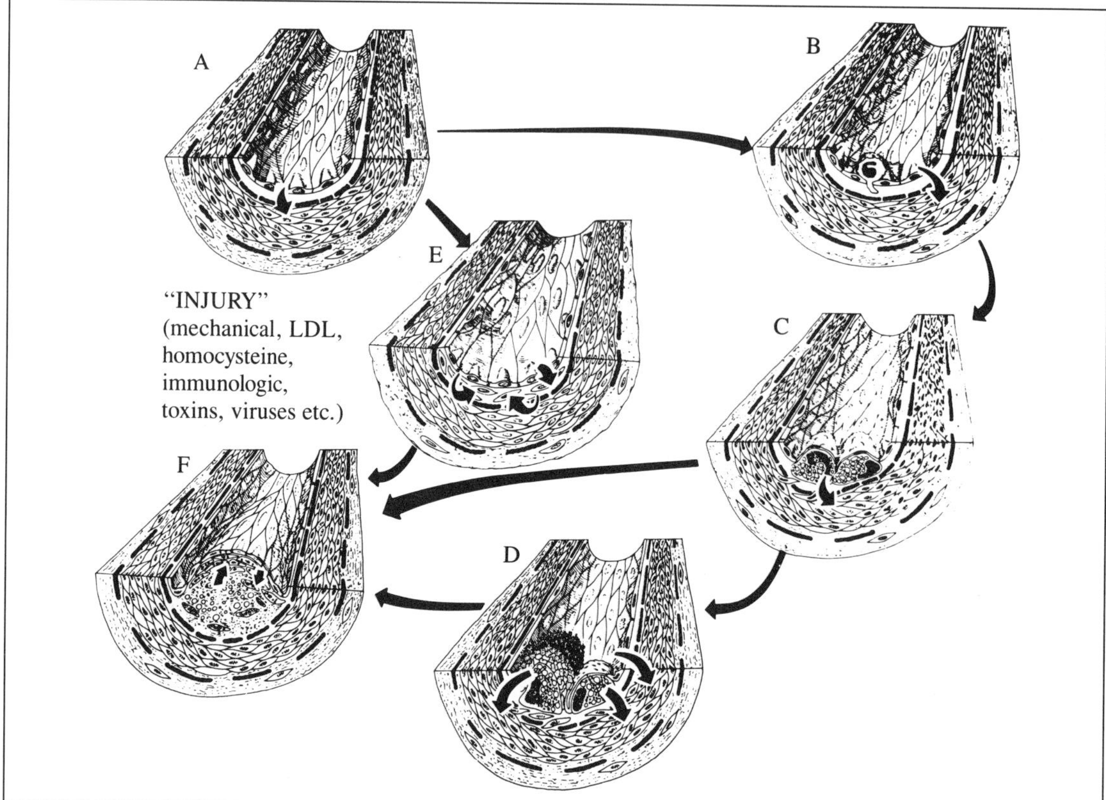

Fig. 1-1
Response of arterial wall to injury: a graphic hypothesis. Atherosclerotic lesions can begin by means of at least two pathways. The pathway demonstrated by the *clockwise, long arrows* is as follows: Injury to arterial endothelium (*A*) may induce growth factor secretion into the arterial media (*short arrows within drawings*). Monocytes attach to the injured endothelium (*B*), which continues to secrete growth factors into the arterial media. Monocytes migrate into the subendothelium and transform into macrophages (*C*), thereby leading to fatty streak formation and further release of growth factors. These fatty streaks may develop directly into fibrous plaques (*long arrow from C to F*) secondary to release of growth factors from macrophages or endothelial cells. Macrophages can also stimulate or injure overlying endothelium. At times, macrophages injure overlying endothelium to such a degree that the endothelium is lost, thereby exposing the underlying fatty streaks to blood flow. Platelet deposition results (*D*), providing yet another source for growth factors stimulation of the subendothelial region. In addition, smooth muscle cells in the proliferating lesion itself (*F*) may secrete growth factors and thereby increase the size of the fibrous plaques. An alternate pathway for the development of advanced atherosclerotic lesions is shown by the *short, clockwise arrows: A–E–F*. Here the endothelium is injured but remains intact. Endothelium secretes growth factor, which stimulates migration of smooth muscle cells from the media into the intima. Further growth factor is produced and released within this zone of injury and cellular migration (*E*). These interactions lead to fibrous plaque formation and further progression of the lesion (*F*). LDL = low-density lipoprotein. (Reprinted by permission from R. Ross, The pathogenesis of atherosclerosis—an update. *N. Engl. J. Med.* 314:488, 1986.)

myocardial cells [4, 5]. With the onset of myocardial ischemia, aerobic mitochondrial function becomes markedly disturbed and ATP production falls off rapidly. Of course some anaerobic production of ATP is possible, but only small quantities are produced, and the end-products of glycolysis inhibit critical enzymes in the glycolytic pathway, thereby further reducing the production of ATP. Thus myocardial cells must have a constant supply of oxygen and nutrients to function.

When myocardial ischemia develops, normal systolic and diastolic function of the myocardium declines within a few seconds. High-energy phosphate compounds (ATP and its "backup" system creatine phosphate) are the source of myocardial cellular energy. Although myocardial tissue ATP levels are maintained for several minutes following cessation of myocardial blood flow, tissue levels of creatine phosphate fall rapidly and are reduced to 20 percent of normal within 2 to 3 minutes of the onset of ischemia [6–8]. Systolic contraction declines rapidly with the onset of ischemia and loss of energy-rich phosphates, ceasing entirely approximately 90 seconds after the interruption of myocardial blood flow [9]. In addition to the loss of high-energy phosphates, other intracellular events contribute to cessation of myocardial cellular function during ischemia. These events include acidosis, reduced sensitivity of contractile proteins to calcium, and accumulation of phosphate and lipid [10–12]. The end result of these intracellular disturbances is rapidly declining systolic and diastolic myocardial cellular function.

Another consequence of myocardial ischemia is alteration in the electrical properties of cardiac muscle. The monophasic action potential of the myocardial cell is altered approximately 16 beats after the onset of ischemia [13]. Ischemia causes myocardial cells to leak potassium into the surrounding extracellular space, resulting in changes in conduction velocity, rate of depolarization, resting membrane potential, and duration of the action potential. Some or all of these alterations in cellular electrophysiology may be involved in the genesis of arrhythmias that arise in the setting of myocardial ischemia.

Studies have documented biochemical alterations in human cardiac metabolism in the setting of myocardial ischemia [14, 15]. Under normal aerobic conditions, human myocardium metabolizes fatty acids and pyruvate in order to produce ATP. In the absence of oxygen, however, the myocardium is incapable of utilizing the latter substrates. In place of fatty acids and pyruvate, the myocardium takes up glucose for anaerobic (glycolytic) generation of ATP [14, 15]. The continued utilization of glucose by cardiac muscle that no longer contracts has been suggested as a marker for "stunned," or *reversibly* injured, myocardium (see below).

With the loss of aerobic metabolic production of ATP, the myocardium shifts to anaerobic glycolysis to slow the depletion of high-energy phosphates. Myocardial generation of these high-energy compounds by anaerobic metabolism is limited [16]. Initially, the rate of anaerobic glycolysis is high, but it rapidly slows within 60 to 90 seconds due to inhibition of glyceraldehyde phosphate dehydrogenase by the high cytosolic reduced nicotinamide adenine dinucleotide–to–nicotinamide adenine dinucleotide (NADH/NAD) ratios, low intracellular pH, and high intracellular lactate levels [16].

After 40 to 60 minutes of ischemia, severely injured myocytes become irreversibly damaged. This phase of myocardial ischemic injury is characterized by very low levels of high-energy phosphate compounds, depressed levels of adenine nucleotides, essentially total cessation of anaerobic metabolism, low myocardial cell pH and glycogen content as well as high inosine and hypoxanthine levels, and markedly increased osmolar load with associated swelling of the cell itself and its organelles [16].

Myocardial Metabolic Demand and Coronary Blood Flow

Myocardial blood flow is coupled to myocardial metabolic demand under normal conditions. With the advent of coronary arterial stenosis or obstruction, myocardial blood flow can no longer increase in the face of myocardial metabolic demand. The result is myocardial ischemia.

Myocardial metabolic demands are dependent on heart rate, systolic blood pressure, left ventricular volume and wall thickness, and myocardial contractility. Increases in heart rate, systolic blood pressure, and myocardial contractility obviously increase myocardial metabolic demand. The product of heart rate times blood pressure is directly proportional to measured myocardial oxygen demand

[17, 18]. Left ventricular wall stress is also a major determinant of myocardial oxygen demand [17, 18]. Wall stress increases (Laplace relation) with increasing ventricular volume and decreases with increasing wall thickness. However, hearts with left ventricular hypertrophy (increased wall thickness) have a larger quantity of functioning myocardium that requires oxygen and nutrients. Thus global left ventricular oxygen demand is augmented with increases in either or both of these two factors, that is, left ventricular mass or left ventricular work. If coronary arterial capacity for blood flow remains unchanged in the face of increasing myocardial mass, ischemia can result even in the absence of major atherosclerotic coronary arterial obstruction (e.g., hypertrophic cardiomyopathy).

There are two major determinants of coronary arterial blood flow: perfusion pressure and coronary vascular resistance. Perfusion pressure is the difference between aortic blood pressure and intramyocardial pressure, which compresses coronary blood vessels. Coronary blood flow is impeded during systole when collapsible vessels are compressed. Thus left ventricular myocardial blood flow occurs primarily during diastole because of high systolic intramyocardial wall tension. Because systolic pressure and wall tension in the right ventricle are much less than those in the left ventricle, systolic compressive forces are less in the right ventricular wall, and myocardial blood flow in the latter is of equal magnitude during systole and diastole. Because left ventricular blood flow occurs primarily during diastole, an increasing heart rate lessens left ventricular coronary blood flow by decreasing diastolic time.

Coronary vascular resistance is determined by blood viscosity and the diameter and length of the coronary arteries (Poiseuille's theorem). Blood viscosity and vessel length vary little from individual to individual. Hence it is the cross-sectional area of the coronary arteries and arterioles that determines coronary vascular resistance. Under normal circumstances, coronary arterial resistance is determined primarily by intramyocardial arterioles. However, when marked atherosclerotic obstruction develops in large epicardial coronary arteries, coronary vascular resistance is determined primarily by these lesions, which encroach on the arterial lumen [19].

Modest coronary arterial stenoses with moderate luminal encroachment do not alter resting coronary arterial blood flow. Stenosis severity must reach an 80 to 90 percent reduction in luminal diameter before resting blood flow is curtailed (Fig. 1-2). When the arterial pressure head beyond a coronary arterial stenosis falls below 55 mm Hg, subendocardial ischemia develops [20]. The more severe the stenotic lesion is, the more transmural in distribution the resulting ischemia is. Ischemia develops first in the subendocardium because myocardial compressive forces resisting myocardial blood flow are greatest here and because the subendocardium is the last site to receive blood flow from the coronary arterial tree, which originates on the epicardial surface of the heart. Therefore when a severe coronary arterial stenosis is present, blood flow goes preferentially to the subepicardium [21, 22]. Imbalance between myocardial metabolic demand and coronary arterial blood flow results in myocardial ischemia. Most episodes of exertional angina are the result of myocardial metabolic demand outstripping blood flow. Episodes of rest or nocturnal angina (unstable angina) are thought to be the result of coronary arterial vasomotion or spasm with conse-

Fig. 1-2
Reduction in resting myocardial blood flow plotted against stenosis of the coronary arterial lumen. Myocardial blood flow is maintained at essentially control levels until the arterial lumen is reduced by approximately 80 percent or more. At this point, myocardial blood flow falls rapidly with increasing stenosis. (From J. S. Alpert. *Physiopathology of the Cardiovascular System.* Boston: Little, Brown, 1984. With permission.)

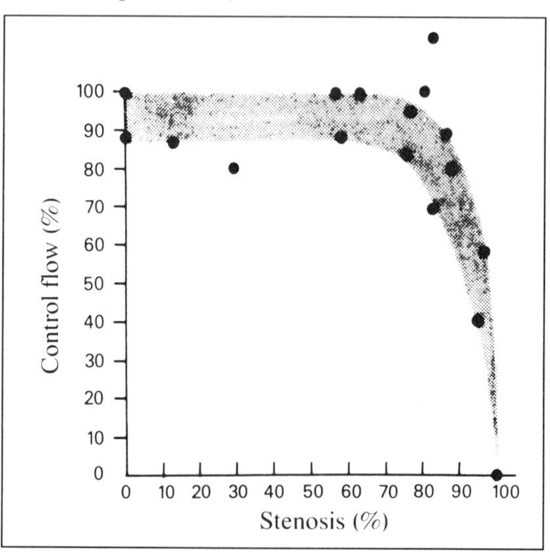

quent marked reduction in coronary arterial blood flow (see below) [23–30].

Coronary vascular smooth muscle tone and hence myocardial blood flow are strongly influenced by the production of various factors produced by the endothelium of the artery itself. Endothelial derived relaxing factor (EDRF), a potent coronary arterial vasodilator, has been shown to be nitric oxide. Apparently, the presence of EDRF in the wall of the coronary artery is required for normal smooth muscle tone. Absence of EDRF predisposes the vessel to vasoconstriction, particularly in the presence of acetylcholine. Atherosclerosis interferes with normal EDRF production, thereby setting the stage for abnormal coronary vascular tone and reduced myocardial blood flow [30–32].

Systolic and Diastolic Myocardial Function

Following abrupt cessation of myocardial blood flow, diastolic and systolic myocardial mechanical dysfunction develops rapidly [33, 34]. Within seconds, diastolic function decreases first as demonstrated by declining negative dP/dt (rate of change of ventricular pressure), rising ventricular end-diastolic pressure, and less-compliant pressure volume curves. Shortly thereafter, ventricular systolic function deteriorates, as judged from progressively abnormal positive dP/dt and cessation of regional myocardial contraction. All myocardial contraction ceases in the ischemic zone within 10 to 15 seconds of the onset of ischemia. Increases in heart rate and systemic arterial blood pressure usually follow, presumably as the result of activation of the sympathetic nervous system. Pulmonary arterial pressures increase pari passu with rising left ventricular diastolic pressure. If coronary blood flow is rapidly restored, diastolic and systolic hemodynamic abnormalities resolve. However, if ischemia is prolonged or occurs repetitively, diastolic or systolic function (or both) may remain abnormal for a more protracted period (see below).

Transition from Ischemia to Necrosis: Stunned Myocardium

Following cessation of coronary arterial blood flow, myocardial ischemia appears first in the subendocardium. Thereafter, ischemia advances transmurally toward the subepicardium [34–39]. Initially, ischemic myocytes are reversibly injured. However, within 15 to 20 minutes of the onset of ischemia and continuing for 3 to 6 hours, a wave of irreversible myocardial cellular injury spreads from the subendocardium to the subepicardium. Along the leading edge of this wave front of myocardial cellular necrosis lie cells that are seriously, but reversibly, injured. Cellular ATP and creatine phosphate levels are low in these injured cells, and cellular volume regulation is abnormal, as noted earlier [39]. Overt membrane damage, however, judged by electron microscopy, is not observed in these reversibly injured cells. Cellular ischemic injury is reversible so long as ATP levels are not depleted below 70 percent of control levels.

Following reestablishment of myocardial blood flow, myocytes gradually replete adenine nucleotides. In general, recovery of myocardial systolic and diastolic function is inversely proportional to the duration of myocardial ischemia [39–45]. After prolonged periods of myocardial ischemia in experimental animals, complete recovery of diastolic and systolic function may take as long as 3 to 7 days. Indeed, myocardial ATP levels are still depressed 4 days after an episode of severe ischemia [46]. Ultrastructural cellular injury can also be observed 3 days after severe myocardial ischemia. Ultrastructural changes noted include the presence of abnormal vacuoles, intermyofibrillar and intermyofilamentous edema, glycogen depletion, and generalized mitochondrial and sarcolemmal damage [16, 46]. Severely, but reversibly, injured myocardium that demonstrates a prolonged functional recovery phase has been referred to as *stunned myocardium* [45].

Abnormalities in systolic and diastolic myocardial function have been observed in models of ischemic myocardial stunning. Stunned myocardium may require only a short period of time before normal contractility is restored, or a considerably longer recovery phase may be observed. In both animal models of myocardial ischemia and humans with myocardial infarction, complete recovery of systolic and diastolic left ventricular function takes 7 to 10 days. The severity and duration of abnormal myocardial function are related to the severity and duration of myocardial ischemia [47–50].

In light of the observations concerning stunned myocardium, the work of Geft and coworkers is of considerable interest. These investigators noted that brief, intermittent periods of myocardial ischemia (5, 10, or 15 minutes of ischemia followed by 15 minutes of reperfusion) produced small, but distinct areas of subendocardial necrosis in dogs. Thus stunned myocardium can be irreversibly injured by further episodes of ischemia [51].

Myocardial Infarction

Ultrastructural and Biochemical Events

As noted earlier, marked biochemical and structural abnormalities develop in myocardial cells following cessation of coronary blood flow or reduction in flow below 15 percent of control values [16, 35]. After approximately 20 to 40 minutes of myocardial ischemia, cellular derangement becomes irreversible and cell death or necrosis ensues. Cell death begins in the subendocardium 1 to 2 mm from the endocardial surface and extends to within 1 to 2 mm of the lateral edge of the ischemic vascular bed [37]. A wave front of cell death moves slowly *from* the subendocardial region *toward* the subepicardial zone where collateral blood flow is greatest. Approximately 3 to 6 hours is required for the wave front of cellular necrosis to reach the subepicardial zone, depending on the extent of collateral blood flow and myocardial oxygen demand (Fig. 1-3) [39].

As noted earlier, high-energy phosphates are rapidly depleted in ischemic myocardial cells. Anaerobic glycolysis is initially employed to produce a modest amount of ATP, but these synthetic pathways are soon inhibited and ATP production ceases [16, 52, 53].

With the onset of irreversible myocardial cellular injury, (1) ATP is almost completely depleted (Fig. 1-4), (2) mitochondria are swollen and contain amorphous matrix densities composed of lipid and protein, and (3) the sarcolemmal membranes develop defects presumably leading to leakage of essential enzymes out of the cell and entrance of calcium ions and water into the cell. Reperfusion of irreversibly injured myocytes is associated with massive cellular edema and influx of Ca^{2+} [39]. Other ultrastructural changes associated with irreversible myocyte injury include clumping of nuclear chromatin plus further swelling and disruption of mitochondria, sarcolemma, and other cell mem-

Fig. 1-3
Wave-front progression of cell death over time following occlusion of the circumflex coronary artery in open-chested dogs. Necrosis occurs first in the subendocardium and then moves in a wave front toward the subepicardium. Thus there is initially a large volume of ischemic but salvageable myocardium soon after coronary occlusion. As time passes, however, less and less viable myocardium remains. AP = anterior; PP = posterior. (From K. A. Reimer and R. B. Jennings, The "wavefront phenomenon" of myocardial ischemic cell death. II. Transmural progression of necrosis within the framework of ischemic bed size [myocardium at risk] and collateral flow. *Lab. Invest.* 40:633, 1979. With permission.)

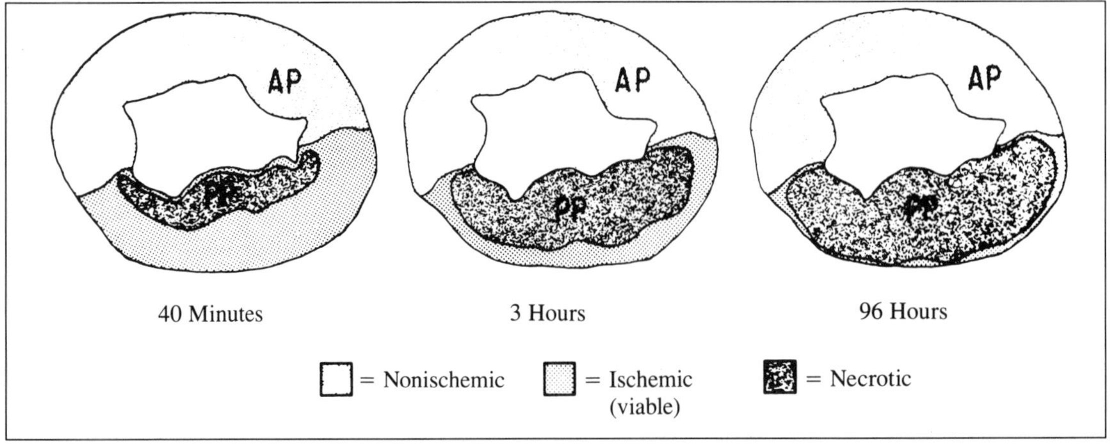

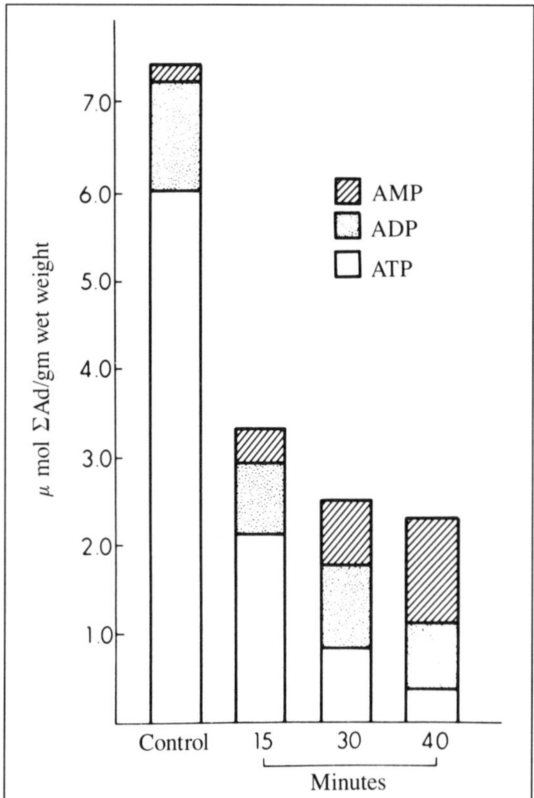

Fig. 1-4
Adenine nucleotide contents of normal and severely ischemic myocardium of dogs following proximal occlusion of the circumflex coronary artery. After 40 minutes of ischemia, when most of the cells in the ischemic zone are irreversibly injured, only 6 percent of the original ATP content remains. Moreover, there was a 69 percent decrease in total adenine nucleotides. AMP = adenine monophosphate nucleotide; ADP = adenine diphosphate nucleotide; ATP = adenine triphosphate nucleotide. (From K. A. Reimer et al., Pathobiology of acute myocardial ischemia: Metabolic, functional, and ultrastructural studies. *Am. J. Cardiol.* 52:72A, 1983. With permission.)

branes. Intramitochondrial calcium crystals accumulate. The myofibrillar apparatus becomes disrupted with the formation of contraction bands. It has been hypothesized that sarcolemmal injury is the critical event in determining the irreversibility of cellular damage. Membrane damage may develop because of activation of endogenous phospholipases, detergent action of acyl carnitine and acyl coenzyme A, oxidation by oxygen free radicals, or failure to resynthesize portions of membranes lost through pinocytosis or other processes [39, 54].

Relation to Coronary Arterial Obstruction

Although contested in the past, it is now generally agreed that coronary arterial thrombosis is the event that initiates myocardial infarction. Coronary thrombi are approximately 1 cm in length and are composed of platelets, fibrin, erythrocytes, and leukocytes [55]. The thrombus may vary in composition at different levels with white thrombus (composed of platelets and fibrin) mixed with red thrombus (composed of erythrocytes, fibrin, platelets, and leukocytes).

Early thrombi are usually nonocclusive and are composed primarily of platelets. Such early thrombi usually overlie a newly generated ulcer or fissure in a long-standing atherosclerotic plaque [56]. This fissuring or ulceration of the plaque apparently exposes underlying thrombogenic material to the circulating blood with resultant thrombogenesis (Fig. 1-5). Presumably, once thrombus formation is initiated, a series of dynamic reactions are set into motion, with endogenous thrombolysis opposing thrombogenesis. If thrombogenesis prevails, an occlusive thrombus totally occludes the coronary arterial lumen.

The sequence of events that causes a previously stable atherosclerotic plaque to rupture, fissure, or ulcerate is still debated at this time. A number of hypotheses have been suggested to explain the etiology of plaque disruption: (1) coronary arterial vasospasm, (2) stress fracture of the plaque secondary to increased plaque wall stress at specific points, (3) injury to coronary arterial vasa vasorum with resultant intramural hemorrhage or plaque necrosis, or (4) platelet aggregation with release of thromboxanes and other vasoactive substances [29, 55–65]. All or none of these processes may be operative simultaneously or sequentially in a particular individual.

A number of investigators have accumulated circumstantial evidence favoring a role for coronary arterial vasospasm in the genesis of coronary arterial thrombosis. Factor and Cho noted the presence of smooth muscle contraction bands consistent with coronary spasm in the medial layer of coronary arteries of patients with fatal myocardial infarction [61]. Angiographic studies in patients with unstable

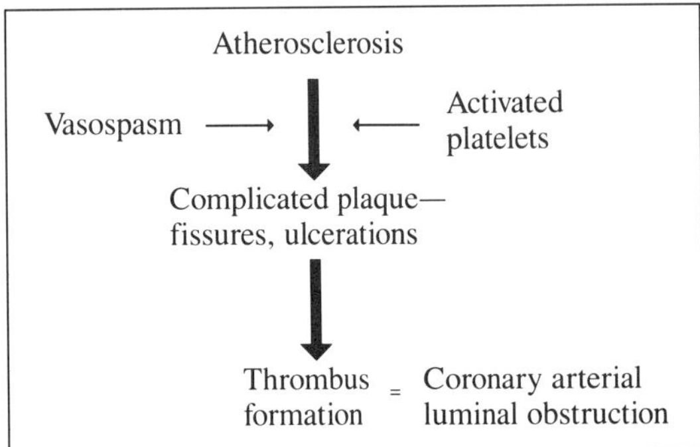

Fig. 1-5
Initiation of myocardial infarction: current hypothesis for the sequence of events leading from a "benign," stable atherosclerotic plaque to a "complicated" plaque to complete coronary arterial obstruction by thrombus.

angina who developed coronary thrombosis and myocardial infarction during catheterization have documented the role of coronary vasospasm in the development of occlusive coronary thrombi [61–65]. Santamore and colleagues developed computer models of atherosclerotic coronary arteries. Their analysis suggests that arterial vasomotion may be an important element in the pathogenesis of plaque rupture [66].

Platelet aggregates in arteriosclerotic arteries are also thought to be important factors in the pathogenesis of AMI [65]. Severe coronary arterial stenosis causes turbulent blood flow and zones of stasis. In addition, the endothelial surface of atherosclerotic coronary arteries is capable of activating the platelet release reaction. Animal studies have documented the presence of platelet aggregates beyond critical coronary arterial stenoses [67, 68]. These platelet aggregates lead to periodic, cyclic reductions in coronary arterial blood flow. Evidence that similar events are occurring within atherosclerotic coronary arteries in humans has come from a number of studies [69–74]. Elevated levels of thromboxane B_2, a stable metabolite of thromboxane A_2, have been observed in coronary venous blood of patients with unstable angina and AMI. Moreover, platelets in such individuals are more easily activated [72, 73], which may, in part, explain activation of platelets in patients with unstable angina despite normal plasma levels of catecholamines. Further support for the concept that abnormal hemostatic function is a causative factor in the development of coronary arterial thrombosis is derived from studies documenting increased levels of fibrinogen and higher maximum rates of fibrin growth, as well as increased prothrombin time, thrombin time, and activated partial thromboplastin time in patients with AMI [74].

Leukocytes may also play a role in the genesis of coronary thrombosis via release of oxidative species or leukotrienes [75]. Expression of granulocyte and monocyte adhesion receptors is also increased in white blood cells taken from patients with unstable angina and AMI. Activation of these leukocytes may induce coronary arterial vasoconstriction and activate platelets, thereby predisposing the individual to coronary thrombosis [76–78]. Leukocyte infiltration into the wall of coronary arteries with ruptured atherosclerotic plaques implicates these cells in the initial phase of the process that leads to coronary arterial thrombosis.

Vasoactive substances such as the ones just mentioned, in combination with thromboxanes, may contribute to or initiate coronary arterial vasospasm. Thus a vicious spiral may be created with coronary vasospasm and vasoactive humoral factors reenforcing an ever-increasing reduction in coronary arterial luminal diameter. Activation of the clotting cascade leading to thrombogenesis further compromises luminal diameter. Eventually, the coronary artery is blocked by a combination of vasospasm and thrombus. Exactly which one of these factors is the primary event in this vicious spiral is unknown. It is even possible that different factors initiate the process leading to thrombogenesis in different individuals.

Falk observed that the risk of rupture depends on plaque composition: Plaques rich in soft extracellular lipid are particularly prone to rupture. Most ruptures are quite small and occur at the periphery of the fibrous cap overlying the atherosclerotic plaque. Furthermore, rupture usually occurs at the point where the fibrous cap is thinnest and most heavily infiltrated by macrophage foam cells, which may predispose the fibrous cap to rupture. Falk believes that plaque vulnerability to rupture is more important than the presence of specific triggers for rupture [79]. A number of investigators have examined shear forces and wall stress in atherosclerotic plaques [80, 81]. The area of highest wall stress within an atherosclerotic plaque is usually the location of plaque rupture.

In summary, angiographic, angioscopic, and pathologic studies have repeatedly documented that patients with acute ischemic syndromes (unstable angina, AMI) have eccentric, irregular lesions in the involved coronary artery. These lesions represent plaque fissures with overlying partially occlusive thrombus. A sequence of events involving coronary arterial vasospasm, plaque wall stress and shear forces, plaque rupture, platelet activation, and thrombogenesis leads to ever-increasing coronary arterial obstruction. If the intrinsic thrombolytic system fails to counterbalance the forces favoring thrombogenesis, total arterial obstruction results [56–83], and myocardial ischemia and eventually necrosis develop.

A number of environmental factors are apparently involved in the genesis of the coronary arterial events just described. A recent respiratory viral infection is a common precursor of AMI [84, 85]. Moreover, there is a circadian rhythm in the occurrence of myocardial infarction: The onset of infarction is most frequent during the early morning hours and least frequent in the evening [86–88]. Platelet aggregatory activity and basal arterial tone are also increased in the early morning hours, again supporting the role of platelets and vascular smooth muscle tone in the onset of AMI [87, 89]. Finally, a number of weather parameters, such as season, barometric pressure, and humidity, correlate with the occurrence of AMI [90].

Collateral Blood Flow

It has been known since the 1930s that total occlusion of a coronary artery is not always followed by myocardial necrosis [91]. Indeed, the volume of collateral blood flow can be sufficient to maintain myocardial cellular viability despite coronary thrombosis. Normal hearts contain an extensive network of small, interarterial anastomotic blood vessels, 40 to 60 μm in diameter. This collateral circulation exists at birth, growing in size along with the rest of the coronary vascular bed. When obstructive coronary artery disease develops, these collateral channels gradually increase in size and blood flow capacity. Considerable variability exists from individual to individual with respect to potential collateral vascular development. Moreover, extensive collateral circulation requires time (perhaps years) to develop. Thus collateral blood flow is highest in older individuals with long-standing coronary artery disease. It is not surprising that well-developed collateral vessels are unusual in patients with AMI, as these patients represent a selected population [92]. The presence of infarction demonstrates that collateral blood flow was not sufficient to maintain myocardial cellular viability. However, significantly better ventricular function is present in regions of the left ventricle supplied by obstructed coronary arteries if extensive collateralization of the diseased coronary artery is present [93]. Congestive heart failure and cardiomegaly occur with greater frequency in infarct patients who lack collateral blood vessels [94]. Moreover, it has frequently been observed in both animals and humans that following coronary occlusion the zone of myocardial infarction is smaller than the area supplied by the occluded vessel if collateral blood vessels are present.

In summary, collateral blood vessels are present from birth and can enlarge in the presence of obstructive coronary artery disease. Collateral blood flow can limit infarct size when total occlusion of a coronary artery develops. Occasionally, the volume of collateral blood flow is sufficient to prevent infarction.

Effect of Infarction on Regional and Global Ventricular Function

Abnormal systolic and diastolic myocardial cellular function develops within a few seconds of cessation of coronary arterial blood flow. Initially, ischemic myocardium expands passively during ventricular filling and emptying. Thus diastolic compliance is initially increased (decreased stiffness) [95–98]. Within a few minutes, however, ischemic myocardium becomes stiffer, and eventually its compliance is less than that of surrounding, viable myocardium [95–98]. This change in diastolic stiffness is probably the result of myocardial contracture, interstitial edema, and leukocyte infiltration during the early phases of AMI. Increased myocardial stiffness during the chronic phase of myocardial infarction is apparently caused by fibrous tissue proliferation and collagen deposition. The left ventricular diastolic pressure increases, and the pressure-volume relation is abnormally shifted by the increase in regional myocardial stiffness that develops after infarction.

Cessation of myocardial blood flow results in four sequential abnormal patterns of myocardial systolic contraction: (1) *dyssynchrony,* or dissociation over the time course of contraction of adjacent segments of myocardium; (2) *hypokinesis,* or reduction in the extent of myocardial shortening; (3) *akinesis,* or cessation of myocardial contraction in affected regions; and (4) *dyskinesis,* or paradoxical systolic expansion of affected myocardial segments [99]. All of these sequential contraction abnormalities occur within seconds to minutes of the cessation of myocardial blood flow.

When a substantial quantity of myocardium becomes ischemic or necrotic (>25 percent of left ventricular myocardium), global left ventricular function deteriorates sufficiently to reduce resting cardiac output, stroke volume, and peak dP/dt [100, 101]. Dyskinetic myocardial segments contribute to the reduction in ventricular stroke output. As edema, cellular infiltration, and ultimately fibrosis develop in ischemic and necrotic myocardial segments, the resultant increased stiffness of these myocardial zones improves left ventricular function by preventing systolic paradoxical wall motion (dyskinesis).

Rackely and coworkers observed a linear relation between left ventricular function and clinical symptoms [102]. The earliest observed abnormality in global left ventricular function is a reduction in diastolic compliance that occurs when 8 percent of the left ventricle is ischemic or necrotic. When the abnormal contracting segment exceeds 10 percent of the left ventricle, global ejection fraction is reduced; once 15 percent of the left ventricle is involved, ventricular end-diastolic pressure and volume increase. Clinical heart failure is evident when 25 percent of the left ventricle ceases to contract. Cardiogenic shock develops when 40 percent of the left ventricular myocardium becomes ischemic or necrotic [102].

Unless infarct extension or expansion develops (see below), some improvement or recovery of global left ventricular function is usually observed [103, 104]. Such improvement occurs over a period of days to weeks and may be the result of improved collateral blood flow, myocardial scar contraction, recovery of stunned myocardium, or myocardial hypertrophy. Such recovery of myocardial function is more common in patients with single-vessel disease than in individuals who have multivessel disease [103]. Patients in whom 20 to 25 percent of the left ventricle fails to contract manifest hemodynamic signs of left ventricular failure regardless of the age of their infarction [105].

Patients with AMI may demonstrate abnormally reduced wall motion in segments of the left ventricle remote from the acutely infarcted zone. Such remote wall motion abnormalities are the result of previous infarction or acute ischemia and are called *ischemia at a distance* [106, 107]. There are two reasons for ischemia at a distance: The noninfarcted myocardial zone is supplied by a critically stenotic coronary artery. Ischemia develops because of (1) increased compensatory myocardial work in the noninfarcted zone secondary to loss of working myocardial segments in the infarct zone, and (2) decreased collateral blood flow to the noninfarcted ischemic zone as a result of the acute coronary arterial thrombosis that produced the initial infarct. Noninfarcted myocardial segments with normal arterial blood supply are often noted to have hypercontractile (compensatory) wall motion.

Infarction Expansion and Ventricular Dilatation

After experimental infarction in dogs, the first 7 days of healing are associated with expansion of the infarct zone and dilatation of the left ventricular cavity [108]. Thereafter, the infarct zone contracts and thins as collagen is deposited. Similar changes have been observed in humans following AMI [109–114]. Marked infarct expansion and left ventricular cavity dilatation are associated with a poor prognosis [109]. Noninfarcted zones develop volume-overload hypertrophy, thereby further contributing to remodeling of the left ventricle after acute infarction [110]. Large infarcts are more likely to expand than small infarcts [112]. Expansion of infarction is the result of slippage of necrotic intramural fibers within the infarct zone. In addition, infarct expansion contributes to left ventricular aneurysm formation.

Electrical Instability

Some form of arrhythmia is almost always present during the acute phase of myocardial infarction.

Ventricular arrhythmias arise in ischemic peri-infarct zones as a result of (1) increased myocardial cell electrical automaticity, often resulting from delayed after-depolarizations; (2) slowing of conduction in specific areas of the heart with resultant reentry and reexcitation loops; and (3) variable shortening or lengthening of the refractory period combined with increased dispersion of refractoriness between ischemic and nonischemic zones [115]. Unidirectional abnormalities of conduction have been observed between ischemic and nonischemic zones of myocardium. Moreover, localized areas of ventricular fibrillation have been noted in experimental animals with AMI. It is thought that these localized zones of fibrillation can spread from the ischemic to the nonischemic segments. Atrial arrhythmias are the result of (1) ischemia or necrosis of atrial myocardium secondary to coronary thrombosis, and (2) atrial dilatation secondary to elevated ventricular filling pressures.

Metabolic products released from ischemic myocardium such as cyclic adenosine monophosphate (AMP), free fatty acids, long-chain fatty acid metabolites, lysophosphoglycerides, lactate, and pyruvate, to mention only a few, have electrophysiologic activity that can be arrhythmogenic [116]. A wide array of atrial and ventricular arrhythmias can occur.

Myocardial Infarction with Normal Coronary Arteries

Approximately 4 percent of patients with AMI have normal coronary arteries documented by coronary angiography. This percentage is even higher, perhaps 10 to 15 percent, in patients under age 35. In some individuals the infarction is the result of a coronary artery disease other than atherosclerosis, for example, coronary arteritis, trauma, or embolism [117]. A number of theories have been developed to explain the etiology of infarction in individuals without an otherwise evident explanation. Coronary arterial vasospasm and small-vessel coronary artery disease are two of the most popular theories. It seems likely that most of these patients do indeed have minimal atherosclerotic plaques within the infarct-related coronary artery. These plaques are so small that they are angiographically invisible [118]. Vasospasm with transient or permanent coronary arterial thrombosis with resultant infarction probably develops at the site of such minimal atherosclerotic change [119].

References

1. Muller, J. E. Coronary artery thrombosis: Historical aspects. *J. Am. Coll. Cardiol.* 3:893, 1983.
2. Ross, R. The pathogenesis of atherosclerosis—An update. *N. Engl. J. Med.* 314:488, 1986.
3. Joris, I., Zand, T., Nunnari, J. J., et al. Studies on the pathogenesis of atherosclerosis. I. Adhesion and emigration of mononuclear cells in the aorta of hypercholesterolemic rats. *Am. J. Pathol.* 113: 341, 1983.
4. Sommer, J. R., and Johnson, E. A. Ultrastructure of cardiac muscle. In R. M. Berne and N. Sperelakis (eds.), *Handbook of Physiology, Sect. 2: The Cardiovascular System.* Bethesda: American Physiological Society, 1979. Pp. 113–186.
5. Wollenberg, A. Responses of the heart mitochondria to chronic cardiac overload and physical exercise. In E. Bajusz and E. Rona (eds.), *Recent Advances in Studies on Cardiac Structure and Metabolism.* Baltimore: University Park Press, 1972. Pp. 213–222.
6. Braasch, W., Gudbjarnason, S., Puri, P. S., et al. Early changes in energy metabolism in the myocardium following acute coronary artery occlusion in anesthetized dogs. *Circ. Res.* 23:429, 1986.
7. Gudbjarnason, S., Mathes, P., and Ravens, K. G. Functional compartmentalization of ATP and creatine phosphate in heart muscle. *J. Mol. Cell. Cardiol.* 1:325, 1970.
8. Wollenberger, A., and Krause, E. G. Metabolic control characteristics of the acutely ischemic myocardium. *Am. J. Cardiol.* 22:349, 1968.
9. Tennant, R., and Wiggers, C. J. The effect of coronary occlusion on myocardial contraction. *Am. J. Physiol.* 112:351, 1935.
10. Tennant, R. Factors concerned in the arrest of contraction in an ischemic myocardial area. *Am. J. Physiol.* 113:677, 1935.
11. Serruys, P. W., Wijns, W., Van den Brond, M., et al. Left ventricular performance, regional blood flow, wall motion and lactate metabolism during transluminal angioplasty. *Circulation* 70:25, 1984.
12. Poole-Wilson, P. A. Haemodynamic and metabolic consequences of angina and myocardial infarction. In K. M. Fox (ed.), *Ischemic Heart Disease.* Norwell, MA: MTP Press, 1987. Pp. 123–148.
13. Donaldson, R. M., Taggart, P., Bennett, J. G., et al. Study of electrophysiological ischemic events during coronary angioplasty. *Texas Heart Inst. J.* 11:23, 1984.
14. Schwaiger, M., Brunken, R., Grover-McKay, M., et al. Regional myocardial metabolism in patients with acute myocardial infarction assessed by posi-

tron emission tomography. *J. Am. Coll. Cardiol.* 8:800, 1986.
15. Camici, P., Araujo, L. I., Spinks, T., et al. Increased uptake of ^{18}F-fluorodeoxyglucose in postischemic myocardium of patients with exercise-induced angina. *Circulation* 74:81, 1986.
16. Jennings, R. B., Murry, C. E., Steenbergen, C., Jr., et al. Development of cell injury in sustained acute ischemia. *Circulation* 82(Suppl II):II-2, 1990.
17. Sarnoff, S. J., Braunwald, E., Welch, G. H., et al. Haemodynamic determinants of oxygen consumption of the heart with special reference to the tension time index. *Am. J. Physiol.* 192:148, 1958.
18. Braunwald, E., Sarnoff, S. J., Case, R. B., et al. Hemodynamic determinants of coronary flow: Effect of changes in aortic pressure and cardiac output on the relationship between oxygen consumption and coronary flow. *Am. J. Physiol.* 192:157, 1958.
19. Sabbah, H. N., and Stein, P. D. Hemodynamics of multiple versus single 50 percent coronary arterial stenoses. *Am. J. Cardiol.* 50:278, 1982.
20. Wyatt, H. L., Forrester, J. S., Tyber, J. V., et al. Effect of graded reductions in the regional coronary perfusion on regional and total cardiac function. *Am. J. Cardiol.* 36:185, 1975.
21. Bache, R. J., and Schwartz, J. S. Effect of perfusion pressure distal to a coronary stenosis on transmural myocardial blood flow. *Circulation* 65:928, 1982.
22. Sabbah, H. N., and Stein, P. D. Effect of acute regional ischaemia in the subepicardium and subendocardium. *Am. J. Physiol.* 242:H240, 1982.
23. Buja, L. M., Hillis, L. D., Petty, C. S., et al. The role of coronary arterial spasm in ischemic heart disease. *Arch. Pathol. Lab. Med.* 105:221, 1981.
24. Gorlin, R. Role of coronary vasospasm in the pathogenesis of myocardial ischemia and angina pectoris. *Am. Heart J.* 103:598, 1982.
25. Yasue, H., Omote, S., Takizawa, A., and Nagao, M. Coronary arterial spasm in ischemic heart disease and its pathogenesis: A review. *Circ. Res.* 52(Suppl 1):147, 1983.
26. Maseri, A., L'Abbate, A., Baroldi, G., et al. Coronary vasospasm as a possible cause of myocardial infarction: A conclusion derived from the study of "preinfarction" angina. *N. Engl. J. Med.* 299: 1271, 1978.
27. Oliva, P. B., and Breckenridge, N. C. Arteriographic evidence of coronary arterial spasm in acute myocardial infarction. *Circulation* 56:366, 1977.
28. Dalen, J. E., Ockene, I. S., and Alpert, J. S. Coronary spasm, coronary thrombosis, and myocardial infarction: A hypothesis concerning the pathophysiology of acute myocardial infarction. *Am. Heart J.* 104:1119, 1982.
29. Maseri, A., Severi, S., Denes, M., et al. "Variant angina": One aspect of a continuous spectrum of vasospastic myocardial ischaemia. *Am. J. Cardiol.* 42:1019, 1978.
30. Lerman, A., and Burnett, J. C., Jr. Intact and altered endothelium in regulation of vasomotion. *Circulation* 86(Suppl III):LLL-12, 1992.
31. Vanhoutte, P. M., and Shimokawa, H. Endothelium-derived relaxing factor and coronary vasospasm. *Circulation* 80:1, 1989.
32. Vane, J. R., Anggard, E. E., and Botting, R. M. Regulatory functions of the vascular endothelium. *N. Engl. J. Med.* 323:27, 1990.
33. Chierchia, S., Burnelli, C., Simonett, I., et al. Sequence of events in angina at rest: Primary reduction in coronary flow. *Circulation* 61:759, 1980.
34. Jennings, R. B., Ganote, C. E., and Reimer, K. A. Ischemic tissue injury. *Am. J. Pathol.* 81:179, 1975.
35. Jennings, R. B., Somers, H. M., Smyth, G. A., et al. Myocardial necrosis induced by temporary occlusion of a coronary artery in the dog. *Arch. Pathol.* 70:68, 1960.
36. Reimer, K. A., and Jennings, R. B. The "wavefront phenomenon" of myocardial ischemic cell death. II. Transmural progression of necrosis within the framework of ischemic bed size (myocardium at risk) and collateral flow. *Lab. Invest.* 40:633, 1979.
37. Reimer, K. A., Lowe, J. E., and Rasmussen, M. M. The wavefront phenomenon of ischemic cell death. I. Myocardial infarct size v. duration of coronary occlusion in dogs. *Circulation* 56:786, 1977.
38. Reimer, K. A., Jennings, R., and Tatum, A. H. Pathobiology of acute myocardial ischemia: Metabolic, functional and ultrastructural studies. *Am. J. Cardiol.* 52:72A, 1983.
39. Heyndrickx, G. R., Baig, H., Nellers, P., et al. Depression of regional blood flow and wall thickening after brief coronary occlusion. *Am. J. Physiol.* 234:H653, 1978.
40. Jennings, R. B., Schaper, J., Hill, M. L., et al. Effect of reperfusion late in the phase of reversible ischemic injury. *Circ. Res.* 56:262, 1985.
41. Puri, P. S. Contractile and biochemical effects of coronary reperfusion after extended periods of coronary occlusion. *Am. J. Cardiol.* 36:244, 1975.
42. Weiner, J. M., Apstein, C. S., and Arthur, J. H. Persistence of myocardial injury following brief periods of coronary occlusion. *Cardiovasc. Res.* 10:678, 1976.
43. Wood, J. M., Hanley, H. G., Entman, M. L., et al. Biochemical and morphological correlates of acute experimental myocardial ischemia in the dog. IV. Energy mechanisms during very early ischemia. *Circ. Res.* 44:52, 1979.
44. Hess, M. L., Barnart, G. R., Crute, S., et al. Mechanical and biochemical effects of transient myocardial ischemia. *J. Surg. Res.* 26:175, 1979.
45. Braunwald, E., and Kloner, R. A. The stunned myocardium: Prolonged postischemic ventricular dysfunction. *Circulation* 66:1146, 1982.
46. Reimer, K. A., Hill, M. L., and Jennings, R. B. Prolonged depletion of ATP and of the adenine nucleotide pool due to delayed resynthesis of adenine nucleotides following reversible myocardial ischemic injury in dogs. *J. Mol. Cell. Cardiol.* 13:229, 1981.
47. Nayler, W. O., Elz, J. S., and Buckley, D. J. The stunned myocardium: Effect of electrical and me-

chanical arrest and osmolality. *Am. J. Physiol.* 254:H60, 1988.
48. Przyklenk, K., and Kloner, R. A. Is "stunned myocardium" a protective mechanism? Effect of acute recruitment and acute beta blockade in recovery of contractile function and high energy phosphate stores at 1 day post reperfusion. *Am. Heart J.* 118:480, 1989.
49. Charlat, M. L., O'Neill, P. G., Hartley, C. J., et al. Prolonged abnormalities of left ventricular diastolic wall thinning in the "stunned" myocardium in conscious dogs: Time course and relation to systolic function. *J. Am. Coll. Cardiol.* 13:185, 1989.
50. Williamson, B. D., Lim, M. J., and Buda, A. J. Transient left ventricular filling abnormalities (diastolic stunning) after acute myocardial infarction. *Am. J. Cardiol.* 66:897, 1990.
51. Geft, I. L., Fishbein, M. C., Ninomiya, K., et al. Intermittent brief periods of ischemia have a cumulative effect and may cause myocardial necrosis. *Circulation* 66:1150, 1982.
52. Gelet, T. R., Altschuld, R. A., and Weissler, A. M. Effects of acidosis on the performance and metabolism of the anoxic heart. IV. *Circulation* 39–40: 60, 1969.
53. Wiliamson, J. R., Schaffer, S., Ford, C., et al. Contribution of tissue acidosis to ischemic injury in the perfused rat heart. *Circulation* 53(Suppl 1):I-13, 1976.
54. Hammond, B., and Hess, M. L. The oxygen free radical system: Potential mediation of myocardial injury. *J. Am. Coll. Cardiol.* 6:215, 1985.
55. Roberts, W. C. Coronary arteries in fatal acute myocardial infarction. *Circulation* 45:215, 1972.
56. Sherman, C. T., Litivack, F., Grundfest, W., et al. Coronary angioscopy in patients with unstable angina pectoris. *N. Engl. J. Med.* 315:913, 1986.
57. Mehta, J., Mehta, P., and Feldman, R. L. Thromboxane release in coronary artery disease: Spontaneous versus pacing-induced angina. *Am. Heart J.* 107: 286, 1984.
58. Bush, L. R., Campbell, W. B., Kern, K., et al. The effects of alpha adrenergic and serotonergic receptor antagonists on cyclic blood flow alternations in stenosed canine coronary arteries. *Circ. Res.* 55:642, 1984.
59. Lewis, H. D., Davis, J. W., Archibald, D. G., et al. Protective effects of aspirin against acute myocardial infarction and death in men with unstable angina. *N. Engl. J. Med.* 309:396, 1983.
60. Barger, A. C., Beeuwkes, R., Lainey, L. L., and Silverman, K. J. Hypothesis: Vasa vasorum and neovascularization of human coronary arteries, a possible role in the pathophysiology of atherosclerosis. *N. Engl. J. Med.* 310:175, 1984.
61. Factor, S. M., and Cho, S. Smooth muscle contraction bands in the media of coronary arteries: A postmortem marker of antemortem coronary spasm? *J. Am. Coll. Cardiol.* 6:1329, 1985.
62. Grollier, G., Scann, P., Commeau, P., et al. Role of coronary spasm in the genesis of myocardial infarction: Study of a case treated by isosorbide dinitrate in situ then by transluminal angioplasty. *Clin. Cardiol.* 8:644, 1985.
63. Naito, H., Yorozu, T., Matsuda, Y., et al. Coronary spasm producing coronary thrombosis in a patient with acute myocardial infarction. *Clin. Cardiol.* 10:275, 1987.
64. Feldman, R. L. Coronary thrombosis, coronary spasm and coronary atherosclerosis and speculation on the link between unstable angina and acute myocardial infarction. *Am. J. Cardiol.* 59:1187, 1987.
65. Conti, C. R., and Mehta, J. L. Acute myocardial ischemia: Role of atherosclerosis, thrombosis, platelet activation, coronary vasospasm, and altered arachidonic acid metabolism. *Circulation* 75(Suppl V):V-84, 1987.
66. Santamore, W. P., Yelton, B. W., and Ogilby, J. D. Dynamics of coronary occlusion in the pathogenesis of myocardial infarction. *J. Am. Coll. Cardiol.* 18:1397, 1991.
67. Uchida, Y., Yoshoimoto, N., and Murao, S. Cyclic fluctuations in coronary blood pressure and flow induced by coronary artery constriction. *Jpn. Heart J.* 16:454, 1975.
68. Folts, J. D., Crowell, E. B., and Rowe, L. L. Platelet aggregation in partially obstructed vessels and its elimination with aspirin. *Circulation* 54:365, 1976.
69. Hirsh, P. H., Hillis, L. D., Campbell, W. B., et al. Release of prostaglandins and thromboxane into the coronary circulation in patients with ischemic heart disease. *N. Engl. J. Med.* 304:685, 1981.
70. Mehta, J., Mehta, P., and Horalek, C. Role of blood platelets and prostaglandins in coronary artery disease. *Am. J. Cardiol.* 48:366, 1981.
71. Mehta, J., Mehta, P., and Feldman, R. L. Severe intracoronary thromboxane release preceding acute coronary occlusion. *Prostaglandins Leukot. Med.* 8:599, 1982.
72. Mehta, J., Mehta, P., and Ostrowski, N. Increase in human platelet alpha-adrenergic receptor affinity for agonist in unstable angina. *J. Lab. Clin. Med.* 106:661, 1985.
73. Born, G. V. R., and Kratzer, M. A. A. Contribution of blood platelets to the pathogenesis of myocardial infarction. *Rev. Med. Brux.* 2:157, 1981.
74. Kostis, J. B., Gaughman, J., and Kuo, P. T. Association of recurrent myocardial infarction with hemostatic factors: A prospective study. *Chest* 81:571, 1982.
75. Werns, S. W., Shea, M. J., and Lucchesi, B. R. Free radical and myocardial injury: Pharmacologic implications. *Circulation* 74:1, 1986.
76. Mehta, J., Dinerman, J., Mehta, P., et al. Neutrophil function in ischemic heart disease. *Circulation* 79:549, 1989.
77. Entman, M. L., and Ballantyne, C. M. Inflammation in acute coronary syndromes. *Circulation* 88:800, 1993.
78. Mazzone, A., DeServi, S., Ricevuti, G., et al. Increased expression of neutrophil and monocyte ad-

hesion molecules in unstable coronary artery disease. *Circulation* 88:358, 1993.
79. Falk, E. Why do plaques rupture? *Circulation* 86(Suppl III):III-30, 1992.
80. Cheng, G. C., Loree, H. M., Kamm, R. D., et al. Distribution of circumferential stress in ruptured and stable atherosclerotic lesions. A structural analysis with histopathological correlation. *Circulation* 87:1179, 1993.
81. Gertz, S. D., and Roberts, W. C. Hemodynamic shear force in rupture of coronary arterial atherosclerotic plaques. *Am. J. Cardiol.* 66:1368, 1990.
82. Ambrose, J. A., Winters, S. L., Stern, A., et al. Angiographic morphology and the pathogenesis of unstable angina pectoris. *J. Am. Coll. Cardiol.* 5:609, 1985.
83. Maseri, A., Chierchia, S., and Davies, G. Pathophysiology of coronary occlusion in acute infarction. *Circulation* 73:233, 1986.
84. Spodick, D. H., Flessas, A. P., and Johnson, M. M. Association of acute respiratory symptoms with onset of acute myocardial infarction: Prospective investigation of 150 consecutive patients and matched control patients. *Am. J. Cardiol.* 53:481, 1984.
85. Spodick, D. H. Acute viral (and other) infection in the onset, pathogenesis, and mimicry of acute myocardial infarction. *Am. J. Med.* 81:661, 1986.
86. Muller, J. E., Stone, P. H., Turi, Z. G., et al. Circadian variation in the frequency of onset of acute myocardial infarction. *N. Engl. J. Med.* 313:1315, 1985.
87. Toffler, G. H., Brezinski, D., Schafer, A. I., et al. Concurrent morning increase in platelet aggregability and the risk of myocardial infarction and sudden cardiac death. *N. Engl. J. Med.* 316:1514, 1987.
88. Muller, J. E., Tofler, G. H., and Stone, P. H. Circadian variation and triggers of onset of acute cardiovascular disease. *Circulation* 79:733, 1989.
89. Panza, J. A., Epstein, S. E., and Quyyumi, A. A. Circadian variation in vascular tone and its relation to alpha-sympathetic vasoconstrictor activity. *N. Engl. J. Med.* 325:986, 1991.
90. Ruhenstroth-Bauer, G., Baumer, H., Burke, E. M., et al. Myocardial infarction and the weather: A significant positive correlation between the onset of heart infarct and 28 KHz atmospherics—a pilot study. *Clin. Cardiol.* 8:149, 1985.
91. Blumgart, H. L., Schlesinger, M. J., and David, D. Studies on the relation of the clinical manifestations of angina pectoris, coronary thrombosis, and myocardial infarction to the pathologic findings with particular reference to the significance of the collateral circulation. *Am. Heart J.* 19:1, 1940.
92. Schwartz, H., Leiboff, R. H., Bren, G. B., et al. Temporal evolution of the human coronary collateral circulation after myocardial infarction. *J. Am. Coll. Cardiol.* 4:1088, 1984.
93. Levin, D. C. Pathways and functional significance of the coronary collateral circulation. *Circulation* 50:831, 1974.
94. Hamby, R. I., Aintablian, A., and Schwartz, A. Reappraisal of the functional significance of the coronary collateral circulation. *Am. J. Cardiol.* 38:304, 1976.
95. Diamond, G., and Forrester, J. S. Effect of coronary artery disease and acute myocardial infarction on left ventricular compliance in man. *Circulation* 45:11, 1972.
96. Forrester, J. S., Diamond, G., Parmley, W., et al. Early increase in left ventricular compliance after myocardial infarction. *J. Clin. Invest.* 51:598, 1972.
97. Pirzada, F. A., Ekong, E. A., Vokonas, P. S., et al. Experimental myocardial infarction. XIII. Sequential changes in left ventricular pressure-length relationships in the acute phase. *Circulation* 53:970, 1976.
98. Smith, M., Ratshin, R. A., Harrel, F. E., et al. Early sequential changes in left ventricular dimensions and filling pressure in patients after myocardial infarction. *Am. J. Cardiol.* 33:363, 1974.
99. Herman, N. V., Heinle, R. A., Klein, M. D., et al. Localized disorders in myocardial contraction. *N. Engl. J. Med.* 227:222, 1967.
100. Pfeffer, M. A., Pfeffer, J. M., Fishbein, M. C., et al. Myocardial infarct size and ventricular function in rats. *Circ. Res.* 44:503, 1979.
101. Forrester, J. S., Wyatt, H. L., DaLuz, P. L., et al. Functional significance of regional ischemic contraction abnormalities. *Circulation* 54:64, 1976.
102. Rackely, C. E., Russell, R. O., Jr., Mantle, J. A., et al. Modern approach to the patient with acute myocardial infarction. *Curr. Probl. Cardiol.* 1:49, 1977.
103. Tamaki, N., Yasuda, T., Leinbach, R. C., et al. Spontaneous changes in regional wall motion abnormalities in acute myocardial infarction. *Am. J. Cardiol.* 58:406, 1986.
104. Sabbah, H. N., Gheorghiade, M., Smith, S. T., et al. Rate and extent of recovery of left ventricular function in patients following acute myocardial infarction. *Am. Heart J.* 114:516, 1987.
105. Klein, M. D., Herman, M. V., and Gorlin, R. G. A hemodynamic study of left ventricular aneurysm. *Circulation* 35:614, 1967.
106. Wynne, J., Sayres, M., Maddox, D. E., et al. Regional left ventricular function in acute myocardial infarction: Evaluation with quantitative radionuclide ventriculography. *Am. J. Cardiol.* 45:203, 1980.
107. Pepine, C. J. New concepts in the pathophysiology of acute myocardial infarction. *Am. J. Cardiol.* 64:2B, 1989.
108. Jugdutt, B. I., and Amy, R. W. Healing after myocardial infarction in the dog: Changes in infarct hydroxyproline and topography. *J. Am. Coll. Cardiol.* 7:91, 1986.
109. Eaton, L. W., Weiss, J. L., Bulkley, B. H., et al. Regional cardiac dilatation after acute myocardial infarction. *N. Engl. J. Med.* 300:57, 1979.
110. McKay, R. G., Pfeffer, M. A., Pasternak, R. C., et al. Left ventricular remodeling after myocardial

infarction: A corollary to infarct expansion. *Circulation* 74:693, 1986.

111. Weisman, H. F., Bush, D. E., Mannisi, J. A., et al. Global cardiac remodeling after acute myocardial infarction: A study in the rat model. *J. Am. Coll. Cardiol.* 5:1355, 1985.
112. Pirolo, J. S., Hutchins, G. M., and Moore, G. W. Infarct expansion: Pathologic analysis of 204 patients with a single myocardial infarct. *J. Am. Coll. Cardiol.* 7:349, 1986.
113. Rumberger, J. A., Behrenbeck, T., Breen, J. R., et al. Nonparallel changes in global left ventricular chamber volume and muscle mass during the first year after transmural myocardial infarction in humans. *J. Am. Coll. Cardiol.* 21:673, 1993.
114. Gaudron, P., Eilles, C., Kugler, I., et al. Progressive left ventricular dysfunction and remodeling after myocardial infarction. Potential mechanisms and early predictors. *Circulation* 87:755, 1993.
115. Levites, R., Bank, V. S., and Helfant, R. H. Electrophysiological effects of coronary occlusion and reperfusion: Observations of dispersion of refractoriness and ventricular automaticity. *Circulation* 52:760, 1975.
116. Opie, L. H. Products of myocardial ischemia and electrical instability of the heart. *J. Am. Coll. Cardiol.* 5:162B, 1985.
117. Alpert, J. S., and Braunwald, E. Acute myocardial infarction: Pathological, pathophysiological, and clinical manifestations. In E. Braunwald (ed.), *Heart Disease* (2nd ed.). Philadelphia: Saunders, 1984. Pp. 1262–1300.
118. Lindsay, J., and Pichard, A. D. Acute myocardial infarction with normal coronary arteries. *Am. J. Cardiol.* 54:902, 1984.
119. Alpert, J. S. Myocardial infarction with angiographically normal coronary arteries. *Arch. Intern. Med.* 154:265, 1994.

2. Triggering of Acute Myocardial Infarction

Otavio C. E. Gebara, James E. Muller, and Geoffrey H. Tofler

Increasing evidence indicates that patients' activities frequently play a prominent role in triggering the onset of acute cardiovascular disease [1]. This evidençe has led to the general hypothesis that atherosclerotic plaque disruption and thrombosis occur at a critical moment when daily stresses produce a combination of hemodynamic, vasoconstrictive, and prothrombotic forces that cause disruption of a vulnerable plaque and development of thrombosis, the final pathway of most myocardial infarctions (MIs) [1]. While the extent of atherosclerosis changes slowly with time and is influenced by chronic risk factors such as hypertension, diabetes mellitus, and elevated cholesterol levels, we hypothesize that hemodynamic, vasoconstrictive, and prothrombotic forces rapidly generated by external stresses can trigger plaque disruption and thrombosis and can be considered acute risk factors. The proposed combined contribution of chronic and acute risk factors required to exceed the threshold to initiate infarction is represented schematically in Figure 2-1.

The importance of acute risk, which until recently was recognized only for anecdotal cases, lies in its potential to fill several gaps in cardiovascular risk assessment that remain despite knowledge gained from studies such as the Framingham Heart Study [2].

The primary data supporting this hypothesis are epidemiologic findings that the onset of acute cardiovascular disease is more likely to occur during the morning hours after arising [3, 4]. Recent studies identified potential triggering activities that could precipitate onset of disease [5–7]. The observation that MI frequently occurs in the absence of severe coronary stenosis [8–10] also supports the importance of acute risk factors in triggering the onset of MI.

Although triggering and circadian variation appear to be new topics of interest, the concepts have strong historical roots.

History of the Triggering Concept

In their original clinical description of acute MI in 1910, Obraztsov and Strazhesko noted, "Direct events often precipitated the disease; the infarct began in one case on climbing a high staircase, in another during an unpleasant conversation, and in a third during emotional distress associated with a heated card game" [11]. In the 1930s, larger studies revealed that MI often occurred without an obvious precipitating event, thus challenging their view. Authors argued for [12, 13] and against [14, 15] the belief that triggers were frequent. The controversy was eventually suspended for many years as Master's conclusion, based on retrospective questionnaires, that "coronary occlusion takes place irrespective of the physical activity being performed or the type of rest taken" gained widespread acceptance [16]. However, studies conducted with modern epidemiologic methods and with the insight provided by new understanding of the pathogenesis of MI indicate that the original concept of Obraztsov and Strazhesko may be correct.

Morning Increase of Myocardial Infarction

The evidence that MI does not occur randomly throughout the day, but shows a prominent increased morning frequency, supports the concept that daily activities are important triggers. Data indicating that the onset of MI is more likely to occur in the morning come from two studies that determined the time of onset of infarction objectively with creatine kinase timing, and from other studies [17, 18] that used onset of pain as the marker for time of MI onset. In the Multicenter Investigation of Limitation of Infarct Size (MILIS) [3] involving 849 patients, the isoenzyme of creatine

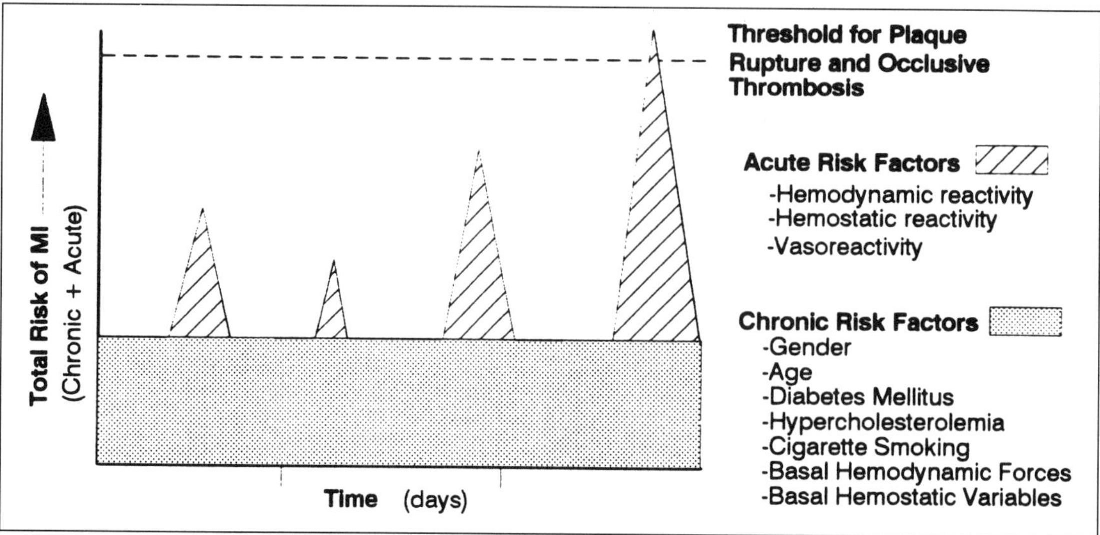

Fig. 2-1
The proposed combined contribution of chronic and acute factors required to exceed the threshold to initiate myocardial infarction (MI). The spikes indicate transient increases in risk resulting from a stress such as anger or physical exertion. These spikes rise from a baseline of chronic risk.

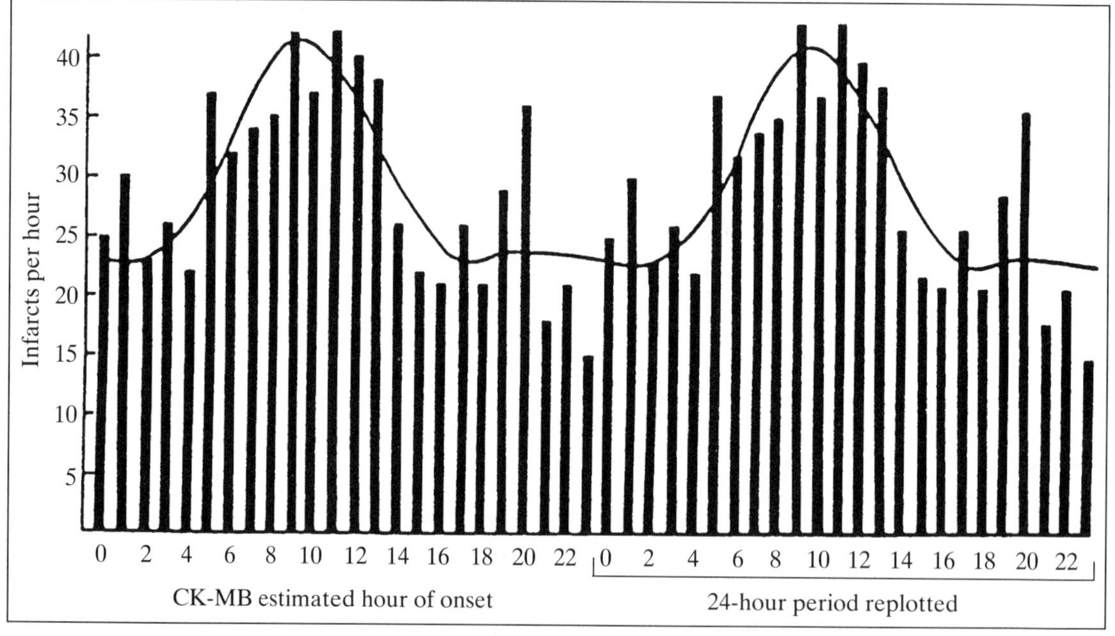

Fig. 2-2
Hourly frequency of onset of myocardial infarction as determined by the creatine kinase (CK)-MB method. The number of infarctions beginning during each of the 24 hours of the day is plotted on the *left side*. On the *right*, the identical data are plotted again to permit appreciation of the relation between the end and the beginning of the day. A two-harmonic regression equation for the frequency of onset of myocardial infarction has been fitted to the data (*curved line*). A primary peak incidence of infarction occurs at 9 a.m. and a secondary peak occurs at 8 p.m. (Reprinted by permission from J. E. Muller et al., Circadian variation in the frequency of onset of acute myocardial infarction. *N. Engl. J. Med.* 313:1315, 1985.)

kinase with muscle and brain subunits (MB) was measured numerous times during the first hours of MI to determine objectively the time of onset of MI. The onset of MI was considered to have occurred 4 hours before the initial elevation of creatine kinase levels. The time of day of onset of MI in the 703 patients for whom complete creatine kinase data were available is shown in Figure 2-2. A marked variation was noted, with a maximum of 45 infarcts occurring between 9 and 10 a.m. and a minimum of 15 between 11 p.m. and midnight. This objective evidence obtained in the MILIS database was confirmed in the database (1741 patients) from the Intravenous Streptokinase in Acute Myocardial Infarction (ISAM) Study [4], which demonstrated that MI was four times more likely to occur between 8 and 9 a.m. than between midnight and 1 a.m.

Goldberg et al. further supported the findings of these two studies. They reported that the increased incidence of MI occurs in the first 4 hours after awakening and onset of activity [18].

Two other cardiovascular diseases, sudden cardiac death and stroke, also have an increased incidence in the morning [19–23]. These findings reinforce the evidence that nonfatal MI has a prominent morning increase in onset. A smaller, evening peak appears in some databases; its cause is not known and requires further investigation.

Epidemiologic Evidence That Activities Trigger Disease Onset

Review of data on possible triggering activities that were collected from 849 patients enrolled in the MILIS [5] revealed that possible triggers were reported by 48.5 percent of patients, 13.6 percent of whom reported two or more triggers. The triggers included emotional upset (18.8 percent), moderate physical activity (14.4 percent), heavy physical activity (8.7 percent), lack of sleep (8.0 percent), overeating (6.9 percent), sexual activity (1.2 percent), surgery (0.4 percent), and others (6.6 percent). These data are similar to those reported by Sumiyoshi et al. [24].

The level of physical activity at onset of MI was determined in 3339 patients entered into the Thrombolysis in Myocardial Infarction (TIMI) II Study [6]. At onset of MI, 18.7 percent of patients were engaged in moderate or marked physical activity, a percentage higher than could be expected to be the usual percentage of the 24 hours that the subjects engage in moderate or marked activity. Independent predictors of MI beginning during activity ($p < .01$) included male gender, no use of calcium antagonists or nitrates in the prior 24 hours, no history of hypertension, and being a nonsmoker.

While these and other studies suggest that triggers of MI are present, and that different subgroups have a different likelihood of their MI being preceded by a potential trigger, all studies suffer from the lack of control data. To assess the relative risk of an MI occurring following a common stressor such as physical exercise, it is essential to estimate the expected level of activity in the hours before the MI. Adjustment for usual exposure is also needed for comparisons of possible triggering between groups because differences clearly exist in the likelihood of patients with specific characteristics, such as older age, performing activities such as heavy physical exertion.

These and other methodological limitations of earlier studies were addressed in the Determinants of Onset of Myocardial Infarction (ONSET) Study, in which more than 1800 patients were interviewed to identify possible triggers of their MI. For the ONSET Study, a case-crossover study design developed by Mittleman and Maclure [7, 25] enabled estimation of the relative risk of an MI following a trigger. This risk is calculated as the observed frequency of the activity during a designated hazard period (the hour prior to the MI) compared with the observed frequency of the activity during a comparable 1-hour period 24 to 25 hours prior to the MI. With this method, it was demonstrated that heavy exertion (exertion estimated to be ≥ 6 metabolic equivalents [METS]) produced a 5.9-fold increase in risk (95 percent confidence interval: 4.6–7.7) of MI in the subsequent hour. The risk of MI onset during heavy exertion was significantly higher in those who were sedentary (107-fold) compared with those who regularly exercised (twofold) [7] (Fig. 2-3).

Although the evidence for psychological stress playing a role in triggering MI is compelling, there have been no controlled studies of this acute phenomenon, and prior studies of anger, hostility, and type A personality as risk factors for MI that focused on chronic risk yielded controversial and sometimes contradictory results [26]. In the ONSET Study, data on outbursts of anger in 1623

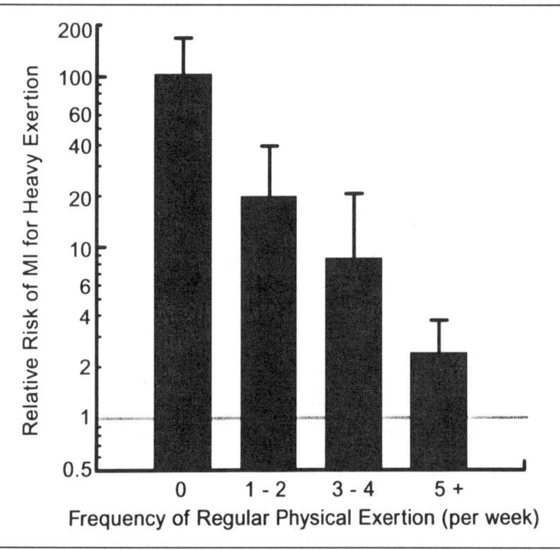

Fig. 2-3
Modification of the relative risk of myocardial infarction (MI) by usual frequency of heavy exertion (defined as ≥ 6 metabolic equivalents [METS]). The relative risks for heavy physical exertion are shown for subgroups of patients whose habitual frequency of heavy physical exertion is less than one, one or two, three or four, and five or more episodes per week. Note that the relative risk is presented on a logarithmic scale. Sedentary individuals experienced an extreme relative risk (107-fold), while those who exerted themselves five or more times per week had an increase in risk only 2.4 times over baseline ($p < .001$). *Error bars* indicate 95% confidence intervals. (Reprinted by permission from M. Mittleman et al., Triggering of acute myocardial infarction by heavy physical exertion: Protection by regular exertion. *N. Engl. J. Med.* 392:1680, 1993.)

patients were collected. Anger corresponding to levels higher than 4 in a 7-level self-report anger scale was reported by 14 percent of patients within 24 hours prior to MI onset. Using the ONSET Study design described above, we found that the risk of MI onset was significantly elevated in the 2 hours following an outburst of anger (level > 4), with a relative risk of 2.3 (95 percent confidence interval: 1.7–3.2) [27].

Autopsy and Angiographic Data Pertinent to Triggering

In 1980, DeWood et al. demonstrated that occlusive coronary artery thrombosis is the cause of most Q-wave MIs [28]. Furthermore, coronary angiographic and angioscopic studies demonstrated a high frequency of nonocclusive coronary thrombosis in patients with unstable angina [29, 30]. Constantinides observed that thrombus had formed over a ruptured atherosclerotic plaque in all the occluded coronary arteries he examined [31]. A recent angiographic finding that contrast media outpouching, indicative of plaque rupture, was observed in patients who had undergone successful thrombolysis supports the importance of plaque rupture in acute coronary syndromes [32].

Although autopsy studies generally reveal severe atherosclerotic stenosis at the base of a fatal coronary thrombus [33], there is angiographic evidence that in many patients surviving an MI, the degree of stenosis is relatively mild and that obstructive thrombus accounts for the majority of the obstruction to blood flow [8–10]. These findings may explain the absence of prior symptoms in many patients presenting with acute MI. Intrinsic plaque characteristics and extrinsic factors that predispose and initiate plaque disruption remain areas of intense investigation. Richardson and coworkers recently reported that in 63 percent of patients, rupture of the plaque occurred at the junction of a lipid pool with normal tissue [34]. Presence of a lipid core, a thin fibrous cap, and macrophage activity seem to be important factors that predispose an atherosclerotic plaque to rupture [35].

Morning Increase of Physiologic Processes That Might Trigger Myocardial Infarction

Physiologic processes that are accentuated in the morning include arterial pressure, blood viscosity, platelet aggregability, and catecholamine secretion. Morning accentuation of physiologic processes to which vulnerable atherosclerotic plaques are exposed, alone or in combination, could account for the morning increase in MI onset (see Fig. 2-1) through a variety of mechanisms.

The morning arterial pressure surge [36] could initiate plaque rupture. The increase in coronary arterial tone [37] could worsen the flow reduction produced by a fixed stenosis. The arterial pressure increase and the coronary tone increase could result in increased shear stress (force directed against the endothelium, the artery's innermost layer, resulting from increased coronary blood flow velocity) [38] predisposing to plaque rupture and increased platelet deposition [39]. The increase in blood viscosity [40], increased platelet aggregability [41] (resulting from assumption of the upright posture) [42], and an insufficient countervailing circadian rise in circulating tissue plasminogen activator activity [43–45] could produce a state of relative hypercoagulability. Such a thrombotic tendency could increase the likelihood that an otherwise harmless mural thrombus overlying a small plaque fissure would propagate and occlude the coronary lumen. Although serum cortisol levels are falling during the period of increased disease onset, they are increased above basal levels [46]. This increase could enhance the sensitivity of the coronary arteries to the vasoconstrictor effects of catecholamines [47], which show a prominent surge after assumption of the upright posture [42].

Although the peak incidence of disease onset occurs in the morning, it is likely that similar physiologic processes trigger disease onset at other times of the day. The peak morning incidence of infarct onset probably results from the synchronization of the population for triggers in the morning, while a secondary evening peak in infarct onset observed in the MILIS data [3] may result from synchronization of the population for an additional trigger, such as the evening meal. For other periods of the day, exposure of the population to potential triggers is random, and no other prominent peaks of incidence are observed.

Effects of Pharmacologic Agents on Timing and Triggers

Evaluation of the effect of medications on the temporal pattern of cardiovascular disease onset may provide a better insight into the mechanism of the disease onset, and also aid in the design of improved preventive strategies.

Beta-adrenergic Blockers

It has been known for some time that beta blockers reduce the incidence of recurrent MI and sudden cardiac death following MI [48, 49]. It has also been reported that these agents are capable of providing primary prevention against MI [50], although this finding has been controversial.

In the MILIS, patients taking beta-blocking agents had no morning peak in onset of acute MI [3]. This finding was confirmed in the ISAM and TIMI II databases [4, 6], which showed that the group undergoing prior beta blockade was the only one among all subgroups not to show a morning increase. Patients who were taking calcium channel blockers prior to their MI exhibited a typical morning increase. A retrospective analysis of the time of day that out-of-hospital sudden cardiac death occurred in the Beta-Blocker Heart Attack Trial (BHAT) [51], a multicenter study involving 3857 patients after MI who were randomized to receive either placebo or propranolol, showed that the major benefit of beta blockade occurred during the morning hours. During this period, there was a 44 percent reduction in the morning incidence of sudden cardiac death in the beta blocker–treated group versus a reduction of just 18 percent at other times of the day. In other studies, an additional beneficial effect of beta blockers has been the morning reduction of silent ischemia episodes, which also have a morning peak of incidence in the nontreated group [52].

Despite extensive study, the mechanism by which beta blockers exert their protective effect has not been identified. It has been particularly difficult to explain the ability of a beta blocker to prevent MI, which is generally caused by coronary thrombosis, since most beta-adrenergic blocking agents have only minimal antiplatelet activity [53]. It is possible that beta blockers exert their protective effect by blunting the morning increase in sympathetic activity. Such blunting would minimize increases in myocardial contractility and arterial pressure, which might increase wall stress [54] and the likelihood of plaque disruption and consequent thrombosis.

Aspirin

Two double-blinded, randomized studies of patients with unstable angina demonstrated that aspirin therapy reduced the incidence of subsequent MI and sudden death by 50 percent [55, 56]. In addition, combined analysis of six large studies on the administration of aspirin to patients after infarction indicated that aspirin reduces postinfarction mortality [57]. The results of these studies on aspirin for secondary prevention were supported by the results of the Physicians' Health Study, which demonstrated the ability of aspirin to provide primary prevention against MI. In the aspirin-treated patients, the morning peak in MI was selectively attenuated (a 59.3 percent reduction in the incidence of infarction during the morning, compared with a 34.1 percent reduction for the remaining hours of the day) [58] (Fig. 2-4). This differential effect may reflect the blunting of a potential triggering mechanism—the morning surge in platelet activity [41].

Fig. 2-4
Prevention of morning myocardial infarction by preventing platelet surge. Proposed contribution of morning platelet surge to morning myocardial infarction and its prevention by aspirin. (*Top*) The ability of aspirin to selectively reduce the morning peak in frequency of myocardial infarction. (From P. M. Ridker et al., Circadian variation of acute myocardial infarction and the effect of low-dose aspirin in randomized trial of physicians. *Circulation* 82:897, 1990. By permission of the American Heart Association. (*Bottom*) The ability of aspirin to abolish the morning increase in platelet aggregability. ADP = adenosine diphosphate. (Modified by permission from G. H. Tofler et al., Concurrent morning increase in platelet aggregability and the risk of myocardial infarction and sudden cardiac death. *N. Engl. J. Med.* 316:1514, 1987.)

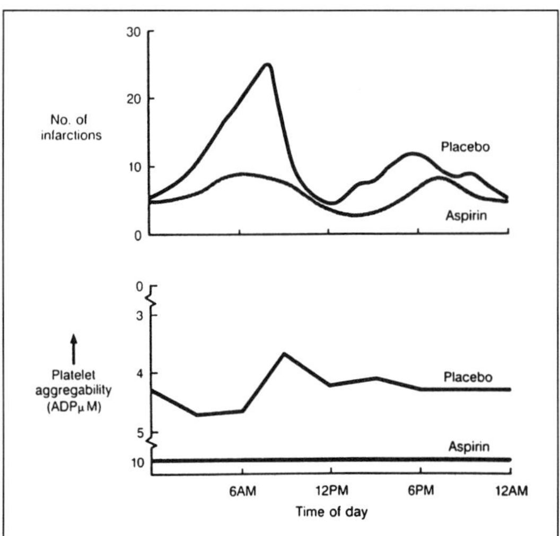

General Theory of Triggering of Coronary Thrombosis

Our group proposed a general hypothesis of the manner in which daily activities might trigger coronary thrombosis [1]. The hypothesis presented in Figure 2-5 adds the concept of triggering activities to the general scheme of the role of thrombosis in the acute coronary syndromes advanced by Falk, Davies and Thomas, and Fuster and Willerson and their respective colleagues [33, 59–62]. It involves three important concepts: *triggers, acute risk factors,* and *vulnerable plaques.* We hypothesize that plaque rupture with occlusive thrombosis occurs at a critical moment when a threshold combination of hemodynamic, prothrombotic, and vasoconstrictive forces (acute risk factors) is rapidly generated by external stressors such as physical exertion or episodes of anger (triggers).

We propose that the initial step in the process leading to coronary thrombosis is the development, with advancing age, of a vulnerable atherosclerotic plaque. Plaque vulnerability is defined functionally as the susceptibility of a plaque to disruption. Development of such vulnerability is a poorly understood process, but is presumably a dynamic, potentially reversible disorder caused by several factors, including changes in plaque constituents or its blood supply via vasa vasorum (blood vessels nourishing the artery wall), and changes in the functional integrity of the overlying endothelium due in part to increased macrophage activity and dissolution of the plaque collagen cap. The new catheterization laboratory techniques of intracoronary angioscopy and ultrasound may, in the future, permit detection of vulnerable plaques.

Onset of MI might begin when a physical or mental stress produces a hemodynamic change that is sufficient to rupture a vulnerable plaque. However, if such a trigger does not occur during a time of plaque vulnerability, the plaque may change and become nonvulnerable. A synergistic combination of triggering activities may account for thrombosis where each activity alone may not exceed the disruption threshold. For example, the combination of physical exertion (producing a minor plaque rupture) followed by cigarette smoking (producing an increase in coronary artery vasoconstriction and a relatively hypercoagulable state) [63] may be needed to cause occlusive thrombosis and disease

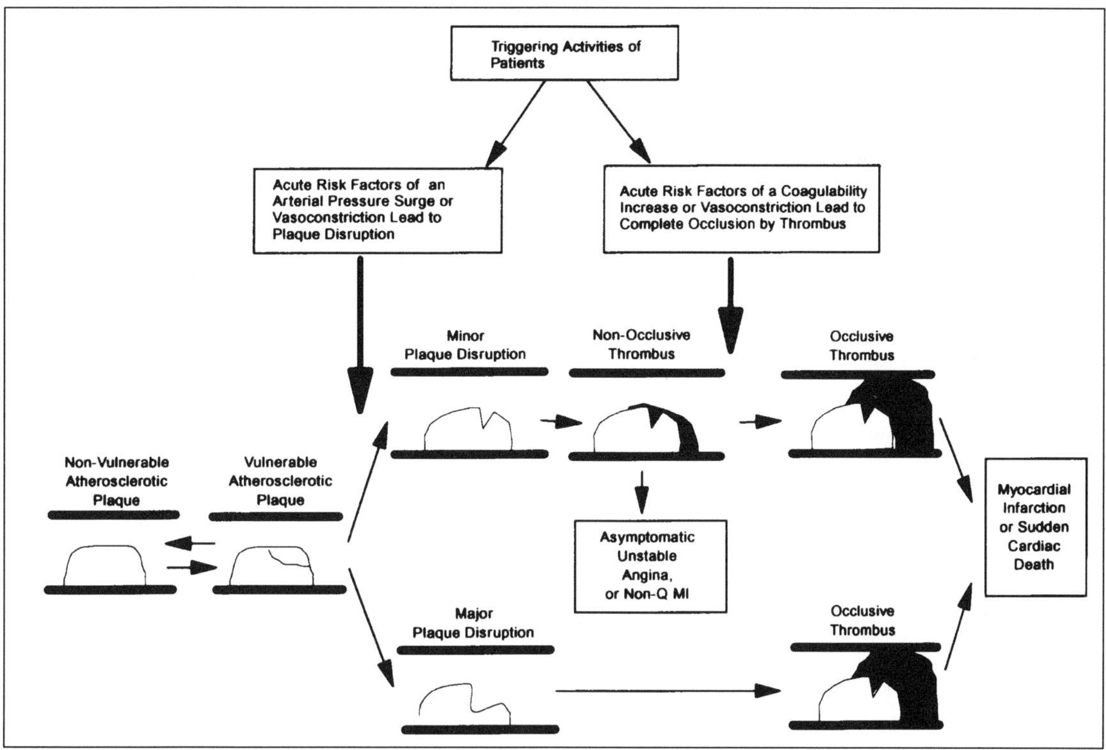

Fig. 2-5
A hypothetic presentation of the manner in which daily activities may trigger coronary thrombosis. Three triggering mechanisms—(1) physical or mental stress producing hemodynamic changes leading to plaque rupture, (2) a coagulability increase, and (3) vasoconstriction—have been added to the well-known scheme depicting the role of coronary thrombosis in unstable angina, myocardial infarction (MI), and sudden cardiac death. See text for detailed discussion. (From J. E. Muller et al., Circadian variation and triggers of onset of acute cardiovascular disease. *Circulation* 79:733, 1989. By permission of the American Heart Association.)

onset. Also, the response to a potential trigger of a healthy individual may differ from that observed in an individual with a condition predisposing to MI. Exaggerated or paradoxical responses may be observed. For example, hypertensive subjects demonstrate a greater increase in forearm vascular resistance after infusion of norepinephrine than do normal subjects [64]. Patients with atherosclerosis may demonstrate a paradoxical vasoconstrictor response in response to acetylcholine infusion [65] and an impaired increase in fibrinolytic potential with exercise [66].

The findings of circadian variation and triggering have also led to the concept of an acute risk factor that supplements the traditional concept of a chronic risk factor. The acute risk factor results from a combination of an external stress (physical or mental) and the individual's reactivity to that stress. While the extent of atherosclerosis changes slowly with time (chronic risk factor), hemodynamic, vasoconstrictive, and prothrombotic forces (acute risk factors) may be rapidly generated by external stresses.

Significance

The primary immediate value of recognition of the circadian variation of acute onset of MI is the emphasis that can be placed on pharmacologic protection during the morning hours for patients already receiving anti-ischemic therapy. Although no data are available to support the hypothesis, it seems reasonable that long-acting anti-ischemic agents would have an advantage over short-acting agents in providing protection against MI in the morning when the effects of short-acting agents taken the night before may begin to attenuate.

Even complete elimination of the morning increase in onset of MI by effective therapy would prevent only a small fraction of the total morbidity and mortality caused by this disease. Although the incidence of disease onset is greatest in the 6 a.m. to noon period, the majority of infarcts occur at other times of the day, and their prevention requires a broader approach. For this reason, it is likely that the primary significance of the recognition of circadian variation of disease onset is the support it provides for the broader concept that the onset of infarction at any time of the day is frequently triggered by activities of the patient.

The finding that MIs appear to be triggered in the morning has raised questions about the desirability of exercise in the morning. At present the evidence that exercise is beneficial in reducing the risk of infarction [67] is substantial. Although theoretic concerns can be raised, there is no evidence that exercise in the morning is more hazardous than exercise at other times of the day. On the contrary, Murray et al. retrospectively studied patients who exercised in the morning and patients who exercised in the afternoon; they found no significant difference in the rate of cardiovascular events [68]. Furthermore, even a tenfold increase in the relative risk of an event caused by morning exertion would produce only a small increase in absolute risk [6]. The absolute risk of having an MI in the hour after exertion might rise from approximately 5 in 1 million to 5 in 100,000. This small absolute risk does not justify a recommendation to avoid morning exertion, particularly when the beneficial effects of regular exertion are taken into consideration. Data from the ONSET Study showing that individuals who regularly exercise have a reduced relative risk of MI triggered by physical activity compared with sedentary individuals (see Fig. 2-3) further support the benefit of regular exercise.

Despite the recent progress in understanding the mechanisms of disease onset, studies ranging from the epidemiologic to the molecular level remain to be done. Insight into triggering and acute risk factors offers a new approach to prevention through identification and treatment of the plaques that are vulnerable to rupture, and through the development of pharmacologic and nonpharmacologic means to sever the linkage between a potential triggering activity and its catastrophic consequences.

References

1. Muller, J. E., Tofler, G. H., and Stone, P. H. Circadian variation and triggers of onset of acute cardiovascular disease. *Circulation* 79:733, 1989.
2. Levy, D., and Kannel, W. B. Cardiovascular risks: New insights from Framingham. *Am. Heart J.* 116: 266, 1988.
3. Muller, J. E., Stone, P. H., Turi, Z. G., et al. Circadian variation in the frequency of onset of acute myocardial infarction. *N. Engl. J. Med.* 313:1315, 1985.
4. Willich, S. N., Linderer, T., Wegscheider, K., et al., the ISAM Study Group. Increased morning incidence of myocardial infarction in the ISAM Study: Absence with prior beta-adrenergic blockade. *Circulation* 80:853, 1989.
5. Tofler, G. H., Stone, P. H., Maclure, M., et al. Analysis of possible triggers of acute myocardial infarction (MILIS study). *Am. J. Cardiol.* 66:22, 1990.
6. Tofler, G. H., Muller, J. E., Stone, P. H., et al. Modifiers of timing and possible triggers of acute myocardial infarction in the Thrombolysis in Myocardial Infarction Study (TIMI II) population. *J. Am. Coll. Cardiol.* 20:1045, 1992.
7. Mittleman, M. A., Maclure, M., Tofler, G. H., et al. Triggering of acute myocardial infarction by heavy physical exertion: Protection by regular exertion. *N. Engl. J. Med.* 329:1677, 1993.
8. Brown, B. G., Gallery, C. A., Badger, R. S., et al. Incomplete lysis of thrombus in the moderate underlying atherosclerotic lesion during intracoronary infusion of streptokinase for acute myocardial infarction: Quantitative angiographic observations. *Circulation* 73:653, 1986.
9. Little, W. L., Constantinescu, M., Applegate, R. J., et al. Can coronary angiography predict the site of a subsequent myocardial infarction in patients with mild-to-moderate coronary artery disease. *Circulation* 78:1157, 1988.
10. Haft, J. I., Haik, B. J., and Goldstein, J. E. Catastrophic progression of coronary artery lesions, the common mechanism for coronary disease progression (Abstract). *Circulation* 76(Suppl IV):IV-168, 1987.
11. Obraztsov, V. P., and Strazhesko, N. D. The symptomatology and diagnosis of coronary thrombosis. In V. A. Vorobeva and M. P. Konchalovski (eds.), *Works of the First Congress of Russian Therapists.* Comradeship Typography of A. E. Mamontov, 1910. Pp. 26–43.
12. Fitzhugh, G., and Hamilton, B. E. Coronary occlusion and fatal angina pectoris. Study of the immediate causes and their prevention. *J.A.M.A.* 100:475, 1933.

13. Sproul, J. A general practitioner's views on the treatment of angina pectoris. *N. Engl. J. Med.* 215:443, 1936.
14. Parkinson, J., and Bedford, D. E. Cardiac infarction and coronary thrombosis. *Lancet* 1:4, 1928.
15. Phipps, C. Contributory causes of coronary thrombosis. *J.A.M.A.* 106:761, 1936.
16. Master, A. M. The role of effort and occupation (including physicians) in coronary occlusion. *J.A.M.A.* 174:942, 1960.
17. Thompson, D. R., Blandford, R. L., Sutton, T. W., and Marchant, P. R. Time of onset of chest pain in acute myocardial infarction. *Int. J. Cardiol.* 7:139, 1985.
18. Goldberg, R., Brady, P., Muller, J. E., et al. Time of onset of symptoms of acute myocardial infarction. *Am. J. Cardiol.* 66:140, 1990.
19. Muller, J. E., Ludmer, P. L., Willich, S. N., et al. Circadian variation in the frequency of sudden cardiac death. *Circulation* 75:131, 1987.
20. Willich, S. N., Levy, D., Rocco, M. B., et al. Circadian variation in the incidence of sudden cardiac death in the Framingham Heart Study population. *Am. J. Cardiol.* 60:801, 1987.
21. French, A. J., and Dock, W. Fatal coronary atherosclerosis in young soldiers. *J.A.M.A.* 124:1233, 1944.
22. Tsementzis, S. A., Gill, J. S., Hitchcock, E. R., et al. Diurnal variation of and activity during the onset of stroke. *Neurosurgery* 17:901, 1985.
23. Marler, J. R., Price, T. R., Clark, G. L., et al. Morning increase in onset of ischemic stroke. *Stroke* 20:473, 1989.
24. Sumiyoshi T., et al. Evaluation of clinical factors involved in onset of myocardial infarction. *Jpn. Circ. J.* 50:164, 1986.
25. Maclure, M. The case-crossover design: A method for studying transient effects on the risk of acute events. *Am. J. Epidemiol.* 133:144, 1991.
26. Eaker, E. D. Use of questionnaires, interviews and psychological tests in epidemiologic studies of coronary heart disease. *Eur. Heart J.* 9:698, 1988.
27. Mittleman, M. A., Maclure, M., Sherwood, J. B., et al. Triggering of myocardial infarction onset by episodes of anger (Abstract). *Circulation* 89:936, 1994.
28. DeWood, M. A., Spores, J., Notske, R., et al. Prevalence of total coronary occlusion during the early hours of transmural myocardial infarction. *N. Engl. J. Med.* 303:897, 1980.
29. Ambrose, J. A., Winters, S. L., Stern, A., et al. Angiographic morphology and the pathogenesis of unstable angina pectoris. *J. Am. Coll. Cardiol.* 5:609, 1985.
30. Sherman, C. T., Litvack, F., Grundfest, W., et al. Coronary angioscopy in patients with unstable angina pectoris. *N. Engl. J. Med.* 315:913, 1986.
31. Constantinides, P. Plaque fissure in human coronary thrombosis. *J. Atheroscler. Res.* 6:1, 1966.
32. Nakagawa, S., Hanada, Y., Koiwaya, Y.,and Tanaka, K. Angiographic features in the infarct-related artery after intracoronary urokinase followed by prolonged anticoagulation: Role of ruptured atheromatous plaque and adherent thrombus in acute myocardial infarction in vivo. *Circulation* 78:1335, 1988.
33. Falk, E. Plaque rupture with severe pre-existing stenosis precipitating coronary thrombosis. *Br. Heart J.* 50:127, 1983.
34. Richardson, P. D., Davies, M. J., and Born, G. V. R. Influence of plaque configuration and stress distribution on fissuring of coronary atherosclerotic plaques. *Lancet* 2:941, 1989.
35. Falk, E. Why do plaques rupture? *Circulation* 86 (Suppl III):III-30, 1992.
36. Millar-Craig, M. W., Bishop, C. N., and Raftery, E. B. Circadian variation of blood pressure. *Lancet* 1:795, 1978.
37. Fujita, M., and Franklin, D. Diurnal changes in coronary blood flow in conscious dogs. *Circulation* 76:488, 1987.
38. Vita, J. A., Treasure, C. B., Ganz, P., et al. Control of shear stress in the epicardial coronary arteries of humans: Impairment by atherosclerosis. *J. Am. Coll. Cardiol.* 14:1193, 1989.
39. Badimon, L., and Badimon, J. J. Mechanisms of arterial thrombosis in nonparallel streamlines: Platelet thrombi grow on the apex of stenotic severely injured vessel wall: Experimental study in pig model. *J. Clin. Invest.* 4:1134, 1989.
40. Ehrly, A. M., and Jung, G. Circadian rhythm of human blood viscosity. *Biorheology* 10:577, 1973.
41. Tofler, G. H., Brezinski, D. A., Schafer, A. I., et al. Concurrent morning increase in platelet aggregability and the risk of myocardial infarction and sudden cardiac death. *N. Engl. J. Med.* 316:1514, 1987.
42. Brezinski, D. A., Tofler, G. H., Muller, J. E., et al. Morning increase in platelet aggregability: Association with assumption of the upright posture. *Circulation* 78:35, 1988.
43. Rosing, D. R., Brakman, P., Redwood, D. R., et al. Blood fibrinolytic activity in man: Diurnal variation and the response to varying intensities of exercise. *Circ. Res.* 27:171, 1970.
44. Andreotti, F., Davies, G. J., Hackett, D. R., et al. Major circadian fluctuations in fibrinolytic factors and possible relevance to time of onset of myocardial infarction, sudden cardiac death, and stroke. *Am. J. Cardiol.* 62:635, 1988.
45. Speiser, W., Langer, W., Pschaick, A., et al. Increased blood fibrinolytic activity after physical exercise: Comparative study in individuals with different sporting activities and in patients after myocardial infarction taking part in a rehabilitation sports program. *Thromb. Res.* 51:543, 1988.
46. Weitzman, E. D., Fukushima, D., Nogeire, C., et al. Twenty-four hour pattern of the episodic secretion of cortisol in normal subjects. *J. Clin. Endocrinol.* 33:14, 1971.
47. Sudhir, K., Jennings, G. L., Esler, M. D., et al. Hydrocortisone-induced hypertension in humans: Pressor responsiveness and sympathetic function. *Hypertension* 13:416, 1989.
48. Norwegian Multicenter Study Group. Timolol in-

duced reduction in mortality and reinfarction in patients surviving acute myocardial infarction. *N. Engl. J. Med.* 304:801, 1981.
49. Beta-blocker Heart Attack Trial Research Group. A randomized trial of propranolol in patients with myocardial infarction: Mortality results. *J.A.M.A.* 247:1707, 1982.
50. Wikstrand, J., Warnold, I., Olsson, G., et al. Primary prevention with metoprolol in patients with hypertension: Mortality results from the MAPHY study. *J.A.M.A.* 259:1976, 1988.
51. Peters, R. W., Muller, J. E., Goldstein, S., et al. Propranolol and the morning increase in the frequency of sudden cardiac death (BHAT study). *Am. J. Cardiol.* 63:1518, 1989.
52. Mulcahy, D., Keegan, J., Cunningham, D., et al. Circadian variation of total ischemic burden and its alteration with anti-anginal agents. *Lancet* 2:755, 1988.
53. Frishman, W. H. Multifactorial actions of beta-adrenergic blocking drugs in ischemic heart disease: Current concepts. *Circulation* 67(Suppl 1):I-11, 1983.
54. Gertz, S. D., and Roberts, W. C. Hemodynamic shear force in rupture of coronary arterial atherosclerotic plaques (Editorial). *Am. J. Cardiol.* 66:1368, 1990.
55. Lewis, H. D., Davis, J. W., Archibald, D. G., et al. Protective effects of aspirin against acute myocardial infarction and death in men with unstable angina: Results of a Veterans Administration Cooperative Study. *N. Engl. J. Med.* 309:396, 1983.
56. Canadian Cooperative Study Group. A randomized trial of aspirin and sulfinpyrazone in threatened stroke. *N. Engl. J. Med.* 299:53, 1978.
57. Hennekens, C. H., Buring, J. E., Sandercock, P., et al. Aspirin and other antiplatelet agents in the secondary and primary prevention of cardiovascular disease. *Circulation* 80:749, 1989.
58. Ridker, P. M., Manson, J. E., Buring, J. E., et al. Circadian variation of acute myocardial infarction and the effect of low-dose aspirin in a randomized trial of physicians. *Circulation* 82:897, 1990.
59. Fuster, V., Badimon, L., Badimon, J. J., and Chesebro, J. H. The pathogenesis of coronary artery disease and the acute coronary syndromes. *N. Engl. J. Med.* 326:242, 1992.
60. Davies, M. J., and Thomas, A. C. Plaque fissuring—the cause of acute myocardial infarction, sudden ischemic death, and crescendo angina. *Br. Heart J.* 53:363, 1985.
61. Fuster, V., Steele, P. M., and Chesebro, J. H. Role of platelets and thrombosis in coronary atherosclerotic disease and sudden death. *J. Am. Coll. Cardiol.* 5(Suppl):175B, 1985.
62. Willerson, J. T., Campbell, W. B., Winniford, M. D., et al. Conversion from chronic to acute coronary artery disease: Speculation regarding mechanisms (Editorial). *Am. J. Cardiol.* 54:1349, 1984.
63. Belch, J. J. F., McArdle, B. M., Burns, P., et al. The effects of acute smoking on platelet behaviour, fibrinolysis, and haemorheology in habitual smokers. *Thromb. Haemost.* 51:6, 1984.
64. Egan, B., Schork, N., Panis, R., and Hinderliter, A. Vascular structure enhances regional resistance responses in mild essential hypertension. *J. Hypertens.* 6:41, 1988.
65. Ludmer, P. L., Selwyn, A. P., Shook, T. L., et al. Paradoxical vasoconstriction induced by acetylcholine in atherosclerotic coronary arteries. *N. Engl. J. Med.* 315:1046, 1986.
66. Khann, P. K., Seth, H. N., Balasubramanian, V., and Hoon, R. S. Effect of submaximal exercise on fibrinolytic activity in ischemic heart disease. *Br. Med. J.* 2:910, 1975.
67. Ekelund, L. G., Haskell, W. L., Johnson, J. L., et al. Physical fitness as a predictor of cardiovascular mortality in asymptomatic North American men. The Lipid Research Clinics Mortality Follow-up Study. *N. Engl. J. Med.* 319:1379, 1988.
68. Murray, P. M., Herrington, D. M., Pettus, C. W., et al. Should patients with heart disease exercise in the morning or the afternoon? *Arch. Intern. Med.* 153:833, 1993.

3. Biochemistry of Acute Myocardial Infarction

Heinrich Taegtmeyer

The success of thrombolytic therapy in acute myocardial infarction is based on the premise that the development of an infarction can be stopped in its tracks. Because successful restoration of blood flow does not always result in a return of contractile function, the biochemical derangements involving the ischemic and infarcting myocardium have come under considerable scrutiny. These derangements are complex and for the most part are not even completely understood. A brief recapitulation of the essence of energy metabolism in normal heart is therefore necessary. I start out with a description of the "chemistry" of the intricate system of metabolic pathways, which is best characterized by the heart's ability to convert chemical into mechanical energy, before I explore the consequences of the sudden interruption of this supply and their clinical implications. For the sake of clarity, the main concepts are emphasized, and only few details are elaborated.

Heart Muscle as Site of Energy Conversion

The functions of metabolism in the heart are easy to understand. The heart is both consumer and provider of energy [1], and the main purpose of all biochemical reactions in the myocardial cell is to supply energy for coordinated contraction. Like any other living tissue, heart muscle captures and utilizes this energy in the form of adenosine triphosphate (ATP). A simple calculation may serve to illustrate the importance of the concept of energy turnover. The tissue content of ATP is normally around 20 μmol/gm of dry weight. At an oxygen consumption rate of about 4.5 μmol/min/gm of dry weight [2] and a phosphorus-oxygen (P/O) ratio of 3, heart muscle utilizes and replenishes about 1500 μmol of ATP/min/gm of dry weight (25 μmol/sec/gm of dry weight). This calculation illustrates that at an undiminished force of contraction, intracellular stores of ATP would be exhausted within a second. Thus ATP must be resynthesized as quickly as it is broken down, a concept that finds its expression in the "ATP cycle," depicted in Figure 3-1. This concept is somewhat oversimplified, as it does not take into account the small stores of phosphocreatine that replenish ATP by the creatinine kinase reaction (phosphocreatine + adenosine diphosphate [ADP] → creatine + ATP) and the action of the adenylate kinase reaction, which restores 1 mol of ATP from 2 mol of ADP (2 ADP → ATP + AMP) (see later discussion). Nonetheless, it can be gleaned that the rate of ATP turnover, rather than the steady-state concentrations of ATP, determines the energy state of the cell. Indeed, a number of studies showed a lack of correlation between ATP tissue content and oxygen consumption as well as contractile function in reperfused myocardium [3–5].

Energy transfer in heart muscle is linked to the flow of energy through a series of moiety-conserved cycles [1]. The main sources of ATP are oxidative phosphorylation of ADP in the respiratory chain and to a lesser extent, phosphorylation of ADP either by substrate-level phosphorylation in the glycolytic pathway and the Krebs cycle, or by the action of creatine kinase. Because oxidative phosphorylation is the major supplier of ATP and because the key enzymes of oxidative metabolism are located in mitochondria, myocardial cells are well endowed with these organelles. Mitochondria make up about one-third of the myocardial cell volume [6]. Not surprisingly, mitochondrial damage appears to be one of the main morphologic and functional consequences of myocardial ischemia and infarction [7–9].

Work from the author's laboratory has been supported by U.S. Public Health Service grant NHL R01-43133.

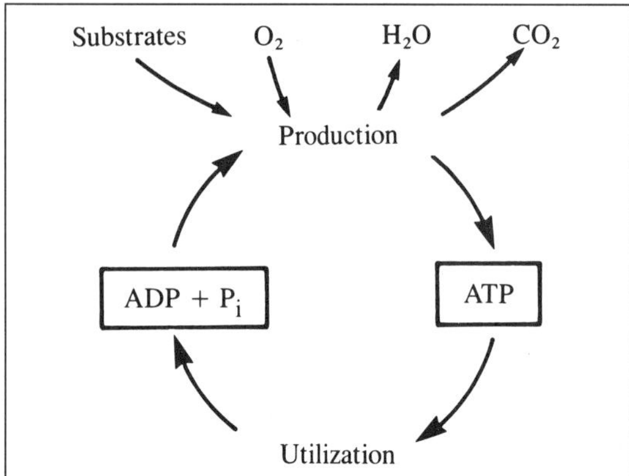

Fig. 3-1
Cycle of cardiac energy metabolism. The myocardial cell captures and utilizes energy in the phosphate bonds of adenosine triphosphate (ATP). Energy is captured in ATP by the conversion of substrates and oxygen to carbon dioxide and water. The energy is liberated through ATPase, causing hydrolysis of ATP to adenosine diphosphate (ADP) and inorganic phosphate (P); ATP is utilized for the various processes involved in contraction and maintenance of cellular homeostasis. An increase in energy utilization results in an instantaneous increase in energy production.

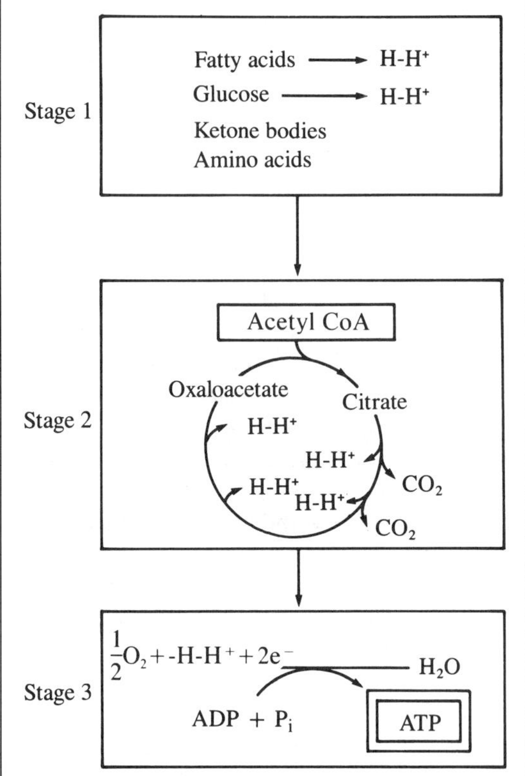

Fig. 3-2
Stages of normal cardiac energy metabolism. In the normal myocardium conversion of energy-providing substrates (fatty acids, glucose, ketone bodies, amino acids) to carbon dioxide and water occurs in a series of complex enzyme-catalyzed reactions, all of which ultimately lead to the production of reducing equivalents for reaction with molecular oxygen in the respiratory chain. All substrates are catabolized to acetyl CoA (stage 1). Acetyl CoA provides the substrate for the citrate synthesis reaction, which commits the compound to combustion in the citric acid cycle. This cycle is the main site for production of reducing equivalents (stage 2). Reducing equivalents react with oxygen in the respiratory chain, the site of oxidative phosphorylation of ADP to ATP (stage 3).

In respiring tissues, oxidative phosphorylation of ADP depends on the production of reducing equivalents (protons) and the passage of electrons along the respiratory chain. Reducing equivalents are produced in the course of substrate catabolism to acetyl coenzyme A (CoA) and the subsequent oxidation of acetyl CoA in the Krebs cycle. As a matter of convenience, it seems reasonable to group the main energy (or proton)-providing reactions into three stages (Fig. 3-2). The first stage comprises all reactions leading to acetyl CoA; the second stage comprises the oxidation of acetyl CoA in the Krebs cycle (producing carbon dioxide as a by-product); and the third stage consists of the flow of electrons down the respiratory chain leading to the release of free energy (producing water as a by-product), which is conserved in the energy-rich phosphate bond of ATP (see Figs. 3-1 and 3-2).

The heart's prodigious requirement for oxygen has been known for more than 100 years. In 1885, Professor Yeo [10] at King's College in London provided the first direct demonstration of oxygen uptake by heart muscle when he perfused a frog heart in a chamber containing hemoglobin, which he analyzed by spectroscopy. Yeo observed not only the reduction of oxyhemoglobin by the heart but also a greater rate of hemoglobin reduction when the heart was electrically stimulated. "Indeed we may conclude," he summarized, "that the absorption of a considerable quantity of oxygen is one of the items essential to the life of the tissue. The greater amount of oxygen used by the contracting heart muscle is so constant that it would appear equally certain that during contraction the oxygen requirement of the tissue notably increases.'' Nearly 20 years later, Winterstein [11] demonstrated the oxygen requirement for the mammalian heart when he showed that isolated rabbit hearts resumed beating as oxygen was readmitted to the perfusion medium after a brief period of anoxia. The first successful reperfusion experiment!

The fuels for oxidative metabolism or respiration of the heart differ with the metabolic environment. Although the heart plays only a minor role in the overall fuel balance of the body, it obeys the same general rules of metabolic regulation as do other tissues [12]. For instance, it has been known for a good number of years that in the fasting state the energy requirements of the heart are met largely by oxidation of fatty acids [13], and that after carbohydrate feeding, the heart switches its preference to glucose [14]. The heart can therefore be regarded as an ''omnivore''; that is, under aerobic conditions it is able to derive energy aerobically from a variety of fuel sources including fatty acids, ketone bodies, glucose, lactate, and even certain amino acids. Depending on the physiologic state of the individual, only plasma glucose levels are relatively constant, whereas levels of lactate, fatty acids, and ketone bodies may vary over a wide range. Not surprisingly, it has been found that the fuel for aerobic energy metabolism in heart muscle varies with the plasma concentration of individual substrates [14, 15] or hormones [16]. Given the large fluctuations in the plasma concentrations of exogenous fuels and the heart's ability to utilize a variety of fuels, Bing [12] viewed the phenomenon as a safety mechanism for the survival of a vital organ. This concept was recently extended [1]. While the metabolism of glucose, lactate, and pyruvate results in the production of acetyl CoA (through decarboxylation of pyruvate) as well as oxaloacetate (through carboxylation of pyruvate), the breakdown of fatty acids yields only acetyl CoA (from beta oxidation). It is therefore appropriate to refer to the carbohydrates glucose, lactate, and pyruvate as *essential fuels* and fatty acids as *nonessential fuels,* because the former provide both oxaloacetate and acetyl CoA for citrate synthesis, while fatty acids contribute acetyl CoA alone. Replenishment of citric acid intermediates (also termed *anaplerosis*) may become an important element of normal and postischemic contractile function [17, 18].

Heart muscle itself is also capable of contributing to the fuels of respiration by releasing both fatty acids and glucose from their storage forms as triglycerides or glycogen. Rates of synthesis and degradation for either storage fuel have not been measured so far, but it is well known that starvation increases the tissue content of both triglycerides and glycogen [19] and that the heart utilizes endogenous triglycerides when perfused with nutrient-free medium [20] or under conditions of increased pressure development [21]. The most striking example of endogenous fuel utilization is, of course, seen with ischemia, when glycogen is rapidly broken down to lactate and alanine.

Metabolic Alterations of Myocardial Ischemia and Infarction

Coupling of Coronary Flow to Metabolic and Mechanical Activity

It cannot be emphasized too strongly that the most characteristic feature of heart muscle is its high rate of energy turnover. Another fact has to be stressed as well: Because almost all of the heart's energy is derived from aerobic metabolism, oxygen consumption by the heart is several times greater than oxygen consumption by other mammalian organs [2], and only a slight perturbance in the supply of oxygen can lead to disastrous consequences for the energy supply of the myocardial cell. Such events are best characterized initially by reduced rates of ATP production (Fig. 3-3) and immediately thereafter by glycogen depletion, as well as the buildup of intermediary metabolites, protons, carbon dioxide, and (under certain conditions) triglycerides. The myocardial protein balance is not affected by the early stages of ischemia.

Because even under resting conditions the heart extracts almost all of the oxygen delivered by arterial blood, there is a tight coupling between blood flow through the coronary arteries and myocardial oxygen consumption. Thus the heart's ability to produce energy aerobically depends on its ability to increase coronary flow in accordance with its energy needs. For example, under resting condi-

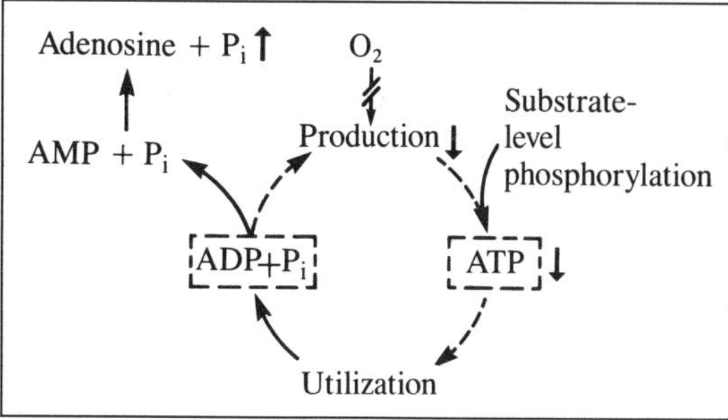

Fig. 3-3
Oxygen deprivation interrupts the cycle of cardiac energy metabolism at the level of energy production. Cellular stores of ATP are minimal, even when replenished by substrate-level phosphorylation. Because ADP is not phosphorylated, it is degraded further to adenosine monophosphate (AMP) and adenosine.

tions coronary flow is about 1 ml/min/gm of wet weight in humans, and it increases in parallel with myocardial oxygen consumption; that is, when oxygen consumption doubles, coronary flow doubles and so on. Conversely, a reduction of coronary flow results in a reduction of myocardial oxygen delivery and a consequential reduction in contractile force. In clinical practice, this relationship manifests itself as stress-induced asynergy or "hibernating myocardium."

Grading of Ischemia and Its Metabolic Response

The earliest forms of ischemia, defined as a lack of oxygen supply due to inadequate blood flow, occur in patients unable to increase coronary flow in responses to increased energy demands. Because resting coronary flow is normal in this setting, this form of ischemia is sometimes referred to as *normal flow ischemia.* By contrast, when coronary flow is reduced at rest, the term *low-flow ischemia* has been used. The extreme form of ischemia is, of course, reached by the complete occlusion of a coronary artery with subsequent necrosis of the tissue supplied. Thus there is a continuum of ischemia, with mild, normal-flow ischemia at one end and the extreme situation of a myocardial infarction at the other end of the spectrum. As will be discussed, the concept of a continuum of ischemia is also borne out by the temporal progression and spatial architecture of an acute myocardial infarction [22], which indicates progression of the zone of irreversible tissue injury from the subendocardium to the subepicardium as the time of ischemia lengthens (see Fig. 1-3).

Ischemia affects myocardial energy metabolism by slowing down the aerobic metabolism of substrates, reducing the tissue content of phosphocreatine and adenine nucleotides, and first increasing and then slowing down anaerobic metabolism of substrates (Table 3-1). Just as there is a continuum of the relative restriction of oxygen delivery, one might expect that there is a continuum of metabolic responses to ischemia. With normal-flow ischemia, heart muscle is still capable of oxidizing fatty acids and glucose under resting conditions. Opie and coworkers [23] showed that as coronary blood flow decreases, the relative contribution of glucose to the residual oxidative metabolism increases and oxidation of glucose accounts for a greater percentage of aerobic ATP production (Table 3-2). Increased uptake of a glucose analog by ischemic myocardium also was found when the energy demand for the heart was increased by pacing or exercise [15, 24]. There is increased lactate release from the stressed myocardium [24, 25] and increased glucose uptake, especially when fatty acid levels are low [26]. Possible reasons for increased glucose uptake with stress and ischemia are as follows: (1) Glucose makes better use of the limited amount of oxygen available to the myocyte. If the blood supply is mildly reduced, the heart switches from fatty acids to glucose as the preferred fuel for respiration. (2) Glycolysis yields a small amount of ATP through substrate-level phosphorylation in the cytosol independent of the availability of oxygen (2 mol of ATP/mol of glucose, whereas 36 mol of ATP is produced per mole of glucose oxidized). (3) Glucose transport is enhanced in oxygen-deprived tissue. Thus more glucose enters the cell, and glucose is preferred over fatty acids as the substrate for energy production.

Table 3-1
Energy metabolism of myocardial ischemia

Aerobic metabolism	↓
Phosphocreatine	↓
Adenine nucleotides	↓
Anaerobic metabolism	↑ (first)
Anaerobic metabolism	↓ (later)

Table 3-2
Relative contributions of glucose, fatty acids, and lactate to ATP production of the aerobic and ischemic dog heart

	ATP (μmol/min/gm)			
Condition	From glucose	From fatty acids	From lactate	Total
Aerobic	1980	2224	468	4672
Mild ischemia	1008–1260	188–257	0	1265–1448
Severe ischemia	677	70	0	747
Total ischemia	0	0	0	0

Source: From L. H. Opie. Effects of regional ischemia on metabolism of glucose and fatty acids. *Circ. Res.* 38(Suppl I):I-52, 1976. With permission of the American Heart Association, Inc.

The regulation of intermediary metabolism of glucose, fatty acids, and amino acids during ischemia is complex and requires further discussion with respect to the accumulation of intermediary metabolites and reversibility of ischemic tissue damage.

When oxygen becomes rate limiting for energy production, flux through the electron transport system of the respiratory chain slows down and the ratio of the reduced form of nicotinamide adenine dinucleotide (NAD) to the oxidized form of NAD ([NADH]/[NAD^+]) increases. This reduced state reflects a lack of ATP production by oxidative phosphorylation, which is accompanied by a loss of contractile function.

The exact biochemical mechanisms responsible for the rapid loss of contractile function are not yet known with certainty. There are those who implicate the loss of ATP [27] and others who implicate the accumulation of potentially toxic intermediary products such as hydrogen ions [28, 29] or lactate [5]. Kübler and Katz [30] thought it unlikely that decreased ATP supplies for energy-consuming reactions in the myocardial cell cause the observed decrease in myocardial contractility because of the low Michaelis constant (K_m) for ATP at the substrate-binding sites of energy-consuming reactions in the heart. In other words, at prevailing concentrations of ATP in the ischemic, noncontracting tissue, enzymes such as myosin-ATPase should still operate at near-maximal velocity. Instead, Kübler and Katz speculated that small changes in ATP may already exert modulatory effects on ion fluxes, and the large amount of inorganic phosphate may form insoluble calcium-phosphate precipitates that trap calcium in the sarcoplasmic reticulum and mitochondria [30]. Another possible explanation for the discrepancy between ATP content and ATP conversion into useful energy for the heart is the trapping, or "compartmentation," of ATP in a compartment not accessible to the enzymes of the contractile apparatus or ion pumps (e.g., mitochondria). Examining the acute effects of ischemia on phosphocreatine and ATP, Gudbjarnason and colleagues [31] found that the breakdown of phosphocreatine was more rapid than the breakdown of ATP. The kinetic heterogeneity of ATP and phosphocreatine depletion seems to indicate an inhibition of transfer of ATP from mitochondria to the cytosol, and it has been speculated that the reduction in the regeneration of cytosolic ATP causes the early cessation of contractile activity in ischemic myocardium. Given the uncertainty of the actual biochemical mechanism for contractile failure in the ischemic and infarcted myocardium, I now examine alterations in the metabolism of individual substrates and attempt a synopsis of the major metabolic derangements.

Glucose Metabolism During Ischemia

Of all substrates used for energy production by the human myocardium, glucose is, with the possible exception of glutamate (see later discussion), the only substrate yielding ATP by anaerobic substrate-level phosphorylation (Fig. 3-4). Intracellular glucose is derived from two sources: extracellular glucose in the plasma and interstitial space, and breakdown of intracellular glycogen (the storage form of glucose, which has also been called "emergency fuel").

Anoxia and ischemia stimulate glucose uptake, glycogenolysis, and glycolysis (Fig. 3-5). The sequence of events can be summarized as follows: Glycogen breakdown is increased as a result of phosphorylase activation (phosphorylation of phosphorylase *b,* giving rise to phosphorylase *a*). For example, with total ischemia in rat heart, glycogen stores fall by 50 percent within 5 minutes and by 70 percent within 20 minutes [3]. Many other investigators [5, 7, 9] made similar observations in many systems. Lack of oxygen enhances the transport of

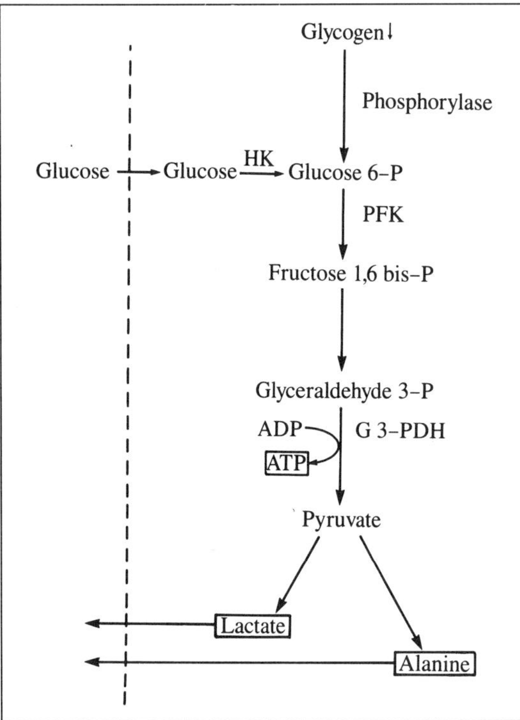

Fig. 3-4
Glucose metabolism in the ischemic heart. Glycogenolysis provides "emergency fuel." Ischemia increases glucose transport across the sarcolemma (*interrupted line*) and increases glycogen breakdown. Both glucose and glycogen are degraded in the glycolytic pathway to lactate and, to a lesser extent, alanine. Glycolysis yields 2 mol of ATP/mol of glucose (whereas the oxidative metabolism of glucose yields 36 mol of ATP). Regulatory enzymes: phosphorylase; HK = hexokinase; PFK = phosphofructokinase; G3-PDH = glyceraldehyde 3-phosphate dehydrogenase.

exogenous glucose, and activities of the glycolytic enzymes, especially hexokinase and phosphofructokinase, are increased. The rapid flux through the glycolytic pathway during early stages of ischemia leads to the intracellular accumulation of lactate, creating a bottleneck at the glyceraldehyde 3-phosphate dehydrogenase reaction [32]. According to Neely and his group, lactate and NADH inhibit the enzyme in both the intact heart [33] and the isolated enzyme preparation [34]. Thus in ischemic heart muscle, energy depletion appears to be further complicated by the accumulation of a product that by itself inhibits the main pathway of anaerobic energy production. Another point needs to be kept in mind: Although ATP production via anaerobic glycolysis may be increased as much as tenfold during the early stages by ischemia, the amount of energy produced still falls short of 90 percent of the energy required for normal cardiac contraction [35].

During reperfusion of reversibly injured ischemic myocardium, lactate is rapidly oxidized, and cardiac function (including myocardial oxygen consumption) returns to normal before ATP or glycogen is restored to preischemic values in the tissue [3]. Thus upon return of oxidative metabolism in the reversibly ischemic myocardium, endogenous substrate (lactate) is utilized first. More importantly, at the high rates of oxygen consumption and substrate utilization found in the heart, the depressed steady-state content of ATP does not correlate with high rates of ATP turnover so long as there is no substantial loss of total adenine nucleotides [36]. Numerous studies in the past suggested a correlation between ATP content and ATP turnover, but these suggestions have not held up to more recent scrutiny [3, 5, 37].

Fatty Acid and Lipid Metabolism During Ischemia

Oxygen deprivation affects fatty acid metabolism in a more devastating way than glucose metabolism. In contrast to glucose, metabolism of fatty acids requires a net investment of ATP in the course of their activation that can only be reclaimed by their oxidative metabolism (Fig. 3-6). Furthermore, unlike glycogen, fatty acids provide no "anaerobic fuel reserve" for a minimal residual ATP production. As a result of decreased electron flux in the respiratory chain, reducing equivalents accumulate. This situation in turn leads first to a slowing and then to the cessation of both beta oxidation and the citric acid cycle, as the rate of beta oxidation is controlled by the availability of (oxidated) NAD^+ [38]. As a consequence of decreased rates of beta oxidation, the tissue content of acetyl CoA declines, and long-chain acyl CoA and long-chain acyl carnitine accumulate. The accumulation of long-chain acyl CoA in the cytosol provides substrate for esterification of fatty acids with α-glycerophosphate, resulting in increased synthesis of triglycerides and in a further decline in cytosolic ATP and accumulation of adenosine monophosphate (AMP) plus inorganic pyrophosphate (see Fig. 3-6). Increased tri-

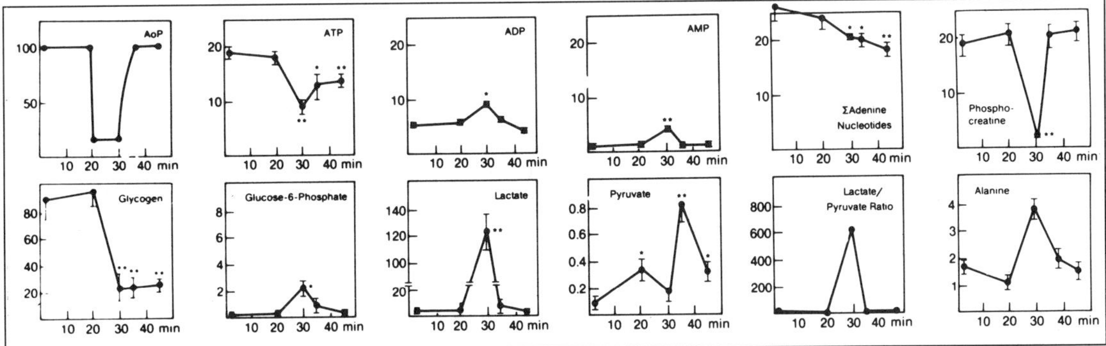

Fig. 3-5
Effects of short-term (10 minutes) ischemia on function and the metabolite content of isolated rat hearts. Hearts were perfused as "working hearts" and subjected to 10 minutes of normothermic total ischemia prior to reperfusion with an oxygenated medium. Recovery of function occurred within 93 seconds and was associated with a disappearance of lactate and restoration of phosphocreatine. Note that both ATP and glycogen levels remained depressed. (From H. Taegtmeyer et al. Energy metabolism in reperfused rat heart. *J. Am. Coll. Cardiol.* 6:864, 1985. With permission.)

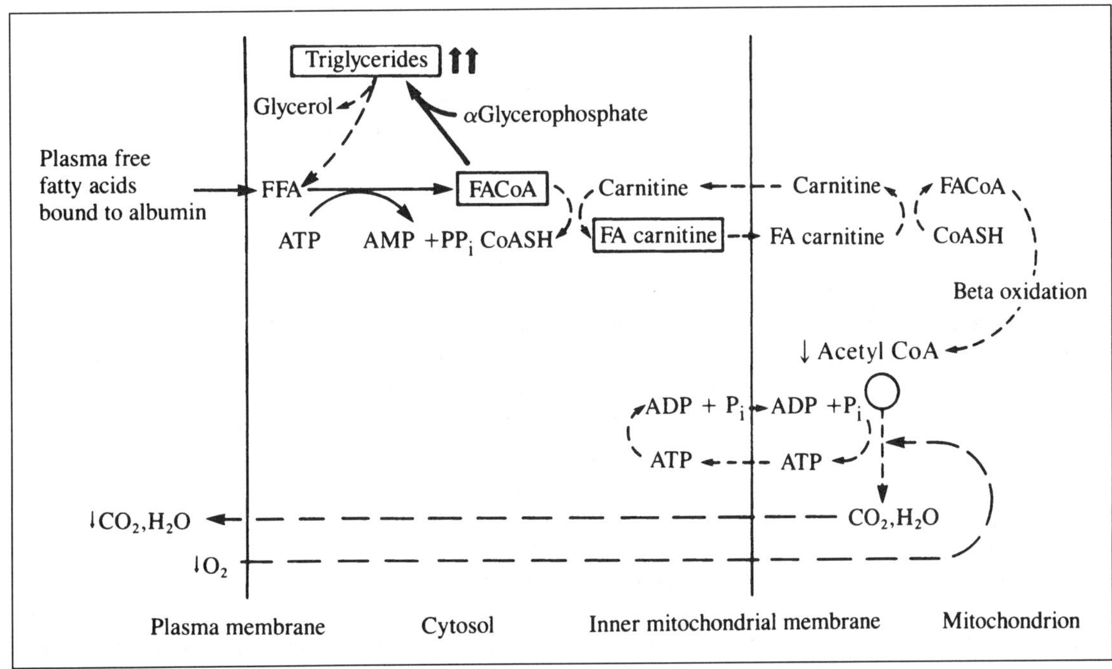

Fig. 3-6
Fatty acid metabolism in the ischemic heart. Lack of oxygen results in the inhibition of both beta oxidation and citric acid cycle activity. Free fatty acids (FFA), fatty acyl CoA (FACoA), fatty acyl carnitine (FA carnitine), and triglycerides accumulate in the ischemic myocardium. CoASH = reduced coenzyme A.

glyceride synthesis in reversibly damaged ischemic myocardium has been demonstrated in the border zone of myocardial infarctions [39] and with positron emission tomography (PET) using ^{11}C-palmitate residue curves [40].

The effects of fatty acids and their intermediates on membranes and enzyme activities are complex. Although not all of these effects are completely understood, a number of physiologically important observations have been made. High concentrations of fatty acyl CoA have been shown to inhibit the adenine nucleotide translocator across the inner mitochondrial membrane [41, 42], although the amount of cytosolic long-chain acyl CoA required to inhibit the transport of adenine nucleotides significantly may be too high to be of physiologic importance. Increased intracellular fatty acid concentrations are also arrhythmogenic [43]. Long-chain acylcarnitine increases intracellular [Ca^{2+}] and induces afterdepolarization in ventricular myocytes [44]. High levels of fatty acyl CoA inhibit the acyl CoA synthesis [45], which in turn leads to decreased uptake of fatty acids. It has been suggested further that the shuttle system for acetyl CoA between cytosol and mitochondria also may be impaired with ischemia [46].

The effects of elevated free fatty acid levels in the plasma on ischemic heart muscle are deleterious in patients, where they may cause arrhythmias [47] although increased free fatty acid levels may be an epiphenomenon of catecholamine-stimulated lipolysis [48]. In the oxygen-deprived heart muscle *in vitro,* fatty acids were found to cause a decrease in myocardial contractility [46, 49–51].

There is increasing evidence that abnormalities in lipid metabolism participate in the pathogenesis of membrane damage in the ischemic myocardium [52–54]. Wood and associates [55] first reported an inhibition of carnitine palmityl CoA transferase by ischemia and then proposed that the accumulation of long-chain fatty acyl carnitines exerts a detergent effect on ion pumps and possibly carrier systems as well [56]. The group at Washington University in St. Louis reported that a breakdown of membrane phospholipids causes an accumulation of lysophospholipids in ischemic myocardium [57] and noted the arrhythmogenic potential of lysophosphoglycerides [58, 59]. Lysophosphotidylcholine increases cytosolic Ca^{2+} in ventricular myocytes by direct action on the sarcolemma [60].

The increased concentrations of free fatty acids and fatty acid esters in the ischemic myocardium and their detergent action may cause either reversible or irreversible membrane damage via inhibition of enzymes, uncoupling of oxidative phosphorylation, and permeability changes [52]. In addition to the detergent effects of lipid-derived substances from either endogenous or exogenous sources, the hydrolysis of membrane phospholipids in early myocardial ischemia has received considerable attention [52, 61]. Because arachidonic acid is a major component of phospholipids, its liberation during ischemia has been taken as a sign of membrane destruction. The significance of the early phospholipid degradation is still uncertain, however, because the total myocardial phospholipid loss is small during the first 3 hours of ischemia [62, 63].

Amino Acid Metabolism in Myocardial Ischemia

Amino acid metabolism during myocardial ischemia was first studied by Mudge and associates [64] and colleagues and I [65, 66]. It was speculated that augmented release of alanine from heart muscle may reflect increased flux through the glycolytic pathway and may be of major energetic importance to myocardial ischemia because of similarities in the release of amino acids from heart muscle [67] and the release of amino acids from skeletal muscle under conditions of relative oxygen deficiency [68]. As illustrated in Figure 3-7, the enzymes lactate dehydrogenase and alanine aminotransferase compete for the same substrate.

Following these observations, transmyocardial differences of amino acids in normal subjects and in patients with coronary artery disease demonstrated augmented myocardial alanine production and glutamate uptake in patients with coronary artery disease [64]. This finding led to a more detailed study of myocardial amino acid metabolism during oxygen deprivation [65, 66, 69–72]. First, it was found that alanine did not arise from proteolysis but from enhanced rates of glucose breakdown [65, 66]. Second, it was learned that alanine production from glucose (see Fig. 3-7) occurs not only in ischemic heart muscle but also in the ischemic brain [73], ischemic rat liver [74], and the blood of diving animals and humans [75, 76]. Because oxygen deprivation is the most potent stimulus for glycolysis, it is plausible that the carbon skeleton of alanine arises from glucose breakdown during anaerobic glycolysis. A portion of alanine accumulating in ischemic heart muscle may also arise from aspartate via coupled transamination and decarboxylation of malate [77], but pyruvate production from other sources (e.g., from oxaloacetate via phospho*enol*-pyruvate carboxykinase) seems unlikely under anaerobic conditions. Although quantitatively much less alanine is produced from pyruvate than lactate,

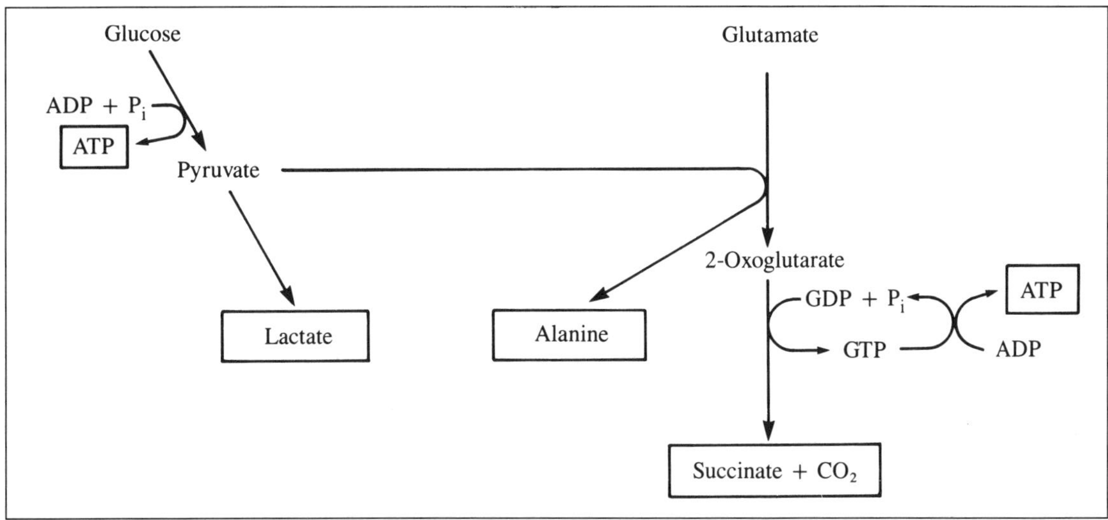

Fig. 3-7
Interaction of glucose and amino acid metabolism. Alanine, succinate, and carbon dioxide accumulate in ischemic myocardium together with lactate. Alanine arises from transamination of pyruvate with glutamate, which in turn is further degraded to succinate. Formation of succinate and carbon dioxide is linked to substrate-level phosphorylation of guanosine diphosphate (GDP), the only anaerobic source of energy other than lactate. GTP = guanosine triphosphate.

the shunting of pyruvate to alanine might be significant when it reduces lactate levels in oxygen-deprived tissue and thus lessens the inhibition of glycolysis that occurs when lactate levels become too high [33]. The physiologic importance of this mechanism is not yet fully understood.

In the proposed scheme of alanine production from the transamination of glutamate and pyruvate, the glycolytic pathway is not in redox balance. If pyruvate is diverted to alanine instead of lactate, NAD^+ must be regenerated by a mechanism that is different from the lactate dehydrogenase reaction. Principally, two cytosolic reactions could be capable of restoring the altered redox balance: (1) the glycerol phosphate dehydrogenase reaction leading to the synthesis of glycerol phosphate and (2) the malate dehydrogenase reaction leading to the synthesis of malate from oxaloacetate. In the latter scheme, oxaloacetate can be derived from aspartate, which in turn is transaminated to form glutamate, one of the substrates for alanine aminotransferase. This pathway would lead to the formation of succinate from oxaloacetate via malate and fumarate and is thought to be one of the key factors in the tolerance of diving mammals to hypoxia [75, 76]. The quantitatively more important source of succinate accumulation during anoxia is glutamate (see Fig. 3-7). As previously discussed, glutamate is transaminated with pyruvate to form alanine. The transamination product, 2-oxoglutarate, is oxidized, and subsequent formation of succinate is associated with substrate-level phosphorylation in the citric acid cycle and production of carbon dioxide. Formation of succinate from the breakdown of the amino acids aspartate and glutamate indeed was demonstrated in the isolated hypoxic papillary muscle of the rabbit [69, 70] and the ischemic isolated perfused rat heart [77]. Formation of carbon dioxide with ischemia and infarction was demonstrated in dog hearts [78]. According to the scheme presented in Figure 3-7, the source of carbon dioxide is most likely glutamate.

Whereas heart mitochondria incubated under aerobic conditions rapidly and completely oxidize glutamate [79], oxygen-deprived heart muscle oxidizes glutamate only in the C1 position to succinyl CoA and succinate [70, 72]. The limited oxidation of glutamate is linked to substrate-level phosphorylation in the citric acid cycle and hence is a source of anaerobic energy.

Two further observations support the view that succinate production by oxygen-deprived myocardium may be the result of anaerobic mitochondrial activity. First, oxidation of fumarate derived from aspartate was observed to be coupled to the synthesis of ATP and succinate in cyanide-treated mitochondrial particles from rat heart [80]. Second, another energy-yielding reaction was found to accompany oxidation of 2-oxoglutarate by mitochondria isolated from kidney and liver when these tissues were incubated under anaerobic conditions [81]. These two observations also support the hypothesis that anaerobic succinate formation is associated with energy production. Quantitative aspects of this nonglycolytic source of energy have not yet been fully evaluated. In hypoxic papillary muscles, succinate and alanine production have been estimated to account for 16 percent of the ATP produced by glycolysis and lactate formation alone [69]. For the clinician, the observation of enhanced glutamate uptake by ischemic myocardium is of interest [82], and most encouraging are the findings that the addition of glutamate to the perfusate seems to lessen the damaging effects of ischemia during cardioplegia [83] and indeed may improve performance of the reperfused ischemic myocardium [84]. Other investigators were unable to substantiate these findings [85].

Protein Synthesis and Degradation

Ever since Schoenheimer's classic observations on the "dynamic state of body constituents" [86], it was recognized that proteins, the basic constituents of all organs in the mammalian body, are continuously synthesized and degraded. Heart muscle is no exception. Although each of the myocardial proteins possesses a different life span, it has been estimated that the mean half-life of all myocardial proteins is only about 5 days and that the proteins of the entire heart are completely exchanged once every 3 weeks [87].

Protein synthesis and degradation are energy-dependent processes and require ATP (Fig. 3-8). It

Fig. 3-8
Protein synthesis and degradation in ischemic myocardium. Protein synthesis and degradation are energy-dependent processes (see *squares*). Oxygen deprivation leads to a greater decrease in protein synthesis (transcription, peptide chain initiation, elongation, and termination) than protein degradation. With few exceptions, amino acids (AA) neither accumulate in nor disappear from ischemic myocardium. Broken lines show energy-dependent pathways. mRNA = messenger RNA; tRNA = transfer RNA.

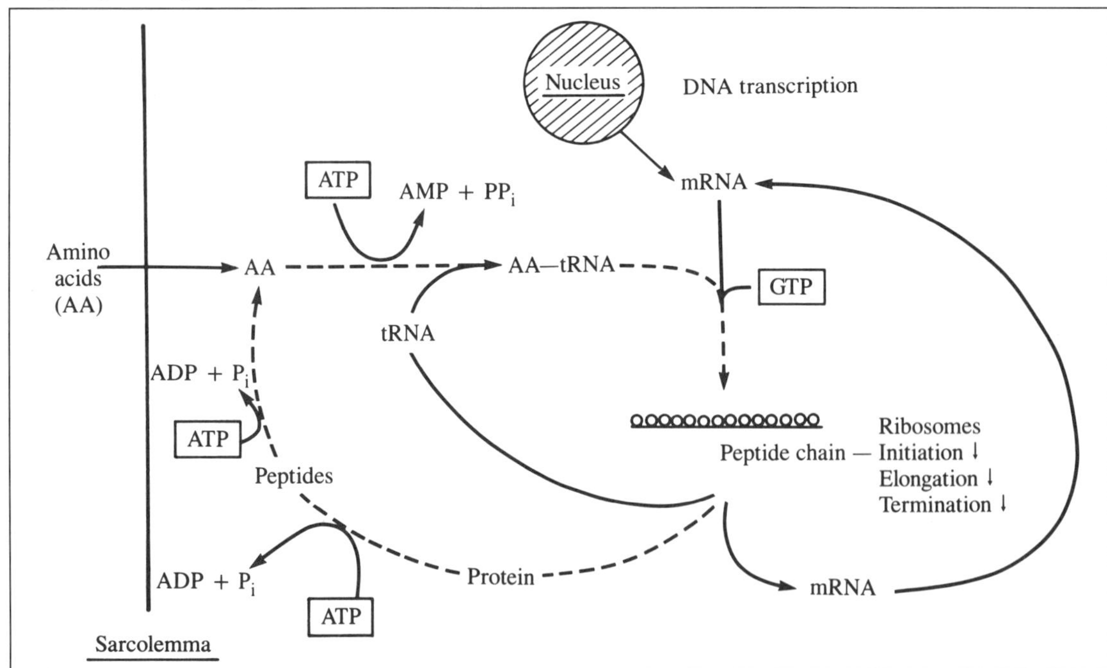

is therefore not surprising that oxygen deprivation slows or inhibits both processes [65, 88, 89]. In ischemic rat heart, protein synthesis and degradation, measured by the incorporation and release of phenylalanine, are both reduced by 80 percent [90]. This observation might explain why release of amino acids from globally ischemic, autolyzing myocardium is delayed by 6 to 12 hours [65].

In oxygen-deprived muscle, protein synthesis is inhibited more than protein degradation. According to Morgan and coworkers [91], such an imbalance between protein synthesis and degradation in energy-depleted heart muscle could lead to a loss of those proteins with rapid rates of turnover and could be a major factor in irreversible damage to ischemic tissue. Indeed, one may take the case one step further and speculate that in molecular terms, there is irreparable damage to the complex system of protein synthesis beginning with gene expression and ending with peptide chain termination, as well as in the ATP-dependent system of protein breakdown [92] (see Fig. 3-7). The exact sites of these damages remain to be elucidated.

Although overall rates of protein degradation are decreased in oxygen-deprived myocardium, the release and activation of several lysosomal enzymes are known to increase [93]. Lysosomes are small cell organelles containing hydrolases and acid proteases, notably cathepsin D. The number of lysosomes in myocytes is relatively small, and specific activities of lysosomal enzymes are relatively low unless the organelle is disrupted by vigorous homogenization, detergent treatment, or notably, ischemia [94]. The "lysosomal hypothesis of ischemic injury" states that ischemia leads to disruption of lysosomal membranes and release of the normally latent lysosomal hydrolases. This reaction results in abnormal degradation of certain cellular constituents because of abnormal contact between hydrolytic enzymes and substrates and lowering of the intracellular pH (i.e., nearer the pH optima of most lysosomal enzymes). If severe enough, this abnormal hydrolysis of cellular constituents could contribute to the development of further cell injury through degradation of structural and enzyme proteins and further activation of latent hydrolases [93]. In other words, a vicious cycle is set up. The lysosomal hypothesis has therefore been particularly attractive because drugs such as the tranquilizer chlorpromazine may limit lysosomal disruption in the liver [95], although the protective effect of chlorpromazine against ischemic damage in heart muscle seems to be small.

Although there is no doubt that lysosomes and lysosomal enzymes undergo major changes during myocardial ischemia, their role in the pathophysiology of early ischemic damage is still undefined. The lysosomal hypothesis may describe a coincidental rather than a causal event [96], and more recent evidence suggests a particular role for lysosomal enzymes in the removal of abnormal, partially degraded proteins [94].

Adenine Nucleotide Metabolism

One of the most devastating effects of reduced oxygen delivery on the myocardium is the loss of adenine nucleotides from the total pool of ATP, ADP, and AMP. An increase in AMP levels leads to increased production of its degradation products, adenosine, inosine, hypoxanthine, and xanthine (Fig. 3-9), as the activity of the rate-determining enzyme 5′-nucleotidase is far greater than that of adenylate deaminase, which competes for the same substrate [97]. The enzyme 5′-nucleotidase assumes a strategic position in the pathway of adenine nucleotide catabolism and deserves more detailed discussion. There are at least two isoforms of the enzyme. The soluble, sarcoplasmic form is physiologically more important than the membrane-bound, sarcolemmal form [98]. According to Swain and Holmes [37], ATP is a potent activator of cytosolic 5′-nucleotidase. It follows that when ATP levels fall during ischemia, the activity of 5′-nucleotidase would also fall. The whole process slows the rate of nucleotide hydrolysis and results in a halt to the drain of nucleotides from the cell. Thus it can easily be envisioned that inhibition of cytosolic 5′-nucleotidase and prevention of adenosine release into the interstitium (as described by Van Belle and coauthors [99]) may be a useful method to preserve myocardial adenine nucleotide pools.

Whereas rephosphorylation of the phosphorylated adenine nucleotides AMP and ADP to ADP and ATP occurs rapidly, the nonphosphorylated compound adenosine and its degradation products may enter a slower "salvage pathway" that eventually restores ATP [100]. More commonly, the degradation products leave the cell and appear in the

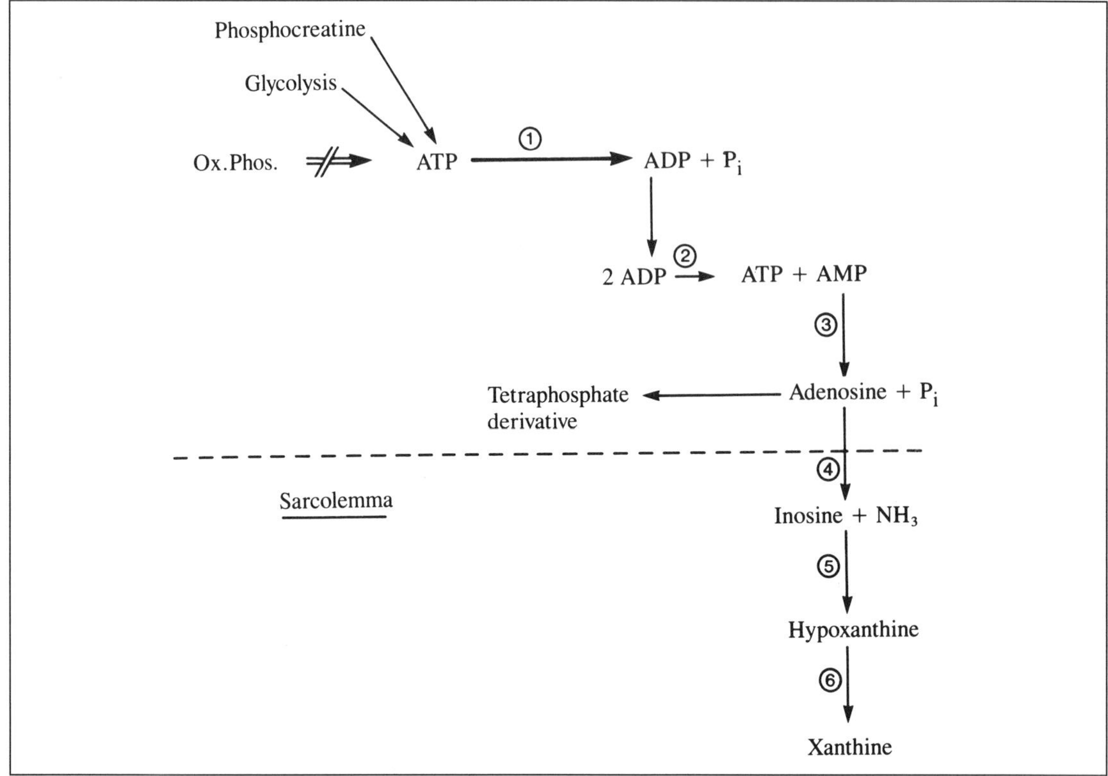

Fig. 3-9
Degradation of adenine nucleotides in ischemic myocardium. With interruption of the main source of ATP (oxidative phosphorylation [Ox. Phos.]). ADP is not quantitatively rephosphorylated. Instead, 1 mol of ATP is recovered from 2 mol of ADP, and AMP is broken down to adenosine. A tetraphosphate derivative of adenosine has been discovered in ischemic tissue [162], but most of the adenosine leaves the cell and is further degraded. Key enzymatic steps: (1) ATPase; (2) adenylate kinase; (3) 5′-nucleotidase; (4) adenosine deaminase; (5) nucleoside phosphorylase; (6) xanthine oxidase.

bloodstream, which results in a net loss of adenine nucleotides. It seems that the supply-demand ratio for oxygen determines adenosine formation by the heart [101]. De novo synthesis of adenine nucleotides is a slow process [102], and it takes hours, if not days, for heart muscle to restore its adenine nucleotide pool [103].

As stated earlier, there is no correlation between adenine nucleotide content and turnover of ATP. Likewise, static measurements of nucleotide pools reflect only the balance between their rate of synthesis and degradation. With ischemia the rate of nucleotide breakdown exceeds the rate of nucleotide synthesis, resulting first in a decline in the cellular content of nucleoside triphosphates (notably ATP) and shortly thereafter in a decline of all phosphorylated nucleosides and adenosine (see Fig. 3-9). Because the washout of catabolites is decreased during ischemia, the metabolites further down in the pathway accumulate. During reperfusion following ischemia, the purine nucleotide content is depressed as a result of metabolite washout [3, 104, 105], although function may have returned to normal or evidence of myocardial necrosis is lacking [106]. However, this does not mean that there is no close relation between a marked depletion in energy-rich phosphates (e.g., ATP $<$ 20 percent of control) and the development of irreversible ischemic injury and necrosis, as it was described by Jennings and coauthors [107]. Thus *severe* adenine nucleotide depletion is inevitably associated with cardiac cell death.

The initial, rapid hydrolysis of ATP to ADP and inorganic phosphate in response to ischemia is probably the main source for protons accumulating in the cytosol [108]. The link between ATP hydrolysis, intracellular acidosis, myocardial cell dysfunction, and cell death [28] awaits further exploration. Similarly, the attractive hypothesis of Ca^{2+} chelation by phosphate, the hydrolysis product of ATP, advanced by Kübler and Katz [30], is still awaiting experimental proof.

Oxygen-Derived Free Radicals

There has been increasing evidence suggesting that oxygen-derived free radicals play an important role in several forms of tissue damage, especially in injuries sustained with ischemia, reperfusion, and stunning [109], but also in injuries associated with intracellular drug metabolism (e.g., anthracycline antibiotics) and with inflammatory responses [110]. A free radical is a molecule or atom that possesses an unpaired electron. Normally, free radicals are produced as intermediates in the mitochondrial electron transport system and during the metabolism of a variety of lipids, including arachidonic acid as well as xanthine in the xanthine oxidase reaction. In heart muscle, molecular oxygen (denoted as the superoxide anion O_2^-) is especially important as an acceptor of electrons in the mitochondrial electron transport system of the respiratory chain.

In an aqueous environment O_2^- is in equilibrium with its protonated form $HO_2^{\cdot}$:

$$H^+ + O_2^- \rightleftharpoons HO_2^{\cdot}$$

Whereas O_2^- is relatively unreactive, $HO_2^{\cdot}$ and other of its derivative products are able to oxidize organic molecules such as membrane lipids and proteins. As shown in Table 3-3, H_2O_2 can be generated by spontaneous dismutation (i.e., rearrangement of electrons) of the reduced form of molecular oxygen (O_2^-) and the protonated form of the superoxide anion ($HO_2^{\cdot}$). This reaction stands in contrast to the xanthine oxidase reaction, in which H_2O_2 can be formed either by reduction of superoxide anions or direct double reduction of O_2. Finally, H_2O_2 can also be generated by an enzyme-catalyzed dismutation of O_2^-. The enzyme superoxide dismutase is able to reduce two molecules of O_2^- to form H_2O_2 and O_2. Because of the different sources of oxygen-derived free radicals, there are also different mechanisms involved in maintaining low intracellular concentrations of oxygen-derived free radicals. Free radicals may be "quenched" by small molecules such as tocopherol, beta carotene, ascorbate, or glutathione. They may also react with lipids, proteins, or DNA. These reactions lead to impairment of cell function and to cell destruction, especially when there is a burst of oxygen-derived free radicals on reperfusion after ischemia. Lastly, a series of enzymes that "scavenge" superoxide and H_2O_2 have evolved. They include superoxide dismutase, catalase, glutathione peroxidase, and glutathione reductase (Fig. 3-10). The latter system serves to lower the steady-state concentrations of free radical species that might otherwise cause excessive damage to the membrane and enzyme systems of the cell.

Table 3-3
Formation of oxygen-derived free radicals

Step 1: Electron reduction of oxygen
$O_2 + e^- \rightarrow O_2^-$
Step 2: Dismutation of O_2^-
$2O_2^- + 2H^+ \rightarrow H_2O_2 + O_2$
Step 3: Haber-Weiss and/or Fenton reactions
$H_2O_2 + O_2^- \rightarrow O_2 + OH^- + OH^{\cdot}$

Although the role of oxygen-derived free radicals in myocardial cell injury and cell death has not yet been completely characterized, a number of studies have shown that superoxide dismutase, catalase, and allopurinol (an inhibitor of the enzyme xanthine oxidase) offer a protective effect against the ravages of myocardial ischemia [111–113] and reperfusion injury after ischemia [114, 115]. Superoxide dismutase, catalase, and glutathione peroxidase can be considered free radical scavengers, because even though H_2O_2 is not a radical species, it is a precursor of the highly toxic protonated form of the superoxide anion $OH^{\cdot}$. The cytotoxic effect of H_2O_2 is therefore a balance of the function of intracellular catalase and glutathione peroxidase, which scavenge H_2O_2 on the one hand, and of the reactions that reduce H_2O_2 to $OH^{\cdot}$ on the other hand. The direct mechanism of tissue damage induced by oxygen-derived free radicals most likely involves protein modifications by $OH^{\cdot}$ (not O_2^-), rendering denatured substrates for accelerated intracellular

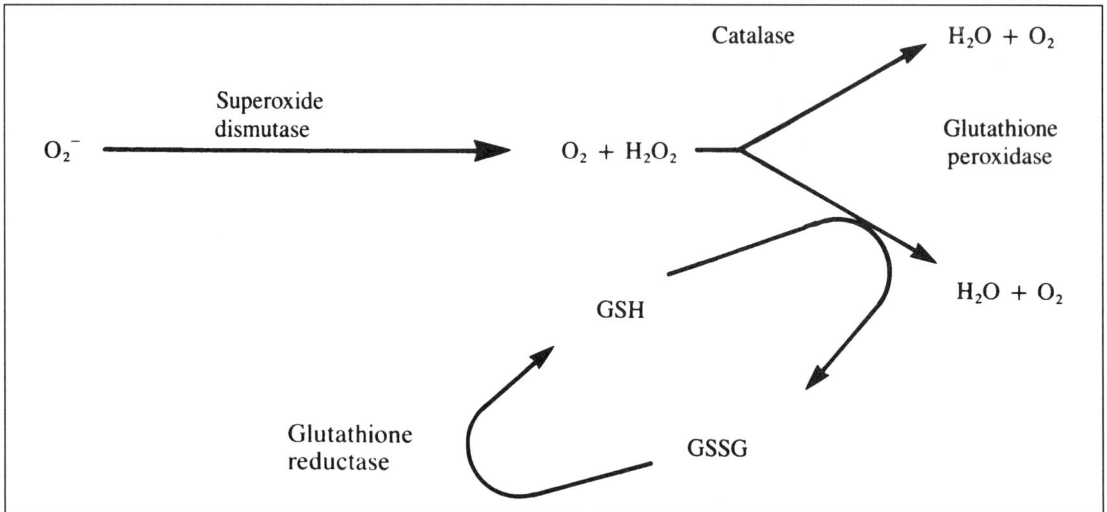

Fig. 3-10
Mechanisms of free radical scavenging. The superoxide anion O_2^-, an intermediate in mitochondrial electron transport systems, may undergo dismutation to O_2 and H_2O_2. H_2O_2 is converted to H_2O and O_2 by either catalase or glutathione peroxidase. GSSG = oxidized glutathione; GSH = reduced glutathione.

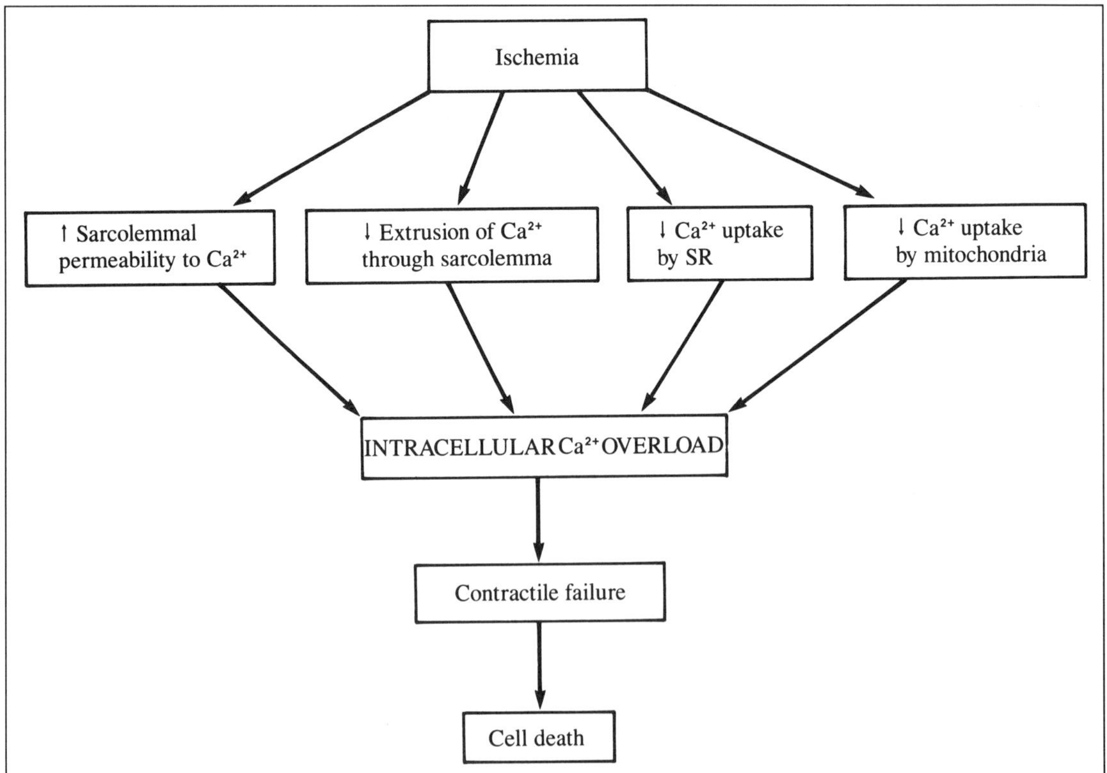

Fig. 3-11
Mechanisms of Ca^{2+} overload in ischemic myocardium. See text for explanation. SR = sarcoplasmic reticulum. (Modified from G. N. Pierce et al. *Heart Dysfunction in Diabetes.* Boca Raton, FL: CRC Press, 1988. With permission.)

proteolysis and lipid peroxidation [116, 117]. It can be expected that the direct assessment of oxygen-derived free radicals in myocardial tissue by spin trap analysis will not only deepen the understanding of the physiologic role of oxygen-derived free radicals but also provide a basis on how protective mechanisms can be enhanced to defend cellular structures from damage caused by oxygen-derived free radicals, especially during reperfusion of ischemic myocardium.

Ca^{2+} Metabolism

The importance of Ca^{2+} for energy metabolism of the heart is easily understood: Ca^{2+} ions are the mediators of excitation-contraction coupling. In addition, most enzymes that hydrolyze ATP are stimulated by Ca^{2+}. Ca^{2+} is a cofactor for the actomyosin cross-bridge formation and for mitochondrial dehydrogenases [118]. Thus, over a wide range of physiologic conditions, Ca^{2+} ions constitute the link between the use and the production of ATP. The cytosolic [Ca^{2+}] changes in the course of the cardiac cycle by two orders of magnitude, from 10^{-7} M during diastole to 10^{-5} M during systole, respectively [119]. The plasma [Ca^{2+}] is at 10^{-3} M, again two orders of magnitude greater than the highest physiologic cystolic [Ca^{2+}], indicating a [Ca^{2+}] gradient between the extracellular and intracellular spaces.

Severe ischemia causes high permeability of the cell membrane to Ca^{2+} [120], decreased extrusion of Ca^{2+} through the sarcolemma, decreased Ca^{2+} uptake by the sarcoplasmic reticulum, decreased Ca^{2+} uptake by mitochondria (all of these, except Ca^{2+} entry into the cell, are energy-dependent processes), and intracellular Ca^{2+} overload leading to contractile failure and ultimately cell death [121–123] (Fig. 3-11).

As depicted in the algorithm in Figure 3-12, the effects of Ca^{2+} overload are overwhelmingly deleterious. Intracellular Ca^{2+} overload activates a number of enzymes (proteases, phospholipase, myofibrillar ATPase), disrupts lysosomal membranes, and "chokes" mitochondrial oxidative phosphorylation because damaged mitochondria

Fig. 3-12
Algorithm of the deleterious effects of Ca^{2+} overload in ischemic myocardium. See text for explanation. (Modified from G. N. Pierce et al. *Heart Dysfunction in Diabetes.* Boca Raton, FL: CRC Press, 1988. With permission.)

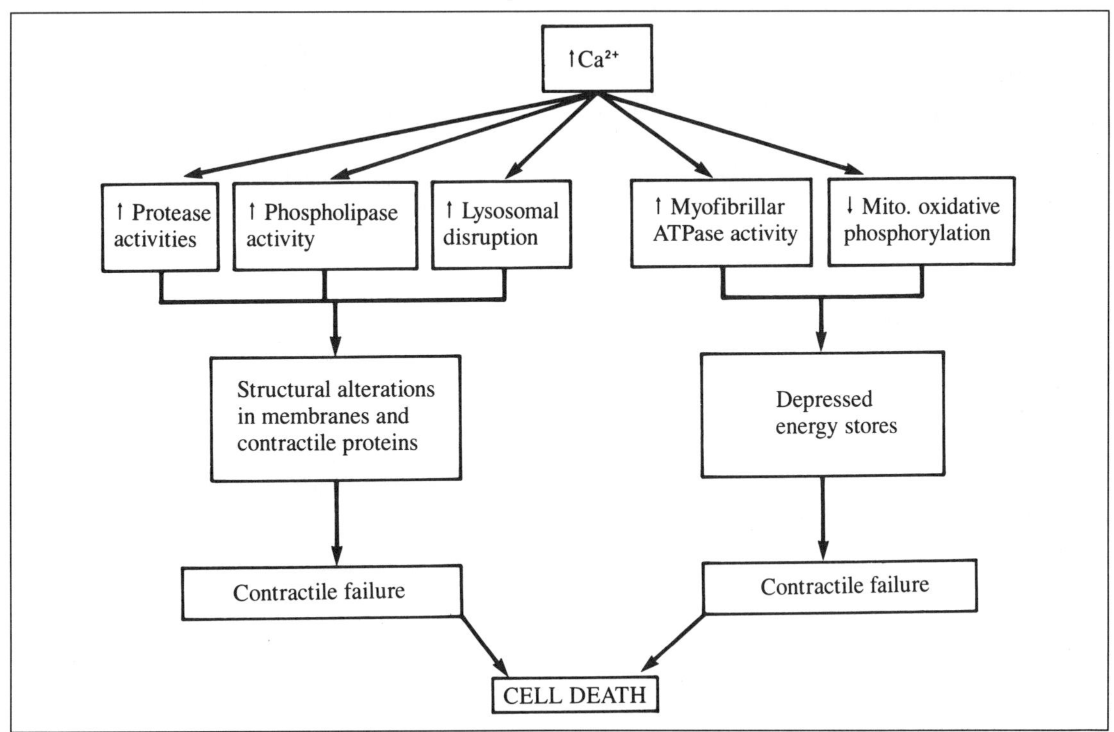

accumulate Ca^{2+} [124–126]. Cell death occurs after a period of contractile failure. One of the earliest unequivocal signs of irreversible ischemic cell injury is the appearance of amorphous matrix densities and granular dense bodies of calcium phosphate in mitochondria on transmission electron micrographs. Accumulation of Ca^{2+} in mitochondria requires a partially functional respiratory chain and ceases after 90 minutes of ischemia [7]. However, if the injury condition disappears before the level of intramitochondrial calcium phosphate becomes too high, the excess Ca^{2+} is dissolved from the precipitates and is released at a rate compatible with the Ca^{2+}-exporting ability of the sarcolemmal systems. According to Carafoli and Bing [127], this process ensures survival of the injured heart cell.

As also discussed by Carafoli and Bing [127], disturbed Ca^{2+} transfer across the sarcolemma, sarcoplasmic reticulum, and mitochondrial membrane is just the "tip of the biochemical iceberg" of myocardial cell dysfunction. The primary target of ischemic tissue injury might well be the enzyme proteins involved in Ca^{2+} metabolism and, vice versa, the Ca^{2+} and cyclic AMP–mediated stimulation of protein kinases.

Integrated Metabolic Responses in Myocardial Ischemia and Infarction; Enzyme Release; Regional Myocardial Metabolism

The multiple metabolic responses to myocardial ischemia and infarction are listed in Table 3-4. It cannot be emphasized strongly enough that the relative contributions of individual factors (discussed earlier in the chapter) to myocardial cell injury in the presence of ischemia and infarction are not known. Each factor is not more than a paradigm, and it is a matter of controversy how the paradigms relate to each other. Even such nondestructive methods as nuclear magnetic resonance spectroscopy have so far failed to determine, for example, to what degree the depletion of energy-rich phosphates or intracellular acidosis or the accumulation of specific intermediary metabolites is responsible for cell dysfunction [128, 129].

Irreversible cell damage and necrosis, on the other hand, are associated with virtual cessation of any form of energy metabolism and protein synthesis; the loss of nucleotides; accumulation of cystolic and mitochondrial Ca^{2+}; destruction of membranes, proteins, and nuclei; and release of enzyme proteins from myocardial cells into the bloodstream. The latter phenomenon is available for direct analysis since the first report by Karmen and colleagues in 1954 [130] that serum glutamate-oxaloacetate (now termed aspartate transaminase) activity is increased in patients with acute myocardial infarction. Increases in cardiac enzyme activities have been used not only for the diagnosis but also for a quantitative assessment of myocardial cell necrosis [131–133]. Although time-activity curves of enzyme release from the tissue are influenced by factors such as reperfusion, inactivation and degradation of enzymes in the lymphatic and systemic circulations, and membrane leakage not associated with irreversible cell damage, the liberation of cytosolic enzymes involved in myocardial energy metabolism

Table 3-4
Loss and gain of metabolites and ions during myocardial ischemia

Loss	Gain
Glycogen	Lactate, alanine
Phosphocreatine	Inorganic phosphate, inorganic pyrophosphate
ATP	Adenosine, inosine, hypoxanthine, xanthine
Adenine nucleotides	Hydrogen ions, ammonia, fatty acyl CoA, triglycerides
Glutamate	Succinate, CO_2
K^+	Ca^{2+}
Phospholipids	Arachidonic acid and lysophosphatides, H_2O_2, free radicals
Structural proteins	Amino acids
Enzymes, myoglobin troponins, fatty acid binding proteins	—
Mitochondrial cristae	Amorphous densities and granular dense bodies
Lysosomes	Cathepsin D and free lysosomal enzymes

such as creatine kinase (CK) MB, aspartate transaminase, alanine aminotransferase, and lactate dehydrogenase (specifically the LDH_1 isozyme) remains one of the three cornerstones for the clinical diagnosis of myocardial infarction, the other two being chest pain and specific changes of the electrocardiogram (ECG).

Given the high degree of functional organization in heart muscle cells, it is not surprising that damaged myocardium releases a multitude of enzymes and low-molecular-weight proteins such as myoglobin, heart fatty acid–binding protein, myosin light chains, and the cardiac troponins I and T (for reviews, see articles by Hearse [27] and Adams and coauthors [134]). For practical purposes, only the aforementioned enzymes have thus gained diagnostic importance. The cardiac troponins, which are complexed to the contractile apparatus and regulate the Ca^{2+}-mediated interaction between actin and myosin, appear to be more sensitive and more specific than conventional enzymes for the diagnosis of myocardial infarction [135, 136]. Table 3-5 lists the serum markers of myocardial injury [134].

When the physical separation between the inside and outside of the cell is removed, not only do low-molecular-weight proteins and enzymes leak out of the cell, but also substances normally excluded from the cell may gain access to the inside of the cell. One such substance is a labeled myosin antibody that binds to the principal protein of the myocardial cell and has been used to localize and quantitate necrotic tissue [137].

In vivo assessment of regional myocardial metabolism by PET has gained increasing importance [138]. Unique features of this imaging modality are the following: (1) the tomographic, three-dimensional images of relatively high resolution; (2) the ability of positron-emitting compounds to trace myocardial blood flow and specific metabolic pathways; and (3) the semiquantitative nature of measuring radioactivity in defined regions of the myocardium [139]. When patients with acute myocardial infarction are studied within 72 hours after the onset of chest pain or asymptomatic ECG changes, PET frequently reveals absent blood flow but persistent glucose-specific metabolic activity in infarcted regions [140]. When radioactivity of the glucose analog tracer [^{18}F]-2-deoxyglucose (FDG) is measured, the tracer, which is phosphorylated but not further metabolized, accumulates to a greater extent in ischemic tissue than in the surrounding, normally perfused myocardium or in infarcted tissues [141]. Conversely, regional oxidation of ^{11}C-palmitate is decreased, presumably because of impaired oxidative metabolism and back-diffusion of tracer from ischemic tissue into the blood. Thus PET techniques are capable not only of tracing metabolic abnormalities but also of distinguishing

Table 3-5
Serum protein markers of myocardial infarction

Marker	Molecular mass (kD)	Range of times to initial elevation (hr)	Mean time to peak elevations (nonthrombolysis)	Time to return to normal range
hFABP	14–15	1.5	5–10 hr	24 hr
Phosphorylase	49.5	1–2	1–2 hr	24 hr
Myoglobin	17.8	1–4	6–7 hr	24 hr
MLC	19–27	6–12	2–4 days	6–12 days
cTnI	23.5	3–12	24 hr	5–10 days
cTnT	33	3–12	12 hr–2 days	5–14 days
MB-CK	86	3–12	24 hr	48–72 hr
MM-CK tissue isoform	86	1–6	12 hr	38 hr
MB-CK tissue isoform	86	2–6	18 hr	Unknown
Enolase	90	6–10	24 hr	48 hr
LDH	135	10	24–48 hr	10–14 days
MHC	400	48	5–6 days	14 days

hFABP = heart fatty acid–binding proteins; MLC = myosin light chain; cTnI = cardiac troponin I; cTnT = cardiac troponin T; MB-CK = MB isozyme of creatine kinase (CK); MM-CK = MM isoenzyme of CK; LDH = lactate dehydrogenase; MHC = myosin heavy chain.

Source: Adapted from J. E. Adams, III, D. R. Abendschein, and A. S. Jaffe. Biochemical markers of myocardial injury. Is MB creatine kinase the choice for the 1990's? *Circulation* 88:750, 1993. With permission of the American Heart Association, Inc.

the activity of different metabolic pathways *in vivo*. In a study by Tillisch and coworkers [142], enhanced FDG uptake by ischemic myocardium was a powerful predictor of tissue viability after revascularization. Future research will show if there are subsets of myocardial infarction with predominantly reversible tissue injury or predominantly irreversible tissue necrosis (as clinically suggested). Future research will also show if myocardial infarct size (and its reduction by therapeutic interventions) can be assessed by PET. The group at Washington University in St. Louis has used the short-chain fatty acid [^{11}C] acetate in conjunction with myocardial blood flow imaging and found the clearance of acetate superior to the retention of FDG in the identification of viable, but poorly contracting myocardium [143]. The same group showed that [^{11}C] acetate imaging could predict recovery of function in hypocontractile myocardium after revascularization [144]. Thus, as the ischemic myocardium cuts back on energy expenditure, PET metabolic tracer techniques hold the promise to distinguish between energy-deprived, surviving myocardium and energy-depleted, necrotic tissue.

Reversible Myocardial Ischemia, Reperfusion, and Reperfusion Injury

In contrast to the well-described phenomenon of altered contractile function during ischemia and reperfusion dating back to the classic studies of Tennant and Wiggers during the 1930s [145] (which denote that the rate of improvement of function in the ischemic region is inversely related to the duration of the occlusion), the understanding of the metabolic basis for reversible myocardial ischemia is still incomplete. The progress in early thrombolysis [146] has brought the concept of the "stunned myocardium" into focus. This concept was first proposed by Braunwald and Kloner [147]. Based on an extensive review of the literature, Braunwald and Kloner concluded that brief occurrences (usually < 20 minutes) of myocardial ischemia are followed by metabolic and functional alterations that may last for days before function returns to normal. It is of interest that even during periods of ischemia longer than 20 minutes, only the core of the tissue may undergo necrosis, whereas the surrounding tissue may be reversibly injured and committed to necrosis only if ischemia continues for a prolonged period [22]. Thus, there is a metabolic "battlefield" surrounding the "bomb crater" of the infarction in the center. Since the reparative processes in heart muscle following myocardial infarction were first discussed by Bing [148], the characterization of this battlefield continues to be the object of much research activity.

According to Braunwald and Kloner [147], a myocardial infarction is characterized by a zone of reversibly injured cells surrounding the center of necrosis that shows delayed recovery of function. Because it is unlikely that any necrotic tissue may regain functional significance, it is reasonable to focus on the metabolic changes occurring in the reversibly injured, viable, yet functionally impaired myocardium. It is the current notion that the metabolism in this reversibly injured myocardium can be restored to normal by reperfusion [149], although the return of function may be delayed by days or even weeks. Besides the observations of an increased uptake of the glucose analog FDG [142], few experimental data exist on the biochemical mechanism(s) underlying the slow recovery of tissue function in the zone of reversible ischemia.

More definitive data are available from reperfused heart muscle preparations after normothermic or hypothermic ischemia because this pathophysiologic state can be more readily assessed in an experimental setting. For instance, numerous studies have shown rapid restoration of the phosphocreatine pool, whereas nucleotide pools remain depleted in functional, postischemic myocardium (for a review, see the work by Swain and Holmes [37]). The rapid increase in phosphocreatine is thought to indicate that mitochondrial energy production is not limited, whereas resynthesis of adenine nucleotides is lagging behind. To date, no studies have unequivocally demonstrated a direct relation between repletion of adenine nucleotide pools and the return of cardiac function. The evidence for a relation between severe (> 80 percent) depletion of adenine nucleotides and cell death is, however, convincing [107, 150], although the exact mechanisms remain to be defined.

The mechanisms of reperfusion injury are complex [151, 152] and still unexplainable. Some investigators pointed out the similarities between reperfusion injury and the "calcium paradox" [153], a phenomenon observed in isolated rat hearts perfused with a Ca^{2+}-free medium. Once Ca^{2+} is readmitted to the perfusate, these hearts go into contracture and show evidence of intracellular Ca^{2+} overload. The exact mechanism for the calcium paradox phenomenon is still unclear.

Other investigators suggested the role of oxygen-derived free radicals as mediators for reperfusion damage [114, 154]. The possible mechanisms for the generation of oxygen-derived free radicals and their effects on cellular proteins were discussed earlier.

Still other investigators believe that lactate accumulation from glycogen breakdown impairs flux through the glycolytic pathway and return of function on reperfusion, whereas others found that preservation of glycogen levels [155] or "glycogen loading" of the heart prior to ischemia [156] lessens the ischemic insult and preserves cardiac function on reperfusion. Decreased tissue content of pyrimidine nucleotide (NAD), and not decreased activity of dehydrogenases, has been found to be a good correlate for the degree of ultrastructural injury and provides the biochemical basis for negative tetrazolium staining of the irreversibly injured tissue [157]. The observations on the protective effects of glucose for the ischemic myocardium are consistent with the earlier work of Sodi-Pallares and coworkers [158] who reported a beneficial effect of the administration of glucose, insulin, and potassium (GIK) on morbidity from arrhythmias and mortality in myocardial infarction and with the experience of Rackley's group [159]. In a controlled study carried out at St. Luke's Episcopal Hospital/Texas Heart Institute, colleagues and I demonstrated that the short-term administration of a concentrated solution of glucose (50%), insulin (80 U/L), and potassium (potassium chloride, 100 mEq/L) given at 1 ml/kg/hr for up to 48 hours improved left ventricular function and reduced 30-day mortality by 75% when it was given postoperatively to patients with refractory left ventricular failure requiring intra-aortic balloon counterpulsation [160].

Schaper and Schaper [161] concluded, probably correctly, that the effects of reperfusion depend on the severity of the ischemic insult at the time of reperfusion. In irreversibly injured myocardium, reperfusion leads to the accelerated demise of the tissue. In reversibly injured myocardium, reperfusion leads to an accelerated return of oxidative metabolism and contractile function. In other words, reperfusion seems beneficial to reversibly injured myocardium and deleterious to irreversibly injured myocardium. The most tantalizing question for both clinicians and biochemists remains how to distinguish the former from the latter while the patient is still alive.

References

1. Taegtmeyer, H. Energy metabolism of the heart: From basic concepts to clinical applications. *Curr. Probl. Cardiol.* 19:57, 1994.
2. Taegtmeyer, H., Hems, R., and Krebs, H. A. Utilization of energy providing substrates in the isolated working rat heart. *Biochem. J.* 186:701, 1980.
3. Taegtmeyer, H., Roberts, A. F. C., and Rayne, A. E. G. Energy metabolism in reperfused rat heart: Return of function before normalization of ATP content. *J. Am. Coll. Cardiol.* 6:864, 1985.
4. Hoffmeister, H. M., Mauser, M., and Schaper, W. Effect of adenosine and AICAR on ATP content and regional contractile function in reperfused canine myocardium. *Basic Res. Cardiol.* 80:445, 1985.
5. Neely, J. R., and Grotyohann, L. W. Role of glycolytic products in damage to myocardium: Dissociation of adenosine triphosphate levels and recovery of function of reperfused canine myocardium. *Circ. Res.* 55:816, 1984.
6. Page, E., and McCallister, L. P. Quantitative electron microscopic description of heart muscle cells. *Am. J. Cardiol.* 31:172, 1973.
7. Jennings, R. B., and Ganote, C. E. Mitochondrial structure and function in myocardial ischemic injury. *Circ. Res.* 38(Suppl I):I-80, 1976.
8. Regitz, V., Raulson, D. J., and Hodack, R. J. Mitochondrial damage during myocardial ischemia. *Basic Res. Cardiol.* 79:207, 1984.
9. Schaper, J., Mulch, J., Winkler, B., and Schaper, W. Ultrastructural, functional and biochemical criteria for estimation of reversibility of ischemic injury: A study on the effect of global ischemia on the isolated dog heart. *J. Mol. Cell. Cardiol.* 11:521, 1979.
10. Yeo, G. F. An attempt to estimate the gaseous interchange of the frog's heart by means of the spectroscope. *J. Physiol. (Lond.)* 6:93, 1885.
11. Winterstein, H. Ueber die Saurstoffatmung des isolierten Säugetierherzens. *Z. Allg. Physiol.* 4:333, 1904.
12. Bing, R. J. The metabolism of the heart. *Harvey Lect.* 50:27, 1955.
13. Goodale, W. T., and Hackel, D. B. Myocardial carbohydrate metabolism in normal dogs, with ef-

fects of hyperglycemia and starvation. *Circ. Res.* 1:509, 1953.
14. Goodale, W. T., Olson, R. E., and Hackel, D. B. The effects of fasting and diabetes mellitus on myocardial metabolism in man. *Am. J. Med.* 27:212, 1959.
15. Schelbert, H. R. The heart. In P. Ell and B. Holman (eds.), *Computed Emission Tomography.* Oxford: Oxford University Press, 1982. P. 91.
16. Merhige, M. E., Ekas, R., Mossberg, K., et al. Catecholamine stimulation, substrate competition, and myocardial glucose uptake in conscious dogs assessed with positron emission tomography. *Circ. Res.* 61(Suppl II):II-124, 1987.
17. Goodwin, G. W., and Taegtmeyer, H. Metabolic recovery of the isolated working rat heart after brief global ischemia. *Am. J. Physiol.* 267:H462, 1994.
18. Russell, R. R., and Taegtmeyer, H. Pyruvate carboxylation prevents the decline in contractile function of rat hearts oxidizing acetoacetate. *Am. J. Physiol.* 30:H756, 1991.
19. Denton, R. M., and Randle, P. J. Concentrations of glycerides and phospholipids in rat heart and gastrocnemius muscles. *Biochem. J.* 104:416, 1967.
20. Olson, R. E., and Hoeshen, R. J. Utilization of endogenous lipid by the isolated perfused rat heart. *Biochem. J.* 103:796, 1967.
21. Crass, M. F., McCaskill, E. S., Shipp, J. C., and Murthy, V. K. Metabolism of endogenous lipids in cardiac muscle: Effect of pressure development. *Am. J. Physiol.* 220:428, 1971.
22. Reimer, K. A., Lowe, J. E., Rasmussen, M. M., and Jennings, R. B. The wave form phenomenon of ischemic cell death. I. Myocardial infarct size vs. duration of coronary occlusion in dogs. *Circulation* 56:786, 1977.
23. Opie, L. H., Owen, P., Thomas, M., and Samson, R. Coronary sinus lactate measurements in assessment of myocardial ischemia: Comparison with changes in lactate/pyruvate and beta-hydroxybutyrate/acetoacetate ratios and with release of hydrogen, phosphate, and potassium from the heart. *Am. J. Cardiol.* 32:295, 1973.
24. Gertz, E. W., Wisneski, J. A., Neese, R. A., et al. Myocardial lactate metabolism: Evidence of lactate release during net chemical extraction in man. *Circulation* 63:1273, 1981.
25. Gertz, E. W., Wisneski, J. A., and Neese, R. Myocardial lactate extraction: Multidetermined metabolic function. *Circulation* 61:256, 1980.
26. Wisneski, J. A., Gertz, E. W., Neese, R. A., et al. Metabolic fate of extracted glucose in normal human myocardium. *J. Clin. Invest.* 76:1819, 1985.
27. Hearse, D. J. Myocardial enzyme leakage. *J. Mol. Med.* 2:185, 1977.
28. Katz, A. M., and Hecht, H. H. The early "pump" failure of the ischemic heart. *Am. J. Med.* 47: 497, 1969.
29. Williamson, J. R., Shaffer, S. W., Ford, C., and Safer, B. Contribution of tissue acidosis to ischemic injury in the perfused rat heart. *Circulation* 53:3, 1976.
30. Kübler, W., and Katz, A. M. Mechanism of early "pump" failure of the ischemic heart: Possible role of adenosine triphosphate depletion and inorganic phosphate accumulation. *Am. J. Cardiol.* 40:467, 1977.
31. Gudbjarnason, S., Mathes, P., and Ravens, K. G. Functional compartmentation of ATP and creatine phosphate in heart muscle. *J. Mol. Cell. Cardiol.* 1:325, 1970.
32. Williamson, J. R. Glycolytic control mechanisms. II. Kinetics of the intermediate changes during the aerobic-anaerobic transition in perfused rat heart. *J. Biol. Chem.* 241:5026, 1966.
33. Rovetto, M. J., Lamberton, W. F., and Neely, J. R. Mechanisms of glycolytic inhibition in ischemic rat heart. *Circ. Res.* 37:742, 1975.
34. Mochizuki, S., and Neely, J. R. Control of glyceraldehyde 3-phosphate dehydrogenase in cardiac muscle. *J. Mol. Cell. Cardiol.* 11:221, 1979.
35. Morgan, H. E., Neely, J. R., and LaNoue, K. F. Biochemical events in ischemic heart. In A. Hjalmarson and L. Wilhelmsen (eds.), *Acute and Long Term Management of Myocardial Ischemia.* Göteberg, Sweden: Astra, 1977. P. 10.
36. Ingwall, J. S. Is cardiac failure a consequence of decreased energy reserve? *Circulation* 87(Suppl VII):VII-58, 1993.
37. Swain, J. L., and Holmes, E. W. Nucleotide metabolism in cardiac muscle. In H. Fozzard et al. (eds.), *The Heart and Cardiovascular System.* New York: Raven Press, 1986. P. 911.
38. Bremer, J., and Wojtzak, A. B. Factors controlling the role of fatty acid beta oxidation in rat liver mitochondria. *Biochem. Biophys. Acta* 280:515, 1972.
39. Biheimer, D. W., Buja, L. M., Parkey, R. W., et al. Fatty acid accumulation and abnormal lipid deposition in peripheral and border zones of experimental myocardial infarcts. *J. Nucl. Med.* 19:276, 1978.
40. Schwaiger, M., Fishbein, M. C., Block, M., et al. Metabolic and ultrastructural abnormalities during ischemia in canine myocardium: Non-invasive assessment by positron emission tomography. *J. Mol. Cell. Cardiol.* 19:259, 1987.
41. Shug, A. L., Shrago, E., Bittar, N., et al. Acyl-CoA inhibition of adenine nucleotide translocation in ischemic myocardium. *Am. J. Physiol.* 228:689, 1975.
42. Ho, C. H., and Pande, S. V. On the specificity of the inhibition of adenine nucleotide translocation by long-chain acyl-coenzyme A esters. *Biochim. Biophys. Acta* 369:86, 1974.
43. Corr, P. B., Gross, R. W., and Sobel, B. E. Arrhythmogenic amphiphillic lipids and the myocardial cell membrane. *J. Mol. Cell. Cardiol.* 14:619, 1981.
44. Fischbach, P. S., Corr, P. B., and Yamada, K. A. Long-chain acylcarnitine increases intracellular

Ca^{2+} and induces afterdepolarization in adult ventricular myocytes. *Circulation* 86:741, 1992.
45. Oram, J. F., Bennetch, S. L., and Neely, J. R. Regulation of fatty acid utilization in isolated perfused rat hearts. *J. Biol. Chem.* 248:5299, 1973.
46. Liedtke, A. J. Alterations of carbohydrate and lipid metabolism in acutely ischemic heart. *Prog. Cardiovasc. Dis.* 23:321, 1981.
47. Oliver, M. F., Kurien, V. A., and Greenwood, T. W. Relation between serum-free fatty acids and arrhythmias and death after acute myocardial infarction. *Lancet* 1:710, 1968.
48. Opie, L. H. Cardiac metabolism—emergence, decline, and resurgence. Part I. *Cardiovasc. Res.* 26:721, 1992.
49. Henderson, A. H., Most, A. S., Parmley, W. W., et al. Depression of myocardial contractility in rats by free fatty acids during hypoxia. *Circ. Res.* 26:439, 1970.
50. Kjekshus, J. K., and Mjos, O. D. Effect of free fatty acids on myocardial function and metabolism in the ischemic dog heart. *J. Clin. Invest.* 51:1767, 1972.
51. Liedtke, A. J., Nellis, S., and Neely, J. R. Effects of excess free fatty acids on mechanical and metabolic function in normal and ischemic myocardium in swine. *Circ. Res.* 43:652, 1978.
52. Katz, A. M. Membrane-derived lipids and the pathogenesis of ischemic myocardial damage. *J. Mol. Cell. Cardiol.* 14:627, 1982.
53. Katz, A. M., and Messineo, F. C. Lipid-membrane interactions and the pathogenesis of ischemic myocardial damage. *Circ. Res.* 48:1, 1981.
54. Katz, A. M., and Messineo, F. C. Fatty acid effects on membranes: Possible role in the pathogenesis of ischemic myocardial damage. *J. Mol. Cell. Cardiol.* 14(Suppl 3):119, 1982.
55. Wood, J. M., Sordahl, L. A., Lewis, R. M., and Schwartz, A. Effect of chronic myocardial ischemia on the activity of carnitine palmityl-coenzyme A transferase in isolated canine heart mitochondria. *Circ. Res.* 32:340, 1973.
56. Wood, J. M., Busch, B., Pitts, B. J. R., and Schwartz, A. Inhibition of bovine heart Na^+/K^+-ATPase by palmityl-carnitine and palmityl-CoA. *Biochem. Biophys. Res. Commun.* 74:677, 1977.
57. Sobel, B. E., Corr, R. B., Robison, A. K., et al. Accumulation of lysophosphoglycerides with arrhythmogenic properties in ischemic myocardium. *J. Clin. Invest.* 62:546, 1978.
58. Corr, P. B., Cain, M. E., Witkowski, F. X., et al. Potential arrhythmogenic derangements in canine Purkinje fibers induced by lysophosphoglycerides. *Circ. Res.* 44:822, 1979.
59. Corr, P. B., Yamada, K. A., Creer, M. H., et al. Lysophosphoglycerides and ventricular fibrillation early after onset of ischemia. *J. Mol. Cell. Cardiol* 19(Suppl V):45, 1986.
60. Woodley, S. L., Ikenouchi, H., and Barry, W. H. Lysophosphotidylcholine increases cytosolic calcium in ventricular myocytes by direct action on the sarcolemma. *J. Mol. Cell. Cardiol.* 23:671, 1991.
61. Chien, K. R., Han, A., Sen, A., et al. Accumulation of unesterified arachidonic acid in ischemic canine myocardium. *Circ. Res.* 54:313, 1984.
62. Reimer, K. A., and Jennings, R. B. Failure of the xanthine oxidase inhibitor allopurinol to limit infarct site after ischemia and reperfusion in dogs. *Circulation* 71:1069, 1985.
63. Steenbergen, C., and Jennings, R. B. Relationship between lysophospholipid accumulation and plasma membrane injury during in vitro ischemia in dog heart. *J. Mol. Cell. Cardiol.* 16:605, 1984.
64. Mudge, G. H., Mills, R. M., Taegtmeyer, H., et al. Alterations of myocardial amino acid metabolism in chronic ischemic heart disease. *J. Clin. Invest.* 58:1185, 1976.
65. Taegtmeyer, H., Ferguson, A. G., and Lesch, M. Protein degradation and amino acid metabolism in autolyzing rabbit myocardium. *Exp. Mol. Pathol.* 26:52, 1977.
66. Taegtmeyer, H., Peterson, M. B., Ragavan, V. V., et al. De novo alanine synthesis in isolated oxygen-deprived rabbit myocardium. *J. Biol. Chem.* 252: 5010, 1977.
67. Carlsten, A., Hallgren, B., Jagenburg, R., and Werko, L. Myocardial metabolism of glucose, lactic acid, amino and fatty acids in healthy individuals at rest and at different work loads. *Scand. J. Clin. Invest.* 13:418, 1961.
68. Felig, P., and Wahren, J. Amino acid metabolism in exercising man. *J. Clin. Invest.* 50:2703, 1971.
69. Taegtmeyer, H. Metabolic responses to cardiac hypoxia: Increased production of succinate by rabbit papillary muscles. *Circ. Res.* 43:808, 1978.
70. Sanborn, T., Gavin, W., Berkowitz, S., et al. Augmented conversion of aspartate and glutamate to succinate during anoxia in rabbit heart. *Am. J. Physiol.* 237:H535, 1979.
71. Rau, E. E., Shine, K. I., Gervais, A., et al. Enhanced mechanical recovery of anoxic and ischemic myocardium by amino acid perfusion. *Am. J. Physiol.* 236:H873, 1979.
72. Peschock, R., and Nunnally, R. L. ^{13}C Magnetic resonance of glutamate metabolism in intact perfused hearts (Abstract). *Circulation* 66(Suppl II):II-109, 1982.
73. Norberg, K., and Siesjo, B. K. Cerebral metabolism in hypoxic hypoxia. II. Citric acid cycle intermediates and associated amino acids. *Brain Res.* 86:45, 1975.
74. Brosnan, J. T., Krebs, H. A., and Williamson, D. H. Effects of ischemia on metabolic concentrations in rat liver. *Biochem. J.* 117:91, 1970.
75. Hochachka, P. W., Owen, T. G., Allen, J. F., Whittow, G. C. Multiple end products of anaerobiosis in diving vertebrates. *Comp. Biochem. Physiol.* B:50, 1975.
76. Hochachka, P. W., and Storey, K. B. Metabolic

consequences of diving in animals and man. *Science* 187:613, 1975.

77. Peuhkurinen, K. J., Takala, T. E. S., Nuutinen, E. M., and Hassinen, I. E. Tricarboxylic acid cycle metabolites during ischemia in isolated perfused rat heart. *Am. J. Physiol.* 244:H281, 1983.
78. Hillis, L. D., Khuri, S. F., Braunwald, E., et al. Assessment of the efficacy of interventions to limit ischemic injury by direct measurement of intramural carbon dioxide tension after coronary artery occlusion in the dog. *J. Clin. Invest.* 63:99, 1979.
79. Krebs, H. A., and Bellamy, D. The interconversion of glutamic acid and aspartic acid in respiring tissues. *Biochem. J.* 75:523, 1960.
80. Wilson, M. A., and Cascarano, J. The energy yielding oxidation of NADH by fumarate in submitochondrial particles of rat tissues. *Biochim. Biophys. Acta* 216:54, 1970.
81. Hunter, F. E. Anaerobic phosphorylation due to coupled oxidation-reduction between alpha-ketoglutaric acid and oxaloacetic acid. *J. Biol. Chem.* 177:361, 1949.
82. Zimmermann, R., Tillmanns, H., Knapp, W. H., et al. Regional myocardial nitrogen-13 glutamate uptake in patients with coronary artery disease: Inverse post-stress relation to thallium-201 uptake in ischemia. *J. Am. Coll. Cardiol.* 11:549, 1988.
83. Lazar, H. L., Buckberg, G. D., Manganaro, A. J., et al. Reversal of ischemic damage with amino acid substrate enhancement during reperfusion. *Surgery* 88:702, 1980.
84. Bittl, J. A., and Shine, K. I. Protection of ischemic rabbit myocardium by glutamic acid. *Am. J. Physiol.* 245:H406, 1983.
85. Taegtmeyer, H., and Russell, R. R. Glutamate metabolism in rabbit heart: Augmentation by ischemia and inhibition with acetoacetate. *J. Appl. Cardiol.* 2:231, 1987.
86. Schoenheimer, R. *The Dynamic State of Body Constituents.* Cambridge, MA: Harvard University Press, 1942.
87. Morgan, H. E., and Neely, J. R. Metabolic regulation and myocardial function. In J. W. Hurst (ed.), *The Heart* (6th ed.). New York: McGraw-Hill, 1986. P. 85.
88. Morgan, H. E., Rannels, D. E., and Kao, R. L. Factors controlling protein turnover in heart muscle. *Circ. Res.* 34, 35(Suppl III):III-22, 1974.
89. Lesch, M., Taegtmeyer, H., Peterson, M. B., and Vernick, R. Studies on the mechanism of the inhibition of myocardial protein synthesis during oxygen deprivation. *Am. J. Physiol.* 230:120, 1976.
90. Chua, B., Kao, R. L., Rannels, D. E., and Morgan, H. E. Inhibition of protein degradation by anoxia and ischemia in perfused rat hearts. *J. Biol. Chem.* 254:6617, 1979.
91. Morgan, H. E., Rannels, D. E., and McKee, E. E. Protein metabolism of the heart. In R. Berne (ed.), *Handbook of Physiology: The Cardiovascular System: The Heart.* Washington, D.C.: American Physiology Society, 1979. P. 845.
92. Hershko, A., Ciechanover, A., Heller, H., et al. Proposed role of ATP in protein breakdown: Conjugation of proteins with multiple chains of the polypeptide of ATP-dependent proteolysis. *Proc. Natl. Acad. Sci. U.S.A.* 77:1783, 1980.
93. Decker, R. S., and Wildenthal, K. Role of lysosomes and latent hydrolytic enzymes in ischemic damage and repair of the heart. In K. Wildenthal (ed.), *Degradative Processes in Heart and Skeletal Muscle.* New York: Elsevier/North Holland, 1980. P. 389.
94. Wildenthal, K., and Crie, J. S. Lysosomes and cardiac protein catabolism. In K. Wildenthal (ed.), *Degradative Processes in Heart and Skeletal Muscle.* New York: Elsevier/North Holland, 1980. P. 113.
95. Seglen, P. O., Grinde, B., and Solheim, A. Z. Inhibition of the lysosomal pathway of protein degradation in isolated rat hepatocytes by ammonia, methylamine, chloroquine and leupeptin. *Eur. J. Biochem.* 95:215, 1979.
96. Wildenthal, K. Lysosomal alterations in ischemic myocardium: Result or cause of myocardial damage? (Editorial). *J. Mol. Cell. Cardiol.* 10:595, 1978.
97. Saleen, Y., Niveditha, T., and Sadasivudu, B. AMP-deaminase, 5′-nucleotidase and adenosine deaminase in rat myocardial tissue in myocardial infarction and hypothermia. *Experientia* 38:776, 1982.
98. Arch, J. R. S., and Newsholme, E. A. Activities and some properties of 5′-nucleotidase, adenosine kinase and adenosine deaminase in tissues from vertebrates and invertebrates in relation to the control of the concentration and the physiological role of adenosine. *Biochem. J.* 174:965, 1978.
99. Van Belle, H., Goossens, F., and Wynants, J. Formation and release of purine catabolites during hypoperfusion, anoxia, and ischemia. *Am. J. Physiol.* 252:H886, 1987.
100. Reibel, D. K., and Rovetto, M. Myocardial adenosine salvage rates and restoration of ATP content following ischemia. *Am. J. Physiol.* 237:H247, 1979.
101. Bardenheuer, H., and Schrader, J. Supply-to-demand ratio for oxygen determines formation of adenosine by the heart. *Am. J. Physiol.* 250: H173, 1986.
102. Zimmer, H. G., Trendelenburg, C., Kammermeier, H., and Gerlach, E. De novo synthesis of myocardial adenine nucleotides in the rat: Acceleration during recovery from oxygen deficiency. *Circ. Res.* 32:637, 1973.
103. Zimmer, H. G. Restitution of myocardial adenine nucleotides: Acceleration by administration of ribose. *J. Physiol. (Paris)* 76:769, 1980.
104. Swain, J. L., Sabina, R. L., McHale, P. A., et al. Prolonged myocardial nucleotide depletion after brief ischemia in the open-chest dog. *Am. J. Physiol.* 242:H818, 1982.
105. Reimer, K. A., Hill, M. L., and Jennings, R. B.

Prolonged depletion of ATP and adenine nucleotide pool due to delayed resynthesis of adenine nucleotides following reversible myocardial ischemia injury in dogs. *J. Mol. Cell. Cardiol.* 13:229, 1981.
106. DeBoer, L. W. V., Ingwall, J. S., Kloner, R. A., and Braunwald, E. Prolonged derangements of canine myocardial purine metabolism after a brief coronary artery occlusion not associated with curatomic evidence of necrosis. *Proc. Natl. Acad. Sci. U.S.A.* 77:5471, 1980.
107. Jennings, R. B., Hawkins, H. K., Lowe, J. E., et al. Relation between high energy phosphate and lethal injury in myocardial ischemia. *Am. J. Pathol.* 92:187, 1978.
108. Gevers, W. Generation of protons by metabolic processes in heart cells. *J. Mol. Cell. Cardiol.* 9:867, 1977.
109. Bolli, R. Mechanism of myocardial "stunning." *Circulation* 82:723, 1990.
110. Freeman, B. A., and Crapo, J. D. Biology of disease: Free radicals and tissue injury. *Lab. Invest.* 47:412, 1982.
111. Burton, K. P., McCord, J. M., and Ghai, G. Myocardial alterations due to free radical generation. *Am. J. Physiol.* 246:H776, 1984.
112. Chambers, D. E., Parks, P. A., Patterson, G., et al. Role of oxygen-derived free radicals in myocardial ischemia. *Fed. Proc.* 42:4696, 1983.
113. Shlafer, M., Kane, P. F., and Kirsh, M. M. Superoxide dismutase plus catalase enhance the efficacy of hypothermic cardioplegia to protect the globally ischemic reperfused heart. *J. Thorac. Cardiovasc. Surg.* 83:830, 1982.
114. Jolly, S. R., Kane, W. J., Bailie, M. B., et al. Canine myocardial reperfusion injury: Its reduction by the combined administration of superoxide dismutase and catalase. *Circ. Res.* 54:277, 1984.
115. McCord, J. M. Oxygen-derived free radicals in post ischemic tissue injury. *N. Engl. J. Med* 312:159, 1985.
116. Davies, K. J. A. Protein damage and degradation by oxygen radicals. I. General aspects. *J. Biol. Chem.* 262:9895, 1987.
117. Davies, K. J. A., and Goldberg, A. L. Oxygen radicals stimulate intracellular proteolysis and lipid peroxidation by independent mechanisms in erythrocytes. *J. Biol. Chem.* 262:8220, 1987.
118. McCormack, J. G., Halestrap, A. P., and Denton, R. M. Role of calcium ions in reperfusion of mammalian intramitochondrial metabolism. *Physiol. Rev.* 70:391, 1990.
119. Fabiato, A., and Fabiato, F. Calcium release from the sarcoplasmic reticulum. *Circ. Res.* 40:110, 1977.
120. Shen, A. C., and Jennings, R. B. Kinetics of calcium accumulative in acute myocardial ischemic injury. *Am. J. Pathol.* 67:441, 1972.
121. Fleckenstein, A., Jahnke, J., Doring, H. J., and Leder, O. Myocardial biology. *Recent Adv. Stud. Cardiac Struct.* 4:563, 1974.
122. Katz, A. M., and Reuter, H. Cellular calcium and cell death. *Am. J. Cardiol.* 44:188, 1979.
123. Katz, A. M., and Tada, M. The "stone heart": A challenge to the biochemist. *Am. J. Cardiol.* 29:578, 1972
124. Dhalla, N. S., Pierce, N. G., Panagia, V., et al. Calcium movements in relation to heart function. *Basic Res. Cardiol.* 77:117, 1982.
125. Lehninger, A. C. Mitochondria and calcium ion transport. *Biochem. J.* 119:129, 1970.
126. Slater, E. C., and Cleland, K. W. The effect of calcium on the respiratory and phosphorylative activities of heart muscle sarcosomes. *Biochem. J.* 55:566, 1953.
127. Carafoli, E., and Bing, R. J. Myocardial failure. *J. Appl. Cardiol.* 3:3, 1988.
128. Bailey, I. A., Radda, G. K., Seymour, A. M., and Williams, S. R. The effects of insulin on myocardial metabolism and acidosis in normoxia and ischemia: A ^{31}P-NMR study. *Biochim. Biophys. Acta* 720:1727, 1982.
129. Ross, B. D., and Freeman, D. Contributions to cardiac biochemistry from magnetic resonance. *J. Appl. Cardiol.* 1:75, 1986.
130. Karmen, A., Wroblewski, F., and Ladue, S. Transaminase activity in human blood. *J. Clin. Invest.* 34:126, 1954.
131. Roberts, R., Parker, C. W., and Sobel, B. E. Detection of acute myocardial infarction by radioimmunoassay for creatine kinase MB. *Lancet* 2:319, 1977.
132. Shell, W. E., Kjeushus, J. K., and Sobel, B. E. Quantitative assessment of the extent of myocardial infarction in the conscious dog by means of analysis of serial changes in serum creatine phosphokinase activity. *J. Clin. Invest.* 50:2614, 1971.
133. Sobel, B. E., Roberst, R., and Larson, K. B. Estimation of infarct size from serum MB creatine phosphokinase activity: Application and limitations. *Am. J. Cardiol.* 37:474, 1976.
134. Adams, J. E., III, Abendschein, D. R., and Jaffe, A. S. Biochemical markers of myocardial injury. Is MB creatine kinase the choice for the 1990's? *Circulation* 88:750, 1993.
135. Katus, H. A., Remppis, A., Neumann, F. J., et al. Diagnostic efficiency of troponin T measurements in acute myocardial infarction. *Circulation* 83:902, 1991.
136. Adams, J. E., III, Sicard, G. A., Allen, B. T. et al. Diagnosis of perioperative myocardial infarction with measurement of cardiac troponin I. *N. Engl. J. Med.* 330:670, 1994.
137. Haber, E. *In vivo* diagnostic and therapeutic uses of monoclonal antibodies in cardiology. *Annu. Rev. Med.* 37:249, 1986.
138. Schelbert, H. R., Phelps, M. E., Hoffman, E., et al. Regional myocardium blood flow, metabolism, and function assessed noninvasively with positron emission tomography. *Am. J. Cardiol.* 46:1269, 1980.
139. Schelbert, H. R., and Schwaiger, M. Positron emis-

sion tomography studies of the heart. In M. Phelps, J. Mazziota, and H. Schelbert (eds.), *Positron Emission Tomography and Autoradiography: Principles and Applications for the Brain and the Heart.* New York: Raven Press, 1986. P. 581.
140. Schwaiger, M., Brunken, R., Crover-McKay, M., et al. Detection of tissue viability in patients with acute myocardial infarction by positron emission tomography. *J. Am. Coll. Cardiol.* 8:800, 1986.
141. Marshall, R. C., Tillisch, J. H., Phelps, M. E., et al. Identification and differentiation of resting myocardial ischemia and infarction in man with positron computer tomography, ^{18}F-labeled fluorodeoxyglucose and ^{13}N ammonia. *Circulation* 67:766, 1983.
142. Tillisch, J., Brunken, R. Marshall, R., et al. Prediction of reversibility of cardiac wall motion abnormalities predicted by positron tomography, ^{18}fluorodeoxyglucose, and $^{13}NH_3$. *N. Engl. J. Med.* 314: 884, 1986.
143. Gropler, R. J., Siegel, B. A., Sampathkumaran, K., et al. Dependence of recovery of contractile function on maintenance of oxidative metabolism after myocardial infarction. *J. Am. Coll. Cardiol.* 19: 989, 1992.
144. Gropler, R. J., Geltman, E. M., Sampathkumaran, K., et al. Functional recovery after coronary revascularization for chronic coronary artery disease is dependent on maintenance of oxidative metabolism. *J. Am. Coll. Cardiol.* 20:569, 1992.
145. Tennant, T., and Wiggers, C. J. Effect of coronary occlusion on myocardial contraction. *Am. J. Physiol.* 112:351, 1935.
146. Bergmann, S. R., Fox, K. A. A., Ter-Pogossian, M. M., et al. Clot-selective coronary thrombolysis with tissue-type plasminogen activator. *Science* 220: 1181, 1983.
147. Braunwald, E., and Kloner, R. A. The stunned myocardium: Prolonged, postischemic ventricular dysfunction. *Circulation* 66:1146, 1982.
148. Bing, R. J. Reparative processes in heart muscle following myocardial infarction. *Cardiology* 50: 314, 1971.
149. Bergmann, S. R., Lerch, R., Fox, K., et al. Temporal dependence of beneficial effects of coronary thrombolysis characterized by positron tomography. *Am. J. Med.* 73:573, 1982.
150. Vary, T. C., Angelakos, E. T., and Schaffer, S. W. Relationship between adenine nucleotide metabolism and irreversible ischemic tissue damage in isolated, perfused rat heart. *Circ. Res.* 45:218, 1979.
151. Becker, L. C., and Ambrosio, G. Myocardial consequences of reperfusion. *Prog. Cardiovasc. Dis.* 30:23, 1987.
152. Poole-Wilson, P. A. Reperfusion damage in heart muscle: Still unexplained but with new clinical relevance. *Clin. Physiol.* 7:439, 1987.
153. Zimmermann, A. N. E., and Hülsmann, W. C. Paradoxical influence of calcium ions on the permeability of the isolated rat heart. *Nature* 211:646, 1960.
154. Ambrosio, G., Weissfeldt, M. D., Jacobus, W. E., and Flaherty, J. T. Evidence of a reversible, radical-mediated component of reperfusion injury: Reduction by recombinant human superoxide dismutase administered at the time of reflow. *Circulation* 75:282, 1987.
155. Lagerstrom, C. F., Walker, W. E., and Taegtmeyer, H. Failure of glycogen depletion to improve left ventricular function of the rabbit heart after hypothermic ischemic arrest. *Circ. Res.* 63:81, 1988.
156. McElroy, D. D., Walker, W. E., and Taegtmeyer, H. Glycogen loading improves left ventricular function of the rabbit heart after hypothermic ischemic arrest. *J. Appl. Cardiol.* 4:455, 1989.
157. Klein, H. H., Puschmann, S., Schaper, J., and Schaper, W. The mechanism of the tetrazolium reaction in identifying experimental myocardial infarction. *Virchows Arch. A Pathol. Anat. Histopathol.* 393:287, 1981.
158. Sodi-Pallares, D., Testelli, M. R., Fishleder, B. L., et al. Effects of intravenous infusion of a potassium-glucose-insulin solution on the electrocardiographic signs of myocardial infarction. *Am. J. Cardiol.* 9:166, 1962.
159. Rogers, W. J., Stanley, A. W., Breing, J. B., et al. Reduction of hospital mortality rate of acute myocardial infarction with glucose-insulin-potassium infusion. *Am. Heart J.* 92:441, 1976.
160. Gradinak, S., Coleman, G. M., Taegtmeyer, H., et al. Improved cardiac function with glucose-insulin-potassium after coronary bypass surgery. *Ann. Thorac. Surg.* 48:484, 1989.
161. Schaper, J., and Schaper, W. Reperfusion of ischemic myocardium: Ultrastructural and histochemical aspects. *J. Am. Coll. Cardiol.* 1:1037, 1983.
162. Mowbray, J., Hutchinson, W. L., Tibbs, G. R., et al. The discovery of a rapidly metabolized polymeric tetraphosphate derivative of adenosine in perfused rat heart. *Biochem. J.* 223:627, 1984.

4. Pathology of Acute Myocardial Infarction

Brooks S. Edwards and Jesse E. Edwards

In considering the pathology of acute myocardial infarction (AMI) we include the pathologic features that underlie the complications, both early and late, of the fundamental condition.

Pathologic Features of Myocardial Infarction

AMI characteristically is observed in patients with chronic coronary arterial obstruction. In some of these, precipitation of the myocardial necrosis is associated with a superimposed acute coronary arterial occlusion from a thrombus. Infarcts so resulting are, in general, more extensive than are those in which acute coronary occlusion is not present.

Two degrees of involvement of the myocardium are recognized. The more extensive disease involves nearly the full thickness of the left ventricular myocardium in the distribution of the underlying coronary disease. Such infarcts tend to be conglomerate. The infarcts with less extensive involvement tend to lie in the subendocardial one-half or one-third of the myocardium, although patchy foci of involvement may lie in the subepicardial half of the myocardium. So-called subendocardial infarcts may be either multifocal or conglomerate. In most instances, regardless of the type of infarct, a layer of myocardium lying immediately underneath the mural endocardium is preserved.

The infarcts of the former type have generally been called transmural, and the latter have been termed subendocardial. Based on electrocardiography, infarcts have been categorized as Q wave infarcts and non-Q wave infarcts. Q wave infarcts tend to be transmural, and non-Q wave infarcts tend to be subendocardial [1]. Although it is beyond the scope of this chapter to enter into lengthy debate relative to the preferential use of the terms mentioned, it should be pointed out that the presence or absence of a Q wave in patients with AMI may be influenced not only by the extent of an infarct but also by its location, the presence or absence of earlier infarction, and delayed intraventricular conduction [2].

The earliest reliable manifestations of AMI, evident microscopically, usually appear at about 8 hours [3, 4]. Early changes include hypereosinophilia of the involved myocardial fibers (Fig. 4-1); in addition, the ischemic myocytes may take on a "wavy" appearance. Thinning of fibers, nuclear loss, and cytoplasmic coagulation may occur within the first 24 hours. The next stage, namely interstitial infiltration with leukocytes, usually polymorphonuclear in nature, is seen at about 24 to 48 hours (Fig. 4-1B). The process of leukocytic infiltration occurs initially at the periphery of the myocardial infarct and proceeds toward the center of the infarct. In large infarcts leukocytic infiltration falls far short of involving the central part of the zone of infarction. After 2 days the leukocytes start showing signs of necrosis, leading to cytoplasmic disruption and nuclear fragmentation of these cells. After about 3 to 4 days, removal of infarcted myocardial fibers begins (Fig. 4-1C). At the early stages of removal the process cannot be identified grossly. Removal of necrotic myocardial fibers is the main process that occurs during the latter half of the first week and all of the second week. The site of this process is identified histologically as a vascular basketwork representing myocardium from which the myocardial fibers have been removed, although the connective tissue and vascular stroma of the cardiac wall remain. Within this tissue may be found fragments of necrotic fibers, phagocytes containing "wear and tear" pigment (lipofuscin), and interstitial leukocytes, principally phagocytes (Fig. 4-1D). The remaining myocytes and the supporting cardiac interstitium become the nidus for infarct expansion and ultimately global ventricular remodeling [25].

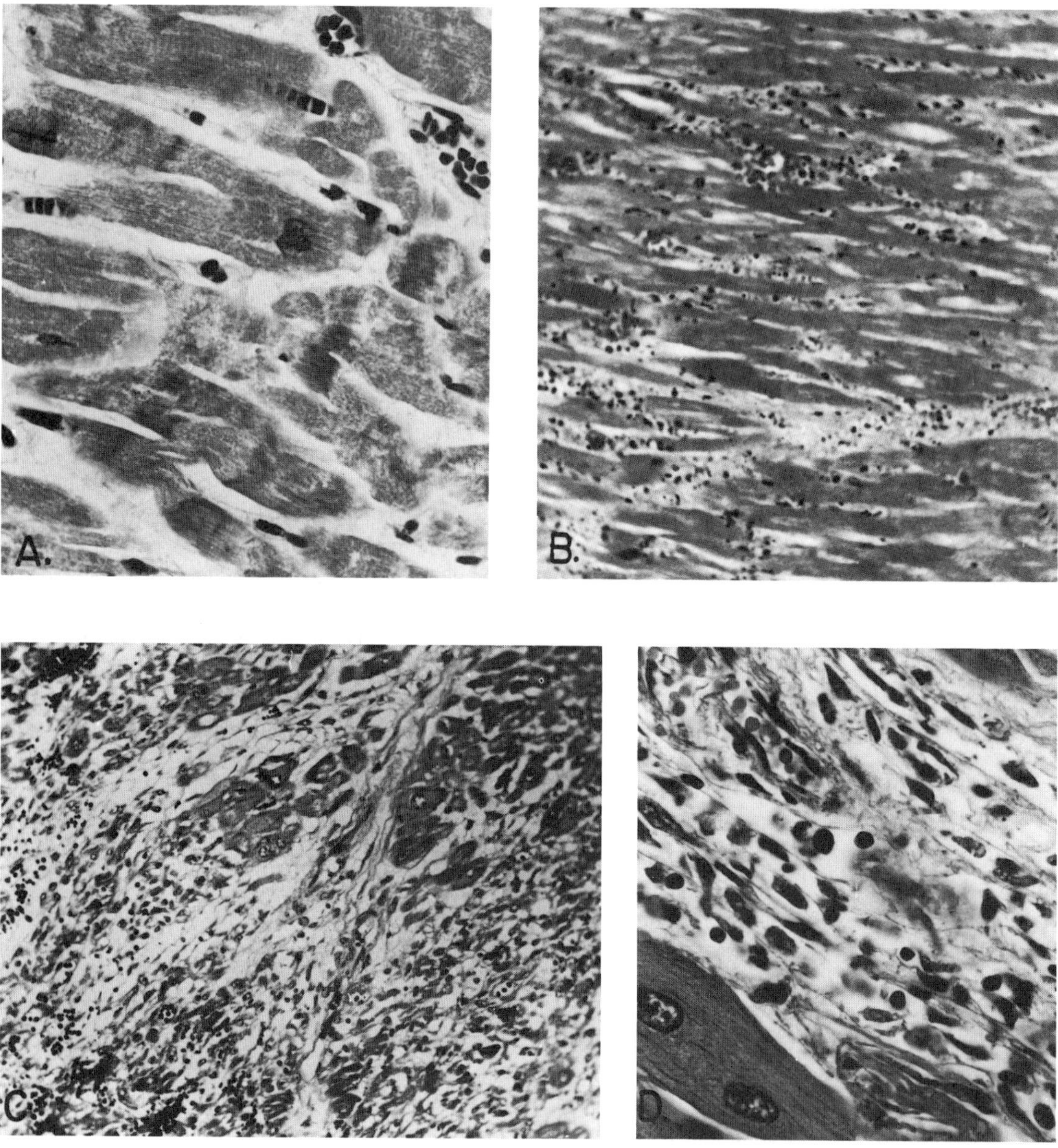

Fig. 4-1
Photomicrographs of myocardial infarcts of various ages. *A.* At 6 to 8 hours after the onset of infarction some fibers have lost their nuclei. There are cytoplasmic irregularities, including coagulation changes and contraction bands. H & E. × 450. *B.* At 2 days, the myocardial fibers stain darkly because of hypereosinophilia. Nuclei have been lost, and there is heavy infiltration interstitially with polymorphonuclear neutrophils. H & E. × 200. *C.* Periphery of the infarct at 5 days. Necrotic fibers are being removed, leaving a basketwork of connective tissue and capillaries of the myocardium. H & E. × 100. *D.* Site of removal of myocardial infarction at 2 weeks. At the center, myocardial fibers have been removed, leaving the capillaries and connective tissue of myocardial stroma. Some interstitial phagocytic cells are also present. H & E. × 450.

During the third week the process of scar formation starts (Fig. 4-2A). It is characterized by fibroblastic proliferation and laying down of delicate collagen. Additional removal of necrotic fibers may occur or is completed by this time. During the fourth week scar formation is evident, the scar having resulted from new production of connective tissue and condensation of stroma (Fig. 4-2B). Scattered phagocytes are present in the early scar.

In older scars, the collagen becomes compact; and at about 6 weeks after the onset of the infarct, elastic fibers may be noted in the scar tissue (Fig. 4-3A). In some scars dilated vessels are present and persist (Fig. 4-3B).

When the scar is established, the infarcted myocardium has usually been removed. Nevertheless, in some large infarcts necrotic muscle may remain for months or years enveloped by scar tissue (Fig. 4-3C). In such instances the remaining necrotic muscle may become calcified.

There are gross findings which correlate with the histologic stages reviewed. Within 6 hours or more the infarcted area may be identified as somewhat cyanotic in nature (Fig. 4-4A). By 1 day the necrotic area is tan, reflecting the color of infarcted myocardium and leukocytes (Fig. 4-4B). When removal of necrotic muscle is established, the zone of removal lying at the edge of the infarcted tissue is characteristically red to purple and depressed (Fig. 4-4C). During the third week the process of removal and early scar formation is represented by a depressed, translucent, ground-glass zone (Fig. 4-4D). The established scar is pale gray to white. Varying degrees of thinning of the wall occur in concert with the proportion of the myocardium that had been infarcted. In many patients scarring may be multifocal, indicating the frequent multifocal distribution of AMI. When the stage of scarring has been reached, thickening of the overlying mural endocardium by gray fibrous tissue (fibroelastosis) may be present. The larger the scar, the greater is the trend for fibroelastosis to develop (Fig. 4-5).

Fig. 4-2
Photomicrographs of myocardial infarcts of various ages. *A*. At 3 weeks. Note the infarcted tissue at the right and the noninfarcted tissue at the left. Between the two zones is a zone from which necrotic myocardium has been removed. Early fibrous changes are occurring, and blood vessels are dilated. H & E. × 100. *B*. Endocardial half of the myocardium in healed myocardial infarction. The black streaks represent scarring. The mural endocardium is at the bottom. A strip of retained muscle is characteristically present immediately underneath the mural endocardium. Elastic tissue stain. × 5.

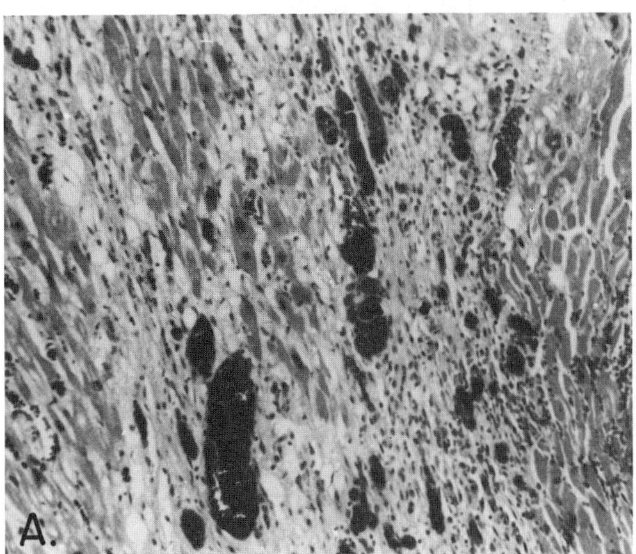

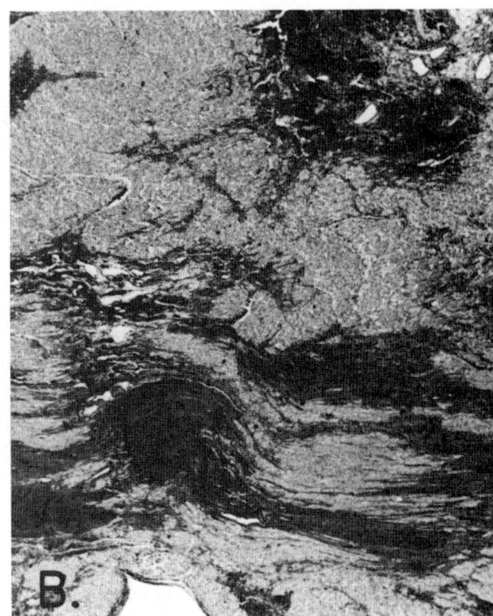

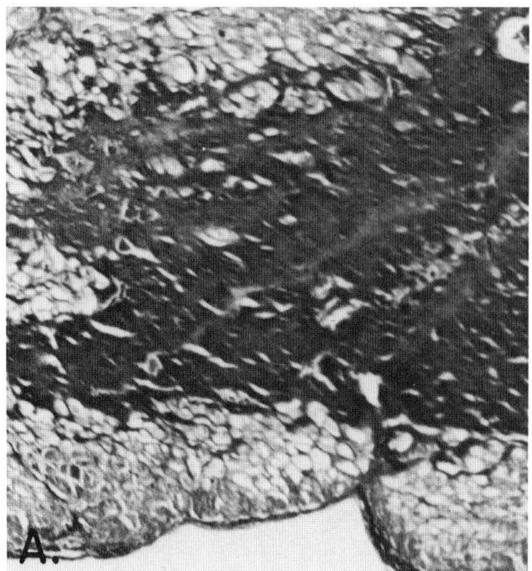

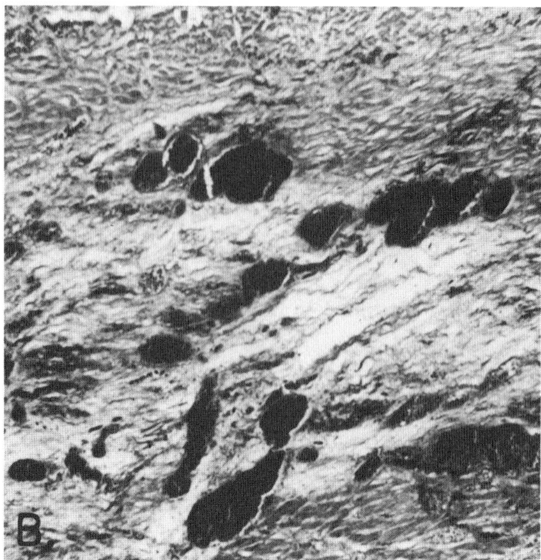

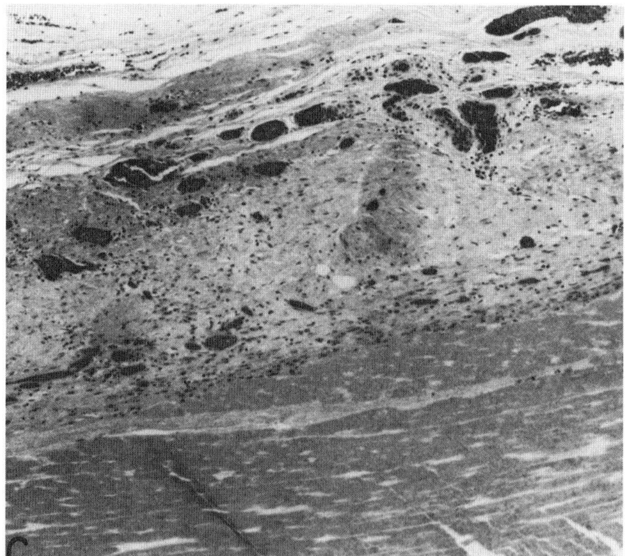

Fig. 4-3
Photomicrographs showing variations in healed myocardial infarction. *A.* Mural endocardium is toward the bottom. Immediately underneath this layer is a zone of retained myocardium. Some of the fibers are vacuolated. Underneath this area is a black area representing dense scar following myocardial infarction. Elastic tissue stain. × 100. *B.* Scar in old myocardial infarction in which numerous wide blood vessels are present. *C.* The scar of the myocardial infarction (upper half) is adjacent to an area of retained necrotic myocardial fibers (lowermost). H & E. × 70.

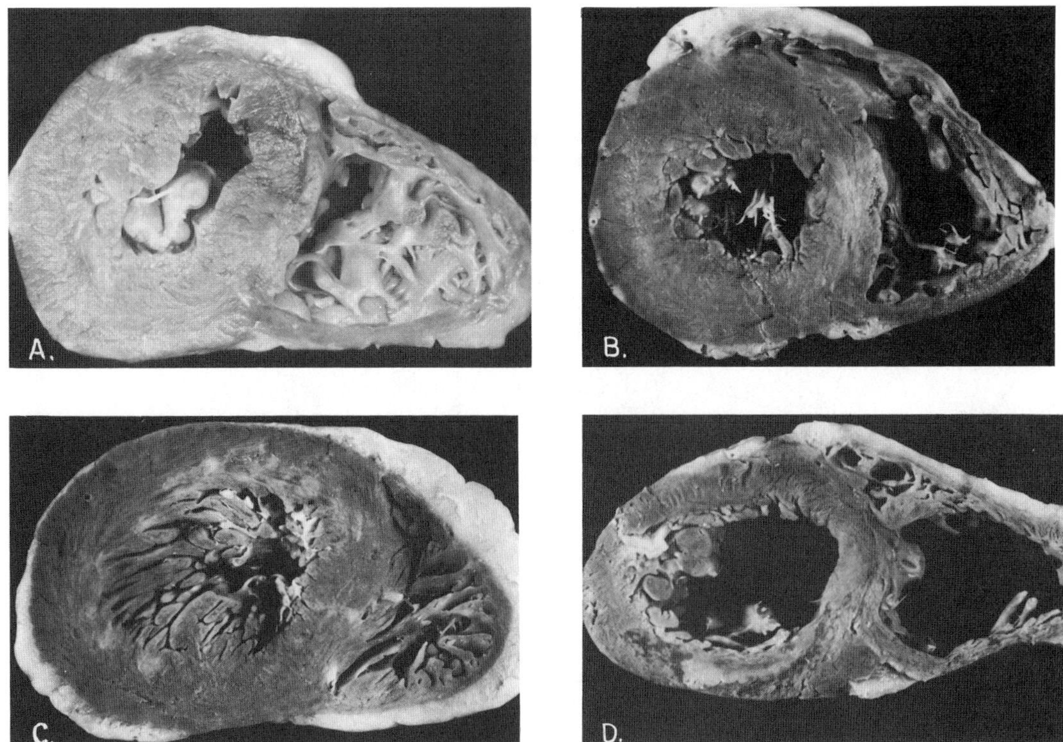

Fig. 4-4
Gross pathology of acute myocardial infarction. In each instance the ventricles have been cut in cross section and are viewed from the basal toward the apical aspect. The upper part of each illustration is anterior and the lower part inferior. The right ventricle lies to the right of the left ventricle in this perspective. *A.* Early anteroseptal infarction. The different texture of the anterior part of the septum and nearby anterior wall reflects a zone that in the fresh state yielded a cyanotic hue. *B.* Anterior infarction of about 4 days' duration. The pale area in the subendocardial half of the anterior wall and the nearby ventricular septum represents acute infarction. Removal is not yet apparent. *C.* Healing infarction in midportion of the ventricular septum. The dark, depressed area represents a zone of removed necrotic muscle. *D.* Transmural acute inferior infarction. The pale area in the inferior wall represents necrotic muscle yet to be removed. Peripheral to this zone is a dark, depressed area representing removal of tissue, characteristic of a 2- to 3-week-old infarct.

Complications

Hypotension and Congestive Heart Failure

The first week following AMI may be complicated by persistent or acute hypotension and the syndrome of congestive heart failure. The etiology of this state (''pump failure'') primarily relates to extensive myocardial ischemia and necrosis or unique sites of myocardial infarction with or without rupture.

Extensive Myocardial Ischemia or Necrosis

It has long been appreciated that extensive myocardial infarction results in severe hemodynamic disturbances and persistent congestive heart failure. The extent of infarction may result from a single AMI (Fig. 4-6); more commonly, though, this myocardial mass is lost during several distinct episodes of AMI (see Fig. 4-5D). In the latter case, it has been demonstrated that the sequential loss of mass results in an additive effect. Autopsy studies have

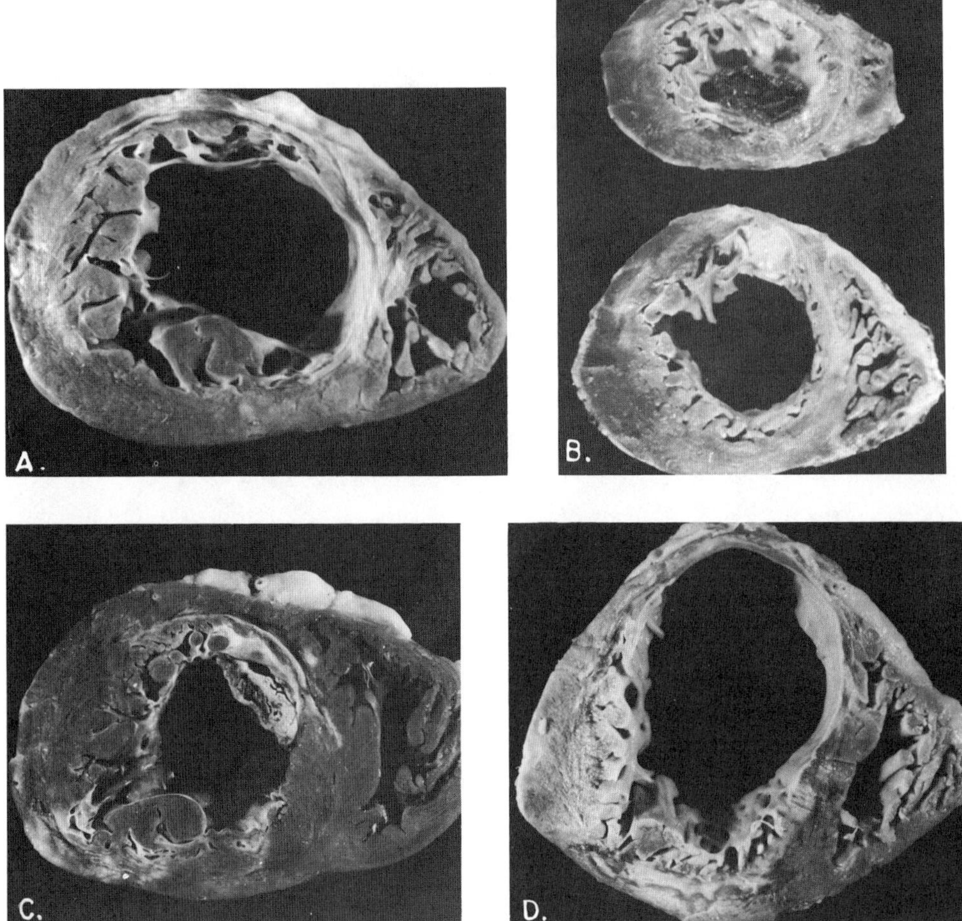

Fig. 4-5
Gross appearances of hearts with healed myocardial infarcts. *A.* Healed extensive anteroseptal infarction. The involved part of the wall is thin. The mural endocardium is thickened by virtue of fibroelastosis. *B.* Two levels of section showing healed anterior infarction with mural thrombosis at the apex. There is endocardial fibroelastosis as well. *C.* Healed conglomerate subendocardial anterior infarction with endocardial fibroelastosis and a mural thrombosis attached. In the inferolateral aspect there is scarring of healed infarction. The papillary muscles are unaffected, however. *D.* Healed extensive anterior infarction and healing inferior infarction. The thin wall and endocardial fibroelastosis are characteristic of a healed extensive anterior infarct, which suggests early aneurysm formation as well. In the inferior wall there is a conglomerate infarct that is undergoing healing. The classic ground-glass appearance of the zone of removal around the pale zone of retained necrotic muscles suggests an age of about 3 weeks.

suggested that when a total of more than 40 percent of myocardial mass is lost, severe pump failure results, and the chances for recovery are remote [5, 6]. Imaging studies utilizing technetium-99m Sestamibi SPECT tomography demonstrated that depending on the state of compensation, more than 50 percent of the left ventricle may be infarcted without resulting end-stage pump failure [26].

Attention has been focused on the so-called stunned myocardium. The stunned myocardium may be characterized by a reversible state of myocardial injury [7]. Under conditions in which perfu-

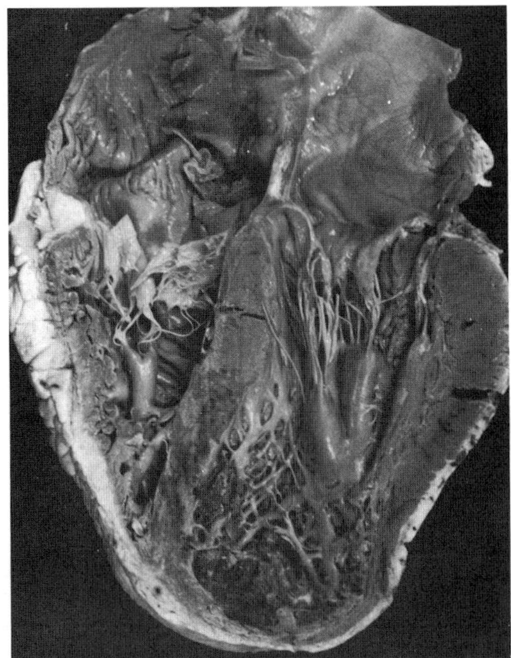

Fig. 4-6
Frontal section through the ventricular septum and ventricles. Extensive infarction of the apical area of the left ventricle extends into the lateral wall and ventricular septum. Note the overlying mural thrombosis.

sion is restored (either naturally or by intervention), that portion of myocardium may resume normal function. Although physiologic imaging studies may suggest the presence of stunned myocardium, there are no unique pathologic markers that identify this condition.

Right Ventricular Infarction

Infarction of the left ventricular inferior wall may extend into the right ventricle [8]. Usually the extent and consequences of this right ventricular infarction are minimal. The relative protection of the right ventricle from infarction may relate to the lower oxygen demands of the thin-walled chamber. Significant right ventricular infarction occurs more commonly in states where the oxygen demand of the right ventricle is increased, which may be seen where there is preexisting pulmonary hypertension and right ventricular hypertrophy. Usually the patients have a dominant right coronary artery with a high-grade proximal stenosis or occlusion. Clinically, the patient may present as hypotensive and volume depleted while undergoing spontaneous diuresis.

Rupture of Ventricular Septum

There are three general types of cardiac rupture that may complicate the acute stages of myocardial infarction [9]. Collectively, they constitute about 15 percent of all deaths resulting from AMI. Rupture may involve the left ventricular free wall (about 85 percent of all ruptures), a papillary muscle, or the ventricular septum, the latter two types constituting about 15 percent of ruptures. Rupture of the left ventricular free wall is considered in greater detail in the section dealing with hemopericardium. Rupture of a papillary muscle is covered in the section on mitral regurgitation.

Rupture of the ventricular septum leads to an acquired left-to-right shunt. Frequently, it is of overwhelming proportion, resulting in early shock followed by a rapidly deteriorating state. When the communication between the two ventricles is restricted in caliber, the shunt may be tolerated for varying periods of time.

There are two types of rupture of the ventricular septum, the simple and the complex [10]. As the name implies, the simple type represents a through-and-through, direct opening between the two ventricles (Fig. 4-7A). The complex type is represented by a tract or several tracts extending through a ventricular septum in a serpiginous manner (Fig. 4-7B,C). The opening(s) into the right ventricle may be some distance from the site of the primary tear. Although exceptions occur, it is usual that the simple type of septal rupture complicates infarcts in the apical half of the left ventricle (usually anterior), whereas the complex type tends to occur in basal infarcts (usually inferior).

Transmural myocardial infarction is virtually always present in individuals with rupture of the ventricular septum. Extensive right ventricular infarction in the presence of septal rupture negatively influences survival [11]. Although some investigators suggested that one-vessel coronary artery disease is common with this entity [31, 32], one study reported significant three-vessel coronary artery disease in 48 of 53 autopsy cases studied [10].

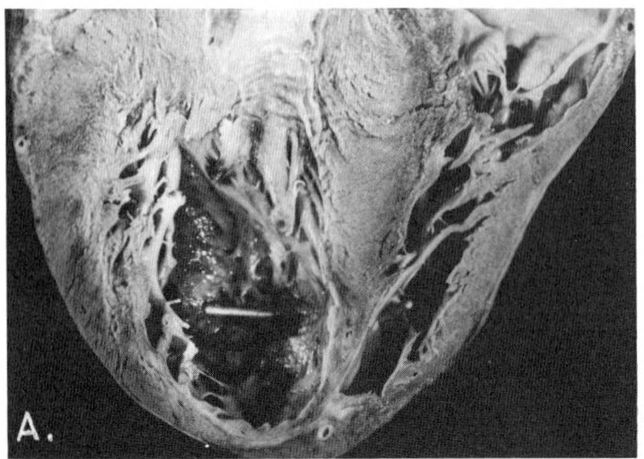

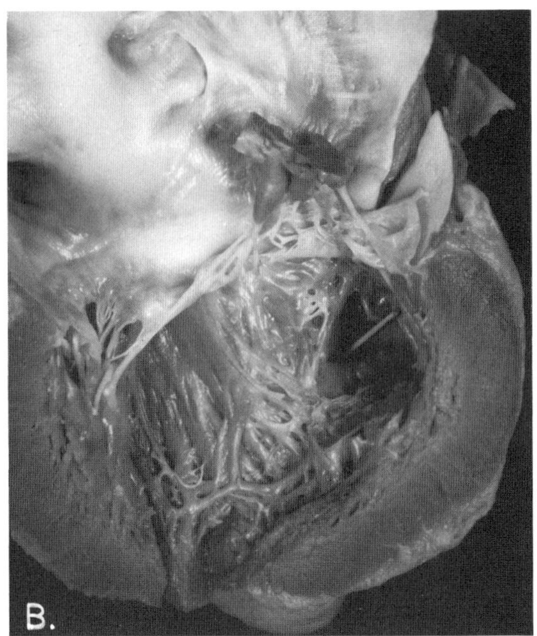

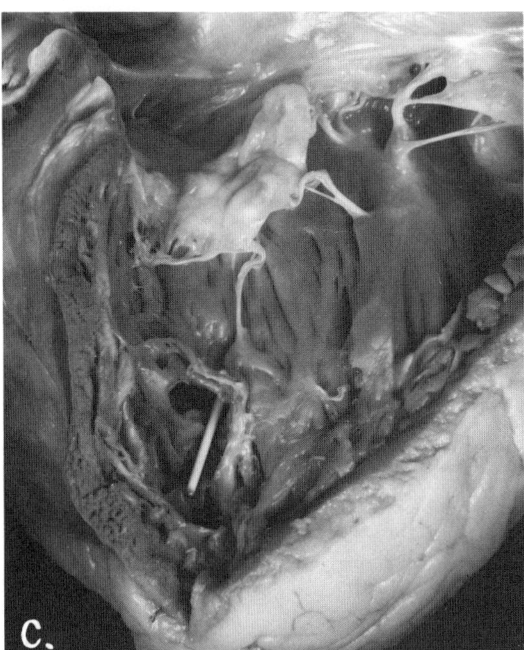

Fig. 4-7
Rupture of the ventricular septum: two types. *A.* Simple type. *B, C.* Complex type. *A.* The ventricular septum has been sectioned in a frontal plane. The ventricles are viewed from behind (left ventricle to the left). There is an acute infarct involving the ventricular septum and the apical portion of the heart. A simple through-and-through tract (probe) extends between the two ventricles. *B.* Left ventricle and atrium. The rupture tract begins at the base of the ventricular septum (probe). *C.* Right atrium and ventricle. The tract (probe) leads into the right ventricle in a more apical location than the initial laceration in the left ventricle.

Associated Conditions Leading to or Intensifying the Degree of Congestive Heart Failure

Especially among the relatively old with myocardial infarction, congestive heart failure, if present, may be caused by the loss of myocardial tissue through infarction (often recurrent) and by the effects of additional conditions. Among the common additional conditions are hypertension, aortic stenosis, chronic obstructive pulmonary disease, and less commonly, extensive forms of senile (cardiac) amyloidosis [12]. Infarct expansion and cardiac remodeling may lead to greater ventricular dysfunction and subsequent development of congestive heart failure [25, 27]. A recent clinical study utilizing angiotensin-converting enzyme inhibitors following AMI demonstrated efficacy in reducing ventricular remodeling and the subsequent development of congestive heart failure [28].

Mitral Regurgitation

Mitral regurgitation may occur during the early phase following AMI and vary in severity from trivial to severe. Because the integrity of the mitral valve depends on the structure and function of not only the valve itself but also the mitral annulus, left atrial wall, left ventricular myocardium, and papillary muscles, mitral insufficiency may result from disruption or malfunction of one or more components [13].

Papillary Muscle Dysfunction or Infarction

Mild and often transient mitral regurgitation is associated with the entity ''papillary muscle dysfunction,'' which may be the result of ischemia of either a papillary muscle or more commonly the left ventricular free wall from which the papillary muscles arise. Whether it represents transient ischemia or a stunned myocardium following infarction of adjacent tissue, the pathologic findings are often nonspecific.

More severe mitral regurgitation results from infarction of papillary muscle and underlying left ventricle (Fig. 4-8).

The posteromedial papillary muscle receives its blood supply from a branch of the posterior descending artery. Because it is an end-artery, collateral circulation is limited and occlusion frequently results in infarction. The anterolateral papillary muscle commonly has dual blood supply from diagonal branches of the anterior descending artery and obtuse marginal branches of the left circumflex coronary artery. The dual supply provides some protective effect, making infarction of the anterolateral papillary muscle less frequent than that of the posteromedial papillary muscle.

Distortion in left ventricular geometry, which may occur following left ventricular infarction, may alter the relations between the two papillary muscles and result in mild to moderate mitral insufficiency. Chronic mitral insufficiency may lead to left atrial enlargement, annular dilatation, and progressively more severe mitral regurgitation [13].

Rupture of Papillary Muscle

Whereas infarction of a part of a papillary muscle system may lead to abnormal coaptation of the mitral leaflets and incompetence, rupture of part or all of a papillary muscle associated with more se-

Fig. 4-8
Two examples of healing myocardial infarction without papillary muscle rupture and with mitral regurgitation. *A.* Cross section of the ventricles. In the inferior wall of the left ventricle is a healing transmural infarct. The related posteromedial papillary muscle is also involved in infarction but is not ruptured. *B.* Photomicrograph of a portion of the posteromedial papillary muscle from a surgically excised mitral valve showing features of healing acute infarction. Rupture of the papillary muscle had not been present. H & E. × 100.

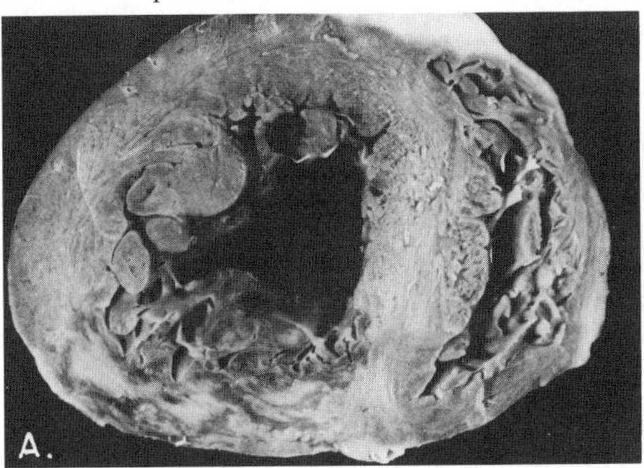

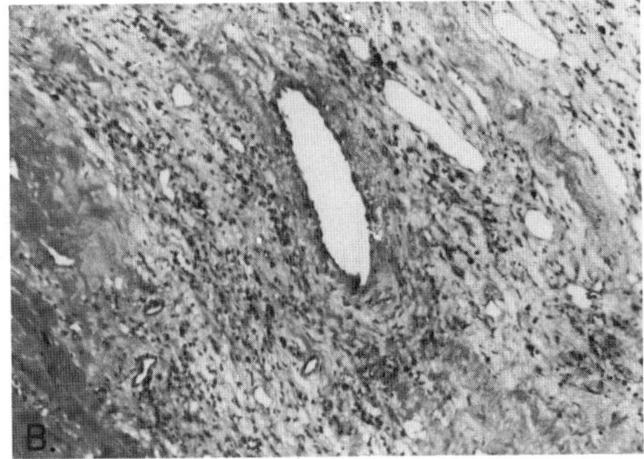

vere mitral regurgitation [14, 15]. Each papillary muscle is composed of a number of heads. Rupture of an individual head may be well tolerated for some time, whereas rupture of an entire papillary muscle complex results in torrential mitral regurgitation and rapid hemodynamic collapse. Rupture of a papillary muscle may occur following a "small," otherwise uncomplicated myocardial infarction. Rupture typically occurs between days 3 and 7 following infarction. Rupture of the posteromedial muscle is four times more common than rupture of the anterolateral muscle (Fig. 4-9).

Hemopericardium

One of the dramatic consequences of AMI is hemopericardium causing acute cardiac tamponade. The most common cause of hemopericardium following AMI is rupture of the free wall of the left ventricle [9]. Less commonly, fatal hemopericardium may result from the late effects of the pericarditis that may accompany transmural AMI [16].

Rupture of the Left Ventricular Free Wall

Rupture of the free wall is usually seen with transmural infarction and usually occurs within the first week after onset of acute infarction (so-called early rupture). The time peak occurs on about the third or fourth day.

Early rupture tends to occur at the periphery of the infarcted site and probably results from a shearing effect between the infarcted and variable myocardium. It is common for ruptured free walls to show histologic evidence of massive leukocytic infiltration. Such a process may cause liquefaction of infarcted myocardium and may represent the primary event leading to gross rupture (Fig. 4-10A,B). The rupture tract extends into and through the epicardium, leading to cardiac tamponade from hemopericardium (Fig. 4-10C). The epicardial lesion is usually a linear break in continuity (Fig. 4-10D). Focal or localized pericarditis may be adjacent to the site of left ventricular rupture. Because a small "sentinel" tear may occur before massive rupture, localized pericarditis may be predictive of impending rupture. A recent clinical study demonstrated unique T wave changes evolving after AMI, indicating localized pericarditis and suggestive of impending cardiac rupture [29].

Among a series of patients with rupture of the free wall, the underlying infarct was equally distributed among anterior, inferior, and lateral locations [9]. Because the lateral wall constitutes the least frequent site of primary infarction, it may be accepted that lateral infarction, once present, is more susceptible to the complication of rupture than are infarcts involving either the anterior or the inferior location. Women are more susceptible to the classic forms of left ventricular rupture than are men.

Uncommonly, rupture of the free wall may occur late, about 2 to 3 weeks after the onset of the underlying infarction. In such patients the rupture is usually a complication of unusually early aneurysm formation (Fig. 4-11). The rupture site shows a "blow-out" type of defect at the center of the developing aneurysm.

Fig. 4-9
Two examples of rupture of a papillary muscle from surgically excised specimens. *A*. The posteromedial papillary muscle (ragged lower edge) has ruptured. *B*. The anterolateral papillary muscle has ruptured.

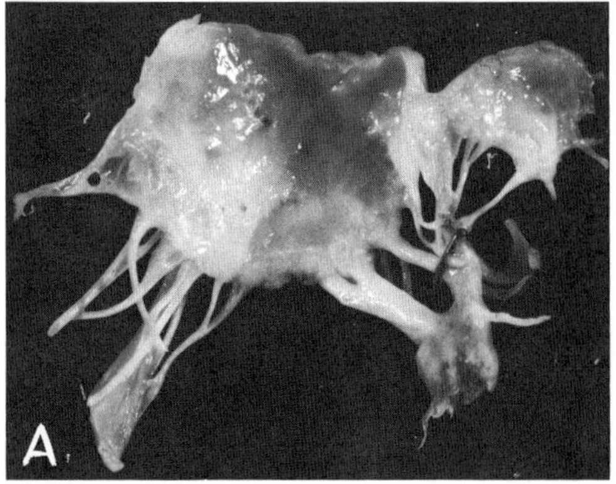

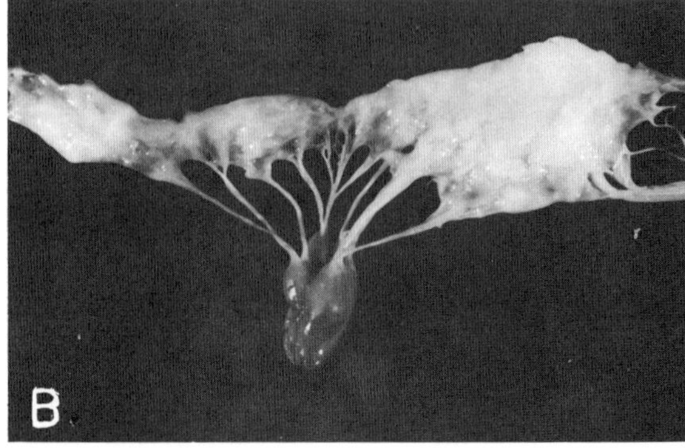

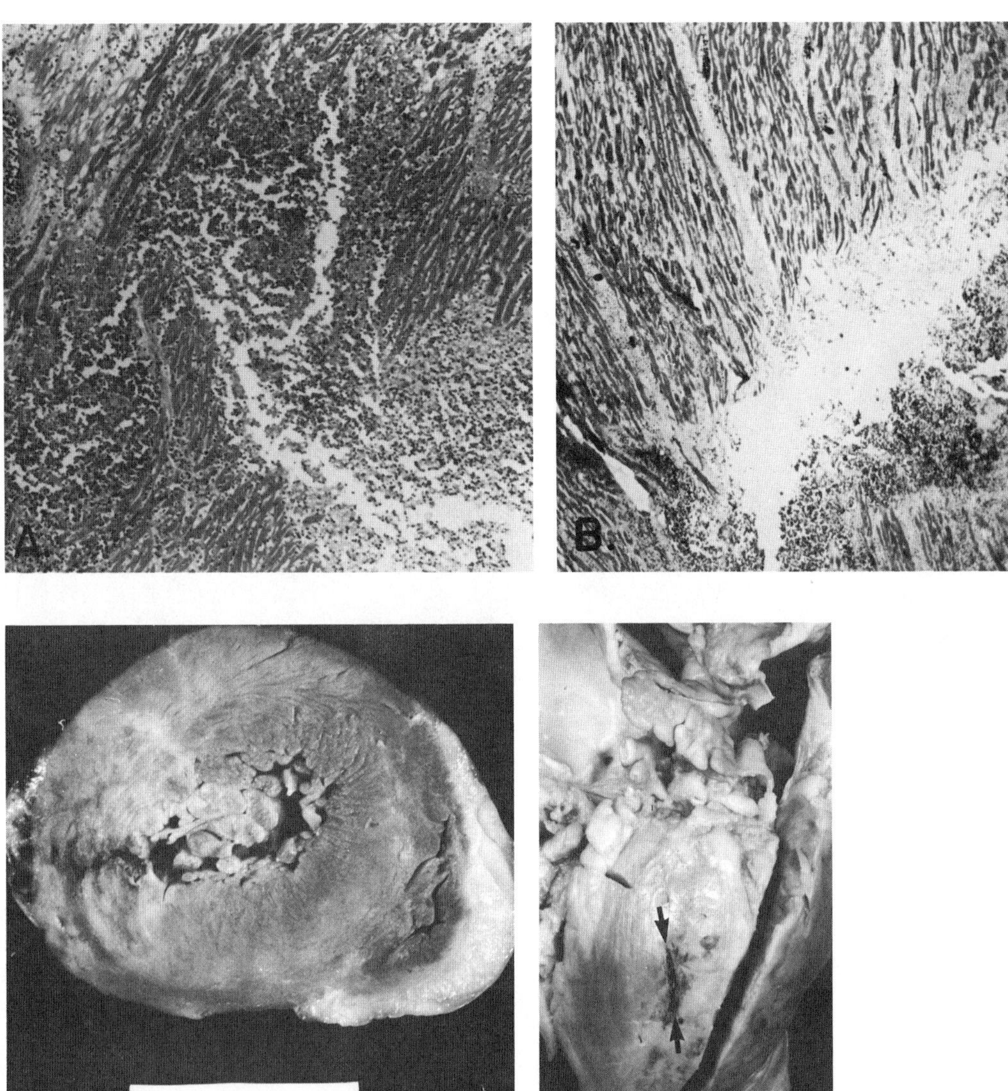

Fig. 4-10
A. Photomicrograph of acute myocardial infarction with unusually heavy leukocytic infiltration. H & E. × 40. *B.* Photomicrograph of acute myocardial infarction with a microlaceration within the left ventricular wall adjacent to a site of heavy leukocytic infiltration. H & E. × 40. *C.* Cross section through the ventricles in an instance of acute lateral infarction with rupture of the free wall. *D.* Acute lateral infarction with rupture of the left ventricular free wall. External view of the heart. The laceration is linear (between *arrows*).

Pericarditis

With AMI, pericarditis is first characterized by fibrinous exudation starting about the second day. The process tends to be localized over the site of infarction and frequently remains in that position. In some patients the fibrinous exudation may be diffuse. In either case, the usual outcome of pericarditis is that it resolves or it becomes organized, the latter process leading to adhesions in the distribution of the fibrinous exudation.

Uncommonly, the process of organization may be a basis for hemopericardium (Fig. 4-12) [16]. The latter is derived from bleeding from capillaries

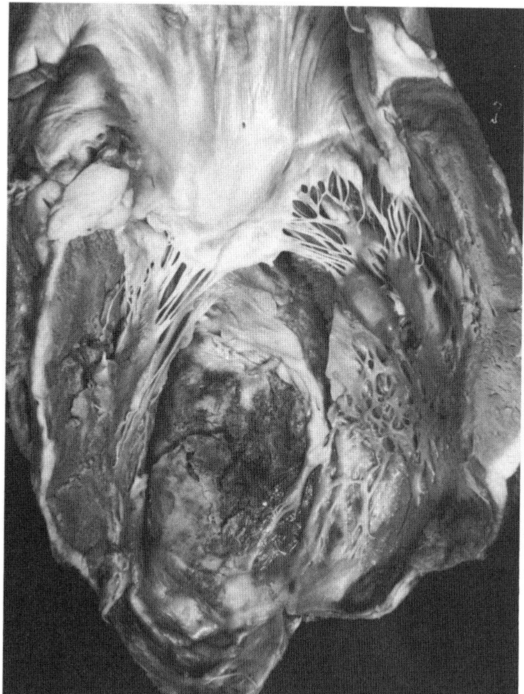

Fig. 4-11
Interior of the left ventricle with a developing aneurysm in early acute myocardial infarction. Rupture of the aneurysm occurred about 3 weeks after the onset of the infarction.

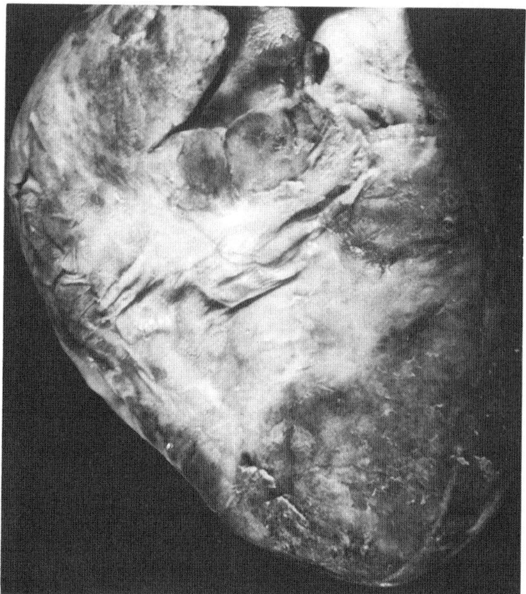

Fig. 4-12
Pericarditis associated with acute anterior myocardial infarction in a patient in whom infarction began 10 days earlier. The discoloration over the apical region may represent early hemorrhage into organizing pericarditis.

of the organizing granulation tissue. The hemorrhagic effusion may be extensive, leading to cardiac tamponade.

This complication, if it appears, tends to occur 2 weeks or more after the onset of the myocardial infarction. It has been suggested that administration of anticoagulant drugs during the period of convalescence for the myocardial infarction makes pericardial hemorrhage more likely than if such drugs were not used.

Thromboembolic Events

The thromboembolic events that complicate AMI are so named because some are truly embolic, whereas others may be either thrombotic or the result of localized arterial disease. In the latter case, ischemic disease of organs supplied by the systemic circulation may result from localized obstructive disease complicated by hypotension related to myocardial infarction.

During the early stage of AMI, ischemic disease of the various organs is likely a result of inadequate perfusion by virtue of hypotension and localized arterial disease. When myocardial infarction has existed for a week or longer, it is likely that ischemic disease results from embolism originating in mural thrombosis of the left ventricle or left atrium [17]. When left ventricular thrombosis complicates myocardial infarction, the thrombosis tends to occur at the apex of the left ventricle regardless of the location of the underlying infarct. Among the exceptions is the occurrence of thrombosis within an aneurysm occupying the inferior aspect of the left ventricle.

Thromboembolic phenomena affecting the lesser circulation are classically those of ileofemoral thrombophlebitis (Fig. 4-13) and pulmonary embolism. With AMI such a phenomenon is now uncommon, probably the consequence of early ambulation of patients with AMI.

In contrast, with healed myocardial infarction the problem of ileofemoral thrombophlebitis and pulmonary embolism persists, particularly in subjects with congestive heart failure. In such patients

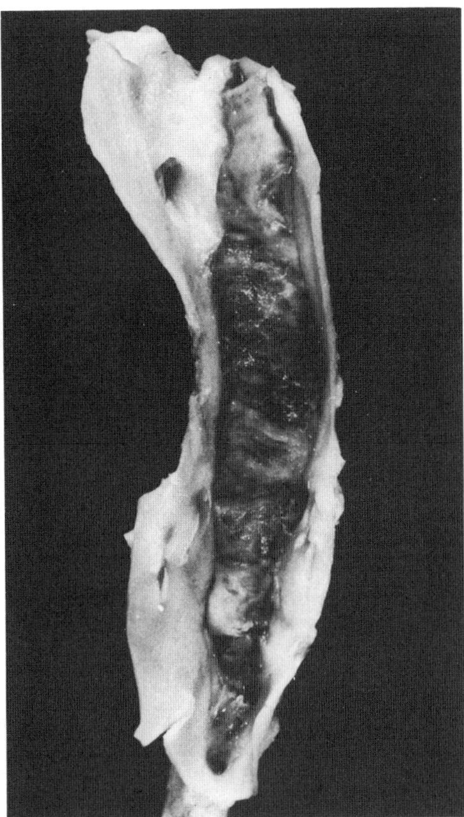

Fig. 4-13
Femoral vein containing thrombus as a complication of congestive heart failure with a potential for pulmonary embolism.

thrombi may also occur in the right ventricle and, particularly, in the right atrial appendage. Even in such instances the principal source of pulmonary embolism is venous thrombosis.

Left Ventricular Aneurysm

Aneurysms complicating myocardial infarction involve the left ventricle, and more commonly anteriorly than inferiorly. Men are more commonly affected than women. Aneurysms are of two types, true and false (pseudoaneurysm) [18].

True aneurysms are derived from extensive myocardial infarcts. As the healing process occurs, the left ventricular wall becomes thin and gradually dilates to become molded into a localized dilatation of the left ventricle (Fig. 4-14). Characteristically, the walls of true aneurysms are mostly fibrotic in nature as scar replaces infarcted wall. The mural endocardium at the aneurysm is thickened with collagen and elastic tissue, a process usually called fibroelastosis (Fig. 4-15). Underneath the thickened endocardium is a layer of preserved, noninfarcted myocardium. It is probable that the ventricular arrhythmias that occur in subjects with left ventricular aneurysm begin in this retained tissue.

False aneurysms, or pseudoaneurysms, of the left ventricle result from contained rupture of the left ventricle complicating infarction without immediate hemopericardium (Fig. 4-16).

Left ventricular aneurysms, whether true or false, frequently harbor mural thrombi. Such thrombi tend to show limited or no organization and are subject to fragmentation and consequent systemic embolism.

Established old true aneurysms do not have a significant tendency to rupture. In contrast, false aneurysms are susceptible to rupture (Fig. 4-16B).

Recurrent Angina or Infarction

Postinfarction angina may result from residual ischemic tissue in the vicinity of the recent myocardial infarction, or it may indicate extensive coronary artery disease with myocardial ischemia remote from the site of recent infarction. An initial non-Q wave infarction may result in a relatively small area of tissue necrosis and typically is associated with a low incidence of occlusive coronary thrombosis [19]. However, this state should be regarded as unstable, possibly characterized by severe coronary artery disease with a large area of viable myocardium in jeopardy. Pathologically, one may observe a large transmural area of AMI with evidence of older subendocardial infarction. Extensive obstructive coronary artery disease is the rule in this situation. The occurrence of dilated vessels in some scars of healed myocardial infarction may represent a low-resistance zone that may function as circulatory steal from intact myocardium. The syndrome of postinfarction angina may be an expression of such a steal.

Postinfarction Arrhythmias and Sudden Death

Following an AMI, arrhythmias of almost all types are known to occur. Some are merely coincidental to the infarct, whereas others are related to it.

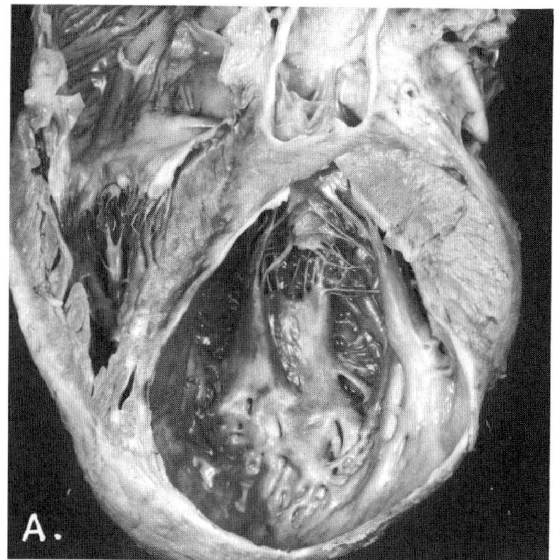

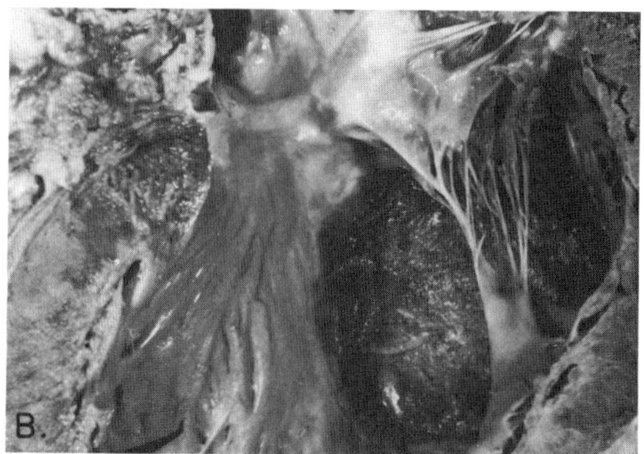

Fig. 4-14
Two examples of true left ventricular aneurysms. *A.* Aneurysm complicating an anterior infarction. The ventricular portion of the heart, cut in frontal section and viewed from in front, shows the left ventricle to the left of the right ventricle. The aneurysm is thin-walled and has a fibroelastic lining. *B.* Interior of the left ventricle with an aneurysm involving the inferior wall of the left ventricle. A large mural thrombus is contained within the aneurysm.

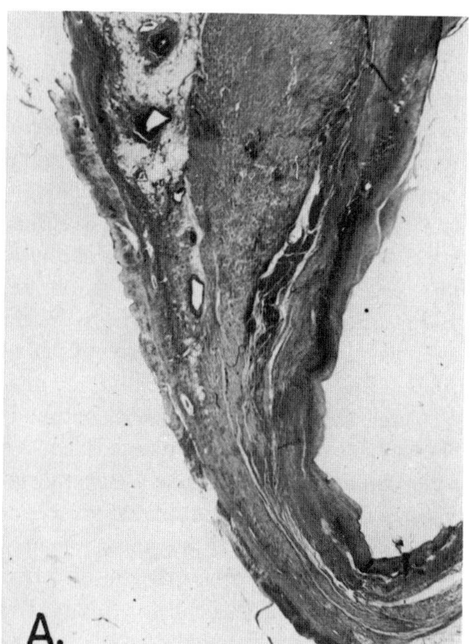

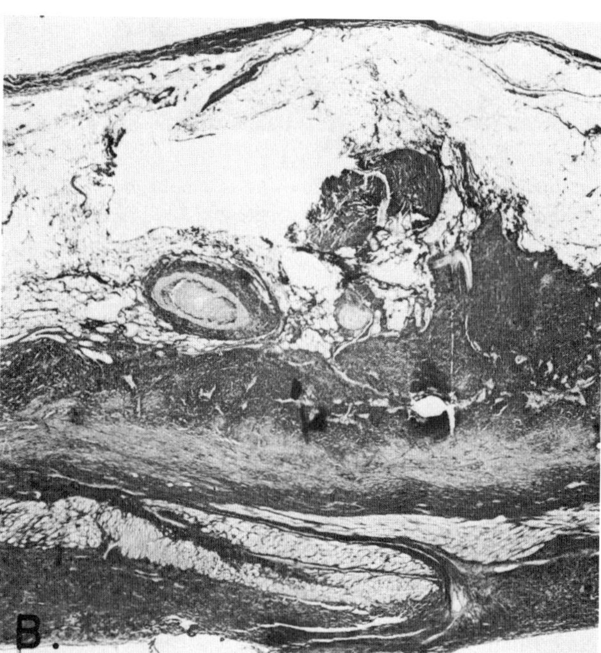

Fig. 4-15
Photomicrographs of true left ventricular aneurysms. *A.* Epicardium is to the left. This low-power view shows virtual molding of the aneurysm at the edge of an infarct. The aneurysm displays endocardial fibroelastosis and some mural thrombosis. Elastic tissue stain. × 5. *B.* Epicardium is above. Low-power view of the wall of the left ventricular aneurysm. Lowermost is a layer of thickened endocardium. Immediately above it, the light area represents a zone of preserved myocardium. More epicardially there is scar, and immediately under the fatty epicardium is a layer of preserved myocardial tissue. Elastic tissue stain. × 5.

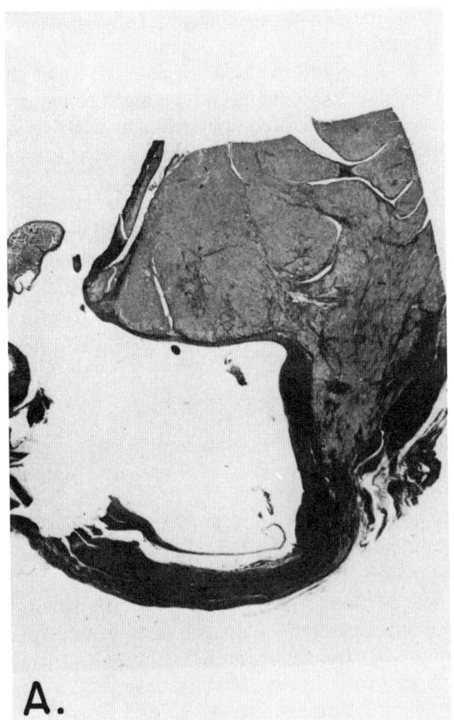

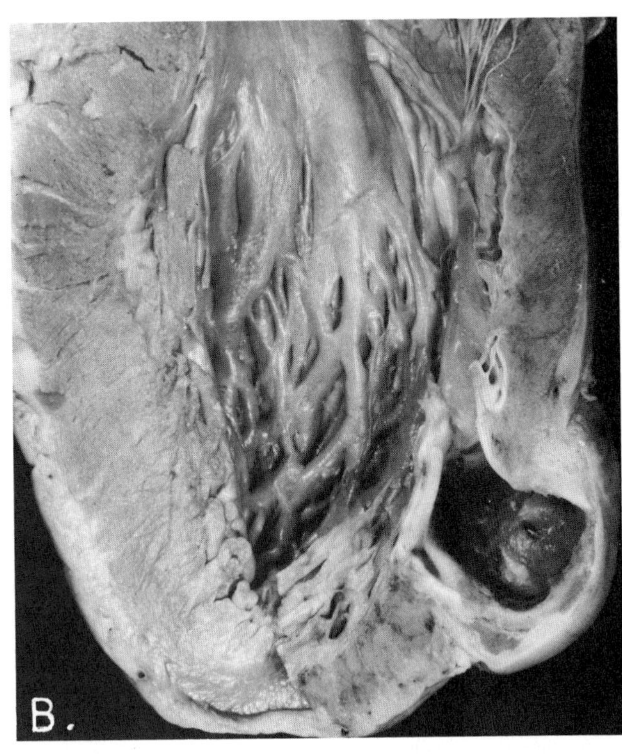

Fig. 4-16
A. Low-power photomicrograph of a false aneurysm of the left ventricle and adjacent tissues. There is an abrupt interruption in the continuity of the ventricular wall representing a site of previous rupture. The dark, thin wall of the false aneurysm represents organized hematoma. Elastic tissue stain. × 5. *B.* Interior of the left venticle with a small false aneurysm at the apical area inferiorly. It had ruptured, leading to a fatal hemopericardium.

Events of atrial fibrillation related to myocardial infarction may reflect left ventricular failure for one of many reasons. Any elevation of ventricular filling pressure with secondary atrial distention may provide the stimulus for atrial fibrillation.

Premature ventricular contractions are common. In instances of large infarcts or left ventricular aneurysm the site of origin of such beats may be the preserved layer of myocardium immediately underneath the endocardium.

Sudden death is the most common type of coronary-related death [20]. In such subjects, the myocardium may be the site of acute ischemic disease with or without acute infarction. In most subjects dying of coronary-related ventricular fibrillation, scarring from a previous infarction is usually present. It should be pointed out that in many cases of sudden coronary death AMI is not present, a concept supported by a follow-up study of survivors of "sudden death," in whom acute infarction does not evolve. Such cases should be considered primary arrhythmogenic deaths and not classified as AMI.

Pathologic Features Following Thrombolytic Therapy

Selected autopsy studies have analyzed the pathologic findings following treatment with thrombolytic therapy [21–23] As one would expect, even in vessels with successful lysis there often remains a significant degree of fixed obstruction. In residual atherosclerotic lesions it is not unusual to observe plaque rupture and hemorrhage; however, these findings may represent the stimulus that initiated thrombosis and not the effect of thrombolytic therapy. Even in the absence of myocardial salvage, there is evidence to suggest that an open artery may provide a beneficial effect limiting infarct expansion [30].

A region of infarcted myocardium is typically present even after successful thrombolysis. The infarcted myocardium may exhibit the classic findings of coagulation necrosis without significant hemorrhage; however, in other spontaneous or drug-induced thrombolysis the infarcted myocardium may be hemorrhagic [21]. The observation of extensive contraction-band necrosis following thrombolytic therapy suggests early reperfusion injury by free radical generation [23]. Caution should be employed when interpreting the presence of contraction bands, as they can be observed in a great variety of situations [24]. Hemorrhagic infarcts typically are observed in situations of delayed reperfusion where small-vessel injury has occurred.

References

1. Freifeld, A. G., Schuster, E. H., and Bulkley, B. H. Nontransmural versus transmural myocardial infarction: A morphologic study. *Am. J. Med.* 75:423, 1983.
2. Phibbs, B. ''Transmural'' versus ''subendocardial'' myocardial infarction: An electrocardiographic myth. *J. Am. Coll. Cardiol.* 1:561, 1983.
3. Mallory, G. K., White, P. D., and Salcedo-Salgar, J. The speed of healing of myocardial infarction: A study of the pathologic anatomy in seventy-two cases. *Am. Heart J.* 18:647, 1939.
4. Fishbein, M. C., Maclean, D., and Maroko, P. R. The histopathologic evolution of myocardial infarction. *Chest* 73:843, 1978.
5. Alonso, D. R., Scheidt, S., Post, M., and Killip, T. Pathophysiology of cardiogenic shock: Quantification of myocardial necrosis, clinical, pathologic and electrocardiographic correlations. *Circulation* 48:588, 1973.
6. Page, D. L., Caulfield, J. B., Kastor, J. A., et al. Myocardial changes associated with cardiogenic shock. *N. Engl. J. Med.* 285:133, 1971.
7. Buckberg, G. D. Studies of controlled reperfusion after ischemia. I. When is cardiac muscle damaged irreversibly? *J. Thorac. Cardiovasc. Surg.* 92:483, 1986.
8. Isner, J. M. Right ventricular myocardial infarction. *J.A.M.A.* 259:712, 1988.
9. Van Tassel, R. A., and Edwards, J. E. Rupture of heart complicating myocardial infarction: Analysis of 40 cases including nine examples of left ventricular false aneurysm. *Chest* 61:104, 1972.
10. Edwards, B. S., Edwards W. D., and Edwards, J. E. Ventricular septal rupture complicating acute myocardial infarction: Identification of simple and complex types in 53 autopsied hearts. *Am J. Cardiol.* 54:1201, 1984.
11. Moore, C. A., Nygaard, T. W., Kaiser, D. L., et al. Postinfarction ventricular septal rupture: The importance of location of infarction and right ventricular function in determining survival. *Circulation* 74:45, 1986.
12. Olson, L. J., Gertz, M. A., Edwards, W. D., et al. Senile cardiac amyloidosis with myocardial dysfunction: Diagnosis by endomyocardial biopsy and immunohistochemistry. *N. Engl. J. Med.* 317:738, 1987.
13. Edwards, J. E., and Burchell, H. B. Pathologic anatomy of mitral insufficiency. *Proc. Mayo Clin.* 33:497, 1958.
14. Nishimura, R. A., Schaff, H. V., Shub, C., et al. Papillary muscle rupture complicating acute myocardial infarction: Analysis of 17 patients. *Am. J. Cardiol.* 51:373, 1983.
15. Vlodaver, Z., and Edwards, J. E. Rupture of ventricular septum or papillary muscle complicating myocardial infarction. *Circulation* 55:815, 1977.
16. Anderson, M. W., Christensen, N. A., and Edwards, J. E. Hemopericardium complicating myocardial infarction in the absence of cardiac rupture: Report of three cases. *Arch. Intern. Med.* 90:634, 1952.
17. Visser, C. A., Kan G., Lie, K. I., and Durrer, D. Incidence and one year follow up of left ventricular thrombus following acute myocardial infarction: An echocardiographic study of 96 patients (Abstract). *J. Am. Coll. Cardiol.* 1:648, 1983.
18. Nakajima, H., and Edwards, J. E. Factors favoring certain complications of acute myocardial infarction: Rupture aneurysm and false aneurysm of left ventricle. *Minn. Med.* 68:291, 1985.
19. DeWood, M. A., Stifter, W. F., Simpson, C. S., et al. Coronary arteriographic findings soon after non-Q-wave myocardial infarction. *N. Engl. J. Med.* 315:417, 1986.
20. Vedin, A., Wilhelmsson, C., Elmfeldt, D., et al. Deaths and non-fatal reinfarctions during two years' follow-up after myocardial infarction: A follow-up study of 440 men and women discharged alive from hospital. *Acta Med. Scand.* 198:353, 1975.
21. Mathey, D. G., Schofer, J., Kuck, K-H., et al. Transmural, haemorrhagic myocardial infarction after intracoronary streptokinase: Clinical, angiographic, and necropsy findings. *Br. Heart J.* 48:546, 1982.
22. Mattfeldt, T., Schwarz, F., Schuler, G., et al. Necropsy evaluation in seven patients with evolving acute myocardial infarction treated with thrombolytic therapy. *Am. J. Cardiol.* 54:530, 1984.
23. Matsuda, M., Fujiwara, H., Onodera, T., et al. Quantitative analysis of infarct size, contraction band necrosis, and coagulation necrosis in human autopsied hearts with acute myocardial infarction after treatment with selective intracoronary thrombolysis. *Circulation* 76:981, 1987.
24. Karch, S. B., and Billingham, M. E. Myocardial

contraction bands revisited. *Hum. Pathol.* 17:9, 1986.

25. Sharpe, N. Ventricular remodeling following myocardial infarction. *Am. J. Cardiol.* 70(10):20C, 1993.
26. McCallister, B. D., Christian, T. F., Gersh, B. J., and Gibbons, R. J. Prognosis of myocardial infarctions involving more than 40% of the left ventricle after acute reperfusion therapy. *Circulation* 88(part 1): 1470, 1993.
27. Hirose, K., Shu, N. H., Reed, J, E., and Rumberger, J. A. Right ventricular dilatation and remodeling the first year after an initial transmural wall left ventricular myocardial infarction. *Am. J. Cardiol.* 72:1126, 1993.
28. Pfeffer, M. A., et al., on behalf of the SAVE Investigators. Effect of captopril on mortality and morbidity in patients with left ventricular dysfunction after myocardial infarction. Results of the Survival and Ventricular Enlargement Trial. *N. Engl. J. Med.* 327:669, 1992.
29. Oliva, P. B., Hammill, S. C., and Edwards, W. D. Cardiac rupture, a clinically predictable complication of acute myocardial infarction: Report of 70 cases with clinicopathologic correlations. *J. Am. Coll. Cardiol.* 22:720, 1993.
30. Lamas, G. A., Pfeffer, M. A., and Braunwald, E. Patency of the infarct-related coronary artery and ventricular geometry. *Am. J. Cardiol.* 68:41D, 1991.
31. Roberts, W. C., Ronan, J. A. Jr., and Harvey, W. P. Rupture of the left ventricular free wall (LVFW) or ventricular septum (VS) secondary to acute myocardial infarction (AMI): An occurrence virtually limited to the first transmural AMI in a hypertensive individual (Abstract). *Am. J. Cardiol.* 35:166, 1975.
32. Radford, M. J., et al. Ventricular septal rupture: A review of clinical and physiologic features and an analyis of survival. *Circulation* 64:545, 1981.

II.
Clinical Diagnosis and Routine Management of Acute Myocardial Infarction

5. History and Physical Examination in Myocardial Ischemia and Acute Myocardial Infarction

David R. Murray, Robert A. O'Rourke, Ann D. Walling, and Richard A. Walsh

History

A thorough, carefully acquired history is an essential component in the evaluation of a patient with suspected myocardial ischemia or infarction. The initial dilemma often faced by the physician is whether or not the presenting complaint is cardiac in origin; if so, the symptoms must be further defined as ischemic or nonischemic in etiology (Fig. 5-1). Economic pressures have intensified the interest in using risk stratification to avoid overuse of expensive coronary care units (CCUs) for patient observation. Prospectively validated algorithms have been proposed to define the cohort of patients with chest pain at low risk for myocardial infarction (MI). These algorithms rely heavily on the character and duration of chest pain as well as prior cardiac events and risk factors [1]. To compound the difficulty of triaging such patients, the history obtained can be misleading because of atypical features, manufactured symptoms, and poorly articulated complaints. However, appropriate decisions concerning patient disposition can be based on sound clinical judgment derived from synthesizing the information gained from the patients' history, physical examination, resting electrocardiogram (ECG), and chest x-ray.

A detailed physical examination is an important adjunct to the history and can aide triage decisions as well as determine therapeutic interventions. Diagnostic clues such as chest wall tenderness, pulmonary lobar consolidation, abdominal tenderness and pleural friction rubs often help sway the physician toward a diagnosis of a noncardiac disorder. Major mechanical complications of MI including left ventricular (LV) decompensation, right ventricular (RV) dysfunction, papillary muscle ischemia/rupture, ventricular septal defect (VSD), and free wall rupture can and should be identified by physical examination to ensure appropriate, aggressive intervention.

Accordingly, the following discussion emphasizes the value and limitations of the history and physical examination in the diagnosis of myocardial ischemia or infarction [2, 3].

Cardiovascular Chest Pain

Cardiac Ischemia

Typical Presentation

The clinical history may be straightforward and diagnostic or atypical and misleading. Symptoms provoked by myocardial ischemia can be perceived, described, and responded to variably by different patients. In a specific patient, however, the pattern is usually fairly predictable and consistent. The typical patient is a middle-aged or elderly man or an older postmenopausal woman. The pain of myocardial ischemia is usually characterized by the abrupt or gradual onset of substernal discomfort, frequently described as deep, dull, and squeezing in nature. It is important to note that many patients deny the presence of chest ''pain'' but readily admit the existence of severe chest ''discomfort'' or ''pressure.'' Other words frequently used by pa-

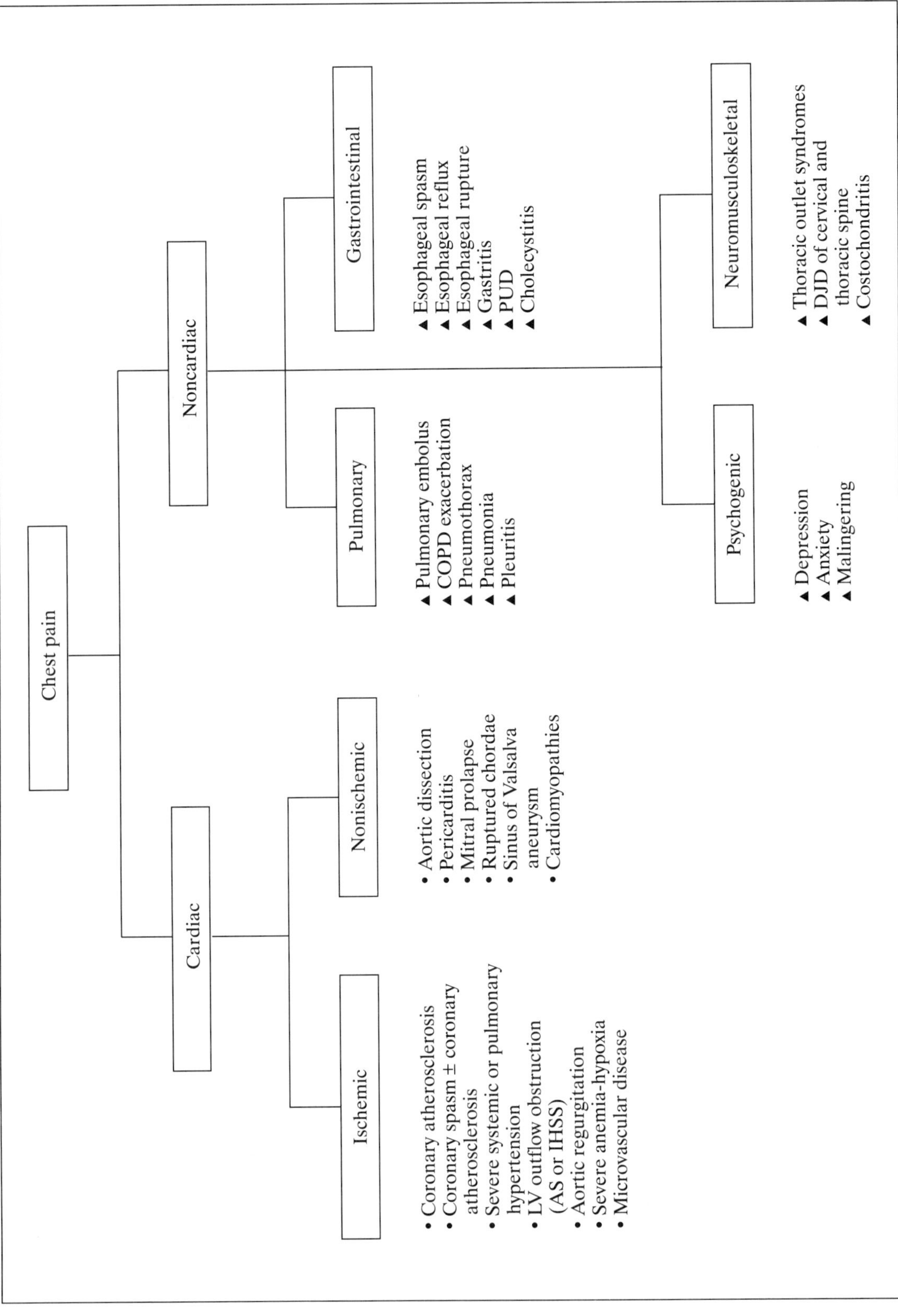

Chest pain
Cardiac
Noncardiac
Ischemic
Nonischemic
Pulmonary
Gastrointestinal
Psychogenic
Neuromusculoskeletal
• Coronary atherosclerosis
• Coronary spasm ± coronary atherosclerosis
• Severe systemic or pulmonary hypertension
• LV outflow obstruction (AS or IHSS)
• Aortic regurgitation
• Severe anemia-hypoxia
• Microvascular disease
• Aortic dissection
• Pericarditis
• Mitral prolapse
• Ruptured chordae
• Sinus of Valsalva aneurysm
• Cardiomyopathies
▲ Pulmonary embolus
▲ COPD exacerbation
▲ Pneumothorax
▲ Pneumonia
▲ Pleuritis
▲ Esophageal spasm
▲ Esophageal reflux
▲ Esophageal rupture
▲ Gastritis
▲ PUD
▲ Cholecystitis
▲ Depression
▲ Anxiety
▲ Malingering
▲ Thoracic outlet syndromes
▲ DJD of cervical and thoracic spine
▲ Costochondritis

tients include "heaviness," "vice-like," "burning," "strangling," "aching," "fullness," or "constricting." Intelligence, education, and sociocultural background may affect the patient's description of precordial discomfort. Facial expressions and gestures [4] should be observed as they may provide additional diagnostic clues. The Levine sign (one or two clenched fists held by the patient over the sternal area) is much more suggestive of ischemic pain than is pointed finger to localized discomfort in the left inframammary region [5]. Brief, sharp, stabbing precordial sensations that are unrelated to exertion are unlikely to be angina. Inspiration and expiration do not influence the quality and intensity of angina.

Typically, the pain of myocardial ischemia is localized to the retrosternal region, at times left-sided, with radiation to one or both inner arms, to the neck and jaw, or to all three areas. Angina also frequently presents as isolated arm, shoulder, neck, or jaw pain. Right-sided chest and arm discomfort are unlikely to be related to angina. Isolated interscapular pain is relatively uncommon; in such cases, aortic dissection must be considered. When jaw pain occurs as a consequence of myocardial ischemia, it is most often mandibular rather than maxillary and can be confused with a "toothache." Angina limited to the epigastrium or subxiphoid region can be confused with gastrointestinal disorders; however, if the discomfort is provoked by exercise and relieved by rest, myocardial ischemia should be suspected. Pain localized to the lower abdomen and periumbilical area is usually not due to myocardial ischemia.

Characteristically, the pain of angina pectoris is of short duration (< 15 minutes), is related to exertion or emotion, and is promptly relieved by rest or nitroglycerin. Both dynamic (isotonic) and static (isometric) exercise can provoke angina. Presumably, as a consequence of excessive sympathoadrenal activation and a more prominent increase in systemic blood pressure and myocardial afterload, the myocardial oxygen demands during static exercise may exceed those during dynamic exercise [6]. A combination of isotonic and isometric exercise, such as walking while carrying out the garbage, may be additive in reaching the anginal threshold. Anger, overt or covert hostility, anxiety, and emotional distress may stimulate coronary vasoconstriction and thus may initiate or aggravate symptoms. Other factors have been implicated in provoking angina and should be elicited in the history. Exposure to the cold may exacerbate angina, especially when associated with exercise (e.g., shoveling snow), presumably because of cold-induced hypertension, tachycardia, and coronary vasoconstriction [7–10]. Exercising in a hot, humid environment can lead to a greater acceleration in heart rate for a given level of exercise [11] and thus increase myocardial oxygen demands. Postprandial angina, especially associated with physical activity, is often misdiagnosed and must be distinguished from a gastrointestinal etiology. Potential mechanisms for this phenomenon include (1) a diversion of blood away from the heart to the gastrointestinal tract, (2) a transient change in viscosity in response to postprandial hyperlipidemia [12, 13], (3) enhanced thromboxane release and subsequent platelet aggregation as a consequence of increased free fatty acid levels [14], and (4) increased heart rate above the usual response with postprandial exercise [15]. Finally, either sexual intercourse, an activity approximately equivalent to 3 to 5 METs on a standard treadmill [16], or cocaine, a drug that causes vasospasm and increased myocardial oxygen demand, can provoke myocardial ischemia and injury.

In some patients, myocardial ischemia occurs predominantly at night. Increased cardiopulmonary blood volume associated with recumbency presumably increases myocardial oxygen demand by enhancing wall tension and reduces subendocardial blood flow by elevating LV end-diastolic pressure. This type of nocturnal angina is often associated with cardiomegaly and LV dysfunction and is re-

Fig. 5-1
Approach to the differential diagnosis of chest pain. LV = left ventricle; AS = aortic stenosis; IHSS = idiopathic hypertrophic subaortic stenosis; COPD = chronic obstructive pulmonary disease; PUD = peptic ulcer disease; DJD = degenerative joint disease. (From R. A. Walsh and R. A. O'Rourke. History and differential diagnosis of acute myocardial infarction. In J. Karliner and G. Gregoratos (eds.), *Coronary Care.* New York: Churchill Livingstone, 1981. P. 170. With permission.)

lieved by vasodilators and diuretics. Another type of nocturnal angina is associated with rapid eye movements and dreaming and is characterized by pronounced fluctuations in heart rate and systemic blood pressure. This form of angina is sporadic, not necessarily accompanied by LV failure, and is often alleviated by treatment with beta-adrenergic blocking agents. Evaluation of LV systolic function is critical for distinguishing between these two types of nocturnal angina [17].

A cardinal feature of myocardial ischemia is prompt improvement, usually within a few minutes, after inciting factors such as activity or stress are eliminated. Nitroglycerin administered sublingually will almost always alleviate angina within 2 to 5 minutes; at times, additional doses may be required. The response to various simple maneuvers, preferably in the presence of a physician, may help discern the difference between ischemic and nonischemic causes of chest discomfort (Fig. 5-2). The Valsalva maneuver may relieve cardiac ischemic rest pain, presumably by reducing LV wall tension via decreased systemic venous return during the strain phase [18]. By inducing vagally mediated bradycardia, carotid massage can decrease myocardial oxygen demand and improve ischemic rest pain. Failure

Fig. 5-2
Summary of baseline data that may be present in the typical patient with acute myocardial infarction. S_4 = fourth heart sound; CHF = congestive heart failure; CO = cardiac output; HR = heart rate; LV = left ventricle; PVC = premature ventricular contraction. (From R. A. Walsh and R. A. O'Rourke. History and differential diagnosis of acute myocardial infarction. In J. Karliner and G. Gregoratos (eds.), *Coronary Care.* New York: Churchill Livingstone, 1981. P. 171. With permission.)

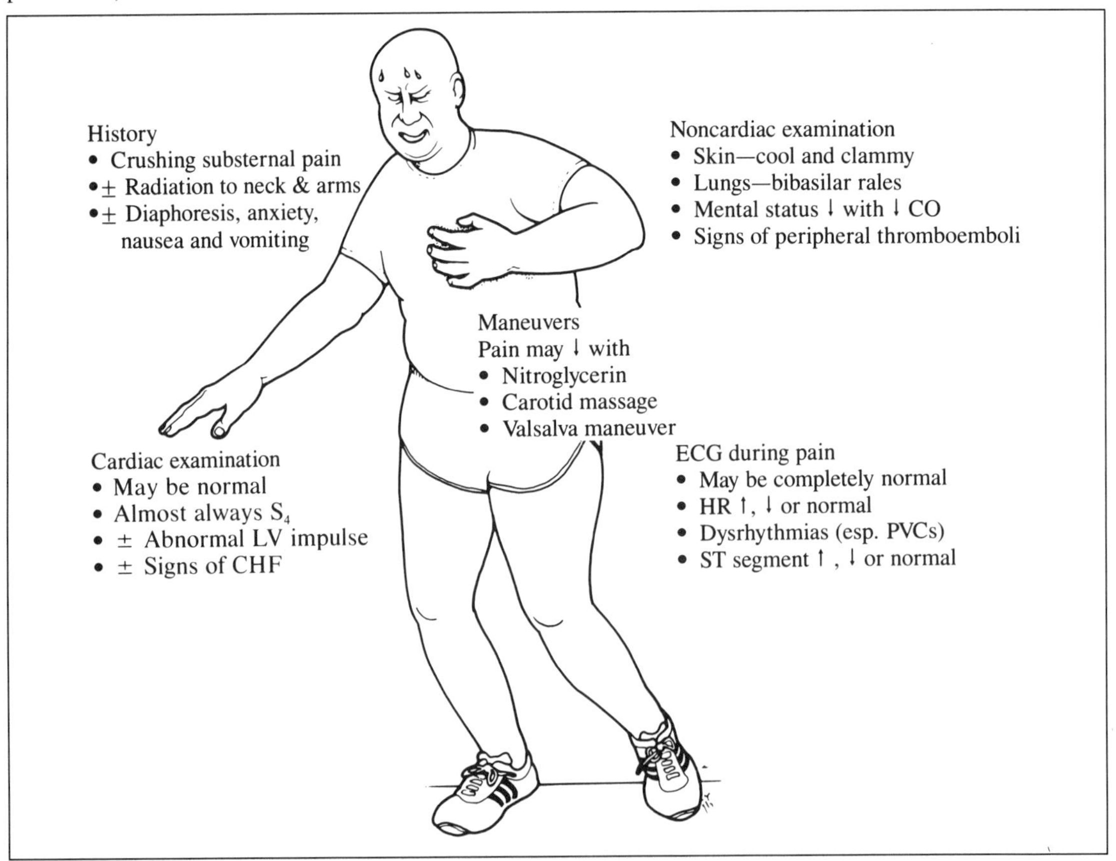

to relieve chest pain by either nitroglycerin or these bedside maneuvers, ideally performed with ECG monitoring, suggests either a noncardiac etiology or pain secondary to acute myocardial infarction (AMI), rather than transient ischemia. These maneuvers should *not* be performed in patients with obvious AMI determined by history or ECG, in those with unstable hemodynamics, or in patients with bradycardia.

In contrast to angina, pain associated with AMI, though of comparable quality and location, is usually more severe, of longer duration (i.e., > 30 minutes), and not relieved by nitroglycerin. Associated symptoms are an integral part of the clinical picture. Nausea and vomiting occur in as many as 40 percent of patients with Q-wave infarction in contrast to less than 5 percent of patients with unstable angina or non-Q-wave infarction [19]. Other common associated symptoms include profuse diaphoresis, a sensation of terror or impending doom, and syncope. The syncopal episodes may be due to tachyarrhythmias (usually ventricular), a vasovagal response to pain, atrioventricular (AV) blockade due to myocardial ischemia affecting the conduction system [20, 21] and nitrate therapy (bradycardic, hypotensive response—especially in volume-depleted patients). Dyspnea often accompanies large infarctions as a consequence of pulmonary venous hypertension resulting from LV dysfunction. Despite these differences, it is often impossible to differentiate the pain of unstable angina from that of AMI.

All interviews of patients with chest pain of possible ischemic etiology should include a careful search for the presence of known risk factors for coronary artery disease. Established independent coronary risk factors include increasing age, male gender, cigarette smoking, diabetes, hypercholesterolemia, hypertension, and family history of premature coronary artery disease. Potential risk factors include obesity, sedentary lifestyle, type A personality, hypertriglyceridemia, and hyperuricemia. The Framingham Study concluded that patients with the combination of increased serum cholesterol, hypertension, and history of cigarette smoking have an incidence of coronary disease eight times that of the general population [22–24]. However, some studies have suggested that up to 40 percent of patients presenting with AMI have no known risk factors. Thus, negative information concerning risk factors may be of little value for an individual patient if the history otherwise suggests myocardial ischemia.

Atypical Presentations

Myocardial ischemia and infarction can present in an atypical manner, mimicking other disorders (Table 5-1) and obscuring the correct diagnosis. AMI must be considered in any patient presenting with pulmonary edema of unknown etiology, especially if the edema is abrupt in onset (''flash'' pulmonary edema). The severe respiratory distress associated with pulmonary congestion may overshadow perception of chest pain. Some patients experience dyspnea as an anginal equivalent, similar to typical angina in terms of provocative and relief factors. In this circumstance, dyspnea may reflect transient ischemic LV dysfunction. Extreme anxiety and nervousness are the predominant symptoms in certain patients. Sometimes these features completely obscure the chest discomfort of AMI. Some patients present with syncope, fatigue, or sudden death resulting from bradycardia, AV block, or ventricular arrhythmias, Nausea, vomiting, and gastric distension with indigestion may occur as a vasovagal response in the setting of acute inferior MI or ischemia. Others present with a stroke due to cerebral embolization from an LV mural thrombus.

Not all episodes of myocardial ischemia and infarction are even symptomatic. ECG evidence of silent ischemia documented on ambulatory ECG recordings in patients with known coronary artery disease and angina is well recognized. Silent in-

Table 5-1
Atypical presentations of myocardial infarction

Nausea and vomiting alone
Atypical location of pain (e.g., arms, back, jaw, occiput only)
Profound fatigue of rapid onset ± syncope
Sudden onset of pulmonary edema
Cerebral or peripheral embolus
Pericarditis
Abnormal ECG in the mentally obtunded patient (e.g., perioperative infarct, diabetic ketoacidosis)
Severe ventricular dysrhythmias

Source: From R. A. Walsh and R. A. O'Rourke. History and differential diagnosis of acute myocardial infarction. In J. Karliner and G. Gregoratos (eds.), *Coronary Care*. New York: Churchill Livingstone, 1981. P. 174. With permission.

farcts occur most often in elderly patients [25], in diabetics [26], and during surgical operations under general anesthesia. The only clue to the diagnosis in the latter setting may be the onset of pulmonary edema, ventricular arrhythmias, or hypotension unexplained by intravascular volume depletion. Data from the Framingham cohort point out that approximately 25 percent of all electrocardiographically documented MIs were found at the time of a routine examination [27, 28]. Of these, almost half were silent and the others were not silent but unrecognized.

In elderly patients, symptoms other than chest pain frequently predominate, including confusion, syncope, stroke, vertigo, weakness, general malaise, abdominal pain, persistent vomiting, and even cough [25]. The sudden onset of dyspnea often dominates the clinical picture. Infarction tends to occur at rest and during sleep more commonly in the elderly [28–30], and a history of prior MI is also more common [25, 28].

Nonischemic Cardiovascular Chest Pain

Nonischemic cardiac causes of chest pain at rest (see Fig. 5-1) are sometimes confused with AMI. The most important consideration in the differential diagnosis is acute aortic dissection. Typically, the pain of aortic dissection occurs suddenly, with the greatest severity at the onset of symptoms—in contrast to pain due to myocardial ischemia, the intensity of which builds gradually with time. The pain is frequently described as "tearing" in quality, interscapular in location, and excruciatingly intense. Depending on the location of the dissection and the degree of luminal compression by the false channel, the pain may radiate to the neck, back, flanks, and legs. Syncope and focal neurologic symptoms may occur when dissection involves the cerebral vessels; mesenteric and limb ischemia may occur when their respective vascular supplies are jeopardized. MI secondary to coronary dissection, cardiac tamponade, and acute aortic regurgitation are recognized complications of type I aortic dissection. Most patients presenting with aortic dissection have a history or clinical evidence of severe, long-standing hypertension. Aortic dissection occurs commonly in Marfan's syndrome and idiopathic cystic medial necrosis, and, although rare, occurs more frequently during pregnancy. The diagnosis can be confirmed by computed automated tomography, magnetic resonance imaging, aortography, or transesophageal echocardiography [31, 32].

Acute pericarditis is another nonischemic cardiac cause of chest pain at rest. The pain is often sharp and cutting in quality but sometimes resembles ischemic pain. The diagnostic hallmark of pain due to pericardial disease is its aggravation by changes in body position (classically alleviated by sitting forward), breathing, and occasionally swallowing. Because of diaphragmatic pleural irritation, pericardial pain can radiate to the shoulders, upper back, and neck, potentially leading to further diagnostic confusion. Given the frequent association of acute pericarditis with MI and aortic dissection, proper diagnosis depends on careful synthesis of the history, physical examination, ECG, and, often, echocardiographic findings.

Chest pain presenting as a feature of the mitral valve prolapse syndrome is usually atypical, occurs at rest—without exacerbation by exercise—and often lasts from several minutes to hours. A careful physical examination may disclose the presence of a midsystolic click, late systolic murmur, or both, to help confirm the diagnosis. The cause-and-effect relationship between mitral valve prolapse and chest pain remains unclear.

Either acute mitral regurgitation (MR) secondary to ruptured chordae tendineae or acute aortic regurgitation secondary to ruptured sinus of Valsalva aneurysm may present with chest pain and acute pulmonary or systemic venous congestion. However, the physical examination coupled with serial ECGs and serum enzyme determinations should readily distinguish these entities from acute MI.

Finally, chest pain can occur in patients with idiopathic dilated cardiomyopathy. Dyspnea associated with pulmonary edema may be misconstrued by such patients as "pain." Patients with focal or generalized myocarditis can present with pain characterized as angina or even MI [33, 34]. Perhaps some patients with idiopathic dilated cardiomyopathy truly have myocardial ischemia. The coronary perfusion pressure may be diminished in the setting of low systemic arterial and elevated LV end-diastolic pressures, leading to a reduction in subendocardial blood flow. Increased wall tension secondary to LV dilatation and increased end-diastolic pressure requires enhanced oxygen delivery.

Thus, subendocardial ischemia might occur despite "normal" epicardial coronary vessels. The presence of significant obstructive coronary disease in this clinical setting would be expected to exacerbate the myocardial supply/demand imbalance.

Noncardiac Chest Pain

Chest Pain of Pulmonary Origin

In most cases, chest pain secondary to pulmonary embolism is readily distinguishable from cardiac ischemia. A history of recent surgery, childbirth, long trips, congestive heart failure, hypercoagulability, unilateral peripheral edema, or deep vein thrombophlebitis helps direct the physician toward the correct diagnosis. The pain is classically acute, sharp, and pleuritic and is associated with dyspnea, tachypnea, diaphoresis, anxiety, and agitation. However, massive pulmonary embolism leading to pulmonary hypertension and low cardiac output can cause pain similar to AMI, probably because of RV ischemia resulting from an increased afterload.

Exacerbations of chronic obstructive pulmonary disease, characterized by dyspnea and wheezing, can be misconstrued for primary cardiac disease. Air hunger, increased work of breathing, and diffuse chest tightness may be interpreted as angina. Parenchymal scarring often causes rales on pulmonary examination and mimics interstitial edema radiographically. To complicate matters, pulmonary venous congestion and subsequent peribronchial edema can induce bronchospasm in patients with reactive airways disease. Right-sided congestive heart failure secondary to pulmonary hypertension may be misinterpreted as biventricular heart failure. Despite these difficulties, the clinical, ECG, and chest x-ray findings usually suggest the correct diagnosis. Other primary pulmonary disorders such as pneumothorax, pneumonia, pleuritis, and malignant lesions present with symptoms quite different from those of cardiac ischemia and are readily diagnosed by chest x-ray and physical examination.

Chest Pain of Gastrointestinal Origin

Diffuse esophageal spasm is the noncardiac condition most frequently confused with ischemic chest pain. The peak incidence, like active coronary disease, is between the ages of 50 and 60 years. Almost always substernal, the pain may be squeezing or aching in quality, and frequently radiates to one or both arms. As with angina, the pain may be precipitated by exercise and relieved by nitroglycerin or calcium channel blockers. A useful differential feature is the frequent association of DES with odynophagia, dysphagia, and regurgitation of gastric contents. The episodes of pain are frequently precipitated by hot or cold drinks or by an emotional upset. The definitive diagnosis of esophageal spasm depends on a demonstration of abnormal esophageal motility on esophagogram or by esophageal manometry.

Esophageal reflux, with or without concomitant spasm, can also mimic angina pectoris. The pain can be localized to the chest or epigastric region and extend to the face, neck, or arms. Symptoms due to esophageal reflux are more likely to occur after heavy meals or soon after the patient assumes a recumbent position, whereas nocturnal angina usually presents 1 to 2 hours after the patient falls asleep. Nocturnal or postprandial eructation and regurgitation of gastric juices are often noted by the patient. Stooping or bending may provoke the symptoms of esophageal reflux; physical exertion in an upright posture induces symptoms less commonly. Many patients are obese and report relief of discomfort by food, antacids, or elevation of the head of the bed. An esophageal acid perfusion test or a barium swallow may be helpful in solidifying the diagnosis. Acute esophageal perforation may produce severe retrosternal pain secondary to chemical mediastinitis caused by leakage of gastric contents. Esophageal rupture usually occurs in the setting of a prolonged bout of wretching or emesis and is a recognized complication of esophageal instrumentation.

Other common gastrointestinal maladies can be mistaken for cardiac ischemia but are usually readily identified on the basis of a thorough history and physical examination. Patients with peptic ulcer disease and gastritis generally present with mid-epigastric, continuous pain at rest, which is not exacerbated by physical activity or relieved by food and antacids. Heavy consumption of alcohol can lead to gastric irritation that can be confused with a cardiac etiology. Finally, chronic cholecystitis can be difficult to distinguish from myocardial ischemia. Recurrent episodes of severe epigastric pain after particularly fatty meals should arouse suspicion of gallbladder disease, especially if the patient feels a need to "walk it off"; patients with angina typically prefer to avoid any activity.

Chest Pain of Emotional Origin

Anxiety is by far the most common cause of chest discomfort. Although anxiety can coexist with, and aggravate, discomfort due to myocardial ischemia, two features help to distinguish the two conditions. First, the chest pain of emotional nature is frequently sharp, left inframammary in location, and well circumscribed. Patients often use the following descriptive words: "needle-like," "knife-like," or "lightning-like." The duration of pain is diagnostically useful, since anxiety related discomfort is frequently either evanescent (seconds to 1 minute) or protracted (sometimes lasting for days). Second, the pain is often noted after, rather than during, activity, or it is experienced during the evening after work. The physician should actively search for indicators of underlying depression, such as a flat or saddened facial expression, retarded motor activity, and hand-wringing coupled with a history of insomnia, loss of appetite, and frequent crying spells. Associated symptoms such as air hunger, circumoral paresthesias, globus hystericus, and multiple somatic complaints suggest a psychogenic basis.

Chest Pain of Neuromuscular Origin

Certain thoracic outlet syndromes may produce symptoms that are confused with cardiac chest pain. Compression of the neurovascular bundle by a cervical rib or the scalenus anterior muscle may cause discomfort radiating to the chest, neck, and ulnar surface of either arm. Helpful differential features from ischemic chest pain include the prominence of associated paresthesias, the lack of a clear association with exercise, and aggravation with certain arm and neck movements.

Degenerative arthritis of the cervical and thoracic vertebrae may cause band-like pain confined to the chest, neck, or back that often radiates to the arms. Radiologic evidence of degenerative disease of the cervical and thoracic vertebrae does not necessarily confirm the diagnostic impression as such findings are often present in asymptomatic elderly adults. Persistence of radicular pain at rest, lack of provocation with exercise, and intensification or production of the pain by movement, sneezing, coughing and positional changes are vital pieces of information to help support the diagnosis of vertebral disease. A careful neuromusculoskeletal examination, perhaps supplemented with nerve conduction studies, is essential.

Shoulder arthropathies such as bursitis, tendonitis, and arthritis are usually distinguished by aggravation with movement of the joint. In certain conditions, such as biceps tendonitis, a localized zone of tenderness may be found. Local injection of an anesthetic agent or corticosteroid may provide relief of symptoms and thus confirm the diagnosis. Tietze's syndrome, or idiopathic costochondritis, causes painful swelling of one or more left costochondral junctions and is relieved by local injection of lidocaine and nonsteroidal anti-inflammatory agents. More commonly, a patient may experience chest wall pain secondary to myofascitis, which often lasts for hours or days and is not consistently exertion-related or relieved by nitroglycerin. Again, certain movements such as twisting, deep breathing, and arm extension/abduction can provoke or exacerbate such pain. However, the demonstration of chest wall tenderness does not rule out the presence of coincident chest discomfort resulting from myocardial ischemia or infarction. Finally, the prevesicular phase of herpes zoster may be characterized by band-like chest pain in a dermatomal distribution. The advanced age of the patient, the presence of hyperesthesia on physical examination, and eventual eruption of typical lesions 3 to 4 days after the onset of symptoms resolve any lingering diagnostic dilemma.

Physical Examination

The physical signs observed in patients during AMI are determined by the temporal relation of the examination to the acute ischemic event and the presence or absence of electrical or mechanical complications. Therefore, the physical findings associated with AMI will be discussed in the following sequence: (1) early uncomplicated MI or myocardial ischemia, (2) early (<48 hours) complicated MI, (3) late (>48 hours) complicated MI, and (4) noncardiac complications associated with AMI [35].

Early Uncomplicated Myocardial Infarction

The overall appearance of the patient presenting with ischemia and possible infarction depends on whether the pain persists and how the patient reacts to the pain when it is present. Most patients do not appear markedly ill, although on close inspection they are usually quiet, fearful, and motionless. The clinical description of the pain is usually brief and is often associated with gestures toward the precordium with the hand or clenched fist. Occasionally, because of the intensity of the pain or the reaction to it, the patient may appear restless and insist on walking. Some patients appear to have acute indigestion and seek relief by belching or vomiting. A few use the bedpan in an attempt to relieve the pain. Fowler [36] postulated that "bedpan deaths" in patients with AMI are coincidental rather than caused by reflex vagal activity while straining. Autonomic dysfunction or transiently reduced LV performance may result in diaphoresis, nausea, vomiting, peripheral cyanosis, and dyspnea [36].

Vital Signs

The heart rate and blood pressure response during AMI depends on when the patient is observed after the onset of symptoms as well as the location and extent of myocardial injury. Autonomic nervous system fluctuations are reported to be more prominent in the first few hours following MI. In a study conducted by Webb et al., only 8 percent of 74 patients evaluated within 30 minutes of the onset of AMI presented with a normal heart rate and blood pressure [37]. The pattern of autonomic response varied, depending on the site of MI. Patients with anterior MIs were more likely to have evidence of sympathetic overactivity than an excessive parasympathetic response, as defined by the finding of tachycardia, hypertension, or both. When extensive, anterior MIs often result in profound hypotension with compensatory tachycardia related to diminished stroke volume in the setting of LV decompensation. Bradycardia secondary to AV blockade can also occur; however, the mechanism has been ascribed to massive anteroseptal injury rather than increased vagal tone. In contrast, most patients (77 percent) with inferior or true posterior MIs demonstrated enhanced parasympathetic tone (heart rate <60 bpm, systolic blood pressure <100 mm Hg, or AV block) [37] attributable to a vasovagal response known as the Bezold-Jarish reflex [38, 39]. The physiology of this reflex has yet to be precisely defined; it is unclear whether the reflex is initiated by stimulation of mechanoreceptors or chemoreceptors in the myocardium, by reperfusion of the occluded vessel, or by all three factors [40–42]. Vagal afferents and efferents are located predominantly in the inferoposterior wall of the left ventricle, accounting for the regional predilection of this reflex. Interestingly, by reducing heart rate and afterload, the Bezold-Jarish reflex can decrease myocardial oxygen demand and, therefore, limit infarct size [43]. Excessive stimulation of this vagal reflex arc, however, can lead to temporary complete AV block and hemodynamic collapse. Finally, the Bezold-Jarish reflex is also likely responsible for the nausea, vomiting, and gastric distention associated with inferior infarctions [44].

The patient is usually afebrile during the first 24 hours of acute infarction. Slight temperature elevation, rarely above 101°F, is common during the first week. With large infarctions, the temperature may reach 103°F. The fever due to myocardial necrosis must be differentiated from that due to other common causes of hyperthermia noted in the CCU, such as aspiration pneumonia following cardiopulmonary arrest, pyelonephritis from indwelling Foley catheters, thrombophlebitis, bacteremia (or both), from indwelling arterial or venous lines, pulmonary emboli, or pericarditis. By producing increased heart rate, metabolic rate and overall oxygen consumption, an elevated body temperature can increase myocardial workload and, thus, can be detrimental to the patient in the midst of an AMI.

Precordial Palpation

In certain patients with AMI, the systolic apical impulse may be diffuse, sustained, or frankly dyskinetic (Fig. 5-3). However, a prominent apical impulse due to abnormal wall motion in AMI may be difficult to distinguish from the sustained systolic impulse of LV pressure overload when coincident hypertension is present. In addition, a palpable LV presystolic filling wave (A wave) that corresponds in timing to an audible fourth heart sound is often

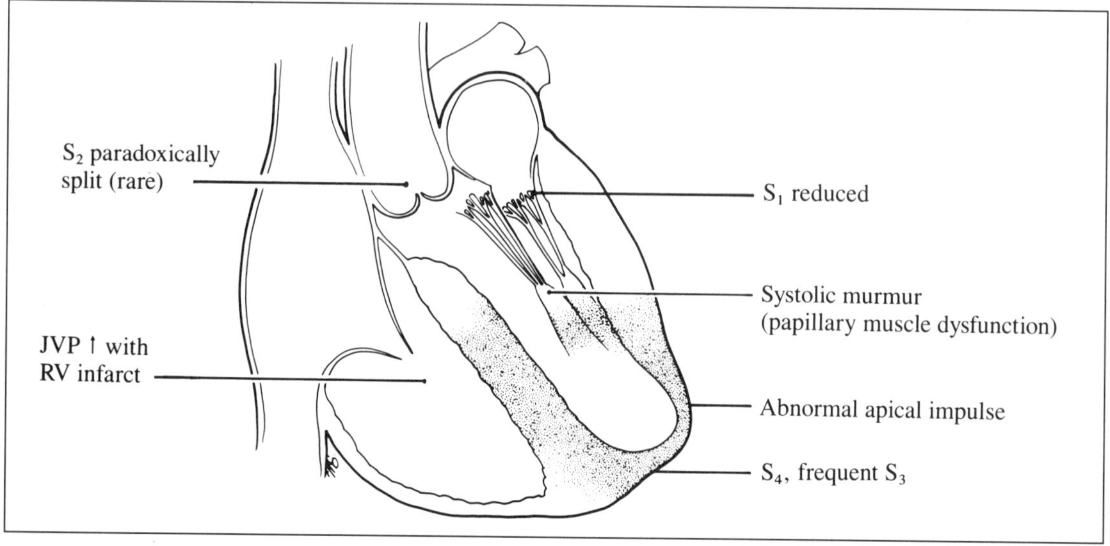

Fig. 5-3
Cardiac physical findings that may be present in uncomplicated acute myocardial infarction. S_1, S_2, S_3, S_4 = first through fourth heart sounds, respectively; JVP = jugular venous pressure; RV = right ventricle. Right ventricular infarction is included to indicate that it is a specific entity, even though it more commonly occurs in patients with a complicated left ventricular infarction. (From R. A. Walsh and R. A. O'Rourke. History and differential diagnosis of acute myocardial infarction. In J. Karliner and G. Gregoratos (eds.), *Coronary Care*. New York: Churchill Livingstone, 1981. P. 179. With permission.)

present. Less frequently, an early LV diastolic rapid filling wave that is associated with an audible third heart sound is palpated. Last, patients with large transmural anterior infarcts often have transient early, mid, or late systolic impulses that are palpable medial and superior to the maximal impulse. Persistence of such dyskinetic areas for more than 8 weeks after MI may indicate the presence of an anteroapical aneurysm.

Jugular Venous Pulse

The jugular venous pulse (JVP) contour and pressure are usually normal in patients with an early uncomplicated infarct (see Fig. 5-3), except in the presence of pulmonary hypertension or associated RV infarction (discussed later). Inspection of the contour of the JVP may reveal the presence and nature of atrial or ventricular arrhythmias. Cannon A waves, reflective of accentuated right atrial pressure as a consequence of right atrial contraction against a closed tricuspid valve, may be observed during rhythm disorders characterized by AV dissociation, AV block, and retrograde atrial activation following ventricular depolarization [45]. For example, rapid regular or regularly irregular cannon A waves would be expected in patients with paroxysmal atrial tachycardia or atrial flutter with variable AV nodal conduction; conversely, intermittent cannon A waves would be seen when AV dissociation accompanies ventricular tachycardia, contingent upon coupling intervals between atrial and ventricular depolarization.

Heart Sounds

The intensity of the first heart sound is diminished in approximately one-fourth of patients with AMI [36] (see Fig. 5-3) and may be caused by the presence of first-degree AV block or decreased LV dP/dt in patients with large infarcts. Paradoxical or reversed splitting of the second heart sound can occur during AMI or reversible ischemia [46]. Two mechanisms are possible for this finding: (1) transient LV conduction delays, and (2) prolongation of electromechanical systole by ischemia or infarction. In our experience, reversed splitting of the second heart sound is rarely observed in ischemic heart disease in the absence of left bundle branch block. The true incidence of this auscultatory finding is unknown. A frequent reason for misdiagnosis of reversed splitting is the disappearance of the pulmonic component of the second heart sound during inspiration in patients with chronic pulmonary disease and increased anteroposterior chest diameters.

Left Ventricular Diastolic Gallop Sounds

LV diastolic gallop sounds are frequently present during transient ischemia or AMI (see Fig. 5-3). These low-pitched sounds are best heard with the bell of the stethoscope lightly applied to the LV apex with the patient turned to the left lateral decubitus position. RV diastolic gallops may be auscultated in the same manner; they are loudest at the left sternal border or subxiphoid area and frequently increase in intensity with inspiration. In one study [47], the fourth heart sound (S_4) was documented in 98 percent of 107 patients evaluated during the first 24 hours after AMI by serial auscultation, phonocardiograms, and simultaneous apexcardiograms. The S_4 is most likely due to reduced ventricular compliance resulting from ischemia or infarction. Thus, the absence of the S_4 on careful auscultation in a patient in sinus rhythm makes the diagnosis of AMI less likely; however, auscultation of the S_4 may be difficult in obese patients and in those with chronic obstructive lung disease.

The third heart sound (S_3) frequently indicates heart failure and likely results from an imbalance between the volume of LV inflow during the rapid filling phase of diastole and the ability of the ventricle to accommodate this increment in volume flow. The S_3 is less common than the S_4 in AMI, occurring in 40 to 65 percent of patients with AMI [47, 48]. Most (60 percent) of the S_3 sounds disappear during the initial 3 days of hospitalization. Presence of an S_3 in the setting of an anterior MI has been associated with twice the mortality of patients presenting with anterior infarctions without an S_3.

At times, the S_3 and S_4 can be difficult to auscultate. Having the patient cough several times can increase pulmonary venous pressure and thereby accentuate LV diastolic gallops. In certain patients in whom precordial auscultation is limited by obesity, increased anteroposterior chest diameter, rhonchi, or wheezing, transmitted diastolic filling sounds can be auscultated over the subclavian and carotid arteries [49]. Up to 50 percent of left-sided fourth heart sounds (S_4) and 25 percent of third heart sounds (S_3) can be detected over the systemic arteries.

Early Complicated Myocardial Infarction

The goals of CCU management during AMI include prevention of recurrent myocardial ischemia and injury, prompt and effective treatment of cardiac arrhythmias, and the early detection of surgically correctable mechanical complications (Fig. 5-4). CCUs and continuous ECG monitoring have considerably reduced the mortality due to arrhythmic consequences of myocardial ischemia and infarction. Mechanical complications are now the most common cause of death in hospitalized patients with AMI or recent MI. The availability of new inotropic agents, external and internal circulatory assist devices, and improved surgical techniques necessitate the early identification of these complications. Careful attention to the physical findings may provide the first clue to their presence.

Right and Left Ventricular Infarction

RV infarction associated with LV infarction has emerged as a distinct clinical entity [50] (see Chapters 13, 16). Studies using ECG, hemodynamic measurements and cardiac radionuclide imaging techniques suggest that significant RV involvement may be present in as many as one-third to one-half of the patients presenting with inferior Q-wave AMI [51–55]. The clinical hallmarks of predominant RV infarction must be promptly recognized in order to rapidly institute appropriate therapy and to judiciously avoid potentially detrimental treatment with diuretics and nitrates. Physical findings associated with RV infarction are listed in Table 5-2. Dell'Italia and colleagues [56] prospectively studied 53 consecutive patients with inferior Q-wave MI to determine whether physical findings could identify patients with and without RV infarction (Table 5-3). Interestingly, many of the patients with hemodynamic evidence of RV infarction (right atrial to pulmonary artery wedge pressure (PCW) ratio of 0.80 or greater) had neither hypotension nor clear lungs as had been previously described [57–60].

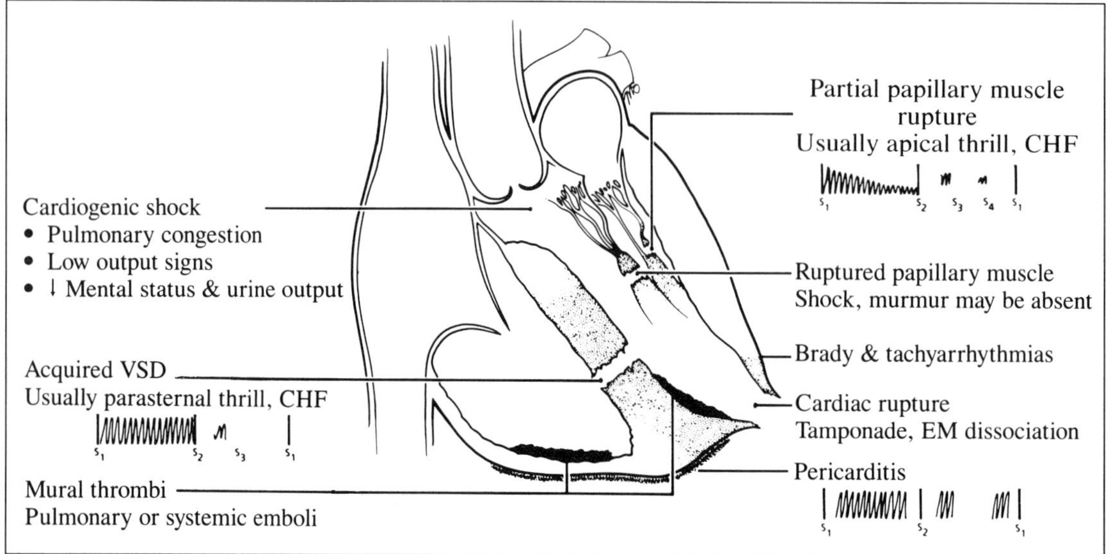

Fig. 5-4
Summary of potential findings in patients with complicated myocardial infarction. CHF = congestive heart failure; EM = electromechanical; VSD = ventriculoseptal defect. (From R. A. Walsh and R. A. O'Rourke. History and differential diagnosis of acute myocardial infarction. In J. Karliner and G. Gregoratos (eds.), *Coronary Care.* New York: Churchill Livingstone, 1981. P. 182. With permission.)

The presence of an elevated JVP (≥8 cm H_2O) and Kussmaul's sign (an increase in JVP during quiet inspiration), either together or in isolation, was found to be highly sensitive and specific for RV injury [56]. However, these physical findings often occur in patients with constrictive pericarditis, advanced cardiac tamponade, severe chronic biventricular failure, pulmonary embolus, and chronic obstructive lung disease with cor pulmonale—diseases that were excluded in the study of Dell'Italia [56]. In order to confirm the diagnosis of predominant RV infarction, the clinical and hemodynamic manifestations should be considered in conjunction with electrocardiography, echocardiography, and cardiac enzyme determination.

Table 5-2
Clinical findings associated with RV infarction

Hypotension
Elevated jugular venous pressure
Kussmaul's sign
Abnormal jugular venous pressure pattern (y ≥ x descent)
Tricuspid regurgitation
Right-sided S_3 and S_4
Pulsus paradoxus
High-grade AV block

Source: From L. J. Dell'Italia and M. R. Starling. Right ventricular infarction: An important clinical entity. *Curr. Probl. Cardiol.* 9(9):16, 1984. With permission.

Left Ventricular Decompensation

The development of CCUs has resulted in a marked decline of deaths primarily attributable to cardiac arrhythmias; LV failure has now emerged as the prime factor responsible for in-hospital death following AMI (see Chapter 16). Cardiogenic shock secondary to marked LV decompensation occurs in 10 to 20 percent of patients with AMI. By definition, patients in cardiogenic shock exhibit evidence of inadequate tissue perfusion as manifested by cool, clammy skin, cyanosis, mental impairment, oliguria, and diminished peripheral pulses (see Fig. 5-4). The physical findings are usually consistent with severe LV dysfunction, for example, hypotension, diastolic gallops (S_3 and S_4), a laterally displaced and frequently dyskinetic apical impulse, and signs of pulmonary congestion. Patients with hypertensive disease may not necessarily present with hypotension but will have at

Table 5-3
Sensitivity and specificity of physical findings for hemodynamically important RV infarction in 53 patients

			Elevated JVP and systemic blood pressure		
Parameter	Elevated JVP*	Kussmaul's sign	Clear lungs	<100 mm Hg and clear lungs	Kussmaul's sign
Sensitivity (%)	88	100	50	25	88
Specificity (%)	69	100	82	96	100

*Jugular venous pressure: ≥8 cm H_2O.
Source: From L. J. Dell'Italia et al. Physical examination of hemodynamically important right ventricular infarction. *Ann. Intern. Med.* 99:608, 1983. With permission.

least a 25 percent decrease in systolic blood pressure accompanied by reflex-mediated signs of systemic arterial hypoperfusion.

Killip and Kimball created a classification scheme to describe the degree of LV failure in patients during AMI [61]. The initial clinical presentation was used to categorize MI patients into four subgroups: class I, no pulmonary rales or S3; class II, bibasilar rales that persist after coughing or S_3; class III, rales over one-half of the lung fields bilaterally with radiographic evidence for pulmonary edema; and class VI, cardiogenic shock. The 2-year mortality rates associated with this classification are 8 percent, 30 percent, 44 percent and 80 to 100 percent for classes I to IV, respectively [61], although emergent coronary angioplasty appears to have made a significant impact in improving the prognosis of the latter group.

Unfortunately, the physical examination can be misleading in an attempt to define the severity of LV dysfunction during AMI [62]. In a study by Forrester et al. [63], patients with AMI were categorized clinically on the basis of the presence or absence of pulmonary congestion, peripheral hypoperfusion, or both. Following right heart catheterization, comparable hemodynamic subsets were established using a PCW of more than 18 mm Hg as an index of increased pulmonary congestion and a cardiac index of less than 2.2 L/min/m^2 as an index of peripheral hypoperfusion. In this study, one-fourth of the patients designated clinically as not having hypoperfusion had a cardiac index of less than 2.2 L/min/m^2. Similarly, pulmonary congestion was not perceived on physical examination in 15 percent of those patients with an elevated pulmonary-capillary pressure [63]. Conversely, rales heard on examination may be secondary to pulmonary parenchymal disease or atelectasis rather than LV dysfunction. Certain clinical maneuvers may help differentiate cardiac from pulmonary rales. Cardiac rales are postural and can be confirmed by placing the patient on one side for 30 minutes resulting in an increase in rales in the dependent lung fields. In contrast, rales of purely pulmonary origin frequently clear during coughing and are independent of posture. Despite the limitations of the physical examination, the degree of pulmonary congestion and peripheral tissue perfusion can often be diagnosed quite accurately without the need for right heart catheterization.

Another bedside clue to the presence of LV dysfunction, commonly severe, is the presence of *pulsus alternans,* a condition in which the amplitude of the arterial pulse oscillates between two levels on a beat-to-beat basis. In patients with LV failure, pulsus alternans is often present transiently after premature beats, although it may be sustained. This finding is best appreciated in the peripheral arterial pulses (e.g., radial or femoral) where the pulse pressure is usually greater than central pulses (e.g., carotids). The mechanism of pulsus alternans remains controversial. A Frank-Starling effect (i.e., volume-dependent LV pressure generation) may be partially responsible: end-diastolic volume alternates between a low and high value leading to smaller and greater LV pressure, respectively. However, load-independent measures of contractility have revealed differences in end-systolic inotropic states between strong and weak beats; thus, changes in end-diastolic volume cannot fully explain the phenomenon of pulsus alternans. Most evidence indicates an alternating failure or attenuation of electromechanical coupling due to diminished internal myocardial calcium stores [64].

Pericarditis Following Acute Myocardial Infarction

A pericardial friction rub associated with postinfarct pericarditis is detected clinically in 10 to 15 percent of patients [65] (see Chapter 17). Yet at autopsy almost all patients with AMI are found to have evidence of localized fibrinous pericarditis overlying the infarction [66]. A characteristic history of positionally related, sharp pleuritic chest pain is obtained in approximately one-half of the patients with evidence of pericarditis. The pericardial rub usually develops during the first 4 days of hospitalization and most often occurs with large infarcts. The rub is heard best by applying firm pressure with the diaphragm of the stethoscope over the precordium while the patient is sitting up and leaning forward; its intensity is influenced by respiratory variation and may be accentuated by having the patient either inhale or exhale maximally. Leathery, scratching, or crunching in quality, the pericardial rub may have three components: (1) the first component occurs during early diastole at the time of rapid passive filling; (2) the second occurs during late diastole at the time of atrial contraction; and (3) the third occurs during ventricular systole (see Fig. 5-4). The hallmark of the pericardial rub associated with AMI is its evanescence—any or all of these components of a pericardial rub may be absent at various times. A single systolic component heard near the apex may be confused with a murmur of MR due to papillary muscle dysfunction or rupture. Serial auscultatory evaluation of patients in various positions in a quiet room is important for detection of the friction rub. Postinfarction pericarditis must be differentiated from acute pulmonary embolism, peptic ulcer disease, and, especially, recurrent myocardial ischemia or infarction. Last, the appearance of a new friction rub more than 10 days after acute infarction probably represents Dressler's syndrome.

Late Complicated Myocardial Infarction

Cardiac Rupture

Rupture of the free wall of the heart is one of the most dreaded complications of AMI because the patient rarely survives (see Fig. 5-4). Cardiac rupture has been reported in approximately 10 percent of fatal cases of AMI [67–69], and it is listed third as a cause of death, after cardiogenic shock and cardiac arrhythmias (see Chapters 4, 16). The classic profile of a patient at increased risk for cardiac rupture is characterized by an elderly (80 years or older) hypertensive woman presenting with a first AMI that is usually complicated by recurrent chest pain suggestive of another infarct or extension [70]. Cardiac rupture usually occurs within the first week after infarction and rarely after the second week.

The clinical symptoms and signs suggesting cardiac rupture may be categorized into three major clinical patterns. The most common presentation is prolonged, recurring chest pain during the initial week after infarction followed by an abrupt onset of dyspnea associated with hypotension and jugular neck vein distention and then rapid deterioration to electromechanical dissociation and death. The prognosis of this rhythm is poor [71], yet one must exclude other etiologies associated with electromechanical dissociation that may be reversible (e.g., tension pneumothorax, severe hypovolemia, pulmonary embolism, hypoxia, acidosis, and tamponade). Failure to produce peripheral pulses during closed-chest resuscitation is also a terminal sign of cardiac rupture.

A less common clinical pattern of cardiac rupture involves more gradual onset of symptoms, suggesting cardiac tamponade. These patients develop distended neck veins, tachycardia, systemic hypotension, and *pulsus paradoxus* (an accentuation of the usual inspiratory decline in systolic arterial pressure by more than 10 mm Hg). When the pulsus paradoxus is more than 20 mm Hg, there is usually a palpable diminution in the peripheral arterial pulses during inspiration. Pulsus paradoxus may not be evident despite cardiac tamponade in the presence of profound systemic hypotension. It is important to understand that pulsus paradoxus does not necessarily indicate cardiac tamponade since this physical finding may occur in patients with acute or chronic respiratory distress, hypovolemic shock, and massive pulmonary embolism as well as in intubated patients undergoing positive-pressure ventilation.

The final presentation of cardiac rupture is characterized by the formation of an LV pseudoaneurysm (see Chapter 4). The LV pseudoaneurysm represents a partially contained cardiac rupture that is usually connected to the left ventricle through a narrow neck. To-and-fro movement of blood through the neck may produce systolic or diastolic murmurs. Rupture of false aneurysms (early or late) usually results in a rapidly accumulating hemopericardium and sudden, unexpected death. Two-dimensional echocardiography and radionuclide blood pool scans are valuable noninvasive techniques for confirming the diagnosis of ventricular pseudoaneurysm [72–75]. The presence of a pseudoaneurysm is an indication for early surgery because of the imminent risk of rupture and death.

New Systolic Murmur Following Myocardial Infarction

The development of a new systolic murmur during AMI is a common occurrence. Heikkila [76] described apical systolic murmurs consistent with MR in 55 percent of patients admitted to the hospital with AMI. In most of this group, the MR was not hemodynamically significant as judged by the absence of congestive heart failure and a stable clinical course. However, determination of the hemodynamic significance of a new systolic murmur in patients with congestive heart failure or shock becomes mandatory. Such a murmur may represent the acute development of a papillary muscle rupture or a ventricular septal rupture, two potentially serious but surgically correctable mechanical complications. In other cases, the murmur may indicate papillary muscle dysfunction due to papillary muscle ischemia or necrosis or spatial derangement of the papillary muscle and chordae tendinae system. The differential diagnosis of a new systolic murmur following AMI also includes tricuspid regurgitation associated with RV infarction, single component friction rub with pericarditis and to-and-fro murmurs with pseudoaneurysms. The ensuing discussion focuses on the specific complications following MI (papillary muscle ischemia/rupture, VSDs) that lead to the development of new systolic murmurs.

Papillary Muscle Dysfunction

The most commonly heard murmur after AMI is that of MR due to papillary muscle dysfunction (see Chapters 4, 16). Burch and colleagues [77–79] first introduced the concept that myocardial ischemia and infarction can result in papillary muscle dysfunction and brief episodes of mitral insufficiency. MR secondary to papillary muscle dysfunction is thought to occur because the papillary muscles are partially or totally unable to develop tension, resulting in slack in the mitral valve apparatus as the apex of the left ventricle moves toward the base [80, 81]. Failure of the chordae to remain tense allows the mitral leaflets to retrovert into the left atrium during systole, producing subsequent regurgitation [82, 83]. The posteromedial papillary muscle is more prone to ischemic dysfunction because it has a single blood supply from either the right or left circumflex coronary artery as opposed to the anterolateral papillary muscle which receives a protective dual blood supply from the left anterior descending and circumflex arteries [84]. Patients with papillary muscle dysfunction are more likely to have recurrent chest pain, heart failure, and death than those who do not have this complication after MI [85].

The murmur of papillary muscle dysfunction was originally described as ''ejection'' in type, with the first sound followed by a silent period that corresponds to isovolumic contraction [77]. This particular variant of MR increases in severity as LV dimension diminishes during contraction, accounting for a graduated intensity of the murmur in mid-systole [86]. To the contrary, Heikkila described a high frequency pansystolic murmur heard best at the apex [76]. Radiation of the murmur toward the sternum or the aortic area often occurs in disorders predominantly affecting the posterior mitral leaflet as the regurgitant jet of blood is directed anteriorly. The murmur in this case may be confused with the murmur of VSD or aortic stenosis. With predominant anterior leaflet involvement, the murmur often radiates posteriorly to the back and is transmitted to the thoracic and cervical spine. The murmur of MR shows little change in intensity despite large alterations in LV volume as occurs with atrial fibrillation and with systole after a premature ventricular beat [87]. By comparison, most mid-systolic murmurs, such as with aortic stenosis, increase in intensity during the cycle following a long diastole because increased LV filling after a long RR interval results in a greater contractile force and an increased gradient across the aortic valve. In the case of MR, the increased LV end-diastolic volume is partially dissipated during early systole by regurgitation into the left atrium. Also, the reduced aortic pressure resulting from the long diastolic period reduces the impedance of LV ejection; therefore, the amount of MR may actually be decreased during the mid to later parts of systole. The murmur of MR varies little with respiration, being slightly louder during held expiration. However, with sudden standing or amyl nitrite inhalation the murmur decreases in intensity, whereas squatting or intravenous phenylephrine administration increases its loudness.

In an attempt to improve the identification of left-sided regurgitant murmurs, Lembo and coworkers [88] evaluated the effectiveness of transient arterial occlusion compared with isometric handgrip exercise, squatting, and amyl nitrite inhalation. Isometric handgrip exercise and squatting increase LV afterload and augment the intensity of these murmurs [89–96]; conversely, amyl nitrite inhalation decreases afterload, thus diminishing intensity [97–100]. By simultaneously inflating blood pressure cuffs on both arms 20 to 40 mm Hg above systolic pressure for 20 seconds, Lembo et al. found that left-sided regurgitant murmurs (mitral and aortic regurgitation, VSD) were intensified. This maneuver was found to be superior to squatting and equal to isometric handgrip exercise and amyl nitrite inhalation. This bedside maneuver can be done quickly and easily on all patients without any limitations or contraindications, as described for the other standard techniques [90–93, 101].

Papillary Muscle Rupture

Papillary muscle rupture, 2.5 times as frequent in patients with inferior wall MI as in those with anterior wall infarction, occurs in 0.4 to 5.0 percent of patients dying with AMI [102, 103] (see Chapters 4, 16). Papillary muscle rupture usually occurs 2 to 4 days after the initial MI and is often associated with severe chest pain, shortness of breath, and a loud systolic murmur. Most patients with this complication after MI suffer from intractable pulmonary edema and cardiogenic shock; others develop pulmonary edema without hemodynamic deterioration as a consequence of partial rupture of the papillary muscle or rupture of the head (and not the entire body) of a papillary muscle (see Fig. 5-4). Ironically, most patients developing cardiogenic shock secondary to papillary muscle rupture have infarction that affects less than 25 percent of the LV myocardium at autopsy.

The systolic murmur associated with papillary muscle rupture may have characteristics observable with acute MR of any etiology. The murmur is usually holosystolic, heard best at the apex, with decreasing intensity during late systole due to equilibration of LV and left atrial (LA) pressures at the time of the LA V wave. Other physical signs include the following: (1) A systolic parasternal lift may be detected at the lower left sternal border. If early and sustained, it may result from a RV impulse due to severe pulmonary hypertension. If it is late and more dynamic, the parasternal lift may be secondary to distention of a noncompliant left atrium by the regurgitant jet. This late parasternal lift corresponds in timing with a large LA V wave at cardiac catheterization. (2) Systolic thrills are rare, but if present they are usually felt at the apex. (3) A fourth heart sound, ascribed to LA "overload" associated with diminished ventricular distensibility, is commonly heard.

Of note, the murmur of papillary muscle rupture may be soft and unimpressive. Because of impaired LA distensibility and adaptability to an acute volume load, the LA pressure increases rapidly in acute MR. Subsequent reduction of the LV/LA pressure gradient early in systole limits the velocity of regurgitant flow. In fact, the velocity rather than the volume of MR determines the intensity of the murmur of MR [104]. Furthermore, because diminished ventricular function and systolic pressure generation is commonly found in the presence of myocardial ischemia, it is not surprising that many holosystolic murmurs are of low intensity even in the presence of considerable MR [105]. Finally, obesity, a thick chest wall, or pulmonary disease may also be responsible for masking the clinical findings of acute MR. Echocardiography with Doppler interrogation should be performed in any patient with the development of cardiogenic shock to rule out the possibility of papillary muscle rupture, even if a distinct new systolic murmur is not appreciated. Urgent surgical intervention is required.

Ventricular Septal Rupture

Ventricular septal rupture [106–108], a rare complication generally occurring 2 to 3 days after the AMI, is found in 0.5 to 1.0 percent of cases of MI (see Chapters 4, 16). The clinical presentation, time course, and auscultatory findings are similar to those in patients with papillary muscle rupture (Fig. 5-4). If no acute surgical correction is undertaken, most patients die within a week. In contrast to congenital VSD, acquired VSD always involves the muscular part of the ventricular septum and not the membranous septum. An associated ventricular aneurysm is present in one-half of the cases. Acquired VSD is more commonly associated with anterior MI, and the ECG frequently shows a right bundle branch block or conduction abnormalities. The systolic murmur is often accompanied by a thrill that is maximal at the lower left sternal border. The thrill may be absent due to severely impaired LV function or the large size of the septal defect. Axillary transmission is distinctly uncommon with VSD; if present, MR should be considered. The diagnosis is confirmed by Doppler echocardiography.

Mural Thrombi

Autopsy studies have shown that endocardial mural thrombosis is a frequent finding in patients dying of MI [109–112] (see Fig. 5-4). Mural thrombi are frequently recognized in patients with extensive anterior Q-wave infarction involving the left ventricle, especially in the presence of severe wall motion abnormalities involving the apex (see Chapters 4, 16).

Clinically, the detection of mural thrombi is difficult without the use of two-dimensional echocardiography [113–117]. Patients may present with a cerebrovascular accident or sudden arterial insufficiency involving the bowel or peripheral extremities. While performing the physical examination, the physician should note any abnormal systolic impulse on palpation that may represent an LV aneurysm. This abnormal impulse is characteristically located superior and medial to the true cardiac impulse and is typified by a prolonged systolic expansile pulsation. This persistent abnormal impulse must be distinguished from the occasional similar impulse found with acute infarction without aneurysm. The latter usually disappears within a few weeks. Patients with an LV aneurysm commonly have an S_3 gallop on auscultation. Frequently a murmur of MR is present, which may be related in part to papillary muscle dysfunction.

Important Noncardiac Physical Findings in the Postinfarct Patient

Careful serial physical examinations are mandatory in the post-MI patient because of various noncardiac problems that may arise during the peri-infarct period (Fig. 5-5). As illustrated, many different organ systems can be adversely affected.

At present, pulmonary embolism occurs much less frequently after AMI because of liberal use of anticoagulant therapy and earlier mobilization of the patient, but it must be considered in the differential diagnosis of chest pain in the CCU. The most common auscultatory finding in patients with documented pulmonary embolism is nonspecific atelectatic rales. Rarely, dullness to percussion at one or both bases due to a hemorrhagic pleural effusion is present in patients with pulmonary infarction. A pleural rub may be heard in this setting or with Dressler's syndrome. Nevertheless, the physical examination in the diagnosis of pulmonary embolism or infarction is much less helpful than are more specific laboratory tests, such as ventilation-perfusion lung scans, impedance plethysmography, and arterial blood gas determinations. The diagnosis of pulmonary embolism should be considered in any patient who has chest pain with associated tachypnea, tachycardia, or fever in the intensive care unit (ICU). Pulmonary infarction is also a recognized complication of indwelling right heart balloon flotation catheters, particularly if the balloon has been inflated or the catheter has been in place for more than 72 hours [118]. Pneumonia is a relatively frequent complication following MI because of prolonged bed rest, atelectasis, retained secretions and, at times, aspiration. Finally, pneumothorax can occur during central venous line placement and must be recognized.

Gastrointestinal discomfort is common in patients hospitalized in the CCU and may arise from multiple causes: (1) gastric distention from nasal oxygen administration, (2) improper endotracheal intubation (left upper quadrant tympany to percussion), (3) constipation and ileus due to bed rest and narcotic analgesics (decreased bowel sounds and fecal masses on abdominal palpation), (4) activation of peptic ulcer disease from stress or thrombolytic therapy, or (5) aggravation of esophageal reflux by recumbency (evidence of pyrosis, epigastric tenderness to palpation, and response to antacids).

Alterations in mental status are common in patients hospitalized in the CCU. Reactive anxiety, depression, denial, ICU psychosis, and hostility are frequent products of the psychogenic stress associated with AMI. These findings must be distinguished from iatrogenically induced mental status changes produced by drugs (e.g., lidocaine-induced hallucinations or seizures, digitalis toxicity, and paradoxical agitation from sedatives or hypnotics

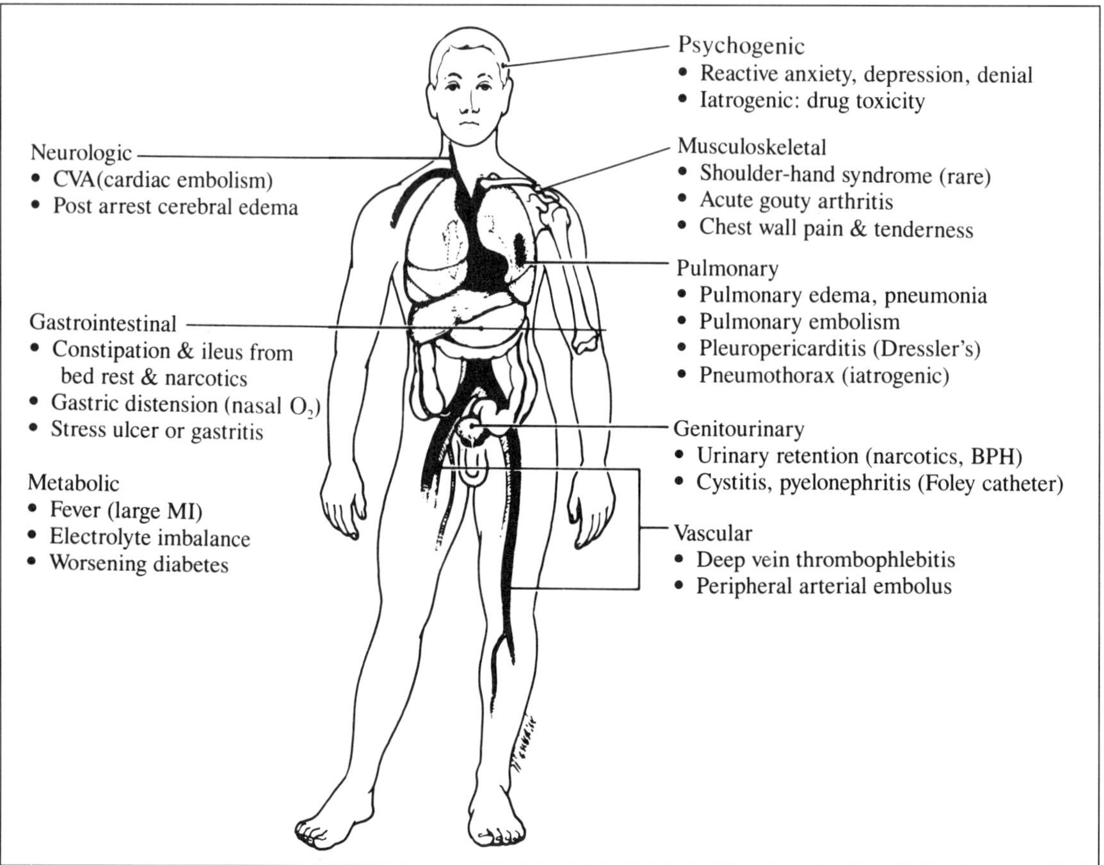

Fig. 5-5
Summary of important noncardiac physical findings that may develop during the peri-infarction period. CVA = cerebrovascular accident; MI = myocardial infarction; BPH = benign prostatic hypertrophy. (From R. A. Walsh and R. A. O'Rourke. History and differential diagnosis of acute myocardial infarction. In J. Karliner and G. Gregoratos (eds.), *Coronary Care*. New York: Churchill Livingstone, 1981. P. 186. With permission.)

in the elderly). Focal neurologic symptoms may arise at any time during the peri-infarction period as a result of decreased cerebral perfusion from low cardiac output in patients with intrinsic cerebrovascular disease or from systemic embolization of a mural thrombus. At times, a reduction in mental alertness is the first sign of deteriorating LV function. Finally, patients who have been resuscitated successfully often have global neurologic findings due to postarrest cerebral anoxia.

The clinical diagnosis of deep vein thrombosis (DVT) has a low specificity and sensitivity and is therefore inaccurate. Studies have shown that most patients who present with signs and symptoms of superficial thrombophlebitis (i.e., pain and tenderness, swelling, redness, palpable cord) do not have concomitant DVT. Unilateral lower extremity edema and tenderness is often related to venous insufficiency and, at times, cellulitis, not DVT. Conversely, other patients may have extensive DVT and few clinical manifestations. Therefore, management decisions in patients suspected of having DVT must rely on objective testing. These tests include (1) contrast venography, the "gold standard"; (2) impedance plethysmography, a noninvasive cost-effective technique relatively sensitive and specific for detection of proximal DVT; (3) ^{125}I-fibrinogen leg scanning, a test that is highly sensitive (95 percent) for detection of calf DVT that has been symptomatic for fewer than 8 days; and (4) Doppler ultrasound, a useful tool to detect proximal DVT (cumulative sensitivity and specificity of approximately 90 percent).

With the advent of thrombolytic therapy (see Chapters 24, 25), bleeding has become the major and most serious noncardiac complication of MI. In general, gastrointestinal bleeding and bleeding at the arterial puncture sites are the most frequent adverse effects. Intracranial, retroperitoneal, or other major bleeding episodes occur in 0.4 to 2.0 percent of patients undergoing thrombolytic treatment. Less serious bleeding disorders include puncture site hematomas, ecchymoses, nosebleeds, purpura, and hematuria. The best approach to the hemorrhagic problem associated with thrombolytic therapy remains proper patient selection.

Genitourinary problems may be encountered because of drug administration or bladder instrumentation. Urinary retention in the elderly male patient with benign prostatic hypertrophy is frequently precipitated by narcotic analgesics. Low urine output may, in fact, be secondary to urinary obstruction; careful suprapubic palpation and percussion may disclose a distended bladder. Cystitis and pyelonephritis are recognized complications of chronic indwelling Foley catheters. Suprapubic tenderness and costovertebral angle tenderness are helpful physical signs that should be elicited if an upper urinary tract infection is suspected.

The reflex sympathetic dystrophy syndrome [119], one of the musculoskeletal complications of MI, is characterized by pain, warmth, and tenderness usually of a distal extremity, and accompanied by signs and symptoms of vasomotor instability, edema, trophic skin changes, and the rapid development of bone demineralization. This syndrome usually affects an entire hand or foot; occasionally, an isolated site such as the patella, hip, or one or two rays of a foot or hand is involved. The contralateral side may be affected in up to 50 percent of patients. Early recognition and treatment are important to prevent permanent disability. Appropriate mobilization of the patient after MI may help to prevent this syndrome. A short course of high-dose prednisone in conjunction with physical therapy helps to alleviate symptoms and improve range of motion. Another musculoskeletal complication of MI, a nonspecific "chest wall syndrome," has been noted in many patients with large infarctions. This poorly understood phenomenon is characterized by generalized tenderness over the left precordium and vague chest pain lasting seconds to days. Last, the usual clinical manifestations associated with acute gouty arthritis and pseudogout may be precipitated by dehydration, medications, and stress experienced after MI.

Metabolic complications are frequent and may be a spontaneous result of the physiologic stress of MI or may be iatrogenically induced. For instance, polydipsia and polyuria may be the first clues to an aggravation of latent or previously controlled diabetes; leg cramps may be the first clue to the presence of diuretic-induced hypokalemia; and changes in mental status may indicate the presence of diuretic-induced hyponatremia. Fevers have been known to occur with large MIs.

Even in today's era of advanced technology, a complete, thoughtful, and careful history and physical examination play an absolutely critical role in the diagnosis and management of myocardial ischemia and infarction. Chest pain can be provoked by many cardiac and noncardiac entities that do not induce myocardial ischemia. The astute clinician should be able to synthesize information obtained in the initial evaluation to determine the likelihood of active myocardial ischemia, infarction, or both, so as to initiate an appropriate therapeutic plan. Cardiac and noncardiac complications of MI can be identified in most cases by simple techniques of inspection, palpation, and auscultation, thereby fostering early aggressive intervention.

References

1. Lee, T. H., Juarez, G., Cook, E. F., et al. Ruling out myocardial infarction: A prospective multicenter validation of a 12-hour strategy for patients at low risk. *N. Engl. J. Med.* 324:1239, 1991.
2. Walsh, R. A., and O'Rourke, R. A. History and Differential Diagnosis of Acute Myocardial Infarction. In J. S. Karliner and G. Gregoratos (eds.), *Coronary Care.* New York: Churchill Livingstone, 1981.
3. Walsh, R. A., and O'Rourke, R. A. Chest Pain. In J. H. Stein (ed.), *Internal Medicine* (3rd ed.). Boston: Little, Brown, 1990.
4. Martin, W. B. Patient's use of gestures in the diagnosis of coronary insufficiency disease. *Minn. Med.* 40:691, 1957.

5. Levine, S. A. Coronary thrombosis—the variable clinical features. *Medicine (Baltimore)* 8:245, 1929.
6. Quarry, V. M., and Spodick, D. H. Cardiac responses to isometric exercise: Comparative effects with different postures and levels of exertion. *Circulation* 49:905, 1974.
7. Lassvik, C., and Areskog, N.-H. Effects of various environmental temperatures on effort angina. *Ups. J. Med. Sci.* 84:173, 1979.
8. Backman, C., Holm, S., and Linderholm, H. Reaction to cold of patients with coronary insufficiency. *Ups. J. Med. Sci.* 84:181, 1979.
9. Hattenhauer, M., and Neill, W. A. The effect of cold air inhalation on angina pectoris and myocardial oxygen supply. *Circulation* 51:1053, 1975.
10. Lassvik, C. T., and Areskog, N.-H. Angina in cold environment: reactions to exercise. *Br. Heart J.* 42:396, 1979.
11. Ansari, A., and Burch G. E. Influence of hot environments on the cardiovascular system: A clinical study of 23 cardiac patients at rest. *Arch. Intern. Med.* 123:371, 1969.
12. Williams, A. V., Higginbotham, A. C., and Knisely, M. H. Increased blood cell agglutination following ingestion of fat, a factor contributing to cardiac ischemia, coronary insufficiency, and anginal pain: A contribution to the biophysics of disease. *Angiology* 8:29, 1957.
13. Regan, T. J., Binak, K., Gordon, S., et al. Myocardial blood flow and oxygen consumption during postprandial lipemia and heparin-induced lipolysis. *Circulation* 23:55, 1961.
14. Lewy, R. I. Effect of elevated plasma-free fatty acids on thromboxane release in patients with coronary artery disease. *Haemostasis* 9:134, 1980.
15. Goldstein, R. E., Redwood, D. R., Rosing, D. R., et al. Alterations in the circulatory response to exercise following a meal and their relationship to postprandial angina pectoris. *Circulation* 44:90, 1971.
16. Hellerstein, H. K., and Friedman, E. H. Sexual activity and the post coronary patient. *Arch. Intern. Med.* 125:987, 1970.
17. Shub, C. Stable angina pectoris. 1. Clinical patterns. *Mayo Clin. Proc.* 64:233, 1990.
18. Pepine, C. J., and Weiner L. Effects of the Valsalva maneuver on myocardial ischemia in patients with coronary artery disease. *Circulation* 59:1304, 1979.
19. Ingram, D. A., Fulton, R. A., Portal, R. W., et al. Vomiting as a diagnostic aid in acute ischaemic cardiac pain. *Br. Med. J.* 281:636, 1980.
20. Cheike, P., and Haist Steff, P. Angina pectoris with syncope due to transient atrioventricular block. *Br. Heart J.* 36:577, 1974.
21. Harper, R., Peter, R., and Hunt, P. Syncope in association with Prinzmetal's variant angina. *Br. Heart J.* 37:771, 1975.
22. Gordon, T., and Kannel, W. B. Multiple risk functions for predicting coronary heart disease: The concept, accuracy, and application. *Am. Heart J.* 103:1031, 1982.
23. Dawber, T. R. *The Framingham Study: The Epidemiology of Atherosclerotic Disease.* Cambridge: Harvard University Press, 1980.
24. Levy, D., Wilson, P. W., Anderson, K. M., et al. Stratifying the patient at risk from coronary disease: New insights from the Framingham Heart Study. *Am. Heart J.* 119 (3, pt. 2):712, 1990.
25. Wei, J. Y., and Gersh, B. J. Heart disease in the elderly. *Curr. Probl. Cardiol.* 12(1):25, 1987.
26. Partamian, J., and Bradley, R. F. Acute myocardial infarction in 258 cases of diabetes: Immediate mortality and five year survival. *N. Engl. J. Med.* 273:455, 1965.
27. Kannel, W. B., and Abbot, R. D. Incidence and prognosis of unrecognized myocardial infarction: An update in the Framingham Study. *N. Engl. J. Med.* 311:1144, 1984.
28. Wei, J. Y. Heart disease in the elderly. *Cardiovasc. Med.* 9:971, 1984.
29. O'Rourke, R. A., Chatterjee, K., and Wei, J. Y. Coronary heart disease. *J. Am. Coll. Cardiol.* 10(2):52A, 1987.
30. Coodley, E. L., and Zebari, D. Characteristics of myocardial infarction in the elderly. In E. L. Coodley (ed.), *Geriatric Heart Disease.* Littleton, MA: PSG Publishing, 1981.
31. Nienaber, C. A., Kodolitsch, Y. V., Nicolas, V., et al. The diagnosis of thoracic aortic dissection by noninvasive imaging procedures. *N. Engl. J. Med.* 328:1, 1993.
32. Cigarroa, J. E., Isselbacher, E. M., DeSanctis, R. W., et al. Diagnostic imaging in the evaluation of suspected aortic dissection: Old standards and new directions. *N. Engl. J. Med.* 328:35, 1993.
33. Narula, J., Khaw, B. A., Dec, G. W., Jr., et al. Recognition of acute myocarditis masquerading as acute myocardial infarction. *N. Engl. J. Med.* 328: 100, 1993.
34. Spodick, D. H. Infection and infarction: acute viral (and other) infection in the onset, pathogenesis, and mimicry of acute myocardial infarction. *Am. J. Med.* 81:661, 1986.
35. Walsh, R. A., and O'Rourke, R. A. The physical examination in acute uncomplicated and complicated myocardial infarction. In J. S. Karliner and G. Gregoratos (eds.), *Coronary Care.* New York: Churchill Livingstone, 1981.
36. Fowler, N. O. Physical signs in acute myocardial infarction and its complications. *Prog. Cardiovasc. Dis.* 10:287, 1968.
37. Webb, S. W., Adgey, A. A., and Pantridge, F. J. Autonomic disturbances at onset of acute myocardial infarction. *Br. Med. J.* 3:89, 1972.
38. Bezold, A., and Hirt, L. Über die physiologischen Wirkungen des Essingsauren Veratrins, *Physiol. Lab. Wurzburg* 1:75, 1867.
39. Jarish, A., and Zotterman, Y. Depressor reflexes

from the heart. *Acta Physiol. Scand.* 16:31, 1948.
40. Mark, A. L., Abboud, F. M., Heistad, D. D., et al. Evidence against the presence of ventricular chemoreceptors activated by hypoxia and hypercapnia. *Am. J. Physiol.* 227:178, 1974.
41. Robertson, D., Hollister, A. S., Forman, M. B., et. al. Reflexes unique to myocardial ischemia and infarction. *J. Am. Coll. Cardiol.* 5:99B, 1985.
42. Wei, J. W., Markis, J. E., Malagold, M., et al. Cardiovascular reflexes stimulated by reperfusion of ischemic myocardium in acute myocardial infarction. *Circulation* 67:796, 1983.
43. Robertson, R. M., and Robertson, D. The Bezold-Jarish reflex: Possible role in limiting myocardial ischemia. *Clin. Cardiol.* 4:75, 1981.
44. Sleight, P. Cardiac vomiting. *Br. Heart J.* 46:5, 1981.
45. Harvey, W. P., and Ronan, J. A. Bedside diagnosis of arrhythmias. *Prog. Cardiovasc. Dis.* 8:419, 1966.
46. Yurchak, P. M., and Gorlin, R. Paradoxic splitting of the second heart sound in coronary artery disease. *N. Engl. J. Med.* 269:741, 1963.
47. Hill, J. C., O'Rourke, R. A., Lewis, R. P., et al. The diagnostic value of the atrial gallop in acute myocardial infarction. *Am. Heart J.* 78:194, 1969.
48. Riley, C. P., Russel, R. O., and Rackly, C. E. Left ventricular gallop sound and acute myocardial infarction. *Am Heart J.* 86:598, 1973.
49. DiDonna, G. J., Karliner, J. S., Peterson, K. L., et al. Transmission of audible precordial gallop sounds to the right supraclavicular fossa. *Br. Heart J.* 37:1277, 1975.
50. Dell'Italia, L. J., and Starling, M. R. Right ventricular infarction: An important clinical entity. *Curr. Probl. Cardiol.* 9(9):27, 1984.
51. Rigo, P., Murray, M., Taylor, D. R., et al. Right ventricular dysfunction detected by gated scintiphotography in patients with acute inferior myocardial infarction. *Circulation* 52:268, 1975.
52. Sharpe, D. N., Botvinick, E. H., Shames, O. M., et al. The non-invasive diagnosis of right ventricular infarction. *Circulation* 57:483, 1978.
53. Wackers, F. J., Lie, K. I., Sokole, E. B., et al. Prevalence of right ventricular involvement in inferior wall infarction assessed with myocardial imaging with thallium-201 and technetium-99m pyrophosphate. *Am. J. Cardiol.* 42:358, 1978.
54. Dell'Italia, L. J., Starling, M. R., Crawford, M. H., et al. Right ventricular infarction: Identification by hemodynamic measurements before and after loading and correlation with non-invasive techniques. *J. Am. Coll. Cardiol.* 4:932, 1984.
55. Zehender, M., Kasper, W., Kauder, E., et al. Right ventricular infarction as an independent predictor of prognosis after acute myocardial infarction. *N. Engl. J. Med.* 328:981, 1993.
56. Dell'Italia, L. J., Starling, M. R., and O'Rourke, R. A. Physical examination for exclusion of hemodynamically important right ventricular infarction. *Ann. Intern. Med.* 99:608, 1983.
57. Cohn, J. N., Guiha, N. H., Broder, M. I., et al. Right ventricular infarction: Clinical and hemodynamic features. *Am. J. Cardiol.* 33:209, 1974.
58. Rotman, M., Ratliff, N. B., and Hawley, J. Right ventricular infarction: A haemodynamic diagnosis. *Br. Heart J.* 36:941, 1974.
59. Lorell, B., Leinback, R. C., Pohost, G. M., et al. Right ventricular infarction: Clinical diagnosis and differentiation from cardiac tamponade and pericardial constriction. *Am. J. Cardiol.* 43:465, 1979.
60. Jensen, D. P., Goolsby, J. P., Jr., and Oliva, P. B. Hemodynamic pattern resembling pericardial constriction after acute inferior myocardial infarction with right ventricular infarction. *Am. J. Cardiol.* 42:858, 1978.
61. Killip, T., and Kimball, J. T. Treatment of myocardial infarction in a coronary care unit: A two year experience with 250 patients. *Am. J. Cardiol.* 20: 457, 1967.
62. Abrams, D. S., Starling, M. R., Crawford, M. H., et al. Value of noninvasive techniques for predicting early complications in patients with clinical class II acute myocardial infarction. *J. Am. Coll. Cardiol.* 2:818, 1983.
63. Forrester, J. S., Diamond, G., Chatterjee, K., et al. Medical therapy of acute myocardial infarction by application of hemodynamic subsets. *N. Engl. J. Med.* 295:1356, 1976.
64. Freeman, G. L., Widman, L. E., Campbell, J. M., et al. An evaluation of pulsus alternans in closed-chest dogs. *Am. J. Physiol.* 262:H278, 1992.
65. Lichstein, E. M., Lieu, H. M., and Gupta, P. Pericarditis complicating acute myocardial infarction: Incidence of complications and significance of electrocardiogram on admission. *Am. Heart J.* 87: 246, 1974.
66. Thadani, V., Chopra, M. P., and Aber Portal, R. W. Pericarditis after acute myocardial infarction. *Br. Med. J.* 2:135, 1971.
67. London, R. E., and London, S. B. Rupture of the heart: A critical analysis of 47 consecutive autopsy cases. *Circulation* 31:202, 1965.
68. Mundth, E. Rupture of the heart complicating myocardial infarction. *Circulation* 46:427, 1972.
69. Bates, R. J., Beutler, S., Resnekov, L., et al. Cardiac rupture—challenge in diagnosis and management. *Am. J. Cardiol.* 40:429, 1977.
70. Schuster, E. H., and Bulkey, B. H. Expansion of transmural myocardial infarction: A pathophysiologic factor in cardiac rupture. *Circulation* 60: 1532, 1979.
71. Raizes, G., Wagner, G. S., and Hackel, D. B. Instantaneous non-arrhythmic cardiac death in acute myocardial infarction: Role of electromechanical dissociation. *Am. J. Cardiol.* 39:1, 1977.
72. Globel, F. L., Visudh-Arom, K., and Edwards, J. E. Pseudoaneurysm of the left ventricle leading

to recurrent pericardial hemorrhage. *Chest* 59:23, 1971.
73. Vlodaver, Z., Coe, J. I., and Edwards, J. E. True and false left ventricular aneurysms: Propensity for the latter to rupture. *Circulation* 51:567, 1975.
74. Aher, B. R., Lewis, M. E., Vargas, A., et al. Noninvasive diagnosis of left ventricular pseudoaneurysm by radioangiography and echocardiography. *Am. Heart J.* 101:236, 1981.
75. Levy, R., Rozanski, A., Charvzi, Y., et al. Complementary roles of two dimensional echocardiography and radionuclide ventriculography in ventricular pseudoaneurysm diagnosis. *Am. Heart J.* 102:1066, 1981.
76. Heikkila, J. Mitral incompetence complicating acute myocardial infarction. *Br. Heart J.* 29:162, 1967.
77. Phillips, J. H., Burch, G. E., and DePasquale, N. P. Syndrome of papillary muscle dysfunction. *Ann. Intern. Med.* 59:508, 1963.
78. Burch, G. E., DePasquale, N. P., and Phillips, J. H. Clinical manifestations of papillary muscle dysfunction. *Arch. Intern. Med.* 112:112, 1963.
79. Burch, G. E., DePasquale, N. P., and Phillips, J. H. The syndrome of papillary muscle dysfunction. *Am. Heart J.* 75:399, 1968.
80. Hirakawa, S., Sasayama, D., Tomoike, H., et al. In situ measurement of papillary muscle dynamics in the dog left ventricle. *Am. J. Physiol.* 233:384, 1977.
81. Ewy, G. A. Isolated papillary muscle dysfunction and infarction. In J. W. Hurst (ed.), *The Heart, Update IV.* New York: McGraw-Hill Book Co., 1979.
82. Roberts, W. C., and Cohen, L. S. Left ventricular papillary muscles: description of the normal and a survey of conditions causing them to be abnormal. *Circulation* 46:138, 1972.
83. Roberts, W. C., and Perloff, J. R. A clinicopathologic survey of the conditions causing the mitral valve to function abnormally. *Ann. Intern. Med.* 77:935, 1972.
84. Estes, E., Dalton, F., and Entmer, M. Anatomy and blood supply of papillary muscles of the left ventricle. *Am. Heart J.* 71:356, 1966.
85. Maisel, A. S., Gilpin, E. A., Klein, L., et al. The murmurs of papillary muscle dysfunction in acute myocardial infarction: clinical features and prognostic implications. *Am. Heart J.* 112:705, 1986.
86. Cheng, T. O. Some new observations on the syndrome of papillary muscle dysfunction. *Am. J. Med.* 47:924, 1969.
87. Karliner, J. S., O'Rourke, R. A., Kearney, D. J., et al. Hemodynamic explanation of why the murmur of mitral regurgitation is independent of cycle length. *Br. Heart J.* 35:397, 1973.
88. Lembo, N., Dell'Italia, J. L., Crawford, M. H., et al. Diagnosis of left-sided regurgitant murmurs by transient arterial occlusion: A new maneuver using blood pressure cuffs. *Ann. Intern. Med.* 105:368, 1986.
89. Lind, A. R., Taylor, S. H., Humphreys, P. W., et al. The circulatory effects of sustained voluntary muscle contraction. *Clin. Sci.* 27:229, 1964.
90. McGraw, D. B., Siegel, W., Stonecipher, H. K., et al. Response of heart murmur intensity to isometric (handgrip) exercise. *Br. Heart J.* 34:605, 1972.
91. Fisher, M.L., Nutter, D. O., Jacobs, W., et al. Haemodynamic responses to isometric exercise (handgrip) in patients with heart disease. *Br. Heart J.* 35:422, 1973.
92. Stefadouros, M. A., Grossman, W., El-Shahawy, M. F., et al. The effect of isometric exercise on the left ventricular volume in normal man. *Circulation* 49:1185, 1974.
93. Sharpey-Schafer, E. P. Effects of squatting on the normal and failing circulation. *Br. Med. J.* 1:1072, 1956.
94. Brotmacher, L. Haemodynamic effects of squatting during repose. *Br. Heart J.* 19:559, 1957.
95. Vogelpoel, L., Nellen, M., Beck, W., et al. The value of squatting in the diagnosis of mild aortic regurgitation. *Am. Heart J.* 77:709, 1969.
96. Nellen, M., Gotsman, M. S., Vogelpoel, L., et al. Effects of prompt squatting on the systolic murmur in idiopathic hypertrophic obstructive cardiomyopathy. *Br. Med. J.* 3:140, 1967.
97. Vogelpoel, L., Nellen, M., Swanepoel, A., et al. The use of amyl nitrite in the diagnosis of systolic murmurs. *Lancet* 2:810, 1959.
98. Perloff, J. K., Calvin, J., DeLeon, A. C., Jr., et al. Systemic hemodynamic effects of amyl nitrite in normal man. *Am. Heart J.* 66:460, 1963.
99. Luisada, A. A., and Madoery, R. J. Functional tests as an aid to cardiac auscultation. *Med. Clin. North Am.* 50:73, 1966.
100. DeLeon, A. C., Jr., and Harvey, W. P. Pharmacological agents and auscultation. *Mod. Concepts Cardiovasc. Dis.* 44:23, 1975.
101. Crawford, M. H., and O'Rourke, R. A. A systematic approach to the bedside differentiation of cardiac murmurs and abnormal sounds. *Curr. Probl. Cardiol.* 1:1, 1977.
102. Cederquist, L., and Soderstrom, J. Papillary muscle rupture in myocardial infarction: A study based upon an autopsy material. *Acta Med. Scand.* 176:287, 1964.
103. Wei, J. Y., Hutchins, G. M., and Bulkey, B. H. Papillary muscle rupture in fatal acute myocardial infarction, a potentially treatable form of cardiogenic shock. *Ann. Intern. Med.* 90:149, 1979.
104. Bruns, D. L. A general theory of the causes of murmurs in the cardiovascular system. *Am. J. Med.* 27:360, 1959.
105. DeBusk, R. F., and Harrison, D. C. The clinical spectrum of papillary muscle disease. *N. Engl. J. Med.* 281:1458, 1969.
106. Selzer, A., Gerln, K., and Kerth, W. J. Clinical,

hemodynamic and surgical considerations of rupture of the ventricular septum after myocardial infarction. *Am. Heart J.* 78:59, 1969.

107. Vlodaver, Z., and Edwards, J. E. Rupture of ventricular septum or papillary muscle complicating myocardial infarction. *Circulation* 55:815, 1977.
108. Hutchins, G. M. Rupture of the interventricular septum complicating myocardial infarction: Pathological analysis of 10 patients with clinically diagnosed perforation. *Am. Heart J.* 97:165, 1979.
109. Hellerstein, H. K., and Martin, J. W. Incidence of thromboembolic lesions accompanying myocardial infarctions. *Am. Heart J.* 33:443, 1947.
110. Phares, W. S., Edwards, J. E., and Burchell, H. B. Cardiac aneurysm: Clinicopathologic studies: *Mayo Clin. Proc.* 28:264, 1953.
111. Dubnow, M. H., Burchell, H. B., and Titus, J. L. Post-infarction ventricular aneurysm in a clinicopathologic and electrocardiographic study of cases. *Am. Heart J.* 70:753, 1969.
112. Davis, R. W., and Ebert, P. A. Ventricular aneurysm: A clinical pathologic correlation. *Am. J. Cardiol.* 29:1, 1972.
113. Van De Bos, A. A., Bletter, W. B., and Hagemeijer, F. Progressive development of left ventricular thrombus: Detection and evolution studied with echocardiographic techniques. *Chest* 74:307, 1978.
114. Stratton, J. R., Lighty, G. W., Jr., Pearlman, A. S., et al. Detection of left ventricular thrombosis in two-dimensional echocardiography: Sensitivity, specificity and causes of uncertainty. *Circulation* 66:156, 1982.
115. Reeder, G. S., Tajik, A. J., and Seward, J. B. Left ventricular mural thrombosis: Two-dimensional echocardiographic diagnosis. *Mayo Clin. Proc.* 56:82, 1981.
116. DeMaria, A. N., Neumann, A., Bomner, W., et al. Left ventricular thrombi identified by cross section echocardiography. *Ann. Intern. Med.* 90:14, 1979.
117. Asinger, R. W., Mikell, F. L., Elsperger, J., et al. Incidence of left ventricular thrombosis after acute transmural infarction: Serial evaluation by two-dimensional echocardiography. *N. Engl. J. Med.* 305:297, 1981.
118. Foote, G. A., Shabel, S. J., and Hodges, M. Pulmonary complications of the flow-directed balloon tipped catheter. *N. Engl. J. Med.* 290:927, 1974.
119. Gilliland, B. C. Miscellaneous arthritides and extra-articular rheumatism. In E. Braunwald, K. J. Isselbacher, R. G. Petersdorf, et al. (eds.), *Harrison's Principles of Internal Medicine.* New York: McGraw-Hill Book Co., 1987.

6. Plasma Enzymes in Acute Myocardial Infarction

Peter R. Puleo and Robert Roberts

The utility of plasma enzymes as molecular markers of acute myocardial infarction (AMI) has undergone a steady evolution. During the 1960s an elevation of one or more of the "cardiac enzymes" was taken as supportive evidence for the diagnosis of AMI. The increased diagnostic specificity that resulted from the recognition and application of myocardium-specific isoenzymes during the 1970s greatly enhanced the clinical usefulness of these assays; today, most clinicians would be reluctant to make the diagnosis of AMI if appropriately timed plasma samples failed to document a rise and fall in MB creatine kinase (CK). Serial analysis of plasma MB-CK has also been employed to accurately quantitate infarct size.

The advent of thrombolytic therapy during the 1980s has created the need for a sensitive and specific marker of AMI that is diagnostic during the initial hours of infarction. In addition, reliable noninvasive indicators of reperfusion might obviate the need for routine diagnostic catheterization following thrombolytic therapy. The subforms MM-CK and MB-CK show promise as early markers of AMI and of successful reperfusion. The role of myoglobin, particularly as a marker of reperfusion, is also promising.

Historical Perspective

Amylase was detected in the serum of normal individuals in 1908 [1]. However, it was not until 1936, when alkaline phosphatase was proposed as a marker of metastatic bone disease [2], that serum enzymes were used diagnostically. The first application of diagnostic enzymology to AMI was in 1954, when La Due et al. [3, 4] reported a rise and fall in serum aspartate transaminase (AST; prior designation SGOT) activity following AMI. One year later, serum lactate dehydrogenase (LD) activity was also shown to be elevated following acute myocardial necrosis [5]. A drawback of using these enzymes as diagnostic markers of AMI is their lack of specificity for myocardial injury: both are released into the blood with injury of muscle, liver, and other tissues. However, in 1957 several groups reported that LD activity in serum could be resolved into several peaks by electrophoresis [6–8], subsequently designated "isoenzymes" [9], with predominance of the fastest migrating peak being specific for AMI [7]. CK was shown to be elevated in the serum of patients with skeletal muscle disease (muscular dystrophy) in 1959 [10]. The following year, elevation of serum CK after AMI was detected [11]. The use of the MB isoenzyme of CK as a specific indicator of AMI was first reported in 1966 [12]. During the subsequent decade, the sensitivity and specificity of plasma MB-CK elevation for acute myocardial necrosis was confirmed in many laboratories, and improved assays for the CK isoenzymes were developed. Today, assay of plasma MB-CK is universally accepted as the most reliable diagnostic test for AMI, and the ratio of MB-CK_2 to MB-CK_1 subforms is evolving as a marker that is highly sensitive and specific for the early diagnosis of acute myocardial infarction.

Biochemical Markers of Acute Myocardial Infarction

Biochemical markers of AMI in current use have in common the property of being present in the intracellular compartment of cardiac myocytes, with release into the blood following the onset of infarction. In the absence of ischemia, the intact sarcolemma maintains the intracellular milieu; the membrane is impermeable to macromolecules, and movement of ions is tightly regulated by intramembrane gates and energy-dependent pumps. Shortly after the onset of ischemia, the ability of the membrane to maintain normal ionic gradients becomes impaired, and intracellular potassium is lost to the interstitium. Whether this reaction is a result of gate/channel dysfunction [13] or due to early loss of integrity of the lipid bilayer itself is unknown. It is also unclear if sufficient impairment of membrane integrity occurs during transient ischemia to allow some loss of macromolecular contents. Several studies have suggested that enzyme release in the animal model (at least in quantities sufficient to result in a discernible rise above baseline blood levels) occurs only with irreversible ischemia [14, 15]; however, the issue remains controversial and difficult to prove or disprove. We observed elevated levels of CK and glycogen phosphorylase in the lymph draining from the hearts of dogs following periods of occlusion as short as 10 to 15 minutes, followed by reperfusion. On histologic examination, there was evidence of minute abnormalities, but not those typical of cardiac necrosis. It is possible that reversible ischemia results in the release of minute amounts of intracellular macromolecules in quantities sufficient to induce an elevation in the lymph but insufficient to raise plasma levels above the normal range [16]. Clinical studies have failed to demonstrate plasma enzyme elevations during transient ischemia (e.g., exercise stress with ischemia or unstable anginal episodes) [17, 18] despite coronary patency, which would favor the appearance of any released enzymes in the blood. In a recent study, ischemia detected by thallium scan after induction by exercise was consistently associated with normal plasma levels of MB-CK and its subforms. In summary, it appears that if leakage of macromolecules from the cell during transient ischemia occurs, it is in quantities insufficient to be detected by currently available assays and as such does not detract from its diagnostic sensitivity and specificity.

Ischemia sustained for more than 30 or 40 minutes results in irreversible cellular injury and subsequent cell death. Membrane integrity is lost, and cellular contents, including macromolecules, are therefore in continuity with the interstitial space. A substantial proportion of cellular enzymes are denatured or degraded in situ; however, a predictable fraction gains entry to the cardiac lymphatics and is transported to the blood. Whether a significant quantity of these proteins enters the bloodstream directly via the cardiac capillaries is unknown; it would depend, among other factors, on the regional myocardial flow (which is usually minimal with a nonreperfused AMI), as well as the molecular size of the protein and the integrity of the capillaries in the infarct region.

It follows from the above discussion that the utility of a protein as a marker of AMI depends on certain factors.

1. Solubility: Molecules having low solubility, such as those that make up the contractile apparatus, move poorly out of the infarcted myocardium.
2. Baseline concentration of the marker molecule in myocardium and in blood: High concentration within myocardial cells and low concentration in normal lymph and blood result in a significant concentration gradient and rapid flux of the marker molecule into the blood following sarcolemma breakdown. Furthermore, a low ambient concentration in normal blood provides a background against which release of the marker molecule into the blood can be readily detected.
3. Molecular weight: Large molecules such as LD [molecular weight (MW) 135,000] diffuse slowly and appear in the blood relatively late, thus precluding early diagnosis; small molecules (e.g., myoglobin, MW 17,800) appear in the blood rapidly.
4. Detectability: The clinical utility of a diagnostic marker depends in part on the reliability, expense, and ease of detection of the marker in a clinical laboratory. The speed with which an assay can be performed is also a consideration for assays whose goal is the early diagnosis of AMI.
5. Specificity: Perhaps most importantly, the usefulness of a marker is determined by the extent to which it is present in myocardium but not in other tissues, so that a rise in plasma levels is specific for myocardial injury.
6. Kinetics of clearance: Ideally, a biochemical marker is cleared from the blood quickly; however, if clearance is too rapid, the time frame during which the diagnosis of AMI can be made may be brief. This situation is the case for myoglobin, which is rapidly cleared into the urine;

with small infarctions, serum levels may return to the normal range by 24 hours after AMI onset.

More than 20 muscle-associated proteins, including enzymes, myoglobin, and contractile proteins, have been evaluated as potential markers of AMI. Most have been of limited diagnostic value because their presence in noncardiac tissue results in elevated plasma levels in the absence of myocardial injury [19]. Three enzymes have been routinely used in the past for the diagnosis of AMI: AST, LD, and CK. Of these, CK and its isoenzymes have proved to be the most reliable and cost-effective biochemical markers of AMI. There is, however, notable interest in myoglobin and Troponin-T.

Creatine Kinase

Characteristics

CK catalyzes the reversible transfer of a high-energy phosphate group from adenosine triphosphate (ATP) to creatine (Cr):

$$\text{Cr} + \text{ATP} \xrightleftharpoons{\text{CK}} \text{Cr-P} + \text{ADP}$$

where Cr-P = creatine phosphate
ADP = adenosine diphosphate

The forward reaction is favored at pH 9.4, and the reverse reaction is favored at pH 7.4.

CK is a dimer [20] of MW 86,000. The cytosolic isoenzymes of CK are formed by the association of M and/or B CK polypeptide subunits in one of three possible combinations: (1) BB-CK, consisting of two B subunits, derives its name from brain tissue, where it is the most abundant form of cytosolic CK synthesized; (2) MM-CK, the predominant form of CK present in skeletal muscle, is composed of two M subunits; (3) MB-CK is a heterodimer composed of one of each of the cytosolic polypeptide chains. The mitochondrial isoenzyme is a homodimer whose two polypeptide chains differ from the M and B chains antigenically, biochemically, and by charge [21–23].

At pH 7.4, mitochondrial CK has a net positive charge, MM-CK is isoelectric, and BB-CK has a net negative charge; MB-CK has charge intermediate between MM-CK and BB-CK. These differences have been exploited to differentially assay the isoenzymes (see below), as well as for the purposes of isoenzyme purification.

Creatine kinase is enzymatically active only in the dimeric form. The three cytosolic isoenzymes can be induced to dissociate and randomly reassociate in solution by quick-freezing and thawing [20]; in this way, all three isoenzymes can be synthesized using any two isoenzymes as the initial substrate. However, mitochondrial CK monomers do not reassociate with the M-CK or B-CK polypeptide [24].

The M, B, and mitochondrial polypeptide chains are each encoded by a separate gene; available evidence suggests that each gene exists as a single copy per haploid human genome [25]. The cDNAs encoding both cytosolic human polypeptides have been cloned in our laboratory, and the full cDNA sequences determined [25, 26]. The genomic nucleotide sequence of the cytosolic forms is currently being elucidated.

Available data implicate CK in the coordination of adenosine triphosphate (ATP) production in the mitochondria with cellular energy demand in the cytoplasm via the "creatine phosphate shuttle" [27–29]. In this facilitated diffusion model, creatine present in mitochondria is phosphorylated by the mitochondrial CK isoenzyme, utilizing ATP generated in the mitochondria by oxidative phosphorylation. The creatine phosphate thus formed diffuses across the mitochondrial membrane into the cytosol, where in the presence of adenosine diphosphate (ADP) and cytosolic CK, ATP and creatine are regenerated in the reverse CK reaction. ATP is then used as an energy source in the cell; creatine diffuses back into the mitochondria. In addition to providing a link between cellular energy demand and ATP production, cytosolic creatine phosphate can act as an energy "buffer" against sudden bursts of energy utilization [29]. Although this model explains a great deal of accumulated experimental evidence [28], direct demonstration of ATP/ADP compartmentation is not yet available [29].

Immunohistochemical and cellular fractionation studies have demonstrated at least some degree of subcellular compartmentation of cytosolic CK. The tail portion of myosin has binding sites for MM-CK [30]; approximately 5 percent of cellular MM-CK activity is associated with the M-line of the sarcomere in both heart and skeletal muscle [31, 32]. In addition, antibodies directed against B-CK bind to the sarcomeric Z-line in heart muscle [33].

Small amounts of MM-CK have also been detected immunochemically and by differential centrifugation in association with the nuclear membrane [34], sarcolemma [35], and sarcoplasmic reticulum [36]. Subcellular compartmentation of "cytosolic" CK may provide optimum localization of ATP regeneration (e.g., at the contractile apparatus or adjacent to sarcolemmal Na^+/K^+-ATPase), in line with its function as the cytosolic limb of the "creatine phosphate shuttle." Mitochondrial CK is localized to the outer surface of the inner mitochondrial membrane [37].

The CK isoenzymes vary significantly in terms of their stability. The cytosolic isoenzymes have been shown to undergo two forms of inactivation [38]: (1) reversible inactivation due to oxidation of thiol groups, which may be prevented (or partially reversed) by storage with a thiol "activator" compound, which acts as a reducing agent; and (2) irreversible inactivation, probably as a consequence of thermal denaturation. MM-CK is the most stable of the isoenzymes; little loss of activity occurs even with storage at room temperature for several days. MB-CK loses activity quickly at room temperature but is stable at −20°C. However, because activity loss occurs with freezing and thawing, storage at 4°C is preferable for preservation of activity for short to intermediate periods (less than 1 week). MB-CK is also subject to photoinactivation; consequently, samples should be shielded from direct light [38]. BB-CK and mitochondrial CK are labile molecules; substantial loss of activity occurs within hours of sample collection; therefore specimens stored without freezing are unlikely to demonstrate these isoenzymes unless assayed immediately after collection.

Samples for CK assay may be collected and stored as either plasma or serum. If an anticoagulant is employed for plasma collection, EGTA should be used rather than EDTA because the latter has a much higher affinity for Mg^{2+}, a required cation for CK activity. In our laboratory, samples are collected in tubes pretreated with β-mercaptoethanol and EGTA so that the final concentration after blood collection is approximately 10 m*M* for both compounds. β-Mercaptoethanol has been shown to be the most effective thiol "activator" agent and is most efficient when added to the sample at the time of collection rather than at the time of assay [38]. Glutathione should not be used as activator, as the serum enzyme glutathione reductase uses this molecule as a proton donor to reduce NADP, yielding false elevations in the CK assay (see below). In addition to serving as an anticoagulant, EGTA affords a protective effect on CK activity independent of mercaptoethanol. Finally, EGTA acts as an inhibitor of serum carboxypeptidase, an important consideration if MM-CK or MB-CK subforms are to be assayed; this subject is discussed at length in the final section.

Creatine kinase molecules of very high molecular weight have been detected in the blood. It is now clear that these "macro-CK" molecules consist of polymerized aggregates of CK. Macro-CK-1, which migrates between MM-CK and MB-CK on gel electrophoresis, is formed by antibody-induced polymerization of CK, most often involving the BB isoenzyme. The antibodies are usually of the immunoglobulin G (IgG) type [39]. Macro-CK-2 consists of polymerized molecules of mitochondrial CK [40]; the mechanism of polymerization is not known. CK-2 migrates close to MM-CK on gel electrophoresis. Both forms of macro-CK have been detected only in the blood of patients; they have not been recovered from cell extracts and therefore represent a post-translational modification rather than a distinct gene product. Other forms of CK include the modified subforms of MM-CK and MB-CK, which are discussed below.

Assay of Total and Isoenzyme Creatine Kinase Activity

Total Creatine Kinase Activity

Assay of total CK enzymatic activity is achieved by a three-step, coupled enzyme system proposed by Oliver [41] and modified by Rosalki [42].

Results of the kinetic CK assay are expressed in international units of activity per liter (IU/L), with 1 IU defined by the International Convention on Biochemistry as the quantity of enzyme required to generate 1 micromole (μmol) of product from 1 μmol of substrate in 1 minute at 30°C. CK activity, like that of most enzymes, is temperature-dependent. Although the temperature at which CK activity is reported is not uniform among clinical laboratories, the relation of any given sample to the reference range is maintained regardless of temperature. CK activity at 37°C may be converted to standard temperature (30°C).

Isoenzyme Assays

The cytosolic CK isoenzymes may be assayed by a wide variety of techniques. The methods may be broadly categorized as those that separate the isoenzymes on the basis of charge differences and those that exploit the antigenic properties of the isoenzymes.

Methods Based on Isoenzyme Charge Differences

The most commonly employed CK isoenzyme assay is electrophoresis on agarose [43]. Serum or plasma is diluted to a uniform total CK activity (usually 300 IU/L), and a small volume is applied to the well of a precast gel; constant voltage is then applied for 15 minutes. The gel acts as an inert support matrix, allowing free movement of water and CK molecules in the electrical field. Migration progresses according to molecular charge (Fig. 6-1); the negatively charged BB isoenzyme, if present in the sample, moves most rapidly toward the positive electrode. MB-CK, having a relative intermediate negative charge, also moves toward the anode, but less rapidly than BB-CK; MM-CK, with little net charge at physiologic pH, remains near the origin. An alternative nomenclature for the cytosolic isoenzymes is based on these charge differences. By convention, isoenzymes are designated by speed of electrophoretic migration toward the positive electrode. Consequently, the most negative isoenzyme (BB-CK) is also designated CK-1, MB-CK as CK-2, and MM-CK as CK-3. After completion of electrophoresis, the gel is uniformly overlaid with the ''Rosalki reagent,'' described above, and incubated for 5 minutes at 37°C. NADPH is generated in situ at the location of the CK isoenzymes on the gel. The intensity of fluorescence of the isoenzyme bands under ultraviolet light is compared by scanning densitometry and expressed as a relative percent. This technique has been improved significantly. Previously, difficulty with standardization of agarose side chains and electroendosmotic force, as well as lack of uniformity of pore size for cellulose acetate, resulted in significant lot-to-lot variability in gel performance. These problems have been resolved, and currently available ''second generation'' gels are uniform in thickness, agarose side chain characteristics, pore size, electroendosmotic force generation, and performance [44, 45]. In contrast to older systems, which were unable to detect MB-CK levels within the normal range (consequently, any detectable serum MB-CK was considered pathologic), present systems are sensitive for MB-CK at levels well within the normal range.

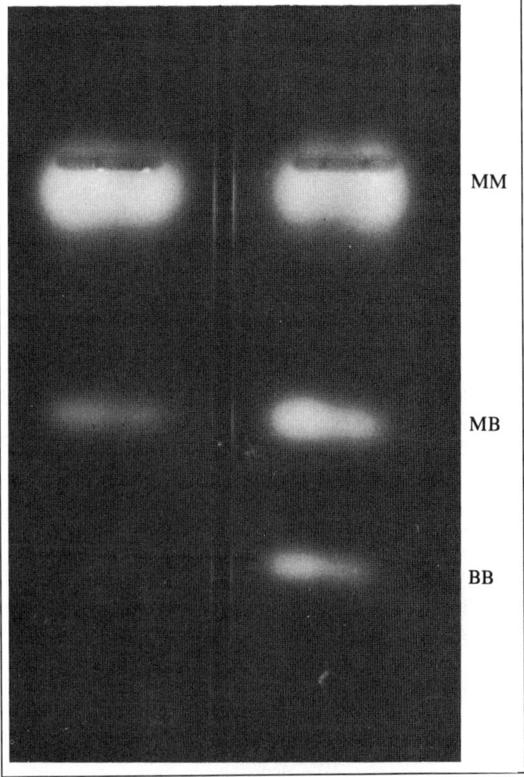

Fig. 6-1
Cytosolic CK isoenzymes detected by agarose gel electrophoresis. Right lane: Control containing heat-inactivated serum and all three purified isoenzymes. MM-CK remains near the origin; BB-CK, having a net negative change, shows the greatest migration toward the anode; and MB-CK is visible between MM-CK and BB-CK. Left lane: Serum from a patient with AMI. Although MM-CK predominates, a definite MB-CK band, constituting 12 percent of the total CK activity, is visible.

Nevertheless, electrophoresis still has several drawbacks compared with other available isoenzyme assays. One consistent problem has been an adequate definition of what constitutes a ''normal'' study. Because of the insensitivity of early electrophoretic systems, the appearance of any activity in the MB-CK range was associated with infarction in most cases. However, with the development of more sensitive systems, MB-CK bands were frequently detected in normal sera; as a result, the definition of a pathologic elevation of MB-CK has been selected as more than 3, 4, or 5 percent (depending on the author) of total CK activity [46]. These cutoff values are clearly adequate to distinguish patients suffering a moderate or large AMI from the normal population.

However, the significance of mild elevations of percent MB-CK (<10 percent of total CK activity) when total CK is only slightly elevated is not clear. In addition, because the electrophoretic assay is not kinetic, it is accurate only when conditions remain in the linear range for both MM-CK and MB-CK. If serum containing high total CK activity is assayed, MM-CK quickly exhausts the Rosalki substrate, whereas MB-CK continues to generate NADPH. Consequently, serum having high total CK activity may yield artifactually elevated MB-CK values. Appropriate dilution of the sample to 300 to 500 IU/L prior to electrophoresis circumvents this problem. Another limitation of electrophoresis is artifact due to naturally fluorescing products in serum, such as albumin-bound bilirubin [47, 48]; a similar effect may be produced by certain drugs (see below). These artifacts do not interfere with kinetic assays, which determine CK activity by the change in ultraviolet absorbance over time; in contrast, electrophoresis provides only a ''snapshot'' of cumulative fluorescence. Non-CK artifact can usually be identified by inspection of the gel, as artifactual bands differ in color from the blue fluorescence of NADPH, and their migration on the gel usually does not correspond exactly with that of MM-CK or MB-CK. Such distinctions may be missed if gels are not examined by an experienced technician prior to densitometry.

The use of controls on each gel to define MB-CK position is helpful for defining artifact. If questions remain as to the source of a band, reagent containing all substrates required for the coupled Rosalki reactions except creatine phosphate, the specific CK substrate, is available; the persistence of a fluorescing band in a gel incubated with this modified reagent identifies its source as non-CK.

Finally, an important problem with electrophoretic detection of MB-CK is the need for individual sample processing by experienced personnel and the long time required to perform the assay (30 to 45 minutes). These factors are largely responsible for the limited frequency with which MB-CK assays are performed in most clinical laboratories; in most laboratories ''stat'' determinations are not available even though these results may be important for patient triage from the coronary care unit (CCU). ''Third generation'' high-voltage systems with robotic sample application, rapid electrophoresis, and automated densitometry may overcome these problems.

Other MB-CK assays based on isoenzyme charge differences rely on the selective binding of the more negatively charged MB isoenzyme to an ion-exchange resin, consisting of a positively charged inert matrix equilibrated with buffer. In the minicolumn assay, the sample is loaded onto a column packed with the positively charged resin; MB-CK and BB-CK electrostatically bind to the matrix, whereas the neutral MM-CK molecules pass directly through the column. Subsequent elutions with higher concentrations of sodium chloride displace MB-CK from the column by competition of the negatively charged B polypeptide with chloride ions for the resin-binding sites. BB-CK may be eluted in the same fashion. CK activity is then assayed in the collected eluate [49]. This assay has not achieved widespread clinical use, in large measure because of problems with carryover of MM-CK into the MB-CK fractions, especially when the applied sample contains high MM-CK activity [17].

The batch absorption assay of Henry et al. [50] employs glass beads coated with an ion-exchange resin. Plasma is mixed with the glass beads, and the resin binds MB-CK; MM-CK is removed by several rinses with low ionic strength buffer. MB-CK is then eluted from the beads by a high salt buffer, and CK activity is assayed by the Rosalki method. Carryover of MM-CK is not a problem because of the multiple low salt washes. This technique is sensitive (95 percent), efficient, precise, and reproducible (coefficient of variation $\pm$ 5 percent) [50, 51], and it can be completed in 5 minutes by personnel with minimal experience. In addition, results are quantitative rather than semiquantitative and are obtained in absolute MB-CK activity (IU/L), rather than as a percent of total CK. Because of these advantages over the more popular electrophoretic assays, we use this method as the standard

CK isoenzyme assay at our institution. We now have experience with more than 200,000 assays using this system; sensitivity and specificity both exceed 95 percent. Samples are routinely analyzed eight times a day, with "stat" tests performed on request. This procedure has allowed more expeditious turnover of patients in the CCU, as patients having serial normal plasma MB-CK activities within 18 to 24 hours of the onset of symptoms may be transferred to less expensive non-CCU beds. It also reduces the incidence of "overflow" of coronary patients to other acute care units. A disadvantage of the glass bead assay is that BB-CK is measured along with MB-CK. However, BB-CK is rarely detectable in plasma by any available assay; when it has been detected by other methods, the level is almost always less than 5 IU/L. Thus even if it is erroneously measured as MB-CK, it is not a sufficient increment to lead to diagnostic confusion [52].

Immunoassays

Immunoassays constitute the second major group of CK isoenzyme assays. The differences in charge, amino acid sequence, and conformation of the M and B polypeptide chains have permitted the development of antibodies that differentially recognize one chain or the other.

Immunoinhibition. Immunoinhibition assays measure MB-CK enzymatic activity by selectively inactivating M-CK subunits with an M-specific antibody. MM-CK and the M subunit of MB-CK are inhibited; consequently, residual activity is attributed to B subunit activity of the MB isoenzyme (as well as BB-CK, if present) [53].

Immunoprecipitation. Immunoprecipitation is similar to immunoinhibition except subunit-specific antibodies are used to precipitate rather than directly inhibit target CK. Anti-M-CK antibody is used to precipitate MM-CK and MB-CK; residual activity is attributed to serum BB-CK. In a separate aliquot, anti-B-CK antibody is employed to precipitate MB-CK and BB-CK; residual activity is due to MM-CK. These two results are then combined to determine MB-CK activity, as total CK activity minus MM-CK and BB-CK activity must equal MB-CK activity [53]. This technique is obviously indirect, and substantial assay-to-assay variability [54] has led to its disuse.

Radioimmunoassay. Radioimmunoassays (RIAs) constitute the most sensitive means available for detecting MB-CK. A radiolabeled ligand (e.g., ^{125}I-labeled BB-CK) is added to the serum sample. A B-subunit-specific antibody is then added, and unlabeled serum MB-CK competes with the labeled BB-CK for antibody binding sites. Higher concentrations of MB-CK in the serum result in more competition with radiolabeled BB-CK for the antibody binding sites; thus less radioactivity is bound and precipitated by the anti-B-CK antibody. Patient samples are assayed in parallel with controls containing known quantities of unlabeled MB-CK. Unlike previously described assays, which quantitate CK in terms of its enzymatic function (expressed in IU/L), the RIA directly quantitates protein mass, expressed as micrograms of CK protein per milliliter (μg/ml). These assays are able to detect as little as 0.2 μg of MB-CK/ml (equivalent to 0.08 IU of CK activity per liter), with an upper limit of normal of 40 μg/L [55], and are precise. However, they have not achieved widespread use because they are somewhat cumbersome and necessitate use of a radionuclide.

ELISA. The enzyme-linked immunosorbent assay, or ELISA, utilizes two antibodies, each recognizing one of the two CK subunits. Anti-M-CK antibody, bound to a solid-phase inert matrix, is exposed to the plasma sample where both MM-CK and MB-CK bind. After washing away unbound CK, the system is flooded with a buffer containing anti-B-CK antibody linked to a "reporter molecule" (alkaline phosphatase or horseradish peroxidase). The labeled second antibody attaches to previously bound MB-CK molecules. The concentration of "sandwiched" MB isoenzyme can be determined by the intensity of a colorimetric reaction mediated by the reporter groups on the second antibody [56].

Monoclonal Antibodies. All polyclonal antibodies developed to date recognize either the M or the B polypeptide subunit and therefore react with both MB-CK and one of the two homodimers. A monoclonal antibody has been developed that recognizes an epitope unique to MB-CK and does not cross react with the MM or BB isoenzymes [57]. This antibody, linked to polystyrene beads, extracts MB-CK from serum, with subsequent assay of the bound isoenzyme using colorimetric detection [57, 58].

The recent development of a monoclonal antibody-based system that reacts specifically to MB-CK has significantly improved both sensitivity and specificity for the diagnosis of myocardial infarction. The monoclonal antibody has been coupled to another enzyme system, making it possible to assay in a colorimetric system—one of the more popular methods uses alkaline phosphotase. With this approach, the assay can be performed in about 10 to 15 minutes and it is possible to automate as well as batch the procedure [152–154]. This approach is most applicable to laboratories processing large volumes and the assays are run in batches rather than individually. This system is now widely used and is rapidly replacing the assays based on polyclonal antibodies and many of the assays based on the immunoassay inhibition system. Each system has its own specific sensitivity and specificity as well as normal range, but in general, most of them have an upper limit of around 9 to 12 ng/ml. It is expected that although many laboratories are still performing electrophoresis, many others will probably switch to this technique because it is rapid, sensitive, specific, and provides a more quantitative approach to assessing serial changes in MB-CK.

Creatine Kinase Isoenzyme Tissue Distribution

Skeletal Muscle

The predominance of MM-CK characteristic of mature skeletal muscle develops relatively late in fetal life. During the first 6 weeks of development only BB-CK is synthesized in fetal skeletal muscle. During the subsequent weeks, M-CK chain synthesis is induced and rapidly supplants B-CK, so that by the eighth week in utero, MB-CK is the most abundant cytosolic isoenzyme, and after the twelfth week MM-CK predominates [59, 60]. By the time of birth, MM-CK constitutes 80 percent of total cystolic CK activity in skeletal muscle [59].

Whether MB-CK is completely absent from adult skeletal muscle or present in small quantities has been the subject of some disagreement. Several investigators have found small quantities of MB-CK in normal adult skeletal muscle [61, 62], whereas others have failed to detect any cytosolic CK other than MM-CK [63, 64]. In a large study by Tsung and Tsung [61], biopsies of normal skeletal muscle were removed from 109 patients at the time of surgery; MB-CK was detected in 44 percent of all muscles tested, usually representing 1 to 3 percent of total CK activity. There was no muscle or muscle group that consistently demonstrated the presence of MB-CK.

Data from several laboratories have demonstrated that injured skeletal muscle synthesizes MB-CK at levels in excess of those reported for normal muscle. Levels of MB-CK representing 7.5 percent or more of total cytosolic CK activity have been detected in muscles affected by chronic exercise [65, 66], inflammation [67], trauma [68]; electrical current [68, 69], or genetic disease [70]. This increased skeletal muscle MB-CK synthesis is also reflected by steady-state plasma MB-CK levels exceeding normal values [67, 71]. The biologic importance of MB-CK synthesis in injured muscle is unknown. It has been postulated that the population of undifferentiated satellite cells, which can differentiate to form mature skeletal myocytes following muscle injury, repeats the developmental program of fetal skeletal muscle [72]. The potential significance of skeletal muscle MB-CK synthesis as a confounding factor in the diagnosis of AMI is discussed below.

Myocardium

Mature human myocardium contains approximately 1600 IU of CK activity/L/gm of tissue. It is the only tissue that harbors a substantial quantity of MB-CK, with 15 to 20 percent of cytosolic CK activity present as the MB isoenzyme; the remaining soluble CK is MM-CK. The adult myocardium of small mammals (rat, mouse, rabbit) contains little or no MB-CK; however, induction of MB-CK synthesis (as well as other proteins characteristic of fetal myocardium) has been observed to accompany pressure-induced hypertrophy. It has been reported that healthy cardiac tissue, like normal skeletal muscle, synthesizes only MM-CK, with MB-CK synthesis occurring only in the presence of cardiac ischemia or hypertrophy [73]. This report has not been substantiated by others and conflicts with earlier data from normal human hearts obtained at necropsy [74]. Other primates studied have approximately 15 percent of myocardial CK activity as the MB isoenzyme [75]. MB-CK in plasma has been observed to rise following catheter-directed fulgurative ablation of atrioventricular nodal bypass tracts in hearts unaffected by ischemia or hypertrophy [76]. Furthermore, we have observed a typical rise and fall of plasma MB-CK following iatrogenic dissection of a normal right coronary artery in a young man undergoing evaluation of a cardiac murmur that was determined to be functional. Thus the weight of data supports a level of 15 percent MB-CK in nondiseased human myocardium. Whether additional accumulation of the MB isoenzyme occurs with hypertrophy remains to be determined.

Other Organs

BB-CK remains the predominant cytosolic isoenzyme in brain from development through adult life [77]. Organs other than heart, brain, and skeletal muscle, including those rich in nonstriated muscle such as the gut, uterus, and urinary bladder, contain relatively low levels of CK per gram of tissue (Fig. 6-2). More importantly from a diagnostic standpoint, none synthesizes significant quantities of MB-CK. However, the brain, gastrointestinal tract, prostate, and uterus are rich in BB-CK (Fig. 6-2); consequently, injury to these organs may result in misdiagnosis of AMI if plasma is assayed by a method that does not discriminate between MB-CK and BB-CK.

The effect of injury or disease on CK content per gram of tissue and CK isoenzyme distribution has been less well studied in tissue other than striated muscle. CK production in neoplasms, most commonly involving the lung, breast, and kidney, has been reported [78]. BB-CK is the isoenzyme most commonly detected in such tumors, but any of the cytosolic isoenzymes may occur. These tumors may cause diagnostic confusion by releasing CK into the blood. The concentration of CK per gram of tissue, predominant isoenzyme synthesized, and level of CK present in the blood do not correlate reliably with the type of tumor or its degree of differentiation.

Creatine Kinase Isoenzymes in Acute Myocardial Infarction

Time Course

Following the onset of AMI, blood levels of total CK and MB-CK do not exceed the normal range until 6 to 10 hours after the onset of symptoms; plasma levels then rise steadily until peak values occur an average of 24 hours after the onset of symptoms. Peak CK occurs somewhat later (28 hours) with Q-wave infarctions and somewhat earlier (15 hours) with non-Q-wave infarctions [79]. Peak values of MB-CK are achieved slightly earlier for MB-CK than for MM-CK, probably because the former is cleared from the blood more rapidly.

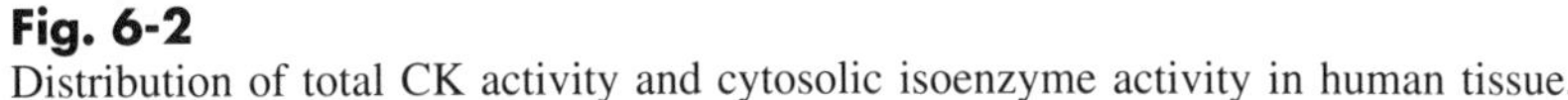
Fig. 6-2
Distribution of total CK activity and cytosolic isoenzyme activity in human tissue.

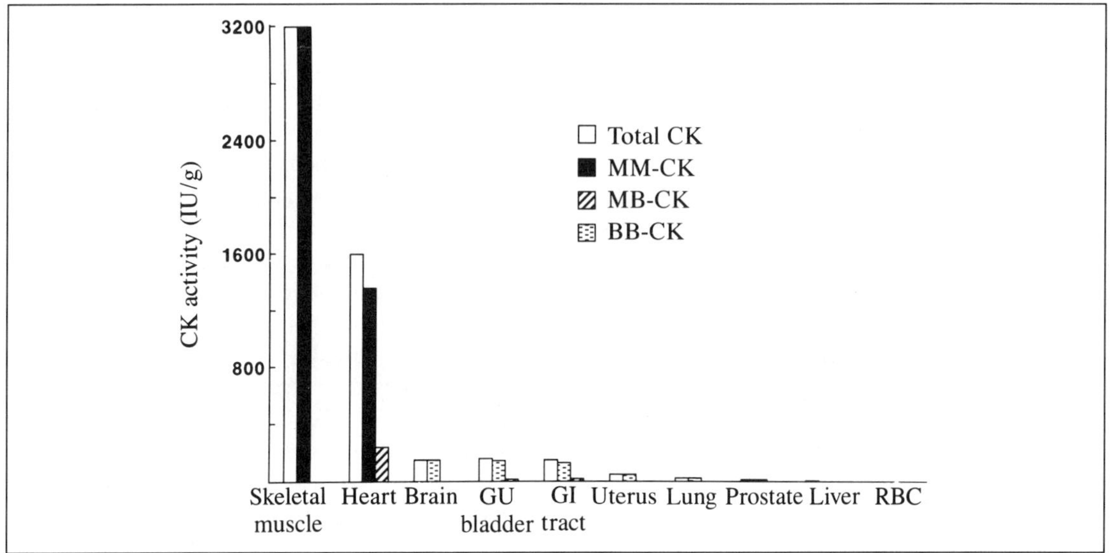

Values then gradually decline, entering the normal range by 48 to 72 hours after the onset of symptoms [19]. The MB-CK/MM-CK ratio (15:85) present in the myocardium is mirrored by a similar proportion in the blood following myocardial release after AMI. This approximate ratio is maintained throughout the CK time–activity curve.

Sensitivity and Specificity

The most important advantage of MB-CK over other biochemical markers of AMI is its great specificity for myocardium [80]. Myocardium is the only tissue that contains substantial levels of MB-CK (Fig. 6-2). The high myocardial CK activity levels, combined with the low concentration of MB-CK activity in normal plasma, which is close to the limit of detection of most assays, result in a high sensitivity of this marker for myocardial necrosis. It is generally agreed that assay of plasma MB-CK affords the most sensitive and specific, as well as cost-effective, means of diagnosing AMI. These parameters, of course, depend in part on the assay used, but for most assays the overall precision exceeds 95 percent [54, 81]. (The immunoprecipitation assays are exceptions and are substantially less reliable.) Use of the total CK assay data alone without isoenzyme study yields a similar sensitivity, but specificity is markedly lower (approximately 70 percent) [82, 83].

With the exception of the immune studies noted above, false-negative results are rare (as suggested by the high sensitivity figures) so long as blood sampling is performed within an appropriate time window. False-positive results, although also unusual, predictably occur in a variety of circumstances.

1. MB-CK may be released from tissue other than the heart. As outlined above, skeletal muscle can be induced to synthesize and release MB-CK by injury. This reaction has been documented in patients having a crush injury [68], an electrical injury [68, 69], dermatomyositis, polymyositis [67], and Duchenne's muscular dystrophy [84], as well as in professional athletes and marathon runners [65, 66]. Elevated levels of MB-CK have been documented not only in the blood of these patients but also directly in the skeletal muscle by analysis of extracts removed on biopsy of affected muscle. A study in our laboratory has demonstrated a late rise of MB-CK to levels above the normal range in 40 percent of individuals undergoing elective direct-current cardioversion of supraventricular arrhythmias, with peak values occurring an average of 40 hours after countershock (unpublished data). This time course corresponds to that observed following other forms of acute muscle injury and presumably reflects new synthesis and release of MB-CK by regenerating skeletal myocytes.

   Release of MB-CK by skeletal muscle is suggested by: (1) An appropriate clinical setting (e.g., skeletal muscle disease or trauma). (2) An atypical time course for AMI: persistent minor degrees of MB-CK elevation in inflammatory disorders, delayed rise of MB-CK (with an immediate rise of MM-CK) following trauma. (3) A low relative percent of MB-CK. Although muscle injury may elevate the absolute plasma MB-CK level, the rise in MB-CK rarely constitutes more than 5 to 10 percent of total CK activity. Note that this figure may be in excess of the electrophoretic definition of myocardial necrosis. (4) A marked elevation of total CK activity. Myocardial infarction rarely increases total CK activity to levels in excess of 20 times the upper limit of normal (about 2500 IU/L in our laboratory); furthermore, a rise of total CK activity in excess of ten times the upper limit of normal on the basis of AMI is usually the result of substantial myocardial necrosis and therefore should be associated with diagnostic electrocardiographic (ECG) changes (usually including Q waves). Absence of these changes should raise suspicion of a nonmyocardial source of MB-CK. It should also be emphasized that certain assays, including electrophoresis and column techniques, are especially vulnerable to artifactual elevation of MB-CK values in the setting of a marked elevation of MM-CK; this situation can be avoided by sample dilution at the time of assay.
2. Apparent MB-CK plasma activity may be elevated in the absence of AMI because of artifact or laboratory error. One cause of this elevation, gel or column overload with MM-CK, has already been discussed. Hemolysis can also lead to artifactually elevated total and MB-CK values due to adenylate kinase interference. A faint band on gel electrophoresis attributable to albu-

min-associated fluorescence [47] is detectable slightly anodal to the expected position of the MB-CK band in most normal plasma samples. Artifactual fluorescence may also be present in patients with renal insufficiency (with or without dialysis) [85] and in those taking drugs that bind serum albumin, including diazepam, chlordiazepoxide, tricyclic antidepressants, and aspirin in high doses. Artifact should be suspected when a band migrates in an unusual position relative to MB-CK controls; such non-MB-CK bands usually also differ in color from the NADPH-generated fluorescence resulting from MB-CK activity.

3. As discussed earlier, several techniques, including ion-exchange methods and immunoassays that recognize the B-CK subunit, may yield false elevations of MB-CK activity because they fail to distinguish between MB-CK and BB-CK activity. This failure occasionally leads to misdiagnosis in patients with injury or surgery involving the prostate, uterus, gastrointestinal tract, or brain [3, 52, 86, 87] and following spontaneous or cesarean delivery [88]. Release of BB-CK is not detectable following uncomplicated ischemic stroke [89], presumably due to the integrity of the blood-brain barrier, but it may be released into the blood after trauma, infection, or diffuse hypoxic brain injury [89, 90]. Finally, tumors may rarely synthesize and release BB-CK [78]. The presence of BB-CK in the plasma is unusual outside these settings; even when detectable, it is usually present in concentrations that are insufficient to result in the spurious elevation of MB-CK activity to levels above the reference range, and it is cleared from the blood rapidly [89].
4. Hypothyroidism has been associated with chronically elevated levels of plasma MM-CK and MB-CK. It is thought to be due to diminished plasma clearance of these isoenzymes by the reticuloendothelial system [91].
5. Macro-CK-1 may be detected as MB-CK in column assays and in immunoassays based on B-chain recognition [39, 92], resulting in a false-positive diagnosis of AMI. Macro-CK-1 is detected most commonly in the blood of elderly women and the chronically ill, with an incidence of 1.6 percent in hospitalized patients [39]. Correct diagnosis may be made by electrophoretic demonstration of band migration intermediate between control MM-CK and MB-CK bands. Macro-CK-2, when detected, is most often found in the blood of severely ill patients, possibly due to cell necrosis in the critically ill, with release of mitochondrial contents into the blood.

Current Role of MB-CK in Diagnosis of Acute Myocardial Infarction

Since the introduction of enzyme markers during the late 1950s, the diagnosis of AMI has traditionally rested on the presence of "two out of three" of the triad of prolonged chest pain, ischemic ECG changes, and elevation of one of the "cardiac enzymes" [93]. However, since that time the accuracy of enzyme diagnosis has improved dramatically, whereas the sensitivity and specificity of clinical symptoms and ECG changes remain relatively poor [81]. Given the excellent sensitivity of the plasma MB-CK assay for the detection of myocardial necrosis, the diagnosis of AMI should not be made in the absence of a diagnostic rise and fall of plasma MB-CK (or LD isoenzymes) provided samples have been obtained at appropriate intervals. Conversely, a rise and fall in MB-CK and total CK in the appropriate proportion and following the typical time course strongly suggests the diagnosis of infarction even when symptoms and ECG changes are not typical. (However, in such cases, spurious elevation of MB-CK due to artifact, BB-CK, macro-CK, or a nonmyocardial source of MB-CK should be sought, as dictated by the clinical setting [94].)

Several protocols have been suggested; for more than a decade we have obtained samples on admission and every 4 hours thereafter for 36 hours. Generally, the diagnosis of acute myocardial infarction is confirmed by 8 to 12 hours; sampling beyond 24 hours is seldom necessary. However, to detect early reinfarction, which is routine particularly in patients who have received thrombolytic therapy, sampling is continued for 36 to 48 hours. The glass bead assay [50] has an upper normal reference value of 14 IU/L. We consider the enzymatic data as positive for AMI if serial plasma samples separated by at least 4 hours exceed the upper reference range or if there is an increase in MB-CK of 50 percent between two samples, with at least one sample exceeding the upper reference limit. If only a single specimen is available, the diagnosis of AMI is made only if MB-CK exceeds the upper reference limit by at least 100 percent. In all cases without reperfusion, the values should return to the normal range within 48 to 72 hours. If successful reperfusion (<6 hours) is achieved with either thrombolysis or angioplasty, values are near normal in 24 to 36 hours.

Between 16 and 43 percent of all CCU patients in whom plasma MB-CK activity exceeds the upper normal range have normal values for total CK activity [95, 96]. Studies suggest that these patients have myocardial necrosis as the source of their MB-CK elevation, as the incidence of typical chest pain, new ECG changes, LD_1/LD_2 "flip," and time course of the MB-CK rise and fall are similar to that seen for AMI with elevated MB-CK *and* total CK activity [96, 97]. Histologic changes of AMI have been documented in one such patient at autopsy [95]. The long-term prognosis in these patients appears to be good in the absence of superimposed severe medical illness [97, 98].

Plasma MB-CK is also useful for the diagnosis of AMI following noncardiac surgery, when MM-CK may be elevated as a result of surgical trauma. In the absence of myocardial necrosis, MB-CK remains within the normal range [99]. Cardiac isoenzymes are not helpful following cardiac surgery, as even minimal surgical manipulation can release MB-CK; however, if MB-CK peak levels exceed 3- to 4-fold, it is highly suggestive. After angioplasty, about 10 to 20 percent of patients will have significant elevation of plasma MB-CK, which is thought to reflect minute myocardial injury. It is estimated that only 1 or 2 gm of myocardial necrosis is necessary to elevate plasma levels of MB-CK above the normal range.

Lactate Dehydrogenase Isoenzymes for the Diagnosis of Acute Myocardial Infarction

Biochemical Properties and Tissue Distribution of Lactate Dehydrogenase

LD is a tetramer of MW 135,000 that catalyzes the reversible reduction of pyruvate to form lactatic acid.

$$\text{Lactate} + \text{NAD} \xrightleftharpoons{\text{LD}} \text{pyruvate} + \text{NADH}$$

LD thus controls an important step in carbohydrate metabolism. Under normal aerobic conditions, pyruvate, a product of glycolysis, is irreversibly converted to acetyl coenzyme A, which then enters the citric acid cycle to generate ATP. However, under the anaerobic conditions that may exist in active muscle, pyruvate accumulates at a rate too rapid for immediate oxidation and is converted to lactate by LD. The lactic acid thus formed in muscle can enter the circulation and be transported to the liver, where it is converted to glucose by gluconeogenesis. Alternatively, the liver can oxidize lactate via LD to re-form pyruvate for oxidative phosphorylation.

Two LD subunit types exist: M type, which is so designated because the homotetramer M_4 is the predominant isoenzyme in skeletal muscle; and H type, which is named for heart tissue, where H_4 is the most abundant LD isoenzyme [100]. In addition to these two homotetramers, all three heterotetramers are found: H_3M_1, H_2M_2, and H_1M_3. Dissociated polypeptide chains are inactive; only the tetramer has enzymatic activity. As is the case for CK, the two polypeptide chains differ in sequence and charge: The H chain is more negatively charged; consequently, H_4 is the fastest-migrating LD isoenzyme by gel electrophoresis, M_4 is the slowest [101], and the three heterotetramers migrate between these two based on their M and H chain content. These facts are the basis of the standard nomenclature for the LD isoenzymes: $H_4 = LD_1$, $H_3M_1 = LD_2, \ldots, M_4 = LD_5$. The isoenzymes also differ in their biochemical characteristics: H_4 has a low K_m for pyruvate and is strongly inhibited by pyruvate; this isoenzyme favors the rapid oxidation of lactate to pyruvate in the heart; pyruvate thus formed can in turn enter the citric acid cycle. M_4 has a higher K_m for pyruvate and is not inhibited by pyruvate; it favors anaerobic metabolism in exercising muscle by converting pyruvate to lactate, which can then be transported to the liver for gluconeogenesis and resolution of the "oxygen debt." The heterotetramers have biochemical properties intermediate between the two homotetramers.

The LD molecule is stable. Enzymatic activity is maximally preserved by storage at room temperature; refrigeration results in loss of activity [102], with relatively greater loss of LD_5 and the other M-containing isoenzymes. Serum is usually assayed rather than plasma, as platelets in plasma are rich in LD activity and may result in spurious elevation.

In addition, red blood cells have abundant LD activity, especially LD_1 and LD_2; therefore it is important that samples not be hemolyzed.

Assay of total LD activity may be achieved by detecting the rate of NADH production (monitored by the rate of change at ultraviolet absorbance: 340 nm) from lactate and NAD in the presence of an aliquot of serum. Isoenzyme assay is by gel electrophoresis and densitometry; no column or immune assays are in current use. The hydroxybutyrate dehydrogenase (HBD) assay gives indirect information on LD isoenzymes. This method employs 2-oxybutyrate rather than lactate as a substrate. Because 2-oxybutyrate is preferentially reduced by LD_1 and LD_2, LD release by myocardium results in substantial HBD assay elevations. This assay is less specific than electrophoresis, as LD_4 and LD_5, although lower in HBD activity than LD_1 and LD_2, do yield some signal. As a result of these drawbacks, this technique is not commonly used. Selective inactivation of LD_4 and LD_5 by heating to 56° to 65°C suffers from similar problems. Consequently, gel electrophoresis is the most widely used method for assay of LD isoenzymes.

Although LD_1 is the most abundant LD isoenzyme present in cardiac tissue, making up about one-half of the LD activity present in myocardium, other tissues are also rich in LD_1: kidney, erythrocytes, pancreas, and gastric smooth muscle contain 30 percent or more of total LD activity as the LD_1 isoenzyme. Consequently, a rise in serum LD_1 activity alone is not specific for myocardial necrosis.

Serum Lactate Dehydrogenase for the Diagnosis of Acute Myocardial Infarction

The LD activity in the blood rises out of the normal range by 10 hours after the onset of AMI. Peak blood levels are reached between 24 and 48 hours after the onset of symptoms. Unlike CK, LD demonstrates a prolonged decline, so that serum levels do not return to the normal range until 10 to 14 days after infarction; consequently, sample collection need not be more frequent than once daily. Clearance of LD from the blood is governed by specific receptors in the surface of the cells of the reticuloendothelial system [103]. The isoenzyme profile in the blood following infarction reflects that seen in myocardium, i.e., predominance of LD_1. The LD_1/LD_2 ratio has been used to distinguish serum LD elevations due to myocardial injury from those arising from other sources. An LD_1/LD_2 ratio that is greater than or equal to 1.0 is generally regarded as the cutoff for the diagnosis of AMI. A ratio of 0.76 has also been recommended; it affords a greater sensitivity but a lower specificity than the higher cutoff [81]. Muscle or liver injury, the most common sources of elevated serum LD activity, are distinguished from cardiac necrosis by the preponderance of LD_4 and LD_5 associated with these conditions. However, injury of skeletal muscle may, in a manner analogous to CK, induce reexpression of LD_1 and LD_2 [104–106], the "fetal" isoenzymes. The effect of this response on the specificity of the LD diagnosis of AMI in the presence of skeletal injury is unclear. LD isoenzyme release patterns due to disease involving the kidney, pancreas, and stomach may be difficult to distinguish from that associated with AMI. Germ cell tumors may also give a false-positive pattern for AMI [107]. Hemolysis, either intravascular or occurring after specimen collection, also releases LD_1. Because of the widespread tissue distribution of LD and the overlap of the isoenzyme profile between tissues, no method can be entirely satisfactory for distinguishing cardiac from noncardiac sources of enzyme release. As a result, when both are available, CK isoenzyme analysis is preferable to LD isoenzyme assay for the diagnosis of AMI. However, if blood samples are not available for the first 48 hours after the suspected myocardial injury, the sustained elevation of serum LD makes assay and isoenzyme fractionation of this marker a more reliable indicator of infarction than CK.

Other Biochemical Markers of Acute Myocardial Infarction

Serum Myoglobin

Myoglobin is a heme-containing protein of MW 17,800. Because of its affinity for molecular oxygen, it is believed to function as an "oxygen reservoir" in striated muscle. Myoglobin is present in high levels in both skeletal and cardiac muscle [108, 109], with no known tissue-specific isoenzymes; thus, it is not a specific marker of AMI. Myoglobin functions as an oxygen carrier rather than as a catalyst; therefore, its activity is measured immunologically by RIA rather than by enzymatic activity. Following AMI, myoglobin rapidly appears in the blood with detectable elevation as early as 1.5 hours after the onset of symptoms [110]. This early rise is probably a result of its low molecular weight and rapid diffusing capacity. Its relatively small molecular size also permits clearance of myoglobin through the glomerular filtration apparatus (hence the danger of myoglobin precipitation in the renal tubules and acute renal failure following massive skeletal muscle injury). Renal clearance of myoglobin is the mechanism for the rapid decline in serum levels after peak concentrations occur at 4 to 6 hours [111]; plasma myoglobin levels often return to the normal range within 24 hours after onset of symptoms [110, 111]. Thus, this marker may be falsely negative within 24 hours of AMI in patients who have sustained a small infarction. The low specificity of myoglobin for cardiac muscle injury remains the major drawback for the use of this molecule as a diagnostic marker of AMI [112, 113]. However, the recent need for a noninvasive marker of reperfusion has rekindled interest in myoglobin. In view of its rapid release and disappearance, studies suggest frequent sampling may provide a rapid increase in plasma levels following successful lysis with thrombolytic therapy as opposed to lack of lysis with thrombolytic therapy. This approach has been limited in part because of the time required to perform the myoglobin assay. Recent developments [155–161] of a rapid assay for myoglobin minimized the limitation and studies are now being performed to determine the specificity and sensitivity of myoglobin as a marker for reperfusion.

In contrast to the radioimmunoassay that required several hours to perform and was often difficult to batch as a clinical laboratory-based assay, several new assays are now available [162]. All these assays are based on an antibody specific for myoglobin; however, they have been extensively modified so that the procedure can be performed within 10 to 15 minutes. The procedure is relatively inexpensive and makes possible obtaining quantitative results over a very broad range of concentrations from 1 to 1,500 μg/L [163–166]. Several techniques have surfaced, all of which use a fluoro detection method of turpidity. The most recent assay, known as immunonephlometric, is suggested for use when qualitative rapid analysis of myoglobin is needed, such as in the emergency room [161]. This test, which takes about 15 minutes and has linearity adequate for about 1,500 μg/L, appears to give reliable results. It is of interest that with this rapid assay, myoglobin may also play a small role in the emergency room since finding very high levels of myoglobin in a patient who does not otherwise have reason to release myoglobin would certainly be suggestive of myocardial infarction. Thus, myoglobin may have a role to play in the future management of patients with myocardial infarction destined for early thrombolytic therapy. In patients undergoing thrombolytic therapy, myoglobin is now being carefully assessed as a possible marker to detect successful reperfusion [165]. Several studies indicate that within 45 to 60 minutes of successful reperfusion, there is a marked elevation of the plasma myoglobin [167, 168]. Samples obtained every 15 to 30 minutes over the subsequent 3 to 4 hours after thrombolytic therapy should provide adequate assessment as to whether reperfusion has occurred. Katus et al. [14] suggest that for those patients treated with thrombolytic therapy within the first 4 hours of onset of symptoms, myoglobin sample delivery within 20 to 30 minutes is likely to provide adequate sensitivity and specificity during the next subsequent hours as a means of determining whether further therapy is required to restore perfusion [165]. It is highly likely that the immunonephlometric assay will become a part of patient management following thrombolytic therapy.

Myosin Light Chains

The myosin light chains (MLCs), which are covalently linked to the myosin heavy chain together with the amino half of the myosin heavy chain make up the "head" region of the molecule. This portion of the myosin molecule is the site of ATPase activity necessary for myofilament sliding and disengagement, a critical element of the contractile apparatus. Apparently, the covalent disulfide linkages joining the two MLC molecules to each myosin heavy chain undergo breakdown following myocardial necrosis, liberating MLC into the circulation. The mechanism of this process is unknown; it has been postulated that enzymes released by inflammatory cells at the site of infarction play a role in this process [114]; acidification of the infarcted region may also be important [115]. MLC-2 appears in the serum following AMI [116], with detectable levels within 6 hours of the onset of

AMI [117]. Peak serum levels, however, do not occur until about 5 days after AMI, presumably due to ongoing liberation of MLC from the contractile apparatus [117]. MLC-1 has also been studied as a marker of AMI [118]. Clearance of these low-molecular-weight (MW 20,000 to 27,000) markers is via the kidney. When separated from the myosin heavy chain, MLC has no enzymatic activity, and thus detection is by RIA. MLC in the diagnosis of AMI is currently under investigation but is not in routine clinical use.

Troponin T

The most recent enzymatic marker being evaluated for myocardial infarction is troponin T. Troponin is part of the tropomyosin protein complex found on the thin filament of the sarcomeric contractile apparatus. Troponin is a complex of three individual proteins with separate functions. Troponin C binds calcium, troponin T binds to myosin and troponin I has an inhibitory function [167–170]. Troponin T in the myocardium is uniquely different from troponin T found in skeletal muscle, which accounts for its cardiac diagnostic specificity. The plasma time-activity profile of troponin T is initially very similar to MB-CK. After myocardial infarction, troponin T is released minimally in the first 4 to 8 hours; levels having diagnostic reliability are reached after 8 to 10 hours. Levels of troponin T peak at 48 to 72 hours and because of its long half-life remain elevated for 2 to 3 weeks. Thus, troponin T has an advantage as a diagnostic marker for late infarction. However, the high background may be prohibitive for diagnosing early reinfarction. Although the cardiac specificity of troponin T has been well documented, troponin T is unlikely to add an advantage over MB-CK since it does not provide an earlier diagnosis and it lacks the sensitivity for early reinfarction. Another disadvantage is that the assay used to detect troponin T, an immunoassay inhibition technique, requires up to 90 minutes for processing.

Infarct Size Determination Using MB-CK Assay

Serial analysis of plasma MB-CK samples has been used to provide accurate estimates of infarct size. The use of enzymatically determined infarct size as an endpoint to assess therapy would permit accumulation of data from each patient; far fewer patients would be required in such a study than in a comparable trial in which death or other infrequent clinical events are monitored as primary endpoints [119].

Studies during the early 1970s in the rabbit model demonstrated that CK is homogeneously distributed throughout the ventricle and that the CK activity detectable in the ventricle following AMI is diminished; furthermore, the magnitude of CK activity depletion is directly proportional to infarct size as determined histologically [120]. Studies in the dog model allowed quantitation of this relation based on plasma CK activity following a series of experimental observations: (1) a region of infarcted myocardium loses 85 percent of endogenous CK activity—the magnitude of this CK depletion from the expected CK activity of the entire ventricle is directly proportional to infarct size; (2) most "depleted" CK is inactivated in situ or in the cardiac lymphatic system; however, a predictable fraction (15 percent) of the depleted CK is released into the blood [121]; (3) serial plasma CK determinations allow accurate quantitation of cumulative CK release into the blood.

Since only a fraction of the CK depleted from the myocardium appears in the blood, a release ratio is used to calculate the amount of CK depleted from the myocardium as a result of the infarction. This estimated ratio based on experimental studies is 15%. The quality of depleted CK activity is subsequently converted to infarct size in grams of tissue, as the CK content of human myocardium is known. This method has been validated by comparing the enzymatic determination of infarct size with gross pathologic results in the animal model [123] and in humans [124]. Furthermore, enzymatic determination of infarct size in humans has been shown to be predictive of postinfarction hemodynamics [125], ejection fraction [126], prognosis [127], and incidence of ventricular arrhythmias [128].

The relations outlined above were developed and confirmed in the experimental and clinical setting of nonreperfused AMI. Reperfusion within 6 hours of the onset of AMI causes a change in the kinetics of myocardial CK release, resulting in an altered CK time–activity curve. Early reperfusion is associated with a reduction in the time from onset of infarction to peak CK, as well as an increase in the magnitude of peak CK relative to total infarct size. This is especially evident with reperfusion occurring less than 4 hours after the onset of AMI. A variety of factors may be responsible for these changes: (1) augmented blood flow to the necrotic region; as a result, a greater proportion of the 85 percent of CK that is "depleted" may enter the blood rather than undergoing local denaturation; (2) reperfusion; as a result, more rapid breakdown of irreversibly injured tissue, possibly due to oxidation injury, may occur.

The net effect of these changes on CK kinetics is to augment the "release ratio"; the quantity of CK depleted from the myocardium is not changed [129]. As a result, enzymatic estimates of infarct size are altered. Definitive experimental or clinical data to validate new parameters for estimating infarct size from plasma enzymes after reperfusion have not been defined [171]. With reperfusion, more CK is released into the circulation because there is less time for myocardial proteolytic digestion and with better flow more CK is rescued from myocardial digestion. This could result in more reliable estimates of infarct size, but studies have not been performed to validate this conclusion.

MM-CK and MB-CK Subforms

Mechanism of Subform Conversion

During the late 1970s, Wevers and his colleagues showed that serum from patients who had suffered an AMI, upon prolonged electrophoresis at 90 volts, exhibited three CK bands in the MM region instead of the expected single band. On the same gels, MB-CK was resolved into two component bands [130, 131]. These multiple bands of a single isoenzyme have been designated sub-bands, and the CK molecules corresponding to each band have been termed subforms or subisoenzymes. The same group also observed a shift in relative sub-band intensity with time after AMI: the slowest migrating (most cathodal) MM-CK and MB-CK sub-bands were most intense during the early hours after infarction; with increasing time after AMI the faster-migrating forms become dominant. Wevers et al. also showed that only the slow-migrating subforms of each isoenzyme, designated MM_3 and MB_2, are present in tissue. The faster-migrating subforms, MB_1-CK, MM_2-CK, and MM_1-CK, are sequentially produced by a modification of the tissue forms after release into the blood. (Like the three cytosolic CK isoenzymes, the subforms can be designated by their relative rate of electrophoretic migration toward the anode: MM_3-CK and MB_2-CK are the slow-migrating forms, MM_1-CK and MB_1-CK are the fast-migrating forms, and MM_2-CK is intermediate between the MM_3 and MM_1 subisoenzymes (Fig. 6-3). This convention is somewhat confusing, as the numeric designation is the reverse of the sequence of appearance following AMI.) Finally, Wevers et al. reproduced the conversion of MM_3-CK to MM_1-CK in vitro by incubating purified tissue MM_3-CK with serum [130]. This conversion can also be demonstrated in vitro with MB_2-CK.

In 1981, using nondenaturing chromatofocusing chromatography, we isolated and purified the three MM subforms [132]. We subsequently demonstrated that subform conversion in the blood is mediated by the plasma enzyme carboxypeptidase-N (CP-N) and reproduced the conversion in vitro in the absence of serum by incubating purified tissue MM_3-CK with CP-N [133]. Using peptide mapping and amino acid sequence analysis, the mechanism of MM_3-CK modification was shown to be via cleavage of the positively charged amino acid lysine

Fig. 6-3
MM-CK and MB-CK subforms in the blood following AMI. Progressive conversion from the tissue subforms (of MM-CK and MB-CK) to the faster-migrating, modified subforms occurs with increasing time after AMI. (Courtesy of Helena Laboratories, Beaumont, Tex.)

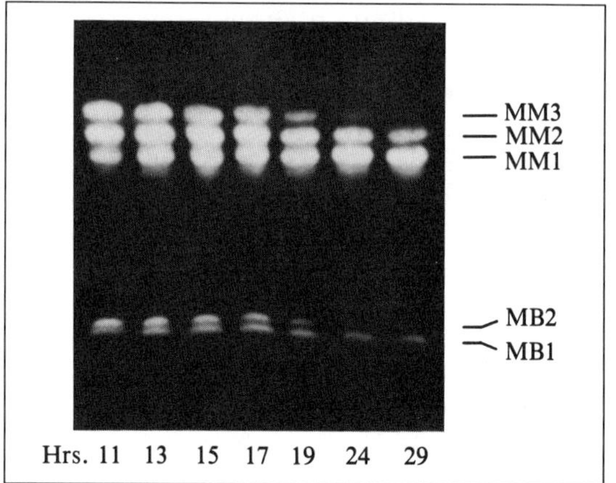

from the carboxyterminus of the M subunit(s); the result is a polypeptide chain having a slightly greater net negative charge (by one unit) and therefore a faster rate of migration toward the positive electrode [133, 134]. The M and B genes have now been cloned and the cDNA sequenced. Both subunits have lysine as the terminal amino acid [172, 173]. The conversion reaction progresses rapidly, both in vivo and in vitro; MM_3-CK is completely converted to MM_1-CK in 2 hours at 37°C [133]. Thus the sequential predominance of the three MM-CK subforms can be explained as follows: initially, release of MM_3-CK from necrotic myocardium makes the tissue form the most abundant plasma MM subform; cleavage of the terminal lysine from one of the two M polypeptides of MM_3-CK by CP-N then yields the heterodimer MM_2-CK, which transiently becomes the predominant subform several hours after the cessation of CK release; removal of the remaining terminal lysine from the second M chain by CP-N produces MM_1-CK (Fig. 6-4), which is the most abundant MM subform after 16 to 20 hours. Stepwise M-chain alteration has been confirmed as the mechanism of subform conversion by dissociation/reassociation experiments, in which the M chains of MM_3-CK and MM_1-CK were split into unpaired single chains by incubation with urea; random reassociation induced by removal of urea via dialysis produced all three subforms; similarly, dissociation and reassociation of the heterodimer MM_2-CK produced all three subforms, as expected. In contrast, dissociation and reassociation of the homodimer MM_1-CK alone yielded only MM_1-CK; MM_3-CK treated alone produced analogous results [133]. Preliminary work in our laboratory implicates a similar mechanism in the conversion of MB_2-CK to MB_1-CK.

Clinical Applications of Subform Analysis

The advent of thrombolytic therapy for AMI and the demonstration of its efficacy in reduction of mortality [135] has underlined the need for both earlier diagnosis of AMI and a noninvasive means to assess reperfusion success.

Early Diagnosis of Acute Myocardial Infarction

The sensitivity of total CK and CK-MB for diagnosis of AMI is low during the early hours of AMI [136]. Myoglobin rises out of the normal range within 2 hours of AMI, but the poor specificity of this marker and the several hours required to perform the radioimmunoassay (RIA) have limited its usefulness. Consequently, no currently available biochemical marker is reliable during the first 10 hours of AMI. Because thrombolytic therapy is most efficacious only when administered within the first 3 to 4 hours of AMI, the decision to initiate

Fig. 6-4
Molecular mechanism of MM-CK subform conversion in the blood. Loss of a single positively charged lysine residue (Lys +) yields a more negatively charged molecule, resulting in faster anodal migration.

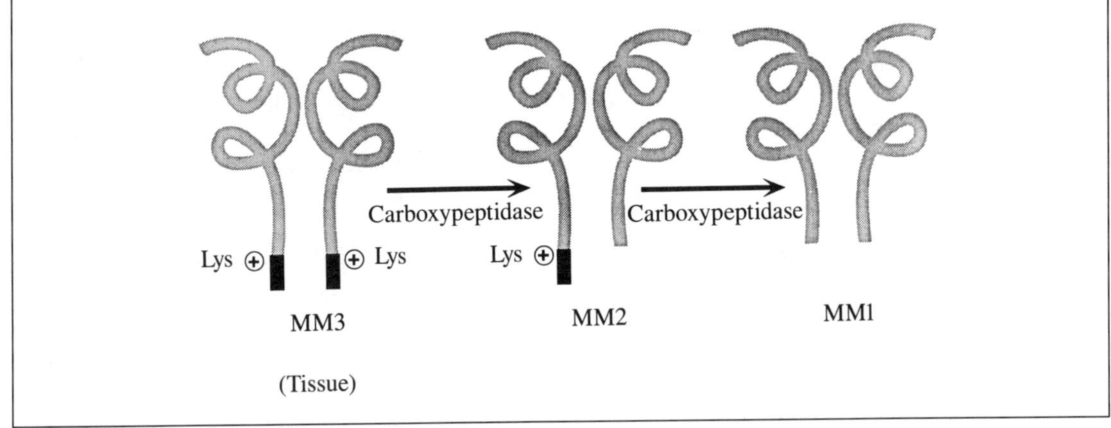

treatment is, of necessity, based on symptoms and ECG findings, which are sensitive but nonspecific [136], as evidenced by the fact that only about 20 percent of patients admitted to the CCU are subsequently shown to have infarction and only about 10 to 14 percent of patients presenting to the emergency room with chest pain are subsequently shown to have acute myocardial infarction [174, 175]. Because thrombolysis carries a small risk of intracranial hemorrhage and other bleeding complications, an early diagnostic marker with a low rate of false positives (i.e., high specificity) would be valuable. This problem of diagnostic uncertainty during the early hours of AMI is further compounded if the indications for thrombolysis are extended to include non-Q-wave infarction, as about 75 percent of these patients present with ST-segment depression, which is nonspecific and similar to the ECG changes of transient ischemia.

CK subform analysis shows promise as an early diagnostic indicator of AMI. At steady state in a normal individual, small amounts of MM-CK from skeletal muscle, and MM-CK and MB-CK from cardiac tissue, are continuously released into the blood, converted to the modified subforms, and cleared from the blood. Because the conversion reaction is rapid, the tissue form, MM_3-CK, contributes only a relatively small percent of the total MM-CK isoenzyme activity (20 to 35 percent). With the onset of AMI, the rate of myocardial MM_3-CK release into the blood quickly exceeds the rate of conversion of MM_3-CK to MM_2-CK and MM_1-CK, and MM_3-CK as a percent of total MM-CK activity rises. A similar rise in the MB_2-CK/MB_1-CK ratio occurs. Thus rapid release of small quantities of MM_3-CK is sufficient to raise the percent MM_3-CK and MB_2-CK before the value for total CK activity is sufficiently increased to exceed the upper limit of normal. For example, if a patient has a baseline MM-CK activity of 60 IU/L, with the upper limit of normal at 120 IU/L, the baseline MM_3-CK activity would be approximately 20 IU/L, i.e., 33 percent of MM-CK activity. An initial release of MM_3-CK early in AMI might raise the MM_3-CK to 60 IU/L but the total only to 100 IU/L, a value within the normal range; however, the MM_3-CK now constitutes 60 percent of MM-CK activity. In effect, each patient's plasma MM-CK activity serves as its own control, with perturbations in steady-state activity readily detectable as changes in subisoenzyme distribution even when CK activity is in the normal reference range.

Initial reports using the MM-CK subform distribution for early diagnosis of AMI in animals [137] and in several studies involving human subjects [138–140] have been promising, with the MM_3-CK/MM_1-CK ratio rising out of the normal range 4 to 6 hours after AMI onset. However, the major drawback for the use of the MM-CK subforms is their lack of specificity. As discussed earlier, assay of total CK activity rather than MB-CK activity for the diagnosis of AMI introduces a 20 to 30 percent false-positive rate due to release of MM-CK from skeletal muscle [82, 83]. Such elevations, due to exercise [141–143] or myositis [144], have been shown to be associated with an increase in percent MM_3-CK [141–144], thus reducing the specificity of this finding.

Because of the lack of specificity of MM-CK subform analysis, we have evaluated the utility of MB-CK subforms in the early diagnosis of AMI. Unlike previous systems used for subform separation, which required 1.5 hours of electrophoresis at 90 volts for adequate resolution, a prototype instrument was developed (Rep; Helena Laboratories, Beaumont, TX) in which electrophoresis is performed at 1400 volts on a dynamically cooled gel [172]. This approach separates the tissue subform, MB_2-CK, from the plasma-modified subform, MB_1-CK, in 14 minutes. The system was validated using purified MB_2-CK and MB_1-CK reconstituted in heat-inactivated serum. The assay is linear for both MB-CK subforms, even at very low levels ($r = .99$ between 1.25 and 30 IU/L, N = 70; upper normal limit 14 IU/L), is highly reproducible and generates the expected MB_2-CK/MB_1-CK ratio when both subforms are present in serum ($r = .95$, N = 144). Sensitivity is 1.0 IU/L; total assay time is 20 minutes.

The ratio of plasma MB_2 and MB_1 under baseline conditions is about 1:1. In preliminary studies [176], we showed that with infarction the ratio changes rapidly from 1.5 to 1 within 2 hours of onset of symptoms of infarction. In a study of over 100 patients with infarction documented over 24 hours by total MB-CK, the MB_2 to MB_1 ratio reliably diagnosed infarction within 4 to 6 hours with a sensitivity and specificity of over 90 percent in contrast to conventional total MB-CK that detected only 57 percent in 6 hours and required 10 hours for 90 percent reliability [177]. Utilizing the ratio equal to or greater than 1.5 of MB_2 to MB_1 as the diagnostic criterion, a prospective study [178] was performed in over 1100 consecutive patients presenting to the emergency room with chest pain and suspected myocardial infarction. There were 121 patients with elevated plasma MB_2 who were subsequently admitted to the CCU, but over 500 patients had normal levels and were discharged home without admission to the hospital. The overall sensitivity and specificity were 96 percent and 93 percent, respectively [179]. Similar diagnostic sensitivity and specificity were observed in patients admitted into TIMI 4, 5, and 6 trials in which the assays were performed without knowledge of the patients' clinical status.

The role of early diagnostic methods in conjunction with thrombolysis will be defined as better methods become widely available. As currently practiced, thrombolysis is administered in the emergency room after physician evaluation. An assay with a 15-minute "turnaround time" might allow collection and reporting of objective data before initiation of therapy. Alternatively, drug therapy might be initiated in patients with a high clinical suspicion of AMI, with termination of drug infusion based on results of subform analysis available within minutes of initiating thrombolytic therapy. The latter course would maximize the potential for myocardial salvage while limiting the risk associated with a full course of therapy to a patient without AMI. A similar protocol might be employed if thrombolytic therapy were initiated by paramedics at the site of initial patient contact "in the field."

Noninvasive Diagnosis of Reperfusion

Initial studies of reperfusion therapy of AMI used intracoronary administration of drug, with coronary angiography to assess therapeutic success as well as to allow for early mechanical intervention in the event of drug failure [145]. More recently, intravenous therapy has been employed to avoid the therapeutic delay associated with acute angiography; however, early angiography was performed to evaluate reperfusion success and to permit early angioplasty in the event of drug failure [146]. Evidence is now accumulating to suggest that angioplasty performed early as an adjunct to thrombolytic therapy confers no advantage over elective angioplasty performed several days later [147]. Therefore many protocols no longer utilize early angiography; as a result, success of therapy remains obscure for several days. If thrombolytic success could be assessed noninvasively, the 30 percent of patients who fail to exhibit clot lysis would not be subjected to catheterization on day 2 or 3 for possible angioplasty, as there is no advantage in late reperfusion. Furthermore, if a noninvasive marker documented lack of success within 1 to 2 hours, mechanical reperfusion might be attempted in selected high-risk patients with failure of drug-induced clot lysis.

The rationale for the use of subforms for detection of reperfusion are twofold: (1) reperfusion is associated with rapid washout of CK from the region of infarction (see above); (2) because MM_3-CK conversion to MM_2-CK and MM_1-CK is rapid, prolonged MM_3-CK elevation represents a marker of persistent CK release and therefore suggests failure of thrombolysis. Observations in patients undergoing thrombolytic therapy have shown that the percent MM_3-CK rises to 75 percent followed by a decline (reflecting rapid MM_3-CK conversion) after MM_3-CK release from tissue has slowed or ceased.

In a study of 103 consecutive patients who underwent attempted reperfusion of AMI at our institutions, we compared the rate of decline of percent MM_3-CK (expressed as the slope in a plot of percent MM_3-CK versus time after the onset of AMI) with reperfusion success [148]. All patients underwent acute angiography to evaluate therapeutic success. Percent MM_3-CK was determined by plasma electrophoresis using a commercially available system. Agarose gels from representative patients are shown in Figure 6-5. The 55 patients with successful reperfusion had an average rate of percent MM_3-CK decline of 4.18 percent per hour, whereas the group of patients with angiographically proved unsuccessful reperfusion had a substantially lower rate of decline, 2.37 percent per hour; the differences between these two groups were highly statistically significant. In addition, using a cutoff value of 3.1 percent per hour, 48 of 55 successfully reperfused patients were above the cutoff, whereas 29 of 39 nonreperfused patients had a slope below the cutoff value. Thus the sensitivity for detection of reperfusion was 87 percent with a specificity of 74 percent. Among 30 patients with AMI in whom no therapy

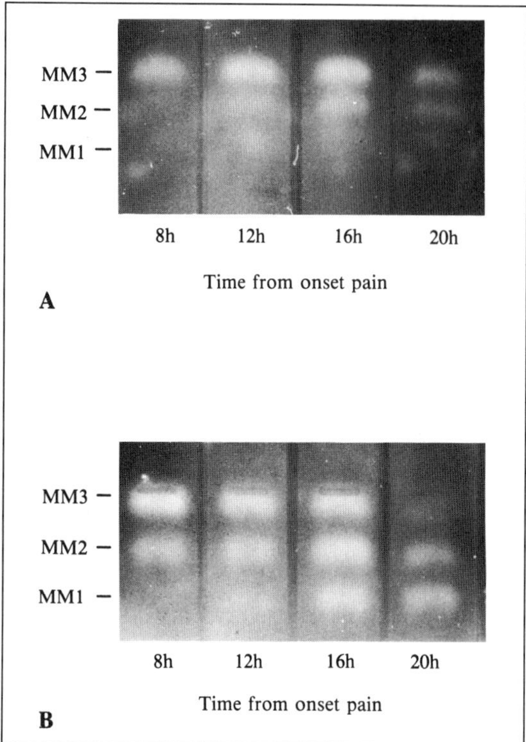

Fig. 6-5
CK-MM subforms in AMI with and without thrombolysis. *A.* Unsuccessful reperfusion is characterized by ongoing MM3-CK release and prolonged MM3-CK predominance. *B.* Successful reperfusion is characterized by cessation of CK release followed by complete conversion to the modified forms.

was attempted, 27 of 30 (90 percent) were below the cutoff values. In contrast, the time from onset of symptoms to peak MB-CK, which has occasionally been used as an index of reperfusion success, demonstrated marked overlap between the two groups; specificity was 49 percent.

Other investigations have reported an earlier time to peak MM_3-CK/MM_1-CK ratio in patients with successful reperfusion than in patients without successful reperfusion [149, 150]; because no "cutoff" times were suggested, the accuracy of this method for detecting reperfusion is not known. Work is currently in progress in our laboratory to detect reperfusion based on the MB-CK rather than the MM-CK subforms. Diagnosis with such a system would be specific, without confounding influence due to MM_3-CK release from skeletal muscle injury due to cardioversion, cardiopulmonary resuscitation, or cardiac catheterization [151].

References

1. Wohlgemuth, J. Unersuchungen über die Diastasen. *Biochem. Z.* 9:10, 1908.
2. Gutman, E. B., Spraul, E. E., and Gutman, A. B. Significance of increased phosphatase activity of bone at the site of osteoblastic metastases secondary to carcinoma of the prostate gland. *Am. J. Cancer* 28:485, 1936.
3. Karmen, A., Wroblewski, F., and La Due, J. Transaminase activity in human blood. *J. Clin. Invest.* 34:126, 1954.
4. LaDue, J. S., Wroblewski, F., and Karmen, A. Serum glutamic oxaloacetic transaminase activity in human acute transmural myocardial infarction. *Science* 120:497, 1954.
5. Wroblewski, F., and LaDue, J. S. Lactic dehydrogenase activity in blood. *Proc. Soc. Exp. Biol. Med.* 90:210, 1955.
6. Sayre, F. W., and Hill, B. R. Fractionisation of serum lactic dehydrogenase by salt concentration gradient elution and paper electrophoresis. *Proc. Soc. Exp. Biol. Med.* 96:695, 1959.
7. Vesell, E. S., and Bearn, A. G. Localization of lactic acid dehydrogenase activity in serum fractions. *Proc. Soc. Exp. Biol. Med.* 94:96, 1957.
8. Wieland, T. H., and Pfleiderer, G. Nachweis der Heterogenitat von Milchsauredehydrogenase verschiedenen ursprungs durch Tragerelektrophorese. *Biochem. Z.* 329:112, 1957.
9. Markert, C. L., and Moller, F. Multiple forms of enzymes: Tissue, ontogenic, and species specific patterns. *Proc. Natl. Acad. Sci. U.S.A.* 45:753, 1959.
10. Ebashi, S., Toyakura, Y., Momoi, H., et al. High creatine phosphokinase activity of sera of progressive muscular dystrophy. *J. Biochem.* 46:103, 1959.
11. Dreyfus, V. C., Schapira, G., Resnais, J., et al. Le creatine-kinase serique dans le diagnostic de l'infarctus myocardique. *Rev. Fr. Etud. Clin. Biol.* 5:386, 1960.
12. Van der Veen, K. J., and Willebrands, A. F. Isoenzymes of creatine phosphokinase in tissue extracts and in normal and pathological sera. *Clin. Chim. Acta* 13:312, 1966.
13. Schwartz, A., Wood, J. M., Allen, J. C., et al. Biochemical and morphologic correlates of cardiac ischemia. I. Membrane systems. *Am. J. Cardiol.* 32:46, 1973.
14. Ahmed, S. A., Williamson, J. R., Roberts, R., et al. The association of increased plasma MB CPK activity and irreversible ischemic myocardial injury in the dog. *Circulation* 54:187, 1976.
15. Siegel, R. J., Said, J. W., Shell, W. E., et al. Identification and localization of creatine kinase B and M in normal, ischemic and necrotic myocardium: An immunohistochemical study. *J. Mol. Cell. Cardiol.* 16:95, 1984.
16. Michael, L. H., Hunt, J. R., Weilbaecher, D., et al. Creatine kinase and phosphorylase in cardiac

lymph: Coronary occlusion and reperfusion. *Am. J. Physiol.* 248(*Heart Circ. Physiol.* 17):H350, 1985.
17. Roberts, R. Diagnostic assessment of myocardial infarction based on lactate dehydrogenase and creatine kinase isoenzymes. *Heart Lung* 10:486, 1981.
18. Shell, W. E., DeWood, M. A., Kligerman, M., et al. Early appearance of MB-creatine kinase activity in nontransmural myocardial infarction detected by a sensitive assay for the isoenzyme. *Am. J. Med.* 71:254, 1981.
19. Roberts, R. Measurement of Enzymes in Cardiology. In R. J. Linden (ed.), *Techniques in Life Sciences.* New York: Elsevier, 1983.
20. Dawson, D. M., Eppenberger, H. M., and Kaplan, N. O. Creatine kinase: Evidence for a dimeric structure. *Biochem. Biophys. Res. Commun.* 21:346, 1965.
21. Roberts, R., and Grace, A. M. Purification of mitochondrial creatine kinase. *J. Biol. Chem.* 255: 2870, 1980.
22. Basson, C. T., Grace, A. M., and Roberts, R. Enzyme kinetics of a highly purified mitochondrial creatine kinase in comparison with cytosolic forms. *Mol. Cell Biochem.* 67:151, 1985.
23. Jacobus, W. E., and Lehninger, A. L. Creatine kinase of rat heart mitochondria. *J. Biol. Chem.* 248: 4803, 1973.
24. Perryman, M. B., Strauss, A. W., Buettner, T. L., et al. Molecular heterogeneity of creatine kinase isoenzymes. *Biochem. Biophys. Acta* 747:284, 1983.
25. Villareal-Levy, G., Ma, T. S., Kerner, S. A., et al. Human creatine kinase: Isolation and sequence analysis of cDNA clones for the B subunit, development of subunit specific probes and determination of gene copy number. *Biochem. Biophys. Res. Commun.* 144:1116, 1987.
26. Perryman, M. B., Kerner, S. A., Bohlmeyer, T. J., et al. Isolation and sequence analysis of a full-length cDNA for human M creatine kinase. *Biochem. Biophys. Res. Commun.* 140:981, 1986.
27. Bessman, S., and Carpenter, C. The creatine-creatine phosphate energy shuttle. *Annu. Rev. Biochem.* 54:831, 1985.
28. Mahler, M. First-order kinetics of muscle oxygen consumption, and an equivalent proportionality between QO_2 and phosphorylcreatine level. *J. Gen. Physiol.* 86:135, 1985.
29. Meyer, R. A., Sweeney, H. L., and Kushmerick, M. J. A simple analysis of the "phosphocreatine shuttle." *Am. J. Physiol.* 246(*Cell Physiol.* 15): C365, 1984.
30. Houk, T. W., and Putnam, S. V. Location of the creatine phosphokinase binding site of myosin. *Biochem. Biophys. Res. Commun.* 55:1271, 1973.
31. Turner, D. C., Maier, V., and Eppenberger, H. M. A protein that binds specifically to the M-line of skeletal muscle is identified as the muscle form of creatine kinase. *Proc. Natl. Acad. Sci. U.S.A.* 70:702, 1973.
32. Wallimann, T., Kuhn, H. J., Pelloni, G., et al. Localization of creatine kinase isoenzymes in myofibrils. II. Chicken heart muscle. *J. Cell. Biol.* 75:318, 1977.
33. Neumeier, D. Subcellular Distribution of Creatine Kinase Isoenzymes. In H. Lang (ed.), *Creatine Kinase Isoenzymes.* New York: Springer-Verlag, 1981.
34. Sharov, V. G., Saks, V. A., Smirnov, V. N., et al. An electron microscopic histochemical investigation of the localization of creatine phosphokinase in heart cells. *Biochim. Biophys. Acta* 468:495, 1977.
35. Saks, V. A., Lipina, N. V., Sharov, V. G., et al. The localization of the MM isozyme of creatine phosphokinase on the surface membrane of myocardial cells and its functional coupling to ouabain-inhibited (Na^+K^+)-ATPase. *Biochim. Biophys. Acta* 465:550, 1977.
36. Baskin, R. J., and Deamer, D. W. A membrane-bound creatine phosphokinase in fragmented sarcoplasmic reticulum. *J. Biol. Chem.* 245:1345, 1970.
37. Scholte, H. R., Weijers, P. J., and Wit-Peeters, E. M. The localization of mitochondrial creatine kinase, and its use for the determination of the sidedness of submitochondrial particles. *Biochim. Biophys. Acta* 291:764, 1973.
38. Morin, L. G. Creatine kinase: Stability, inactivation, reactivation. *Clin. Chem.* 23:646, 1977.
39. Urdal, P., and Landaas, S. Macro creatine kinase BB in serum, and some data on its prevalence. *Clin. Chem.* 25:461, 1979.
40. Lang, H., and Wurzburg, U. Creatine kinase, an enzyme of many forms. *Clin. Chem.* 28:1439, 1982.
41. Oliver, I. T. A spectrophotometric method for the determination of creatine phosphokinase and myokinase. *Biochem. J.* 61:116, 1955.
42. Rosalki, S. B. An improved procedure for creatine phosphokinase determination. *J. Lab. Clin. Med.* 69:696, 1967.
43. Boone, D. J., Duncan, P. H., MacNeil, M. L., et al. Results of a nationwide survey of analyses for creatine kinase and creatine kinase isoenzymes. *Clin. Chem.* 30:33, 1984.
44. Buzas, Z., and Chrambach, A. Un-supercoiled agarose with a degree of molecular sieving similar to that of crosslinked polyacrylamide. *Electrophoresis* 3:130, 1982.
45. Cook, R. B., and Witt, H. J. Agarose composition, aqueous gel, and method of making same. U. S. Patent 4,290,911, 1981.
46. Lott, J. A., and Stang, J. M. Serum enzymes and isoenzymes in the diagnosis and differential diagnosis of myocardial ischemia and necrosis. *Clin. Chem.* 26:1241, 1980.
47. Aleyassine, H., and Tonks, D. B. Albumin-bound fluorescence: A potential source of error in fluorometric assay of creatine kinase BB isoenzyme (Letter). *Clin. Chem.* 24:1849, 1978.
48. Massey, T. H., and Barta, J. S. Creatine kinase isoenzymes in neonate plasma by cellulose acetate electrophoresis: Albumin and adenylate kinase artifacts. *Clin. Chem.* 28:1174, 1982.

49. Mercer, D. W. Separation of tissue and serum creatine kinase isoenzymes by ion-exchange column chromatography. *Clin. Chem.* 20:36, 1974.
50. Henry, P. D., Roberts, R., and Sobel, B. E. Rapid separation of plasma creatine kinase isoenzymes by batch absorption on glass beads. *Clin. Chem.* 21:844, 1975.
51. Morin, L. G. Evaluation of current methods for creatine kinase isoenzyme fractionation. *Clin. Chem.* 23:205, 1977.
52. Apple, F. S., Greenspan, N. S., and Dietzler, D. N. Elevation of creatine kinase BB CK in hospitalized patients. *Ann. Clin. Lab. Sci.* 12:398, 1982.
53. Wurzburg, U. Measurement of creatine kinase isoenzyme activity by immunological methods. In H. Lang (ed.), *Creatine Kinase Isoenzymes.* New York: Springer-Verlag, 1981.
54. Lott, J. A. Serum enzyme determinations in the diagnosis of acute myocardial infarction. *Hum. Pathol.* 15:706, 1984.
55. Ritter, C. S., Mumm, S. R., and Roberts, R. Improved radioimmunoassay for creatine kinase isoenzymes in plasma. *Clin. Chem.* 27:1878, 1981.
56. Chan, D. W., Taylor, E., Frye, R., et al. Immunoenzymetric assay for creatine kinase MB with subunit-specific monoclonal antibodies compared with an immunochemical method and electrophoresis. *Clin. Chem.* 31:465, 1985.
57. Vaidya, H. C., Maynard, Y., Dietzler, D. N., et al. Direct measurement of creatine kinase-MB activity in serum after extraction with a monoclonal antibody specific to the MB isoenzyme. *Clin. Chem.* 32:657, 1986.
58. Landt, Y., Vaidya, H. C., Porter, S. E., et al. Semi-automated direct colorimetric measurement of creatine kinase isoenzyme MB activity after extraction from serum by use of a CK-MB-specific monoclonal antibody. *Clin. Chem.* 34:575, 1988.
59. Foxall, C. D., and Ermery, A. E. Changes in creatine kinase and its isoenzymes in human fetal muscle during development. *J. Neurol. Sci.* 24:483, 1975.
60. Tzvetanova, E. Creatine kinase isoenzymes in muscle tissue of patients with neuromuscular diseases and human fetuses. *Enzyme* 12:279, 1971.
61. Tsung, J. S., and Tsung, S. S. Creatine kinase isoenzymes in extracts of various human skeletal muscles. *Clin. Chem.* 32:1568, 1986.
62. Wilhelm, A. H., Albers, K. M., and Todd, J. K. Creatine phosphokinase isoenzyme distribution in human skeletal and heart muscles. *I.R.C.S. Med. Sci.* 4:418, 1976.
63. Yasmineh, W. G., Ibrahim, G. A., Abbasnezhad, M. A., et al. Isoenzyme distribution of creatine kinase and lactate dehydrogenase in serum and skeletal muscle in Duchenne muscular dystrophy, collagen disease, and other muscular disorders. *Clin. Chem.* 24:1985.
64. Roberts, R., Henry, P. D., Witteveen, S. A. G. J., et al. Quantification of serum creatine phosphokinase isoenzyme activity. *Am. J. Cardiol.* 33:650, 1974.
65. Apple, F. S., Rogers, M. A., Sherman, W. M., et al. Profile of creatine kinase isoenzymes in skeletal muscles of marathon runners. *Clin. Chem.* 30:413, 1984.
66. Siegel, A. J., Silverman, L. M., and Evans, W. J. Elevated skeletal muscle creatine kinase MB isoenzyme levels in marathon runners. *J.A.M.A.* 250: 2835, 1983.
67. Keshgegian, A. A., and Feinberg, N. V. Serum creatine kinase MB isoenzyme in chronic muscle disease. *Clin. Chem.* 30:575, 1984.
68. Shahanglan, S., Ash, O. W., Wahlstrom, N. O., et al. Creatine kinase and lactate dehydrogenase isoenzymes in serum of patients suffering burns, blunt trauma, or myocardial infarction. *Clin. Chem.* 30:1332, 1984.
69. McBride, J. W., Labrosse, K. R., and McCoy, H. G., et al. Is serum creatine kinase-MB in electrically injured patients predictive of myocardial injury? *J.A.M.A.* 255:764, 1986.
70. Goto, I., Nagamine, M., and Katsuki, S. Creatine phosphokinase isozymes in muscles. *Arch. Neurol.* 20:422, 1969.
71. Staubli, M., Roessler, B., Kochli, H. P., et al. Creatine kinase and creatine kinase MB in endurance runners and in patients with myocardial infarction. *Eur. J. Appl. Physiol.* 54:40, 1985.
72. Sadeh, M., Stern, L. Z., Czyzewski, K., et al. Alterations of creatine kinase, ornithine decarboxylase, and transglutaminase during muscle regeneration. *Life Sci.* 34:483, 1984.
73. Ingwall, J. S., Kramer, M. F., Fifer, M. A., et al. The creatine kinase system in normal and diseased human myocardium. *N. Engl. J. Med.* 313:1050, 1985.
74. Marmor, A., Margolis, T., and Alpan, G., et al. Regional distribution of the MB isoenzyme of creatine kinase in the human heart. *Arch. Pathol. Lab. Med.* 104:425, 1980.
75. Yasmineh, W. G., Pyle, R. B., and Nicoloff, D. M. Rate of decay and distribution volume of MB isoenzyme of creatine kinase, intravenously injected into the baboon. *Clin. Chem.* 22:1095, 1976.
76. Baraka, M., Deveaux, N., Frank, R., et al. Creatine kinase MB isoenzyme activity after endocardial catheter fulguration (Abstract). *Circulation* 76(Suppl IV):IV-174, 1987.
77. Eppenberger, H. M., Eppenberger, M. E., Richterich, R., et al. The ontogeny of creatine kinase isoenzymes. *Dev. Biol.* 10:1, 1964.
78. Tsung, S. H. Creatine kinase activity and isoenzyme pattern in various normal tissues and neoplasms. *Clin. Chem.* 29:2040, 1983.
79. Roberts, R. Recognition, pathogenesis, and management of non-Q-wave infarction. *Mod. Concepts Cardiovasc. Dis.* 56:17, 1987.
80. Roberts, R., Gowda, K. S., Ludbrook, P. A., et al. Specificity of elevated serum MB creatine phosphokinase activity in the diagnosis of acute myocardial infarction. *Am. J. Cardiol.* 36:433, 1975.

81. Lee, T. H., and Goldman, L. Serum enzyme assays in the diagnosis of acute myocardial infarction. *Ann. Intern. Med.* 105:221, 1986.
82. Grande, P., Christiansen, C., Pedersen, A., et al. Optimal diagnosis in acute myocardial infarction. *Circulation* 61:723, 1980.
83. Klein, M. S., Shell, W. E., and Sobel, B. E. Serum creatine phosphokinase (CPK) isoenzymes after intramuscular injections, surgery, and myocardial infarction. *Cardiovasc. Res.* 7:412, 1973.
84. Somer, H., Dubowitz, V., and Donner, M. Creatine kinase isoenzymes in neuromuscular diseases. *J. Neurol. Sci.* 29:129, 1976.
85. Jaffe, A. S., Ritter, C., Meltzer, V., et al. Unmasking artifactual increases in creatine kinase isoenzymes in patients with renal failure. *J. Lab. Clin. Med.* 104:193, 1984.
86. Kimler, S. C., and Sandhu, R. S. Circulating CK-MB and CK-BB isoenzymes after prostate resection. *Clin. Chem.* 26:55, 1980.
87. Tsung, S. H. Several conditions causing elevation of serum CK-MB and CK-BB. *Am. J. Clin. Pathol.* 75:711, 1981.
88. Laboda, H. M., and Britton, V. J. Creatine kinase isoenzyme activity in human placenta and in the serum of women in labor. *Clin. Chem.* 23:1329, 1977.
89. Somer, H., Kaste, M., Troupp, H., et al. Brain creatine kinase in blood after acute brain injury. *J. Neurol. Neurosurg. Psychiatry* 38:572, 1975.
90. Kaste, M., Somer, H., and Konttinen, A. Brain-type creatine kinase isoenzyme. *Arch. Neurol.* 34:142, 1977.
91. Goldman, J., Matz, R., Montimer, R., et al. High elevations of creatine phosphokinase in hypothyroidism: An isoenzyme analysis. *J.A.M.A.* 238: 325, 1977.
92. Bayer, P. M., Boehm, M., Hajdusich, P., et al. Immunoinhibition and automated column chromatography compared for assay of creatine kinase isoenzyme MB in serum. *Clin. Chem.* 28:166, 1982.
93. WHO: *Hypertension and Coronary Heart Disease: Classification and Criteria for Epidemiological Studies.* World Health Organization Technical Series 168. WHO, Geneva, 1959.
94. Roberts, R. The two out of three criteria for the diagnosis of infarction: Is it passe? (Editorial). *Chest* 86:511, 1984.
95. Dillon, M. C., Calbreath, D. F., Dixon, A. M., et al. Diagnostic problem in acute myocardial infarction: CK-MB in the absence of abnormally elevated total creatine kinase levels. *Arch. Intern. Med.* 142:33, 1982.
96. Heller, G. V., Blaustein, A. S., and Wei, J. Y. Implications of increased myocardial isoenzyme level in the presence of normal serum creatine kinase activity. *Am. J. Cardiol.* 51:24, 1983.
97. Yusuf, S., Collins, R., Lin, L., et al. Significance of elevated MB isoenzyme with normal creatine kinase in acute myocardial infarction. *Am. J. Cardiol.* 59:245, 1987.
98. White, R. D., Grande, P., Califf, L., et al. Diagnostic and prognostic significance of minimally elevated creatine kinase-MB in suspected acute myocardial infarction. *Am. J. Cardiol.* 55:1478, 1985.
99. Roberts, R., and Sobel, B. E. Elevated plasma MB creatine phosphokinase activity. *Arch. Intern. Med.* 136:421, 1976.
100. Appella, E., and Markert, C. L. Dissociation of lactate dehydrogenase into subunits with guanidine hydrochloride. *Biochim. Biophys. Acta* 6:171, 1961.
101. Wieland, T., and Pfleiderer, G. Chemical differences between multiple forms of lactic acid dehydrogenase. *Ann. N.Y. Acad. Sci.* 94:691, 1961.
102. Kreutzer, H. H., and Fennis, W. H. S. Lactic dehydrogenase isoenzymes in blood serum after storage at different temperatures. *Clin. Chim. Acta* 9:64, 1964.
103. Smit, M. J., Duursma, A. M., and Bouma, J. M. W., et al. Receptor-mediated endocytosis of lactate dehydrogenase M_4 by liver macrophages: A mechanism for elimination of enzymes from plasma. *J. Biol. Chem.* 262:13020, 1987.
104. Brody, I. A. Effect of denervation on the lactate dehydrogenase isozymes of skeletal muscle. *Nature* 205:196, 1965.
105. Emery, A. E. H. Electrophoretic pattern of lactic dehydrogenase in carriers and patients with Duchenne muscular dystrophy. *Nature* 201:1044, 1964.
106. Schapira, F., Dreyfus, J. C., and Schapira, G. Fetal-like patterns of lactic-dehydrogenase and aldolase isoenzymes in some pathological conditions. *Enzym. Biol. Clin.* 7:98, 1966.
107. McKenzie, D., Henderson, A. R., Gordesky, S. E., et al. Electrophoresis of lactate dehydrogenase isoenzymes. *Clin. Chem.* 29:189, 1983.
108. Kagen, L. J. *Myoglobin: Biochemical, Physiological and Clinical Aspects.* New York: Columbia University Press, 1972. P. 79.
109. Roberts, R. Myoglobinemia as an index to myocardial infarction. *Ann. Intern. Med.* 87:788, 1977.
110. Granadier, E., Keidar, S., Kahana, L., et al. The roles of serum myoglobin, total CPK, and CK-MB isoenzyme in the acute phase of myocardial infarction. *Am. Heart J.* 105:408, 1983.
111. Groth, T., Hakman, M., and Sylven, C. Prediction of myocardial infarct size from early serum myoglobin observations. *Scand. J. Clin. Lab. Invest.* 47:599, 1987.
112. Norregaard-Hensen, K., Petersen, P. H., Hangaard, J., et al. Early observations of S-myoglobin in the diagnosis of acute myocardial infarction: The influence of discrimination limit, analytical quality, patient's sex and prevalence of disease. *Scand. J. Clin. Lab. Invest.* 46:561, 1986.
113. Roxin, L. E., Cullhed, I., Groth, T., et al. The value of serum myoglobin determinations in the early diagnosis of acute myocardial infarction. *Acta Med. Scand.* 215:417, 1984.

114. Bird, J. W. C., Carter, J. H., Triemer, R. E., et al. Proteinases in cardiac and skeletal muscle. *Fed. Proc.* 39:20, 1980.
115. Smitherman, T. C., Dycus, D. W., and Richards, E. G. Dissociation of myosin light chains and decreased myosin ATPase activity with acidification of synthetic myosin filaments: Possible clues to the fate of myosin in myocardial ischemia and infarction. *J. Mol. Cell. Cardiol.* 12:149, 1980.
116. Nagai, R., Ueda, S., and Yazaki, Y. Radioimmunoassay of cardiac myosin light chain II in the serum following experimental myocardial infarction. *Biochem. Biophys. Res. Commun.* 86:683, 1979.
117. Katus, H. A., Diederich, K. W., Schwarz, F., et al. Influence of reperfusion on serum concentrations of cytosolic creatine kinase and structural myosin light chains in acute myocardial infarction. *Am. J. Cardiol.* 60:440, 1987.
118. Isobe, M., Nagai, R., Ueda, S., et al. Quantitative relationship between left ventricular function and serum cardiac myosin light chain I levels after coronary reperfusion in patients with acute myocardial infarction. *Circulation* 76:1261, 1987.
119. Sobel, B. E., Roberts, R., and Larson, K. B. Estimation of infarct size from serum MB creatine phosphokinase activity: Applications and limitations. *Am. J. Cardiol.* 37:474, 1976.
120. Kjekshus, J. K., and Sobel, B. E. Depressed myocardial creatine phosphokinase activity following experimental myocardial infarction in rabbit. *Circ. Res.* 27:403, 1970.
121. Roberts, R., Henry, P. D., and Sobel, B. E. An improved basis for enzymatic estimation of infarct size. *Circulation* 52:743, 1975.
122. Sobel, B. E., Markham, J., Karlsberg, R. P., et al. The nature of disappearance of creatine kinase from the circulation and its influence on enzymatic estimation of infarct size. *Circ. Res.* 41:836, 1977.
123. Shell, W. E., Kjekshus, J. K., and Sobel, B. E. Quantitative assessment of the extent of myocardial infarction in the conscious dog by means of analysis of serial changes in serum creatine phosphokinase (CPK) activity. *J. Clin. Invest.* 50:2614, 1971.
124. Hackel, D. B., Reimer, K. A., Ideker, R. E., et al. Comparison of enzymatic and anatomic estimates of myocardial infarct size in man. *Circulation* 70:824, 1984.
125. Bleifeld, W., Mathey, D., Hanrath, P., et al. Infarct size estimated from serial serum creatine phosphokinase in relation to left ventricular hemodynamics. *Circulation* 55:303, 1977.
126. Rogers, W. J., McDaniel, H. G., Smith, L. R., et al. Correlation of CPK-MB and angiographic estimates of infarct size in man. *Circulation* 56:199, 1977.
127. Sobel, B. E., Bresnahan, G. F., Shell, W. E., et al. Estimation of infarct size in man and its relation to prognosis. *Circulation* 46:640, 1972.
128. Roberts, R., and Husain, R. Relation between infarct size and ventricular arrhythmia. *Br. Heart J.* 37:1169, 1975.
129. Roberts, R., and Ishikawa, Y. Enzymatic estimation of infarct size during reperfusion. *Circulation* 68(Suppl I):83, 1983.
130. Wevers, R. A., Delsing, M., Klein, A., et al. Postsynthetic changes in creatine kinase isoenzymes. *Clin. Chim. Acta* 86:323, 1978.
131. Wevers, R. A., Olthuis, H. P., Van Niel, J. C. C., et al. A study on the dimeric structure of creatine kinase. *Clin. Chim. Acta* 75:377, 1977.
132. Sims, H. S., Ritter, C. S., Fukuyama, T., et al. Characterization of the modification of creatine kinase following its release into plasma after infarction (Abstract). *Clin. Res.* 29:242A, 1981.
133. George, S., Ishikawa, Y., Perryman, M. B., et al. Purification and characterization of naturally occurring and in vitro induced multiple forms of MM creatine kinase. *J. Biol. Chem.* 259:2667, 1984.
134. Perryman, M. B., Knell, J. D., and Roberts, R. Carboxypeptidase-catalyzed hydrolysis of C-terminal lysine: Mechanism for in vivo production of multiple forms of creatine kinase in plasma. *Clin. Chem.* 30:662, 1984.
135. Gruppo Italiano per lo Studio della Streptochinasi nell'Infarto Miocardico (GISSI). Effectiveness of intravenous thrombolytic treatment in acute myocardial infarction. *Lancet* 1:397, 1986.
136. Lee, T. H., Gregory, W. R., Weisberg, M. C., et al. Sensitivity of routine clinical criteria for diagnosing myocardial infarction within 24 hours of hospitalization. *Ann. Intern. Med.* 106:181, 1987.
137. Hashimoto, H., Abendschein, D. R., Strauss, A. W., et al. Early detection of myocardial infarction in conscious dogs by analysis of plasma MM creatine kinase isoforms. *Circulation* 71:363, 1985.
138. Jaffe, A. S., Serota, H., Grace, A., et al. Diagnostic changes in plasma creatine kinase isoforms early after the onset of acute myocardial infarction. *Circulation* 74:105, 1986.
139. Morelli, R. L., Carlson, C. J., Emilson, B., et al. Serum creatine kinase MM isoenzyme sub-bands after acute myocardial infarction in man. *Circulation* 67:1283, 1983.
140. Wu, A. H. B., Gornet, T. G., Wu, V. H., et al. Early diagnosis of acute myocardial infarction by rapid analysis of creatine kinase isoenzyme-3 (CK-MM) subtypes. *Clin. Chem.* 33:358, 1987.
141. Apple. F. S., Heilsten, Y., and Clarkson, P. M. Early detection of skeletal muscle injury by assay of creatine kinase MM isoforms in serum after acute exercise. *Clin. Chem.* 34:1102, 1988.
142. Apple, F. S., Rogers, M. A., and Ivy, J. L. Creatine kinase isoenzyme MM variants in skeletal muscle and plasma from marathon runners. *Clin. Chem.* 32:41, 1986.
143. Clarkson, P. M., Apple, F. S., Byrnes, W. C., et al. Creatine kinase isoforms following isometric exercise. *Muscle Nerve* 10:41, 1987.
144. Annesley, T. M., Strongwater, S. L., and Schnitzer, T. J. MM subisoenzymes of creatine kinase as an index of disease activity in polymyositis. *Clin. Chem.* 31:402, 1985.

145. Rentrop, P., Blanke, H., Kostering, K., et al. Acute myocardial infarction: Intracoronary application of nitroglycerine and streptokinase in combination with transluminal recanalization. *Clin. Cardiol.* 5:354, 1979.
146. Chesebro, J. H., Knatterud, G., Roberts, R., et al. Thrombolysis in myocardial infarction (TIMI) trial, phase I: A comparison between intravenous tissue plasminogen activator and intravenous streptokinase. *Circulation* 76:142, 1987.
147. Califf, R. M., Topol, E. J., Kereiakes, D. J., et al. Long-term outcome in the thrombolysis and angioplasty in myocardial infarction trial (Abstract). *Circulation* 76(Suppl IV):IV-260, 1987.
148. Puleo, P. R., Perryman, M. B., Bresser, M. A., et al. Creatine kinase isoform analysis in the detection and assessment of thrombolysis in man. *Circulation* 75:1162, 1987.
149. Apple, F. S., Sharkey, S. W., Werdick, M., et al. Analyses of creatine kinase isoenzymes and isoforms in serum to detect reperfusion after acute myocardial infarction. *Clin. Chem.* 33:507, 1987.
150. Morelli, R. L., Emilson, B., and Rapaport, E. MM-CK subtypes diagnose reperfusion early after myocardial infarction. *Am. J. Med. Sci.* 293:139, 1987.
151. Roberts, R., Ludbrook, P. A., Weiss, E. S., et al. Serum CPK isoenzymes after cardiac catheterization. *Br. Heart J.* 37:1144, 1975.
152. Landt, T. Y., Vaida, H. C., Porter, S. E., et al. Semiautomated direct colorimetric measurement of creatine kinase isoenzyme-BM activity after extraction from serum by use of a CK-MB specific monoclonal antibody. *Clin. Chem.* 34:575, 1988.
153. Butch, A. W., Goodnow, T. T., and Brown, W. S. STRATUS automated creatine kinase-MB assay evaluated: Identification and elimination of falsely elevated results associated with a high molecular-mass form of alkaline phosphatase. *Clin. Chem.* 35:2048, 1989.
154. Eisenberg, P. R., Shaw, D., Schaab, C., et al. Concordance of creatine kinase-MB activity and mass. *Clin. Chem.* 35:440, 1984.
155. Konings, C. H., Funke-Kupper, A. J., and Verheugt, F. W. A. Comparison of two latex agglutination test kits for serum myoglobin in the exclusion of acute myocardial infarction. *Ann. Clin. Biochem.* 26:254, 1989.
156. Apple, F. S. Diagnostic markers for detection of acute myocardial infarction and reperfusion. *Lab. Med.* 23:298, 1992.
157. Schultz, A., Larsen, C. E., Kristensen, S. D., et al. Serum myoglobin measured by latex agglutination: rapid test for exclusion of acute myocardial infarction. *Am. Heart J.* 112:609, 1986.
158. Kricka, L. J. Myoglobin—An early marker of myocardial damage. *A.A.C.C. Endo.* 10:1, 1991.
159. Vaidya, H. C. Myoglobin. *Lab. Med.* 23:306, 1992.
160. Massoubre, C., Chivot, L., Mainard, F., et al. Immunonephelometric assay of myoglobin. *Clin. Chim. Acta* 201:223, 1991.
161. Delanghe, J. R., Chapelle, J. P., and Vanderschueren, S. C. Quantitative nephelometric assay for determining myoglobin evaluated. *Clin. Chem.* 36:1675, 1990.
162. CME-TV Study Guide. *Serum Cardiac Markers: Toward the Earlier Diagnosis of AMI.* Hagerman, Idaho: CME-TV, Inc., 1993.
163. Silva, D. P., Jr., Landt, Y., Porter, S. E., et al. Development and application of monoclonal antibodies to human cardiac myoglobin in a rapid fluorescence immunoassay. *Clin. Chem.* 37:1356, 1991.
164. Uji, Y., Okabe, H., Sugiuchi, H., et al. Measurement of serum myoglobin by a turbidimetric latex agglutination method. *J. Clin. Lab. Anal.* 6:7, 1992.
165. Katus, H. A., Diederich, K. W., Scheffold, T., et al. Non-invasive assessment of infarct reperfusion: The predictive power of the time to peak value of myoglobin, CKMB, and CK in serum. *Eur. Heart J.* 9:619, 1988.
166. Hoberg, E., Katus, H. A., Diederich, K. W., et al. Myoglobin, creatine kinase-B isoenzyme, and myosin light chain release in patients with unstable angina pectoris. *Eur. Heart J.* 8:989, 1987.
167. Adams, J. E. III, Abendschein, D. R., and Jaffe, A. S. Biochemical markers of myocardial injury: Is MB creatine kinase the choice for the 1990s? *Circulation* 88:750, 1993.
168. Roberts, R., and Kleiman, N. S. Earlier diagnosis and treatment of acute myocardial infarction necessitates the need for a "new diagnostic mind set." *Circulation* 89:872, 1993.
169. Katus, H. A., Looser, S., Hallermayer, H., et al. Development and in vitro characterization of a new immunoassay of cardiac troponin T. *Clin. Chem.* 38:386, 1992.
170. Zabel, M., Hohnloser, S. H., Koster, W., et al. Analysis of creatine kinase CK-MB, myoglobin, and troponin T time-activity curves for early assessment of coronary artery reperfusion after intravenous thrombolysis. *Circulation* 87:1542, 1993.
171. Roberts, R. Enzymatic estimation of infarct size. Thrombolysis induced its demise: Will it now rekindle its renaissance? *Circulation* 81:707, 1990.
172. Villarreal-Levy, G., Ma, T. S., Kerner, S. A., et al. Human creatine kinase: Isolation and sequence analysis of cDNA clones for the B subunit, development of subunit specific probes and determination of gene copy number. *Biochem. Biophys. Res. Commun.* 144:1116, 1987.
173. Perryman, M. B., Kerner, S. A., Bohlmeyer, T. J., et al. Isolation and sequence analysis of a full-length cDNA for human M creatine kinase. *Biochem. Biophys. Res. Commun.* 140:981, 1986.
174. Selker, H. P. Coronary care unit triage decision aids: How do we know when they work? *Am. J. Med.* 87:491, 1989.
175. Goldman, L., Cook, E. F., Brand, D. A., et al. A computer protocol to predict myocardial infarction in emergency department patients with chest pain. *N. Engl. J. Med.* 318:797, 1988.
176. Puleo, P. R., Guadagno, P. A., Roberts, R., et al.

A sensitive and rapid assay for the plasma subforms of MB creatine kinase. *Clin. Chem.* 35:1452, 1989.
177. Puleo, P. R., Guadagno, P. A., Roberts, R., et al. Early diagnosis of acute myocardial infarction based on assay for subforms of creatine kinase-MB. *Circulation* 82:759, 1990.
178. Puleo, P. R., Guadagno, P. A., Scheel, M. V., et al. Rapid and convenient assay of MB creatine kinase (CK) subforms in the initial hours of myocardial infarction (Abstract). *Circulation* 80:II, 1989.
179. Puleo, P. R., Wathen, C., Tawa, C. B., et al. Diagnosis or exclusion of acute myocardial infarction in the emergency room utilizing rapid MB creatine kinase subform assay. *N. Engl. J. Med.* (in press).

7. Routine Management of Acute Myocardial Infarction

Gary S. Francis

Early symptoms of ill health or prodromal chest pain are reported in 60 to 70 percent of patients ultimately diagnosed with acute myocardial infarction (AMI). *Prodromata* can be defined as a constellation of new symptoms, a sign of health deterioration, or a worsening or change in a stable pattern of symptoms or signs that occur in proximity to the myocardial infarction. Somewhat unexpectedly, a lack of college education is significantly related to the patient's recognition of prodromata [1]. In general, less educated patients tend to report a greater incidence of prodromata [1].

New or accelerated angina is one of the most common symptoms (35 percent), along with dyspnea (39 percent) and fatigue–weakness (42 percent) [1]. The most common response to prodromal symptoms is lay consultation (77 percent), with medical consultation being obtained by only 36 percent of patients prior to coming to the emergency ward [1]. Older individuals (65 years or older) are far more likely to consult a physician [1]. It is a somewhat disappointing fact that only 22 percent of patients who experience prodromata and consult their physician are evaluated within 24 hours, and only 56 percent are evaluated within 1 week [1]. The classic study of myocardial infarction prodromata by Alonzo and colleagues was conducted during the early 1970s, however, and there may be wider appreciation today by both lay people and physicians of the importance of prompt attention to the symptoms of a possible heart attack.

It is important to recognize that prodromal symptoms may be mild, intermittent, and ambiguous. The transcience of the symptoms may encourage "benign" neglect. Patients who have an established relationship with a physician are more likely to seek his or her advice [1]. Public education programs do heighten awareness, despite the medical community's apprehensions, and do not appear to inundate emergency rooms and physicians' offices with false and unjustified complaints [1]. Given our current ability to deal with early myocardial infarction, we owe it to our patients to carefully and quickly evaluate complaints that might serve as prodromata for myocardial infarction. Today this process is most expeditiously done in emergency wards, which should be staffed with experienced and qualified personnel.

Classic crescendo angina seems to be clearly related, retrospectively, to myocardial infarction [2, 3]. We now have substantial data that such patients are often undergoing a change in their coronary artery lesions [4–8], usually rupture of a plaque with intermittent thrombosis [9]. These patients should be promptly hospitalized and treated with anticoagulants and nitrates. Early coronary arteriography is necessary if pain is not readily responsive to therapy.

Of course, not all patients with prodromal symptoms progress to myocardial infarction. In fact, the Stanford group has reported that prodromata are equally reported by patients who develop myocardial infarction and those with myocardial ischemia who subsequently "rule out" [3]. The latter group, however, is well known to have a similar 18-month prognosis and should be vigorously investigated [10]. A "rule out" is not license to simply discharge the patient with a "clean bill of health." These patients, once "ruled out," should undergo a discharge exercise test and be considered for coronary angiography if the test is abnormal or if they continue to have evidence of myocardial ischemia at rest [10] (Fig. 7-1).

The real key to success lies in educating the public about coming to the hospital as soon as they have warning symptoms of AMI. Patients who

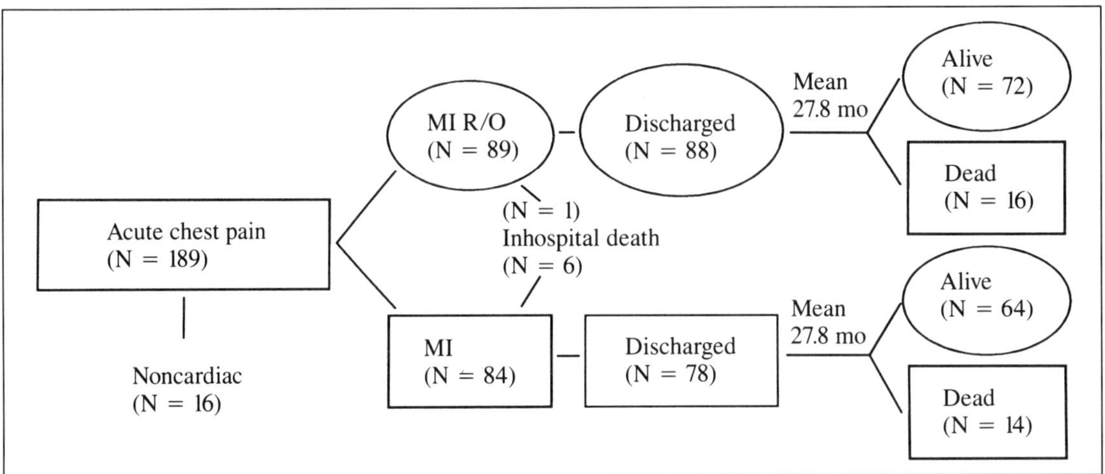

Fig. 7-1
Distribution and follow-up of 189 patients admitted with acute chest pain suspected to be a myocardial infarction. MI R/O = myocardial infarction ruled out. (From J. S. Schroeder et al. Do patients in whom myocardial infarction is ruled out have a better prognosis after hospitalization than those surviving infarction? *N. Engl. J. Med.* 303:1, 1980. Reprinted by permission.)

arrive early (within 2 hours of chest pain) have a significantly better prognosis during a 2-year follow-up than patients who arrive late (Fig. 7-2). Unfortunately, patients at relatively high risk of death after AMI (those with preexisting diabetes mellitus, systemic hypertension, or congestive heart failure), along with women and older patients tend to arrive significantly later in the emergency ward than patients without these characteristics [11].

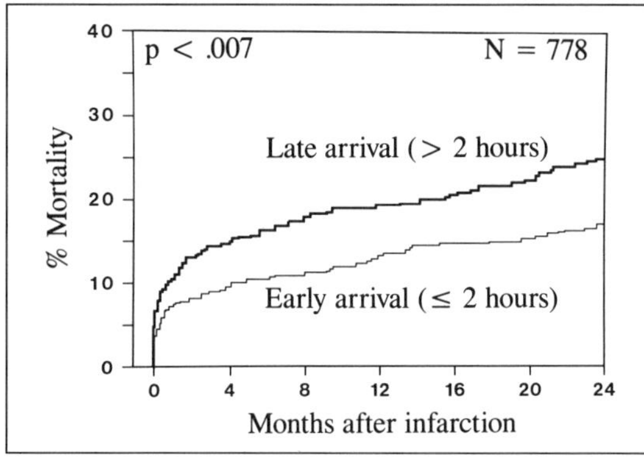

Fig. 7-2
Mortality over a 2-year period for early (within 2 hours) and late (more than 2 hours) arriving patients to the emergency ward with AMI. These data were collected prior to the thrombolysis era (August 1978 to December 1983). (From Z. G. Turi et al. Implications for acute intervention related to time of hospital arrival in acute myocardial infarction. *Am. J. Cardiol.* 58:203, 1986. With permission.)

Emergency Room Strategies

The management of AMI continues to evolve rapidly. There is now a firm consensus that transmural infarction is due to coronary artery thrombosis [12], after years of debate on this topic [13]. Reperfusion of an occluded artery, performed during the first few hours of evolving infarction, may reduce infarct size and improve survival [12–15]. Most of the clinical experience with reperfusion has been with streptokinase [14–17], but recombinant tissue-type plasminogen activator (rt-PA), a relatively fibrin-specific agent, appears to have a superior coronary recanalization rate [18]. Several points have become clear when considering these data: (1) Time is critical—the sooner the artery is recanalized, the more striking the improvement in survival [14]; and (2) more benefit is derived from reperfusing arteries subtending large amounts of myocardial tissue. These changes in the management of AMI have profound implications for emergency care physicians [19].

Nearly 50 percent of patients with AMI who present to the emergency room have a normal or nondiagnostic electrocardiogram (ECG). To improve diagnostic accuracy, serial ECGs should be obtained every 30 minutes while the patient with chest pain is evaluated in the emergency room. When the diagnosis is clinically secure, thrombolytic therapy should be given without hesitation. The promise of thrombolytic therapy remains largely unfulfilled; it is estimated that only 10 percent of patients with AMI currently receive thrombolytic therapy. Patients who are judged clinically as unsuitable for thrombolytic therapy have a higher risk for adverse cardiovascular events [20].

To achieve beneficial results of thrombolytic therapy, a well organized and efficient emergency care system is required. Processes that ordinarily delay care, including waiting for blood tests, sending the patient for x-ray examinations, and extensive consultation, must be avoided. Instead, emphasis must be placed on the rapid and accurate diagnosis of AMI. This approach requires cardiologists to become more intimately involved with the activities of the emergency ward. In certain situations, the need for transfer of a well defined subset of patients to more specialized hospitals is necessary, but community hospitals can clearly participate [21].

Because thrombolytic therapy is not without risk, contraindications to this form of therapy must be clearly understood. The most serious complication is intracranial bleeding, which occurred with a frequency of 0.2 percent in the Gruppo Italiano per lo Studio della Streptochinasi nell'Infarto Miocardico (GISSI) trial [14], 0.46 percent in the Intravenous Streptokinase in Acute Myocardial Infarction (ISAM) trial [17], and 1.6 percent in the Thrombolysis in Myocardial Infarction (TIMI) trial using 150 mg of rt-PA for 6 hours and 0.6 percent when 100 mg was given for 6 hours [22]. The frequency of cerebral hemorrhage related to streptokinase in the second International Study of Infarct Survival (ISIS-2) trial was 0.1 percent [23]. Therefore, patients with AMI who receive thrombolytic therapy have a small risk of stroke. Those treated with tissue plasminogen activator (t-PA) have a small but significant excess of stroke as compared with those who receive streptokinase (1.33 versus 0.94 percent, GISSI-II) [24]. There was also a significant excess of strokes with t-PA in ISIS-3 (1.39 t-PA versus 1.04 streptokinase, $p < .01$) [25]. Subcutaneous heparin used in conjunction with a thrombolytic agent does not appear to increase the risk of stroke (risk with heparin 1.13% versus 1.14% without subcutaneous heparin, GISSI-II). However, older age, a higher Killip class, and the occurrence of anterior myocardial infarction significantly increase the risk of stroke.

It is important for each emergency care system to develop a uniform protocol for managing AMI. In general, the decision to use thrombolytic therapy for AMI and its initiation should be carried out in the emergency ward. As it now stands, patients who present with ECG evidence of AMI (ST segment elevation) and who have no contraindications should be considered for thrombolytic therapy in the emergency ward prior to transport to the coronary care unit (CCU) (Fig. 7-3). The time window is narrow and not clearly defined, but our current understanding suggests that most improvement occurs when lytic therapy is begun within 4 hours of the onset

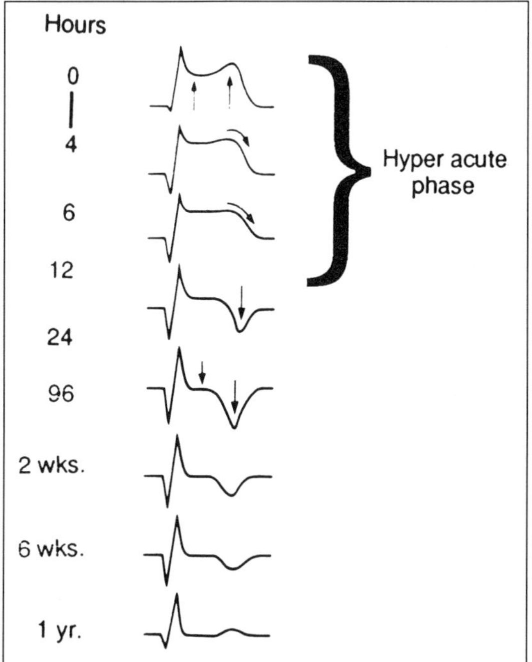

Fig. 7-3
Evolution of electrocardiographic changes observed in myocardial infarction. Serial changes are depicted. (From G. T. Gau. Electrocardiography and Vectorcardiography. In R. O. Brandenburg, V. Fuster, E. R. Giuliani et al. [eds.], *Cardiology: Fundamentals and Practice* [Vol. I]. Chicago: Year Book Medical Publishers, 1987. P. 268. By permission of the Mayo Foundation.)

of pain; this window can probably be extended to 12 hours or longer in patients who continue to have unrelenting chest pain. In fact, there is a growing body of evidence that suggests that a patent infarct-related artery may be beneficial even beyond the time that patency may salvage myocardium [23, 26].

In addition to the history and physical examination, the ECG remains the most useful tool in the rapid and accurate diagnosis of AMI. The sensitivity and specificity of the ECG are excellent in patients with documented anterior AMI (86.7 percent sensitive and 89.5 percent specific in one study [27]). When left bundle branch block and paced rhythm are excluded, it is the most useful early test available for establishing the correct diagnosis [28]. Patients admitted to the hospital to "rule out myocardial infarction" despite a negative ECG often go on to infarction on follow-up (17 percent in the study by Behar et al. [29]), so that clinical judgment remains the pivotal process. Remarkably, data by Lee and colleagues [30] indicated that only 4 percent of patients with AMI are misdiagnosed and discharged from the emergency ward. About one-half the missed AMIs could have been diagnosed by improved ECG reading skills [30], further emphasizing the need for cardiologists to interact with emergency care physicians.

An ECG is always performed for any patient presenting to the emergency ward with symptoms possibly due to ischemic heart disease. A completely normal ECG makes AMI unlikely [31]. Only 1 percent of such patients have AMI, and only 4 percent of this group eventually are diagnosed as having unstable angina. Most patients (60 percent) with AMI have *new* findings of ST segment elevation or Q waves, and almost all others show *new* changes of ischemia. About 15 percent of patients with AMI present to the emergency room with an abnormal ECG but no *new* changes. One need not prove that the ECG changes are new—only that they are not known to be old. A common mistake is to assume that ECG changes are old, when there is no former ECG that shows those findings. One should not rely too heavily on telephone descriptions, which are often unreliable.

The initial ECG can be helpful for determining triage options: a CCU, an intermediate care unit, or discharge [31]. Patients with ECGs that show evidence of infarction, ischemia, strain, left ventricular hypertrophy, left bundle branch block, or paced rhythm are far more likely to have a life-threatening complication (ventricular fibrillation, sustained ventricular tachycardia, or heart block) when the clinical diagnosis of AMI is suspected, and these patients should be sent to the CCU. Such complications are 23 times more likely to occur, according to Brush et al. [31]. Alternatively, a normal ECG in the face of suspected AMI portends a good prognosis (0.6 percent chance of life-threatening complication), and these patients can be admitted to an intermediate care unit. This protocol would reduce admissions to a CCU by 36 percent and thereby save considerable hospital costs without compromising patient care.

Patients with AMI and severe hypotension (shock) or hemodynamic instability should be sent immediately to the cardiac catheterization laboratory for percutaneous transluminal coronary angioplasty (PTCA).

Data produced in the GISSI-II and ISIS-2 trials indicate that the elderly derive a clear, favorable benefit-to-risk ratio for thrombolytic treatment [32]. The data also demonstrate that t-PA is associated with a higher rate of hemorrhagic stroke in the elderly, but the risk can be modulated favorably if the dose is adjusted for weight [33].

Recent evidence suggests that "front-loaded" or accelerated infusions of t-PA may be more effective than the currently approved standard dose [34, 35]. The recently concluded Global Utilization of Streptokinase and t-PA for Occluded Coronary Arteries (GUSTO) Trial supports the following approach [126]:

1. Aspirin 160-mg oral dose immediately.
2. Intravenous heparin 5,000-unit bolus immediately.
3. Intravenous heparin infusion 1,000 units per hour (1200 units for patients >80 kg) adjusted to keep partial thromboplastin time (PTT) 60–85 seconds and continued for 3 to 5 days.
4. Intravenous t-PA 15-mg bolus followed by an infusion of 0.75 mg/kg for 30 minutes, not to exceed 50 mg, followed by 0.5 mg/kg to 35 mg for 60 minutes. The t-PA dose should be weight adjusted.
5. Intravenous atenolol 5 mg for 5 minutes; after 10 minutes an additional 5 mg intravenously for 5 minutes; after another 10 minutes a 50-mg oral

dose. Beta-adrenergic blockers are contraindicated in patients with heart block, severe left ventricular dysfunction with overt heart failure or cardiogenic shock, a history of asthma, or severe chronic obstructive lung disease.

When the patient has previously received streptokinase, urokinase or anistreplase (anisoylated plasminogen streptokinase activator complex [APSAC]) or if the patient is modestly bradycardic or hypotensive, t-PA is preferred. Front-loaded t-PA may be preferred in young patients who present very early with anterior myocardial infarction. The standard, approved dose of t-PA is a 10-mg bolus followed by a 1-hour infusion of 50 mg. Twenty milligrams is then given for the second hour, with the final 20 mg given during the third hour (total dose of t-PA = 100 mg during 3 hours). When streptokinase is chosen, 1.5 million units is given for 60 minutes. For APSAC, a 30-unit bolus is given intravenously. For urokinase, 3 million units is given for 45 to 60 minutes.

There are reasonable bedside markers of reperfusion following thrombolytic therapy [36]. A rapid and progressive decrease in pain and ST elevation are reliable indicators, but frequent fluctuations of both are common. Accelerated idioventricular rhythm and episodes of sinus bradycardia are generally specific for reperfusion, but do not always occur when the heart is reperfused.

There is now sufficient evidence the "window" for thrombolytic therapy can be extended to at least 12 hours. The Late Assessment of Thrombolytic Efficacy trial (LATE) demonstrated an 8.9 percent mortality rate in the t-PA group versus 11.97 percent in the placebo group for patients treated within 12 hours [127]. A sizable group present after 6 hours. In ISIS-3, 22 percent of patients presented after 6 hours [25]. After 12 hours, patients who may benefit the most, such as the elderly, patients with large infarction, and those with continuing pain, should be considered for thrombolytic therapy [37]. Improvement in global and regional systolic function is more closely related to the initial extent of acutely depressed ventricular function than the time to thrombolytic therapy [38]. However, opening the occluded artery in the absence of overt ischemia may not benefit left ventricular function at 6 weeks [39].

The risks and benefits of adding intravenous heparin to aspirin and thrombolysis are still debated. The routine administration of full dose heparin as adjunctive therapy to aspirin and thrombolysis has not been tested fully in a large-scale randomized trial [128]. In general, intravenous heparin is recommended when giving t-PA. Data in support of giving intravenous heparin with streptokinase are lacking. Future studies with new thrombin inhibitors, such as hirudin and hirulog, may provide important new information about this unresolved clinical question.

Because of the cost of t-PA, controversy continues over the issue of streptokinase versus t-PA. Front-loaded t-PA, as given in GUSTO, was associated with an excess of hemorrhagic strokes compared to the use of streptokinase ($p = .03$). However, GUSTO showed that front-loaded t-PA has a mortality benefit of about 1 percent, at a cost differential of about $2400. Young patients with an anterior myocardial infarction who arrive at the hospital early will benefit most from front-loaded t-PA. There is much less confidence about older patients with inferior myocardial infarctions who arrive late. Very early institution of therapy is far more important than the type of thrombolytic agent used. More attention to the concept of very early treatment is essential.

Control of Pain, Sedation, and Hypertension

The relief of pain in patients with AMI remains an important priority. Generally, two strategies are employed: (1) reduction of ischemia and (2) direct analgesia.

Relief of Myocardial Ischemia

Although once considered contraindicated for AMI, nitroglycerin can decrease myocardial oxygen demand by decreasing preload and afterload and decreasing left ventricular wall tension [40–42]. Nitrates may also improve collateral flow to the ischemic myocardium [43, 44]. Nitrates are generally safe and well tolerated. Although mononitrate did not reduce mortality in ISIS-4, nitrates continue to be widely used in the routine management of AMI. Patients with AMI should be considered for treatment with sublingual nitroglycerin provided hypotension is not present [45]. In fact, sublingual nitroglycerin (20 to 25 mg) is comparable to intravenous morphine for pain relief and has a more favorable effect on ECG estimates of myocardial necrosis (Fig. 7-4) [45]. However, hypotension can occur with sublingual nitroglycerin (Fig. 7-5), and the patient should be observed carefully for clinical improvement or changes in hemodynamics. If the initial dose is well tolerated, intravenous nitroglycerin should be administered with careful monitoring of blood pressure [46]. The dose may vary from 10 to 200 μg/min and should be titrated so as not to allow the systolic blood pressure to fall below 90 mm Hg. Long-acting oral nitrates should be avoided during very early myocardial infarction because there is far less control over the hemodynamic response. Patients with inferior myocardial infarction are more prone to develop hypotension and bradycardia following nitroglycerin [47]; it should be used cautiously in these patients. This complication can be reversed by raising the patient's legs and giving intravenous atropine (Figs. 7-6 and 7-7) [47]. Patients with presumed right ventricular myocardial infarction should probably not be given nitroglycerin, as they are much more dependent on an increased preload to maintain stroke volume [48].

Although substantial reductions in blood pressure may be well tolerated by patients with acute myocardial infarction given nitroglycerin [49, 50], it is prudent to achieve a reduction in mean arterial pressure of only 10 percent [51, 52]. Severe hypotension and bradycardia, which occur in about 10 percent of patients given nitroglycerin in the setting of AMI, can occur even with the intravenous preparation (Figs. 7-5 and 7-6) [47].

Nitroglycerin appears to be most useful in patients with anterior AMI who have persistent or recurrent chest pain or heart failure. It should be initiated at a dose of 10 μg/min and increased by 10 μg/min every 10 minutes to achieve a 10 percent reduction in systolic blood pressure; heart rate should not be allowed to increase by more than 20 percent, and systolic blood pressure should not be allowed to go below 90 mm Hg. Doses beyond 200 μg/min are rarely necessary.

Sodium nitroprusside, because of its more balanced effect on preload and afterload, may be a logical alternative to nitroglycerin. This hypothesis was tested in the large Veterans Administration trial [53] that required patients to have a left ventricular

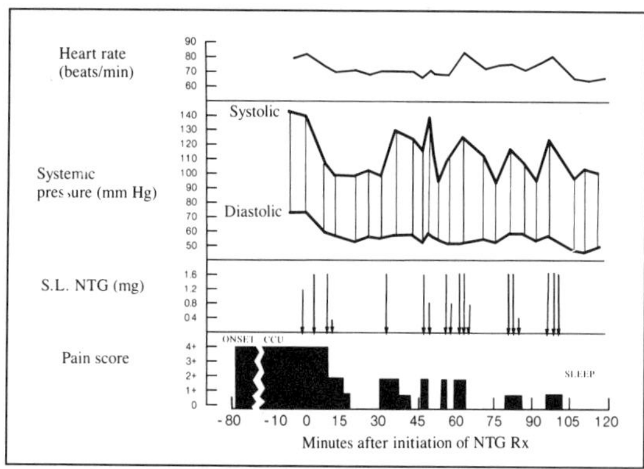

Fig. 7-4
A patient with AMI was treated with high-dose sublingual nitroglycerin (S.L. NTG). *Arrows* denote the amount and time of administration. The effects of high-dose sublingual nitroglycerin on ST segment change and pain are comparable to those of morphine sulfate [32]. (From Y. I. Kim and J. F. Williams, Jr. Large dose sublingual nitroglycerin in acute myocardial infarction: Relief of chest pain and reduction of Q-wave evolution. *Am. J. Cardiol.* 49:842, 1982. With permission.)

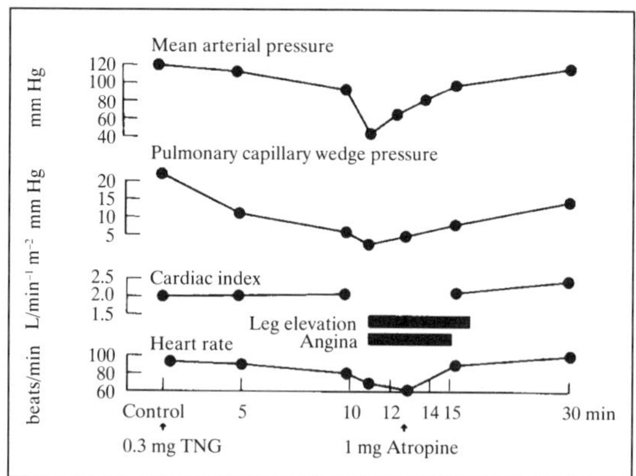

Fig. 7-5
Hemodynamic effects of 0.3 mg sublingual nitroglycerin in a patient who developed a precipitous fall in mean arterial pressure. The patient's symptoms and hypotension were relieved by raising the legs and administration of 1 mg of intravenous atropine. (From C. E. Delgado et al. Role of sublingual nitroglycerin in patients with acute myocardial infarction. *Br. Heart J.* 37:392, 1975. With permission.)

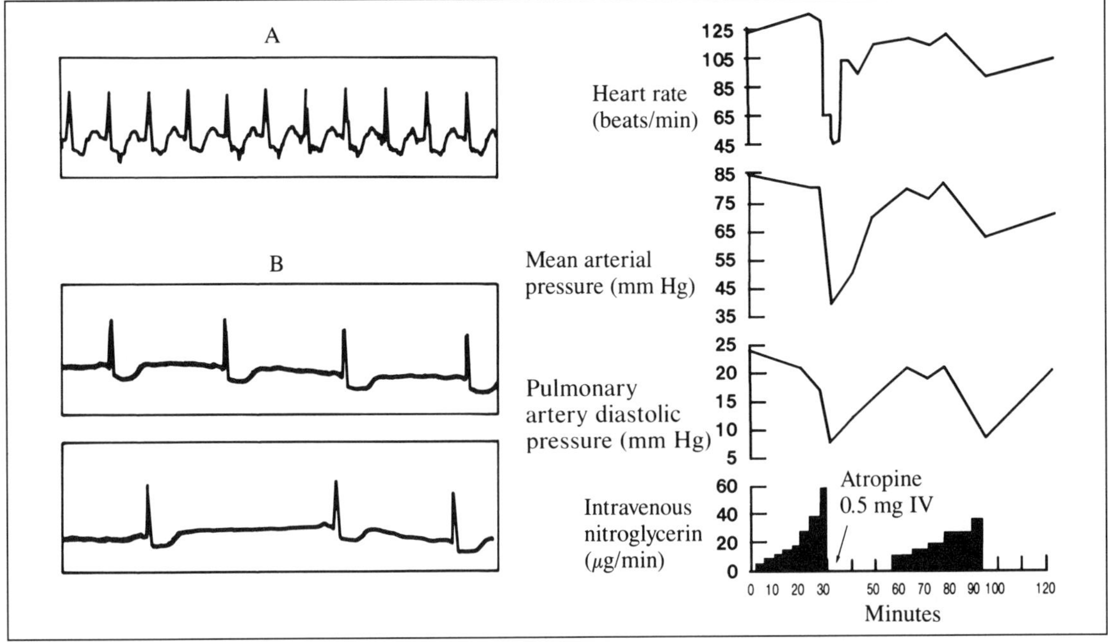

Fig. 7-6
ECG recordings (*left panel*) from a patient with acute anteroseptal myocardial infarction and sinus tachycardia (*A*). Intravenous nitroglycerin (*right panel*) caused bradycardia (*B*) and severe arterial hypotension at 20 to 40 μg/min. It was responsive to 0.5 mg of intravenous atropine but recurred following the reinstitution of intravenous nitroglycerin. (From P. C. Come and B. Pitt. Nitroglycerin induced severe myocardial infarction. *Circulation* 54:624, 1976. By permission of the American Heart Association, Inc.)

filling pressure of 12 mm Hg or more to enter the protocol. In fact, early use of nitroprusside actually increased mortality compared with placebo (24 percent versus 13 percent). Patients with pump dysfunction persistent beyond 9 hours after onset of symptoms may benefit from nitroprusside [53], but nitroglycerin infusion is now preferred to nitroprusside early after acute infarction.

Analgesia

Morphine sulfate remains the standard analgesic for patients with AMI. Meperidine and pentazocine can be substituted in patients with well documented hypersensitivity to morphine. Morphine is usually given in doses of 4 to 8 mg intravenously and repeated every 5 to 15 minutes in doses of 2 to 8 mg until pain is relieved. Occasionally, large, cumulative doses (2 to 3 mg/kg) are required to relieve pain. Hypotension, bradycardia, nausea, and vomiting can occur, as well as respiratory depression. A rather pronounced peripheral venodilator effect occurs that reduces preload and is helpful in patients with pulmonary edema [54, 55]. However, despite peripheral venous dilation, left ventricular filling pressure does not change strikingly with morphine, and the mechanism whereby it relieves cardiac dyspnea is not understood [56]. When combined with other vasodilators (e.g., nitroglycerin), the hypotensive action of morphine may be exaggerated. This reaction can also occur in patients who are hypovolemic, which is often the case in patients with AMI. In the event of morphine-induced respiratory depression, naloxone hydrochloride should be administered in 0.4-mg increments intravenously to a total dose of 1.4 mg. Occasionally, a patient may need artificial ventilation.

Hypertension

Blood pressure elevation early during the evolution of AMI is common, occurring in 30 to 40 percent

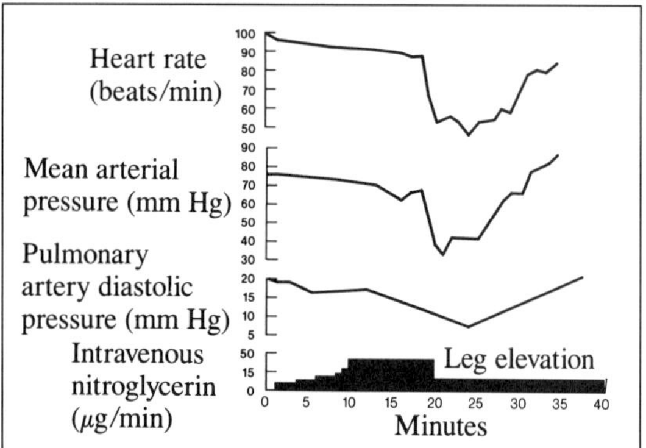

Fig. 7-7
Hemodynamic changes in a patient with acute non-Q-wave myocardial infarction given intravenous nitroglycerin. In this case, the hypotension responded to leg elevation. Nitroglycerin-induced hypotension and bradycardia can occur with the sublingual or intravenous preparation in patients with Q-wave or non-Q-wave infarction, or anterior or inferior infarction, although it is more commonly observed in patients with inferior myocardial infarction. (From P. C. Come and B. Pitt. Nitroglycerin induced severe myocardial infarction. *Circulation* 54:624, 1976. By permission of the American Heart Association, Inc.)

of patients, depending on the criteria used [57]. However, because an elevated blood pressure may improve perfusion to areas supplied by partially obstructed vessels, but also increases myocardial oxygen demand by increasing left ventricular wall stress, it is difficult to predict the overall effects of altering arterial pressure on myocardial oxygen supply and demand. Increasing mean arterial pressure in experimental myocardial infarction from 110 mm Hg to 145 mm Hg clearly results in extension of ischemic injury [58]. In patients with chronic coronary artery disease, at similar increases in myocardial oxygen consumption, the stress of increased heart rate results in more myocardial ischemia than the stress of increased afterload [59]. In the dog with acute coronary artery occlusion, an increase in systemic arterial pressure exerts an influence on the severity of myocardial ischemic injury that is related directly to the magnitude of systemic arterial hypertension: a mild increase of pressure (diastolic pressure 95 to 115 mm Hg) reduces ischemic injury; a moderate increase (diastolic pressure 116 to 140 mm Hg) exerts no consistent effect on ischemia; and a marked increase (diastolic pressure >140 mm Hg) worsens ischemic injury [60]. However, 24 hours of mildly increased aortic pressure accentuates end-diastolic wall thinning and results in failure to return to control values [61]. Patients with long-standing systemic hypertension and left ventricular hypertrophy may be at particular risk during AMI. Experimental coronary occlusion in animals with hypertension and left ventricular hypertrophy is associated with reduced collateral flow to the area at risk [62]. Moreover, infarct size relative to the area at risk is increased significantly with left ventricular hypertrophy [62].

Given these experimental findings, it seems reasonable to control excessively elevated blood pressure in patients with AMI. No precise guidelines can be stated, but a persistently elevated systolic blood pressure (>150 mm Hg), diastolic blood pressure (>110 mm Hg), or both, should probably be treated if the pressure does not readily respond to analgesics and sedation. Treatment regimens vary with local policy. Nitroprusside (10 to 300 μg/min) usually controls blood pressure sufficiently. Intravenous labetalol (20 mg IV slowly), repeated as necessary, also is useful and usually prevents reflex tachycardia. Intravenous nitroglycerin and beta blockers can be used to control systemic hypertension. Precipitous lowering of blood pressure by agents such as nifedipine or hydralazine should be avoided.

Lidocaine

The routine use of prophylactic lidocaine in patients with suspected AMI should be avoided where facilities for resuscitation are available [63, 64]. Its use should be restricted to patients with suspected AMI who have premature ventricular beats that are frequent (>6/min), closely coupled (R-on-T), multiform in configuration, and occur in short bursts of 3 or more in succession. It should also be used in patients with ventricular tachycardia or ventricular fibrillation. An initial intravenous injection of 1 mg/kg, not to exceed 100 mg, should be given, with additional injections of 0.5 mg/kg every 8 to 10 minutes if necessary, to a total of 4 mg/kg. A maintenance dose of 1.4 to 3.5 mg/min in a 70-kg patient is usually sufficient. The loading dose and maintenance dose should be markedly reduced in patients with heart failure, shock, liver disease, and in the elderly. Patients with AMI observed from 1970 to 1990 showed a declining incidence of primary ventricular fibrillation.

Atropine

Patients with AV block or symptomatic sinus bradycardia should be given 0.5 mg atropine intravenously, repeated every 5 minutes for a total dose of no more than 2 mg. Doses less than 0.5 mg may cause paradoxical slowing; excessive doses are associated with sinus tachycardia, urinary retention, and adverse central nervous system effects. Pacemaker insertion is the treatment of choice for symptomatic bradycardia not responding promptly to atropine administration.

Calcium Channel Blockers

Calcium channel blockers reduce myocardial oxygen demand by lowering blood pressure and can improve coronary blood flow by dilating coronary arteries. Nevertheless, they have no role in the routine management of patients with AMI. Reflex tachycardia, myocardial depression, and diversion of blood from ischemic zones may account for their lack of benefit. A large meta-analysis has demonstrated that prophylactic use of calcium channel blockers is not likely to be beneficial and may be potentially harmful in some high-risk patients with AMI [66].

Magnesium

Several small clinical trials have demonstrated that intravenous magnesium has a favorable effect on patients with AMI. In addition to its well-known antiarrhythmic effects, magnesium produces systemic vasodilation, reducing myocardial oxygen demand, improves coronary blood flow, decreases platelet aggregation, and protects against excessive catecholamine effects on the heart [67]. Results of the recent Leicester Intravenous Magnesium Intervention Trial (LIMIT-2) indicate that intravenous magnesium sulfate (8 m*M* for 5 minutes followed by 65 m*M* for 24 hours) reduced early mortality in AMI by 24 percent, but there was no apparent antiarrhythmic effect [68]. However, this was not confirmed in ISIS-4, demonstrating that small trials can be misleading. Magnesium cannot be routinely recommended for the treatment of AMI. It may benefit occasional patients who demonstrate hypomagnesemia.

ACE Inhibitors

The results of the Survival and Ventricular Enlargement (SAVE) trial suggest that captopril, when started, on average, 11 days after myocardial infarction, may improve survival in patients with a transmural AMI who have an ejection fraction of 0.40 or less and no overt heart failure [124]. The drug, a widely used angiotensin-converting enzyme (ACE) inhibitor, is begun at 6.25 mg tid, and gradually titrated over several weeks to 50 mg tid. The mechanism of its favorable effect is not entirely clear, but patients assigned to captopril had fewer myocardial ischemic events and less need for angioplasty or coronary artery bypass surgery. Although the precise timing of when to initiate captopril and how to define which patient population benefits most are not yet clear, a strong case can be made for using captopril in patients after the acute phase of myocardial infarction, provided there is an observable reduction in left ventricular ejection fraction ($\leq$0.40) and no contraindication for its use. These observations recently have been confirmed by the Acute Infarction Ramipril Efficacy (AIRE) trial, which demonstrated that ramipril titrated to 5 mg bid when given to patients with clinical evidence of either transient or ongoing heart failure after myocardial infarction (day 2 to day 9) was associated with a substantial survival benefit [125]. This benefit was apparent across all subgroups, and occurred as early as 30 days into the trial. In ISIS-4, patients who received captopril had a small but significant decrease in mortality that persisted at 6 months. A small reduction in mortality was also observed with the use of lisinopril in GISSI-III, indicating the ACE inhibitors have a very consistent beneficial role in patients with AMI.

Other Routine Measures of Care

A soft or liquid diet is usually prescribed during the first 24 hours following AMI. Stable patients can be given a 1200-calorie, low-sodium, low-cholesterol diet. Caffeine and other stimulants are avoided. A stool softener is traditionally given to prevent straining at stool, and patients should be advised to use a bedside commode if possible from day 1.

Nearly all patients with AMI are hypoxemic [70, 71]. The mechanism of the hypoxemia is poorly understood but is probably related to small airway dysfunction secondary to elevated pulmonary capillary wedge pressure [72] and reduced lung volume [73]. Oxygen is routinely administered at a dose of 2 to 4 L/min for the first 3 to 4 days following AMI.

Chest Radiograph

A chest radiograph should be obtained on admission in all patients, as there is a good relation between left ventricular hemodynamics and the radiographic findings [74–76]. The heart size and extent of pulmonary vascular markings offer important prognostic information [77]. In the absence of pulmonary congestion, according to Thomas et al. [74], there is a 94 percent 1-month survival and 88 percent 1-year survival. When the heart size is also normal, there is a 96 percent 1-month survival and a 91 percent 1-year survival. With diffuse alveolar edema present on the initial chest radiograph, there is an 18 percent 1-month survival and no 1-year survivals. Therefore, the degree of pulmonary vascular congestion and left heart size on the initial chest radiograph after AMI are useful for defining high-risk and low-risk groups.

Drug Interactions

An inventory of what medications the patient already is taking at the time of the myocardial infarction must be carefully determined. Those drugs that are known to put the patient at further risk should be discontinued. For example, if the patient presents with AMI and severe congestive heart failure or complete heart block and is taking a beta-adrenergic blocker, the beta blocker should be stopped. Contrary to widespread concern that the sudden withdrawal of beta-adrenoceptor blocking drugs may result in a rebound adrenergic hypersensitivity state, this appears not to be a major problem in patients with AMI [78]. Likewise, one would also likely discontinue other drugs known to interfere with atrioventricular (AV) nodal conduction, such as verapamil (which could also aggravate heart failure) or diltiazem, in patients with severe heart failure or heart block.

Drug interactions must be carefully assessed. For example, diltiazem, cimetidine [79], and lidocaine [80–83] can cause sinus node arrest in patients with underlying sinus node dysfunction. Any combination of these drugs, particularly if a beta-adrenergic blocker is also being used, might be expected to cause sinus node standstill. Cimetidine also increases the biologic half-life of propranolol by reducing liver blood flow [84], thereby enhancing its negative inotropic and chronotropic properties. The frequency of bradyarrhythmias, when the combination of diltiazem and a beta blocker is used, has been particularly noticeable. The risk-benefit ratio of virtually every medication prescribed in the setting of AMI must be carefully weighed: How will it influence loading conditions, electrical conduction, myocardial oxygen demand, and coronary blood flow? What is the possible interaction with other agents?

Electrocardiogram

The admission ECG should always be carefully evaluated. Repeat ECGs should be ordered routinely each morning and should be obtained *during chest pain* and whenever there is a change in the patient's clinical course. Pseudoinfarct patterns may occur in healthy young athletes as well as patients with idiopathic dilated cardiomyopathy, subarachnoid hemorrhage, idiopathic hypertrophic subaortic stenosis, and preexcitation syndromes [85]. Although upright tall T waves appear simultaneously with ST segment elevation in patients with AMI [86], the T waves may be the earlier ECG sign of myocardial injury [87]. ST segment elevation does not necessarily signify subsequent myocardial necrosis [88]. Marked transient giant R waves can be seen before or after ventricular fibrillation [89]. Lead III is most likely to have ST segment elevation in patients with inferior AMI (94 percent), whereas lead V_2 has the highest incidence of ST segment elevation in patients with an anterior AMI [90]. Although the ECG is a good indicator of the general location of a myocardial infarction, detailed ECG classification schemes to locate infarctions precisely are not useful [91, 92]. ECG-diagnosed anterior, posterior, and apical myocardial infarctions generally correlate with pathologic anatomy, however [93]. Circumflex coronary artery occlusion can perhaps be identified by ST segment elevation in one or more inferior leads (II, III, aVF) with ST segment elevation in one or more lateral leads (aVL, V_5, or V_6) without ST segment depression in lead I [94]. ST segment elevation (V_2) may occur when the left anterior descending coronary artery is occluded and no collateral circulation is present, whereas a similar occlusion may cause ST segment depression when collateral function is adequate [95]. In general, however, it is treacherous to attempt to define precisely the pathologic coronary substrate based on the initial ECG.

The pathogenic implications of precordial ST segment depression during an acute inferior transmural myocardial infarction are controversial [96, 97]. Two hypotheses have been advanced to explain these ECG findings: (1) reciprocal changes due to the representation of the ischemic ST segment vector in leads opposite the area of ischemia; and (2) adjacent or distant ischemia related to multiple-vessel disease. Despite the fact that this ST segment depression may not always represent "ischemia at a distance" [98], it is now reasonably clear that *persistent* precordial lead ST segment depression observed with a pattern of acute transmural inferior infarction predicts clinical and hemodynamic left ventricular dysfunction [99], and the prognosis is accordingly influenced [99, 100].

Non-Q-Wave Myocardial Infarction

Myocardial infarction has been conventionally referred to as transmural (Q wave) and nontransmural (non-Q-wave) [101]. It was not until 1944, with the introduction of the precordial leads, that the Q wave was thought to be associated with "coronary thrombosis." However, it was soon recognized that the Q wave, although rather sensitive, was lacking in specificity. Moreover, careful postmortem examinations indicated that about one-half of "subendocardial infarcts" generated pathologic Q waves, whereas one-half of the transmural infarcts did not [102]. It has been suggested that the terms *Q wave* and *non-Q-wave* do not precisely relate to the previous terms *transmural* and *nontransmural* infarction [103]. In contrast to Q-wave infarction, total coronary occlusion of the infarct-related vessel is unusual in the early hours of non-Q-wave infarction, although it tends to increase over subsequent days [104]. Non-Q-wave infarction may be related to a marginally preserved blood supply that is still sufficient to cause tissue necrosis. Although patients with non-Q-wave infarction may have a somewhat more benign in-hospital course compared with patients having a Q-wave myocardial infarction, their long-term prognosis is similar or even somewhat worse [101]. They are at risk for early reinfarction, angina, and bypass surgery [105, 106]. The presence of complex ventricular arrhythmias at the time of hospital discharge is an important predictor of 1-year mortality in the presence of non-Q-wave infarction [107]. Because these patients are more prone to recurrent ischemic events, they frequently undergo angiography and surgery. It has been demonstrated in patients with non-Q-wave infarction that diltiazem (90 mg every 6 hours) effectively prevents early reinfarction and severe angina [108].

Myocardial Infarct Extension and Expansion

The complication of myocardial infarction extension, as defined by a rise in plasma MB creatine kinase (MB-CK), occurs in 8 to 9 percent of patients [109]. Hospital mortality for these patients is increased fourfold (Fig. 7-8) but is not different for nonextension patients once they leave the hospital. Cardiogenic shock is experienced more than three times as often in patients with extension, thereby contributing to the markedly increased hospital mortality. Extension can occur early, before the return of plasma MB-CK to baseline or, more often, late (days 5 to 7), after the return of plasma MB-CK to baseline (Fig. 7-9). Less than one-half of patients with extension have recurrent ischemic pain or ECG changes, implying that this complication is likely to be missed unless frequent sampling of enzymes is performed. Important clinical events or findings have also been shown to have predictive value with regard to myocardial extension, however. Patients with recurrent ischemic pain during

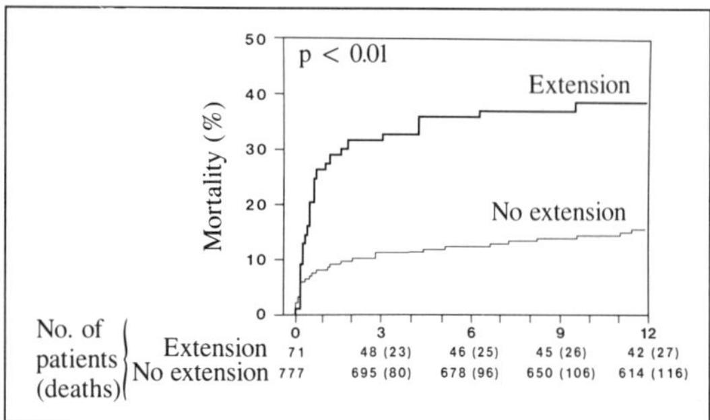

Fig. 7-8
Cumulative mortality in patients with and without myocardial infarct extension. There is a significant increase in early mortality in patients with extension ($p<.01$). The subsequent mortality of the two groups is not significantly different. (From J. E. Muller et al. Myocardial infarct extension: Occurrence, outcome, and risk factors in the multicenter investigation of limitation of infarct size. *Ann. Intern. Med.* 108:1, 1988. With permission.)

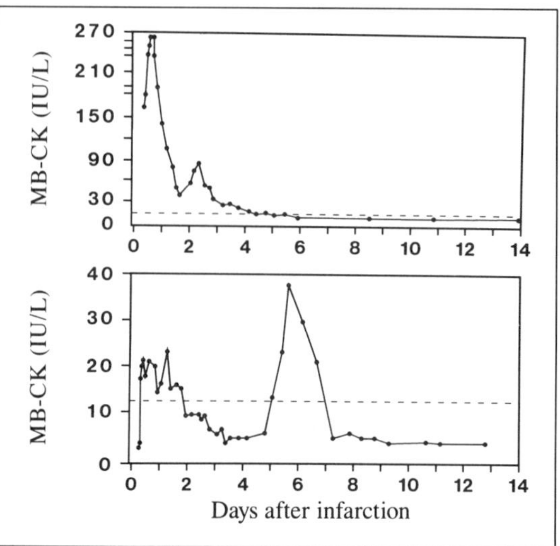

Fig. 7-9
MB creatine kinase (MB-CK) time-activity curves for a patient in whom the myocardial extension occurred before return of plasma MB-CK to baseline (*top*) and a patient in whom extension occurred after return of MB-CK to baseline (*bottom*). The area below the *dashed line* represents the normal range of MB-CK values. (From J. E. Muller et al. Myocardial infarct extension: Occurrence, outcome, and risk factors in the multicenter investigation of limitation of infarct size. *Ann. Intern. Med.* 108:1, 1988. With permission.)

the second hospital day, those with a history of previous myocardial infarction, and those with ST segment depression on the admission ECG (non-Q-wave infarction) are more likely to experience extension [109]. Such patients, known to be at risk for extension, should be considered for early coronary arteriography and possible interventions to reduce the high early-hospital mortality.

Myocardial infarct expansion, a fixed, permanent, disproportionate regional thinning and dilation of the infarct zone, occurs with 35 to 40 percent of anterior transmural infarctions [110–114]. It does not occur in non-Q-wave myocardial infarction. Patients with a history of systemic hypertension are at greater risk for this serious complication [115], which often leads to progressive and chronic ventricular enlargement and congestive heart failure. Anti-inflammatory agents may contribute to infarct expansion [114]. There are experimental data from the rat model of myocardial infarction that captopril may reduce myocardial remodeling and thereby improve survival when given prophylactically soon after the acute injury [116]. Infarct expansion has also been shown to be reduced by administering oral nifedipine (120 mg daily) beginning on the day of infarction and continuing for 10 days [117]. Despite the severity of this complication, however, one should be cautious about applying any form of "routine" therapy. The effects of calcium channel blockers on survival after myocardial infarction have tended to favor a small excess mortality in the treated group [118]. Further study is necessary before we can know the true influence of pharmacologic and reperfusion therapy on myocardial expansion with acute infarction. Infarct expansion, extension, and reinfarction are compared in Table 7-1.

Management Beyond the First Day

Aspirin should probably be used in every patient with AMI, unless contraindicated. If t-PA therapy is used, it should be followed by an initial 5000-unit bolus of intravenous heparin, given at the start of the infusion, with a continuous infusion of heparin begun within 1 hour at a rate of 1000 U/hr. The dose of heparin should then be adjusted to maintain the activated partial thromboplastin time between 1.5 and 2 times the control. Aspirin should be given

Table 7-1
Comparison of infarct expansion, extension, and reinfarction

Expansion	Extension	Reinfarction
INCIDENCE		
Up to 70% of all fatal infarctions About 35–45% of anterior transmural infarctions Lower incidence seen at other sites	About 15–20% of fatal infarctions Clinical incidence varies according to diagnostic criteria and patient selection, but probably is between 10% and 20% in the general population	About 10–20% in most studies; higher incidence among women
TIME COURSE		
Hours to several days after infarction	Arbitrarily defined as occurring between 24 hours and completion of the in-hospital postinfarction course	Arbitrarily defined as occurring after the in-hospital postinfarction course
PATHOLOGIC FEATURES		
Gross pathology Infarct thinning and dilatation Secondary global dilatation (possibly) Histology Myocyte slippage	Gross pathology: healing myocardial infarction with surrounding foci of more recent necrosis usually within the same vascular risk region Histology: contraction band necrosis present in the newer foci of necrosis	Gross and histologic pathology: remote healed myocardial infarction with new infarction in the same or a different vascular risk region
CONSEQUENCES		
Congestive heart failure Increased mortality Left ventricular dilatation (regional and global) Mural thrombus Cardiac ruputure Left ventricular aneurysm Infarct extension? Postinfarction angina?	Actual increase in infarct size Congestive heart failure Cardiogenic shock Increased mortality Infarct expansion?	Increase in total infarct mass Congestive heart failure Cardiogenic shock Increased mortality

Source: From H. F. Weisman and B. Healy. Myocardial infarct expansion, infarct extension, and re-infarction: Pathophysiological concepts. *Prog. Cardiovasc. Dis.* 30:73, 1987. With permission.

(325 mg/day) for at least 6 days and then decreased to 80 mg/day. On day 6, intravenous heparin should be replaced by subcutaneous heparin (10,000 U q12h), which should be continued until hospital discharge. Sometimes intravenous heparin is given for only 4 days. Heparin should not be stopped unless the patient is receiving aspirin. Gradual discontinuation of heparin, as opposed to abrupt cessation, is sometimes preferred. There appears to be no advantage to early PTCA in terms of reduction in mortality or reinfarction than to a more conservative strategy [119]. Coronary arteriography is recommended for patients who demonstrate recurrent ischemia in the hospital or during the predischarge exercise test. The results of phase II of the National Institutes of Health-sponsored Thrombolysis in Myocardial Infarction trial (TIMI II) demonstrate a stunning 6-week mortality rate of 4.7 percent when t-PA in combination with aspirin and heparin is used in patients with AMI of less than 4 hours duration [119]. This stands in sharp contrast to hospital mortality rates in excess of 20 percent reported in the early days of coronary care [120, 121].

Patients not on treatment with beta blockers, verapamil, or diltiazem should be considered candidates for a beta blocker. Relative contraindications to beta blocker therapy include a ventricular rate less than 55 bpm, a systolic blood pressure less than 90 mm Hg, moist rales extending above the lower third of the lung fields, advanced AV block, or a history of asthma or severe chronic lung disease. Data from the TIMI II trial indicate that beta blockers lower the incidence of nonfatal reinfarction and recurrent ischemic events during hospitalization [119]. Patients considered at low risk may not benefit from long-term beta blocker use [122], whereas high-risk patients will accrue the greatest benefit from long-term beta blockers.

Patients who have severe resting ischemia in the hospital beyond the first 24 hours or those with a history of MI and clinical or radiographic signs of left ventricular failure in the hospital should be considered for coronary angiography [123]. The remaining patients, most of whom will perform an exercise test, should be considered for coronary arteriography if they demonstrate an ischemic response during exercise or a poor workload (less than 4 metabolic exercise equivalents [METs] where 1 MET equals the amount of oxygen used at rest). If exercise testing cannot be done, a resting radionuclide left ventriculogram is recommended, and coronary angiography should be performed if the ejection fraction lies between 0.20 and 0.44 [123]. These guidelines will identify patients at an increased 1-year risk (average mortality rate 16 percent), who make up about one-half of the postinfarction population.

It is clear to experienced physicians that there is no "routine" management of AMI in the present era. Every patient is different, and management varies accordingly. As we grow closer to understanding the mechanisms of infarction, treatments will change. We have come a great deal closer to this goal in recent years. We can now reperfuse the myocardium, abolish the residual stenosis, and limit the ischemic burden in many patients who present early in the phases of acute infarction. Most patients continue to come too late after the onset of symptoms, however. Reperfusion is not a realistic option in these patients. Nevertheless, we can still optimize left ventricular loading conditions and heart rate. We can predict which patients are likely to develop pump dysfunction and can act accordingly. The proper management of the patient with AMI requires knowledge of physiology, pathology, pharmacology, anatomy, and psychology. There is perhaps no other medical emergency that draws so completely on our role as physician and patient advocate.

References

1. Alonzo, A. A., Simon, A. B., and Feinleib, M. Prodromata of myocardial infarction and sudden death. *Circulation* 52:1056, 1975.
2. Pitt, B. Natural history of myocardial infarction and its prodromal syndromes. *Circulation* 53(Suppl I):I-132, 1976.
3. Schroeder, J. S., Lamb, I. H., and Hu, M. Prodromal characteristics as indicators of cardiac events in patients hospitalized for chest pain. *Clin. Cardiol.* 2:33, 1979.
4. Ambrose, J. A., et al. Angiographic morphology and the pathogenesis of unstable angina. *J. Am. Coll. Cardiol.* 5:609, 1985.
5. Breshahan, D. R., et al. Angiographic occurrence and clinical correlates of intraluminal coronary artery thrombosis: Role of unstable angina. *J. Am. Coll. Cardiol.* 6:285, 1985.
6. Ambrose, J. A., et al. Angiographic evolution of coronary artery morphology in unstable angina. *J. Am. Coll. Cardiol.* 7:472, 1986.
7. Falk, E. Unstable angina with fatal outcome: Dynamic coronary thrombosis leading to infarction and/or sudden death. *Circulation* 71:699, 1985.
8. Wilson, R. F., Holida, M. D., and White, C. W. Quantitative angiographic morphology of coronary stenosis leading to myocardial infarction or unstable angina. *Circulation* 73:286, 1986.
9. Sherman, C. T., et al. Coronary angioscopy in patients with unstable angina. *N. Engl. J. Med.* 315: 913, 1986.
10. Schroeder, J. S., Lamb, I. H., and Hu, M. Do patients in whom myocardial infarction is ruled out have a better prognosis after hospitalization than those surviving infarction? *N. Engl. J. Med.* 303: 1, 1980.
11. Turi, Z. G., et al. Implications for acute intervention related to time of hospital arrival in acute myocardial infarction. *Am. J. Cardiol.* 58:203, 1986.
12. DeWood, M. A., et al. Prevalence of total coronary occlusion during the early hours of transmural myocardial infarction. *N. Engl. J. Med.* 303:897, 1980.
13. Chandler, A. B., et al. Coronary thrombosis in myocardial infarction. *Am. J. Cardiol.* 34:823, 1974.
14. G.I.S.S.I. Trial. Effectiveness of intravenous thrombolytic treatment in acute myocardial infarction. *Lancet* 1:397, 1986.
15. Simoons, M. L., et al. Improved survival after early thrombosis in acute myocardial infarction. *Lancet* 2:578, 1985.
16. Kennedy, J. W., et al. Western Washington randomized trial of intracoronary streptokinase in acute myocardial infarction. *N. Engl. J. Med.* 309:1477, 1983.
17. I.S.A.M. Study Group. A prospective trial of intravenous streptokinase in acute myocardial infarction (I.S.A.M.). *N. Engl. J. Med.* 314:1465, 1986.
18. T.I.M.I. Study Group. The thrombolysis in myocardial infarction (T.I.M.I.) trial: Phase I findings. *N. Engl. J. Med.* 312:932, 1985.
19. Kennedy, J. W., et al. Recent changes in management of acute myocardial infarction: Implications for emergency care physicians. *J. Am. Coll. Cardiol.* 11:446, 1988.
20. Pfeffer, M. A., Moyé, L. A., Braunwald, E., et al.

Selection bias in the use of thrombolytic therapy in acute myocardial infarction. *J.A.M.A.* 266:528, 1991.

21. Topol, E. J., et al. Community hospital administration of intravenous plasminogen activator in acute myocardial infarction: Improved timing, thrombolytic efficacy and ventricular function. *J. Am. Coll. Cardiol.* 10:1173, 1987.
22. The TIMI Trial (Letter). *J. Am. Coll. Cardiol.* 10:970, 1987.
23. ISIS 2 Collaborative Group. Randomized trial of intravenous streptokinase, oral aspirin, both, or neither among 17,187 cases of suspected acute myocardial infarction: ISIS 2. *Lancet* 2:871, 1988.
24. Maggioni, A. P., Franzosi, M. G., Santoro, E., et al. The risk of stroke in patients with acute myocardial infarction after thrombolytic and antithrombotic treatment. *N. Engl. J. Med.* 327:1, 1992.
25. ISIS-3 (Third International Study of Infarct Survival) Collaborative Group. ISIS-3: A randomised comparison of streptokinase vs tissue plasminogen activator vs anistreplase and of aspirin plus heparin vs aspirin alone among 41,299 cases of suspected acute myocardial infarction. *Lancet* 339:1, 1992.
26. Braunwald, E. Myocardial reperfusion, limitation of infarct size, reduction of left ventricular dysfunction, and improved survival: Should the paradigm be expanded? *Circulation* 79:441, 1989.
27. Yasuda, T., et al. Accuracy of localization of acute myocardial infarction by 12 lead electrocardiography. *J. Electrocardiol.* 15:181, 1982.
28. McQueen, M. J., Holder, D., and El-Maraghi, N. R. H. Assessment of the accuracy of serial electrocardiograms in the diagnosis of myocardial infarction. *Am. Heart J.* 105:258, 1983.
29. Behar, S., et al. Evaluation of electrocardiogram in emergency room as a decision-making tool. *Chest* 71:486, 1977.
30. Lee, T. H., et al. Clinical characteristics and natural history of patients with acute myocardial infarction sent home from the emergency room. *Am. J. Cardiol.* 60:219, 1987.
31. Brush, J. E., et al. Use of the initial electrocardiogram to predict in-hospital complications of acute myocardial infarction. *N. Engl. J. Med.* 312:1137, 1985.
32. Krumholz, H. M., Pasternak, R. C., Weinstein, M. C., et al. Cost effectiveness of thrombolytic therapy with streptokinase in elderly patients with suspected acute myocardial infarction. *N. Engl. J. Med.* 327:7, 1992.
33. Topol, E. J., and Califf, R. M. Thrombolytic therapy for elderly patients. *N. Engl. J. Med.* 327:45, 1992.
34. Neuhaus, K.-L., Von Essen, R., Tebbe, U., et al. Improved thrombolysis in acute myocardial infarction with front-loaded administration of alteplase: Results of the rt-PA-APSAC Patency Study (TAPS). *J. Am. Coll. Cardiol.* 19:885, 1992.
35. Vaughan, D. E., and Braunwald, E. Front-loaded accelerated infusions of tissue plasminogen activator: Putting a better foot forward. *J. Am. Coll. Cardiol.* 19:1076, 1992.
36. Shah, P. K., Cercek, B., Lew, A. S., et al. Angiographic validation of bedside markers of reperfusion. *J. Am. Coll. Cardiol.* 21:55, 1993.
37. White, H. D. Thrombolytic therapy for patients with myocardial infarction presenting after six hours. *Lancet* 340:221, 1992.
38. Harrison, J. K., Califf, R. M., Woodlief, L. H., et al. Systolic left ventricular function after reperfusion therapy for acute myocardial infarction. An analysis of determinants of improvement. *Circulation* 87: 1531, 1993.
39. Ellis, S. G., Mooney, M. R., George, B. S., et al. Randomized trial of late elective angioplasty versus conservative management for patients with residual stenoses after thrombolytic treatment of myocardial infarction. *Circulation* 86:1400, 1992.
40. Smith, E. R., et al. Coronary artery occlusion in the conscious dog: Effects of alterations in arterial pressure produced by nitroglycerin, hemorrhage, and alpha adrenergic agonists on the degree of myocardial ischemia. *Circulation* 47:51, 1973.
41. Epstein, J. E., et al. Reduction of ischemic injury by nitroglycerin during acute myocardial infarction. *N. Engl. J. Med.* 292:29, 1975.
42. Gerry, J. L., Jr., et al. Effects of nitroglycerin on regional myocardial ischemia induced by atrial pacing in dogs. *Circ. Res.* 48:569, 1981.
43. Jugdutt, B. I., et al. Effect of intravenous nitroglycerin on collateral blood flow and infarct size in the conscious dog. *Circulation* 63:17, 1981.
44. Fukuyama, T., Schectman, K. B., and Roberts, R. The effects of intravenous nitroglycerin on hemodynamics, coronary blood flow and morphologically and enzymatically estimated infarct size in conscious dogs. *Circulation* 62:1227, 1980.
45. Kim, Y. I., and Williams, J. F., Jr. Large dose sublingual nitroglycerin in acute myocardial infarction: Relief of chest pain and reduction of Q wave evolution. *Am. J. Cardiol.* 49:842, 1982.
46. Mikolich, J. R., et al. Relief of refractory angina with continuous intravenous infusion of nitroglycerin. *Chest* 77:375, 1980.
47. Come, P. C., and Pitt, B. Nitroglycerin induced severe hypotension and bradycardia in patients with acute myocardial infarction. *Circulation* 54:624, 1976.
48. Ferguson, J. J., et al. Nitroglycerin induced hypotension with acute myocardial infarction: A marker of right ventricular involvement? *Circulation* 72(Suppl III):III-460, 1985.
49. Flaherty, J. T., et al. Effects of intravenous nitroglycerin on left ventricular function and ST changes in acute myocardial infarction. *Br. Heart J.* 38: 612, 1976.
50. Flaherty, J. T., et al. Intravenous nitroglycerin in acute myocardial infarction. *Circulation* 51:132, 1975.
51. Flaherty, J. T., et al. A randomized prospective trial

of intravenous nitroglycerin in patients with acute myocardial infarction. *Circulation* 68:576, 1983.
52. Jugdett, B. I., et al. Persistent reduction in left ventricular asynergy in patients with acute myocardial infarction by intravenous infusion of nitroglycerin. *Circulation* 68:1264, 1983.
53. Cohn, J. N., et al. Effect of short-term infusion of sodium nitroprusside on mortality rate in acute myocardial infarction complicated by left ventricular failure: Results of a Veterans Administration Cooperative Study. *N. Engl. J. Med.* 306:1129, 1982.
54. Thomas, A. D., et al. Haemodynamic effects of morphine in patients with acute myocardial infarction. *Br. Heart J.* 27:863, 1965.
55. Timmis, A. D., et al. Haemodynamic effects of intravenous morphine in patients with acute myocardial infarction complicated by severe left ventricular failure. *B.M.J.* 280:980, 1980.
56. Ryan, W. F., Henning, H., and Karliner, J. S. Effect of morphine on left ventricular dimensions and function in patients with previous myocardial infarction. *Clin. Cardiol.* 2:417, 1979.
57. Gibson, T. C. Blood pressure levels in acute myocardial infarction. *Am. Heart J.* 96:475, 1978.
58. Watanabe, T., et al. Effects of increased arterial pressure and positive inotropic agents on the severity of myocardial ischemia in the acutely depressed heart. *Am. J. Cardiol.* 30:371, 1972.
59. Loeb, H. S., et al. Effects of pharmacologically induced hypertension, myocardial ischemia and coronary hemodynamics in patients with fixed coronary obstruction. *Circulation* 57:41, 1978.
60. Hillis, L. D., et al. Effect of various degrees of systemic arterial hypertension on acute canine myocardial ischemia. *Am. J. Physiol.* 240:H855, 1981.
61. Roan, P. G., et al. Effects of systemic hypertension on ischemic and non-ischemic regional left ventricular function in awake, unsedated dogs after experimental coronary occlusion. *Circulation* 65:115, 1982.
62. Koyanagi, S., et al. Increased size of myocardial infarction in dogs with chronic hypertension and left ventricular hypertrophy. *Circ. Res.* 50:55, 1982.
63. Yusuf, S., Sleight, P., Held, P., et al. Routine medical management of acute myocardial infarction. Lessons from overviews of recent randomized controlled trials. *Circulation* 82(Suppl II):II-117, 1990.
64. Singh, B. N. Routine prophylactic lidocaine administration in acute myocardial infarction. An idea whose time is all but gone? *Circulation* 86:1033, 1992.
65. Antman, E. M., and Berlin, J. A. Declining incidence of ventricular fibrillation in myocardial infarction. Implications for the prophylactic use of lidocaine. *Circulation* 86:764, 1992.
66. Held, P., Yusuf, S., and Furberg, C. Effects of calcium antagonists on initial infarction, reinfarction and mortality in acute myocardial infarction and unstable angina. *B.M.J.* 299:1187, 1989.
67. Horner, S. M. Efficacy of intravenous magnesium in acute myocardial infarction in reducing arrhythmias and mortality. Meta-analysis of magnesium in acute myocardial infarction. *Circulation* 86:774, 1992.
68. Woods, K. L., Fletcher, S., Roffe, C., et al. Intravenous magnesium sulphate in suspected acute myocardial infarction: Results of the second Leicester Intravenous Magnesium Intervention Trial (LIMIT-2). *Lancet* 339:1553, 1992.
69. Shechter, M., Kaplinsky, E., and Rabinowitz, B. The rationale of magnesium supplementation in acute myocardial infarction. A review of the literature. *Arch. Intern. Med.* 152:2189, 1992.
70. Rebuck, A. S., Cade, J. F., and Campbell, E. J. M. Pulmonary aspects of myocardial infarction. *Mod. Concepts Cardiovasc. Dis.* 42:17, 1973.
71. Fillmore, S. J., et al. Blood-gas changes and pulmonary hemodynamics following acute myocardial infarction. *Circulation* 45:583, 1972.
72. Hales, C. A., and Kazemi, H. Small-airways function in myocardial infarction. *N. Engl. J. Med.* 290:761, 1974.
73. Gray, B. A., et al. Alterations in lung volume and pulmonary function in relation to hemodynamic changes in acute myocardial infarction. *Circulation* 59:551, 1979.
74. Harrison, M. O., Conte, P. J., and Heiztman, E. F. Radiological detection of clinically occult cardiac failure following myocardial infarction. *Br. Radiol.* 44:265, 1971.
75. McHugh, T. J., et al. Pulmonary vascular congestion in acute myocardial infarction: Hemodynamic and radiologic correlations. *Ann. Intern. Med.* 76:29, 1972.
76. Kostuk, W., et al. Correlations between the chest film and hemodynamics in acute myocardial infarction. *Circulation* 48:624, 1973.
77. Battler, A., et al. The initial chest x-ray in acute myocardial infarction: Prediction of early and late mortality and survival. *Circulation* 61:1004, 1980.
78. Croft, C. H., et al. Abrupt withdrawal of β-blockade therapy in patients with myocardial infarction: Effects on infarct size, left ventricular function, and hospital course. *Circulation* 73:1281, 1986.
79. Lineberger, A. S., Sprague, D. H., and Battaglini, J. W. Sinus arrest associated with cimetidine. *Anesth. Analg.* 64:554, 1985.
80. Lippestad, C. Th., and Forfang, K. Production of sinus arrest by lignocaine. *B.M.J.* 1:537, 1971.
81. Cheng, T. O., and Wadhwa, K. Sinus standstill following intravenous lidocaine administration. *J.A.M.A.* 223:790, 1973.
82. Dhingra, R. C., et al. Electrophysiologic effects of lidocaine on sinus node and atrium in patients with and without sinoatrial dysfunction. *Circulation* 57:448, 1978.
83. Manyari-Ortega, D. E., and Brennan, F. J. Lidocaine-induced cardiac asystole. *Chest* 74:227, 1978.

84. Feely, J., Wilkinson, G. R., and Wood, A. J. Reduction of liver blood flow and propranolol metabolism by cimetidine. *N. Engl. J. Med.* 304:723, 1981.
85. Goldberger, A. L. Recognition of ECG pseudoinfarct patterns. *Mod. Concepts Cardiovasc. Dis.* 49:13, 1980.
86. Pardee, H. E. B. An electrocardiographic sign of coronary artery obstruction. *Arch. Intern. Med.* 26: 244, 1920.
87. Dressler, W., and Roseler, H. High T waves in the earliest stage of myocardial infarction. *Am. Heart J.* 34:627, 1947.
88. Blumgart, H. L., et al. Experimental studies on the effect of temporary occlusion of coronary arteries in producing persistent electrocardiographic changes. *Am. J. Med. Sci.* 194:493, 1937.
89. Madias, J. E., and Krikelis, E. N. Transient giant R waves in the early phase of acute myocardial infarction: Association with ventricular fibrillation. *Clin. Cardiol.* 4:339, 1981.
90. Aldrich, H. R., et al. Identification of the optimal electrocardiographic leads for detecting acute epicardial injury in acute myocardial infarction. *Am. J. Cardiol.* 59:20, 1987.
91. Sullivan, W., et al. Correlation of electrocardiographic and pathological findings in healed myocardial infarction. *Am. J. Cardiol.* 42:724, 1978.
92. Roberts, W. C., and Gardin, J. M. Location of myocardial infarcts: A confusion of terms and definitions. *Am. J. Cardiol.* 42:868, 1978.
93. Savage, R. M., et al. Correlation of post mortem anatomic findings with electrocardiographic changes in patients with myocardial infarction. *Circulation* 55:279, 1977.
94. Bairey, C. N., et al. Electrocardiographic differentiation of occlusion of the left circumflex versus the right coronary artery as a cause of acute inferior myocardial infarction. *Am. J. Cardiol.* 60:456, 1987.
95. Macdonald, R. G., Hill, J. A., and Feldman, R. L. ST segment response to acute coronary occlusion: Coronary hemodynamic and angiographic determinants of direction of ST segment shift. *Circulation* 74:973, 1986.
96. Ferguson, D. W., et al. Angiographic evidence that reciprocal ST-segment depression during acute myocardial infarction does not indicate remote ischemia: Analysis of 23 patients. *Am. J. Cardiol.* 53:55, 1984.
97. Little, W. C., Rogers, E. W., and Sodums, M. T. Mechanism of anterior ST-segment depression during acute inferior myocardial infarction: Observations during coronary thrombolysis. *Ann. Intern. Med.* 100:226, 1984.
98. Crawford, M. H., O'Rourke, R. A., and Grover, F. L. Mechanism of inferior electrocardiographic ST-segment depression during acute anterior myocardial infarction in a baboon model. *Am. J. Cardiol.* 54:1114, 1984.
99. Lembo, N. J., et al. Clinical and prognostic importance of persistent precordial (V_1-V_4) electrocardiographic ST segment depression in patients with inferior transmural myocardial infarction. *Circulation* 74:56, 1986.
100. Shah, P. K., et al. Noninvasive identification of a high risk subset of patients with acute inferior myocardial infarction. *Am. J. Cardiol.* 46:915, 1980.
101. Roberts, R. Recognition, pathogenesis, and management of non-Q-wave infarction. *Mod. Concepts Cardiovasc. Dis.* 56:17, 1987.
102. Raunio, H., et al. Changes in the QRS complex and ST segment in transmural and subendocardial myocardial infarctions: A clinical pathologic study. *Am. Heart J.* 98:176, 1979.
103. Phibbs, B. "Transmural" versus "subendocardial" myocardial infarction: An electrocardiographic myth. *J. Am. Coll. Cardiol.* 1:561, 1983.
104. DeWood, M. A., et al. Coronary arteriographic findings soon after non-Q-wave myocardial infarction. *N. Engl. J. Med.* 315:417, 1986.
105. Pratt, C. M., et al. Design of a multicenter, double-blind study to assess the effects of prophylactic diltiazem on early re-infarction after a non-Q-wave acute myocardial infarction: Diltiazem re-infarction study. *Am. J. Cardiol.* 58:906, 1986.
106. Gibson, R. S., et al. The prevalence and clinical significance of residual myocardial ischemia 2 weeks after uncomplicated non-Q-wave infarction: A prospective natural history study. *Circulation* 73:1186, 1986.
107. Maisel, A. S., et al. Complex ventricular arrhythmias in patients with Q wave versus non-Q wave myocardial infarction. *Circulation* 72:963, 1985.
108. Gibson, R. S., et al. Diltiazem and reinfarction in patients with non-Q-wave myocardial infarction: Results of a double-blind, randomized, multicenter trial. *N. Engl. J. Med.* 315:423, 1986.
109. Muller, J. E., et al. Myocardial infarct extension: Occurrence, outcome, and risk factors in the multicenter investigation of limitation of infarct size. *Ann. Intern. Med.* 108:1, 1988.
110. Hutchins, G. M., and Bulkley, B. H. Infarct expansion versus extension: Two different complications of acute myocardial infarction. *Am. J. Cardiol.* 41:1127, 1978.
111. Eaton, L. W., et al. Regional cardiac dilatation after acute myocardial infarction: Recognition by two-dimensional echocardiography. *N. Engl. J. Med.* 300:57, 1979.
112. Erlebacher, J. A., et al. Late effects of acute infarct dilation on heart size: A two dimensional echocardiographic study. *Am. J. Cardiol.* 49:1120, 1982.
113. McKay, R. G., et al. Left ventricular remodeling after myocardial infarction: A corollary to infarct expansion. *Circulation* 74:693, 1986.
114. Weisman, H. F., and Healy, B. Myocardial infarct expansion, infarct extension, and reinfarction: Patho-

physiological concepts. *Prog. Cardiovasc. Dis.* 30:73, 1987.

115. Plerard, L. A., et al. Hemodynamic profile of patients with acute myocardial infarction at risk of infarct expansion. *Am. J. Cardiol.* 60:5, 1987.
116. Pfeffer, J. M., Pfeffer, M. A., and Braunwald, E. Hemodynamic benefits and prolonged survival with long-term captopril therapy in rats with myocardial infarction and heart failure. *Circulation* 75(Suppl I):I-149, 1987.
117. Gottlieb, S. O., et al. Nifedipine reduces early infarct expansion: Results of a double blind, randomized trial (Abstract). *Circulation* 72(Suppl 3):274, 1985.
118. Yusuf, S., and Furberg, C. D. Effects of calcium channel blockers on survival after myocardial infarction. *Cardiovasc. Drugs Ther.* 1:343, 1987.
119. The TIMI Study Group. Comparison of invasive and conservative strategies after treatment with intravenous tissue plasminogen activator in acute myocardial infarction: Results of the thrombolysis in myocardial infarction (TIMI) phase II trial. *N. Engl. J. Med.* 320:618, 1989.
120. Killip, T., and Kimball, J. T. Treatment of myocardial infarction in a coronary care unit: A two-year experience with 250 patients. *Am. J. Cardiol.* 20: 457, 1967.
121. Henning, H., et al. Prognosis after acute myocardial infarction: A multivariate analysis of mortality and survival. *Circulation* 59:1124, 1979.
122. Viscoli, C. M., Horwitz, R. I., and Singer, B. H. Beta-blockers after myocardial infarction: Influence of first-year clinical course on long-term effectiveness. *Ann. of Intern. Med.* 118:99, 1993.
123. Ross, J., Jr., et al. A decision scheme for coronary angiography after acute myocardial infarction. *Circulation* 79:292, 1989.
124. Pfeffer, M. A., Braunwald, E., Moyé, L. A., et al. Effect of captopril on mortality and morbidity in patients with left ventricular dysfunction after myocardial infarction. Results of the Survival and Ventricular Enlargement Trial. *N. Engl. J. Med.* 327:669, 1992.
125. The Acute Infarction Ramipril Efficacy (AIRE) Study Investigators. Effect of ramipril on mortality and morbidity of survivors of acute myocardial infarction with clinical evidence of heart failure. *Lancet* 342:821, 1993.
126. The GUSTO Investigators. An international, randomized trial comparing four thrombolytic strategies for acute myocardial infarction. *N. Engl. J. Med.* 329:673, 1993.
127. EMARAS Collaborative Group. Randomized trial of late thrombolysis in patients with suspected acute myocardial infarction. *Lancet* 342:767, 1993.
128. Ridiker, P. M., Hebert, P. R., Fuster, V., et al. Are both aspirin and heparin justified as adjuncts to thrombolytic therapy for acute myocardial infarction? *Lancet* 341:1574, 1993.

8. Hemodynamic Monitoring of Acute Myocardial Infarction

Joel M. Gore and Peter L. Zwerner

The flow-directed pulmonary artery (PA) catheter introduced by Swan and associates in 1970 [1] has found widespread use in the clinical management of patients with acute myocardial infarction (AMI). Hemodynamic monitoring is a procedure that is now performed daily in most hospitals throughout the United States. The ability to measure pulmonary capillary wedge pressure and cardiac output provides hemodynamic information that can be invaluable for evaluating myocardial performance. This information may aid in classifying and treating various hemodynamic abnormalities encountered in patients with AMI.

The use of the PA catheter in AMI patients has been increasing over the years [2]. It is estimated that in 1986 500,000 PA catheters were placed, 100,000 in patients with AMI. The use of PA catheters has spawned a $2 billion industry in the United States. It is important for the clinician to remember that the catheter is not a therapy but, rather, a device to guide therapy. There is a potential to overuse the PA catheter, and this fact must be kept in perspective. The clinician should be wary not to succumb to the pressure of modern technology. The insertion of the catheter must not delay therapy nor should it replace the bedside clinical evaluation of patients.

Clinicians who employ hemodynamic monitoring should understand the fundamentals of the insertion technique, the equipment utilized, and the data that can be generated before insertion is undertaken [3]. The hemodynamic data obtained must be fully evaluated or significant information may be missed. Frequently, only two parameters are utilized—"wedge" pressure and cardiac output—whereas other parameters, including right atrial, right ventricular, and pulmonary artery pressures, are given only cursory attention. In addition, the catheter is often left in place for inappropriately long periods of time [4]. Catheters should always be removed when the data collected are no longer being used to direct the management of the patient.

Indications

Numerous indications for insertion of the PA catheter are now accepted (Table 8-1). Critically ill patients in whom the changing function of the heart is an essential factor during treatment are candidates for hemodynamic monitoring. Hemodynamic monitoring in patients with AMI has four central objectives: (1) to assess left and/or right ventricular function; (2) to monitor changes in hemodynamic status; (3) to guide treatment with a variety of pharmacologic and nonpharmacologic agents; and (4) to provide prognostic data.

One of the most common indications for hemodynamic monitoring is the management of patients with various complications of myocardial infarction. Hypotension is common in the setting of AMI and may be secondary to a variety of conditions. Dehydration due to overly aggressive diuretic therapy, vomiting, diarrhea, or profuse diaphoresis may produce hypotension. In contrast, hypotension may be the first manifestation of cardiogenic shock. Patients with right ventricular infarction may also be hypotensive, and the diagnosis and treatment of this clinical entity can be greatly aided by hemodynamic monitoring.

Hemodynamic monitoring is useful for the diagnosis of individuals with severe left ventricular failure and a loud systolic murmur who may have suffered a ventricular septal rupture or acute mitral regurgitation. In other individuals, marked left ventricular failure is secondary to extensive infarction without a mechanical complication. Hemodynamic

Table 8-1
Indications for hemodynamic monitoring of AMI

Management of complicated AMI
Hypovolemia vs. cardiogenic shock
Ventricular septal rupture vs. acute mitral regurgitation
Severe left ventricular failure
Right ventricular failure
Refractory ventricular tachycardia
Differentiating severe pulmonary disease from left ventricular failure
Assessment of cardiac tamponade
Assessment of therapy in selected individuals
Afterload reduction in patients with severe left ventricular failure
Inotropic agents
Beta blockers
Temporary pacing (ventricular vs. atrioventricular)
Intra-aortic balloon counterpulsation
Mechanical ventilation

and oximetry evaluation aid in distinguishing these various entities.

Patients with refractory ventricular arrhythmias or postinfarction angina may have underlying unrecognized left ventricular failure secondary to extensive infarction or ischemia. Hemodynamic monitoring discloses the severity of left ventricular dysfunction and aids in management. In addition, cardiac arrhythmias can often cause recognizable changes in the atrial pressure tracings that can be used to both diagnose the arrhythmia and understand the hemodynamic consequences of the rhythm disturbance [5].

Coexisting pulmonary and cardiac diseases represent a difficult diagnostic and therapeutic dilemma. A confirmed pulmonary artery wedge pressure is a key hemodynamic variable. An elevated pulmonary capillary wedge pressure indicates left ventricular dysfunction, whereas a normal wedge pressure with an elevated PA diastolic pressure indicates pulmonary disease or pulmonary vasoconstriction.

Hemodynamic monitoring can be useful for assessing and maximizing therapy with various pharmacologic agents. Afterload reduction in patients with severe left ventricular failure and hypotension can be optimized with hemodynamic monitoring. In addition, the hemodynamic effects of inotropic agents and beta blockers can be continuously monitored.

The effect of various other forms of therapy can be evaluated with hemodynamic monitoring. Therapy using various modes of temporary pacing (ventricular versus atrioventricular), the intra-aortic balloon counterpulsation device, and mechanical ventilation with or without positive end-expiratory pressure can be directed utilizing hemodynamic data.

Pericardial effusion can be easily diagnosed with echocardiography, although cardiac tamponade can present with varying amounts of pericardial fluid. Hemodynamic measurements determine the physiologic significance (if any) of a specific volume of pericardial effusion. The response to therapy in these patients can be followed by means of hemodynamic monitoring.

Indications for hemodynamic monitoring in patients with AMI must be individualized. When the decision to use a PA catheter is made, one must consider the fact that it is not an innocuous procedure; the risks must be weighed against the potential benefits. Instituting hemodynamic monitoring should not delay therapy and must not replace good clinical judgment.

Hemodynamic Monitoring Equipment

Pulmonary Artery Catheters

Pulmonary artery catheters are available in a variety of sizes and offer a range of features. The catheters are generally constructed of polyvinyl chloride, which has flexibility characteristics ideal for flow-directed catheters. Polyvinyl chloride has a high thrombogenicity, and therefore the catheters are generally coated with heparin. This heparin bonding process has been shown to be effective in reducing thrombus formation on the catheter [6, 7]. The hydrophilic properties of polyvinyl chloride have been reported to result in the absorption of certain drugs commonly utilized in the coronary care unit (CCU) setting [8, 9]. Therefore, the potential for delayed drug delivery during infusion exists, and it is recommended that drug therapy always be titrated to the patient's clinical response.

The outside diameter of cardiac catheters is measured in French (Fr) gauge with 1 Fr = 0.335 mm (0.013 in.). The PA catheters utilized in the intensive care unit usually have an outside dimension of 5 to 7 Fr and are 110 cm in length. An inflatable balloon is positioned 1 to 2 cm from the tip of the catheter to allow flow direction. The balloon capacity varies according to the catheter size, and the operator must be aware of the individual balloon's maximal inflation volume, as prescribed by the manufacturer. In general, air should be used as the inflation medium. Filtered carbon dioxide may be utilized when there is a risk that balloon rupture would result in the introduction of air into the arterial system. This situation would be the case in patients with right-to-left intracardiac shunts, such as those with an atrial septal or a ventricular septal defect.

Pulmonary artery catheters are available with a number of lumens. The double-lumen catheter has a lumen for balloon inflation and a lumen for distal pressure monitoring or blood sampling. The 7-Fr triple-lumen catheter has an additional lumen 20 to 30 cm from the distal tip of the catheter that allows simultaneous measurement of central venous (right atrial) and pulmonary artery pressures. The most commonly employed PA catheter in the CCU setting is the four-lumen, 7.5-Fr thermodilution catheter (Fig. 8-1). This catheter has a thermistor placed 4 cm proximal to the catheter tip, in addition to the three previously described lumens. The fourth lumen is utilized for placement of the electrical leads required for coupling the thermistor to the cardiac output computer. This apparatus allows thermodilution cardiac output measurements.

A five-lumen catheter is also available that, in addition to the features of the four-lumen catheter, employs a fifth lumen opening 40 cm from the catheter tip. This lumen allows additional central venous access for fluid or drug infusions. This catheter is recommended when peripheral venous access is limited, volume resuscitation is required, or drugs requiring infusion into a large vessel (e.g., dopamine, epinephrine) are being utilized.

Fig. 8-1
Four-lumen PA catheter. A = connection to thermodilution cardiac output computer; B = connection to distal lumen; C = connection to proximal lumen; D = stopcock connected to balloon at the catheter tip for balloon inflation; E = thermistor; F = balloon. Note that the catheter is marked in 10-cm increments. (From J. M. Rippe et al. (eds.), *Intensive Care Medicine.* Boston: Little, Brown, 1985. P. 44. With permission.)

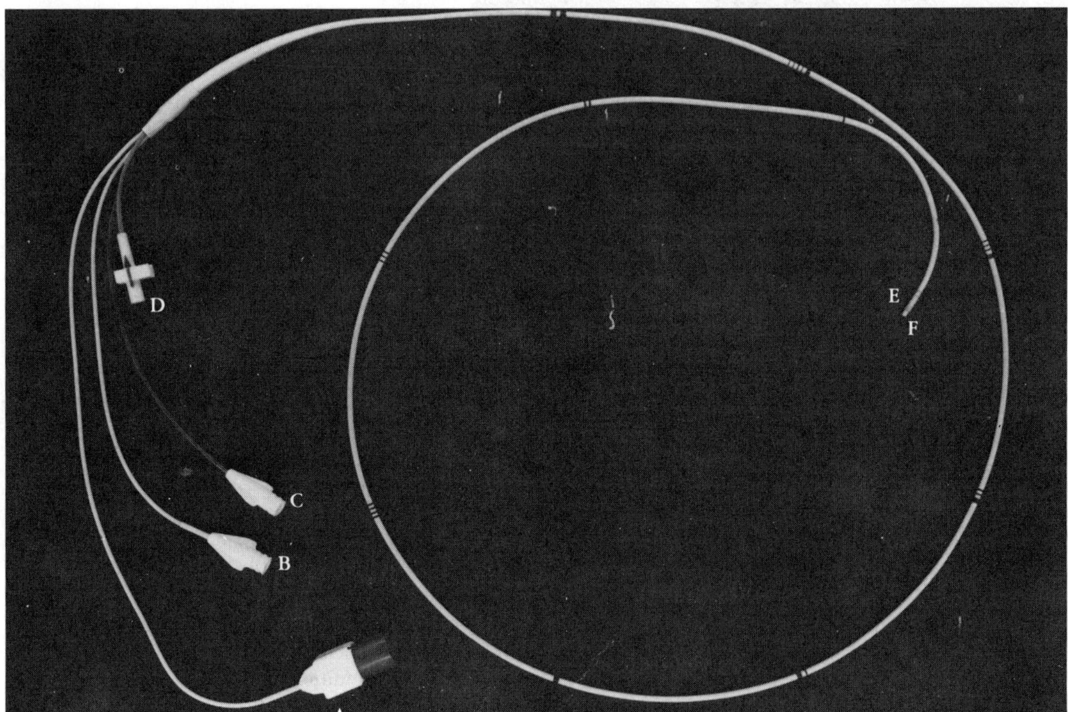

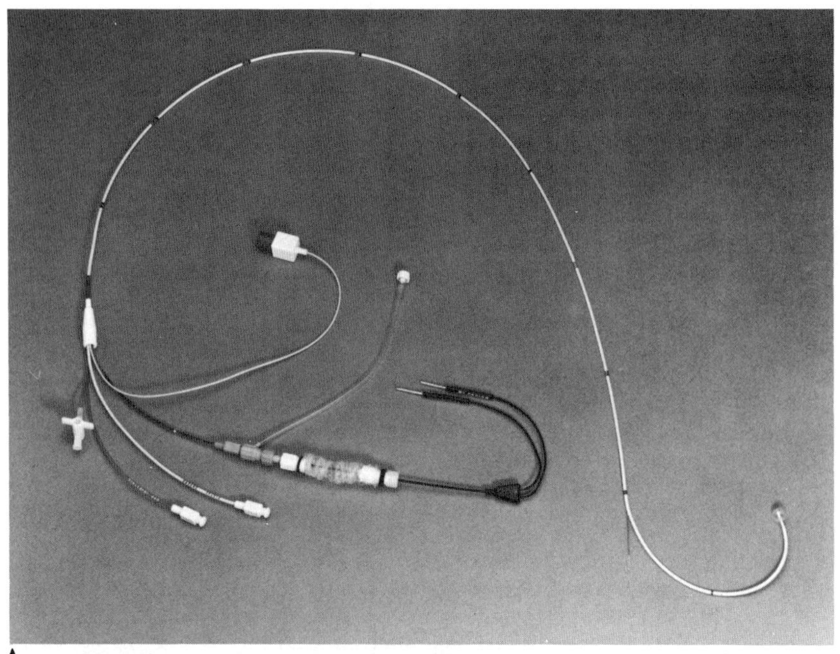

A

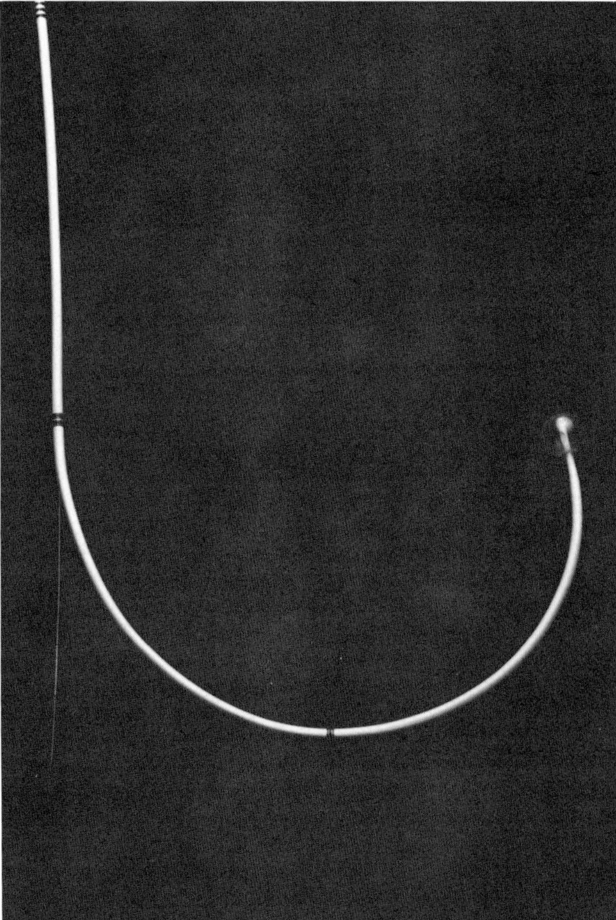

B

Fig. 8-2
A. Five-lumen ''right ventricular Paceport'' catheter; the fifth lumen, located 19 cm from the distal tip, can be used for pressure monitoring or for passage of a specially designed pacing electrode. *B.* Close-up view of the catheter with a pacing electrode extending out the additional lumen.

Several special-purpose PA catheters are available. The "pacing PA catheter" incorporates two groups of electrodes externally on the catheter surface (six total: two ventricular, four atrial), an arrangement that enables intracardiac eletrocardiographic (ECG) recording or temporary cardiac pacing. These catheters are utilized for emergency temporary cardiac pacing, although it is often difficult to position the catheter for reliable simultaneous cardiac pacing and PA pressure monitoring. The Paceport right ventricular catheter (C. R. Bard Inc., Billerica, MA), a five-lumen catheter, is designed with the fifth lumen located 19 cm from the distal tip. This lumen position allows passage of a specially designed pacing electrode through the catheter into the right ventricular apex (Fig. 8-2). Rapid emergency temporary intracardiac pacing can be accomplished without need for a separate central venous puncture. In addition, simultaneous PA pressure may be measured. When a pacing probe is not being used, the fifth lumen provides additional central access or the opportunity to monitor right ventricular pressure continuously.

The ability to continuously measure and record mixed venous oxygen saturation in vivo is clinically available through the use of a fiberoptic reflectance oximetry system incorporated into a five-lumen PA catheter. This catheter has an additional lumen that contains optical fibers that allow transmission of light to and from the bloodstream (Fig. 8-3). Alternating pulses of three wavelengths are emitted from three diodes. Hemoglobin absorbs this transmitted light, which is then refracted back to a second optical detector. The amount of desaturated hemoglobin relative to oxyhemoglobin can be measured because the absorption of light by desaturated hemoglobin and oxyhemoglobin varies as a function of wavelength. The optical signal is converted to an electrical signal and transmitted to a data processor. The calculated hemoglobin oxygen saturation is averaged over a 5-second period and displayed.

Pressure Transducers

Hemodynamic monitoring depends on a system that converts changes in pressure to an electrical signal suitable for interpretation. Transducers are devices that are connected through a fluid-filled tubing system to a catheter placed in an intravascular space (Fig. 8-4). The transducer has a dome that is a fluid-filled chamber directly connected to the fluid-filled catheter. Intravascular pressure changes are transmitted through the fluid-filled catheter to the fluid-filled dome. There is a diaphragm in the chamber that is connected to the pressure transducer. The diaphragm is displaced by the transmitted intravascular pressure changes, and a series of resistance wires are deformed. These wires are connected to form a Wheatstone bridge, which allows changes in resistance to induce a current. The current produced is proportional to the deformation of the diaphragm. These current changes are amplified and displayed as a waveform on a cathode ray tube and in numerical terms on a pressure meter.

Fig. 8-3
Fiberoptic reflectance oximetry system incorporated into a five-lumen PA catheter.

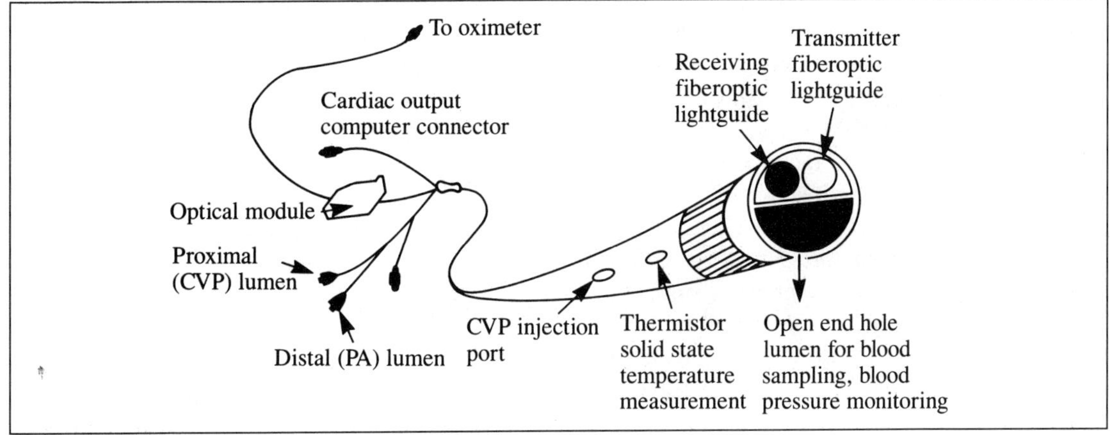

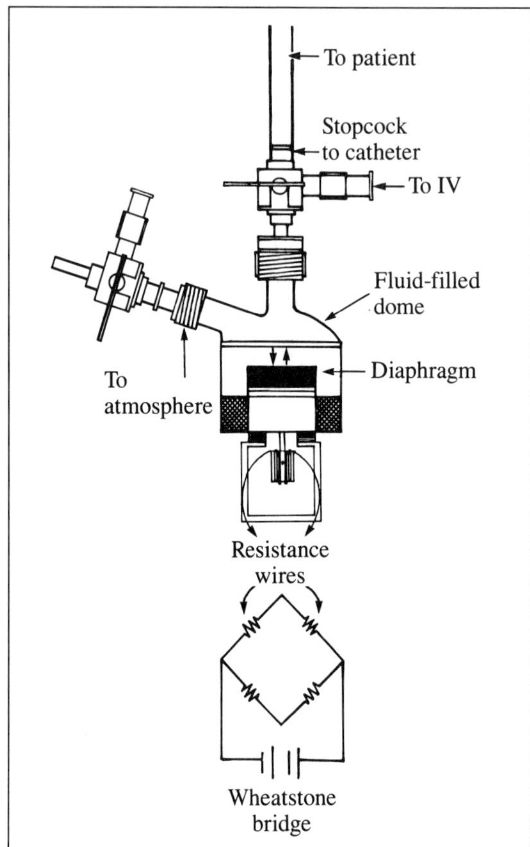

Fig. 8-4
Transducer/Wheatstone bridge.

It allows continuous instantaneous measurement of intravascular pressure changes.

Most systems allow either systolic, diastolic, or mean pressure numerical representation. Newer systems provide simultaneous recording of all three variables. It is recommended that the ECG be displayed simultaneously with the pressure tracing in order to time the various components of the pressure trace (e.g., A wave, V wave).

The pressure amplifier requires an integrated electronic calibration circuit and a zero control. It is essential that the pressure amplifier provide a hard-copy printout of the pressure waveform and simultaneous ECG in order to properly analyze the pressure tracing. The system should allow various recording speeds, usually 25, 50, and 100 mm/sec. Rapid speeds "expand" the recorded waveform for analysis, and slow speeds allow continuous recording.

Currently produced pressure monitors are less prone to drift, although they must be periodically calibrated and balanced. Calibration is generally accomplished against an internal electronic reference, although occasional balancing by manometry is recommended.

The ability to obtain clinically meaningful hemodynamic data depends on the fidelity of the pressure recording. *Damping* is a term referring to the property of a system to return to its resting point. Overdamping of the pressure tracing is commonly encountered in hemodynamic pressure monitoring. The usual source of overdamping is air in the pressure tubing. Reflushing the tubing system to remove air bubbles usually remedies this problem. Damping of the tracing is often caused by having the distal port of the PA catheter opposed to an intracardiac surface. Slight repositioning, inflation of the balloon, or reflushing of the catheter may correct this condition. The PA catheter has a tendency to migrate into the pulmonary vasculature periphery, leading to "overwedging" of the catheter. Caution must be exercised regarding the position of the catheter tip. Radiologic assessment of catheter position prior to balloon inflation is recommended to avoid vascular trauma due to overinflation of the balloon within the pulmonary vasculature.

Excessively exaggerated pressure waveforms may also be encountered. The length of tubing affects the damping properties. Long tubing may cause more oscillations in the pressure tubing system, resulting in underdamping of the pressure tracing. Utilizing shorter lengths of connecting tubing may ameliorate this condition.

Pressure signal quality is maximized if there is minimal distance between the transducer and the signal source. The most precise signals can be obtained with catheter tip manometers. The current generation of catheter tip micromanometers are impractical for routine CCU use owing to expense, rigidity, and drift. The expected new generations of catheter tip manometers may eliminate the problems experienced with the current devices and allow routine use of micromanometer technology.

Insertion Techniques

Equipment Preparation

Adequate preparation is essential when performing invasive procedures, and a team approach involving the physician and nursing staff is required. The operator must be assured that the necessary equipment is present, accessible, and in operating condition prior to initiating the procedure. A careful explanation of the procedure to the patient is necessary to allay anxiety. Patients who are unable to cooperate must receive adequate sedation so invasive procedures can be performed with minimum risk. Regardless of the indications for hemodynamic monitoring, an uncooperative patient is not a candidate for introducing large-gauge intravenous devices. Once the patient has been fully informed of the procedure, he or she must be placed in as comfortable a position as possible to ensure continued cooperation. In addition, it is imperative that the person who performs the procedure assume a comfortable position in order to minimize operator fatigue.

Central Venous Access

Measurement of right heart pressures is contingent on safe and reliable access to the central venous system. Five sites are commonly utilized for insertion of PA catheters: subclavian vein, internal jugular vein, femoral vein, basilic vein, and external jugular vein. The axillary vein has also been reported to be a safe and simple alternate route for placement of PA catheters [10]. Various cannulation techniques are possible for each site. The internal jugular may be cannulated via an anterior, central, or posterior approach. The subclavian vein is reached via an intra- or supraclavicular route; the basilic vein is cannulated via a percutaneous entry or by direct visualization via a cutdown technique. It must be emphasized that no one technique is "superior," and that physicians practicing in the intensive care setting must be familiar with several approaches.

Numerous commercially prepared kits are available that contain the necessary equipment for gaining central venous access and for insertion of PA catheters (Fig. 8-5). Care should be taken to follow manufacturer's instructions regarding the specifics of the equipment utilized.

Excellent references exist for detailed explanations of various central venous catheter insertion techniques [11–13]. The internal jugular approach is the one most commonly utilized in our institution, and a detailed explanation of catheter insertion via this route follows.

1. Figure 8-6 shows the surface anatomy of the jugular region and various approaches to internal jugular vein cannulation.
2. The patient and operator must be in a comfortable position with the patient placed in Trendelenburg position to maximize central venous pressure and venous distention. The operator should be at the head of the bed with the patient's head positioned as close to the head of the bed as possible and turned 30 to 45 degrees opposite the side of cannulation.
3. The area to be cannulated is scrubbed with antibacterial solution and widely draped with sterile barriers.
4. Local anesthesia is obtained by infiltrating the skin with lidocaine using a 25-gauge needle.
5. Deeper anesthesia is accomplished utilizing a 1.5-in. 21-gauge needle. The internal jugular vein can now be located with this needle, which is attached to a syringe. Once the vein is entered, the 21-gauge needle may be kept in place to act as a guide for vessel locations.
6. A syringe is now attached to the 18-gauge needle-cannula, which is inserted into the previously located internal jugular vein while continuously gently aspirating for free venous flow. When free flow appears, the Teflon cannula is moved over the needle into the vein using a circular motion. The needle is then removed and a syringe placed on the cannula to check for continued free venous flow. If flow is inadequate or arterial pulsations occur, the cannula is withdrawn and pressure is applied to the area for approximately 5 minutes.
7. If free venous flow occurs, the *soft* J tip of the guidewire is advanced through the cannula. The guidewire should meet no resistance when being threaded through the cannula. Continuous ECG monitoring is necessary at this stage, as the guidewire can advance into the right ventricle and cause electrical irritability. When the guidewire is in position, the cannula can be withdrawn, leaving the guidewire in place. The guidewire must be secured (a hand on the wire) at all times to avoid loss of the guidewire into the central venous circulation.
8. A small incision in the skin is made with a scalpel at the point of the guidewire entry. This measure allows ease of placement of the vessel dilator/sheath apparatus through the skin.
9. The dilator/sheath should be placed over the

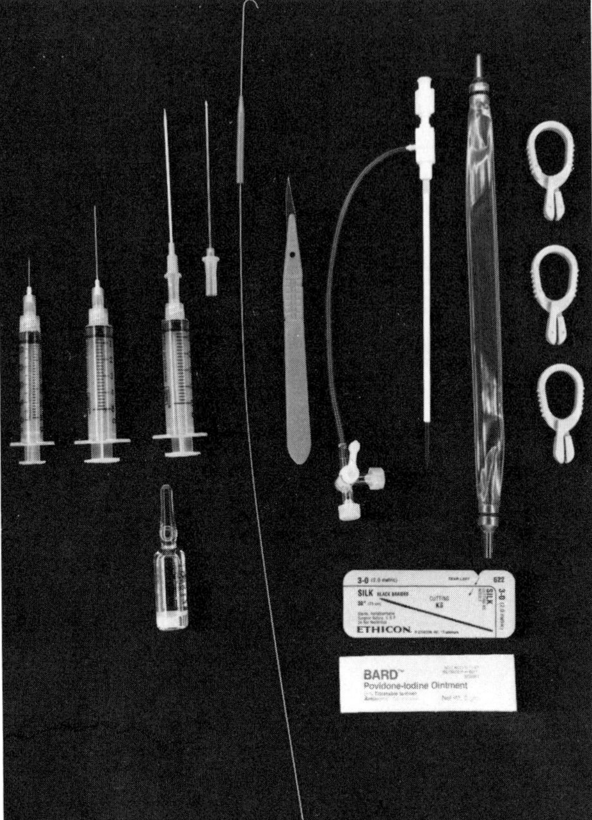

Fig. 8-5
Equipment available in a commercially supplied kit for PA catheter introduction. Supplies shown include (clockwise from left) 3-cc syringe with 25-gauge needle for anesthetizing the skin; 5-cc syringe with 1.5-in. 21-gauge needle for anesthetizing superficial tissues and locating the vein to be cannulated; 5-cc syringe with catheter-over-needle; 25-cm guidewire; scalpel; introducer and sheath; sterile sheath for catheter; towel clips: 3-0 suture for fixing catheter in place; iodine ointment; and 1% lidocaine (Xylocaine). (From J. M. Rippe et al. (eds.), *Intensive Care Medicine.* Boston: Little, Brown, 1985. P. 47. With permission.)

guidewire and advanced through the skin into the vessel using a circular motion. Care should be taken to secure the guidewire at all times. The dilator/sheath should pass smoothly into the vessel once the skin has been penetrated.

10. The dilator and guidewire are removed, leaving the introducer sheath in place. The side arm of the introducer sheath is aspirated to establish the presence of free venous blood flow. The side arm is then intermittently flushed with heparinized saline or attached to a continuous infusion to maintain patency.

Pulmonary Artery Catheter Preparation

1. Flush all lumens except the balloon lumen with sterile solution.
2. Inflate the balloon with an appropriate volume of air to check for balloon integrity and the presence of leaks.
3. Attach tubing from the transducer to all ports of the catheter and flush with saline. Turn the distal stopcock to ''pressure'' and check that the pressure-monitoring equipment is opera-

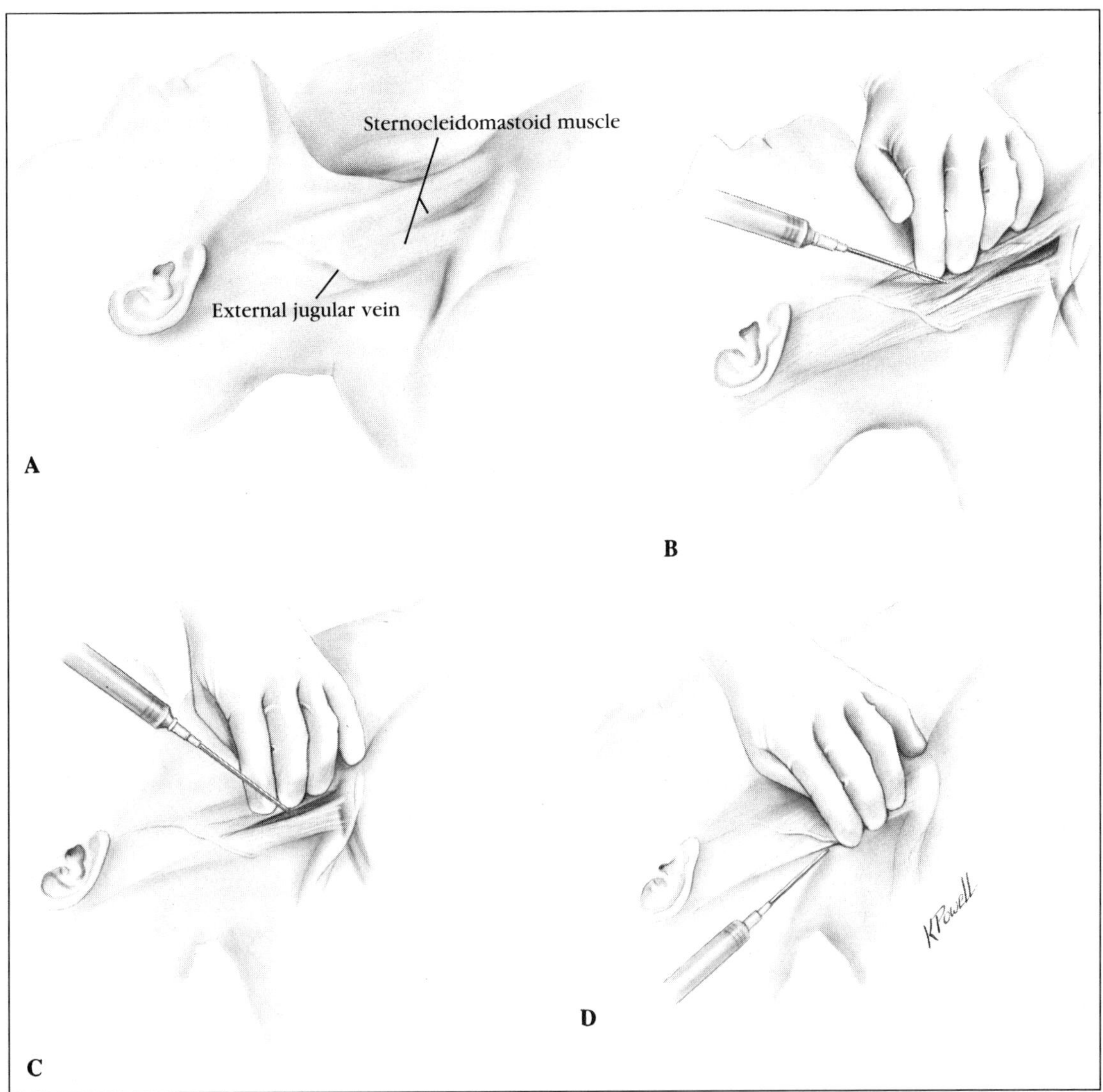

Fig. 8-6
Surface anatomy and various approaches to cannulation of the internal jugular vein. *A.* Surface anatomy. *B.* Anterior approach. *C.* Central approach. *D.* Posterior approach. (From J. M. Rippe et al. (eds.), *Intensive Care Medicine.* Boston: Little, Brown, 1985. P. 22. With permssion.)

tional by moving the distal end of the catheter and observing for simultaneous pressure changes on the oscilloscope.

4. Place a sterile sleeve on the catheter, ensuring that the proper end is positioned to engage the introducer.
5. Gently advance the catheter into the internal jugular vein, superior vena cava, and right atrium under continuous pressure monitoring (each band mark on the catheter represents 10 cm). The right atrium is usually reached at a distance of 10 to 20 cm.
6. Obtain right atrial oxygen saturation.
7. Inflate the balloon, and under continuous pressure and ECG monitoring, advance the catheter through the right atrium until a right ventricular pressure tracing appears. Record this value and obtain the oxygen saturation. Arrhythmia moni-

toring is critical at this stage, as the catheter may produce serious ventricular arrhythmias while in the right ventricle.

8. Advance the catheter until a PA pressure is observed. Gently continue to advance the catheter until a pulmonary capillary pressure wedge tracing is obtained. Deflate the balloon under continuous hemodynamic monitoring and record a return to a PA pressure waveform. Obtain and record the oxygen saturation. Inflation of the balloon with the prescribed amount of air should reproduce the pulmonary capillary wedge waveform, which may be recorded. Test to see that the catheter is properly positioned in the pulmonary artery by deflating the balloon completely and observing the change from a wedge pressure tracing to a PA pressure tracing.
9. Suture the introducer and PA catheter into place and extend the sterile sleeve to its maximum length. Apply sterile dressing.
10. Obtain a chest radiograph in the semiupright position immediately to check for catheter position and for the presence of a pneumothorax.

Special Considerations

Physicians are likely to encounter several conditions in the CCU that require special consideration when hemodynamic monitoring is to be used. An individualized approach is necessary to ensure safety for any given patient. The following section discusses several situations in which the approach to hemodynamic monitoring may vary from the routine.

Anticoagulated Patients

Anticoagulants are commonly prescribed for a variety of cardiac disorders. Patients in the CCU are frequently receiving either intravenous heparin or oral warfarin (Coumadin) therapy. The approach to venous access in this setting requires special attention to minimize the risk of serious hemorrhagic complications.

In general, it is recommended that patients have normal coagulation parameters before central venous access is attempted. Anticoagulants are discontinued when possible, and sufficient time is allowed to pass prior to the procedure to allow coagulation times to return to normal. In patients receiving intravenous heparin, the drug may be discontinued 3 to 4 hours prior to the procedure to allow normalization of the partial thromboplastin time. Protamine also can acutely reverse the effect of heparin. Intravenous heparin therapy may be restarted once central venous access is obtained and the procedure is complete.

Warfarin has a protracted half-life, and discontinuance of the drug has little acute effect on the prothrombin time. The effects of this drug may be acutely reversed with infusion of fresh frozen plasma. Vitamin K also reverses the effects of warfarin, although it may take several days to normalize bleeding parameters.

In many patients it is either ill-advised or impractical to reverse the anticoagulant effects of heparin or warfarin. These patients therefore have a coagulopathy prior to PA catheter insertion. This situation represents a relative contraindication to PA monitoring, although several techniques may be utilized to minimize the risk of serious bleeding in these patients. It is recommended that the basilic vein be utilized in all patients with abnormal bleeding parameters. Visualization of the vessel via a cutdown is recommended. This approach allows direct access to the site of catheter entry and enables the operator to control sites of potential bleeding.

Central venous access via the external or internal jugular vein is a secondary choice in patients with coagulopathies. The anatomy of this region allows direct compression of potential sites of bleeding. Inadvertent puncture of the carotid artery must be avoided. If a carotid artery puncture does occur, direct pressure over the vessel usually controls excessive bleeding.

The subclavian vein as a site for central venous access should be avoided in this patient population. The subclavian vessels lie under the clavicle; and in the event of uncontrolled bleeding or inadvertent puncture of the subclavian artery, the vessels would be inaccessible to direct compression.

Thrombolytic Therapy

Thrombolytic therapy has become commonplace for the treatment of AMI. Frequently, patients require invasive hemodynamic monitoring during the perithrombolytic period. Thrombolytic therapy is not an absolute contraindication for performing invasive procedures. Central venous and arterial access may be obtained with relative safety if certain guidelines are followed.

It is well established that early initiation of thrombolytic therapy is essential to have a favorable impact on AMI. It must be emphasized that it is rarely necessary to delay thrombolytic therapy in order to obtain invasive hemodynamic monitoring. Peripheral venous access for blood sampling and drug and fluid infusion should be established prior to initiating thrombolytic therapy. A peripheral arterial catheter may be placed after therapy has been initiated, in order to monitor blood pressure and aid in obtaining blood samples. At the University of Massachusetts Medical Center, peripheral arterial catheters have been placed in more than 800 patients following thrombolytic therapy with few complications. It is recommended that the use of intra-arterial catheters in general be reserved for patients who require continuous arterial blood pressure monitoring or frequent blood sampling.

Pulmonary artery catheters may be placed in patients receiving thrombolytic therapy, although caution must be exercised. When there is an indication for PA monitoring in these patients, the thrombolytic drug infusion must be immediately discontinued. Tissue plasminogen activator has a half-life of 8 to 9 minutes, which allows rapid reversal of the thrombolytic effects of this drug. Steptokinase has a longer half-life, approaching 20 minutes, and induces a fibrinolytic state that may last 24 hours following infusion due to depletion of clotting factors. Patients receiving streptokinase therapy require fresh frozen plasma in addition to discontinuation of the drug to help normalize bleeding parameters. The concomitant use of heparin may further contribute to bleeding complications following invasive procedures, and heparin should be discontinued prior to initiating invasive hemodynamic monitoring in patients receiving thrombolytic therapy.

The approach to central venous access in the setting of thrombolytic therapy should be similar to the techniques utilized for patients receiving anticoagulants. The brachial approach via a cutdown technique is the procedure of choice; other easily compressible sites can be utilized.

Pulmonary Hypertension, Right Ventricular Dilatation, and Low Cardiac Output

In patients with severe pulmonary hypertension, dilatation of the right atrium or ventricle, or low cardiac output states, it may be difficult to place a flow-directed catheter into the right ventricle, pulmonary artery, or pulmonary capillary wedge position. Fluoroscopic guidance may be required to aid in positioning the catheter for such patients. Occasionally, it is beneficial to stiffen the catheter by infusing 5 to 10 ml of cold sterile solution via the distal lumen. Alternatively, under fluoroscopic guidance, a 0.025-cm guidewire (length 145 cm) may be placed through the distal lumen of a 7-Fr PA catheter. This maneuver makes the catheter more rigid and aids in control and placement. A guidewire should always be placed by an experienced operator under fluoroscopic guidance, as stiff catheters increase the risk of right heart perforation. In rare circumstances, it is necessary to utilize a non-flow-directed PA catheter (e.g., Cournand) because of its increased rigidity. These catheters have a potential for perforating the right heart and must always be placed via fluoroscopic guidance by a physician experienced in cardiac catheterization techniques.

Patients with right heart failure from any cause have excessively elevated central venous pressure, which places them at risk for hemorrhagic complications from central venous cannulation. It is recommended that central venous access be obtained via sites readily accessible to compression or that the brachial approach via a cutdown technique be utilized.

Mechanical Ventilation

Patients undergoing positive-pressure ventilation are at increased risk for complications of invasive hemodynamic monitoring. Hyperinflation of the lungs may predispose to pneumothorax. Ventilator-dependent patients with preexisting respiratory compromise are least likely to tolerate the consequences of a pneumothorax. A pneumothorax in these patients is under tension and requires placement of a chest tube for adequate treatment.

Central venous access via the subclavian approach is associated with the highest incidence of pneumothorax. Pneumothorax accounts for 25 percent of all complications when this route of central venous access is utilized. The internal jugular vein approach appears to have a much lower incidence of pneumothorax formation and should be utilized, when practical, in patients on mechanical ventilators.

Normal Physiologic Data

Hemodynamic monitoring requires careful attention to the accuracy of the data obtained. The physician must be familiar with the calibration and balancing of manometers and amplifiers, and must be able to recognize, understand, and differentiate the pressure tracings obtained from the right atrium, right ventricle, pulmonary artery, and pulmonary capillary wedge positions (Fig. 8-7).

The technical aspects of placing flow-directed catheters are not difficult to master, although the interpretation and synthesis of the data obtained required special training. The foundation of hemodynamic monitoring is built on the knowledge of normal physiologic parameters (Table 8-2). Pressure data obtained from hemodynamic monitoring are rarely specific for a particular disease, and patients may have more than one abnormality. In addition to the pressure data, analysis of the waveform is useful for recognition of certain cardiac conditions.

Table 8-2
Normal resting right heart pressures

Cardiac chamber	Pressure (mm Hg)
RIGHT ATRIUM	
Range	0–5
Mean	3
RIGHT VENTRICLE	
Systolic	17–30
Diastolic	0–6
PULMONARY ARTERY	
Systolic	15–30
Diastolic	5–13
Mean	10–18
PULMONARY CAPILLARY WEDGE	
Mean	2–12

Right Atrium

The normal right atrial pressure is 0 to 6 mm Hg. Two major positive atrial pressures, the A and V waves, can usually be recorded from the right atrium (Figs. 8-8 and 8-9). The A wave is due to atrial contraction and follows the P wave on the ECG. The V wave is due to venous filling of the left and right atrium during ventricular systole when the mitral and tricuspid valves are closed. The peak of the V wave occurs at the end of ventricular systole at a time when the two atria are maximally filled. The x descent, occurring after the A wave, reflects atrial relaxation and the sudden downward motion of the atrioventricular valves. The y descent is due to rapid atrial emptying following opening of the mitral and tricuspid valves. During inspira-

Fig. 8-7
Pressure tracing obtained from a PA catheter.

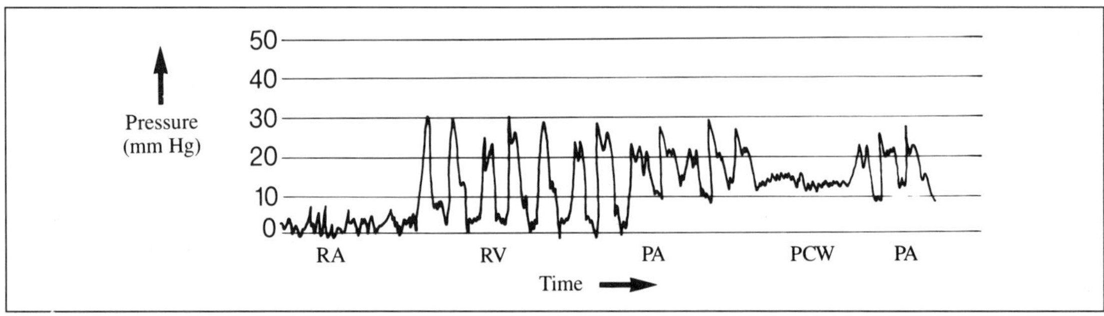

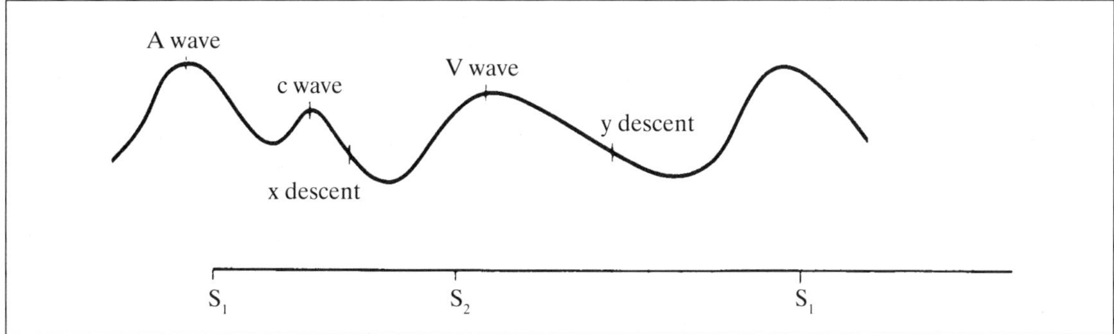

Fig. 8-8
Stylized representation of a right atrium waveform in relation to heart sounds. (See text for discussion A, c, and V waves and x and y descents.)

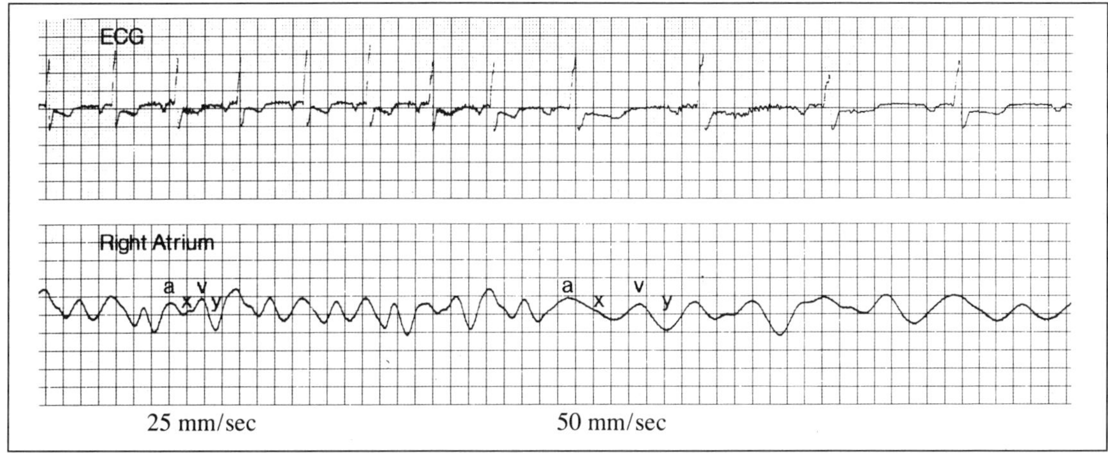

Fig. 8-9
Right atrial tracing recorded at two paper speeds.

tion, the mean right atrial pressures decline (because of the decrease in intrathoracic pressure), whereas the A and V waves frequently become more prominent.

Right Ventricle

The right ventricle pressure and waveform are the result of both the right atrial and pulmonary artery pressures. The normal range is 17 to 30/0 to 6 mm Hg. The right ventricular pressure should equal the PA pressure during systole while the pulmonary valve is open. The right ventricular diastolic pressure should equal the mean right atrial pressure during diastole while the tricuspid valve is open. In the past, right ventricular hemodynamic data were not used clinically, as the catheters did not allow continuous monitoring of this chamber. The introduction of the right ventricular pacing catheter has enabled continuous observation of right ventricular hemodynamics through the port in the right ventricle. With selected disease entities, such as tricuspid regurgitation, ventricular septal rupture, cardiac tamponade, right ventricular infarction, and pulmonary embolism, monitoring the right ventricle may be beneficial.

Pulmonary Artery

The PA waveform is characterized by a systolic peak and diastolic through with a dicrotic notch due to closure of the pulmonic valve. The normal

PA pressure is 15 to 30/5 to 13 mm Hg, with a normal mean of 10 to 18 mm Hg. A mean PA pressure of more than 20 mm Hg signifies the presence of pulmonary hypertension. The peak of the PA systolic wave occurs within the T wave of a simultaneously recorded ECG. The PA diastolic pressure is virtually equal to pulmonary capillary pressure when pulmonary vascular resistance is normal.

The morphology of the PA pressure waveform is of value for the diagnosis of conditions resulting in large volumes filling a noncompliant left atrium. In this instance, the tracing is often distorted by a V wave transmitted backward through the low-resistance pulmonary vascular bed (Fig. 8-10). The V wave may, in fact, resemble the PA waveform, and the operator may not notice that the catheter has gone from the PA position into the wedge posi-

Fig. 8-10
PA and pulmonary capillary wedge pressure tracings from two patients with a giant V wave distorting the PA pressure tracing.

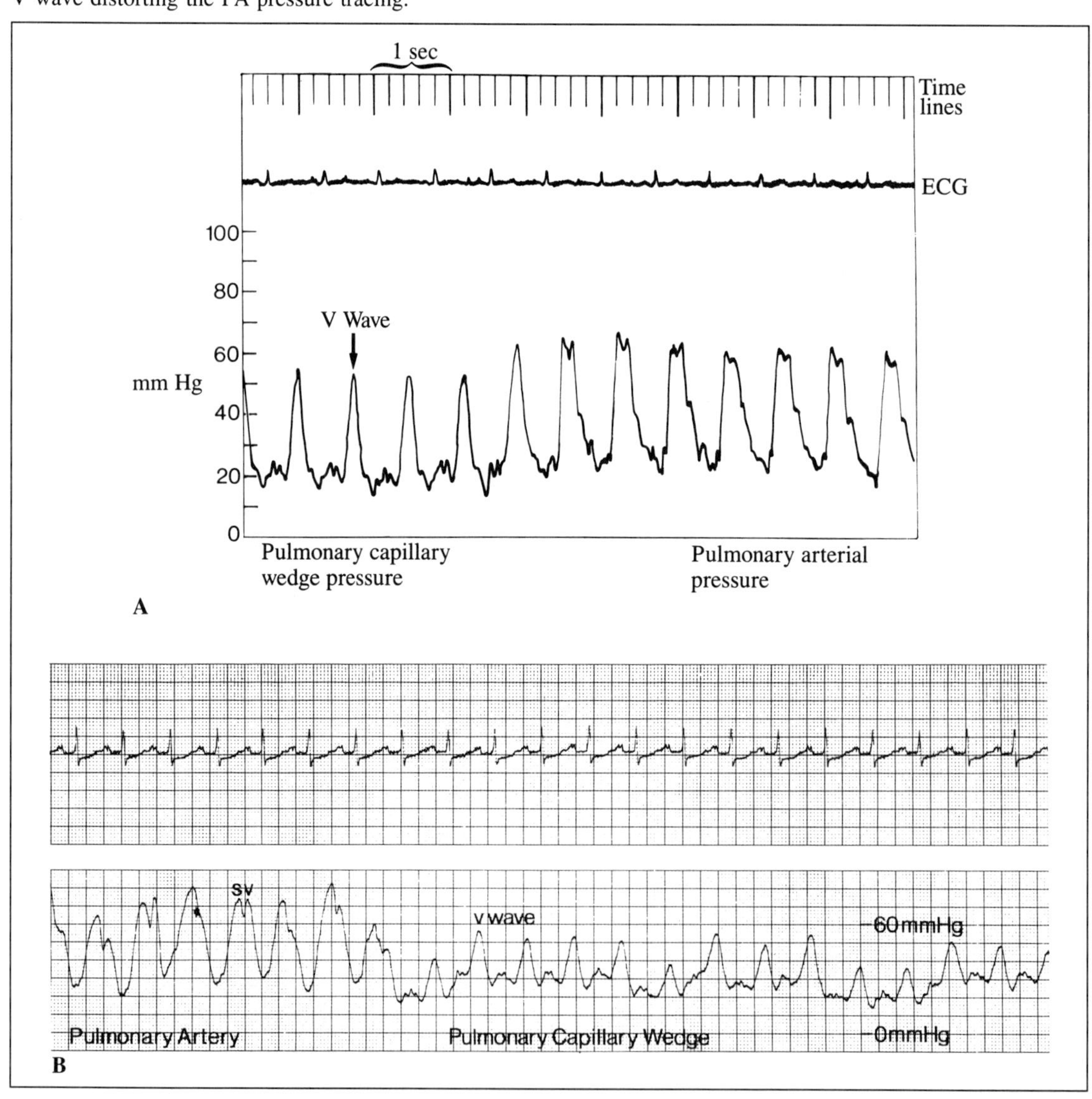

tion. This move can result in permanent wedging of the catheter.

Pulmonary Capillary Wedge

The pulmonary capillary wedge pressure is a phase-delayed and amplitude-damped version of left atrial pressure. The pressure waveform is bifid and of low magnitude. Pulmonary capillary pressure is obtained when the PA catheter is in a ''PA-occluded'' position. The inflated balloon prevents flow between this branch of the pulmonary artery and the left atrium, as there is no pressure drop along this vascular segment. The distal tip of the catheter is therefore monitoring left atrial pressure. The pressure obtained is more properly called the PA-occluded pressure. The mean PA-occluded pressure is normally 2 to 12 mm Hg. It should average 2 to 7 mm Hg below by the mean PA pressure.

The waveform of the PA-occluded pressure is markedly damped relative to that of the pulmonary artery. In contrast to the right atrial waveform, the normal PA-occluded waveform demonstrates a V wave that is slightly larger than the A wave.

Confirmation that the catheter is truly measuring PA-occluded or pulmonary capillary wedge pressure is obtained by withdrawing a sample of blood from the catheter tip and measuring oxygen saturation. Satisfactory ''wedge'' position is indicated by obtaining a 1- to 2-ml catheter-tip blood specimen with an oxygen saturation nearly equivalent to that of the patient's arterial blood. During procurement of the blood specimen, it is important to have the patient breathe slowly and deeply to ensure that the lung segment from which the sample is being obtained is well ventilated.

Cardiac Output

Cardiac output is an integral part of the data obtained from hemodynamic monitoring. Right-sided heart pressures should be analyzed along with the cardiac output. The thermodilution technique is the mostly commonly used bedside means of measuring cardiac output. This technique employs the principle of indicator dilution. A known quantity of cold solution is introduced into the circulation and adequately mixed by passage through two cardiac chambers (right atrium and right ventricle). A thermistor mounted on the distal tip of the PA catheter measures the temperature of PA blood, and the resulting cooling curve allows calculation of blood flow. Cardiac output is proportional to the integral of the time versus temperature curves. Cardiac output is usually calculated by a computer using a complicated formula incorporating the area under the thermodilution curve (change in temperature versus time). It can be useful to inspect the thermodilution temperature curve to ensure that the computer-derived measurement is accurate (Fig. 8-11).

The thermodilution cardiac output can be inaccurate in the presence of several clinical conditions. Thermodilution cardiac output is less accurate in low output states, tricuspid regurgitation, and atrial or ventricular septal defects. The most accurate clinical method for measuring cardiac output is the Fick technique that employs arteriovenous (AV) difference of blood oxygen content and total body oxygen consumption. The normal AV oxygen content difference is 3.0 to 5.0 ml/dl. As cardiac output declines, the peripheral tissues extract more oxygen from hemoglobin and the AV oxygen difference increases. The opposite occurs with an increase in cardiac output. Thus the AV oxygen difference can be used to follow cardiac output. Cardiac output is defined by the following formula.

$$\text{Cardiac output} = \frac{\text{oxygen consumption}}{\text{arterial } O_2 \text{ content} - \text{mixed venous } O_2 \text{ content}}$$

If one assumes that arterial oxygen saturation and total body oxygen consumption are relatively stable over short periods of time, by applying the Fick principle one may observe changes in mixed venous oxygen saturation (SVO_2) reflecting changes in cardiac output. The fiberoptic reflectance oximetry catheter allows continuous measurement of mixed venous oxygen saturation. Changes in SVO_2 are proportional to changes in cardiac output, and this system allows continuous monitoring of this variable.

Other Variables

The hemodynamic pressure measurements directly obtained from right heart catheterization represent only a small portion of the data that can be generated. Additional information can be obtained by

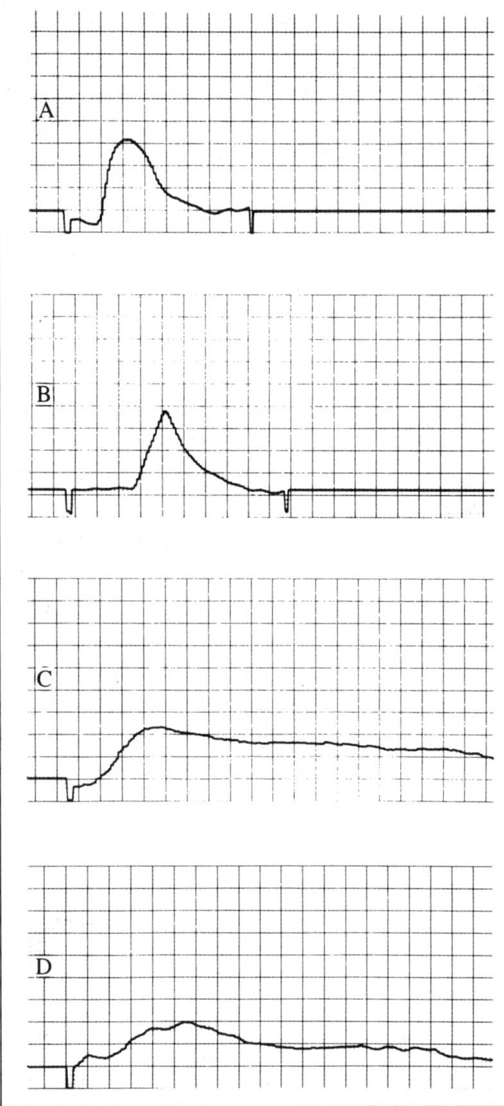

Fig. 8-11
Thermodilution temperature curves generated to determine cardiac output. *A.* Normal cardiac output. *B.* High cardiac output. *C.* Low cardiac output. *D.* Inaccurate cardiac output due to erratic injection of saline.

Table 8-3
Hemodynamic formulas

Cardiac output (CO)	HR × SV
Cardiac index (CI)	CO/BSA
Stroke volume (SV)	CO/HR
Stroke index (SI)	SV/BSA or CI/HR
Left ventricular stroke work index (LVSWI)	$\frac{1.36 \times (\text{MAP} - \text{PCWP}) \times \text{SI}}{100}$
Systemic vascular resistance (SVR)	$\frac{(\text{MAP} - \text{RAP})}{\text{CO}} \times 80$
Pulmonary vascular resistance (PVR)	$\frac{(\text{PAP} - \text{PCWP})}{\text{CO}} \times 80$
Mean arterial pressure (MAP)	$\frac{(2 \times \text{diastolic}) + \text{systolic}}{3}$
Ejection fraction (EF)	$\frac{\text{SV}}{\text{end-diastolic volume}} \times 100$

HR = heart rate, SV = stroke volume, BSA = body surface area, MAP = mean arterial pressure, PCWP = pulmonary capillary wedge pressure, RAP = right atrial pressure, PAP = mean pulmonary artery pressure.

Table 8-4
Selected hemodynamic values

Cardiac output	4–6 L/min
Cardiac index	2.5–4.0 L/min/m^2
Stroke volume	60–90 ml
Stroke index	40 ± 7 ml/beat/m^2
Left ventricular stroke work index	45–60 g-m/beat/m^2
Systematic vascular resistance	800–1200 dyne/sec/cm^{-5}
Pulmonary vascular resistance	50–150 dyne/sec/cm^{-5}
Mean arterial pressure	70–100 mm Hg
Arteriovenous oxygen difference	4.5–6.0 vol. %

making calculations based on the basic hemodynamic data that have been recorded. Tables 8-3 and 8-4 include some commonly derived variables and their normal values.

Until recently, accurate assessment of PA pressure has been obtainable only with invasive right heart catheterization. In general, noninvasive techniques lack sensitivity and are limited in their ability to detect and quantify mild to moderate elevation of PA pressures. The introduction of Doppler echocardiography has enabled the PA pressure to be measured noninvasively. Measurement of the gradient across the tricuspid valve by quantification of the velocity of the jet of tricuspid regurgitation allows one to estimate right ventricular systolic pressure and thereby the systolic PA pressure. In addition, various indexes of pulmonary flow velocity correlate with PA pressure.

Hemodynamics in Common Clinical Situations

Acute Myocardial Infarction

It has been shown that there is a good correlation between the clinical and hemodynamic profile of patients with AMI (Table 8-5). Forester et al. [14] developed a classification method relating the clinical presentation of AMI patients to specific hemodynamic determinants of left ventricular pump performance.

Group I. Patients with an uncomplicated MI, no pulmonary congestion or peripheral hypoperfusion, normal capillary wedge pressure, and normal cardiac index.

Group II. Patients with modest left-ventricular failure as manifested by an S_3 gallop and bibasilar rales. Hemodynamics reveal an elevated capillary wedge pressure (>18 mm Hg), a minimally depressed cardiac index, and normal systemic blood pressure.

Group III. Patients without clinical evidence of pulmonary edema but with evidence of low cardiac output and fatigue, usually in the presence of decreased renal function as evidenced by rising blood urea nitrogen (BUN) and creatinine levels. Blood pressure is usually low in these patients. Hemodynamic monitoring reveals a slightly elevated wedge pressure (12–28 mm Hg) and a reduced cardiac index (<2.2 L/min/m^2). In addition, systemic vascular resistance is usually increased (>1500 dyne/sec/cm^{-5}).

Group IV. This group includes patients with cardiogenic shock that manifests clinically as hypotension, fatigue, mental obtundation, and pulmonary congestion. These patients are acidotic and hypoxic, and they have deteriorating renal function (increasing BUN and creatinine levels). Hemodynamic monitoring reveals an elevated wedge pressure (18–25 mm Hg) with evidence of pulmonary hypertension (mean PA pressure >35 mm Hg), decreased cardiac index (CI) (<2.0 L/min/m^2), and elevated systemic vascular resistance.

Appropriate therapy is guided by the hemodynamic data. In general, hemodynamic monitoring is most useful in patients in group IV in whom it is important to exclude the presence of a mechanical lesion. During the clinical course of myocardial infarction there are times when there is a discrepancy between the clinical appearance of the patient and the hemodynamic picture. It is at this time also that hemodynamic monitoring may be useful.

Acute Mitral Regurgitation

Acute mitral regurgitation (MR) can present in a variety of ways. A patient with this condition may have sudden, unexplained dyspnea with minimal cardiac auscultatory findings. The chest radiograph may reveal florid pulmonary edema with a normal heart size. It is more common for acute MR to occur in the setting of an inferior myocardial infarction,

Table 8-5
Hemodynamic patterns for common clinical conditions

	Chamber pressures (mm Hg)				
Cardiac condition	RA	RV	PA	PAOP	CI
Normal	0–6	25/0–6	25/0–12	6–12	≥2.5
AMI without LVF	0–6	25/0–6	30/12–18	≤18	≥2.5
AMI with LVF	0–6	30–40/0–6	30–40/18–25	>18	>2.0
Biventricular failure	>6	50–60/>6	50–60/25	18–25	>2.0
RVMI	12–20	30/12–20	30/12	≤12	<2.0
Cardiac tamponade	12–16	25/12–16	25/12–16	12–16	<2.0
Pulmonary embolism	12–20	50–60/12–20	50–60/12	<12	<2.0

RA = right atrium, RV = right ventricle, PA = pulmonary artery, PAOP = pulmonary artery occlusion pressure, CI = cardiac index, LVF = left ventricular failure, RVMI = right ventricular myocardial infarction.

although it can be seen with anterior AMI. In the setting of AMI, acute MR usually occurs 24 to 48 hours after the onset of infarction with sudden onset of dyspnea. The individual is usually hypotensive and tachycardic. A murmur is usually but not always present and can be nondescript.

Hemodynamic monitoring reveals a giant V wave in the wedge pressure tracing (Fig. 8-10). It results from the left ventricle ejecting blood into a normal-sized, relatively noncompliant left atrium. As mentioned, a large V wave is not definitely diagnostic of acute MR, as it can occur whenever the left atrium is distended and noncompliant, as with ventricular septal rupture or left ventricular failure of any cause [15–17]. The giant V wave of acute MR is often transmitted to the PA tracing, which yields a bifid PA waveform composed of the PA systolic wave and the V wave. As the catheter is wedged, the PA systolic wave disappears but the V wave remains. It is useful to remember that the PA systolic wave occurs earlier in relation to the QRS (between the QRS and T wave) than does the V wave (end of the T wave). Acute MR is the rare instance when the PA end-diastolic pressure may be lower than the mean pulmonary capillary wedge pressure. PA blood oxygen saturation is generally decreased because of a reduction in cardiac output; however, in rare cases the giant left atrial V wave is accompanied by transient reversal of pulmonary blood flow with highly oxygenated blood entering the pulmonary artery. This situation may result in overestimation of cardiac output (if one uses the Fick method) or incorrect diagnosis of a left-to-right shunt. The systemic vascular resistance is frequently elevated, and prerenal azotemia develops.

Ventricular Septal Rupture

Rupture of the ventricular septum causes acute volume overload of the right ventricle. This complication of AMI occurs 2 to 5 days after the initial event and may be found with both inferior and anterior infarction. The first clue to its appearance is the development of biventricular failure. The clinical examination usually reveals a loud holosystolic murmur along the sternum with wide radiation, an S_3 gallop, and, frequently, elevated jugular venous pressure.

The diagnosis of acute ventricular septal rupture is made by finding a significant increase in oxygen saturation of blood between the right atrium and the pulmonary artery. The oxygen saturation value from the right atrium must be interpreted carefully, as it may be misleadingly decreased if blood is sampled near the coronary sinus. The mean right atrial, pulmonary artery, and pulmonary capillary wedge pressures are all significantly elevated. A prominent V wave may be seen in the wedge tracing [17], but this finding is usually not as striking as that which occurs with acute mitral regurgitation.

In the setting of acute ventricular septal defect, the systemic cardiac output is less than the thermodilution-determined cardiac output. The thermodilution method measures right-sided cardiac output, i.e., pulmonary blood flow, which reflects left-to-right shunting. ''Normal'' thermodilution cardiac output in a patient with an acute ventricular septal defect usually reflects a severe reduction in systemic blood flow. When following Fick cardiac outputs in patients with acute ventricular septal rupture, a fall in PA blood saturation may actually represent less left-to-right shunting and an improvement in forward cardiac output. In a patient with an acute ventricular septal defect, mixed venous oxygen saturation is calculated using inferior and superior vena caval blood oxygen saturation.

Cardiac Tamponade

When pericardial fluid accumulates, it may result in increased pericardial pressure, which can impair ventricular diastolic filling. Severe impairment of diastolic filling may result in cardiac tamponade. Clinically, the patient is tachycardic, hypotensive, and dyspneic. Examination reveals clear lung fields and a quiet precordium. Radiographically, the lungs are clear and the cardiac silhouette enlarged. The combination of a small, quiet heart, increased central venous pressure, and hypotension constitute *Beck's triad.*

The hemodynamic hallmarks of cardiac tamponade are elevation and equalization of the right atrial, right ventricular diastolic, PA diastolic, and mean pulmonary capillary wedge pressures. Arterial waveform analysis reveals pulsus paradoxus. Close examination of the right atrial pressure can be informative. There is a dominant x descent due to the diminished cardiac volume at this time. The y descent is frequently absent, which results in a unimodal right atrial pressure recording. Even in the presence of severe cardiac tamponade, inspiration is accompanied by a small drop in intrapericardial pressure, and therefore in right atrial pressure, which can be detected at the bedside by an inspiratory fall in the level of the jugular venous pressure. This decline in right atrial pressure can be helpful for distinguishing cardiac tamponade from other conditions that result in elevated right-sided diastolic pressure, restriction or right ventricular infarction.

Right Ventricular Infarction

Clinically important right ventricular infarction usually occurs in the setting of inferior myocardial infarction. It is frequently accompanied by hypotension, increased jugular venous pressure, clear lung fields, and bradyarrhythmias. Right-side ECG can be useful for making the diagnosis. The hemodynamic findings are characteristic, although they may be confused with constrictive pericarditis or cardiac tamponade. The right atrial pressure is elevated (usually >10 mm Hg) with relatively low right ventricular and PA systolic pressures. The right atrial pressure is often disproportionately increased relative to the wedge pressure. With significant elevation of right atrial pressure, shunting can occur across a patent foramen ovale leading to arterial desaturation. The right atrial waveform reveals prominent x and y descents. During inspiration, the right atrial pressure usually does not decline and may actually increase (Kussmaul's sign). An increase in right atrial pressure may also be seen with compression of the liver. Right ventricular end-diastolic pressure is elevated, and the pulse pressure is narrowed in both right ventricle and pulmonary artery. Tricuspid regurgitation due to papillary muscle dysfunction and right ventricle dilatation may complicate right ventricular infarction.

Therapy is directed toward elevating the right ventricular diastolic and right atrial pressures, often to 20 mm Hg, by infusing volume in order to move blood through the right side of the heart in the face of decreased right ventricular contractility.

Pulmonary Hypertension

Pulmonary hypertension is present when the mean PA pressure is more than 20 mm Hg. The cause can be either passive (''upstream'' increase in pressure) or reactive (local increase in pressure). The difference between the mean PA pressure and the pulmonary capillary wedge pressures is used to make this determination. A difference of more than 12 mm Hg, indicates *reactive pulmonary hypertension;* a difference of 12 mm Hg or less indicates *passive hypertension.* Pulmonary hypertension can result from a combination of passive and reactive causes.

Pulmonary hypertension is usually referred to as primary or secondary, based on the underlying etiology. *Primary pulmonary hypertension* has an unknown etiology, whereas *secondary pulmonary hypertension* occurs in patients with long-standing intracardiac shunts, chronic lung disease, or chronic left ventricular failure. Pulmonary hypertension can also be classified as *passive* (upstream increase in pressure leading to increased pulmonary pressures) or *reactive* (local increase in pressure). The pulmonary capillary wedge pressure is usually normal with reactive pulmonary hypertension (primary pulmonary hypertension, pulmonary hypertension due to lung disease) and abnormal with passive pulmonary hypertension (left ventricular failure). With passive pulmonary hypertension, the PA diastolic pressure increases passively, in keeping with the elevated wedge pressure. With pulmonary hypertension of either etiology (reactive or passive), the mean PA pressure, by definition, is elevated, often exceeding 50 mm Hg. The right ventricular end-diastolic pressure is normal until late in the course of the disease. Long-standing pulmonary hypertension can lead to right ventricular dilatation with resulting tricuspid regurgitation. The right atrial pressure tracing of tricuspid regurgitation reveals accentuated V waves with steep y descents. The mean right atrial pressure is elevated. The right atrial V wave of tricuspid regurgitation is not as pronounced as the left atrial V wave of acute mitral regurgitation. With tricuspid regurgitation, Kussmaul's sign may be present, i.e., a rise in mean right atrial pressure with inspiration. Pulmonary hypertension with a dilated right ventricle and tricuspid regurgitation often presents difficulties for placement of the PA catheter. Tricuspid regurgitation interferes with the measurement of thermodilution cardiac output because of the back and forth flow of the indicator (saline) between the right atrium and right ventricle.

Massive Pulmonary Embolism

Massive pulmonary embolism is invariably manifested by unexplained acute dyspnea with arterial blood oxygen desaturation, low cardiac output, and elevated jugular venous pressure. The ECG usually demonstrates acute cor pulmonale. Hemodynamic monitoring reveals markedly elevated right atrial pressure (often more than 10 mm Hg). Right ventricular and PA systolic pressures are elevated but rarely exceed 40 to 50 mm Hg, as the normal right ventricle cannot generate a high PA pressure acutely. The right ventricle generally dilates and fails once right ventricular systolic pressure reaches 50 to 60 mm Hg. Higher PA pressures suggest a chronic component to the pulmonary hypertension. The pulmonary capillary wedge pressure is usually low, as is the cardiac output. The PA end-diastolic pressure remains significantly higher than the mean wedge pressure. The A and V waves of the wedge tracing are frequently absent, as the abnormal pulmonary vasculature does not allow retrograde transmission of these pressure waves from the left atrium to the distal catheter lumen. Pulmonary vascular resistance is elevated.

In patients with respiratory distress from any cause, large swings in intrathoracic pressure can occur that can be transmitted to the pulmonary capillary wedge tracing. These wide swings in intrathoracic pressure reduce the accuracy of the capillary wedge pressure as a measure of left ventricular filling pressure. It is possible for left ventricular filling pressure to be overestimated in this setting. Attempts should be made to take measurements at end expiration.

Complications of Hemodynamic Monitoring

The ability to monitor PA pressures has increased our understanding of the pathophysiology of cardiac disease. This procedure is not without risk, and the precise role in the monitoring of patients in the CCU remains controversial. Numerous case reports have described specific complications associated with the use of PA catheters, although large-scale studies are lacking. In a series of more than 500 patients, serious complications occurred in approximately 4 percent [18]. Other estimates of the incidence of significant morbidity range from 23 to 50 percent. A rate of 15.8 percent was reported when data from several series were pooled [19, 20].

Complications may be divided into three categories: (1) those associated with obtaining venous access; (2) those occurring during PA catheter insertion; and (3) those developing with the catheter in situ. Most complications are avoidable when the operator is aware of the potential pitfalls and exercises careful attention to detail.

Complications of Central Venous Access

Local vascular complications can be associated with insertion of the central venous catheter. Common complications include local hematomas, inadvertent entry into the arterial system, and invasion of the pleural space with subsequent pneumothorax formation [20–26].

Hematoma formation is usually not clinically significant and can often be controlled with local pressure. Serious hematoma formation with significant bleeding or compression of mediastinal structures, with airway compromise, can occur, particularly in patients with an underlying coagulopathy [27]. Inadvertent arterial puncture is not uncommon [28]. The incidence of inadvertent carotid artery puncture with attempted internal jugular vein cannulation has been reported to be approximately 4.8 percent [29]. Reports of AV fistula and pseudoaneurysm formation have also been described [30, 31].

Structures adjacent to vascular sites can be damaged, and there are reports of thoracic duct injury with resultant chylothorax formation [32]. Pneumothorax formation can be a serious complication of catheter insertion, although the incidence is low [29, 33]. The incidence of pneumothorax is increased by using the subclavian approach; hence, the internal jugular approach is the preferred route in patients unlikely to tolerate a pneumothorax.

Sheared plastic catheter embolization has been reported, and caution must be exercised regarding the position of the needle and plastic cannula before insertion of the introducer [34]. Air embolism can also occur if the catheter or introducer is left open and negative thoracic pressure is generated [35]. Careful attention to covering open ports in the venous system minimizes air entry into the right heart.

Arrhythmias

Insertion of PA catheters is associated with a variety of cardiac arrhythmias. Premature atrial and ventricular beats are common as the catheter passes through the right atrium and right ventricle, respectively [29, 36]. Catheter-induced atrial fibrillation and atrial flutter have been described [36]. Nonsustained ventricular tachycardia can occur as the catheter passes through the right ventricle, although the incidence of sustained ventricular tachycardia and ventricular fibrillation is low [37]. Normal electrolyte levels prior to catheter insertion minimize the potential for serious ventricular arrhythmias.

Abnormalities in electrical conduction can be encountered when right heart catheters engage the interventricular septum. Reports of transient right bundle branch block are not uncommon [38, 39], and complete heart block may also be produced [38]. Because of the potential for inducing right bundle branch block and complete heart block, it is recommended that prophylactic temporary transvenous pacing be employed prior to right heart catheterization in patients with preexisting left bundle branch block.

Pulmonary Artery Trauma

Various injuries to the pulmonary artery have been associated with the use of PA catheters. Rupture of the pulmonary artery with fatal hemorrhage has been reported [40, 41]. The onset of hemoptysis during catheter insertion signals this complication, although hemoptysis is not always present. Emergency surgical repair of the pulmonary artery or pneumonectomy may be required. PA rupture usually occurs when there is overinflation of the balloon that has migrated to a distal position. Patients with pulmonary hypertension are at increased risk for this complication. Careful consideration of catheter position prior to balloon inflation and limiting the number of balloon inflations can minimize the likelihood of PA trauma. The balloon should always be inflated with the least amount of air necessary to obtain a pulmonary capillary wedge pressure tracing.

Pulmonary artery infarction due to persistent undetected wedging of the catheter can occur [42, 43]. It may be a result of inadvertent persistent balloon inflation, or more commonly, caused by distal migration of the catheter tip. These lesions are usually not clinically evident, although chest radiographs may demonstrate abnormalities in the region of the catheter tip. Careful attention to the position of the catheter tip and continuous monitoring of the pressure waveform minimize this complication.

Knotting

Knotting of flow-directed catheters can occur, although it is uncommon when proper technique is utilized [44]. It occurs when the catheter is advanced without the distal tip proceeding through the cardiac chambers. It is recommended that the catheter never be advanced farther than the appropriate distance for each cardiac chamber, as directed by the pressure waveform. In addition, the balloon should routinely be inflated during catheter advancement to maximize flow direction of the catheter. If the catheter fails to advance into the next heart chamber, it should be removed to the preceding chamber and readvanced.

Thrombotic Complications

Thrombosis is a well described complication associated with the use of PA catheters. Thrombotic complications can be the result of a thrombus that forms on the catheters, either proximally or distally, or within the catheter lumen with subsequent embolization to the pulmonary circulation. Thrombosis may therefore manifest clinically as either pulmonary embolism [20, 45, 46] or occlusive vascular thrombosis [45, 47]. The incidence of clinical thrombosis is uncertain; however, previously placed PA catheters have been examined at the time of open heart surgery, and the incidence of catheter thrombus formation approaches 100 percent [6, 7]. Chastre and Gilbert [48] reported a 66 percent incidence of asymptomatic thrombosis of the internal jugular vein in patients with PA catheters. Numerous cases of central venous thrombosis associated with the use of PA catheters have been reported [47, 49], as have cases of catheter-related septic central venous thrombosis [50].

Thrombosis may involve the distal tip of the PA catheter, affecting fidelity of the pressure tracing. Continuous infusion through the various catheter lumens should always be utilized to minimize this potential problem.

Infections

The use of invasive hemodynamic monitoring has been associated with both local and systemic infections [20, 22, 23, 51, 52]. The infection rate for indwelling catheters appears to be between 2 and 4 percent [24, 53, 54]. The rate may rise to 8 percent for a second catheter placed over a guidewire [53]. A large-scale prospective study of PA catheterization in patients undergoing cardiac surgery found that 18 (2.3 percent) of 794 cultured catheter tips were positive. An in situ time of more than 72 hours was associated with a significantly higher percentage (7.2 percent) of positive tip cultures [27].

Numerous factors influence the likelihood of catheter-related infection. The duration of use, care of insertion site, care of stopcocks, transducers, and infusion fluid, in addition to the patient baseline immune status, affect the rates of infection. It must be emphasized that PA catheters should be removed immediately when the hemodynamic data are no longer necessary for patient care.

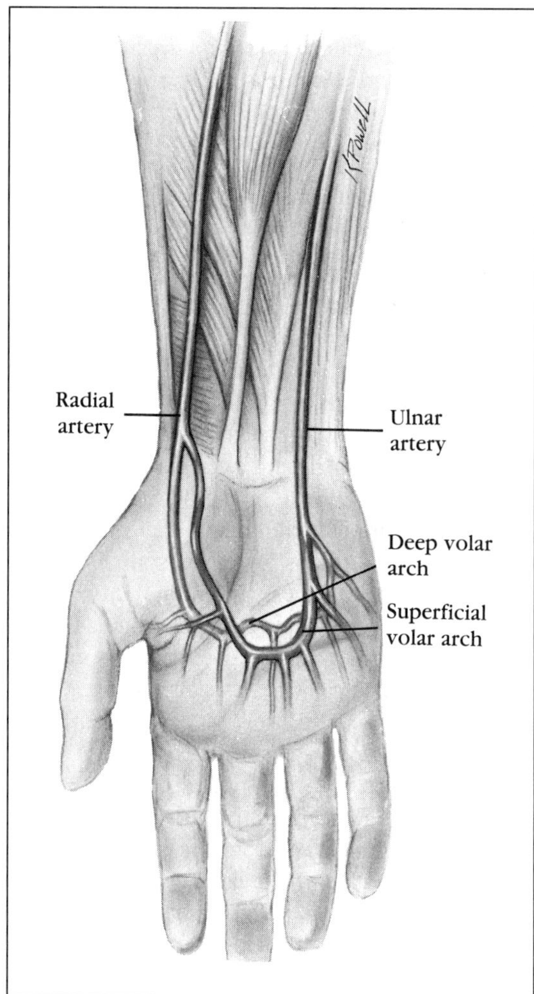

Fig. 8-12
Anatomy of the radial artery. Note the collateral circulation to the ulnar artery through the deep volar arterial arch and dorsal arch. (From J. M. Rippe et al. (eds.), *Intensive Care Medicine.* Boston: Little, Brown, 1985. P. 36. With permssion.)

Systemic Arterial Monitoring

Reliable assessment of the systemic arterial blood pressure is required in patients in the CCU. It is most often achieved by the use of the blood pressure cuff and auscultation of Korotkoff sounds.

Portable vital sign monitors can noninvasively and automatically measure systolic, diastolic, and mean arterial pressures. These automatic blood pressure cuff monitors operate on alternate-current line voltage or batteries and cycle automatically at operator-programmed intervals between 1 and 90 minutes. The most important consideration when obtaining indirect blood pressure measurements is use of a correctly sized cuff. A cuff that is too wide leads to underestimation of blood pressure, whereas an inappropriately narrow cuff leads to erroneously high measurements.

In most patients these indirect methods adequately assess blood pressure. There is a subset of patients in whom continuous assessment of systemic arterial pressure is required. Patients with labile blood pressure with either hyper- or hypotension constitute such a group. In these "unstable" patients, minute-by-minute assessment of blood pressure is required to determine efficacy of therapeutic interventions. Arterial cannulation and direct systemic blood pressure monitoring allow beat-to-beat monitoring of blood pressure in this critically ill population.

Multiple arterial sites are available for catheter insertion. Most common sites include the radial, dorsalis pedis, brachial, and femoral arteries. Arterial catheters may be placed either percutaneously or via a cutdown technique. Descriptions of arterial catheter replacement are available [11, 55].

In general, it is recommended that a $2^1/2$ in. plastic cannula be inserted percutaneously into the radial artery. The radial artery is the preferred site because of its superficial location and the presence of collaterals with the ulnar artery via the deep and superficial volar arches (Fig. 8-12). The Allen test should always be used prior to catheter insertion to minimize the potential for compromised arterial circulation to the hand.

References

1. Swan, H. J. C., Ganz, W., Forrester, J., et al. Catheterization of the heart in man with use of a flow-directed balloon-tipped catheter. *N. Engl. J. Med.* 283:447, 1970.
2. Gore, J. M., Goldberg, T. J., Spodick, D. H., et al. A community wide assessment of the use of pulmonary artery catheters in patients with acute myocardial infarction. *Chest* 92:721, 1987.
3. Gore, J. M., Alpert, J. S., Benotti, J. R., et al. *Handbook of Hemodynamic Monitoring.* Boston: Little, Brown, 1984.
4. Robin, E. D. The cult of the Swan-Ganz catheter: Overuse and abuse of pulmonary flow catheters. *Ann. Intern. Med.* 103:445, 1985.
5. Sharkey, S. W. Beyond the wedge: Clinical physiology and the Swan-Ganz catheter. *Am. J. Med.* 83: 111, 1987.
6. Hoar, P. F., Wilson, R. M., and Mangano, J. T. Heparin bonding reduces thrombogenicity of pulmonary artery catheters. *N. Engl. J. Med.* 305:993, 1981.
7. Mangano, D. T. Heparin bonding long-term protection against thrombosis. *N. Engl. J. Med.* 307:894, 1982.
8. D'Arcy, P. F. Drug interactions and reactions update. *Drug Intell. Clin. Pharm.* 17:726, 1983.
9. Jacobi, J., et al. Loss of nitroglycerin to central venous pressure catheters. *Drug. Intell. Clin. Pharm.* 16:331, 1982.
10. Martin, C., Auffray, J. P., Saux, P., et al. The axillary vein: An alternate approach to percutaneous pulmonary artery catheterization. *Chest* 90:694, 1986.
11. VanderSalm, T. J., Cutler, B. S., and Wheeler, H. B. *Atlas of Bedside Procedures.* Boston: Little, Brown, 1979.
12. Seneff, M. G., and Rippe, J. M. Central venous catheters. In J. M. Rippe et al. (eds.), *Intensive Care Medicine.* Boston: Little, Brown, 1985. Pp. 16–33.
13. Seneff, M. G. Central venous catheterization: A comprehensive review. *J. Intensive Care Med.* 2:163, 218, 1987.
14. Forrester, J. F., Diamond, G., Chatterjee, K., and Swan, H. J. C. Medical therapy of acute myocardial infarction by application of hemodynamic subsets (Parts I & II). *N. Engl. J. Med.* 24:1356, 1404, 1976.
15. Fuchs, R. M., Heuser, R. R., Yin, F. C., and Brinker, J. A. Limitations of pulmonary wedge V waves in diagnosing mitral regurgitation. *Am. J. Cardiol.* 49:849, 1982.
16. Pichard, A. D., Kay, R., Smith, H., et al. Large V waves in the pulmonary wedge tracing in the absence of mitral regurgitation. *Am. J. Cardiol.* 50:1044, 1982.
17. Downes, T. R., Hackshaw, B. T., Kahl, F. R., et al. Frequency of large V waves in the pulmonary artery wedge pressure in ventricular septal defect of acquired (during acute myocardial infarction) or congenital origin. *Am. J. Cardiol.* 60:415, 1987.
18. Boyd, K. D., Thomas, S. J., Gold, J., and Boyd, A. D. A prospective study of complications of pulmonary artery catheterization in 500 consecutive patients. *Chest* 84:245, 1983.
19. Sprung, C. L., Jacobs, L. J., Caralis, P. V., and Karpf, M. Ventricular arrhythmias during Swan-Ganz catheterization of the critically ill. *Chest* 79:413, 1981.
20. Elliott, C. G., Zimmerman, G. A., and Clemmer, T. P. Complications of pulmonary artery catheterization in the care of critically ill patients. *Chest* 76:647, 1979.
21. Katz, J. D., Cronau, L. H., Barash, P. G., and Mandel, S. D. Pulmonary artery flow guided catheters in the perioperative period: Indications and complications. *J.A.M.A.* 237:2832, 1977.
22. Puri, V. K., Carlson, R. W., Bander, J. J., and Weil, M. H. Complications of vascular catheterization in the critically ill: A prospective study. *Crit. Care Med.* 8:495, 1980.
23. Sise, M. J., Hollingsworth, P., Brimm, J. E., et al. Complications of the flow-directed pulmonary-artery catheter: A prospective analysis in 219 patients. *Crit. Care Med.* 9:315, 1981.
24. Davies, M. J., Cronin, K. D., and Domaingue, C. M. L. Pulmonary artery catheterization: An assessment of risks and benefits in 220 surgical patients. *Anaesth. Intensive Care* 10:9, 1982.
25. Rao, T. L. K., Gorski, D. W., Laughlin, S., and El-Etr, A. A. Safety of pulmonary artery catheterization. *Anesthesiology* 57:A116, 1982.
26. Barash, P. G., Nardi, D., Hammon, G., et al. Catheter-induced pulmonary artery perforation: Mechanisms, management and modifications. *J. Thorac. Cardiovasc. Surg.* 82:5, 1981.
27. Knoblanche, G. E. Respiratory obstruction due to hematoma following internal jugular vein cannulation. *Anaesth. Intensive Care* 7:286, 1979.

28. Silver, G. M., Bogerty, S. A., Hayashi, R. M. et al. Arterial complications of attempted Swan-Ganz insertion. *Am. J. Cardiol.* 53:340, 1984.
29. Damen, J., and Bolton, D. A prospective analysis of 1,400 pulmonary-artery catheterizations in patients undergoing cardiac surgery. *Acta Anaesthesiol. Scand.* 30:386, 1986.
30. Hansbrough, J. F., Narrod, J. A., and Rutherford, R. Arteriovenous fistulas following central venous catheterization. *Intensive Care Med.* 9:287, 1983.
31. Sheild, C. F., Richardson, J. D., Buckley, C. J., et al. Pseudoaneurysm of the brachiocephalic arteries: A complication of percutaneous internal jugular vein catheterization. *Surgery* 78:190, 1975.
32. Khalil, K. G., Parker, F. B., Jr., Mukherjee, N., et al. Thoracic duct injury: A complication of jugular vein catheterization. *J.A.M.A.* 221:908, 1972.
33. Patel, C., Laboy, V., Verus, B., et al. Acute complications of pulmonary artery catheter insertion in critically ill patients. *Crit. Care Med.* 14:195, 1986.
34. Doering, R. B., Stommer, E. A., and Connolly, J. E. Complications of indwelling venous catheters with particular reference to catheter embolism. *Am. J. Surg.* 114:259, 1967.
35. Horrow, J. C., and Laucks, S. O. Coronary air embolism during venous cannulation. *Anesthesiology* 56:212, 1982.
36. Geha, D. G., Davis, N. J., and Lappas, D. G. Persistent atrial arrhythmias associated with placement of Swan-Ganz catheter. *Anesthesiology* 39:651, 1973.
37. Cairns, J. A., and Holder, D. Ventricular fibrillation due to passage of Swan-Ganz catheter. *Am. J. Cardiol.* 35:589, 1975.
38. Thomson, I. R., Dalton, B. C., Lappas, D. G., et al. Right bundle branch block and complete heart block caused by the Swan-Ganz catheter. *Anesthesiology* 51:359, 1979.
39. Luck, J. C., and Engel, T. R. Transient right bundle branch block with Swan-Ganz catheterization. *Am. Heart J.* 92:263, 1976.
40. Pape, L. A., Haffajee, C. I., Markis, J. E., et al. Fatal pulmonary hemorrhage after the use of the flow-direct balloon-tipped catheter. *Ann. Intern. Med.* 90:344, 1979.
41. Golden, M. S., Pinder, T., Anderson, W. T., et al. Fatal pulmonary hemorrhage complicating use of a flow-direct balloon-tipped catheter in a patient receiving anticoagulant therapy. *Am. J. Cardiol.* 32: 865, 1973.
42. Foote, G. A., Schabel, S. I., and Hodges, M. Pulmonary complications of the flow-directed balloon tipped catheter. *N. Engl. J. Med.* 290:927, 1974.
43. Goodman, D. J., Rider, A. K., Billingham, M. E., et al. Thromboembolic complications with balloon-tipped pulmonary arterial catheter. *N. Engl. J. Med.* 291:777, 1974.
44. Lipp, H., O'Donoghue, K., and Resnekov, L. Intracardiac knotting of a flow directed balloon catheter. *N. Engl. J. Med.* 284:220, 1971.
45. Bradway, W., Bronde, R. J., Koufman, J. C., et al. Internal jugular thrombosis and pulmonary embolism. *Chest* 80:335, 1981.
46. Goldstein, M. T., Nestko, P., Olshan, A. R., et al. Superior vena cava thrombosis and pulmonary embolus. *Arch. Intern. Med.* 142:1726, 1982.
47. Yorra, F. H., Oblath, R., Jaffee, H., et al. Massive thrombosis associated with use of a Swan-Ganz catheter. *Chest* 65:682, 1974.
48. Chastre, J., and Gilbert, C. Thrombosis as complications of pulmonary artery catheterization via the internal jugular vein. *N. Engl. J. Med.* 306:1487, 1982.
49. Gore, J. M., Matsumoto, A. H., Layden, J. J., et al. Superior vena cava syndrome, its association with indwelling balloon-tipped pulmonary artery catheters. *Arch. Intern. Med.* 144:506, 1984.
50. Kaufman, J., Demas, C., Stark, K., and Flancbaum, L. Catheter-related septic central venous thrombosis—current therapeutic options. *West. J. Med.* 145: 200, 1986.
51. Applefield, J. J., Caruthers, T. E., and Reno, R. J. Assessment of the sterility of long-term cardiac catheterization using the thermodilution Swan-Ganz catheter. *Chest* 74:377, 1978.
52. Myers, M. L., Austin, T. W., and Silobald, W. J. Pulmonary artery catheter infections. *Ann. Surg.* 201: 237, 1985.
53. Senagore, A., Waller, S. D., Bonnell, B. W., et al. Pulmonary artery catheterization: A prospective study of internal jugular and subclavian approaches. *Crit. Care Med.* 15:35, 1987.
54. Plit, M. L., Rumbak, M. J., Lipman, J., and Eidelman, J. Invasive vascular catheterization in the critically ill. *S. Afr. Med. J.* 72:245, 1987.
55. Liebowitz, R. S., and Rippe, J. M. Arterial line placement and care. In: J. M. Rippe et al. (eds.), *Intensive Care Medicine.* Boston: Little, Brown, 1985. Pp. 33–42.

III.
Electrical Complications of Acute Myocardial Infarction: Diagnosis and Treatment

9. Approach to Patients with Asymptomatic Ventricular Arrhythmias After Myocardial Infarction

Eric N. Prystowsky

Sudden cardiac death is a major health problem that is estimated to occur nearly once every minute in the United States [1]. Cardiac catheterization data as well as postmortem studies demonstrate that most victims have significant coronary artery disease [2–5]. Through the efforts of Cobb and colleagues in association with the Seattle Fire Department, emergency care systems have been shown to decrease the mortality of cardiac arrest victims through on-the-scene cardiopulmonary resuscitation of patients who have collapsed from a malignant ventricular arrhythmia [6]. However, only a few patients with out-of-hospital ventricular fibrillation are successfully defibrillated and subsequently discharged from the hospital [6]. Clearly, a better approach would be to identify and provide prophylactic therapy for those individuals with coronary artery disease who are at high risk for future occurrences of a sustained ventricular tachyarrhythmia.

Numerous investigations demonstrated that ventricular arrhythmias, in addition to the presence and severity of coronary artery disease and left ventricular (LV) dysfunction, are risk factors for sudden cardiac death [7–19]. The presence of nonsustained ventricular tachycardia (VT-NS) has been defined as an independent risk factor for subsequent arrhythmic death after acute myocardial infarction (AMI), and the risk appears to extend beyond the first year after myocardial infarction (MI) [19]. Califf and coworkers [20] analyzed the prognostic implications of ventricular arrhythmias in patients who were undergoing cardiac catheterization for presumed coronary artery disease. These authors found that the severity of ventricular arrhythmias was closely associated with the extent of coronary artery disease and LV dysfunction. Of patients who had VT-NS, 71 percent had an LV ejection fraction (LVEF) of less than 0.40, and 16 percent of patients with an EF of less than 0.40 had VT-NS. Although patients with more severe ventricular arrhythmias, quantitated using a modified Lown grading system, had a decreased survival rate during a 2-year follow-up period, the ventricular arrhythmia score added no additional significant prognostic information once all the information from cardiac catheterization was included in the analysis. Thus, the presence of VT-NS has been demonstrated to be an independent risk factor for sudden cardiac death in some but not all studies.

CAST, CAST II, and Amiodarone Drug Trials

Identification of a group of patients at high risk for subsequent sudden cardiac death would be useful if appropriate antiarrhythmic therapy prevented the fatal arrhythmic event. Several studies have addressed this issue.

Cardiac Arrhythmia Suppression Trial

The Cardiac Arrhythmia Suppression Trial (CAST) was a multicenter study that tested whether suppression of nonsustained ventricular arrhythmias that caused no or only mild symptoms after MI reduces arrhythmic death [21]. Patients were eligible if they were within 6 days to 2 years of a documented MI and had six or more premature ventricular complexes (PVCs) per hour on a 24-hour qualifying Holter recording. An LVEF of 0.55 or less was required if the Holter monitoring was performed within 90 days after infarction, or an LVEF of 0.40 or less if the monitoring was performed later. Patients who met the criteria and had no exclusions underwent an open-label drug titration phase, during which as many as three drugs (encainide, flecainide, and moricizine) were evaluated. Suppression of arrhythmia was defined as reduction of 80 percent or more for PVCs and 90 percent or more for runs of VT-NS measured on a 24-hour Holter recording. Patients with successful arrhythmia suppression were randomly assigned to receive placebo or the successful drug. Overall, 1455 patients received encainide, flecainide, or placebo; moricizine or placebo was given to 272 patients.

The Data and Safety Monitoring Board for CAST I met on April 16 and 17, 1989, and recommended that the use of encainide and flecainide be discontinued. During a 10-month-average follow-up, patients receiving encainide or flecainide had a higher arrhythmic mortality than those taking placebo. For encainide and flecainide there were 4.5 percent arrhythmic deaths and nonfatal cardiac arrests, compared with 1.2 percent for the placebo group; the relative risk was 3.6 for active drug. There was also a higher total mortality with encainide and flecainide. Of note, the base-line characteristics were similar for the placebo and active drug groups. Too few data were available for moricizine, which was continued in CAST II [22].

Cardiac Arrhythmia Suppression Trial II

CAST II had several protocol changes from CAST I, including testing of only moricizine compared with control [22]. In addition, patients had to be within 90 days of qualifying MI, have an LVEF of 0.40 or less, and there was an initial controlled trial to establish the risks of starting low-dose (600 mg/day) moricizine. The early, randomized phase of CAST II included 1325 patients; the long-term phase evaluated 1155 patients with adequate suppression of ventricular arrhythmias. There was also a substudy that randomized 219 patients who had partial arrhythmia suppression in the early phase to control or active drug.

The Data and Safety Monitoring Board recommended premature termination of CAST II. In the initial 2-week phase, death or cardiac arrest occurred in 17 of 665 patients given moricizine compared with 3 of 660 placebo-treated patients ($p < .02$); the relative risk was 5.6. All 3 patients taking placebo died from an arrhythmia. Arrhythmic mortality occurred in 9 moricizine-treated patients; cardiac arrest occurred in 5 such patients. Further, the data from the long-term study indicated that a survival benefit from moricizine was highly unlikely.

In summary, CAST I and CAST II showed that, after myocardial infarction, suppression of asymptomatic nonsustained ventricular arrhythmias with flecainide, encainide, or moricizine is unwise, and leads to increased arrhythmic mortality. Proarrhythmia is often an early event that occurs during drug titration with many agents. Thus, in patients with symptomatic ventricular arrhythmias who require suppressive treatment, in-hospital initiation of drug therapy is recommended.

Amiodarone Trials

Several trials have evaluated the effects of amiodarone on survival of patients after MI [23–27]. No study has enough patients to provide definitive data, although the overall results are promising. The Basel Antiarrhythmic Study of Infarct Survival (BASIS) enrolled patients with complex ventricular arrhythmias noted on a 24-hour electrocardiographic recording after AMI before hospital discharge. Ninety-eight patients received amiodarone and 114 had no antiarrhythmic therapy. During a 1-year follow-up, sudden death and sustained ventricular tachycardia or ventricular fibrillation occurred significantly less often in patients taking amiodarone. A subsequent analysis showed that the apparent survival benefit of amiodarone was confined to patients with LVEF of 0.40 or more [25].

Today, there are at least two prospective large-scale trials evaluating the prophylactic use of amiodarone in patients after AMI. Recommendations for such prophylactic use depend on the trial results.

Risk Factor Analysis

The prophylactic use of antiarrhythmic drugs in patients after MI requires an analysis of the risks and benefits of such therapy to the patient. However, previous data regarding risk factor analysis for subsequent arrhythmic events after AMI have been obtained in patients undergoing traditional care during the AMI period. Notably, some studies suggest that revascularization of infarcting myocardium improves survival during long-term follow-up [28–30], although the reason for the improved survival is not fully understood. Markers of electrical instability do seem to improve with reperfusion as noted by a loss of late potentials identified by signal-averaged electrocardiography [31]. Furthermore, inducibility of ventricular tachycardia at electrophysiologic study appears to occur more frequently in patients without acute reperfusion than in those who have received thrombolytic therapy [32, 33]. Nevertheless, results from Gruppo Italiano per lo Studio della Streptochinasi nell'Infarto Miocardico II (GISSI-2) showed that frequent PVCs were a significant independent risk factor for total and sudden death in the six months after MI [34]. Clearly, more data are needed on the effect of successful reperfusion during AMI on traditional risk factors.

Nonsustained Ventricular Tachycardia

The relation of VT-NS to sudden cardiac death is uncertain. In some patients VT-NS triggers the onset of sustained ventricular tachycardia or ventricular fibrillation. In others, the VT-NS may become sustained at a given point. This transformation is not common in our experience, however, and the heart rate associated with VT-NS is often dissimilar from the rates seen with sustained ventricular tachycardia in a given patient (Fig. 9-1) [35]. In many patients it is also possible that VT-NS merely serves as a marker of a ventricle that is capable of supporting more serious arrhythmias. In this instance there would be no cause-and-effect relation between the nonsustained and the sustained ventricular arrhythmia.

Asymptomatic patients who have VT-NS tend to show rather characteristic features of their arrhythmia. Episodes of tachycardia are usually three to five complexes in duration, occur fewer than

Fig. 9-1
Ambulatory ECG recording of nonsustained (*A*) and sustained (*B*) ventricular tachycardia. The patient was undergoing in-hospital evaluation of his arrhythmia at the time of the sustained ventricular arrhythmia and was cardioverted successfully.

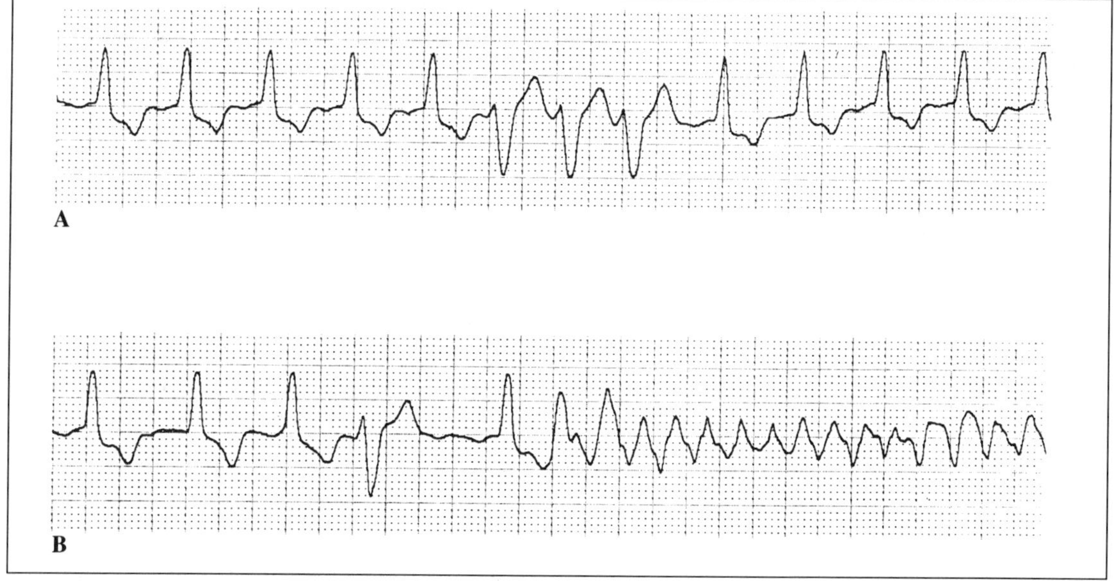

five times daily, and have a rate of 160 per minute or less. Several investigators have evaluated characteristics of VT-NS as predictors for the subsequent occurrence of a sustained arrhythmia, but most have failed to show any correlation. One exception was a study conducted by Meinertz and others [36] in which there did appear to be an association between the frequency of either VT-NS or ventricular pair episodes and the subsequent clinical outcome. Other investigations have not been able to support these observations. It appears that an asymptomatic patient with three to four beats of ventricular tachycardia at a rate of 130 beats per minute (bpm) is at a risk similar to a patient who has six to eight beats of tachycardia at a rate of 180 bpm. The rate of ventricular tachycardia is often variable in these patients (see Fig. 9-1). Kammerling and associates [35] showed that there was only a minimal correlation between the rate of VT-NS and the rate of sustained ventricular tachycardia in the same patient and that the more frequent the episodes of ventricular tachycardia, the more marked the variability in tachycardia rate. Thus, a lack of correlation between the rate of tachycardia and subsequent sudden cardiac death is not surprising. As stated earlier, no study has definitely shown that antiarrhythmic drug therapy prolongs life in patients with asymptomatic nonsustained ventricular tachycardia after myocardial infarction.

Signal-Averaged Electrocardiography

Signal-averaged electrocardiography (SAECG) is used to reduce noise, most importantly skeletal muscle activity, so that low-amplitude electrical signals from the heart can be detected. SAECG usually is obtained as follows [37]: Three surface bipolar ECG leads (X,Y,Z) are acquired for 100 to 200 heart beats, and the voltage of the ECG is fed through a high-gain (× 1000) amplifier. A computer averages the signal, and a high-pass filter is used to minimize the contribution of the large-amplitude low-frequency content. The high-pass filter most commonly used is either 25 or 40 Hz. The X, Y, and Z leads are combined into a vector magnitude referred to as the filtered QRS complex (Fig. 9-2).

Three specific measurements of the filtered QRS complex are used to identify patients most likely to develop sustained ventricular tachycardia or ventricular fibrillation. These measurements are the root-mean-square voltage of the last 40 msec of the filtered QRS complex, the duration of the filtered QRS complex, and the duration of the low-amplitude signals at the end of the filtered QRS complex that are less than 40 μV [37–41]. The criteria for an abnormal SAECG vary among laboratories, but a primary goal has been to identify ventricular late potentials, which are high-frequency, low-amplitude signals that are continuous with the end of the QRS complex. These late potentials most likely represent areas of slow conduction in a damaged ventricle that may be associated with potential reentrant tachycardia circuits [42–51]. It is interesting to note that ventricular late potentials may disappear after successful ventricular tachycardia surgery [48, 50, 52–54], whereas, in my experience, successful antiarrhythmic drug therapy to control ventricular tachycardia does not seem to result in loss of late potentials. Indeed, with successful drug treatment, in some patients there is a prolongation of ventricular conduction time with the appearance of late potentials.

Several studies have demonstrated that the SAECG is a useful test to predict which patients after MI are most likely to develop sustained ventricular tachyarrhythmias. Kanovsky and coworkers [55] analyzed results from SAECG, 24-hour ECG recording, and cardiac catheterization to determine whether SAECG provided independent information to identify patients with a history of sustained ventricular tachycardia. The patient population included 76 individuals who had coronary artery disease and who were undergoing routine cardiac catheterization and 98 patients referred because of documented sustained ventricular tachycardia. All patients had MI, but the median age of infarction differed between the patient groups; it was 8 weeks for the control patients and 46 weeks for those with a history of sustained ventricular tachycardia. Multivariate logistic regression analysis identified three parameters that were independently significant: positive SAECG, peak premature ventricular contractions of more than 100 per hour, and the presence of an LV aneurysm. Notably, combinations of these abnormal tests provided better predictive value than use of a single test. If an aneurysm was excluded from the model, an LVEF of less than 0.40 was noted to be a significant independent variable.

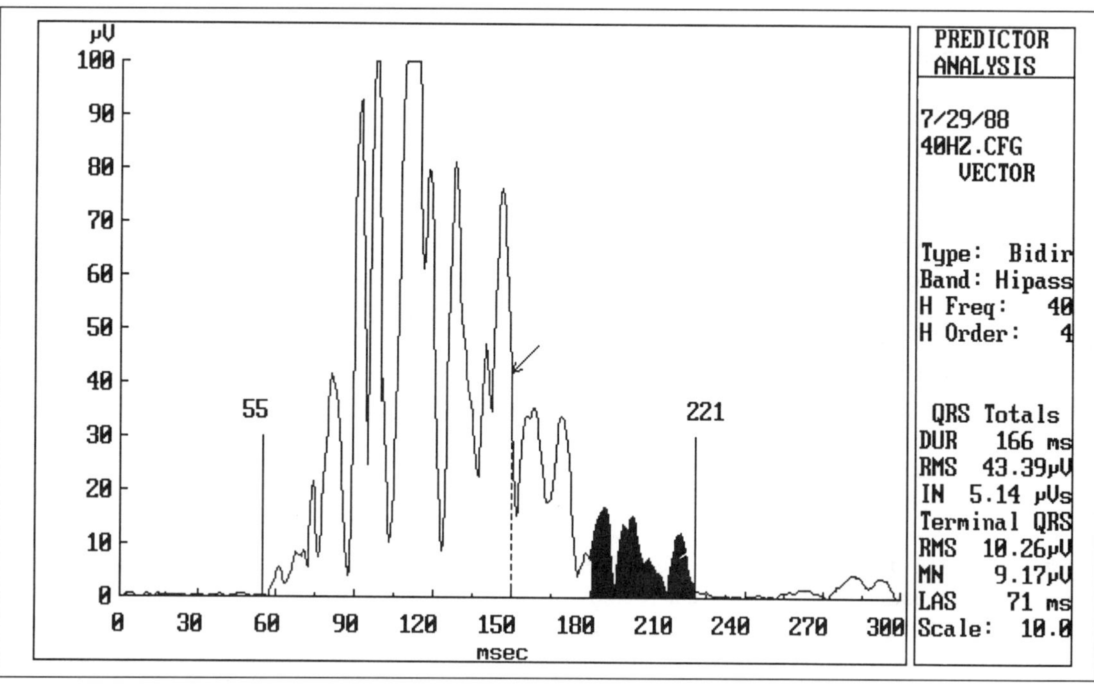

Fig. 9-2
Abnormal signal-averaged electrocardiogram. The filtered QRS duration is 166 msec, which is markedly prolonged. The root-mean-square (RMS) voltage of the terminal 40 msec (*blackened area*) is abnormally low (10.26 μV) and constitutes a positive late potential. Arrow point = 40 μV.

A prospective study of Gomes and colleagues [41] analyzed the prognostic significance of the SAECG, LVEF, and 24-hour ambulatory ECG recording in 102 patients after AMI. The SAECG was obtained 10 ± 6 days after MI, and the other tests were performed within 72 hours of each other. The follow-up period was 12 ± 6 months; during this time 15 patients had either sustained ventricular tachycardia or sudden cardiac death. Arrhythmic events occurred in 29 percent of patients with an abnormal SAECG versus 3.5 percent of patients with a normal SAECG ($p < .003$); 13 of 15 patients with sustained ventricular arrhythmias were identified with this technique. Abnormal results with LVEF and spontaneous ventricular arrhythmias recorded during the ambulatory ECG also presaged life-threatening arrhythmias. A high-risk subset of patients was identified when all three tests were abnormal, and 8 of 16 (50 percent) of these patients had an arrhythmic event during follow-up. However, although the false-positive rate was lower, this combination of tests did not identify seven patients with a subsequent event.

In a follow-up study, Gomes and coworkers [56] investigated the relative predictive value of a 25-Hz versus a 40-Hz high-pass filter, as well as the relative predictive value of the SAECG and LVEF in anterior wall versus inferior wall MI. The sensitivity of the SAECG was slightly better at 40-Hz filtering but depended somewhat on which SAECG variable was being tested. Using 40-Hz filtering, the authors noted that patients who had inferior wall infarctions had a 100 percent sensitivity but a low (50 percent) specificity. In patients with an anterior wall MI, the sensitivity was 75 percent and the specificity 80 percent. Thus, as has been noted in other studies of patients with chronic coronary artery disease, the SAECG has greater sensitivity in patients with an inferior versus an anterior wall MI. It is of note that the sensitivity of an LVEF of less than 0.40 was high (87 percent) with a low specificity (38 percent) in patients with an anterior infarction, whereas the sensitivity was only 50 percent with a higher specificity (71 percent) in patients with an inferior wall MI. Thus, the predictive value of the SAECG was superior to that of the

LVEF in patients with an anterior infarction, but in patients with an inferior infarction there was no difference between the two tests.

Two other investigations deserve comment. Kuchar and coworkers [57] prospectively evaluated 210 consecutive patients after AMI using the SAECG, 24-hour ambulatory ECG recording, and radionuclide left ventriculogram. During a median follow-up period of 14 months, seven patients had sustained ventricular tachycardia, and eight additional patients died suddenly. One patient who died suddenly had bundle branch block and did not undergo signal averaging. Of the remaining 14 patients who had an arrhythmic event after hospital discharge, 13 had an abnormal SAECG, whereas only 1 patient (1 percent) with a normal tracing had an arrhythmic event during follow-up. By stepwise logistic regression, an abnormal SAECG, LVEF of less than 0.40, and complex ventricular ectopy were noted to be independently significant; the LVEF was the most powerful variable in the model. Importantly, with regard to future arrhythmic events, the combination of an abnormal SAECG and LVEF was associated with a sensitivity of 80 percent and a specificity of 89 percent. The combination of these variables was superior to the combination of SAECG and complex ventricular arrhythmias.

Denniss and coworkers [58] studied the prognostic significance of sustained ventricular tachycardia and of ventricular fibrillation induced by programmed electrical stimulation and the presence of late potentials on SAECG in 403 patients after AMI. Patients who had late potentials had a higher incidence of inducible ventricular tachycardia. Patients who had inducible ventricular tachycardia had a probability of remaining free from subsequent arrhythmic events of 84 percent for the first year and 78 percent for 2 years. This rate was much worse than the event rate noted in patients in whom either no ventricular tachycardia was induced or ventricular fibrillation was initiated. Analysis of SAECG data showed that the probability of remaining free from an arrhythmic event was 85 percent at 1 year and 79 percent at 2 years with positive late potentials versus probabilities of 98 percent and 96 percent, respectively, when no late potentials were present. Multiple logistic regression analysis demonstrated that inducible ventricular tachycardia and the presence of late potentials were not independent predictors of subsequent sustained ventricular tachyarrhythmic events. However, although the positive predictive accuracy of SAECG or programmed ventricular stimulation was rather low using a single variable or a combination of variables, the negative predictive accuracy was more than 95 percent.

In our experience, the SAECG is often falsely positive in patients after MI. Its negative predictive value is good, especially in patients with an inferior wall MI. Newer techniques such as spectrotemporal mapping may improve the predictive accuracy of the SAECG [59].

Autonomic Testing

Schwartz and associates [60] have investigated the relation between baroreceptor reflexes in conscious dogs and the development of ventricular fibrillation during exercise stress testing in a unique ischemic model. Results from this laboratory have now been reported on baroreflex sensitivity and subsequent cardiovascular mortality in patients after AMI [61]. The preliminary data suggest that patients with a markedly low baroreflex sensitivity are at risk for subsequent cardiac death. Patients with low baroreflex sensitivity scores presumably have decreased parasympathetic tone, which may in some way be related to the subsequent occurrence of sustained ventricular tachyarrhythmias since several lines of evidence suggest that enhanced parasympathetic tone may be antiarrhythmic. Although these data are intriguing, they need to be extended and confirmed in a large, prospective, multicenter study.

Heart rate variability (HRV) is another test of autonomic function that evaluates sympathovagal balance [62, 63]. Changes in sinus rate can be evaluated by a variety of methods, including breathing at a fixed rate of 5 to 6/min, calculation of the Valsalva index, and, more recently, time and frequency domain analysis [64, 65]. Although some investigators report that abnormalities of HRV are useful to identify patients at risk for sudden death after AMI [64, 65], others have been unable to detect any unusual trends in HRV before ventricular fibrillation recorded during ambulatory monitoring [66]. In my opinion, HRV is a promising investigational tool that is not yet ready for routine clinical use.

Proposed Approach to High-Risk Patients

At this time no large prospective randomized clinical trials have demonstrated that antiarrhythmic therapies decrease the incidence of sudden death or the occurrence of sustained ventricular tachycardia in patients who appear to be at high risk for development of sustained ventricular tachyarrhythmias. Two prospective trials, the Multicenter Unsustained Tachycardia Trial (MUSTT) and the Multicenter Automatic Defibrillator Implantation Trial (MADIT) are evaluating risk-stratification with electrophysiologic testing [67].

The MUSTT includes patients with VT-NS after MI who have an LVEF of 0.40 or less. Patients who meet entrance criteria undergo electrophysiologic testing using as many as three extrastimuli from the right ventricular apex and outflow tract [68]. Patients with sustained monomorphic ventricular tachycardia induced with any pacing cadence, or with ventricular fibrillation initiated by use of fewer than three extrastimuli are randomized to treatment with antiarrhythmic therapy, including use of an implantable cardioverter defibrillator, or to no therapy. Patients who do not meet induction criteria are not treated. MUSTT is approved and funded by the National Institutes of Health, and over 50 centers in the United States and Canada are involved in MUSTT.

We encourage physicians to enroll eligible patients in these prospective trials. As data become available, a more definitive strategy for these patients can be formulated.

References

1. Gillum, P. R. Sudden coronary death in the United States, 1980–1985. *Circulation* 79:756, 1989.
2. Kuller, L., Lilienfeld, A., and Fisher, R. Epidemiological study of sudden and unexpected deaths due to arteriosclerotic heart disease. *Circulation* 34:1056, 1966.
3. Liberthson, R. R., Nagel, E. L., Hirschman, J. C., et al. Pathophysiologic observations in prehospital ventricular fibrillation and sudden cardiac death. *Circulation* 49:790, 1974.
4. Reichenbach, D. D., Moss, N. S., and Meyer, E. Pathology of the heart in sudden cardiac death. *Am. J. Cardiol.* 39:865, 1977.
5. Weaver, W. D., Lorch, G. S., Alvarez, H. A., et al. Angiographic findings and prognostic indicators in patients resuscitated from sudden cardiac death. *Circulation* 54:895, 1976.
6. Cobb, L. A., Weaver, W. D., Fahrenbruch, C. E., et al. Community-based interventions for sudden cardiac death. Impact, limitations, and changes. *Circulation* 85(Suppl I):I98, 1992.
7. Prystowsky, E. N. Antiarrhythmic therapy for asymptomatic ventricular arrhythmias. *Am. J. Cardiol.* 61:102A, 1988.
8. Chiang, B. N., Perlman, L. V., Ostrander, L. D., Jr., et al. Relationship of premature systoles to coronary heart disease and sudden death in the Tecumseh epidemiologic study. *Ann. Intern. Med.* 70:1159, 1969.
9. The Coronary Drug Project Research Group. Prognostic importance of premature beats following myocardial infarction: Experience in the Coronary Drug Project. *J.A.M.A.* 223:1116, 1973.
10. Fisher, R. D., and Tyroler, H. A. Relationship between ventricular premature contractions on routine electrocardiography and subsequent death from coronary artery disease. *Circulation* 47:712, 1973.
11. Vismara, L. A., Amsterdam, E. A., and Mason, D. T. Relation of ventricular arrhythmias in the late hospital phase of acute myocardial infarction to sudden death after hospital discharge. *Am. J. Med.* 59:6, 1975.
12. Schulze, R. A., Strauss, H. W., and Pitt, B. Sudden death in the year following myocardial infarction: Relation to ventricular premature contractions in the last hospital phase and left ventricular ejection fraction. *Am. J. Med.* 62:192, 1977.
13. Ruberman, W., Weinblatt, E., Goldberg, J. D., et al. Ventricular premature beats and mortality after myocardial infarction. *N. Engl. J. Med.* 297:750, 1977.
14. Moss, A. J., David, H. T., DeCamilla, J., et al. Ventricular ectopic beats and their relation to sudden and nonsudden cardiac death after myocardial infarction. *Circulation* 60:998, 1979.
15. Kotler, M. N., Tabutznik, B., Mower, M. M., et al. Prognostic significance of ventricular ectopic beats with respect to death in the late postinfarction period. Circulation 47:959, 1973.
16. Ruberman, W., Weinblatt, E., Goldberg, J. D., et al. Ventricular premature complexes in prognosis of angina. *Circulation* 61:1172, 1980.
17. Bigger, J. T., Fleiss, J. L., Kleiger, R., et al. The relationships among ventricular arrhythmias, left ventricular dysfunction, and mortality in the two years after myocardial infarction. *Circulation* 69:250, 1984.
18. Homes, J., Kubo, S. H., Code, R. J., et al. Arrhythmias in ischemic and nonischemic dilated cardiomyopathy: Prediction of mortality of ambulatory electrocardiography. *Am. J. Cardiol.* 55:146, 1985.
19. Bigger, J. T., Fleiss, J. L., Orlinitzky, L. M., et al. Prevalence, characteristics and significance of ven-

tricular tachycardia detected by 24-hour continuous electrocardiographic recordings in the late hospital phase of acute myocardial infarction. *Am. J. Cardiol.* 58:1151, 1986.

20. Califf, R. M., McKinnis, R. A., Burks, J., et al. Prognostic implications of ventricular arrhythmias during 24-hour ambulatory monitoring in patients undergoing cardiac catheterization for coronary artery disease. *Am. J. Cardiol.* 50:23, 1982.
21. The Cardiac Arrhythmia Suppression Trial (CAST) Investigators. Preliminary report: Effect of encainide and flecainide on mortality in a randomized trial of arrhythmia suppression after myocardial infarction. *N. Engl. J. Med.* 321:406, 1989.
22. The Cardiac Arrhythmia Suppression Trial II Investigators. Effect of the antiarrhythmic agent moricizine on survival after myocardial infarction. *N. Engl. J. Med.* 327:227, 1992.
23. Burkart, F., Pfisterer, M., Kiowski, W., et al. Effect of antiarrhythmic therapy on mortality in survivors of myocardial infarction with asymptomatic complex ventricular arrhythmias: Basel antiarrhythmic study of infarct survival (BASIS). *J. Am. Coll. Cardiol.* 16:1711, 1990.
24. Pfisterer, M., Kiowski, W., Brunner, H., et al. Long-term benefit of 1-year amiodarone treatment for persistent complex ventricular arrhythmias after myocardial infarction. *Circulation* 87:309, 1993.
25. Pfisterer, M., Kiowski, W., Burckhardt, D., et al. Beneficial effect of amiodarone on cardiac mortality in patients with asymptomatic complex ventricular arrhythmias after acute myocardial infarction and preserved but not impaired left ventricular function. *Am. J. Cardiol.* 69:1399, 1992.
26. Cairns, J. A., Connolly, S. J., Gent, M., et al. Post-myocardial infarction mortality in patients with ventricular premature depolarizations. *Circulation* 84: 550, 1991.
27. Ceremuzynski, L., Kleczar, E., Krzeminska-Pakula, M., et al. Effect of amiodarone on mortality after myocardial infarction: A double-blind, placebo-controlled, pilot study. *J. Am. Coll. Cardiol.* 20:1056, 1992.
28. Rothbaum, D. A., Linnemeier, T. J., Landin, R. J., et al. Emergency transluminal percutaneous coronary angioplasty in acute myocardial infarction: A 3-year experience. *J. Am. Coll. Cardiol.* 10:264, 1987.
29. Gruppo Italiano Per Lo Studio Della Streptochinasi Nell'Infarto Miocardico (GISSI). Effectiveness of intravenous thrombolytic treatment in acute myocardial infarction. *Lancet* 1:397, 1986.
30. Stack, R. S., Califf, R. M., Hinohara, T., et al. Survival and cardiac event rates in the first year after emergency coronary angioplasty for acute myocardial infarction. *J. Am. Coll. Cardiol.* 11:1141, 1988.
31. Irwin, J. M., Smith, P. M., Stack, R. S., et al. Successful reperfusion of infarcting myocardium is associated with reversal of electrical predictors of sudden cardiac death. *J. Am. Coll. Cardiol.* 2(II):183, 1988.
32. Kersschot, I. E., Brugada, P., Ramentol, M., et al. Effects of early reperfusion in acute myocardial infarction on arrhythmias induced by programmed stimulation: A prospective, randomized study. *J. Am. Coll. Cardiol.* 7:1234, 1986.
33. Sager, P. T., Perlmutter, R. A., Rosenfeld, L. E., et al. Electrophysiologic effects of thrombolytic therapy in patients with a transmural anterior myocardial infarction complicated by left ventricular aneurysm formation. *J. Am. Coll. Cardiol.* 12:19, 1988.
34. Maggioni, A. P., Zuanetti, G., Franzosi, M. G., et al. Prevalence and prognostic significance of ventricular arrhythmias after acute myocardial infarction in the fibrinolytic era: GISSI-2 results. *Circulation* 87:312, 1993.
35. Kammerling, J. M., Miles, W. M., Zipes, D. P., et al. Characteristics of spontaneous nonsustained ventricular tachycardia poorly predict rate of sustained ventricular tachycardia. *Clin. Res.* 34:312A, 1986.
36. Meinertz, T., Hofmann, T., Kasper, W., et al. Significance of ventricular arrhythmias in idiopathic dilated cardiomyopathy. *Am. J. Cardiol.* 53:902, 1984.
37. Simson, M. B., and MacFarlane, P. W. The signal-averaged electrocardiogram. In P. W. MacFarlane and T. D. V. Lawrie (eds.), *Comprehensive Electrocardiography.* New York: Pergamon Press, 1989, Pp. 1199–1218.
38. Simson, M. B. Use of signals in the terminal QRS complex to identify patients with ventricular tachycardia after myocardial infarction. *Circulation* 64: 235, 1981.
39. Breithardt, G., Borggrefe, M., Quantius, B., et al. Ventricular vulnerability assessed by programmed ventricular stimulation in patients with and without late potentials. *Circulation* 68:275, 1983.
40. Denes, P., Santarelli, P., Hauser, R. G., et al. Quantitative analysis of the high-frequency components of the terminal portion of the body surface QRS in normal subjects and in patients with ventricular tachycardia. *Circulation* 67:1129, 1983.
41. Gomes, J. A., Winters, S. L., Stewart, D., et al. A new noninvasive index to predict sustained ventricular tachycardia and sudden death in the first year after myocardial infarction: Based on signal-averaged electrocardiogram, radionuclide ejection fraction and Holter monitoring. *J. Am. Coll. Cardiol.* 10(II): 349, 1987.
42. Boineau, J. P., Cox, J. L. Slow ventricular activation in acute myocardial infarction: A source of reentrant premature ventricular contraction. *Circulation* 48: 702, 1973.
43. Waldo, A. L., and Kaiser, G. A. A study of ventricular arrhythmias associated with acute myocardial infarction in the canine heart. *Circulation* 47:1222, 1973.
44. El-Sherif, N., Scherlag, B. J., Lazzara R., et al. Reentrant ventricular arrhythmias in the late myocardial infarction period. I. Conduction characteristics in the infarction zone. *Circulation* 55:686, 1977.
45. Simson, M. B., Untereker, W. J., Spielman, S. R., et al. Relation between late potentials on the body

surface and directly recorded fragmented electrograms in patients with ventricular tachycardia. *Am. J. Cardiol.* 51:105, 1983.
46. Simson, M. B., Euler, D., Michelson, E. L., et al. Detection of delayed ventricular activation on the body surface in dogs. *Am. J. Physiol.* 241:H363, 1981.
47. Berbari, E. J., Scherlag, B. J., Hope, R. R., et al. Recording from the body surface of arrhythmogenic ventricular activity during the ST segment. *Am. J. Cardiol.* 41:697, 1978.
48. Rozanski, J. J., Mortara, D., Myerburg, R. J., et al. Body surface detection of delayed depolarization in patients with recurrent ventricular tachycardia and left ventricular aneurysm. *Circulation* 63:1172, 1981.
49. Fontaine, G., Guiraudon, G., Frank, R., et al. Stimulation studies and epicardial mapping in ventricular tachycardia: Study of mechanisms and selection for surgery. In H. Kulbertus (ed.), *Reentrant Arrhythmias.* Lancaster: MTP, 1977. Pp. 334–350.
50. Breithardt, G., Becker, R., Seipel, L., et al. Noninvasive detection of late potentials in man—a new marker for ventricular tachycardia. *Eur. Heart J.* 2:1, 1981.
51. Richards, D. A., Blake, G. J., Spear, J. F., et al. Electrophysiologic substrate for ventricular tachycardia: Correlation of properties in vivo and in vitro. *Circulation* 69:369, 1984.
52. Uther, J. B., Dennett, C. J., and Tan, A. The detection of delayed activation signals of low amplitude in the vectorcardiogram of patients with recurrent ventricular tachycardia by signal averaging. In E. Sandoe, D. J. Julian, and J. W. Bell (eds.), *Management of Ventricular Tachycardia—Role of Mexiletine.* Amsterdam: Excerpta Medica, 1978. Pp. 80–82.
53. Breithardt, G., Seipel, L., Ostermeyer, J., et al. Effects of antiarrhythmic surgery on late ventricular potentials recorded by precordial signal averaging in patients with ventricular tachycardia. *Am. Heart J.* 104:996, 1982.
54. Marcus, N. H., Falcone, R. A., Harken, A. H., et al. Body surface late potentials: Effects of endocardial resection in patients with ventricular tachycardia. *Circulation* 70:632, 1984.
55. Kanovsky, M. S., Falcone, R. A., Dresden, C. A., et al. Identification of patients with ventricular tachycardia after myocardial infarction: Signal-averaged electrocardiogram, Holter monitoring, and cardiac catheterization. *Circulation* 70:264, 1984.
56. Gomes, J. A., Winters, S. L., Martinson, M., et al. The prognostic significance of quantitative signal-averaged variables relative to clinical variables, site of myocardial infarction, ejection fraction and ventricular premature beats: A prospective study. *J. Am. Coll. Cardiol.* 13:377, 1989.
57. Kuchar, D. L., Thorburn, C. W., and Sammel, N. L. Prediction of serious arrhythmic events after myocardial infarction: Signal-averaged electrocardiogram, Holter monitoring and radionuclide ventriculography. *J. Am. Coll. Cardiol.* 9:531, 1987.
58. Denniss, R. A., Richards, D. A., Cody, D. V., et al. Prognostic significance of ventricular tachycardia and fibrillation induced at programmed stimulation and delayed potentials detected on the signal-averaged electrocardiograms of survivors of acute myocardial infarction. *Circulation* 74:731, 1986.
59. Haberl, R., et al. Top-resolution frequency analysis of electrocardiogram with adaptive frequency determination: Identification of late potentials in patients with coronary artery disease. *Circulation* 82:1183, 1990.
60. Schwartz, P. J., Vanoli, E., Stramba-Badiale, M., et al. Autonomic mechanisms and sudden death: New insights from analysis of baroreceptor reflexes in conscious dogs with and without a myocardial infarction. *Circulation* 78:969, 1988.
61. LaRovere, M. T., Specchia, G., Mortara, A., et al. Baroreflex sensitivity, clinical correlates, and cardiovascular mortality among patients with a first myocardial infarction: A prospective study. *Circulation* 78:816, 1988.
62. Lombardi, F., et al. Heart rate variability as an index of sympathovagal interaction after acute myocardial infarction. *Am. J. Cardiol.* 60:1239, 1987.
63. Saul, J. P., et al. Assessment of autonomic regulation in chronic congestive heart failure by rate spectral analysis. *Am. J. Cardiol.* 61:1292, 1988.
64. Kleiger, R. E., et al. Decreased heart rate variability and its association with increased mortality after acute myocardial infarction. *Am. J. Cardiol.* 59:256, 1987.
65. Farrell, T. G., et al. Risk stratification for arrhythmic events in postinfarction patients based on heart rate variability, ambulatory electrocardiographic variables and the signal-averaged electrocardiogram. *J. Am. Coll. Cardiol.* 18:687, 1991.
66. Vybiral, T., et al. Conventional heart rate variability analysis of ambulatory electrocardiographic recordings fails to predict imminent ventricular fibrillation. *J. Am. Coll. Cardiol.* 22:557, 1993.
67. Prystowsky, E. N., Knilans, T. K., and Evans, J. J. Diagnostic evaluation and treatment strategies for patients at risk for serious cardiac arrhythmias, Part 2: Ventricular tachyarrhythmias and Wolff-Parkinson-White syndrome. *Mod. Concepts of Cardiovasc. Dis.* 60(10):55, 1991.
68. Prystowsky, E. N., et al. Induction of ventricular tachycardia during programmed electrical stimulation: Analysis of pacing methods. *Circulation* 73 (Suppl II):32, 1986.

10. Heart Block in Acute Myocardial Infarction

Robert W. Peters

Disorders of atrioventricular (AV) and intraventricular conduction are relatively common complications of acute myocardial infarction (AMI). The pathophysiology, prognosis, and therapy of these disorders vary considerably depending on the location of the infarct and the clinical setting in which it occurs. Advances in clinical electrophysiology have provided an important means of investigating conduction system disease. In this chapter, the functional anatomy and histopathology of the specialized conduction system are reviewed along with the clinical aspects of conduction system disease, including diagnosis and therapy, in patients with AMI.

Specialized Conduction System

Functional Anatomy

In order to elucidate the consequences of compromised coronary blood flow, it is important to review those aspects of anatomy that are most relevant to the development conduction disorders in AMI (Table 10-1). More detailed descriptions of coronary anatomy and blood supply are well reviewed in other texts [1].

The AV node is a small ovoid structure formed by convergence of specialized atrial tracts within the subendocardial aspect of the right side of the interatrial septum. The proximal portion of the AV node has an abundant blood supply, primarily from the origin of the large AV nodal artery, which emanates from the posterior descending artery—a branch of the right coronary artery in 90 percent of cases and the left circumflex coronary artery in the other 10 percent. Important collateral circulation to the proximal AV node may be provided by septal branches of the left anterior descending coronary artery. In contrast, the distal portion of the AV node receives a relatively scanty blood supply. There is extensive autonomic innervation to the AV node.

The common (His) bundle arises as a strand of Purkinje fibers that originate in the AV node and gradually converge to form a narrow tubular structure that courses through the membranous interventricular septum until it divides into the bundle branches and fascicles, usually near the crest of the muscular septum. Within the common bundle, Purkinje fibers are arranged in parallel strands divided into morphologically separate compartments by a collagenous framework. The blood supply, usually the same as that of the distal AV node, is derived from branches of the AV nodal artery or septal branches of the left anterior descending coronary artery. There is relatively little autonomic innervation of the common bundle.

There is considerable interindividual variation in the separation of the common bundle into the bundle branch system. In general, the right bundle branch tends to originate as a thin group of fibers that remains intact until it branches at the base of the anterior papillary muscle into anterior, lateral, and posterior aspects. The left bundle branch usually spreads out across the left side of the interventricular septum in a fan-like fashion which, at least in some individuals, is clearly divisible into anterior (superior), posterior (inferior), and septal portions. The bundle branch system, in general, has an abundant blood supply including branches from the AV nodal artery, septal perforating branches of the left anterior descending coronary artery, Kugel's artery, septal branches of the posterior descending artery, and variable contributions from more remote branches. However, the anterior (superior) fascicle of the left bundle branch often has only a single arterial supply, rendering it the component most vulnerable to ischemic insult. The ventricular specialized conduction system has relatively little autonomic innervation.

Table 10-1
Blood supply and innervation of the specialized conduction system

Area	Blood supply	Specific arteries supplying the area	Autonomic innervation
Proximal AV node	++	AVN, LAD	++
Distal AV node	+	AVN, LAD	++
His bundle	+	AVN, LAD	–
RBB	++	LAD, PDA, AVN	–
LASF	+	LAD	–
LPIF	++	LAD, PDA, AVN	–

AVN = AV nodal artery (a branch of the posterior descending coronary artery that comes from the right coronary artery in 90% of cases); LAD = septal perforating branches of the left anterior descending coronary artery; PDA = posterior descending coronary artery; ++ = very abundant; + = less abundant; – = negligible; RBB = right bundle branch; LASF = left anterior (superior) fascicle; LPIF = left posterior (inferior) fascicle.

Histopathology of Acute Myocardial Infarction

In most cases of acute inferior or inferoposterior wall myocardial infarction (MI), the conduction system pathology is confined to the AV node, a not unexpected finding in light of the minor role that the right coronary artery plays in the blood supply to the lower aspects of the conduction system. Most clinicopathologic studies of patients with inferior wall infarction complicated by AV block report little structural damage to the AV node, even in cases of complete AV block, suggesting that reversible factors such as hypoxia are responsible.

In contrast is a study by Bilbao and coworkers. They carefully dissected the specialized conduction system in 44 patients who died from inferoposterior MI and demonstrated that almost all patients with AV block had necrosis of the prenodal atrial myocardial fibers, whereas most patients without AV block did not [2]. These authors noted that the supranodal atrial myocardium is supplied by a single vessel in contrast to the abundant blood supply of the AV node. It is of particular interest that patients with prenodal atrial necrosis tended to be resistant to pharmacologic therapy of AV block, whereas those without necrosis were not.

Also of note is the report of Bassan and associates that patients with inferior wall MI and obstruction of the left anterior descending coronary artery have a sixfold greater incidence of high-grade AV block than similar patients without left anterior descending obstruction [3]. Their findings support the importance of collateral blood supply to the AV node from the left anterior descending system.

In contrast to inferior wall MI, anterior wall infarction complicated by high-grade AV block is usually accompanied by extensive necrosis of the His bundle and bundle branches in the setting of severe left ventricular dysfunction. Okabe and associates performed careful dissections of the conduction system in ten patients with right bundle branch block complicating acute anterior wall MI [4]. They found extensive necrosis of the intramyocardial portion of the right bundle branch in nine, the only exception being an individual with a transient conduction defect. In contrast, necrosis was not seen in the hearts of ten patients dying from acute anterior wall MI not complicated by right bundle branch block. The AV node is usually unaffected in anterior wall infarction.

Electrocardiographic Features of Heart Block with Myocardial Infarction

Atrioventricular Block

The most important aspect of the electrocardiographic (ECG) evaluation of AV block with AMI (Table 10-2) is determining the site of block within the conduction system. When impaired AV conduction occurs during anterior wall infarction, the site is likely to be the His-Purkinje system because the left anterior descending coronary artery furnishes most of the blood supply to the interventricular septum, whereas inferior/inferoposterior wall MI usually affect the AV node. First-degree AV block

Table 10-2
AV block in acute myocardial infarction

Severity of block	Inferior wall infarct (usually narrow QRS)	Anterior wall infarct (usually wide QRS)
First degree	PR prolongation	PR prolongation
Second degree	Type I	Usually type II
Third degree	Usually junctional escape rhythm at 50–60 bpm; may respond to pharmacologic agents	Idioventricular escape rhythm at <40 bpm; tends to be unreliable, making temporary pacing mandatory

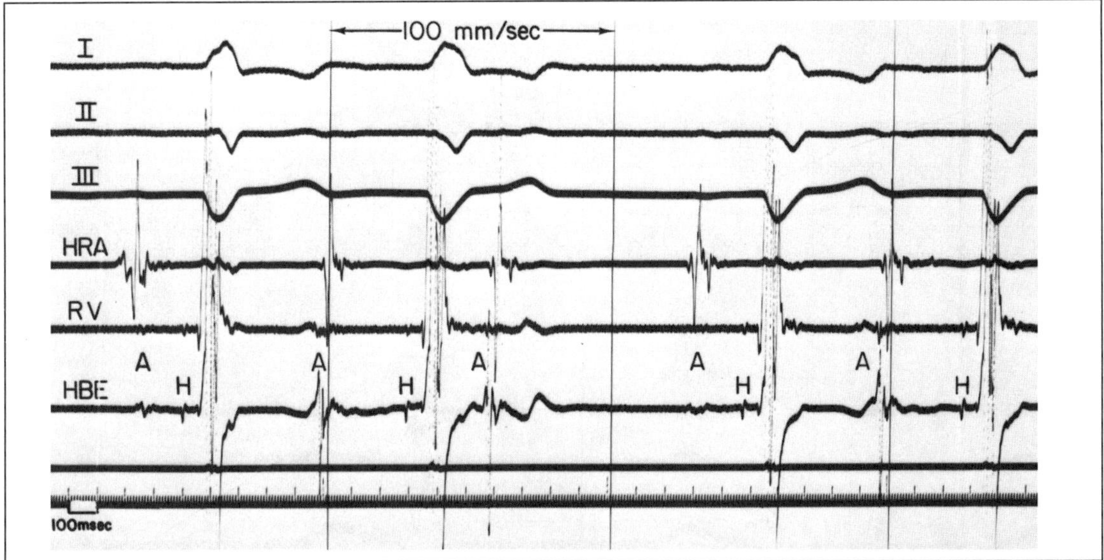

Fig. 10-1
Surface ECG leads and accompanying intracardiac recordings illustrating type I second-degree AV block in a 54-year-old man with acute inferior wall myocardial infarction. The arrhythmia developed abruptly 6 hours after the onset of symptoms and was not associated with hemodynamic compromise. It resolved spontaneously 24 hours later. I, II, III = standard ECG leads I, II, III; HRA = high right atrial lead; RV = right ventricular lead; HBE = His bundle lead; A = atrial depolarization; H = His bundle potential.

may occur with MI of any location, and the site of the infarction may help localize the area of conduction delay. Type I second-degree AV block (Wenckebach phenomenon) (Fig. 10-1), or complete AV block in the setting of inferior wall MI is typically AV nodal in origin. In contrast, type II second-degree AV block, or complete AV block with a wide complex escape rhythm complicating anterior wall infarction (Fig. 10-2), is virtually always infranodal. With 2:1 AV block, the presence of a narrow QRS complex suggests that the block is located at the AV node, whereas a wide QRS favors infranodal block.

Exceptions to these general rules are not uncommon, however. For example, a preexisting intraventricular conduction defect makes the QRS width an unreliable index of the site of AV block. Similarly, type I second-degree AV block complicating inferior wall MI has been reported within the distal conduction system [5]. In some individuals, the proximal portion of the right bundle branch is supplied solely by the right coronary artery, so right bundle branch block may occur in the setting of inferior wall infarction. Hypervagotonia, relatively common early in the course of inferior infarction, may mimic type II second-degree AV block (Fig.

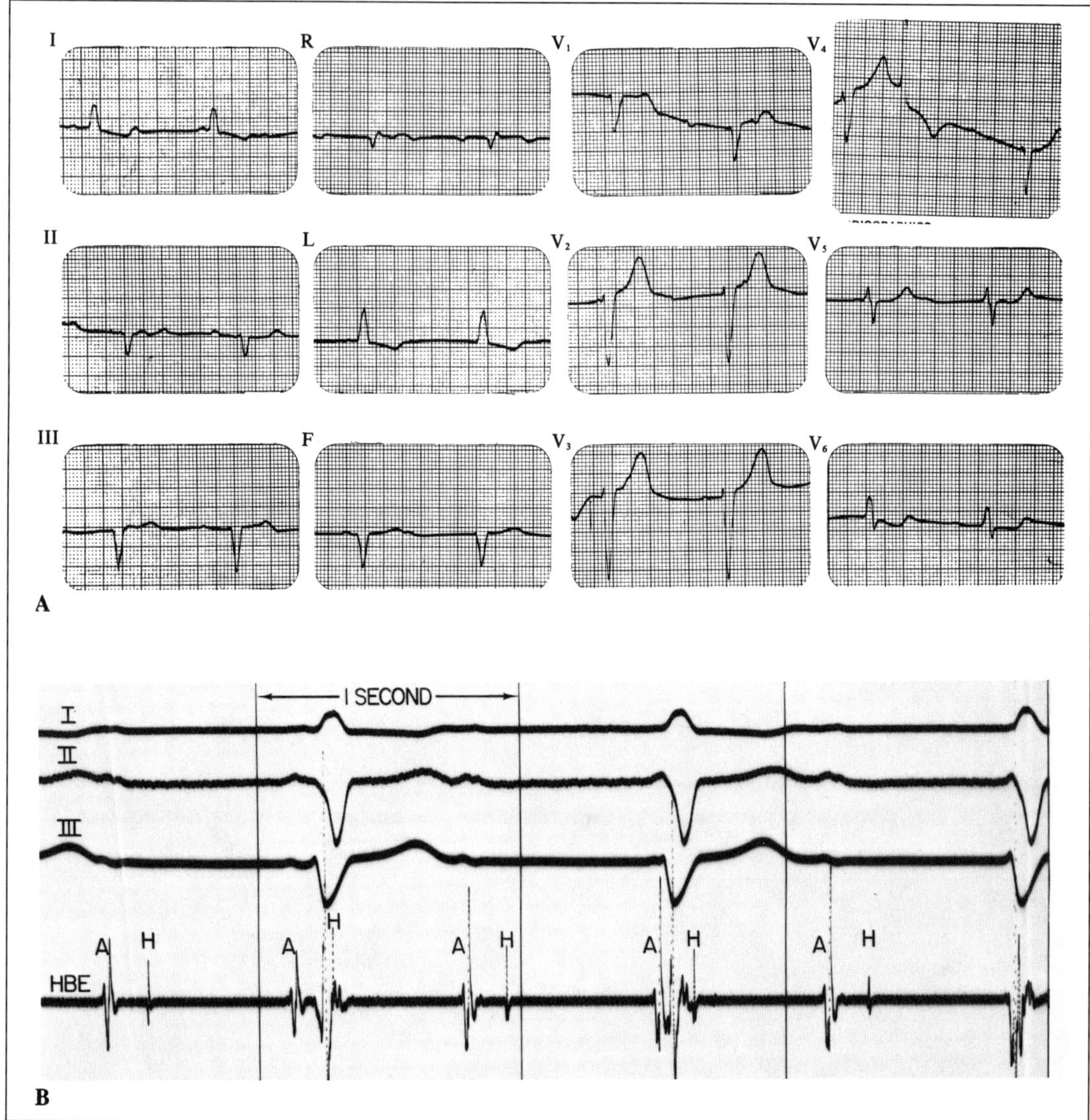

Fig. 10-2

A. Standard 12-lead ECG in a 64-year-old man with anterior wall myocardial infarction complicated by acute pulmonary edema. Complete AV block (shown here) developed 12 hours after the onset of symptoms and was preceded by left bundle branch block and first-degree AV block. Because of the slow ventricular rate and unreliability of the escape focus, immediate temporary pacemaker insertion was mandatory. *B.* His bundle electrogram recorded from the same patient during temporary pacemaker insertion. Block occurs below the His bundle, a pattern characteristic of anterior wall myocardial infarction. I, II, III = standard ECG leads I, II, III; HBE = His bundle lead; A = atrial depolarization; H = His bundle potential.

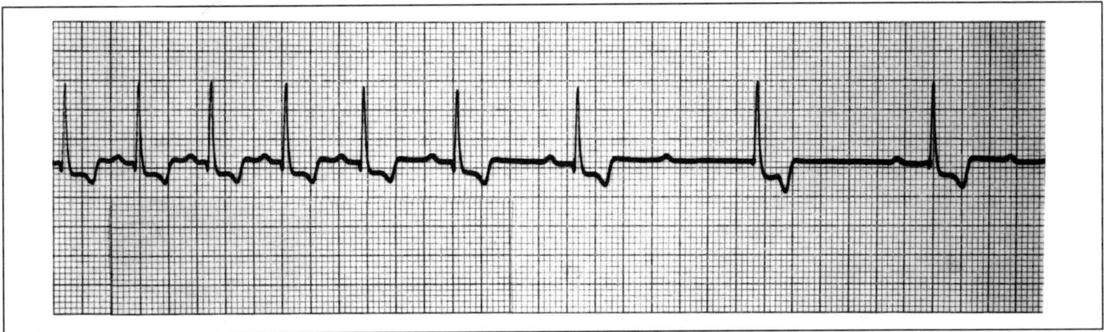

Fig. 10-3
Standard ECG lead I showing the onset of complete AV block with an idioventricular escape rhythm in a 71-year-old woman with an otherwise uncomplicated inferior wall myocardial infarction. The simultaneous occurrence of sinus slowing and AV block is diagnostic of hypervagotonia. The dysrhythmia resolved spontaneously within 30 seconds.

10-3), the key to the diagnosis being simultaneous sinus slowing and nonconducted P waves [6]. In situations where the level of AV block is uncertain but clinically relevant (e.g., 2:1 AV block in the setting of anterior wall infarction) an electrophysiologic study including a recording of the His bundle electrogram can be helpful (see Figs. 10-1 and 10-2).

Intraventricular Conduction Defects

ECG diagnosis of the various types of intraventricular conduction defects is well described in standard textbooks [1]. However, it is appropriate to begin with a brief review of ventricular activation as it is affected by MI. Normal ventricular depolarization is initiated in one or more locations along the left side of the ventricular septum. Septal activation then proceeds rightward, anteriorly and inferiorly. With right bundle branch block, septal activation is normal, so the characteristic Q waves of acute MI are often well visualized (Fig. 10-4). In contrast, with left bundle branch block, the initial forces are altered (with the septum being depolarized from right to left) so the diagnosis of AMI is often not possible from the ECG alone. Because both left and right bundle branch block affect ventricular repolarization, the ECG diagnosis of non-Q-wave infarction is often uncertain. The fascicular blocks alter the pattern of ventricular activation and may complicate the ECG diagnosis of MI. With left anterior (superior) fascicular block, initial forces are inferior and posterior, potentially masking inferior infarction and mimicking anterior wall infarction (Fig. 10-5). Conversely, with left posterior (inferior) fascicular block, initial forces are anterior, superior, and leftward, simulating inferior wall infarction and masking lateral wall infarction.

Clinical Aspects of Atrioventricular Block in Acute Myocardial Infarction

The significance of AV block in AMI must be assessed in light of the clinical setting. The location of the block, the patient's hemodynamic status, the use of cardioactive medication, and other factors such as autonomic tone may be more important than the degree of the block. AV block may occur in up to 30 percent of patients with acute inferior wall infarction [7] and is especially common during the first few hours after the onset of symptoms. As would be expected from the blood supply of the inferior wall and the high degree of vagal activity accompanying inferior wall infarction, most conduction disturbances in this setting are AV nodal in origin. Accordingly, the QRS complex is usually narrow and the junctional escape rhythm stable at a reasonable rate (50–60 beats per minute [bpm]) so that even complete AV block may not require specific therapy. Although some studies have found

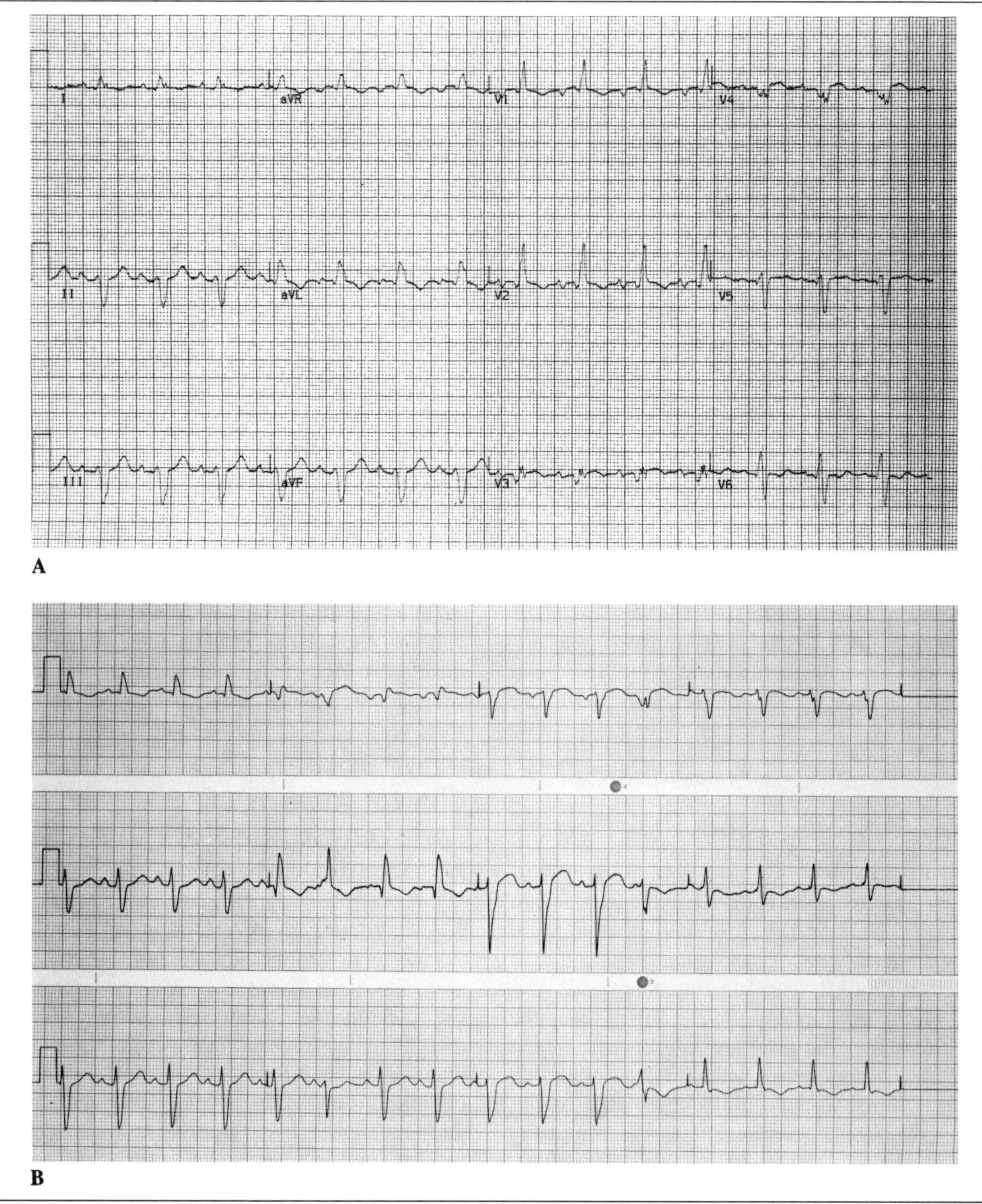

Fig. 10-4
Two ECGs from a 48-year-old man with an anteroseptal myocardial infarction complicated by left ventricular failure. *A.* Despite the presence of right bundle branch block and left anterior fascicular block, large Q waves indicative of anterior wall infarction are visible in the precordial leads. The development of new bilateral bundle branch block is an indication for temporary pacing because of the risk of high-grade AV block, but even with pacing the prognosis remains poor. *B.* Approximately 20 minutes later, the left bundle branch block developed and obscured the infarct pattern. This ''alternating'' bundle branch block pattern usually indicates severe infranodal disease.

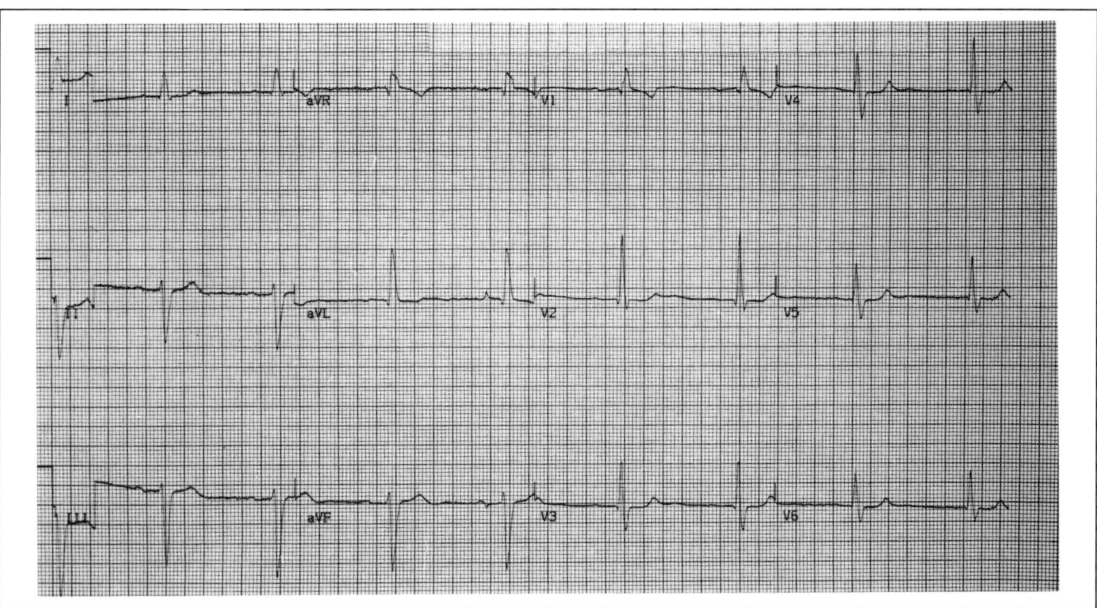

Fig. 10-5
Right bundle branch block and left anterior fascicular block in a 64-year-old woman without coronary artery disease. The small Q waves in leads V_1–V_3 are due to left anterior fascicular block (mimicking anteroseptal myocardial infarction).

that high-grade AV block in inferior wall infarction is associated with more extensive myocardial damage and a higher mortality rate, others have failed to confirm this finding [8–10]. Regardless of the ventricular escape rate, patients with high-grade AV block and inferior wall infarction who exhibit signs or symptoms of hypoperfusion may benefit from an increase in heart rate. (In addition to conventional findings such as hypotension or oliguria, some consider ventricular ectopy a sign of hypoperfusion.)

Pharmacologic measures include vagolytic drugs such as atropine or sympathomimetic agents such as isoproterenol. If atropine is used, intravenous therapy is preferable because of its rapid onset of action and because absorption may be erratic, especially in the presence of heart failure or hypotension. To avoid potentially deleterious tachycardia, relatively low doses of atropine (0.5 or 0.6 mg) should be used and may be repeated after several minutes if ineffective. Adverse effects of atropine include tachyarrhythmias (usually sinus tachycardia), urinary retention, central nervous system disturbances, dry mouth, and, if very low doses (0.3 mg or less) are used, paradoxical bradycardia. These adverse effects are relatively common in elderly patients and may persist for several hours, so atropine is best avoided in the presence of such conditions as prostatic enlargement and disorientation.

Intravenous isoproterenol offers the advantage of almost immediate onset of action and dissipation of effects once the infusion is discontinued. In addition, it may increase myocardial contractility in situations where this effect is desired. Isoproterenol can be initiated starting at a dose as low as 1 μg/min and titrated up to the desired increase in heart rate or hemodynamic response. Adverse effects of isoproterenol include tachyarrhythmias (potentially serious ventricular arrhythmias are not infrequent) and worsening of myocardial ischemia. Intravenous aminophylline may also improve AV conduction in at least some individuals with inferior wall MI, but experience with this drug is limited.

If pharmacologic therapy is ineffective or undesirable, temporary transvenous pacing offers a satisfactory alternative. Pacing has the advantage of avoiding pharmacologic side effect but is invasive and has the potential for causing infection, thrombophlebitis, cardiac perforation, and arrhythmias.

Several groups have investigated the problem of AV block in the setting of inferior wall MI with the intention of defining the mechanism and identifying subgroups who might benefit from a particular type of therapy. In a group of 144 patients with inferior wall infarction complicated by high-grade AV block, Tans and coworkers found that those with signs of low cardiac output and heart rates below 50 bpm seemed to benefit from temporary pacing, whereas patients with hypoperfusion and higher heart rates uniformly fared poorly regardless of therapy [9].

Feigl and associates, in a similar group of 34 patients, found that those who developed high-grade block suddenly (without antecedent first-degree AV block) and within 6 hours of onset of symptoms had transient block that was responsive to atropine [11]. Individuals who developed AV block later (usually more than 24 hours after symptom onset) generally had antecedent first-degree AV block and were resistant to atropine; many required temporary pacing for block that often lasted several days. In four patients, the resolution of "early" AV block was followed by the appearance of "late" AV block with its characteristic resistance to atropine. The authors postulated the "early" AV block is due to hypervagotonia whereas "late" block is ischemically mediated and may resolve gradually as ischemia lessens.

In support of this hypothesis is a case, reported by Wesley and associates, of a 62-year-old woman with a recent inferior wall MI who developed high-grade AV block. It was resistant to atropine but dramatically responsive to aminophylline, a competitive adenosine antagonist, in doses lower than that required to release catecholamines or increase cyclic adenosine monophosphate (cAMP) [12]. Adenosine, an endogenous metabolite known to accumulate during periods of ischemia, depresses AV nodal conduction [13, 14].

In contrast, Strasberg and coworkers studied the effects of similar doses of aminophylline in a group of 15 patients with second- or third-degree AV block occurring "late" (2 to 6 days) after the onset of AMI [15]. They found that facilitation of AV conduction occurred primarily in those with type I second-degree AV block but no beneficial effects were noted in those with 2:1 or complete AV block. The sinus rate actually decreased, suggesting that the dose of aminophylline employed did not alter serum catecholamine concentration. The authors hypothesized that perhaps only milder degrees of AV block were capable of being reversed by the dose of aminophylline that they used but that a higher-grade block might require an increase in serum catecholamine concentration.

Lewin and coworkers described 12 patients with alternating (multilevel) Wenckebach periods in the setting of acute inferior wall infarction [16]. They found a relatively high incidence of hemodynamic deterioration (especially during the periods of AV block) and a high mortality rate (25 percent). Atropine increased the degree of AV block, actually precipitating the multilevel Wenckebach periods in three patients, and isoproterenol had no effect. Thus temporary pacing was required in all.

A number of recent, large series have examined the prognosis of patients with inferior wall MI complicated by high-grade AV block [17–20]. In general, these investigations have found that these patients tend to be older and sicker with larger infarcts and lower ejection fractions, leading to higher in-hospital mortality. In one series, excess mortality was accounted for solely by the coexistence of right ventricular infarction [20]. However, those patients with high-grade block who survive to be discharged from the hospital appear to have a long-term prognosis that is comparable to those without AV block. Thus, this information may help to identify a high-risk subset of patients with inferior wall MI who may benefit from very early intervention.

High grade AV block complicating anterior wall MI is considerably less common than that complicating inferior wall infarction. However, in contrast to inferior wall infarction, high-grade AV block complicating anterior wall MI is usually located within the His-Purkinje system (see Fig. 10-2). Transition from a first nonconducted sinus P wave to complete AV block is often abrupt, and the resulting idioventricular escape rhythm is slow and unreliable. Conducted beats almost always have a wide QRS complex. Interruption of the abundant septal blood supply, sufficient to cause high-grade AV block, usually causes severe left ventricular dysfunction so that mortality is high. Emergency temporary pacing (and probably permanent pacing) of these individuals is mandatory but may not improve survival appreciably.

Clinical Aspects of Intraventricular Conduction Defects with Acute Myocardial Infarction

In general, isolated fascicular block in AMI does not appreciably increase mortality or incidence of progression to high-grade AV block, although there may be a more severe degree of left ventricular dysfunction [21].

A number of studies have examined the clinical course of patients with bundle branch block and AMI (Table 10-3) [22–39]. All attest to the high incidence of severe left ventricular failure and the resulting high mortality, although there is considerable controversy as to whether temporary or permanent pacing alters this poor prognosis. Because of the feasibility of early intervention in some of these patients, it has become increasingly important to identify subgroups which are at especially high risk. Of interest is a recent series described by Dubois and colleagues who found that transient bundle branch block in AMI has the same poor prognosis as a permanent conduction defect [40]. Also of note is a large study by Ricou and coworkers who were able to identify a substantial minority of patients with right bundle branch block (those without left ventricular failure) whose mortality rate was no different from comparable patients without the conduction defect [41].

Regarding the issue of temporary pacing, two studies are worth discussing in detail because of the large number of patients involved. The multicenter study of Hindman et al. retrospectively reviewed the clinical course of 494 patients with documented AMI and bundle branch block [15, 16]. Sixty-two patients developed conduction defects in the setting of cardiogenic shock and were excluded from further analysis. Hospital mortality in the remain-

Table 10-3
Intraventricular conduction defects and progression to high-grade AV block with acute myocardial infarction

First author	No. of patients	Conduction defect	MI site	Mortality (%)	Progression to HDB (%)	Mortality of HDB patients (%)	Temporary pacing recommended
Hindman [22,23]	432	BBB	Any	28	22	47	See Table 10-4
Lamas [24]	?/698*	IVCD	Any	—	5.4	42	See Table 10-4
Dominghetti [25]	59	IVCD	Any	30	10	83	+ (BB)
Hollander [26]	49	BBB	Any	—	30	—	+ (AS MI & BB or LBBB)
Gann [27]	292	IVCD	Any	53	4.4	69	+ (Preexisting RBBB)
Waugh [28]	198	IVCD	Any	28	11.6	30	+ (BB and P–R prolongation)
Scanlon [29]	28	BB	Any	36	21	33	+
Atkins [30]	28	BB	Any	30	25	37	+
Nimetz [31]	71	BBB	Any	31	42	57	(−)
Godman [32]	68	BBB	Any	56	31	86	(−)
Godman [33]	100	BB	Any	70	47	85	(−)
Scheinman [34]	97	IVCD	Any	38	25	—	(−)
Lichstein [35]	14	BB	AS	50	21	67	(−)
Lie [36]	70	RBBB or BB	AS	74	26	—	+ (BB with prolonged H–V)
Waters [37]	27	BB	Any	44	56	—	(−)
Kubis [38]	63	BB	—	60	46	—	(−)
Hauer [39]	42	BBB	Any	57	7	0	(−)

BBB = bundle branch block; IVCD = intraventricular conduction defect; MI = myocardial infarction; HDB = high-degree block; RBBB = right bundle branch block; LBBB = left bundle branch block; LAFB = left anterior fascicular block; LPFB = left posterior fascicular block; BB = bifascicular block; AS = anteroseptal; + = temporary pacing recommended; (−) = temporary pacing not recommended; P–R = P–R interval on ECG; H–V = infranodal conduction time on intracardiac electrogram.
*Number of patients with IVCD not specified.

ing 432 patients (28 percent) was most closely related to severity of heart failure, although the development of high-grade AV block (22 percent of patients) was also a predictor. Specific risk factors for advanced AV block during the acute phase were bilateral bundle branch involvement, first-degree AV block, and new or indeterminate onset of the conduction defect (Table 10-4). The presence of two of these risk factors was associated with a 19 to 31 percent (depending on which two) incidence of progression to high-grade block, which certainly warrants temporary pacing (see Fig. 10-4).

The Multicenter Investigation of the Limitation of Infarct Size (MILIS) study group analyzed data from 698 patients with AMI to determine risk factors for the development of complete heart block [24]. A total of 38 patients (5.4 percent) had documented complete heart block; and in general, this group was characterized by a high incidence of congestive heart failure and a high mortality. Specific risk factors for complete heart block (detailed in Table 10-3) each counted a single point. Patients with 3 points or more comprised a high-risk group (at least a 25 percent incidence of progression), and those with 2 points were at intermediate risk; pacing was considered (depending on the clinical situation) in these patients but was not mandatory. Their findings were then tested in two other retrospectively derived populations—one from a combination of six studies in the medical literature and the other from the Duke data bank—with similar results. An important limitation of both the MILIS and Hindman studies is that data were analyzed regardless of infarct location (indeed, in patients with left bundle branch block the site may not have been known). Because the clinical presentation and prognosis of patients with high-grade AV block and inferior wall MI may be different from that of anterior wall infarction, their data should be applied with caution to any individual patient. Indeed, 19 patients classified as having type II second-degree AV block had narrow QRS complexes, many in inferior wall MI. In the absence of intracardiac recordings, the site of block is unknown and, as recently pointed out by Barold, there is reason to believe that in many of these patients, it was located at the AV node [42].

The issue of permanent pacing for patients with intraventricular conduction defects and MI who sur-

Table 10-4
Risk of progression to high-grade AV block with acute myocardial infarction

Multicenter retrospective study [22,23]		
Risk factor(s)	Risk of high-grade AV block (%)	
(a) 1° AV block	13	
(b) New or indeterminate onset of BBB	11	
(c) Bilateral BBB	10	
(a) and (b)	19	
(b) and (c)	31	
(a) and (c)	20	
(a), (b), and (c)	38	
MILIS [24]		
Risk factor(s)	No. of risk factors	Risk of 3° AV block (%)
1° AV block	None	1.2
Type I 2° AV block	One	7.8
Type II 2° AV block	Two	25.0
LAFB	Three	36.4
LPFB		
RBBB		
LBBB		

BBB = bundle branch block; LAFB = left anterior fascicular block; LPFB = left posterior fascicular block; 1°, 2°, 3° = first-, second-, third-degree AV block, respectively.

vive to leave the coronary care unit has also been the subject of a number of reports (Table 10-5) [22, 23, 25, 28, 30, 37–39, 43, 44]. The 1-year follow-up provided by Hindman et al. in the multicenter retrospective study is foremost among them because of its large numbers [22, 23]. In their data, patients who experienced transient high-grade AV block during the hospitalization (regardless of whether they fulfilled the criteria for temporary pacing) had a 28 percent incidence of recurrent block, sudden cardiac death, or both over the next 12 months (compared with only 6 percent for those without high-grade block). Of particular note were a small subset of patients who experienced recurrence of high-grade block late in the hospitalization, after their temporary pacemakers had been removed, because of restoration of normal AV conduction. Thus once the decision to implant a permanent pacemaker has been made, patients should have continuous cardiac monitoring and temporary pacing until it is carried out.

Somewhat at variance with the above study is the Birmingham (England) Trial in which 50 patients who survived 2 weeks after MI complicated by either right bundle branch block with or without concomitant anterior fascicular block or left posterior fascicular block alone were randomized to a permanent pacemaker or a control group [45]. Specifically excluded were patients requiring permanent pacing (because of symptomatic bradycardia or persistent high-grade block). Over the follow-up period (up to 5 years), there was no difference between groups in terms of total mortality or sudden death and no observed progression of conduction system disease. Ventricular arrhythmias were an important cause of death in both groups. It is difficult to compare these data to those of Hindman et al., however, because the incidence of transient high-grade block prior to randomization is not specified. Along similar lines, Lie and associates found a high incidence of late (up to 6 weeks) in-hospital ventricular fibrillation in a large group of patients with anteroseptal MI complicated by right or left bundle branch block [39].

The advent of intracardiac electrophysiologic studies has provided a potentially important instrument for evaluating patients with intraventricular conduction defects and MI (Table 10-6) [35, 46–50]. It has been hypothesized that marked prolongation of infranodal conduction time (HV interval) might be predictive of subsequent progression to high-grade AV block [51]. Initial studies, however, have been disappointing. Most have found that, although HV prolongation may identify a group with more severe heart disease and a high mortality, most of the deaths have been due to ventricular arrhythmias and not high-grade AV block. Most of the patients studied have had only mild-to-moderate HV prolongation, however (perhaps because patients with marked HV prolongation do not survive), so the application of these data to patients with markedly impaired infranodal conduction may not be warranted. Cortadellas et al. recently described a group of nine patients with right bundle branch block in anterior wall MI whose conduction defect was normalized by distal His bundle pacing, suggesting that the level of block was within the His bundle [52]. This group had a high mortality, comparable to other series of patients with bundle branch block complicating MI, and three progressed to high-grade AV block, despite the fact that HV was normal in all nine patients.

From the above considerations, it seems clear that patients with acute anterior wall MI complicated by intraventricular conduction defects have a high mortality due to left ventricular failure. However, a substantial number of these individuals do not die from heart failure alone, and it becomes imperative to avoid mortality from preventable causes such as high-grade AV block. The large studies of Hindman et al. and Lamas and associates (MILIS) have delineated high-risk groups who may benefit from temporary pacing [22–24]. Although they were compiled retrospectively, it is unlikely that a large prospective study will ever be undertaken. Similarly, the data from Hindman et al. provide helpful guidelines for the use of prophylactic permanent pacing in survivors of the acute period. Although it seems clear from the work of Watson and associates, Lie and coworkers, and others that most sudden deaths following MI are due to ventricular arrhythmias, even in patients with extensive conduction system disease, it seems prudent to implant prophylactic permanent pacemakers in individuals who have experienced transient high-degree block, especially if an intraventricular conduction defect or first-degree AV block persists. Further studies are needed to determine if intracardiac electrophysiologic studies would be of help in this population.

Table 10-5
Follow-up data in survivors of acute myocardial infarction complicated by intraventricular conduction defects

First author	No. of patients	Conduction defect	MI site	Follow-up (mo)	Discharged with permanent pacemaker (no.)	Mortality (%)	Sudden death (no.)	Prophylactic permanent pacing recommended
Hindman [22,23]	311	BBB	Any	2	40	28	45	+ (with transient HDB)
Atkins [30]	20	BB	Any	11 (mean)	8	50	7	+ (with transient HDB)
Dominghetti [25]	36	IVCD	Any	19 (mean)	0	25	5	+ (RBBB, LPFB)
Waugh [28]	386	IVCD	Any	12	0	9	32	+ (1° AVB and BB or LBB)
Ginks [43]	25	BBB & transient HDB	AS	49 (mean)	4	36	5	(−)
Ritter [44]	18	BB & transient HDB	Any	18 (mean)	12	28	5	+
Waters [37]	15	BB*	Any	16	3	7	0	(−)
Kubis [38]	25	BB	Any	18	11	40	4	+
Watson [45]	50	BB	Any	Up to 60	23	50	12	(−)
Hauer [39]	18	BBB	AS	13 (mean)	1	6	0	(−)

MI = myocardial infarction; BBB = bundle branch block; BB = bifascicular block; HDB = high-degree block; IVCD = intraventricular conduction defect; RBBB = right bundle branch block; LPFB = left posterior fascicular block; LBBB = left bundle branch block; 1° AVB = first-degree AV block; + = prophylactic permanent pacing recommended; (−) = not recommended.
*Six had transient high-degree block that regressed in the hospital.

Table 10-6
Studies involving intracardiac electrophysiologic studies in patients with acute myocardial infarction complicated by intraventricular conduction defects

First author	No. of patients	Conduction defects	MI site	Prolonged H–V (%)	Follow-up (mo)	Progression to HDB (%)	Predictive value of H–V: Mortality	Predictive value of H–V: HDB
Pagnoni [46]	59	IVCD	Any	24	Up to 18	2	(+)	(−)
Watson [45]	50	BB	Any	62	Up to 60	0*	(−)	(−)
Lie [47]	35	BB	AS	46	In-hospital	35	(+)	(+)
Schoenfeld [48]	14	BBB	Any	86	Up to 12	43		
Lichstein [35]	15	New BB	Any	60	Up to 6		(+)	
Gould [49]	14	BBB	Any	40	Up to 6	0	(−)	
Harper [50]	32	BBB	Any	50	Up to 3	30	(+)	

MI = myocardial infarction; H–V = infranodal conduction time; HDB = high-grade AV block; SD = sudden cardiac death; AS = anteroseptal; + = H–V has positive predictive value; (−) = H–V does not have predictive value.
*There were 23/50 patients paced prophylactically.

Therapeutic Advances: Effects on the Conduction System

No chapter would be complete without a brief discussion of some of the developments in the therapy of AMI and the effects of these interventions on the conduction system. Antiarrhythmic drugs, beta blockers, calcium channel blockers, and reperfusion techniques have the potential to affect intracardiac conduction in patients with AMI.

Antiarrhythmic Drugs

Antiarrhythmic drugs are widely utilized during the peri- and postinfarction periods because of the prevalence and potentially malignant nature of ventricular arrhythmias. However, many of these drugs have the potential to depress AV and intraventricular conduction. Although good prospective data are not available, a large retrospectively compiled series found no adverse effects of these drugs in patients with normal AV conduction and those with first-degree AV block or type I second-degree AV block [53]. Until more definitive information is available, however, antiarrhythmic drugs, especially some of the newer and more potent ones, should be used with caution in patients with significant conduction system disease, particularly in the setting of moderate or severe left ventricular dysfunction.

Beta Blockers

Several large randomized double-blind placebo-controlled studies have demonstrated that the administration of beta blockers in therapeutic doses following AMI reduces mortality by 25 to 30 percent over a follow-up period of up to 2 years [54–56]. Because beta blockers may impair AV nodal conduction, patients with second- or third-degree AV block were excluded unless the block resolved within the randomization window. In all three studies there was no significant difference between treatment and placebo groups in terms of the incidence of high-grade AV block. Thus beta blockers appear generally safe to use during the peri- or postinfarction period in the absence of second- or third-degree AV block.

Calcium Channel Blockers

The Diltiazem Reinfarction Study was a randomized double-blind placebo-controlled trial of diltiazem, 360 mg daily, in patients with acute subendocardial (non-Q-wave) MI [57]. Therapy was initiated 24 to 72 hours after the onset of symptoms and was continued for 21 days. High-grade AV block developed in 11 of 287 diltiazem-treated patients compared with 2 of 289 patients receiving placebo. Therapy needed to be discontinued in only 3 patients, all in the diltiazem group. Although the difference between groups did not achieve statistical significance (perhaps because the trial was relatively small), it seems advisable to administer diltiazem with caution (in a monitored setting) until more definitive information becomes available.

Reperfusion Techniques

Heart block has been reported in association with Prinzmetal's angina [58, 59], raising the possibility that reperfusion might adversely affect AV conduction. Although there is little specific information addressing this issue, in the large Gruppo Italiano per lo Studio della Streptochinasi nell'Infarto Miocardico (GISSI-I) study control patients actually had a slightly higher incidence of AV block (although the difference was not statistically significant) than did the thrombolysis group [60], suggesting that temporary pacing would not be of benefit.

With this background and in light of the increasing use of various reperfusion techniques, a brief discussion of the effects of these interventions upon the conduction system is warranted. There is now considerable evidence that at least some conduction defects occurring in AMI are due to disruption of the blood supply and may resolve when flow is reestablished [61, 62]. For example, Roth and associates describe eight patients with anterior wall MI complicated by right bundle branch block, six of whom also developed left anterior fascicular block [61]. Thrombolytic therapy resulted in prompt (<2 hours) resolution of the conduction defect in all. Most of these patients had clinical evidence of congestive heart failure with a mean predischarge ejection fraction of 0.38, suggesting that this group is fairly representative of patients with anterior wall MI complicated by conduction defects.

In contrast, Wiseman et al. describe a patient with acute anterior wall MI who developed bifascicular block just as the infusion of recombinant tissue plasminogen activator was begun [62]. Cardiac catheterization revealed complete occlusion of the left anterior descending coronary artery just distal to the first septal perforating branch. Coronary angioplasty was successful in restoring flow and the conduction defect resolved rapidly, but complete heart block with ventricular asystole occurred abruptly 30 hours later. After appropriate resuscitative measures, including use of a temporary transvenous pacemaker, were carried out, repeat cardiac catheterization revealed a patent artery (Thrombolysis in Myocardial Infarction (TIMI) grade 3 flow). Thus, reperfusion must be approached cautiously in this instance since the factors that govern resolution and reappearance of conduction defects are poorly understood.

The issue of high-grade AV block in inferior wall MI treated with thrombolytic agents has been examined in two large recent trials. The Thrombolysis and Angioplasty in Myocardial Infarction (TAMI) study group examined the clinical course of 373 patients with inferior wall MI given thrombolytic therapy within 6 hours of symptom onset [63]. The patients who developed complete AV block (50/373, 13 percent) had larger infarcts, a higher reocclusion rate, and a higher in-hospital mortality. Multivariate analysis showed that the development of complete AV block was a strong predictor of in-hospital mortality, although very few of the deaths were due to AV block. In the TIMI II trial, the investigators studied 1786 patients with inferior wall MI who received thrombolytic therapy within 4 hours of symptom onset [64]. High-grade AV block was present on admission in 6.3 percent and developed within 24 hours of thrombolysis in another 5.7 percent. Heart block was transient in all patients, but those who developed block had larger infarcts and their mortality was approximately three times higher than those without heart block. Thus, in inferior wall MI, reperfusion may reverse conduction defects without improving overall prognosis. These patients comprise a high-risk group that should be considered for early intervention.

References

1. Schlant, R. C., and Silverman, M. E. Anatomy of the heart. In J. W. Hurst (ed.), *The Heart* (6th ed.). New York: McGraw-Hill, 1986. Pp. 16–37.
2. Bilbao, F. J., Zabalza, I. E., Vilanova, J. R., and Froufe, J. Atrioventricular block in posterior acute myocardial infarction: A clinicopathologic correlation. *Circulation* 75:733, 1987.
3. Bassan, R., Maia, I., Dozza, A., et al. Atrioventricular block in acute inferior wall myocardial infarction: Harbinger of associated obstruction of the left anterior descending coronary artery. *J. Am. Coll. Cardiol.* 8:733, 1986.
4. Okabe, M., Fukuda, K., Nakashima, Y., et al. A quantitative histopathological study of right bundle branch block complicating acute anteroseptal myocardial infarction. *Br. Heart J.* 65:317, 1991.
5. Strasberg, B., Sclarovsky, S., and Agmon, J. Wenck-

ebach block in the distal conduction system complicating a non-Q wave acute myocardial infarction. *Chest* 92:745, 1987.

6. Massie, B., Scheinman, M. M., Peters, R., et al. Clinical and electrophysiologic findings in patients with paroxysmal slowing of the sinus rate and apparent type II atrioventricular block. *Circulation* 58: 305, 1978.
7. Rotman, M., Wagner, G. S., and Wallace, A. G. Bradyarrhythmias in acute myocardial infarction. *Circulation* 45:149, 1972.
8. Opolski, G., Kraska, T., Ostrzychi, A., et al. The effect of infarct size on atrioventricular and intraventricular conduction disturbance in acute myocardial infarction. *Int. J. Cardiol.* 10:141, 1986.
9. Tans, A. C., Lie, K. I., and Durrer, D. Clinical setting and prognostic significance of high degree atrioventricular block in acute inferior myocardial infarction. *Am. Heart J.* 99:4, 1980.
10. Rotman, M., Wagner, G. S., and Waugh, R. A. Significance of high degree atrioventricular block in acute posterior myocardial infarction. *Circulation* 45:257, 1973.
11. Feigl, D., Ashkenazy, J., and Kishon, Y. Early and late atrioventricular block in acute inferior myocardial infarction. *J. Am. Coll. Cardiol.* 4:35, 1984.
12. Wesley, R. C., Lerman, B. B., DiMarco, J. P., et al. Mechanism of atropine-resistant atrioventricular block during inferior myocardial infarction; possible role of adenosine. *J. Am. Coll. Cardiol.* 8:1232, 1986.
13. Belardinelli, L., Belloni, F. L., Rubio, R., and Berne, R. M. Atrioventricular conduction disturbance during hypoxia: Possible role of adenosine in rabbit and guinea pig heart. *Cir. Res.* 47:684, 1980.
14. Dimarco, J. P., Sellers, T. P., Berney, R. M., et al. Adenosine: Electrophysiologic effects and therapeutic use for terminating paroxysmal supraventricular tachycardia. *Circulation* 68:1254, 1983.
15. Strasberg, B., Bassevich, R., Mager, A., et al. Effects of aminophylline on atrioventricular conduction in patients with late atrioventricular block during inferior wall acute myocardial infarction. *Am. J. Cardiol.* 67:527, 1991.
16. Lewin, R. F., Kasniec, J., Sclarovsky, S., et al. Alternating Wenckebach periods in acute inferior myocardial infarction: Clinical, electrocardiographic, and therapeutic characterization. *PACE* 9:468, 1986.
17. DuBois, C., Piérard, L. A., Smeets, J.-P., et al. Long-term prognostic significance of atrioventricular block in inferior acute myocardial infarction. *Eur. Heart J.* 10:816, 1989.
18. Nicod, P., Gilpin, E., Dittrich, H., et al. Long-term outcome in patients with inferior myocardial infarction and complete atrioventricular block. *J. Am. Coll. Cardiol.* 12:589, 1988.
19. McDonald, K., O'Sullivan, J. J., Conroy, R. M., et al. Heart block as a predictor of in-hospital death in both acute inferior and acute anterior myocardial infarction. *Quarterly J. Med.* 74:277, 1990.
20. Mauric, Z., Zaputovich, L., Matana, A., et al. Prognostic significance of complete atrioventricular block in patients with acute inferior myocardial infarction with and without right ventricular involvement. *Am. Heart J.* 119:823, 1990.
21. Sugiwra, T., Iwasaka, T., Hasegawa, T., et al. Factors associated with persistent and transient fascicular blocks in anterior wall acute myocardial infarction. *Am. J. Cardiol.* 63:784, 1989.
22. Hindman, M. C., Wagner, G. S., Jaro, M., et al. The clinical significance of bundle branch block complicating acute myocardial infarction. 1. Clinical characteristics, hospital mortality, and one-year follow-up. *Circulation* 4:679, 1978.
23. Hindman, M. C., Wagner, G. S., Jaro, M., et al. The clinical significance of bundle branch block complicating acute myocardial infarction. 2. Indications for temporary and permanent pacemaker insertion. *Circulation* 4:689, 1978.
24. Lamas, G. A., Muller, J. E., Turi, Z. G., et al. A simplified method to predict occurrence of complete heart block during acute myocardial infarction. *Am. J. Cardiol.* 57:1213, 1986.
25. Dominghetti, G., and Perret, C. Intraventricular conduction disturbances in acute myocardial infarction: Short- and long-term prognosis. *Eur. J. Cardiol.* 11:51, 1980.
26. Hollander, G., Nadiminti, V., Lichstein, E., et al. Bundle branch block in acute myocardial infarction. *Am. Heart J.* 105:738, 1983.
27. Gann, D., Balachandran, P. K., El Sherif, N., and Samet, P. Prognostic significance of chronic versus acute bundle branch block in acute myocardial infarction. *Chest* 67:298, 1975.
28. Waugh, R. A., Wagner, G. S., Haney, T. L., et al. Immediate and remote prognostic significance of fascicular block during acute myocardial infarction. *Circulation* 47:765, 1973.
29. Scanlon, P. J., Pryor, R., and Blount, S. G. Right bundle branch block associated with acute myocardial infarction. *Circulation* 42:135, 1970.
30. Atkins, J. M., Leshin, S. J., Blomquist, G., and Mullins, C. B. Ventricular conduction blocks and sudden death in acute myocardial infarction: Potential indications for pacing. *N. Engl. J. Med.* 288:281, 1973.
31. Nimetz, A. A., Scubroooks, S. J., Hutter, A. M., and DeSanctis, R. W. The significance of bundle branch block during acute myocardial infarction. *Am. Heart J.* 90:439, 1975.
32. Godman, M. J., Lassers, B. W., and Julian, D. G. Complete bundle-branch block complicating acute myocardial infarction. *N. Engl. J. Med.* 282:237, 1970.
33. Godman, M. J., Alpert, B. A., and Julian, D. G. Bilateral bundle-branch block complicating acute myocardial infarction. *Lancet* 2:345, 1971.
34. Scheinman, M., and Brenman, B. Clinical and anatomic complications of intraventricular conduction blocks in acute myocardial infarction. *Circulation* 46:753, 1972.
35. Lichstein, E., Gupta, P. K., Chadda, K. D., et al. Findings of prognostic valve in patients with incomplete bilateral bundle branch block complicating

acute myocardial infarction. *Am. J. Cardiol.* 32: 913, 1973.
36. Lie, K. I., Wellens, H. J., and Schuilenburg, R. M. Bundle branch block and acute myocardial infarction. In H. J. J. Wellens (ed.), *The Conduction System of the Heart: Structure, Functions and Clinical Indications.* Philadelphia: Lea & Febiger, 1976.
37. Waters, D. D., and Mizgala, H. F. Long-term prognosis of patients with incomplete bilateral bundle branch block complicating acute myocardial infarction: Role of cardiac pacing. *Am. J. Cardiol.* 34:1, 1974.
38. Kubis, M., and Suejda, J. Indication of permanent pacing after acute myocardial infarction complicated by combined intraventricular block. *Cor Vasa* 24: 295, 1982.
39. Hauer, R. N. W., Lie, K. I., Lier, K. L., and Durrer, P. Long-term prognosis in patients with bundle branch block complicating acute anteroseptal infarction. *Am. J. Cardiol.* 49:1581, 1982.
40. DuBois, C., Piérard, L. A., Smoets, J.-P., et al. Short and long-term prognostic importance of complete bundle-branch block complicating acute myocardial infarction. *Clin. Cardiol.* 11:292, 1988.
41. Ricou, F., Nicod, P., Gilpin, E., et al. Influence of right bundle branch block on short and long-term survival after acute anterior myocardial infarction. *J. Am. Coll. Cardiol.* 17:858, 1991.
42. Barold, S. S. Narrow QRS Mobitz II second-degree atrioventricular book in acute myocardial infarction: True or false? *Am. J. Cardiol.* 67:1291, 1991.
43. Ginks, W. R., Sutton, R., Oh, W., and Leatham, A. Long-term prognosis after acute anterior infarction with atrioventricular block. *Br. Heart J.* 39:186, 1977.
44. Ritter, W. A., Atkins, J. M., Blomquist, C. G., and Mullins, C. B. Permanent pacing in patients with transient trifascicular block during acute myocardial infarction. *Am. J. Cardiol.* 38:205, 1976.
45. Watson, R. S. D., Glover, D. R., Page, A. J. F., et al. The Birmingham trial of permanent pacing in patients with intraventricular conduction disorders after myocardial infarction. *Am. Heart J.* 108:496, 1984.
46. Pagnoni, F., Finzia, A., Valentini, R., et al. Long-term prognostic significance and electrophysiological evolution of intraventricular conduction disturbances complicating acute myocardial infarction. *PACE* 9:91, 1986.
47. Lie, K. I., Wellens, H. J., Schuilenburg, R. S., et al. Factors influencing prognosis of bundle branch block complicating acute antero-septal infarction: The value of His bundle recordings. *Circulation* 50: 935, 1974.
48. Schoenfeld, C. D., Mascarenhas, E., Bhardwaj, P., et al. Clinical and electrophysiologic significance of bundle branch block in acute myocardial infarction. *PACE* 2:428, 1979.
49. Gould, L., Reddy, V. V. R., Kim, S. G., and Oh, K. C. His bundle electrogram in patients with acute myocardial infarction. *PACE* 2:428, 1979.
50. Harper, R., Hunt, D., Vohra, J., et al. His bundle electrogram in patients with acute myocardial infarction complicated by atrioventricular or intraventricular conduction disturbances. *Br. Heart J.* 37: 705, 1975.
51. Aranda, J. M., Befeler, B., and Castellanos, A. His bundle recordings, bundle branch block and myocardial infarction. *Ann. Intern. Med.* 86:106, 1977.
52. Cortadellas, J., Cinca, J., Moya, A., and Rius, J. Clinical and electrophysiologic findings in acute ischemic intraHisian bundle-branch block. *Am. Heart J.* 119:23, 1990.
53. Scheinman, M. M., Remedios, P., Cheitlin, M. D., et al. Effects of antiarrhythmic drugs on atrioventricular conduction in patients with acute myocardial infarction. *Circulation* 62:20, 1980.
54. Beta-Blocker Heart Attack Trial Research Group. A randomized trial of propranolol in patients with acute myocardial infarction. I. Mortality results. *J.A.M.A.* 247:1707, 1982.
55. Norwegian Multicenter Study Group. Timolol-induced reduction in mortality and reinfarction in patients surviving acute myocardial infarction. *N. Engl. J. Med.* 304:801, 1981.
56. Hjalmerson, A., Herlitz, J., Malek, I., et al. Effect on mortality of metoprolol in acute myocardial infarction. *Lancet* 2:823, 1981.
57. Gibson, R. S., Boden, W. E., Theroux, P., et al. Diltiazem and reinfarction in patients with non-Q-wave myocardial infarction. *N. Engl. J. Med.* 315: 423, 1986.
58. Selzer, A., Langston, M., Ruggeroli, C., and Cohn, K. Clinical syndrome of variant angina with normal coronary arteriograms. *N. Engl. J. Med.* 295:1343, 1976.
59. Plotnick, G. D., Carliner, N. H., Fisher, M. L., et al. Rest angina with transient S-T segment elevation: Correlation of clinical features with coronary anatomy. *Am. J. Med.* 65:257, 1978.
60. Italian Group for the Study of Streptokinase in Myocardial Infarction (GISSI). Effectiveness of intravenous thrombolytic treatment in acute myocardial infarction. *Lancet* 1:397, 1986.
61. Roth, A., Miller, H. I., Glick, A., et al. Rapid resolution of new right bundle branch block in acute myocardial infarction patients after thrombolytic therapy. *PACE* 16:13, 1993.
62. Wiseman, A., Ohman, E. M., Wharton, J. M. Transient reversal of bifascicular block during acute myocardial infarction with reperfusion therapy: A word of caution. *A. Heart J.* 117:1381, 1989.
63. Clemmenson, P., Bates, E. R., Califf, R. M., et al. Complete atrioventricular block complicating inferior wall acute myocardial infarction treated with reperfusion therapy. *Am. J. Cardiol.* 67:225, 1991.
64. Berger, P. B., Ruocco, N. A., Jr., Ryan, T. J., et al. Incidence and prognostic implications of heart block complicating inferior myocardial infarction treated with thrombolytic therapy: Results from TIMI II. *J. Am. Coll. Cardiol.* 20:533, 1992.

11. Treatment of Ventricular Arrhythmias in Acute Myocardial Infarction

Raymond L. Woosley and Jean T. Barbey

The focus of the coronary care unit (CCU) is to minimize myocardial damage during acute myocardial infarction, as well as to monitor and treat disturbances of cardiac rhythm. In recent years, efforts to minimize myocardial injury have predominated and there has been less of a role for antiarrhythmic therapy per se. Our understanding of whether and how to treat arrhythmias has changed: For example, there is disagreement over the significance of "warning arrhythmias," and the risk-benefit ratio of lidocaine therapy for patients with acute myocardial infarction is now in question. These issues must be resolved before one can be dogmatic about the role of antiarrhythmic drugs in acute myocardial infarction. For many years lidocaine was recommended as prophylactic therapy for any patient thought to be having a myocardial infarction [1]. A meta-analysis of the controlled trials with lidocaine in patients with acute myocardial infarction found that lidocaine did not improve mortality [2]. Another analysis of trials found that the incidence of ventricular fibrillation had fallen to less than 0.35 percent in 1990, a level at which drug efficacy would be difficult to detect [3]. This observation and the results of the Cardiac Arrhythmia Suppression Trial (CAST) [4, 5] conducted in patients with ventricular arrhythmias after recovery from myocardial infarction led physicians to reserve antiarrhythmic drugs for patients who are highly symptomatic or arrhythmias that are clearly life-threatening, that is, ventricular tachycardia or fibrillation [2, 3, 6]. Analysis of the risk-benefit ratio of antiarrhythmic drugs has become of prime concern in patients with arrhythmias [6].

When one is considering antiarrhythmic therapy for patients with myocardial infarction, the initial evaluation should include the following:

1. Several ancillary factors may underlie or provoke arrhythmias following heart attack; among them are hypoxia, electrolyte disturbance, and digitalis toxicity. Each of these possible contributors should be corrected prior to consideration of antiarrhythmic drug therapy.
2. The specific diagnosis of the arrhythmia should be made, keeping in mind that analysis of the surface electrocardiogram (ECG) alone may lead to misdiagnosis, with the potential for lethal consequences.
3. The promptness with which therapy must take effect should be assessed, with the realization that the onset of action for some agents (e.g., lidocaine) can occur within minutes, whereas others (e.g., procainamide) require 20 to 30 minutes or more for the safe administration of loading dosages.

In extremely urgent situations, as when patients have recurring episodes of ventricular tachycardia or fibrillation after cardioversion, lidocaine is considered the drug of first choice; it can be given safely as a bolus injection and can be effective within seconds. If the patient fails to respond to adequate dosages of lidocaine and the arrhythmia still requires urgent therapy, bretylium is the next alternative. Many physicians continue the lidocaine infusion and add bretylium using a series of loading boluses and a maintenance infusion (see below).

When more time is available, such as for treatment of a patient with sustained ventricular tachycardia who is stable hemodynamically, we prefer intravenous procainamide to convert or suppress the arrhythmia. Lidocaine also can be effective in this setting, but bretylium is not a reasonable choice because it does not provide an option for chronic oral therapy and is poorly tolerated, with orthostatic hypotension being an almost universal adverse effect [7].

Once a patient has passed the acute phase of myocardial infarction and continues to have or develop ventricular arrhythmias, the goals of therapy are considerably different. If the arrhythmias are symptomatic, such as nonsustained or sustained ventricular tachycardia, medications that have an oral formulation and are likely to be well tolerated must be considered. Lidocaine and bretylium are no longer candidates except that they may be useful for controlling arrhythmias while one is trying to identify an effective oral regimen. Likewise, procainamide is not the optimal selection for therapy that is anticipated to last for several months or years because of the high incidence of patient withdrawal due to adverse reactions including allergy and a lupus erythematosus syndrome. Some of the newer agents such as sotalol are better tolerated for chronic therapy and may be considered.

The development of recurrent, sporadic, sustained ventricular tachycardia during the convalescent phase of acute myocardial infarction or afterward should prompt the physician to consider the use of programmed ventricular stimulation (PVS) as the means to evaluate the effectiveness of therapy. If ventricular tachycardia recurs soon after cardioversion, PVS may not be needed to evaluate therapy; however, in many patients the recurrence of tachycardia is sporadic, and for optimal drug evaluation and therapy it must be induced by PVS to be studied. There was controversy over how to manage patients with symptomatic ventricular tachycardia and high-frequency ventricular ectopy until the Electrophysiology Study Versus Electrocardiographic Monitoring (ESVEM) trial was completed. This study compared Holter ECG recordings with PVS in patients who qualified for management using either approach [8]. The investigators found a similar overall outcome with the two methods but ambulatory monitoring identified an effective antiarrhythmic drug regimen almost twice as often as did PVS (45 versus 77 percent). There also has been a lack of consensus concerning the role of implantable cardioverter-defibrillators for chronic therapy of patients with life-threatening arrhythmias. The National Institutes of Health (NIH)–sponsored Antiarrhythmics Versus Implantable Devises (AVID) trial will hopefully answer questions concerning the relative merit of antiarrhythmic drugs and these newer devices in the treatment of patients with life-threatening ventricular arrhythmias [9]. Unfortunately, there are no controlled trials available to suggest that these patients benefit from antiarrhythmic therapy and there is clear evidence that some agents increase mortality [4, 5].

Early intervention with beta-adrenergic receptor–blocking drugs (in patients without contraindications) can decrease subsequent mortality, although the mechanism by which this is achieved is not understood [10–13]. One possibility is that they lessen metabolic demand on the myocardium and thus reduce damage and preserve function. However, although therapy with beta-adrenergic receptor antagonists soon after myocardial infarction will appreciably lower the risk of subsequent sudden cardiac death, patients at the highest risk for this event are generally difficult candidates for beta-adrenergic blockade because of heart failure.

Polymorphic ventricular tachycardia has become increasingly recognized in the peri-infarction setting as well as in others. When this rhythm is associated with prolongation of cardiac repolarization (as in torsades de pointes), quinidine-like drugs are implicated as causal factors, and the initiating mechanism may well be bradycardia-dependent triggered automaticity in the form of early afterdepolarizations [14, 15]. Treatment with pacing, magnesium, and isoproterenol is effective when the syndrome is recognized. On the other hand, polymorphic ventricular tachycardia that occurs in the setting of a normal QT interval must be distinguished because it can be treated with local anesthetic antiarrhythmic drugs. The term *torsades de pointes* should not be applied to all polymorphic ventricular tachycardias. The two forms described here are different, and we restrict the use of the term *torsades de pointes* to the syndrome that includes the arrhythmia in the presence of a markedly prolonged QT interval [16].

A discussion of general pharmacologic principles important in the use of antiarrhythmic drugs is followed by a more detailed consideration of specific agents. Unfortunately, despite advances in the elucidation of the mechanisms involved in the genesis of arrhythmias, drug therapy remains largely empiric.

Principles of Management

Pharmacokinetic Principles

The following is a brief review of pharmacokinetic principles as they apply to therapy with antiarrhythmic agents. For more extensive information, the reader is referred to a detailed review of the pharmacokinetics of antiarrhythmic drugs [17].

The goal is to attain myocardial drug concentrations within the range necessary for suppressing or converting an arrhythmia without reaching toxic concentrations at any site in the body. Rapid attainment of an antiarrhythmic effect is best accomplished by an intravenous loading regimen, but loading doses have the attendant disadvantage of rapidly changing drug levels in the plasma and vital organs. Thorough understanding of drug distribution, metabolism, and elimination in both normal individuals and patients with renal, cardiac, or hepatic dysfunction is necessary to arrive at initial estimates for dosage regimens, which are then individualized for the patient to be treated. The physician must be well versed in the principles of pharmacokinetics, have available the pharmacokinetic data for the drug to be administered, be familiar with the clinical condition of the patient, and understand how this condition pertains to the available pharmacokinetic data. Then, being prepared to adjust for any errors in predictions, the physician must monitor therapy using all of the clinical tools available, including ECG and plasma concentration monitoring.

After intravenous administration many antiarrhythmic drugs follow what is described as a two-compartment, open pharmacokinetic model. These ''compartments'' are not anatomic entities; rather, they are calculated theoretical volumes. Nonetheless, these concepts are a valuable aid to designing individualized therapy. With intravenous administration, the drug is first delivered into a central compartment, which reflects the concentration in the plasma, myocardium, and central nervous system. The drug then distributes fairly rapidly into peripheral tissues (Fig. 11-1). Elimination, a slower process, generally takes place from the central compartment. Immediately following intravenous injection, therapeutic concentrations may be attained in the plasma and the myocardium; however, this effect may be short-lived because of redistribution into other tissues.

Fig. 11-1
Biexponential decay of plasma concentration of lidocaine after intravenous injection of a 50-mg dose in a normal individual. The initial rapid fall in concentration indicates distribution of lidocaine out of the central compartment into the peripheral compartment. The second phase, represented by a more gradual drop in plasma concentration, reflects elimination. Cp = plasma concentration; $t_{1/2}$ = half-life. (From R. L. Woosley. Lidocaine therapy. *Cardiac Impulse* 8:No. 2, 1987. With permission.)

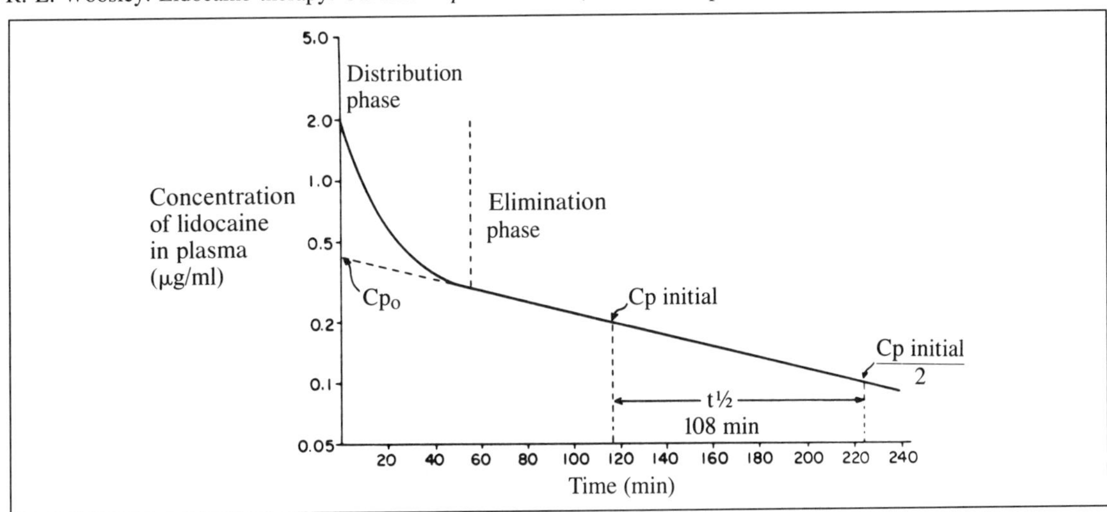

Volume of Distribution

The volume of distribution of a drug is a theoretical volume based on the original dose given and its subsequent plasma concentration. The volume of distribution (V_d) may be regarded as that theoretical volume within which a drug would be distributed in order to achieve the plasma concentration measured.

Immediately following administration of an intravenous bolus into a central compartment, the plasma concentration achieved is equal to the dose divided by the volume of distribution (of the central compartment). Volume of distribution generally does not correspond to any physiologic space and may (because of plasma levels being reduced when drug is bound to tissue) exceed the total volume of the body. However, it provides a guide to choosing an initial dose and is one of the determinants of elimination half-life.

The volume of distribution can change in patients who develop congestive heart failure. For example, the volume of distribution for lidocaine in patients with heart failure is approximately one-half that for normal individuals.

Clearance

Clearance is a rate term describing the process of drug elimination and is expressed as milliliters of blood cleared of drug per minute. For most antiarrhythmic drugs, clearance is a "first-order process," which means that the amount of drug eliminated depends on the concentration of drug in the central compartment. Dosage and clearance determine the ultimate steady-state plasma concentration (Cp_{ss}) achieved during maintenance intravenous therapy:

$$Cp_{ss} = \text{infusion rate/clearance}$$

Total clearance is the sum of renal and nonrenal clearance. An example of nonrenal clearance for most drugs is hepatic metabolism.

Half-Life

Half-life is a convenient way to characterize processes such as elimination and distribution that proceed on a first-order basis. For instance, after an intravenous bolus of a rapidly distributed drug such as lidocaine is given, 50 percent of the process of distribution is complete after one distribution half-life, 75 percent after two half-lives, 87.5 percent after three half-lives, and so on (Fig. 11-2). Such processes can therefore be regarded as nearly complete after four to five half-lives. Because lidocaine's *distribution* half-life is usually approximately 8 minutes, *distribution* is complete 32 to 40 minutes after a bolus. Similarly, *elimination* is essentially complete after four to five *elimination* half-lives (8 to 10 hours for lidocaine in usual patients whose elimination half-life is approximately

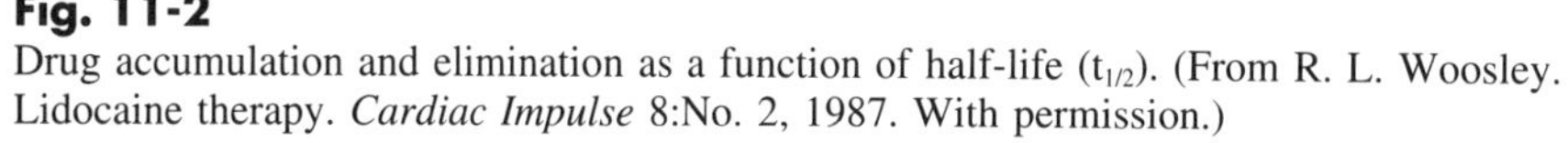
Fig. 11-2
Drug accumulation and elimination as a function of half-life ($t_{1/2}$). (From R. L. Woosley. Lidocaine therapy. *Cardiac Impulse* 8:No. 2, 1987. With permission.)

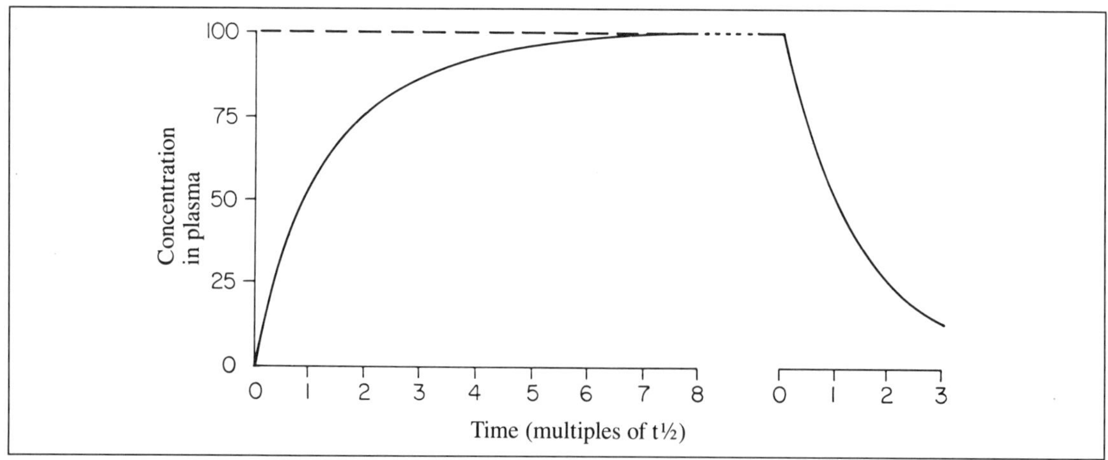

2 hours). In addition, the time required to reach steady-state conditions following initiation of chronic therapy (by any route) is four to five elimination half-lives and is dependent on the volume of distribution and clearance:

Half-life = $(0.693 \times V_d)$/clearance

Loading doses are sometimes used with the mistaken concept that they hasten the time to reach steady-state equilibrium. Although they may shorten the time needed to attain *therapeutic plasma levels,* the time required to reach steady-state equilibrium is always four to five half-lives and is unaffected by the use of loading doses.

Bioavailability

Bioavailability is the fraction of an oral dose reaching the systemic circulation when compared to the amount available (100 percent) following intravenous administration. Only a portion of an orally administered dose may be absorbed, or metabolism of a drug can take place prior to its entry into the systemic circulation. The latter can occur in the intestinal lumen, the intestinal wall, or most commonly, the liver. Several drugs undergo such extensive "first-pass" hepatic metabolism before reaching the systemic circulation that dosing recommendations must be considerably adjusted depending on the route of administration. For instance, the ranges of respective intravenous and oral dosages for propranolol are 1 to 10 mg and 40 to 80 mg. Alterations in drug disposition due to disease states (e.g., acute myocardial infarction, congestive heart failure, hepatic or renal disease) may be conceptualized in terms of alterations of volumes of distribution, clearance, and elimination half-life. Disease states may alter volume of distribution or clearance alone (and thus alter elimination half-life) or may change both volume of distribution and clearance. Note that if clearance and volume of distribution are reduced to the same degree, elimination half-life is unaltered. This is particularly applicable to the use of lidocaine in patients with congestive heart failure. The volume of distribution for lidocaine is approximately one-half that for normal individuals, and a reduced loading dose is required [18]. A reduced maintenance dose is also required because of reduced clearance, but the half-life may be within the usual range because both the volume of distribution and the clearance have changed proportionately.

Transition to Chronic Oral Therapy

Chronic treatment with antiarrhythmic drugs has changed dramatically in recent years. The results of the CAST led to restriction of oral drug therapy to patients with life-threatening or highly symptomatic arrhythmias. If a patient clearly requires chronic therapy, a full understanding of the clinical pharmacology of the available drugs is essential for optimal response. Oral therapy should start at low doses, and each dose schedule should be continued, if possible, until steady-state conditions are achieved (four to five elimination half-lives). If arrhythmia is still present or inducible by PVS and side effects are absent, a higher dosage regimen can then be tried. Plasma concentrations should be monitored to ensure the presence of adequate drug, to establish a baseline for future patient care, to warn of possible impending toxicity, and to confirm any clinical suspicion of drug toxicity. No drug can truly be declared a therapeutic failure unless arrhythmia persists in the face of side effects.

Plasma Concentration Monitoring

The monitoring of antiarrhythmic drug plasma concentrations is often a valuable guide for adjusting therapy. For lidocaine, plasma concentrations parallel the effect, suggesting that the "effector" tissue site and plasma are in the same pharmacokinetic compartment [19]. This rule does not apply to some drugs such as bretylium and amiodarone. Immediately following parenteral administration of the latter agents, plasma concentrations are high, although the antiarrhythmic effect may be negligible [20, 21]. This observation implies that for these agents plasma and myocardium are in different compartments, and time is needed for distribution of the drug or development of effect. For procainamide, long-term therapy is complicated by the production of the potentially active metabolite *N*-acetylprocainamide (NAPA) [22]. NAPA concentrations in plasma exceed those of procainamide in about 50 percent of the population [23]. Nevertheless, plasma concentration monitoring can be useful for these agents once equilibrium between plasma concentration and effector site concentration is achieved [24].

Antiarrhythmic drug actions

Drug	Channels						Receptors				Pumps	Clinical effects			ECG effects		
	Na			Ca	K	I_f	α	β	M_2	P	Na/K ATPase	LV FX	Sinus rate	Extra cardiac	PR	QRS	JT
	Fast	Med	Slow														
Lidocaine	○											→	→	◍			↓
Mexiletine	○											→	→	◍			↓
Tocainide	○											→	→	●			↓
Moricizine	Ⓘ											↓	→	○		↑	
Procainamide		Ⓐ			◍							↓	→	●	↑	↑	↑
Disopyramide		Ⓐ			◍				○			↓	→	◍	↑↓	↑	↑
Quinidine		Ⓐ			◍		○		○			→	↑	◍	↑↓	↑	↑
Propafenone			Ⓐ					◍				↓	↓	○	↑	↑	
Flecainide			Ⓐ		◍							↓	→	○	↑	↑	
Encainide			Ⓐ									↓	→	○	↑	↑	
Bepridil	○			●	◍							?	↓	○			↑
Verapamil	○			●			◍					↓	↓	○	↑		
Diltiazem				◍								↓	↓	○	↑		
Bretylium					●		▲	▲				→	↓	○			↑
Sotalol					●			●				↓	↓	○	↑		↑
Amiodarone	○			○	●		◍	◍				→	↓	●	↑		↑
Alinidine					◍	●						?	↓	●			
Nadolol								●				↓	↓	○	↑		
Propranolol	○							●				↓	↓	○	↑		
Atropine									●			→	↑	◍	↓		
Adenosine										△		?	↓	○	↑		
Digoxin									△		●	↑	↓	●	↑		↓

Therapeutic ranges for plasma concentrations of antiarrhythmic drugs should be regarded only as rough guidelines and a plasma concentration must be evaluated within the clinical setting. Although the lower limit of the published therapeutic range is the plasma concentration that is likely to produce an effect, some patients may respond to even lower concentrations [25]. Similarly, the upper limit of the therapeutic range is the concentration beyond which an additional therapeutic benefit is unlikely to occur and the incidence of side effects rises. Again, some patients may require higher concentrations to achieve a therapeutic effect and may tolerate higher concentrations without adverse effects [25]. Thus therapeutic ranges of plasma concentrations are no substitute for clinical judgment. Clearly, monitoring plasma concentrations during chronic therapy is useful for both verifying compliance and establishing a baseline should the patient's clinical status change (e.g., should congestive heart failure develop). It is also important to ascertain that the plasma concentration being measured is the appropriate one. Some drugs have active metabolites that may produce the predominant, or a different, pharmacologic action. Examples include procainamide, whose active metabolite NAPA may accumulate to antiarrhythmic concentrations in patients with renal failure [26], and propafenone, which is converted to the 5-hydroxy metabolite that contributes to arrhythmia suppression [27]. Clearly, measuring parent drug concentrations in these settings may not be helpful and may in fact be misleading.

Fig. 11-3

Summary of the potentially most important actions of antiarrhythmic drugs. The drugs are listed in order of their primary in vitro action so that the symbols on the diagonal (top left to bottom right) represent this action. Drugs with multiple actions (e.g., amiodarone) have symbols that depart strikingly from the diagonal. The drug actions are in two major groups: in vitro actions and clinical actions. The in vitro actions are subdivided into the effects on channels, receptors, and pumps, that is, the major determinants of cardiac electrophysiology. The actions of drugs on the sodium, calcium, potassium, and I_f (the funny current) channels are indicated. Sodium channel blockade is subdivided into three groups of actions characterized by fast (<200 msec), medium (200 to 1500 msec), and slow (>1500 msec) time constants for recovery from block. This parameter is a measure of use dependence and predicts the likelihood that a drug will decrease the conduction velocity in normal sodium-dependent tissues of the heart and perhaps the propensity of a drug for causing bundle branch block or proarrhythmia. Blockade in the inactivated (I) or activated (A) state is indicated. Information on the state dependency of the block caused by moricizine, propafenone, encainide, and flecainide is especially limited and may be altered with additional research. Drug interaction with receptors (alpha- and beta-adrenergic, muscarinic subtype [M_2], and adenosine or purinergic [P]) and drug effects on the sodium-potassium pump (Na, K-ATPase) are indicated. Circles indicate antagonist or inhibitory actions; unfilled triangles indicate direct- or indirect-acting agonists or stimulators. The darkness of the symbol increases with the intensity of the action. Filled triangles for bretylium indicate its biphasic action to initially stimulate alpha and beta receptors by release of norepinephrine followed by subsequent block of norepinephrine release and indirect antagonism of these receptors. The likelihood of clinically effective doses of the drugs to alter left ventricular function (LV FX), sinus heart rate, and ECG intervals (PR, QRS, or JT) is shown with arrows. Where clinical experience is limited or contradictory, a question mark is indicated. Shaded circles are used to indicate the relative potency for extracardiac side effects such as hepatitis or other organ toxicity. Note that proarrhythmic potential is not listed. The major reasons for not including this information are that there are very limited comparative data available and all antiarrhythmic drugs have this potential in some patients. In many cases, it is related more to the individual patient than it is to the specific drug. (From Task Force of the Working Group on Arrhythmias of European Society of Cardiology. The Sicilian Gambit: A new approach to the classification of antiarrhythmic drugs based on their actions on arrhythmogenic mechanisms. *Circulation* 84:1831, 1991. Reproduced with permission of the American Heart Association, Inc.)

Drug present in plasma may exist either free or protein bound. Because only the free drug is available to exert pharmacologic activity, a change in the free drug concentration produces a proportional change in the effects seen. A pertinent example of these principles occurs with lidocaine. During the acute phases of myocardial infarction, the plasma concentration of alpha-1-acid glycoprotein (AAG), the binding protein for lidocaine, becomes elevated [28]. Some antiarrhythmic agents, most notably lidocaine, bind extensively to this protein, and hence their total plasma concentration is affected by changing AAG concentrations [29]. Assays for plasma lidocaine measure both protein-bound and free lidocaine and thus do not give a true picture of the amount of free drug available. Shortly after infarction, apparent plasma lidocaine levels tend to rise, reflecting lidocaine bound to higher levels of AAG; however, the concentration of free lidocaine may change little [30]. In this case, the lidocaine dosage should not be reduced to compensate for the higher total plasma concentration so long as the patient displays no adverse effects. Subsequent decreases in AAG concentration in the days following myocardial infarction influence measurement of the apparently available lidocaine levels as well, only in the opposite direction. Quinidine is another antiarrhythmic agent that binds to AAG, and increased levels of this protein in plasma explain the increase in total drug levels of quinidine seen after infarction that are not associated with excess drug effect [31, 32]. Monitoring of *free* drug levels in this setting is of unproved value but theoretically should be more reliable than the current practice of measuring total drug (bound and free) in plasma for guiding therapy.

Reducing Empiricism in Therapy

Unfortunately, we do not understand the mechanism of most arrhythmias occurring in the setting of myocardial ischemia. Therefore, therapy is of necessity empiric. However, some of the empiricism can be reduced by utilizing a systematic approach and a thorough understanding of the pharmacology of the drugs to be used. Until recently, the Vaughan Williams classification was the primary framework for organizing an increasing list of available drugs [33]. However, its limitations and the potential for being clinically misleading prompted cardiologists to seek another approach. The Sicilian Gambit was proposed as a replacement for the outdated Vaughan Williams classification [34]. The Sicilian Gambit emphasizes that drugs have many actions and the clinical outcome may depend on more than one of these actions interacting with a complex arrhythmia substrate. Figure 11-3 is a reproduction of the framework the Task Force of the Working Group on Arrhythmias recommended for considering the actions of the antiarrhythmic drugs on channels, receptors, and membrane pumps. The major value of the Sicilian Gambit approach is that it provides all of the clinically relevant information instead of truncating valuable information. For example, the two additional actions listed for quinidine, blockade of potassium channels and alpha receptors, are virtually ignored in the Vaughan Williams classification. Pronouncing that quinidine is a class "IA" drug is only informative to those who have also memorized the "code." Even then it will not warn one to expect hypotension mediated by alpha blockade or alert one to the higher risk of torsades de pointes compared to other "IA" drugs. Similarly the anticholinergic actions of disopyramide would be unanticipated. The Sicilian Gambit offers an approach for joining knowledge about the mechanism of arrhythmias with an up-to-date understanding of the pharmacology of the drugs.

Basic to an understanding of the mechanism of action of antiarrhythmic agents is an understanding of the cardiac sodium channel. Hodgkin and Huxley proposed that sodium channels exist in three distinct states [35]. According to the modulated receptor hypothesis of cardiac sodium channel regulation proposed by Hille [36] and Hondeghem and Katzung [37], each of the three states of the sodium channel (open, closed, inactivated) has a different affinity for any given drug that blocks sodium channels. By combining drugs such as lidocaine (which rapidly dissociates from the sodium channel and allows rapid recovery from block) with a drug such as quinidine (which dissociates from the sodium channel more slowly and requires more time for recovery from block), synergistic blockade of sodium channels (particularly during tachycardia or with premature beats) should be possible [38, 39]. The treatment of acute and chronic ventricular arrhythmias frequently necessitates combination therapy owing to the low efficacy of single agents. By combining drugs with differing kinetics of interaction with the sodium channel, one may produce a broader range of antiarrhythmic actions and, hopefully, increased drug efficacy. Additionally, drugs whose antiarrhythmic activity results from different mechanisms of action can be synergistic. A simple example is the combination of a drug that alters conduction velocity (sodium channel blockade) with one that prolongs repolarization and refractoriness (potassium channel blockade).

Arrhythmia Exacerbation

It is increasingly recognized that antiarrhythmic therapy can be associated with arrhythmia exacerbation. It can range from a marked increase in the frequency of ventricular ectopic depolarizations to the new onset or increased frequency of sustained ventricular tachycardia. The latter is not necessarily associated with marked QT prolongation, particularly with the use of drugs that markedly slow conduction velocity (e.g., propafenone and flecainide). The incidence of such arrhythmia exacerbation may be as high as 20 percent in patients with severely depressed left ventricular function, coronary artery disease, and a history of sustained ventricular tachycardia when flecainide-like agents are administered [40]. The incidence of torsades de pointes is difficult to estimate for most drugs, but it is certainly seen more commonly with agents such as quinidine, sotalol, procainamide, and disopyramide. Predisposing factors such as bradycardia and hypokalemia have been identified, and in a study of 24 patients, Roden et al. found these factors to be present in 83 percent of those who developed torsades de pointes [41]. In the population with less severe arrhythmias, the incidence of arrhythmia aggravation has been estimated to be 2 to 12 percent with currently available drugs.

Specific Antiarrhythmic Agents

Lidocaine

Indications

Lidocaine is usually the drug of first choice for the acute suppression of serious ventricular arrhythmias. However, its use has changed in recent years, as discussed earlier in this chapter. It is clearly indicated for patients who develop ventricular tachycardia or fibrillation and require cardiopulmonary resuscitation. It is no longer recommended as prophylactic therapy in patients at risk for ventricular arrhythmias. In spite of its ability to decrease the incidence of primary ventricular fibrillation in patients with documented acute myocardial infarction, it has not been found to improve mortality [2]. In fact, a meta-analysis of studies previously published in the literature [2] found a trend toward an increased mortality. A sound understanding of lidocaine's pharmacokinetics is necessary so that therapy can be individualized for each patient. The dosage and the means for monitoring response are very different for a patient receiving lidocaine during cardiopulmonary resuscitation than for a patient who is awake and in a sustained and hemodynamically stable ventricular tachycardia (see below). Even among stable patients, the effective dosage varies tremendously and monitoring the clinical response is essential. An excellent example of using clinical response rather than fixed dosages or drug concentrations to evaluate therapy was reported by Alderman and coworkers [25]. Of nine patients who were apparently resistant to standard doses of lidocaine, three in fact had arrhythmias responsive at higher doses (blood levels were still within the therapeutic range), and four had arrhythmias resistant to lidocaine at usual blood levels but responsive at levels of 5 to 9 μg/ml. Only two of the nine patients were, in fact, resistant and demonstrated mild central nervous system side effects without an antiarrhythmic effect.

Pharmacology: In Vitro and Animal Data

In concentrations similar to those attained during clinical use, lidocaine's sodium channel–blocking action reduces the rate of the rise of phase 0 and produces shortening or no change in action potential duration (APD) and effective refractory period (ERP) of normal Purkinje fibers [42, 43]. It contrasts with other sodium channel blockers such as quinidine and procainamide, which produce lengthening of the APD. Though it has minimal effects in normal tissue, lidocaine prolongs refractoriness and slows conduction in ischemic tissue during transient coronary artery occlusion in dogs [44]. This is consistent with its greater effects on sodium channels in the inactivated state (as would be seen during ischemia).

Some indications of a potential proarrhythmic action of lidocaine in certain animal models have been reported [45–47], and it is of interest that Adgey et al. [48] suggested that lidocaine was not a particularly effective drug for suppressing ventricular ectopic depolarizations early during myocardial infarction. In contrast, both Borer et al. [49] and Spear et al. [50] showed that lidocaine increased ventricular fibrillation thresholds in acutely ischemic dogs. Lidocaine has almost no effect on atrial tissue in vitro [51], consistent with the clinical observation that it is of little use for supraventricular tachyarrhythmias.

Clinical Electrophysiology

Lidocaine has little effect on the electrophysiology of the normal conduction system. Studies on the effect of lidocaine in patients with conduction system abnormalities have produced variable results. Kunkel et al. [52] showed no change in the AH, HV, or QRS interval following lidocaine administration to ten patients with bundle branch block; similar results were reported by Bekheit et al. [53]. Gupta et al. [54], however, showed that lidocaine could potentiate infranodal block in patients at high risk (prolonged HV interval or 2:1 infranodal block), and Aravindakshan et al. [55] reported abrupt slowing of the ventricular rate following lidocaine administration in 5 of 18 patients with stable atrioventricular (AV) block. In addition, the potential for advanced degrees of sinus node dysfunction has been reported in isolated instances [56, 57]. No systematically obtained data are available on the effects of lidocaine administration to patients with conduction system disturbances acquired during acute myocardial infarction. In this group, particularly in those with abnormalities involving conduction below the AV node, lidocaine (and all antiarrhythmic drugs) should be administered cautiously, if at all, unless a temporary pacemaker is inserted.

In studies carried out in patients without acute myocardial ischemia or infarction, lidocaine had inconsistent effects on atrial and AV nodal refractory periods, although it did shorten refractoriness of the His-Purkinje system [58].

Absorption, Distribution, Metabolism, and Elimination

Lidocaine undergoes extensive first-pass hepatic metabolism to the deethylated forms, monoethyl glycine xylidide and glycine xylidide, that are excreted by the kidneys. These metabolites have less antiarrhythmic potency than the parent drug and may contribute to the production of central nervous system side effects seen with lidocaine.

Lidocaine clearance is well approximated by measuring the liver blood flow [59, 60]. Thus although oral lidocaine is well absorbed, adequate amounts of the active parent drug cannot reach the systemic circulation without generation of toxic concentrations of the metabolites. For this reason, only intravenous lidocaine therapy is useful for arrhythmia suppression. Following intravenous administration, lidocaine disposition is well represented by the two-compartment open model (see Fig. 11-1) [18]. The half-life of lidocaine distribution between the central compartment and peripheral tissues is approximately 8 minutes. Because antiarrhythmic activity is correlated with lidocaine's concentration in the central compartment, this activity falls rapidly following administration of a single intravenous bolus. Little therapeutic effect is evident at lidocaine plasma concentrations below 1.5 μg/ml, whereas increasing toxicity occurs at concentrations above 5 μg/ml. In some patients, however, concentrations in the 5 to 9 μg/ml range may be required for arrhythmia suppression and can be achieved safely with cautious drug administration [25].

Toxicity

The most frequent side effects during lidocaine administration are central nervous system symptoms (especially tinnitus). If a bolus of lidocaine is administered too rapidly, seizures are likely to ensue. With more gradual attainment of excessive plasma levels, symptoms are usually limited to drowsiness, dysarthria, disorientation, and dysesthesia; the occurrence of such symptoms may in fact be useful for bedside assessment of the adequacy of lidocaine dosing in the face of recurrent arrhythmia. Excessive lidocaine can also cause coma and enters into the differential diagnosis of post–cardiac arrest encephalopathy. Likewise, excessive dosages of lidocaine can depress cardiac function. A vicious cycle can occur, as depressed cardiac function decreases lidocaine clearance, thereby causing an even greater increase in the plasma concentration. In a small subset of patients, lidocaine can also unpredictably provoke or exacerbate conduction system disturbances, as discussed already.

Dosage and Administration

Lidocaine's primary use as an antiarrhythmic agent is for the acute suppression of tachyarrhythmia. In these circumstances a prompt effect is obviously desirable. Single intravenous boluses achieve therapeutic effects only transiently because the drug is rapidly distributed out of the plasma and myocardium. Increasing the size of the bolus dose is likely to produce central nervous system adverse effects. Therefore, to promptly achieve and maintain therapeutic plasma concentrations, a loading regimen of multiple doses or infusions should be used. Pharmacokinetic analyses [61] suggest and clinical studies [62] confirm that in a stable patient a total loading dose of lidocaine is approximately 3 to 4 mg/kg administered over 20 to 30 minutes. In addition, ''boluses'' should be administered slowly (over 2 to 3 minutes) while the patient is continuously observed for the presence of side effects; should side effects occur, further loading should be stopped.

There have been several attempts to standardize but still individualize lidocaine therapy based on pharmacokinetic principles and data. A logical and easily applied approach was proposed by Benowitz [61]. This dosing regimen involves a loading bolus injection designed to initially fill the central compartment to a concentration in the usual therapeutic range, followed by a series of smaller injections to replace drug as it distributes to the peripheral compartment. Once the loading process is started, the patient should be placed on maintenance infusion calculated from the expected clearance but adjusted for anticipated alterations in clearance due to heart failure or liver disease. This approach was tested clinically in several studies and reduced the fluctuations and variability in plasma levels obtained [62, 63].

Loading Infusions

Table 11-1 describes the concepts and the equation to calculate the magnitude of a loading dose when the volume of distribution and the desired concentration are known. The equation is based on the definition of concentration (i.e., mass per unit volume). Multiplication of the volume of distribution by the desired concentration yields the mass of drug required or ''dosage.'' A loading dose would ideally be adequate to produce a concentration of 3 μg/ml when the drug has totally distributed throughout the body. However, for a 75-kg person with normal hemodynamics and organ function, the total volume of distribution of lidocaine at steady-state averages 100 liters. However, this calculation would result in a loading dose of 300 mg of lidocaine, a dose that would be extremely toxic if given at one time. We know that lidocaine, when administered intravenously, behaves according to the kinetics of a linear two-compartment model system. Initial concentrations after a rapid injection indicate that the volume of the central compartment is approximately 33 liters, approximately one-third of the total volume of distribution. If one administers one-third of the total loading dose, it should produce a plasma level of 3 μg/ml in the central compartment and then decline with a *distribution* half-life

Table 11-1
Protocol to rapidly provide plasma lidocaine concentrations of 3 μg/ml*

		Load by body weight	
Time	Dose	Normal patient	Patient with heart failure
0	1st bolus—loads central compartment	1.5 mg/kg	0.9 mg/kg
8 min	2nd bolus—replaces loss in 1st $t^1/_2$	0.8 mg/kg	0.4 mg/kg
16 min	3rd bolus — replaces loss in 2nd $t^1/_2$	0.8 mg/kg	0.4 mg/kg
24 min	4th bolus—replaces loss in 3rd $t^1/_2$	0.8 mg/kg	0.4 mg/kg
	Total body load	3.9 mg/kg	2.1 mg/kg

*Based on Loading dose = volume of distribution × desired plasma concentration = 1.32 L/kg × 3 μg/ml = 3.9 mg/kg.

of 8 minutes. After 8 minutes the level should fall to 1.5 μg/ml in the central compartment and then decline to 1.5 μg/ml because half of the initial dose (50 mg) has distributed into the peripheral compartment. Replacement with a 50-mg injection should return the concentration to 3 μg/ml. If no additional loading dose were given at this time, the plasma concentration would fall below the usual therapeutic range. The maintenance dose should accumulate to reach the therapeutic range in several hours. However, during this period the patient's arrhythmia may recur and the patient may be mistakenly labeled "refractory" to lidocaine. As shown in Table 11-1, a series of loading injections every 8 minutes will prevent the plasma concentration from falling below the usual therapeutic range and thereby prevent the patient from becoming vulnerable to the development of lethal arrhythmias. Table 11-2 displays a simplified version of this approach that is easy to remember and appropriate for most patients of average size. Both Tables 11-1 and 11-2 list the reduction in loading doses necessary for patients with heart failure in whom the volume of distribution is usually reduced to 50 percent of normal.

Another effective and well-tolerated loading regimen was outlined by Wyman et al. [63]: For a 75-kg person, an initial bolus of 75 mg is given, followed by 50 mg every 5 minutes to a total dose of 225 mg. This regimen usually achieves and maintains plasma concentrations within the usual guidelines (1.5 to 5.0 μg/ml). A priming dose of 75 mg (1 mg/kg) followed by a loading infusion of 150 mg (2 mg/kg) over 18 minutes also has been used successfully [62].

It must be emphasized that these guidelines are based on average values and there is a large variance in the distribution and elimination of lidocaine. For example, the volume of the central compartment varies from 33 to 60 liters. This means that the peak plasma concentration after a bolus injection will vary up to twofold in normal individuals. For this reason, one should choose the lower value of 33 liters to calculate the initial loading bolus dose. Awareness of this variability is essential and requires that the patient be evaluated continuously while receiving lidocaine. During the loading process, the patient's cardiogram, blood pressure, and mental status should be monitored, and at the first sign of excessive lidocaine administration, the loading process should be stopped.

Maintenance Therapy

The selection of a maintenance dose is based on the concept that at steady state the amount of drug cleared from the body must be replaced. If we know the volume of plasma cleared of drug per minute (clearance) and the plasma concentration (target), multiplication of these values yields the mass of drug cleared per minute. Tables 11-3 and 11-4 demonstrate how this calculation can guide the selection of an infusion rate that can be individualized for patients with heart failure or liver disease. Table 11-3 lists the calculated dosages based on body weight in kilograms and Table 11-4 gives a simplified dosing regimen estimated for an average 75-kg adult. A maintenance infusion designed to replace ongoing losses due to drug elimination should be started in the range of 15 to 60 μg/kg/min (1 to 4 mg/min). If symptomatic arrhythmias persist in the face of an adequate loading dosage (as assessed by

Table 11-2
Lidocaine load for average patient

Time	0	8 min	16 min	24 min
Normal patient	100 mg	50 mg	50 mg	50 mg
Patient with congestive heart failure	50 mg	25 mg	25 mg	25 mg

Stop load for: CNS symptoms, hypotension, heart block, or bradycardia

Table 11-3
Protocol to maintain plasma lidocaine concentration of 3 μg/ml*

Patient	Infusion rate
Normal (clearance = 10 ml/min/kg)	30 μg/kg/min
Heart failure (clearance = 6 ml/min/kg)	18 μg/kg/min

*Based on Dose = desired plasma concentration × clearance. For example, dose = 3 μg/ml × 10 ml/min/kg = 30 μg/kg/min.

Table 11-4
Lidocaine maintenance therapy for average patients

Normal patients	2–3 mg/min	*or*	30 μg/kg/min
Heart failure	1–3 mg/min	*or*	19 μg/kg/min
Liver disease	0.5–1.0 mg/min	*or*	10 μg/kg/min

plasma concentrations of more than 7 μg/ml, or the presence of side effects, or both), other agents should be used.

Regardless of the loading regimen employed, the lidocaine concentration eventually reached at steady state is dependent only on the drug infusion rate and clearance. The time required to reach steady-state conditions is four to five elimination half-lives (approximately 8 to 10 hours in normal individuals). If the plasma concentration achieved at steady state is excessive, symptoms of lidocaine toxicity (most notably cardiac conduction and central nervous system disturbances) may occur many hours after the initiation of effective therapy and may be misinterpreted as "CCU psychosis." On the other hand, if the eventual steady-state level is too low, many hours after the institution of seemingly effective therapy, arrhythmia may recur, and it may be misinterpreted as "lidocaine resistance." Assuming that side effects are absent, the appropriate action is the following: (1) If the patient's clinical condition permits, obtain a plasma sample for measurement of lidocaine concentration (for future reference); (2) administer a small bolus (25 to 50 mg over 2 minutes); and (3) increase the maintenance infusion rate by 25 to 50 percent. Increasing the maintenance infusion rate without the incremental bolus may not lead to effective plasma concentrations until 8 to 10 hours later. If the arrhythmia recurs before steady state has been reached, it might be advisable to simply administer a bolus and keep the same maintenance infusion. Again, plasma level monitoring assists in these decisions.

The practice of "tapering" lidocaine infusion rates is based on the misconception that lidocaine is eliminated rapidly. In fact, the rapid dissipation of lidocaine's effects early after an intravenous bolus is due to distribution, not elimination. Once steady-state conditions have been achieved, terminating a lidocaine infusion results in a gradual decline in plasma levels over the next 8 to 10 hours as elimination occurs. Not only is there no reason to taper lidocaine infusions, if oral antiarrhythmic therapy is to be initiated, tapering prolongs the period during which unpredictable additive effects may occur between lidocaine and newly initiated oral therapy. Likewise, tapering makes it difficult to predict when lidocaine levels have fallen below the range expected to be effective.

It is possible to predict when the plasma lidocaine concentration will fall below usually therapeutic levels by determining the plasma lidocaine concentration at the time the infusion is terminated and calculating the half-life from the equation in Figure 11-4 and estimating the number of half-lives required for the concentration to fall to approximately 1.5 μg/ml.

Modification of Dosage in Disease States

The effects of heart, liver, and renal disease on lidocaine disposition were reported by Thomson et al. [18]. Initial loading regimens are dependent on volume of distribution and should be decreased by about 50 percent in the presence of heart failure, whereas no adjustment is necessary for renal or liver disease. Clearance is decreased by approximately 40 percent in the presence of heart failure or liver disease; therefore intravenous maintenance infusions must be decreased in the presence of these disease states. It is important to note that in the presence of congestive heart failure, both the central volume of distribution *and* clearance are decreased; therefore elimination half-life is often unchanged

Fig. 11-4
Estimation of the half-life of lidocaine. By determining the plasma concentration of lidocaine at the time an infusion is terminated, one can estimate the time needed to reach the lower limit of the therapeutic range. V_d = volume of distribution; $t_{1/2}$ = half-life. (From R. L. Woosley. Lidocaine therapy. *Cardiac Impulse* 8:No. 2, 1987. With permission.)

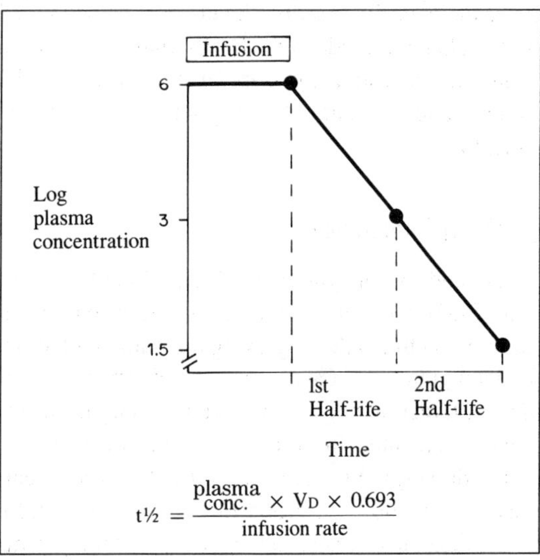

from that found in normal individuals (see earlier discussion on clearance). Thus the time required to achieve steady-state conditions following institution of a maintenance infusion is still often 8 to 10 hours, even in the presence of congestive heart failure (but plasma concentrations will be higher due to reduced clearance and volume of distribution). Conversely, because clearance is predominantly altered in liver disease, with little change in the volume of distribution, the half-life of elimination is markedly prolonged (almost 5 hours) and steady-state conditions are not achieved until 20 to 25 hours after institution of an intravenous infusion. Despite the fact that lidocaine metabolites are excreted by the kidneys, renal disease has not been reported to exert any significant effect on lidocaine dosing regimens, although binding of lidocaine to plasma proteins is decreased in patients with chronic renal failure.

In post–myocardial infarction patients receiving lidocaine infusions for more than 24 hours, plasma lidocaine levels can increase and the elimination phase half-life can show a marked increase (to over 3 hours) [64]. The mechanism by which it occurs is poorly understood. Suggestions include inhibition of lidocaine metabolism by accumulation of metabolites or changes in lidocaine binding to plasma proteins, perhaps due to changes in acute-phase reactants such as AAG [30]. Monitoring lidocaine concentrations in patients remaining on therapy for more than 24 to 48 hours may help detect the patients with increasing drug concentrations. However, because AAG levels may be higher in these patients, the free drug level may be unchanged and higher total lidocaine levels may actually be required and tolerated. Careful evaluation of the patient and the patient's response to therapy is essential.

Drug Interactions

An additive or synergistic depression of myocardial function or intracardiac conduction may occur during combined therapy using lidocaine with other antiarrhythmic agents [65]. A pharmacokinetic drug interaction between propranolol and lidocaine was documented in an anesthetized dog in which beta-adrenergic blockade caused a decrease in cardiac output and liver blood flow. As a result, lidocaine clearance was reduced, and lidocaine plasma concentrations were subsequently increased [66]. A similar phenomenon was noted in humans [67].

Cimetidine reportedly decreases lidocaine's volume of distribution, decreases splanchnic (and hence liver) blood flow, and inhibits the enzymes responsible for lidocaine deethylation. All three effects serve to raise lidocaine plasma concentrations, and both loading and maintenance dosages may require downward adjustment in patients receiving cimetidine [68].

Occasionally patients have an excellent response to lidocaine but with continued therapy fail to respond. One possible explanation could be a decrease in free levels of lidocaine caused by increases in the concentration of AAG. However, another possibility was proposed by Bennett et al. [69]. These authors found that a major metabolite of lidocaine, glycine xylidide, under certain in vitro conditions can antagonize sodium channel blockade produced by lidocaine. Such interactions call attention to the structurally specific interactions of drugs and metabolites that can occur at the receptor that regulates sodium channel function.

Procainamide

Indications

Procainamide is effective acute parenteral therapy for ventricular arrhythmias and, unlike lidocaine, can be administered orally. Procainamide also has electrophysiologic characteristics that make it useful for the treatment of supraventricular tachyarrhythmias. However, as is the case with all drugs that prolong cardiac repolarization (procainamide, quinidine, disopyramide, and sotalol), procainamide should not be used in patients with a long QT interval syndrome, hypokalemia, or a history of torsades de pointes because of the possibility of arrhythmia aggravation.

Pharmacology

The major effects of procainamide (and quinidine or disopyramide) on atrial tissue, ventricular muscle, and Purkinje fibers are prolongation of the APD and refractoriness, a decrease in phase 4 depolarization (automaticity) in pacemaker cells, and a decrease in conduction velocity [70]. In patients, intravenous procainamide increased the ventricular

ERP (VERP) as well as the ratio of VERP to the QT interval; the increase in this ratio might account for procainamide's efficacy in suppressing reentrant tachyarrhythmias [71]. Procainamide also might prolong conduction in depressed portions of reentrant pathways, thereby creating bidirectional block and terminating tachycardia [72].

Procainamide can convert atrial flutter or fibrillation to sinus rhythm; however, patients with atrial flutter should usually receive digitalis or other AV nodal blockers prior to therapy with any of the antiarrhythmic drugs. In the nondigitalized patient these agents may actually precipitate an increase in ventricular response. This increase is probably due to a combination of a direct drug effect, slowing of the flutter rate (which had been maintaining the AV node in a refractory state), and an indirect anticholinergic action accelerating conduction across the AV node.

When procainamide was administered to 16 patients with intraventricular conduction delay, AH intervals did not change, but HV intervals increased by a mean of 18 percent. Procainamide-induced sinus node depression was noted in one of these patients [73].

Absorption, Distribution, Metabolism, and Elimination

Absorption of procainamide is rapid and almost complete (75 to 90 percent) following oral administration. However, because of differences in rate of absorption coupled with rapid elimination, plasma concentrations vary widely within a group of patients. Plasma concentration monitoring, as will be discussed, can help guide dosage selection [24], although it is essential to remember that plasma concentration monitoring data must be interpreted with caution, as procainamide undergoes conversion to a potentially active metabolite.

Following intravenous administration, procainamide, like lidocaine, follows a two-compartment, open kinetic model. However, the concentration in plasma may not directly reflect the myocardial effects. Galeazzi et al. [74] showed a dissociation between QT interval prolongation and plasma procainamide concentration during the first 6 hours after acute intravenous administration. Late production of NAPA, a potent blocker of potassium channels, may be responsible for the change in QT interval. NAPA has little, if any, effect on sodium channels and therefore has a very different electrophysiologic profile than its parent.

Approximately 15 to 50 percent of a dose of procainamide is metabolized by hepatic *N*-acetyltransferase to NAPA. The presence of this metabolic pathway is genetically determined and is expressed in a bimodal distribution in humans [23]. Approximately 45 percent of Caucasian and 20 percent of Oriental populations have deficient *N*-acetyltransferase activity and are slow acetylators of procainamide and several other drugs. In rapid acetylators, most of a procainamide dose is converted to NAPA, and the plasma concentration of NAPA exceeds that of procainamide at steady state. NAPA is eliminated almost exclusively by the kidneys. The mean elimination half-life of procainamide is 3.5 hours in patients with normal renal and hepatic function, and the elimination half-life of NAPA is approximately 6 to 8 hours. Half-lives of both compounds are prolonged in patients with diminished creatinine clearance.

To achieve an antiarrhythmic effect, a procainamide plasma level of at least 4 μg/ml is needed for most patients [24]. An increase in both the incidence and the severity of side effects, primarily gastrointestinal symptoms, is seen when plasma concentrations exceed 8 to 10 μg/ml. Plasma concentrations of NAPA are variable but are usually about equal to those of procainamide. Individuals with normal renal function and plasma NAPA-procainamide ratios of more than 1 can be defined as rapid acetylators of procainamide. NAPA has been administered to patients with arrhythmias, and its "therapeutic range" appears to be between 9 and 19 μg/ml [22]. Side effects are common during NAPA therapy, and some of the adverse effects during chronic procainamide administration are probably due to the presence of this metabolite.

Plasma concentrations or procainamide and NAPA should be monitored under certain circumstances. In patients with renal failure, NAPA accumulates and may be the compound responsible for therapeutic effect or toxicity [26]. In rapid acetylators, excessive NAPA concentrations may be responsible for side effects, or the combined concentrations of parent drug and metabolite may produce toxicity. Because of their different pharmacologic actions, the concentrations must be considered separately and not together as some have advocated.

Toxicity

The major dose-related side effects accompanying oral procainamide therapy are gastrointestinal symptoms. Excessively rapid intravenous administration can cause hypotension, possibly due to ganglionic blockade, and depression of myocardial contractility as well as heart block.

The drug-induced lupus erythematosus syndrome is the most common severe reaction during chronic procainamide therapy. It occurs earlier and more frequently in slow acetylators of procainamide [75], and virtually any of the symptoms usually associated with systemic lupus erythematosus (e.g., rash, pericarditis, arthritis) may be present (although nephritis is exceedingly rare). The syndrome resolves if procainamide therapy is stopped. One hypothesis suggests that procainamide is oxidatively transformed into a reactive metabolite, which then interacts with nuclear histone protein and elicits antinuclear antibody formation [76]. This theory is supported by the observation that patients who are able to rapidly acetylate the drug are relatively protected. Another line of evidence suggesting that acetylation is a protective pathway is that patients who have developed symptomatic drug-induced lupus erythematosus during chronic procainamide therapy can experience a remission during NAPA therapy [22]. Although virtually all patients receiving therapeutic dosages of procainamide for more than a year develop antinuclear antibodies, it alone is not an indication to stop procainamide therapy because only about 20 percent of patients develop the lupus syndrome. Procainamide therapy has been associated with the development of agranulocytosis (0.2 percent incidence), and the manufacturer recommends careful monitoring of white blood cell counts after initiating therapy.

Dosage and Administration

Procainamide can be administered intravenously or orally. When procainamide is used for the acute treatment of ventricular or supraventricular tachyarrhythmias, intravenous administration using a loading regimen is preferred. If the situation is less urgent, a maintenance oral dosage can be started without a "loading dose."

Loading regimens for procainamide (500 to 1000 mg) are administered either in boluses of 100 mg every 5 minutes [77] or as a constant-rate infusion at 250 to 300 μg/kg/min [78]. Close monitoring of the patient's ECG, blood pressure, and pulse is mandatory during loading. If no antiarrhythmic effect is seen after 1000 mg of procainamide has been administered, a further 500 mg can be given if no hypotension or excessive QRS or QT interval prolongation is present. Although it is unlikely that dosages of more than 1.5 gm will produce an antiarrhythmic effect when lower doses have failed, plasma concentrations should be checked to ensure that adequate drug has been given. Depending on cardiac and renal function, the maintenance dose is 15 to 60 μg/kg/min administered as a continuous intravenous infusion. Because the elimination half-life varies from 3 to 5 hours, steady-state conditions are approached within 12 to 25 hours, regardless of the loading regimen used. Thus it is possible that many hours after the institution of effective therapy with a loading dose, plasma concentrations may reach either excessive or subtherapeutic levels. In addition, 48 hours or more may be required for maximum accumulation of NAPA.

If conversion to oral procainamide therapy is desired, it should be remembered that procainamide is rapidly absorbed from the gastrointestinal tract. Adverse effects due to excessive plasma concentrations may develop if an oral dose is given too early after the intravenous infusion is stopped. The appropriate approach in this situation is to determine the plasma concentration and estimate the appropriate time to wait after stopping the intravenous infusion before starting a chronic oral dosing regimen without a loading dose (because loading has already been accomplished). Because of the relatively narrow margin between therapeutic and toxic effects, and because of relatively rapid elimination, procainamide must be given every 6 hours in a sustained-release formulation. The initial dosage is 500 mg every 6 to 8 hours and is adjusted upward as necessary, guided by antiarrhythmic effects, the occurrence of side effects, and plasma concentration monitoring.

Modification of Dosage in Disease States

For patients with acute myocardial infarction, procainamide loading doses generally should be lower than for normal individuals, and maintenance dosages also must be reduced to avoid accumulation to toxic levels. Although the half-life, and therefore the time to steady state, is not markedly different in these patients, total body clearance is reduced up to 40 percent, suggesting a concomitant decrease in volume of distribution [79]. Similar dosage reductions appear to be necessary in patients with heart failure. With renal disease, there is a reduction in the elimination of both procainamide and NAPA. Maintenance dosages must be decreased, and often doses of procainamide as low as 375 mg can be administered every 8 to 12 hours with an antiarrhythmic effect in these individuals, possibly due to NAPA accumulation [26].

Drug Interactions

In an experimental setting, the combination of lidocaine and procainamide exerts synergistic adverse hemodynamic effects (disproportionate hypotension) [65]. This problem has particular relevance for therapy in the CCU where patients refractory to the first drug chosen may require additional antiarrhythmic therapy.

Bretylium

Indications

Bretylium is indicated for the treatment of recurrent ventricular fibrillation, or ventricular tachycardia in an intensive care or coronary care setting [80]. Intravenous administration appears to act within minutes to suppress ventricular fibrillation, although in some patients there may be a delay of 20 minutes to 2 hours in the onset of antiarrhythmic action. This delay may be due to use of initial dosages lower than needed for an antiarrhythmic effect or delayed attainment of adequate myocardial tissue levels. Of particular interest are reports that bretylium can effectively reverse ventricular tachyarrhythmias refractory to lidocaine following myocardial infarction [81, 82]. Moreover, Holder et al. [83] reported bretylium to be effective in 20 of 27 patients with ventricular fibrillation refractory not only to lidocaine but to DC countershock, with 12 of these 20 patients surviving to be discharged from the hospital. Rapid bretylium injection alone, in the absence of cardioversion, restored sinus rhythm in five of seven patients with ventricular fibrillation [84].

Pharmacology

Following intravenous administration, bretylium exerts two distinct pharmacologic actions on the autonomic nervous system. It is initially taken into adrenergic neurons via a norepinephrine pump. This action produces release of norepinephrine, resulting in tachycardia, hypertension, and occasionally increased arrhythmias. Following this brief phase (usually <15 minutes but occasionally longer) further release of norepinephrine is blocked, and orthostatic hypotension is commonly present. A third effect is due to bretylium's potassium channel–blocking action, which prolongs APD and the effective refractory period, thereby decreasing dispersion of refractoriness, particularly between normal and infarcted tissue [85]. Bretylium can also hyperpolarize Purkinje fibers that have low resting potentials [86], with a resultant increase in conduction velocity. It is unclear which of these many actions are responsible for its clinical efficacy; however, there is evidence in patients that the adrenergic neuron–blocking effect and the antiarrhythmic effect of bretylium can be dissociated in some patients [87].

Absorption, Distribution, Metabolism, and Elimination

Bretylium is usually administered by intravenous infusion. It is eliminated by the kidneys without undergoing metabolism [88], with an elimination half-life (following intravenous dosage) calculated to be 13.6 hours. A description of the time course of myocardial drug accumulation and antifibrillatory effects following intravenous dosage in dogs demonstrated a parallel between electrophysiologic effects and myocardial drug concentrations, with peak effects occurring 3 to 6 hours after an intravenous bolus [89]. A therapeutic range of bretylium plasma concentrations (which would parallel myocardial drug concentrations once steady state was achieved) has not been established.

Toxicity

Adverse effects during bretylium administration are usually a direct consequence and extension of its pharmacologic actions. Thus transient hypertension, tachycardia, and arrhythmia worsening are occasionally seen closely following intravenous administration, and orthostatic hypotension is almost universally present a few minutes later. Bretylium does not adversely affect cardiac output or left ventricular filling pressure in patients with recent myocardial infarction [90]. Although bretylium decreases pulmonary vascular resistance, it increased pulmonary vascular resistance in patients with mitral valve disease following surgery [91]. Excessively rapid intravenous administration has been associated with nausea and vomiting; these effects can be reduced or prevented by decreasing the rate of administration. Postural hypotension can be managed most easily by leaving the patient in the supine position. If supine hypotension develops, the treatment of choice is volume expansion: patients receiving bretylium therapy are in a functionally denervated state and may be particularly sensitive to exogenous pressor agents such as dobutamine or norepinephrine.

Dosage and Administration

Like lidocaine and procainamide, bretylium should be administered intravenously with a loading regimen followed by a maintenance infusion. Bretylium's pharmacokinetics have not been intensively studied, and dose-response relations have not been clearly identified because of the difficult nature of the clinical setting in which it is used; hence exact dosing regimens have not been worked out. Additionally, as noted already, maximal antifibrillatory effects may not be obvious for several hours following the institution of therapy. One intravenous loading regimen involves administration of 5 to 10 mg/kg over 15 to 30 minutes followed by maintenance infusions of 2 to 4 mg/min. If rhythm control is not established, further loading doses (up to a total of 20 to 30 mg/kg) can be administered. The patient should be supine while bretylium is administered; hypotension is not an indication to stop therapy because although very low dosages block autonomic neuron function, higher dosages are required for an antiarrhythmic effect. Bretylium has also been administered intramuscularly with intermittent injections. However, this method is not recommended because absorption is uncertain and injection sites must be varied to avoid tissue necrosis.

Modifications in Disease States

Bretylium clearance is markedly reduced in the presence of renal disease [92] and the drug should be administered in the lowest effective dosage in patients with renal insufficiency. No data are available on dosage adjustments required in other conditions such as congestive heart failure or liver disease, but it is unlikely that the dosage should be adjusted for these individuals. Bretylium therapy should be avoided in patients in whom a marked drop in systemic vascular resistance may be deleterious (e.g., those with valvular aortic stenosis) and in those with pulmonary hypertension.

Drug Interactions

Because of the initial norepinephrine release induced by bretylium and the attendant risk of worsening arrhythmias, bretylium should probably be administered with caution to patients who are receiving digitalis. Once norepinephrine uptake by adrenergic neurons is blocked, a state of functional denervation hypersensitivity exists; and at this stage patients are sensitive to exogenous pressor amines. Because reversal of the antiadrenergic actions allows arrhythmia recurrence in some individuals, further evaluation of this observation in a larger patient population is needed before it is widely adopted. The interaction between bretylium and tricyclic antidepressants has already been discussed (see Pharmacology).

Beta-Adrenergic Receptor–Blocking Agents

One of the most significant advances in cardiovascular therapy was the conclusion of a number of large-scale clinical trials of drugs evaluating beta-receptor antagonists in the post–myocardial infarction population. In well-conducted, double-blind, placebo-controlled trials, timolol, propranolol, metoprolol, alprenolol, and practolol decreased the incidence of recurrent myocardial infarction and sudden cardiac death by 25 to 50 percent [10–13]. This effect does not appear to be related to the characteristics that differ among these drugs such as membrane stabilization and cardioselectivity. Although some early therapeutic trials using beta-receptor antagonists showed variable effects on the recurrence of myocardial infarction and sudden cardiac death, those results most likely reflected inadequate dosages or poor study design. It is important, therefore, that the practicing physician be aware of the dosages and patient subsets that produced results in these trials. Clearly, use of any other agent or of any other dosage of these agents remains of unproved value. Although the mechanism by which these drugs exert a protective action remains speculative, there is no question that beta-receptor antagonists can exert antiarrhythmic effects in certain settings, but it is equally possible that these agents exert their protective actions through some other mechanism. A number of trials also studied the effects of early intervention with beta-adrenergic receptor–blocking drugs in an attempt to modify infarct size. Early treatment with metoprolol (15 mg intravenously followed by 100 mg orally twice daily thereafter) was studied by Hjalmarson [10], who found a 36 percent reduction in mortality due to sudden cardiac death. Use of beta-receptor antagonists soon after myocardial infarction is currently accepted as being of benefit to patients who can tolerate these agents (i.e., those with reasonably good left ventricular function). The use of beta-adrenergic receptor antagonists for ventricular tachycardia during the early myocardial infarction period should be discouraged.

Magnesium

The role of magnesium in acute coronary care has been the focus of research in recent years. Until recently, most considered magnesium therapy to be effective only when deficiency was at the root of arrhythmia. However, in vitro studies indicated that magnesium had calcium channel–blocking activity and suggested a primary therapeutic role in certain arrhythmias [93]. When administered in pharmacologic concentrations, magnesium demonstrated multiple actions that may benefit patients with acute myocardial infarction. These include reduction in ventricular and supraventricular arrhythmias, systemic and coronary vasodilation, decreased platelet aggregation, improved myocardial metabolism, and reduction of myocardial infarct size [93]. These observations served as the impetus for several small clinical trials that suggested that early mortality could be decreased in patients with suspected myocardial infarction [94]. The results of these trials, performed in the prethrombolytic era, were grouped in two meta-analyses [95, 96] that further strengthened the impression that intravenous magnesium would be a safe and effective way to reduce mortality after acute myocardial infarction.

In 1992, the results of the prospective second Leicester Intravenous Magnesium Intervention Trial (LIMIT-2) were published [97]. In this study, 2316 patients with suspected acute myocardial infarction received either intravenous magnesium sulfate (8 mmol over 5 minutes followed by 65 mmol over 24 hours) or normal saline solution. The primary outcome measure was 28-day mortality, which was 7.8 percent in the treatment group and 10.3 percent in the placebo group. Magnesium was protective in all subgroups of patients, including the 35 percent who received thrombolytics.

However, more recently, the results of the fourth International Study of Infarct Survival (ISIS-4) became available [98]. In this study, 75 percent of patients received fibrinolytics and no benefit from magnesium therapy was noted. This raised questions regarding the exact role of magnesium in the thrombolytic era, although favorable reports continue to appear [99].

Calcium Channel Antagonists

Clinical trials have evaluated the acute short-term use of the calcium channel–blocking agents nifedipine, verapamil, and diltiazem. These agents were given within hours after the onset of suspected myocardial infarction and generally demonstrated no beneficial influence on infarct size, progression to acute myocardial infarction, or mortality [100, 101].

References

1. Harrison, D. C. Should lidocaine be administered routinely to all patients after acute myocardial infarction? (Editorial). *Circulation* 58:581, 1978.
2. MacMahon, S., Collins, R., Peto, R., et al. Effects of prophylactic lidocaine in suspected acute myocardial infarction. *J.A.M.A.* 260:1910, 1988.
3. Antmann, E. M., and Berlin, J. A. Declining incidence of ventricular fibrillation in myocardial infarction. Implications for the prophylactic use of lidocaine. *Circulation* 86:764, 1992.
4. CAST Investigators. Preliminary report: Effect of encainide and flecainide on mortality in a random-

ized trial of arrhythmia suppression after myocardial infarction. *N. Engl. J. Med.* 321:406, 1989.

5. CAST-II Investigators. Effect of the antiarrhythmic agent moricizine on survival after myocardial infarction. *N. Engl. J. Med.* 327:227, 1992.
6. Jaffe, A. S. Prophylactic lidocaine for suspected acute myocardial infarction. *Heart Dis. Stroke* 1: 179, 1992.
7. Woosley, R. L., Reele, S. B., Roden, D. M., et al. Pharmacologic reversal of hypotensive effect complicating antiarrhythmic therapy with bretylium. *Clin. Pharmacol. Ther.* 32:313, 1982.
8. Mason, J. W., and ESVEM Investigators. A comparison of seven antiarrhythmic drugs in patients with ventricular tachyarrhythmias. *N. Engl. J. Med.* 329:452, 1993.
9. Epstein, A. E. AVID necessity. *PACE Pacing Clin. Electrophysiol.* 16:1773, 1993.
10. Hjalmarson, A. Early intervention with a beta-blocking drug after acute myocardial infarction. *Am. J. Cardiol.* 54(Suppl):11E, 1984.
11. Hansteen, V. Beta blockade after myocardial infarction: The Norwegian propranolol study in high-risk patients. *Circulation* 67:157, 1983.
12. Beta-blocker Heart Attack Trial Research Group. A randomized trial of propranolol in patients with acute myocardial infarction: I. Mortality results. *J.A.M.A.* 247:1707, 1982.
13. Norwegian Multicenter Study Group. Timolol-induced reduction in mortality in reinfarction in patients surviving acute myocardial infarction. *N. Engl. J. Med.* 304:801, 1981.
14. Brachmann, J., Scherlag, B. J., Rosenshtraukh, L. V., and Lazzara, R. Bradycardia-dependent triggered activity: Relevance to drug-induced multiform ventricular tachycardia. *Circulation* 68:846, 1983.
15. Roden, D. M., and Hoffman, B. F. Action potential prolongation and induction of abnormal automaticity by low quinidine concentrations in canine Purkinje fibers. Relationship to potassium and cycle length. *Circ. Res.* 56:857, 1985.
16. Tzivoni, D., Keren, A., and Stern, S. Torsades de pointes versus polymorphous ventricular tachycardia (Editorial). *Am. J. Cardiol.* 52:639, 1983.
17. Woosley, R. L. Antiarrhythmic drugs. In R. C. Schlant, R. W. Alexander, R. A. O'Rourke, et al. (eds.), *The Heart.* New York: McGraw-Hill, 1994. Pp. 775–805.
18. Thomson, P. D., Melmon, K. L., Richardson, J. A., et al. Lidocaine pharmacokinetics in advanced heart failure, liver disease and renal failure in humans. *Ann. Intern. Med.* 78:499, 1973.
19. Gianelly, R., von Der Groeben, J. O., Spivak, A. P., and Harrison, D. C. Effects of lidocaine on ventricular arrhythmias in patients with coronary heart disease. *N. Engl. J. Med.* 277:1215, 1967.
20. Anderson, J. L., Brodine, W. N., Patterson, E., et al. Serial electrophysiologic effects of bretylium in man and their correlation with plasma concentrations. *J. Cardiovasc. Pharmacol.* 4:871, 1982.
21. Heger, J. J., Solow, E. B., Prystowsky, E. N., and Zipes, D. P. Plasma and red blood cell concentrations of amiodarone during chronic therapy. *Am. J. Cardiol.* 53:912, 1984.
22. Roden, D. M., Reele, S. B., Higgins, S. B., et al. Antiarrhythmic efficacy, pharmacokinetics and safety of *N*-acetylprocainamide in human subjects: Comparison with procainamide. *Am. J. Cardiol.* 46:463, 1980.
23. Reidenberg, M. M., Drayer, D. E., Levy, M., and Warner, H. Polymorphic acetylation of procainamide in man. *Clin. Pharmacol. Ther.* 17:722, 1975.
24. Koch-Weser, J., and Klein, S. W. Procainamide dosage schedules, plasma concentrations, and clinical effects. *J.A.M.A.* 215:1454, 1971.
25. Alderman, E. L., Kerber, R. E., and Harrision, D. C. Evaluation of lidocaine resistance in man using intermittent large-dose infusion techniques. *Am. J. Cardiol.* 34:342, 1974.
26. Drayer, D. E., Lowenthal, D. T., Woosley, R. L., et al. Cumulation of *N*-acetylprocainamide, an active metabolite of procainamide, in patients with impaired renal function. *Clin. Pharmacol. Ther.* 22:63, 1977.
27. Funck-Brentano, C., Kroemer, H. K., Pavlou, H, et al. Genetically-determined interaction between propafenone and low dose quinidine: Role of active metabolites in modulating net drug effect. *Br. J. Clin. Pharmacol.* 27:435, 1989.
28. Barchowsky, A., Shand, D. G., Stargel, W. W., et al. On the role of alpha-1-acid glycoprotein in lignocaine accumulation following myocardial infarction. *Br. J. Clin. Pharmacol.* 13:411, 1982.
29. Routledge, P. A., Stargel, W. W., Wagner, G. S., et al. Increased alpha-1-acid glycoprotein and lidocaine disposition in myocardial infarction. *Ann. Intern. Med.* 93:701, 1980.
30. Routledge, P. A., Shand, D. G., Barchowsky, A., et al. Relationship between alpha 1-acid glycoprotein and lidocaine disposition in myocardial infarction. *Clin. Pharmacol. Ther.* 30:154, 1981.
31. Edwards, D. J., Axelson, J. E. E., Slaughter, R. L., et al. Factors affecting quinidine protein binding in man. *J. Pharm. Sci.* 73:1264, 1984.
32. Garfinkel, D., Mamelok, R. D., and Blaschke, T. F. Altered therapeutic range for quinidine after myocardial infarction and cardiac surgery. *Ann. Intern. Med.* 107:48, 1987.
33. Vaughan Williams, E. M. Classification of antiarrhythmic drugs. In E. Sandoe, E. Flensted-Jensen, and K. H. Olsen (eds.), *Symposium on Cardiac Arrhythmias.* Sodertalje, Sweden: Astra, 1970. Pp. 449–472.
34. Task Force of the Working Group on Arrhythmias of the European Society Cardiology. The Sicilian Gambit: A new approach to the classification of antiarrhythmic drugs based on their actions on arrhythmogenic mechanisms. *Circulation* 84:1831, 1991.
35. Hodgkin, A. L., and Huxley, A. F. A quantitative description of membrane current and its application

to conduction and excitation in nerve. *J. Physiol* 117:500, 1952.
36. Hille, B. Local anesthetics: Hydrophilic and hydrophobic pathways for the drug receptor reaction. *J. Gen. Physiol.* 69:497, 1977.
37. Hondeghem, L. M., and Katzung, B. G. Time- and voltage-dependent interactions of antiarrhythmic drugs with cardiac sodium channels. *Biochim. Biophys. Acta* 474:373, 1977.
38. Hondeghem, L. M., and Katzung, B. G. Test of a model of antiarrhythmic drug action: Effects of quinidine and lidocaine on myocardial conduction. *Circulation* 61:1217, 1980.
39. Duff, H. J., Mitchell, L. B., Manyari, D., and Wyse, D. G. Mexiletine-quinidine combination: Electrophysiologic correlates of a favorable antiarrhythmic interaction in humans. *J. Am. Coll. Cardiol.* 10: 1149, 1987.
40. Morganroth, J., and Horowitz, L. N. Flecainide: Its proarrhythmic effect and expected changes on the surface electrocardiogram. *Am. J. Cardiol.* 53(Suppl):89B, 1984.
41. Roden, D. M., Woosley, R. L., and Primm, R. K. Incidence and clinical features of the quinidine-associated long QT syndrome: Implications for patient care. *Am. Heart J.* 111:1088, 1986.
42. Bigger, J. T., Jr., and Mandel, W. J. Effect of lidocaine on the electrophysiological properties of ventricular muscle and Purkinje fibers. *J. Clin. Invest.* 49:63, 1970.
43. Davis, L. D., and Temte, J. V. Electrophysiological actions of lidocaine on canine ventricular muscle and Purkinje fibers. *Circ. Res.* 24:639, 1969.
44. Kupersmith, J. Electrophysiological and antiarrhythmic effects of lidocaine in canine acute myocardial ischemia. *Am. Heart J.* 97:360, 1979.
45. Gamble, O. W., and Cohn, K. Effect of propranolol, procainamide, and lidocaine on ventricular automaticity and reentry in experimental myocardial infarction. *Circulation* 46:498, 1972.
46. Carson, D. L., Cardinal, R. Savard, P. et al. Relationship between an arrhythmogenic action of lidocaine and its effects on excitation patterns in acutely ischemic porcine myocardium. *J. Cardiovasc. Pharmacol.* 8:126, 1986.
47. Patterson, E., Gibson, J. K., and Lucchesi, B. R. Electrophysiologic actions of lidocaine in a canine model of chronic myocardial ischemic injury—Arrhythmogenic actions of lidocaine. *Circulation* 64(Suppl):IV-123, 1981.
48. Adgey, A. A. J., Allen, J. D., Geddes, J. S., et al. Acute phase of myocardial infarction. *Lancet* 2:501, 1971.
49. Borer, J. S., Harrison, L. A., Kent, K. M., et al. Beneficial effect of lidocaine on ventricular electrical stability and spontaneous ventricular fibrillation during experimental myocardial infarction. *Am. J. Cardiol.* 37:860, 1976.
50. Spear, J. F., Moore, E. N., and Gerstenblith, G. Effect of lidocaine on the ventricular fibrillation threshold in the dog during acute ischemia and premature ventricular contractions. *Circulation* 46:65, 1972.
51. Mandel, W. J., and Bigger, J. T., Jr. Electrophysiologic effects of lidocaine on isolated canine and rabbit atrial tissue. *J. Pharmacol. Exp. Ther.* 178: 81, 1971.
52. Kunkel, F., Rowland, M., and Scheinman, M. M. The electrophysiologic effects of lidocaine in patients with intraventricular conduction defects. *Circulation* 49:894, 1974.
53. Bekheit, S., Murtagh, J. G., Morton, P., and Fletcher, E. Effect of lignocaine on conducting system of human heart. *Br. Heart J.* 35:305, 1973.
54. Gupta, P. K., Lichstein, E., and Chadda, K. D. Lidocaine-induced heart block in patients with bundle branch block. *Am. J. Cardiol.* 33:487, 1974.
55. Aravindakshan, V., Kuo, C.-S., and Gettes, L. S. Effect of lidocaine on escape rate in patients with complete atrioventricular block. *Am. J. Cardiol.* 40:177, 1977.
56. Cheng, T. O., and Wadhwa, K. Sinus standstill following intravenous lidocaine administration. *J.A.M.A.* 223:790, 1973.
57. Marriott, H. J. L., and Phillips, K. Profound hypotension and bradycardia after a single bolus of lidocaine. *J. Electrocardiol.* 7:79, 1974.
58. Josephson, M. E., Caracta, A. R., Lau, S. H., et al. Effects of lidocaine on refractory periods in man. *Am. Heart J.* 84:778, 1972.
59. Stenson, R. E., Constantino, R. T., and Harrison, D. C. Interrelationships of hepatic blood flow, cardiac output, and blood levels of lidocaine in man. *Circulation* 43:205, 1971.
60. Zito, R. A., and Reid, P. R. Lidocaine kinetics predicted by indocyanine green clearance. *N. Engl. J. Med.* 298:1160, 1978.
61. Benowitz, N. L. Clinical applications of the pharmacokinetics of lidocaine. *Cardiovasc. Clin.* 6:77, 1974.
62. Stargel, W. W., Shand, D. G., Routledge, P. A., et al. Clinical comparison of rapid infusion and multiple injection methods for lidocaine loading. *Am. Heart J.* 102:872, 1981.
63. Wyman, M. G., Slaughter, R. L., Farolino, D. A., et al. Multiple bolus technique for lidocaine administration in acute ischemic heart disease. II. Treatment of refractory ventricular arrhythmias and the pharmacokinetic significance of severe left ventricular failure. *J. Am. Coll. Cardiol.* 2:764, 1983.
64. LeLorier, J., Grenon, D., Latour, Y. Pharmacokinetics of lidocaine after prolonged intravenous infusions in uncomplicated myocardial infarction. *Ann. Intern. Med.* 87:700, 1977.
65. Cote, P., Harrison, D. C., Basile, J., and Schroeder, J. S. Hemodynamic interaction of procainamide and lidocaine after experimental myocardial infarction. *Am. J. Cardiol.* 32:937, 1973.
66. Branch, R. A., Shand, D. G., Wilkinison, G. R., and Nies, A. S. The reduction of lidocaine clearance by *dl*-propranolol: An example of hemodynamic

drug interaction. *J. Pharmacol. Exp. Ther.* 184: 515, 1973.

67. Ochs, H. R., Carstens, G., and Greenblatt, D. J. Reduction in lidocaine clearance during continuous infusion and by coadministration of propranolol. *N. Engl. J. Med.* 303:373, 1980.
68. Feeley, J., Wilkinson, G. R., McAllister, C. B., and Wood, A. J. J. Increased toxicity and reduced clearance of lidocaine by cimetidine. *Ann. Intern. Med.* 96:592, 1982.
69. Bennett, P. B., Woosley, R. L., and Hondeghem, L. M. Competition between lidocaine and one of its metabolites, glycylxylidide, for cardiac sodium channels. *Circulation* 78:692, 1988.
70. Hoffman, B. F., Rosen, M. R., and Wit, A. L. Electrophysiology and pharmacology of cardiac arrhythmias. VII. Cardiac effects of quinidine and procaine amide. *Am. Heart J.* 90:117, 1975.
71. Kastor, J. A., Josephson, M. E., Guss, S. B., and Horowitz, L. N. Human ventricular refractoriness. II. Effects of procainamide. *Circulation* 56:462, 1977.
72. Giardina, E.-G. V., and Bigger, J. T., Jr. Procaine amide against re-entrant ventricular arrhythmias. *Circulation* 48:959, 1973.
73. Scheinman, M. M., Weiss, A. N., Shafton, E., et al. Electrophysiological effects of procaine amide in patients with intraventricular conduction delay. *Circulation* 49:522, 1974.
74. Galeazzi, R. L., Benet, L. Z., and Scheiner, L. B. Relationship between the pharmacokinetics and pharmacodynamics of procainamide. *Clin. Pharmacol. Ther.* 20:278, 1976.
75. Woosley, R. L., Drayer, D. E., Reidenberg, M. M., et al. Effect of acetylator phenotype on the rate at which procainamide induces antinuclear antibodies and the lupus syndrome. *N. Engl. J. Med.* 298: 1157, 1978.
76. Freeman, R. W., Uetrecht, J. P., Woosley, R. L., et al. Covalent binding of procainamide in vitro and in vivo to hepatic protein in mice. *Drug Metab. Dispos.* 9:188, 1981.
77. Giardina, E.-G.V., Heissenbuttel, R. H., and Bigger, J. T., Jr. Intermittent intravenous procainamide to treat ventricular arrhythmias. Correlation of plasma concentration with effect on arrhythmia, electrocardiogram and blood pressure. *Ann. Intern. Med.* 78:183, 1973.
78. Funck-Brentano, C., Light, R. T., Lineberry, M. D., et al. Pharmacokinetic and pharmacodynamic interaction of *N*-acetyl procainamide and procainamide in humans. *J. Cardiovasc. Pharmacol.* 14:364, 1989.
79. Lalka, D., Wyman, M. G., Goldreyer, B. N., et al. Procainamide accumulation kinetics in the immediate post-myocardial infarction period. *J. Clin. Pharmacol.* 18:397, 1978.
80. Koch-Weser, J. Drug therapy: Bretylium. *N. Engl. J. Med.* 300:473, 1979.
81. Dhurandhar, R. W., Teasdale, S. J., and Mahon, W. A. Bretylium tosylate in the management of refractory ventricular fibrillation. *Can. Med. Assoc. J.* 105:161, 1971.
82. Terry, G., Vellani, C. W., Higgins, M. R., and Doig, A. Bretylium tosylate in treatment of refractory ventricular arrhythmias complicating myocardial infarction. *Br. Heart J.* 32:21, 1970.
83. Holder, D. A., Sniderman, A. D., Frazer, G., and Fallen, E. L. Experience with bretylium tosylate by a hospital cardiac arrest team. *Circulation* 55: 541, 1977.
84. Sanna, G., and Arcidiacono, R. Chemical ventricular defibrillation of the human heart with bretylium tosylate. *Am. J. Cardiol.* 32:982, 1973.
85. Cardinale, R., and Sasyniuk, B. I. Electrophysiological effects of bretylium tosylate on subendocardial Purkinje fibers from infarcted canine hearts. *J. Pharmacol. Exp. Ther.* 204:159, 1978.
86. Wit, A. L., Steiner, C., and Damato, A. N. Electrophysiologic actions of bretylium tosylate on single fibers of the canine specialized conducting system and ventricle. *J. Pharmacol. Exp. Ther.* 173:344, 1970.
87. Woosley, R. L., Reele, S. B., Roden, D. M., et al. Pharmacologic reversal of hypotensive effect complicating antiarrhythmic therapy with bretylium. *Clin. Pharmacol. Ther.* 32:313, 1982.
88. Anderson, J. L., Patterson, E., Wagner, J. G., et al. Oral and intravenous bretylium disposition. *Clin. Pharmacol. Ther.* 28:468, 1980.
89. Anderson, J. L., Patterson, E., Conlon, M., et al. Kinetics of antifibrillatory effects of bretylium: Correlation with myocardial drug concentrations. *Am. J. Cardiol.* 46:583, 1980.
90. Chatterjee, K., Mandel, W. J., Vyden, J. K., et al. Cardiovascular effects of bretylium tosylate in acute myocardial infarction. *J.A.M.A.* 233:757, 1973.
91. Cotev, S., Merin, G., Stern, S., et al. Effect of bretylium on the pulmonary and systemic circulation in patients with mitral valve disease after cardiopulmonary bypass. *J. Clin. Pharmacol.* 11:409, 1971.
92. Adir, J., Narang, P. K., Josselson, J., and Sadler, J. H. Pharmacokinetics of bretylium in renal insufficiency (Letter). *N. Engl. J. Med.* 300:1390, 1979.
93. Woods, K. L. Possible pharmacological actions of magnesium in acute myocardial infarction. *Br. J. Clin. Pharmacol.* 32:3, 1991.
94. Rasmussen, H. S., Norregard, P., Lindeneg, O., et al. Intravenous magnesium in acute myocardial infarction. *Lancet* 1:234, 1986.
95. Teo, K. K., Yusuf, S., Collins, R., et al. Effects of intravenous magnesium in suspected acute myocardial infarction: Overview of randomised trials. *B. M. J.* 303:1499, 1991.
96. Horner, S. M. Efficacy of intravenous magnesium in acute myocardial infarction in reducing arrhythmias and mortality. *Circulation* 86:774, 1992.
97. Woods, K. L., Fletcher, S., Roffe, C., and Haider,

Y. Intravenous magnesium sulphate in suspected acute myocardial infarction: Results of the Second Leicester Intravenous Magnesium Intervention Trial (LIMIT-2). *Lancet* 339:1553, 1992.
98. ISIS Collaborative Group. ISIS-4: Randomized study of intravenous magnesium in over 50,000 patients with suspected acute myocardial infarction. *Circulation* 88(4, Part 2):I-292, 1993.
99. Schechter, M., Hod, H., Kaplinsky, E., and Rabinowitz, B. Magnesium as alternative therapy in acute myocardial infarction patients unsuited for thrombolysis. *Circulation* 88(4, Part 2):I-395, 1993.
100. Multicenter Diltiazem Postinfarction Trial Research Group. The effect of diltiazem on mortality and reinfarction after myocardial infarction. *N. Engl. J. Med.* 319:385, 1988.
101. Furberg, C. D. Overview of completed sudden death trials: US experience. *Cardiology* 74:24, 1987.

12. Treatment of Supraventricular Arrhythmias in Acute Myocardial Infarction

Borys Surawicz and John D. Slack

To clarify the management of supraventricular arrhythmias associated with myocardial infarction, we must first recognize the general characteristics of these arrhythmias. Therefore, this topic is covered first, followed by a discussion of the mechanisms of the interventions that have been found to be useful for treating patients with these supraventricular arrhythmias. General guidelines for such treatment are then outlined, and finally specific first-line approaches to the management of the supraventricular arrhythmias in myocardial infarction patients are proposed.

Characteristics of Supraventricular Arrhythmias in Patients with Acute Myocardial Infarction

Sinus Tachycardia

Sinus tachycardia occurs in about one-third of patients [1], and is attributed to sympathetic overactivity, particularly when associated with hypertension [2]. Persistence of sinus tachycardia for more than several days usually signifies ventricular failure, and represents an unfavorable prognostic sign. [1]. Also, sinus tachycardia may be a precursor of primary ventricular fibrillation in the coronary care unit.

Bradycardia

Bradycardias that are secondary to atrioventricular (AV) conduction disturbances are discussed elsewhere in this book. The prevailing cause of bradyarrhythmias and the accompanying hypotension in patients with myocardial infarction is vagal hyperactivity [3]. In one study, bradycardia was present in 55 percent of patients seen within 30 minutes after the onset of acute myocardial infarction [2]. In several series of patients admitted to coronary care units, the incidence of sinus bradycardia ranged from 10 to 41 percent [1, 3].

Another cause of bradycardia is acute ischemia of the sinoatrial node that may follow occlusion of the right coronary or left circumflex artery proximal to the takeoff of the sinus node artery [3]. However, the incidence of sinus node dysfunction precipitated by coronary occlusion is low. In one study of 431 patients admitted to a coronary care unit, sinus node dysfunction was present in 4.6 percent [4], mostly in the presence of inferior wall myocardial infarction. In about two-thirds of these patients, sinus bradycardia subsided following treatment with atropine or temporary pacing [4]. The remaining had a less benign syndrome of tachycardia-bradycardia, frequently requiring continuing treatment with antiarrhythmic drugs or pacing or both. If needed, AV sequential pacing may improve hemodynamic parameters if ventricular pacing alone does not provide a satisfactory result [5]. The most common mechanism of tachycardia-bradycardia syndrome in these patients is a combination of a slow AV junctional escape rhythm with bouts of AV nodal reentrant tachycardia, atrial flutter, or atrial fibrillation. Unlike AV block, sinus bradycardia does not appear to predispose to ventricular fibrillation [6].

Acute reperfusion of the area of myocardial injury, either with thrombolytic agents or with percutaneous transluminal coronary angioplasty (PTCA), may provoke immediate brady-tachyarrhythmia, especially when the infarct-related vessel supplies the inferoposterior wall of the heart [7]. Often, significant hypotension accompanies these arrhythmias. This is attributed to stimulation of the myocardial mechanoreceptors (Bezold-Jarisch reflex).

Atrial Premature Complexes and Multiform Atrial Tachycardia

Isolated atrial premature complexes occur commonly in patients with acute myocardial infarction but because of a high prevalence of this arrhythmia in the general population, the role of myocardial infarction in their pathogenesis is not always obvious. Increasing frequency of atrial premature beats often heralds the onset of atrial fibrillation, and may require treatment with an agent that slows AV conduction or stabilizes the atrial rhythm (vide infra), particularly if the rapid heart rate worsens ischemia or contributes to hemodynamic instability.

Multiform atrial tachycardia, that is, a supraventricular tachycardia with P waves of variable morphology, may be due to a multifocal ectopic activity or to unifocal impulses with variable intra-atrial conduction. This arrhythmia occurs more frequently in elderly patients with chronic lung disease. In most patients with acute myocardial infarction, this arrhythmia lasts less than a few days but may be recurrent or chronic. Sometimes multiform atrial tachycardia evolves into atrial flutter or atrial fibrillation.

Monomorphic Atrial Tachycardia

Atrial tachycardia may be due to reentry but this mechanism is rare. A more commonly postulated mechanism of this arrhythmia is nontriggered or triggered automaticity. In patients with automatic ectopic atrial tachycardia, the onset is usually precipitated by a late atrial premature complex, the P-wave configuration of a tachycardia-initiating complex is identical to the P wave of succeeding complexes, and the PR interval is not prolonged. Afterward the cycle first shortens progressively (warm-up phenomenon) but once tachycardia becomes established, the PP intervals do not vary by more than 50 msec, unless an exit block is present. However, the rate of tachycardia tends to vary appreciably from day to day, being influenced by such factors as posture, exercise, and anxiety.

In two studies, the reported incidence of atrial tachycardia in patients with myocardial infarction ranged from 0 in 400 [8] to 32 (27 percent) of 119 [9]. In three other studies the incidence of transient atrial tachycardias was 4 to 8 [10], 3.8 [11], and 2 percent [12]. The variability of these values may be due to the differences in methodology of monitoring because brief and infrequent episodes can be readily missed. Another variable is the number of patients treated with digitalis, which is the most common factor precipitating this arrhythmia. The arrhythmia is usually benign, and is not associated with an increased incidence of congestive heart failure, pericarditis, or atrial infarction [9]. In one study [9], arrhythmia lasted longer than 5 minutes only in 3 of 32 patients. Because of the transient nature and short duration, treatment of this arrhythmia is seldom required.

Reentrant Atrioventricular Nodal Tachycardia

Tachycardias dependent on dual AV nodal conduction or a concealed AV bypass are uncommon in patients with acute myocardial infarction [3]. When present, the arrhythmias may contribute to hypotension and low cardiac output.

Nonparoxysmal Atrioventricular Junctional Tachycardia

This arrhythmia is attributed to an abnormal automaticity, or to triggered activity associated with delayed after-depolarizations, that is, a mechanism similar to AV junctional tachycardia associated with digitalis toxicity [13]. During routine monitoring, nonparoxysmal AV junctional tachycardia was found in 3 to 16 percent of patients [14–16]. However, continuous tape recording of patients in a coronary care unit revealed this arrhythmia in 12 (40 percent) of 30 patients during the first 24 hours [14]. Subsequently, the incidence decreased to 13 percent at 48 hours, and to 3 percent at 72 hours [14]. In this study, nonparoxysmal AV junctional tachycardia was associated with sinus arrhythmia. Although AV junctional tachycardia rarely produces changes in the clinical status [15], the arrhythmia appears to be an independent prognostic marker for cardiogenic shock [17]. The overall mortality of patients with nonparoxysmal junctional tachycardia is higher than in the remaining patients [14, 15]. The rate of tachycardia is more rapid and mortality is higher in patients with anterior than in those with inferior infarction [14, 15].

Atrial Flutter

Atrial flutter occurs as the first arrhythmia in 1 to 3 percent of patients with acute myocardial infarction [9, 11, 12]. Because of clinical deterioration associated with the persistence of this arrhythmia, intravenous drug administration or cardioversion is frequently indicated (Fig. 12-1) [11]. When diagnosis is uncertain, right atrial electrography may be helpful in confirming the diagnosis of atrial flutter. Also, the right atrial electrode can be used for atrial overdrive pacing to terminate the atrial flutter [18].

Atrial Fibrillation

Atrial fibrillation is the most common new supraventricular arrhythmia in patients with acute myocardial infarction. The reported incidence in different studies ranged from 5 to 18 percent [12, 19–24]. The higher figures usually include individuals with preexisting atrial fibrillation. The incidence of new atrial fibrillation is closer to about 5 percent [12, 19]. Atrial fibrillation usually appears during the first 48 to 72 hours [22, 23] and in 90 percent of patients within the first 4 days [11], but is believed to be rare during the earliest stage of infarction. In the study of Hod et al. [25], atrial fibrillation was present in 7 (3 percent) of 214 patients admitted within 3 hours after the onset of pain. These patients had inferior myocardial infarction, and in each the circumflex coronary artery was occluded proximal to the left atrial circumflex branch. In five of these patients, myocardial infarction was caused by occlusion of the circumflex artery and in the remaining two, by occlusion of the right coronary artery that supplied collaterals to the previously occluded left circumflex artery. In each of these seven patients, the right coronary artery was also occluded proximal to the origin of the AV nodal artery. Thus, the appearance of atrial fibrillation during the earliest stage of infarction required the combination of occluded proximal circumflex artery and impaired perfusion of the AV node. When the reperfusion was successful, atrial fibrillation subsided rapidly but in a patient in whom reperfusion was not achieved, atrial fibrillation persisted for 16 hours [25]. Atrial fibrillation is also frequently associated with the presence of right ventricular infarction [26].

Fig. 12-1
Electrocardiogram of a 65-year-old woman with acute anteroseptal wall myocardial infarction and atrial flutter with 2:1 atrioventricular block. Intravenous administration of verapamil (10 mg) failed to convert atrial flutter to sinus rhythm. DC cardioversion with 30 joules established sinus rhythm.

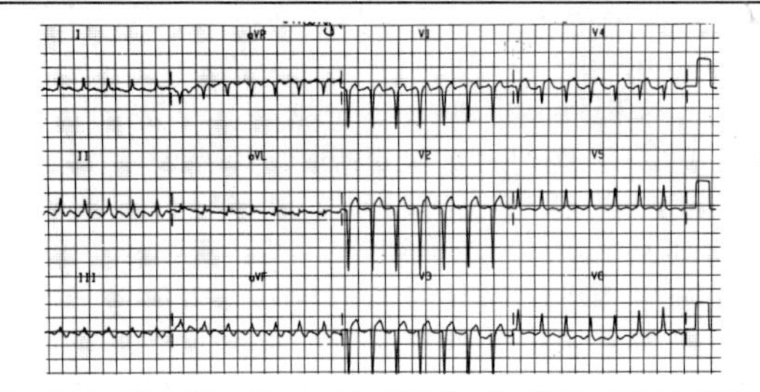

In about one-half of patients with atrial fibrillation, the onset can be traced to an atrial premature complex [12, 27] and in another half, to atrial flutter [23]. Factors believed to contribute to the appearance of atrial fibrillation in the setting of acute myocardial infarction included atrial infarction, release of catecholamines, acute pericarditis, preexisting atrial muscle disease, chronic lung disease, acute hypoxia, drugs, and hypokalemia [28].

In about one-half of all patients, the episodes of atrial fibrillation are single and in another half, multiple [20, 21]. In 50 percent of patients with single episodes, the ventricular rate was higher than 120 bpm. Multiple episodes of atrial fibrillation tend to be of shorter duration [20]. Atrial fibrillation lasted less than 2 hours in about 50 percent [20, 21], less than 4 hours in 74 percent, and less than 24 hours in 90 percent of patients [23]. When studied within 3 months after hospital discharge, only 6 of 77 patients still had atrial fibrillation, and in 3 of those chronic atrial fibrillation had been present before the onset of myocardial infarction [27]. The reported persistence of atrial fibrillation in as many as 33 percent of patients at the time of hospital discharge [19] may reflect the inclusion of patients with chronic atrial fibrillation predating the infarction.

In a large number of studies atrial fibrillation was associated with advanced age [12, 19–21, 24, 29], congestive heart failure, poor left ventricular function [12, 19, 24, 29–31], and extensive myocardial infarction [21, 22]. Other associated conditions included mitral regurgitation [19], pericarditis [11, 29, 30], increased incidence of ventricular tachycardia, ventricular fibrillation, right bundle branch block [20], and left bundle branch block [30]. The presence of atrial fibrillation was not related to the site of myocardial infarction [11, 19, 20] and was not linked causally to atrial infarction [20]. Transient atrial fibrillation did not contribute to an increased incidence of emboli unless the arrhythmia persisted.

Atrial fibrillation is a marker of poor prognosis. The arrhythmia is associated with an increased in-hospital [17, 20–23] and posthospital [20, 31] mortality. This increase in mortality is not attributed to the atrial fibrillation per se [11] but to a greater extent of myocardial infarction, presence of congestive heart failure [23], more advanced age, and other complicating factors [24]. However, in patients with mild congestive heart failure, the presence of atrial fibrillation appears to worsen the prognosis [32].

Preexcitation

Myocardial infarction may unmask the presence of a previously nonfunctioning AV bypass tract. In one report of such event in three patients [33], one had Wolff-Parkinson-White (WPW) pattern and two a short PR interval, associated with supraventricular tachycardia. In the patient with the WPW pattern, autopsy revealed a bypass tract, and in one of the two patients with short PR interval, the interval became normal during convalescence. The authors postulated that infarction activates latent accessory pathways, possibly due to increased sympathetic stimulation. The same mechanism was proposed in two other patients [34] in whom the WPW pattern and supraventricular tachycardia appeared during the acute stage of infarction and disappeared after recovery.

Drugs and Procedures Used in Therapy of Supraventricular Arrhythmias

Digitalis

In this country, digoxin is by far the most commonly used digitalis preparation, though in some regions digitoxin is the favorite drug. Digitalis may cause slowing of the ventricular rate by several mechanisms. The vagal and antiadrenergic effects of digitalis cause slowing of the ventricular rate during atrial fibrillation or flutter by blocking the conduction in the AV node. The same action may terminate AV nodal reentrant tachycardia. Administration to patients with congestive heart failure may decrease sinus rate indirectly, due to a decreased sympathetic tone as a result of an improved ventricular function.

After oral administration of digoxin, approximately 70 to 85 percent of the drug is absorbed from the gastrointestinal tract. The half-life of digoxin is about 36 hours in the presence of normal renal function. Most laboratories have established therapeutic levels at between 0.5 and 2.2 ng/ml. In patients not treated with digitalis in the recent past, these levels can be achieved using digoxin 0.25 mg daily by mouth within 6 to 8 days. When rapid digitalization is required, the drug is given intravenously, beginning with a dose of 0.75 mg followed by 0.25 mg every 2 to 4 hours until the desired effect or the maximum dose (1.5 mg) has been reached.

It is commonly believed that patients with acute myocardial infarction exhibit increased sensitivity to digitalis; that is, the margin between the therapeutic and the toxic dose in these patients is reduced. This may be due to an increased myocardial oxygen demand caused by the positive inotropic effect of the drug, or to a loss of intracellular potassium from ischemic myocardium. Also the presence of high sympathetic tone may inhibit the vagal effects of digitalis on the AV node [35]. For these reasons many clinicians no longer consider digitalis as the drug of choice for the treatment of supraventricular tachyarrhythmias in patients with acute myocardial infarction. Nevertheless, in the patient with significant left ventricular dysfunction, digoxin remains a very useful agent.

Treatment with digitalis requires careful attention to potassium replacement. Excessive doses must be avoided if cardioversion is contemplated. Accumulation of digitalis can be prevented by the use of short-acting preparations such as intermittent administration of ouabain intravenously [36], but this method is seldom applied in current practice.

Although administration of 1.5 mg of digoxin intravenously reverses atrial fibrillation of short duration to sinus rhythm in the majority of patients [37], this occurrence may be fortuitous because in most patients the attacks of atrial fibrillation subside spontaneously, and because conversion to sinus rhythm that follows digoxin administration is seldom preceded by an appreciable slowing of ventricular rate [37].

Numerous studies suggested that digitalis may have an adverse effect on survival during follow-up after myocardial infarction [38]. However, after adjusting for atrial fibrillation, left ventricular failure, and several other independent variables, higher mortality of patients treated with digitalis was not related to digitalis per se but to the condition of patients treated with digitalis [38, 39].

Atropine

Atropine is a muscarinic receptor–blocking agent that inhibits the action of endogenous acetylcholine. Atropine (0.6 to 2.0 mg intravenously) is useful in the treatment of sinus and junctional bradycardia, especially when it is complicated by hypotension during the early phase of acute myocardial infarction. Administration of small doses (< 0.3 mg of atropine sulfate intravenously) may cause a paradoxical slowing of heart rate attributed to a stimulating effect on the central nervous system. Atropine may cause urinary retention, especially in patients with an enlarged prostate, and is contraindicated in patients with closed-angle glaucoma. Administration of atropine may interrupt the antifibrillatory effect of elevated vagal tone, and pacing may be a prudent option if repetitive doses of atropine are required [40].

Beta-Adrenergic Blocking Agents

By competitive inhibition of adrenergic stimulation, beta blockers depress automaticity (phase 4 diastolic depolarization) of the sinoatrial node, AV junction, and His-Purkinje fibers [41]. Beta blockers also increase the AH interval, and prolong the effective and functional refractory periods of the AV node [42]. At concentrations of 50 to 100 times higher than the therapeutic levels, certain beta blockers (e.g., propranolol) also produce sodium channel–blocking effects but these are of questionable clinical significance.

The first commercially available beta-adrenergic blocker, propranolol, is well absorbed from the gastrointestinal tract but its systemic availability is less than 30 percent due to the first-pass effect [41]. Peak levels are reached within 1 to 2 hours after oral administration. The half-life is 2 to 4 hours, but increases to 4 to 6 hours during chronic oral administration. Therapeutic blood levels range from 40 to 100 ng/ml but severalfold differences in plasma levels may be present in patients treated with the same dose of propranolol [43].

Oral administration of propranolol (40 to 360 mg/day) or other beta-adrenergic blockers in equivalent doses is helpful in controlling the ventricular rate in patients with chronic atrial fibrillation, especially in combination with digitalis. Side effects include aggravation of congestive heart failure, excessive bradycardia, fatigue, bronchospasm, sleep disturbance, and hypoglycemia in diabetics.

Other beta-adrenergic blockers include the nonselective beta blocker timolol with a half-life of 5.5 hours, and the cardioselective beta blockers metoprolol and atenolol. The long-acting beta blockers include nadolol, atenolol, and sustained-release preparations of propranolol and metoprolol. Some beta-adrenergic blockers (e.g., pindolol and acebutolol) possess the properties of a partial beta agonist. The ultrashort-acting beta blocker esmolol with a half-life of less than 10 minutes, if used with caution, is useful in the acute treatment of supraventricular arrhythmias [44, 45].

The treatment of acute arrhythmias with the beta-adrenergic blockers in patients with myocardial infarction is based on the assumption that their negative inotropic effect is outweighed by the benefit of slowing the ventricular rate. In most cases this assumption is valid.

The synergistic effect of beta blockers and digitalis on the impulse transmission through the AV node may be either advantageous or deleterious, depending on the doses and other circumstances (Fig. 12-2). Bradycardia occurring during treatment with a beta-adrenergic blocker alone or in combination with digitalis may be reversed by prompt intravenous administration of atropine sulfate (1.0 to 1.5 mg), or isoproterenol solution (0.2 mg in 250 ml of 5% dextrose in water) at a rate of 1 to 5 ml/min.

To slow the ventricular rate during supraventricular tachyarrhythmia, small doses (e.g., 0.5 mg) of propranolol may be administered intravenously every 2 minutes up to an average dose of 4 to 5 mg [46]. Not infrequently, such treatment will result in conversion to sinus rhythm. Other beta-adrenergic blockers may be administered, in patients with

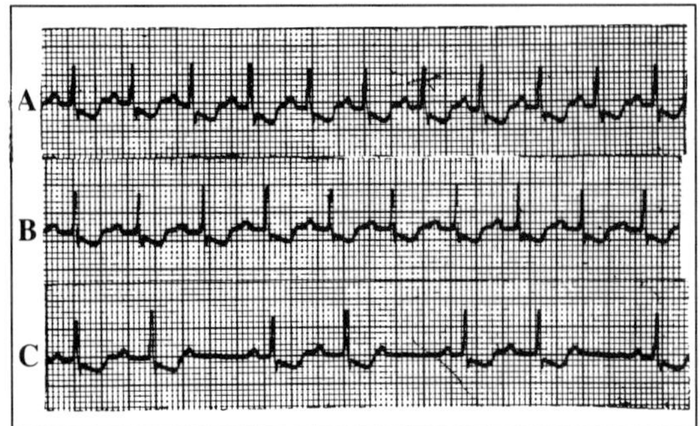

Fig. 12-2
Synergistic effect of digitalis and propranolol on atrioventricular conduction. *A.* Sinus rhythm while receiving digoxin, 0.25 mg orally daily. *B.* Three minutes after intravenous administration of propranolol (2 mg). Note the slower rate and longer PR interval. *C.* One minute later, Mobitz type 1 atrioventricular block.

atrial fibrillation or supraventricular tachycardia, as follows:

Atenolol: 1.0 mg intravenously every 5 minutes up to a total of 5 to 15 mg [47, 48], followed by an oral dose of 50 to 100 mg daily.

Metoprolol: 15 mg in three divided doses 5 minutes apart as needed, followed by 50 to 100 mg orally every 12 hours [49].

Alprenolol: 0.1% solution administered at a rate of 1 mg/min up to a total of 20 mg [50].

Nadolol: 0.05 mg/kg given at rate of 1 mg/min; oral administration of 20 to 160 mg/day for long-term therapy [51].

Esmolol, an ultrashort-acting beta-adrenergic blocker with an elimination half-life of about 9 minutes, is of potential advantage because of ultrashort action [45, 52]. The drug is rapidly gaining acceptance as the beta blocker of choice for supraventricular arrhythmias in patients with acute myocardial infarction. The infusion rate is titrated to control the heart while avoiding hypotension. Transient asymptomatic hypotension occurs in approximately 50 percent of individuals, but discontinuation rather than downward dosage adjustment is required in only about 10 percent [53]. The infusion of esmolol is begun by a 1-minute loading dose of 500 μg/kg/min followed by a titration infusion of 50 μg/kg/min. After 5 minutes, a repeated loading dose of 500 μg/kg/min is given followed by an increase in the titration infusion rate of 50 μg/kg/min. Once appropriate control of the heart rate is achieved, oral agents can be started to enable the discontinuation of intravenous esmolol infusion within 12 to 24 hours. Up to 50 percent of patients with new-onset atrial fibrillation or flutter convert to sinus rhythm shortly after beginning treatment with esmolol [54]. Precipitation of bronchospasm or aggravation of congestive heart failure seldom occurs if a careful titration protocol is followed.

Calcium Channel Blockers

Verapamil and diltiazem are the two commonly used calcium channel blockers for the treatment of supraventricular arrhythmias. Both drugs depress automaticity of the sinoatrial node, slow conduction through the AV node, and terminate AV nodal reentry in a high proportion of patients. These drugs also depress slow channel-dependent depolarizations in other tissues but have little effect on the normal His-Purkinje fibers and myocardium [55]. However, they may be effective in terminating arrhythmias caused by triggered automatic activity in the atria or the AV junction. Verapamil is largely metabolized in the liver; the bioavailability is only 35 percent due to first-pass elimination [56]. The mean half-life of verapamil after a single oral dose is 6 hours but it increases to 12 hours during chronic therapy [57].

Verapamil consistently slows the ventricular rate in atrial fibrillation and flutter but reestablishes sinus rhythm only in about 10 percent of patients. Verapamil can precipitate ventricular tachycardia or ventricular fibrillation in patients with WPW syndrome and atrial fibrillation when the impulses are conducted anterogradely through the bypass [58].

The usual dose of verapamil is 5 to 10 mg or 0.145 mg/kg of body weight administered intravenously within 1 to 2 minutes; this dose can be repeated after 10 minutes, if necessary. Caution should be exercised using a combination of verapamil with beta blockers because such combination entails the risk of AV block or significant left ventricular dysfunction [59].

Verapamil was formerly a drug of choice for terminating paroxysmal supraventricular tachycardia [60, 61]. When it is administered at a rate of 1 mg/min up to a total dose of about 20 mg, the success rate is 80 to 90 percent. However, in about one-half of patients a dose of less than 5 mg is sufficient [62]. Verapamil also frequently converts atrial flutter to sinus rhythm but seldom restores sinus rhythm in patients with atrial fibrillation [63]. In this condition the usual goal of therapy with verapamil is slowing the ventricular rate. The effectiveness of verapamil in slowing the ventricular rate lessens when the sympathetic tone is increased as a result of congestive heart failure, infection, or fever (Fig. 12-3) [35]. If rate control but not cardioversion occurs, a continuous infusion of verapamil at a rate of 5 to 15 mg/hr titrated to control the ventricular response can be used.

Other calcium channel–blocking drugs used intravenously to terminate supraventricular tachycardia or to slow the ventricular rate in patients with atrial fibrillation or flutter are diltiazem at 0.25 mg/kg over 2 minutes [64] and tiapamil at 1 mg/kg [65]. Diltiazem is given as a bolus of 0.25 mg/kg over 2 minutes. It may be repeated at a dose of 0.35 mg/kg 15 minutes later if the initial bolus is ineffective. Rate control, or rarely cardioversion, occurs in about 5 minutes. If successful, the initial bolus injections may be followed by a continuous infusion of 5 to 15 mg/hr as needed to control the ventricular response. The effect may persist for 0.5 to 7.0 hours after the infusion is stopped [66]. Like verapamil, caution must be used if the patient has a marginal blood pressure, as hypotension may occur. These calcium channel–blocking agents should not be used in the patient with short PR or sick sinus syndrome. Cautious use with lower doses is recommended if the patient has received concomitant therapy with a beta blocker, as greatly elevated calcium channel blocker levels result in this setting.

Fig. 12-3
The effectiveness of verapamil in slowing the ventricular rate depends on the patient's sympathetic tone. Strips of electrocardiogram (lead II) before and after verapamil administration in the same patient in the presence (12/77) and in the absence (3/78) of congestive heart failure and fever. Note the differences in dose, plasma concentration of verapamil, and response of ventricular rate in the presence of atrial fibrillation. (From J. Dominic et al. Verapamil plasma levels and ventricular rate response in patients with atrial fibrillation and flutter. *Clin. Pharmacol. Ther.* 26:710, 1979. With permission.)

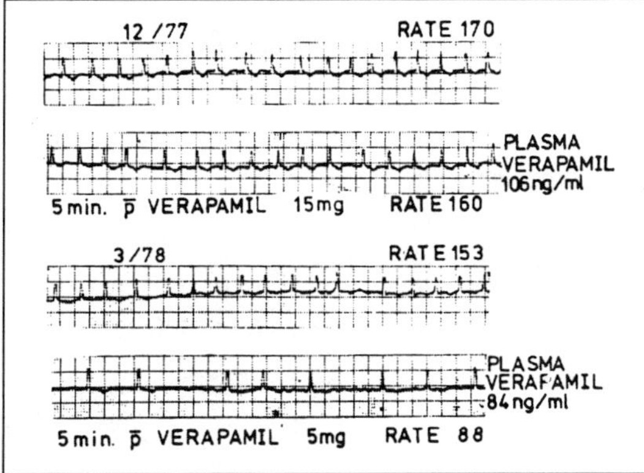

Calcium channel–blocking drugs appear to be well tolerated in most patients with acute myocardial infarction but their administration should not be continued in the presence of hypotension or increased pulmonary capillary wedge pressure [67]. An abrupt withdrawal of verapamil causes no manifestations of "withdrawal syndrome" and does not exacerbate angina pectoris [68]. Combining verapamil with digitalis to slow the ventricular rate requires caution because verapamil may increase the blood digoxin concentration [69].

In patients with adequate ventricular function the combination of calcium channel blockers and beta blockers may be more effective than either drug alone [70]. Using a single oral dose of diltiazem (120 mg) and propranolol (160 mg), Yeh et al. [71, 72] converted supraventricular tachycardia to sinus rhythm in the majority of patients within an average period of 39 to 49 minutes. For the prevention of paroxysmal supraventricular tachycardia, the usual oral maintenance dose of verapamil is about 240 mg, and that of diltiazem about 180 mg administered daily as a sustained-release preparation.

In patients with ventricular preexcitation, verapamil and diltiazem may increase the number of complexes conducted through the AV bypass tract by shortening the refractory period of the bypass tract, presumably as a result of a sympathetic reflex-evoked hypotension [73].

Adenosine

Adenosine has become the drug of choice for pharmacologic cardioversion of reentrant supraventricular tachycardias that incorporate the AV node into the reentrant pathway. The onset and duration of action of adenosine, measured in seconds, provide a larger margin of safety than other agents whose onset and duration of action are measured in minutes and hours. Although little information is available regarding the use of adenosine in the setting of acute myocardial infarction, experiences in other settings suggest that it also may be the safest drug for pharmacologic cardioversion in patients with myocardial infarction [74, 75].

Adenosine is an endogenous nucleoside formed as a product of the enzymatic breakdown of either adenosine triphosphate (ATP) or *S*-adenosylhomocysteine. Adenosine is a potent coronary artery vasodilator and has antiadrenergic and negative chronotropic actions. It activates specific extracellular adenosine receptors. Its principal electrophysiologic action on supraventricular tissues is mediated by the stimulation of an outward potassium current. This is accompanied by hyperpolarization of atrial and sinus node myocytes, a decrease in the duration of action potentials, and a decrease in the rate of phase 4 (diastolic) depolarization. The upstroke velocity of the AV node cells is also decreased, contributing to the negative dromotropic action [76].

Adenosine is administered intravenously as a bolus of 6 mg. This dose may be doubled after 1 minute if the initial dosage is ineffective. The onset of action is determined by the circulation time from the site of injection to the heart. Side effects of flushing, dyspnea, and chest pain occur with similar rapidity. These side effects, as well as transient bradycardia, last only 20 to 30 seconds.

Bronchospasm may occur in a susceptible individual and may last for a longer period of time, requiring treatment with aminophylline, which blocks adenosine receptors (50 to 200 mg intravenously). Therefore, adenosine should not be used in patients with a history of asthma.

In addition to its ability to terminate AV nodal or AV reentrant tachycardias, adenosine may be used as a diagnostic tool to clarify the mechanism of both narrow and wide QRS complex tachycardias. Its ability to block AV conduction may uncover underlying atrial activity (e.g., flutter). In wide QRS complex tachycardia, adenosine has no effect on ventricular tachycardia, but the brief duration of adenosine's action will cause no harmful delay in initiating appropriate treatment after the mechanism is clarified. Although seldom relevant to the treatment of tachycardia in the setting of myocardial infarction, administration of adenosine may uncover preexcitation (Fig. 12-4) [77].

Wide QRS complex tachycardia in the setting of acute myocardial infarction should be assumed to be ventricular in origin. However, both supraventricular tachycardia with aberrancy or preexcitation can cause diagnostic problems (Fig. 12-5). Rapid administration of adenosine in the setting of wide QRS complex tachycardia has a sensitivity of 90 percent and a specificity of 93 percent with a positive predictive value of 92 percent in discriminating the site of origin [74]. This compares favorably with the analysis of the common electrocardiographic markers in both speed and accuracy [78].

Class I (Sodium Channel–Blocking) Antiarrhythmic Drugs

On the basis of their effect on the electrocardiogram, sodium channel–blocking drugs can be subdivided conveniently into three classes. Class IA drugs prolong both the QRS complex and the JT (QT–QRS) intervals. They include quinidine, procainamide, and disopyramide. Amiodarone, though seldom listed as a member of this class of drugs,

Fig. 12-4
Prompt interruption of supraventricular tachycardia by adenosine. Atrioventricular nodal bypass tract is exposed in the second complex from the right.

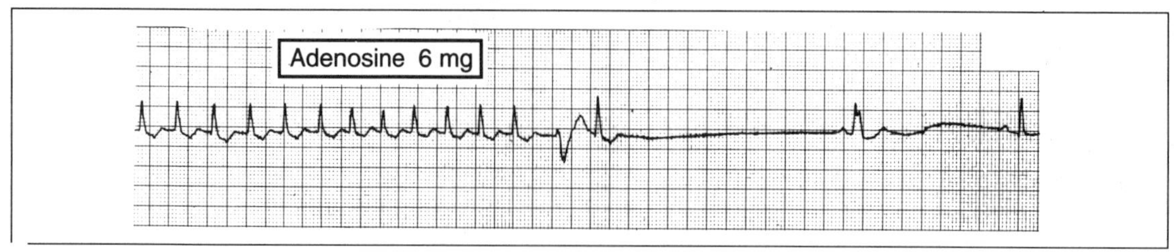

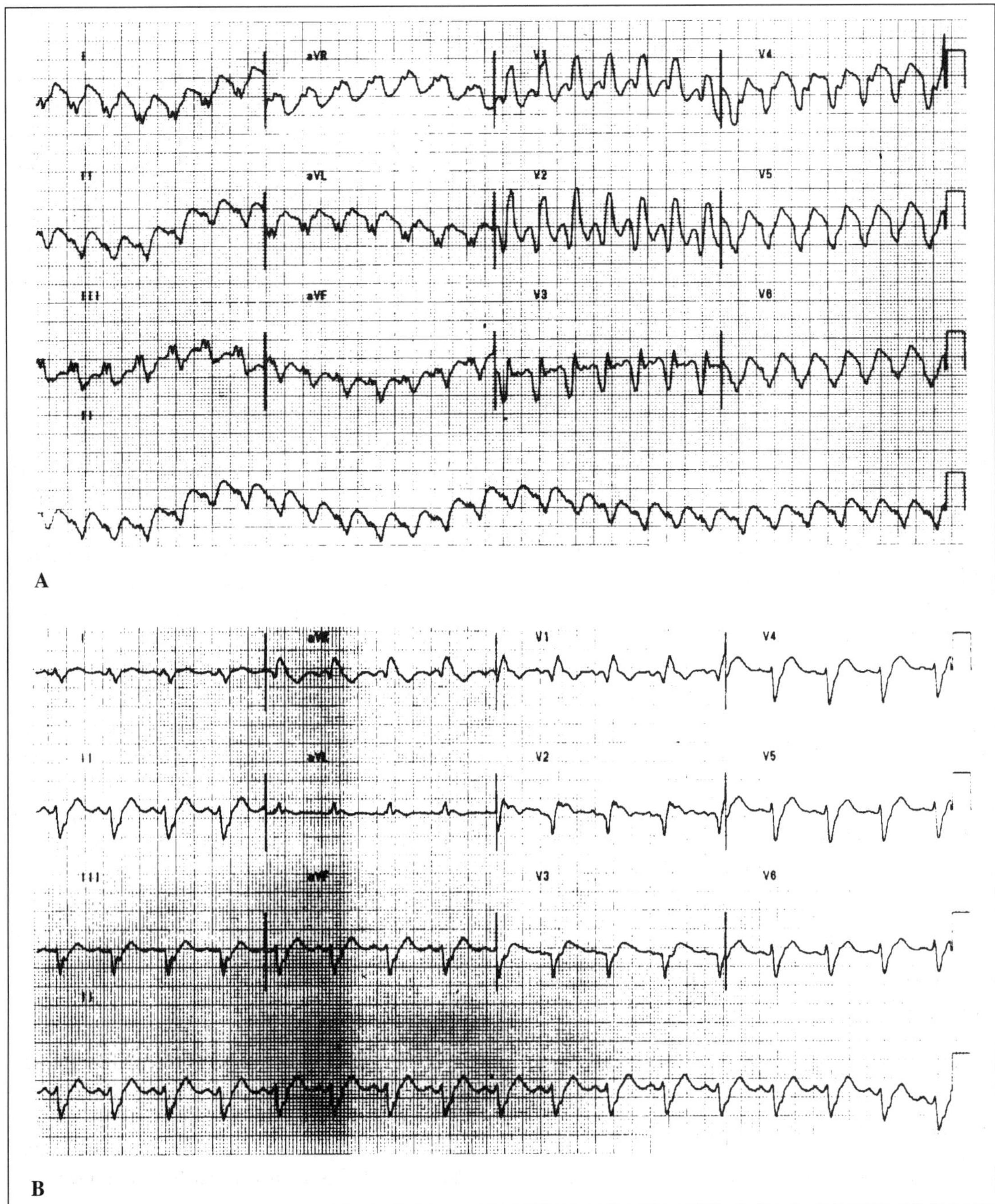

Fig. 12-5
A. Supraventricular wide QRS complex tachycardia with an aberration initially misdiagnosed as ventricular tachycardia based on morphology. *B.* The same pattern of intraventricular conduction disturbance in the setting of anterior myocardial infarction during sinus rhythm.

has some of the same properties. Class IB drugs have no discernible effect on the duration of either the QRS or the JT interval. The representatives of this group are lidocaine, tocainide, mexiletine, and phenytoin. Class IC drugs include flecainide, encainide, and propafenone. They prolong the QRS duration but not the JT interval.

Quinidine

The three commonly used quinidine preparations are quinidine sulfate, quinidine gluconate, and quinidine polygalacturonate. Of these, quinidine sulfate is more rapidly absorbed, reaching a peak plasma level within 1 to 2 hours with a bioavailability of 60 to 100 percent. Quinidine gluconate is more slowly absorbed, reaching a peak plasma level within about 4 hours, and has bioavailability of 40 to 90 percent [79]. Quinidine polygalacturonate is absorbed most slowly, and has the lowest bioavailability. The content of quinidine base in these three preparations is 83 percent in the sulfate, 62 percent in the gluconate, and 60 percent in the polygalacturonate preparation [80]. The principal application of quinidine is for the purpose of maintaining sinus rhythm after conversion to atrial fibrillation. In one study of patients treated with a long-acting quinidine sulfate preparation (0.6 gm twice daily in patients weighing < 80 kg, and 0.8 gm twice daily in patients weighing > 80 kg), sinus rhythm was maintained in 51 percent of patients versus 28 percent in those not receiving quinidine [81]. In another study [82], 1 year after cardioversion, sinus rhythm was maintained in 50 percent of patients treated with quinidine, 30 percent of those treated with digoxin, and 23 percent of untreated patients. The safety of long-term administration of quinidine to maintain sinus rhythm has been questioned because of higher mortality in the quinidine-treated patients compared to those not treated with quinidine [83].

The most dreaded complication of quinidine therapy is the development of polymorphic or monomorphic ventricular tachycardia. Since these arrhythmias usually occur at the beginning of therapy, monitoring the treatment during the first 5 days in the hospital is advisable. Also, a test 0.2-gm dose is usually given before the onset of therapy to detect a possible idiosyncrasy. The most common reason for discontinuing quinidine is diarrhea that can be ameliorated with aluminum-containing antacids.

Because of its anticholinergic action, quinidine may cause acceleration of the ventricular rate during atrial flutter or atrial fibrillation. To prevent this, the drug is frequently administered concomitantly with digitalis, verapamil, or a beta-adrenergic blocker. In patients receiving digitalis, quinidine increases the plasma digoxin concentration and enhances the probability of digitalis toxicity. The reduction of digoxin dose by 30 to 40 percent has been recommended for when both drugs are administered together [84].

Procainamide

Procainamide may be effective in the conversion of atrial fibrillation to sinus rhythm when it is administered intravenously at a rate of 15 to 20 mg/min up to 1000 mg. The most important determinant of the successful cardioversion is the short duration of arrhythmia [85]. When intravenous procainamide is used, close attention must be given to the QT interval, blood pressure, and ambient ventricular ectopic activity.

Orally administered procainamide for maintenance therapy is rapidly absorbed. Peak concentrations are reached usually within 1.0 to 1.5 hours after administration, and bioavailability is in excess of 80 percent. The half-life of procainamide is only about 3 hours but the use of sustained-release preparations (e.g., Procan SR) enables the administration of the drug every 6 to 8 hours. Procainamide is partly metabolized in the liver into *N*-acetylprocainamide that has an antiarrhythmic property, and is almost exclusively eliminated by the kidneys.

Disopyramide

This drug is probably as effective in the suppression of supraventricular arrhythmias as procainamide but the strong anticholinergic and the negative inotropic effects diminish the usefulness of disopyramide in patients with myocardial infarction.

Other Drugs Used for the Termination of Supraventricular Tachycardias

Most of the information available about the drugs listed in this section stems from the observations in patients with conditions other than myocardial infarction. Propafenone has been used in doses of

2 mg/kg intravenously [86]. Oral administration of 150 mg twice daily to 300 mg every 8 hours may be used for chronic suppression of supraventricular arrhythmias without any apparent increase in long-term mortality [87]. Flecainide is administered in doses of 0.5 to 2.0 mg/kg intravenously, followed by 200 to 300 mg/day orally, and encainide in doses of 0.3 to 2.0 mg/kg intravenously, followed by 100 to 225 mg/day orally. Both flecainide and encainide depress myocardial function and should be used cautiously in patients with acute myocardial infarction [88–91]. Their long-term use appears relatively contraindicated based on the findings of the Cardiac Arrhythmia Suppression Trial (CAST) in which they were administered for suppression of ventricular premature complexes after myocardial infarction [92]. Amiodarone can be given intravenously in a dose of 150 mg within 5 minutes, followed by 600 mg/day for 3 to 4 days [93]. Similar effects on supraventricular tachycardia can be achieved using amiodarone orally, either as a single dose of 15 mg/kg [94] or 100 to 400 mg/day in divided doses. Similar to flecainide and encainide, amiodarone can depress myocardial function [95]. Sotalol may be used in the treatment of supraventricular arrhythmias. Infusion of 1.5 mg/kg over 10 minutes terminated supraventricular tachycardia in 83 percent of patients [96]. Oral administration of 80 to 160 mg of sotalol twice daily has been effective in preventing recurrent supraventricular tachycardia [97, 98].

Miscellaneous Drugs

In the treatment of supraventricular tachycardia, adenosine has largely replaced the intravenous administration of two drugs commonly used in the past: edrophonium, a cholinesterase inhibitor (10 mg), and phenylephrine (1 mg/min up to 10 mg) [99]. The effectiveness of these drugs was frequently enhanced by combining the treatment with carotid sinus stimulation.

When the tachycardias are caused by AV nodal or AV reentry, the reentry pathways can be transiently interrupted by intravenous administration of magnesium salts [100]. Intravenous infusion of 2 gm of magnesium sulfate solution over 15 seconds terminated supraventricular tachycardia in 6 of 14 patients. The side effects are similar to those of adenosine but are more severe. Magnesium slows conduction not only in the AV node but also in the accessory pathways and ventricular myocardium.

Electrical Cardioversion

Synchronized DC cardioversion can terminate most of the arrhythmias due to reentry but the energy required to terminate the tachycardias varies according to the type of arrhythmias. Thirty to fifty joules may be sufficient to terminate paroxysmal tachycardia and atrial flutter. However, higher energy levels (100 to 400 joules) are usually needed for atrial fibrillation. The delivered energy is inversely related to the square root of the resistance. The latter can be minimized by the use of electrode gels. The electrode paddle positions are no longer considered as important modifiers of resistance, and there is no apparent advantage in using the anteroposterior as opposed to the anterolateral paddle placement [101].

Cardioversion should be performed after at least 6 hours of fasting. Standby cardiopulmonary resuscitation equipment such as oxygen, ventilation bag, suction tubing, and endotracheal tube should be available. Before the shock is delivered, amnesia is induced by means of intravenously administered diazepam (Valium), midazolam (Versed), or one of the short-acting barbiturates such as thiopental sodium (Pentothal) or methohexital sodium (Brevital). Diazepam is usually given as 5 mg intravenously every minute until the patient becomes unresponsive to verbal command. The total amount of intravenously administered diazepam varies from 15 to 40 mg (0.16 to 0.32 mg/kg), depending on the age and body weight of the patient. If excessive dosage appears to have been given, flumazenil can be administered in a dose of 0.2 to 1.0 mg to rapidly reverse the sedating effects of diazepam and the other benzodiazepines. Oxygen by mask is usually administered for a few minutes before and after cardioversion. Because of the drug's long half-life (30 hours), somnolence may persist for a few hours. The new water-soluble benzodiazepine midazolam has pharmacologic properties similar to those of diazepam but is a more potent anesthetic with a shorter half-life (1.3 to 2.2 hours), allowing for a more rapid recovery of psychomotor functions. Methohexital (Brevital), a new ultrashort-acting barbiturate, is three times more potent than thiopental and has a shorter half-life.

In patients with atrial flutter, slowing the ventricular rate or conversion to sinus rhythm using digoxin or quinidine may be difficult and time-consuming. In contrast, in most cases, a low-energy (i.e., 30 to 50 joules) shock can accomplish rapid cardioversion to sinus rhythm. Thus, even in patients with acute myocardial infarction the electrical shock is an accepted initial treatment of atrial flutter.

In the absence of digitalis toxicity or uncorrected hypokalemia, digitalis need not be discontinued for more than 1 or 2 days before cardioversion. However, DC cardioversion may precipitate ventricular arrhythmias and cause a prolonged period of sinus arrest or marked sinus bradycardia in patients with sick sinus syndrome or digitalis toxicity. In most patients, bradycardia is at least partially reversible after intravenous atropine administration (1.0 to 2.0 mg).

Because of the 1 to 3 percent risk of embolization after cardioversion [102], we recommend anticoagulation whenever feasible, for a period of 1 month after the procedure. If the procedure is elective, anticoagulants should be given also for a period of 3 weeks before cardioversion. However, transesophageal echocardiography may identify individuals at low risk of embolization if they have no clots or echo-dense contrast material swirling in the left atrium, including the appendage and the pulmonic veins [103].

Prophylactic pacing is recommended in patients with suspected sinus node malfunction. An alternative to cardioversion in patients with atrial flutter is rapid atrial pacing. In one recent study, this procedure successfully converted atrial flutter to sinus rhythm in 89 percent of trials in 46 consecutive patients [104]. Internal cardioversion was effective when external cardioversion of atrial fibrillation failed to restore sinus rhythm [105].

General Guidelines for the Treatment of Supraventricular Arrhythmias

Barring an emergency that may require an immediate action, a number of preliminary steps must be made before antiarrhythmic therapy is initiated. We recommend in each patient to (1) establish the mechanism of arrhythmia; (2) consider the role of possible precipitating or aggravating factors such as hypoxia, pulmonary insufficiency, poorly controlled diabetes, administration of a sympathomimetic agent, diuretics, antiarrhythmic drugs, treatment with digitalis, presence of systemic or pulmonary emboli, anemia, hyperthyroidism, and pericarditis; (3) correct hypokalemia, even though there is no convincing evidence that it constitutes an independent cause of supraventricular arrhythmia (in contrast to well-established evidence for aggravating effect on ventricular arrhythmias in patients with myocardial infarction) [106]; (4) establish possible effects of arrhythmias on hemodynamics and myocardial perfusion; (5) estimate the natural course and the expected duration of untreated arrhythmia in question; and (6) define the therapeutic goal, for example, suppression of arrhythmia, slowing ventricular rate, increase in contribution of atrial contraction, and so on.

Specific First-Line Approaches to the Management of Supraventricular Arrhythmias

Although therapeutic decisions should be based on the understanding of the arrhythmia mechanism and the antiarrhythmic drug action (discussed already), it may be helpful to list the preferred first-line approaches recommended by us.

Sinus bradycardia: Atropine sulfate is given intravenously, occasionally with temporary atrial or ventricular pacing.

Sinus tachycardia: The underlying cause (e.g., anxiety, fear, pain, low cardiac output, hypotension) should be treated. In rare cases administration of low doses of beta-adrenergic blockers is helpful.

Frequent premature atrial complexes: Treatment is seldom required. Occasionally one of the class I antiarrhythmic drugs (e.g., procainamide or quinidine) may be used.

Reentrant AV nodal or AV tachycardia: Adenosine is now the initial drug of choice unless it is contraindicated by a history of bronchial asthma. If adenosine is ineffective or if episodes of tachycardia recur, verapamil or diltiazem is used intravenously. If these drugs are contraindicated or are ineffective, beta-adrenergic blockers are given intravenously. Beta-adrenergic blockers should be used cautiously if they are administered before the calcium channel blockers are eliminated from the body. If arrhythmia remains refractory, amiodarone is given intravenously, and if the condition is hemodynamically unstable, electrical cardioversion may be necessary.

Atrial and AV junctional tachycardia: Digitalis toxicity should be ruled out. The general approach is the same as for AV nodal reentrant tachycardia.

Multifocal atrial tachycardia: The underlying cause, usually pulmonary insufficiency, should be treated. The drug of choice, if needed, is verapamil.

Atrial flutter: If the patient is hemodynamically stable, beta-adrenergic blockers or calcium channel blockers are given intravenously to slow the ventricular response. Attempt of pharmacologic cardioversion using intravenous procainamide is a second approach. If the patient is hemodynamically unstable, electrical cardioversion or rapid atrial pacing may be needed.

Atrial fibrillation: Intravenous verapamil, diltiazem, or a beta blocker may be given to quickly slow the ventricular rate. In patients with left ventricular dysfunction, digoxin is often the drug of choice. If arrhythmia persists and causes hemodynamic instability, electrical cardioversion is applied followed by preventive therapy and anticoagulation. For the prevention of recurrences, quinidine, procainamide, or disopyramide, with either digitalis, verapamil, or low doses of beta-adrenergic blockers, can be used. Anticoagulants are recommended in patients with recurrent, protracted, or established atrial fibrillation unless there is a bleeding tendency or other contraindications. The question of whether or not to use anticoagulants in the presence of pericarditis is unsettled. There is an independent association between atrial fibrillation and pericarditis both during and after the hospital course of myocardial infarction [107–109], and the continuation of anticoagulants in this condition entails a small risk of hemopericardium that may be equal to the risk of embolic complications in patients not treated with anticoagulants.

Atrial tachyarrhythmias with rapid anterograde conduction through the AV bypass tract: Digitalis and calcium channel blockers must be avoided. Intravenous administration of amiodarone or procainamide [110] or electrical cardioversion or both are used for acute treatment. Oral amiodarone is given for prevention.

References

1. Yu, P. N. The acute phase of myocardial infarction. *Cardiovasc. Clin.* 7:45, 1975.
2. Webb, S. W., Adgey, A. A., and Pantridge, J. F. Autonomic disturbance at onset of acute myocardial infarction. *B.M.J.* 3:89, 1972.
3. Hindman, M. C., and Wagner, G. S. Arrhythmias during myocardial infarction: Mechanisms, significance, and therapy. *Cardiovasc. Clin.* 11:81, 1980.
4. Parameswaran, R., Ohe, T., and Goldberg, H. Sinus node dysfunction in acute myocardial infarction. *Br. Heart J.* 38:93, 1976.
5. Murphy, P., Morton, P., Murtagh, J. J., et al. Hemodynamic effects of different temporary pacing modes for the management of bradycardias complicating acute myocardial infarction. *PACE Pacing Clin. Electrophysiol.* 15:391, 1992.
6. Lie, K. I., Wellens, H. J., Downar, E., and Durrer, D. Observations on patients with primary ventricular fibrillation complicating acute myocardial infarction. *Circulation* 52:755, 1975.
7. Hohnloser, S. H., Zabel, M., Olschewski, M., et al. Arrhythmias during the acute phase of reperfusion therapy for acute myocardial infarction: Effects of beta-adrenergic blockade. *Am. Heart J.* 123: 1530, 1992.
8. Vazifdar, J. P., and Levine, S. A. Rarity of atrial tachycardia in acute myocardial infarction and in thyrotoxicosis. *Arch. Intern. Med.* 118:41, 1966.
9. Lesser, L. Atrial tachycardia in acute myocardial infarction. *Ann. Intern. Med.* 86:582, 1977.
10. Chung, E. K. Tachyarrhythmias associated with acute myocardial infarction: Diagnosis, frequency, and significance. *Cardiovasc. Clin.* 7:157, 1975.
11. Liberthson, R. R., Salisbury, K. W., Hutter, A. M., and DeSanctis, R. W. Atrial tachyarrhythmias in acute myocardial infarction. *Am. J. Med.* 60:956, 1976.
12. Lofmark, R., and Orinius, E. Supraventricular tachyarrhythmias in acute myocardial infarction. *Acta Med. Scand.* 203:517, 1978.
13. Rosen, M. R., Fisch, C., Hoffman, B. F., et al. Can accelerated atrio-ventricular junctional escape rhythms be explained by delayed afterdepolarizations? *Am. J. Cardiol.* 45:1272, 1980.
14. Knoebel, S. B., Rasmussen, S., Lovelace, D. E., and Anderson, G. J. Nonparoxysmal junctional

tachycardia in acute myocardial infarction: Computer-assisted detection. *Am. J. Cardiol.* 35:825, 1975.
15. Fishenfeld, J., Desser, K. B., and Benchimol, A. Non-paroxysmal AV junctional tachycardia associated with acute myocardial infarction. *Am. Heart J.* 86:754, 1973.
16. Konecke, L. L., and Knoebel, S. B. Nonparoxysmal junctional tachycardia complicating acute myocardial infarction. *Circulation* 45:367, 1972.
17. Madsen, E. B., Hougaard, P., and Gilpin, E. Dynamic evaluation of prognosis from time-dependent variables in acute myocardial infarction. *Am. J. Cardiol.* 51:1579, 1983.
18. Hii, J. T., Mitchell, B. L., Duff, H. J., et al. Comparison of atrial overdrive pacing with and without extrastimuli for termination of atrial flutter. *Am. J. Cardiol.* 70:463, 1992.
19. Helmers, C., Lundman, T., Mogensen, L., et al. Atrial fibrillation in acute myocardial infarction. *Acta Med. Scand.* 193:39, 1973.
20. Hunt, D., Sloman, G., and Penington, C. Effects of atrial fibrillation on prognosis of acute myocardial infarction. *Br. Heart J.* 40:303, 1978.
21. Cristal, N., Peterburg, I., and Szwarcberg, J. Atrial fibrillation developing in the acute phase of myocardial infarction. Prognostic implication. *Chest* 70:8, 1976.
22. Sugiura, T., Iwasaka, T., Ogawa, A., et al. Atrial fibrillation in acute myocardial infarction. *Am. J. Cardiol.* 56:27, 1985.
23. Klass, M., and Haywood, L. J. Atrial fibrillation associated with acute myocardial infarction: A study of 34 cases. *Am. Heart J.* 79:752, 1970.
24. Beck, O. A., and Hochrein, H. Atrial fibrillation and flutter as a complication of acute myocardial infarction. *Dtsch. Med. Wochenschr.* 101:1148, 1976.
25. Hod, H., Lew, A. S., Keltai, M., et al. Early atrial fibrillation during evolving myocardial infarction: A consequence of impaired left atrial perfusion. *Circulation* 75:146, 1987.
26. Rechavia, E., Strasberg, B., Mager, A., et al. The incidence of atrial arrhythmias during inferior wall myocardial infarction with and without right ventricular involvement. *Am. Heart J.* 124:387, 1992.
27. Loewy, E. H. Effects of atrial fibrillation on prognosis of acute myocardial infarction. *Br. Heart J.* 41:255, 1979.
28. Harrison, D. C. Atrial fibrillation in acute myocardial infarction. Significance and therapeutic implications. *Chest* 70:3, 1976.
29. McLean, K. H., Bett, J. N., and Saltups, A. Tachyarrhythmias in acute myocardial infarction. *N.J. Med.* 5:3, 1975.
30. Flugelman, M. Y., Hasin, Y., Shefer, A., et al. Atrial fibrillation in acute myocardial infarction. *Isr. J. Med. Sci.* 22:355, 1986.
31. Siltanen, P., Pohjola-Siktonen, S., Haapakoski, J., et al. The mortality predictive power of discharge electrocardiogram after first acute myocardial infarction. *Am. Heart J.* 109:1231, 1985.
32. Liem, K. L., Lie, K. I., Durrer, D., and Wellens, H. J. Clinical setting and prognostic significance of atrial fibrillation complicating acute myocardial infarction. *Eur. J. Cardiol.* 4:59, 1976.
33. Gavrilescu, S., Gavrilescu, M., and Luca, C. Accelerated atrioventricular conduction during acute myocardial infarction. *Am. Heart J.* 94:21, 1977.
34. Goel, B. J., and Han, J. Manifestation of the Wolff-Parkinson-White syndrome after myocardial infarction. *Am. Heart J.* 87:633, 1974.
35. Dominic, J., McAllister, R. G., Kuo, C. S., et al. Verapamil plasma levels and ventricular rate response in patients with atrial fibrillation and flutter. *Clin. Pharmacol. Ther.* 26:710, 1979.
36. Jewitt, D. E., Balcon, R., Raftery, E. B., and Oram, S. Incidence and management of supraventricular arrhythmias after acute myocardial infarction. *Lancet* 2:734, 1967.
37. Weiner, P., Bassan, M. M., Jarchousky, J., et al. Clinical course of acute atrial fibrillation treated with rapid digitalization. *Am. Heart J.* 105:223, 1983.
38. Bigger, J. T., Fleiss, J. L., Rolnitzky, L. M., et al. Effect of digitalis treatment on survival after acute myocardial infarction. *Am. J. Cardiol.* 55:623, 1985.
39. Byington, R., and Goldstein, S. Association of digitalis therapy with mortality in survivors of acute myocardial infarction: Observations in the Beta-blocker Heart Attack Trial. *J. Am. Coll. Cardiol.* 6:976, 1985.
40. Ferrari, G. M., Salvati, P., Grossoni, M., et al. Pharmacologic modulation of the autonomic nervous system in the prevention of sudden cardiac death. *J. Am. Coll. Cardiol.* 21:283, 1993.
41. Frishman, W. H. *Clinical Pharmacology of the Beta Adrenoreceptor Blocking Drugs* (2nd ed.). Norwalk, CT: Appleton-Century-Crofts, 1984.
42. Wit, A. L., Hoffman, B. F., and Rosen, M. R. Electrophysiology and pharmacology of cardiac arrhythmias. IX. Cardiac electrophysiology effects of beta adrenergic receptor stimulation and blockade. Part C. *Am. Heart J.* 90:795, 1975.
43. Shand, D. G. Individualization of propranolol therapy. *Med. Clin. North Am.* 58:1063, 1974.
44. Swerdlow, C., Peterson, J., Liem, L. B., and Blake, K. Electropharmacology of flestolol in patients with supraventricular tachyarrhythmias. *J. Am. Coll. Cardiol.* 9:247A, 1987.
45. Kirshenbaum, J. M., Kloner, R. A., Antman, E. M., and Braunwald, E. Use of ultra-short acting beta-blocker in patients with acute myocardial ischemia. *Circulation* 72:873, 1985.
46. Lemberg, L., Castellanos, A., and Arcebal, A. G. The use of propranolol in arrhythmias complicating acute myocardial infarction. *Am. Heart J.* 80:479, 1970.
47. Ramsdale, D. R., Faragher, E. B., Bennett, D. H.,

et al. Ischemic pain relief in patients with acute myocardial infarction by intravenous atenolol. *Am. Heart J.* 103:459, 1982.

48. Schley, G., Beckmann, R., and Hengstebeck, W. The treatment of acute cardiac dysrhythmias with atenolol (Tenormin) particularly after myocardial infarction. *Z. Kardiol.* 67:280, 1978.
49. The Miami Trial Research Group. Metoprolol in acute myocardial infarction. Arrhythmias. *Am. J. Cardiol.* 56:35G, 1985.
50. Lemberg, L., Arcebal, A. G., Castellanos, A., and Slavin, D. Use of alprenolol in acute cardiac arrhythmias. *Am. J. Cardiol.* 30:77, 1972.
51. Saksena, S., Klein, G. J., Kowey, P. R., et al. Electrophysiologic effects, clinical efficacy and safety of intravenous and oral nadolol in refractory supraventricular tachyarrhythmias. *Am. J. Cardiol.* 59:307, 1987.
52. Morganroth, J., Horowitz, L. N., Anderson, J., and Turlapaty, P. Comparative efficacy and tolerance of esmolol to propranolol for control of supraventricular tachyarrhythmia. *Am. J. Cardiol.* 56:33F, 1985.
53. Gray, R. J., Bateman, T., Czer, L. S., et al. Esmolol: A new ultrashort-acting beta-adrenergic blocking agent for rapid control of heart rate in postoperative supraventricular tachyarrhythmias. *J. Am. Coll. Cardiol.* 5:1451, 1985.
54. Platia, E. V., Michelson, E. L., Porterfield, J. K., and Das, G. Esmolol versus verapamil in the acute treatment of atrial fibrillation or atrial flutter. *Am. J. Cardiol.* 63:925, 1989.
55. Singh, B. M., Eilrodt, G., and Peter, C. T. Verapamil: A review of its pharmacological properties and therapeutic use. *Drugs* 15:169, 1978.
56. Kates, R. E., Keefe, D. L. D., Schwartz, J., et al. Verapamil dispositions: Kinetics in chronic atrial fibrillation. *J. Clin. Pharmacol. Ther.* 30:44, 1981.
57. Schwartz, J. B., Keefe, D. L. D., Kirsten, E., et al. Prolongation of verapamil elimination kinetics during chronic oral administration. *Am. Heart J.* 104:198, 1982.
58. McGovern, B., Garan, H., and Ruskin, J. N. Precipitation of cardiac arrest by verapamil in patients with Wolff-Parkinson-White syndrome. *Ann. Intern. Med.* 104:791, 1986.
59. Packer, M., Meller, J., Medina, N., et al. Hemodynamic consequences of combined beta adrenergic and slow calcium channel blockade in man. *Circulation* 65:660, 1982.
60. Rikenberger, R. L., Prystowsky, E. N., Heger, J. J., et al. Effects of intravenous and chronic oral verapamil administration in patients with supraventricular tachycardias. *Circulation* 62:996, 1980.
61. Krikler, D. M. Verapamil in arrhythmia. *Br. J. Clin. Pharmacol.* 21:183S, 1986.
62. Waxman, H. L., Myerburg, R. J., Appel, R., and Sung, R. J. Verapamil for control of ventricular rate in paroxysmal supraventricular tachycardia and atrial fibrillation or flutter. *Ann. Intern. Med.* 94:1, 1981.
63. Platia, E. V., Michelson, E. L., Porterfiled, J. K., and Das, G. Esmolol versus verapamil in the acute treatment of atrial fibrillation or atrial flutter. *Am. J. Cardiol.* 63:925, 1989.
64. Waleffe, A., Hastir, F., and Kulbertus, H. E. Effects of intravenous diltiazem administration in patients with inducible tachycardia. *Eur. Heart J.* 6:882, 1985.
65. Strozzi, C., Sfrisi, C., Laütenesser, F., et al. Tiapamil in the management of supraventricular arrhythmias occurring after acute myocardial infarction. *Cardiology* 69(Suppl):187, 1982.
66. Ellenbogen, K. A., Dias, V. C., Plumb, V. J., et al. A placebo-controlled trial of continuous intravenous diltiazem infusion for 24 hour heart rate control during atrial fibrillation and atrial flutter: A multicenter study. *J. Am. Coll. Cardiol.* 18:891, 1991.
67. Hagemeijer, F. Verapamil in the management of supraventricular tachyarrhythmias occurring after a recent myocardial infarction. *Circulation* 57:751, 1978.
68. The Danish Study Group on Verapamil in Myocardial Infarction. Abrupt withdrawal of verapamil in ischaemic heart disease. *Eur. Heart J.* 5:529, 1984.
69. Klein, H. O., and Kaplinsky, E. Verapamil and digoxin. Their respective effects on atrial fibrillation and their interaction. *Am. J. Cardiol.* 50:894, 1982.
70. Yee, R., Gulamhusein, S. S., and Klein, G. J. Combined verapamil and propranolol for supraventricular tachycardia. *Am. J. Cardiol.* 53:757, 1984.
71. Yeh, S. J., Lin, F. C., Chou, Y. Y., et al. Termination of paroxysmal supraventricular tachycardia with a single oral dose of diltiazem and propranolol. *Circulation* 71:104, 1985.
72. Yeh, S. J., Fu, M., Lin, F. C., et al. Serial electrophysiologic studies of the effects of oral diltiazem on paroxysmal supraventricular tachycardia. *Chest* 87:639, 1985.
73. Gulamhusein, S., Ko, P., Carruthers, G., and Kelin, G. J. Acceleration of the ventricular response during atrial fibrillation in the Wolff-Parkinson-White syndrome after verapamil. *Circulation* 65:348, 1982.
74. Camm, A. J., and Garratt, C. J. Adenosine and supraventricular tachycardia. *N. Engl. J. Med.* 325:1621, 1991.
75. DiMarco, J. P., Miles, W., Akhtar, M., et al. Adenosine for paroxysmal supraventricular tachycardia: Dose ranging and comparison with verapamil. *Ann. Intern. Med.* 113:104, 1990.
76. Freilich, A., and Tepper, D. Adenosine and its cardiovascular effects. *Am. Heart J.* 123:1324, 1992.
77. Garratt, C. J., Antonin, A., Griffith, M. J., et al. Use of intravenous adenosine in sinus rhythm as a diagnostic test for latent preexcitation. *Am. J. Cardiol.* 65:868, 1990.
78. Akhtar, M., Shenasa, M., Jazayer, M., et al. Wide

QRS complex tachycardia. *Ann. Intern. Med.* 109:905, 1988.
79. Greenblatt, D. J., Pfeifer, H. J., Ochs, H. R., et al. Pharmacokinetics of quinidine in humans after intravenous, intramuscular and oral administration. *J. Pharmacol. Exp. Ther.* 202:365, 1977.
80. Woosley, R. R., and Shand, D. G. Pharmacokinetics of antiarrhythmic drugs. *Am. J. Cardiol.* 41:986, 1978.
81. Sodermark, T., Jonsson, B., Olsson, A., et al. Effect of quinidine on maintaining sinus rhythm after conversion of atrial fibrillation or flutter. A multicenter study from Stockholm. *Br. Heart J.* 37:486, 1975.
82. Grande, P., Sonne, B., and Pedersen, A. A controlled study of digoxin and quinidine in patients DC reverted from atrial fibrillation to sinus rhythm. Circulation 74(Suppl II):101, 1986.
83. Coplen, S. E., Antman, E. M., Bevlin, J. A., et al. Efficacy and safety of quinidine therapy for maintenance of sinus rhythm after cardioversion. *Circulation* 82:1106, 1990.
84. Doering, W. Quinidine-digoxin interactions. Pharmacokinetics, underlying mechanism, and clinical implication. *N. Engl. J. Med.* 301:400, 1979.
85. Fenster, P. E., Comess, K. A., Marsh, R., et al. Conversion of atrial fibrillation to sinus rhythm by acute intravenous procainamide infusion. *Am. Heart J.* 106:501, 1983.
86. Shen, E. N., Keuns, E., Huyck, E., et al. Intravenous propafenone for termination of reentrant supraventricular tachycardia. A placebo controlled, randomized double-blind, crossover study. *Ann. Intern. Med.* 105:655, 1986.
87. Manz, M., Steinbeck, G., and Luderitz, B. Usefulness of programmed stimulation in predicting efficacy of propafenone in long-term antiarrhythmic therapy for paroxysmal supraventricular tachycardia. *Am. J. Cardiol.* 56:593, 1985.
88. Sonnhag, C., Kallryd, A., Nylander, E., and Ryden, L. Long term efficacy of flecainide in paroxysmal atrial fibrillation. *Acta Med. Scand.* 224:563, 1988.
89. Cockrell, J. L., Scheinman, M. M., Titus, C., et al. Safety and efficacy of oral flecainide therapy in patients with atrioventricular re-entrant tachycardia. *Ann. Intern. Med.* 114:189, 1991.
90. Suttorp, M. J., Herre Kingma, J., Jessurun, E. R., et al. The value of class IC antiarrhythmic drugs for acute conversion of paroxysmal atrial fibrillation or flutter to sinus rhythm. *J. Am. Coll. Cardiol.* 16:1722, 1990.
91. Chimienti, M., Bergolis, M. L., Moizi, M., and Salerno, J. A. Electrophysiologic and clinical effects of oral encainide in paroxysmal atrioventricular node reentrant tachycardia. *J. Am. Coll. Cardiol.* 14:992, 1989.
92. Echt, D. S., Liebson, P. R., Mitchell, L. B., et al. Mortality and morbidity in patients receiving encainide, flecainide, or placebo. *N. Engl. J. Med.* 324:781, 1991.
93. Leak, D. Intravenous amiodarone in the treatment of refractory life-threatening cardiac arrhythmias in the critically ill patient. *Am. Heart J.* 111:456, 1986.
94. Escoubet, B., Coumel, P., Poirier, J. M., et al. Suppression of arrhythmias within hours after a single oral dose of amiodarone and relation to plasma and myocardial concentration. *Am. J. Cardiol.* 55:696, 1985.
95. Gosselink, A. T. M., Crijns, H. J. G. M., Van Gelder, K., et al. Low dose amiodarone for maintenance of sinus rhythm after cardioversion of atrial fibrillation or flutter. *J.A.M.A.* 267:3289, 1992.
96. Jordaens, L., Gorseis, A., Stroobandt, R., et al. Efficacy and safety of intravenous sotalol for termination of paroxysmal supraventricular tachycardia. *Am. J. Cardiol.* 68:35, 1991.
97. Juul-Moller, S., Edvardsson, N., and Rehnqvist-Ahlberg, R. Sotalol versus quinidine for the maintenance of sinus rhythm after direct current conversion of atrial fibrillation. *Circulation* 82:1932, 1990.
98. Luderitz, B., and Manz, M. Pharmacologic treatment of supraventricular tachycardia: The German experience. *Am. J. Cardiol.* 70:66A, 1992.
99. DiMarco, J. P., Sellers, T. D., Lerman, B. B., et al. Diagnostic and therapeutic use of adenosine in patients with supraventricular tachyarrhythmias. *J. Am. Coll. Cardiol.* 6:417, 1985.
100. Viskin, S., Belhassen, B., Sheps, D., and Laniado, S. Clinical and electrophysiologic effects of magnesium sulfate on paroxysmal supraventricular tachycardia and comparison with adenosine triphosphate. *Am. J. Cardiol.* 70:879, 1992.
101. Kerber, R. E., Jensen, S. R., Grayzel, J., et al. Electric cardioversion: Influence of paddle electrode location and size on success rate and energy requirement. *N. Engl. J. Med.* 305:658, 1981.
102. Mancini, G. B., and Goldberger, A. L. Cardioversion of atrial fibrillation: Consideration of embolization, anticoagulation, prophylactic pacemaker, and long-term success. *Am. Heart J.* 104:617, 1982.
103. Manning, W. S. J., Silverman, D. I., Gordon, S. P. F., et al. Cardioversion from atrial fibrillation without prolonged anticoagulation with the use of transesophageal echocardiography to exclude the presence of atrial thrombi. *N. Engl. J. Med.* 328: 750, 1993.
104. Greenberg, M. L., Kelly, T. A., Lerman, B. B., and DiMarco, J. P. Atrial pacing for conversion of atrial flutter. *Am. J. Cardiol.* 58:95, 1986.
105. Levy, S., Lauribe, P., Dolla, E., et al. A randomized comparison of external and internal cardioversion of chronic atrial fibrillation. *Circulation* 86:1415, 1992.
106. Nordrehaug, J. E., and von der Lippe, G. Serum potassium concentrations are inversely related to ventricular, but not to atrial, arrhythmias in acute myocardial infarction. *Eur. Heart J.* 7:204, 1986.
107. Liem, K. L., Durrer, D., Lie, K. I., and Wellens,

H. J. Pericarditis in acute myocardial infarction. *Lancet* 2:1004, 1975.

108. Dubois, C., Smeets, J. P., Demoulin, J. C., et al. Frequency and clinical significance of pericardial friction rubs in the acute phase of myocardial infarction. *Eur. Heart J.* 6:766, 1985.

109. Henrard, L., and Lisin, N. Myocardial infarction and late pericarditis. *Arch. Mal. Coeur Vaiss.* 72:862, 1979.

110. Cowan, J. C., Gardiner, P., Reid, D. S., et al. A comparison of amiodarone and digoxin in the treatment of atrial fibrillation complicating suspected acute myocardial infarction. *J. Cardiovasc. Pharmacol.* 8:252, 1986.

IV.
Mechanical Complications of Acute Myocardial Infarction: Diagnosis and Treatment

13. Hemodynamic Profiles of Pump Disturbances in Acute Myocardial Infarction: Management Strategies

Kanu Chatterjee

Hemodynamic disturbances following acute myocardial infarction range from little or no change to severe abnormalities. The extent, location, and rapidity of myocardial necrosis are the major determinants of the severity of hemodynamic derangements. The magnitude of left ventricular dysfunction resulting from previous myocardial infarction also contributes to the overall functional and hemodynamic impairment. Ischemic myocardium, in addition to infarcted myocardium, compromises ventricular performance and produces hemodynamic abnormalities. At the onset of myocardial infarction, the extent of ischemic but viable myocardium is relatively greater than the extent of necrosis. With prompt relief of ischemia, recovery of function of the ischemic myocardium may be associated with rapid hemodynamic improvement. In contrast, progressive deterioration in hemodynamics occurs with infarct extension and expansion.

Hyperfunctioning noninfarcted myocardial segments compensate for the loss of function of the ischemic and infarcted segments [1–3]. With adequate compensation there may be little or no hemodynamic derangement. However, profound hemodynamic disturbances may occur with inadequate, or failure of, compensations to maintain cardiac performance.

Peripheral circulatory changes in response to pump failure following myocardial infarction contribute to sustain perfusion (arterial) pressure to the vital organs and for the economic and effective distribution of decreased cardiac output. Enhanced systemic and regional sympathetic activity and stimulation of the renin-angiotensin-aldosterone system increase systemic vascular resistance and maintain arterial pressure [4]. Increased peripheral venous tone promotes venous return to the heart and increases intracardiac volume, which enhances forward stroke volume by the Frank-Starling mechanism. Thus arterial pressure and cardiac output may remain normal despite the loss of function of ischemic and infarcted myocardium. However, these compensatory peripheral circulatory changes may also exert adverse effects on cardiac performance and hemodynamics. Marked sympathetic activation may induce tachycardia, which is associated with increased myocardial oxygen consumption. Increased systemic vascular resistance also increases left ventricular outflow resistance, which decreases stroke volume, as an inverse relation exists between left ventricular stroke volume and its outflow resistance [5]. Ventricular diastolic pressures usually increase along with increased volume, and thus pulmonary and systemic venous pressures also increase—the hemodynamic determinants of the congestive symptoms. Furthermore, myocardial oxygen consumption increases along with increased left ventricular volume. The net changes in systemic hemodynamics therefore result from a number of interacting central and peripheral adjustments accompanying acute myocardial infarction. Mechanical complications such as mitral regurgitation or ventricular septal rupture produce specific hemodynamic abnormalities. Predominant right ventricular infarction is also associated with hemodynamic abnormalities different from those that result from predominant left ventricular infarction. Thus the mechanisms of hemodynamic derangements in severe pump failure following acute myocardial infarction result from complex interactions between systolic and diastolic dysfunction due to myocardial ischemia and injury and altered peripheral hemodynamics mediated by activated neuroendocrine systems. The compensatory increases in adrenergic and renin-angiotensin-aldosterone systems that contribute to maintain arterial pressure and intravascular and intracardiac blood volume also cause vasoconstriction, increase preload and afterload, and contribute to impaired organ perfusion. Thus a vicious cycle may be established, involving neuroendocrine, peripheral, and central hemodynamics that cause progressive deterioration in these patients [65].

This chapter reviews first the general functional derangements of acute myocardial ischemia and infarction and then the hemodynamic consequences of the specific complications of acute myocardial infarction.

Systolic Dysfunction in Acute Myocardial Infarction

Total thrombotic occlusion at the site of atheromatous plaque in the infarct-related artery is the mechanism of transmural myocardial infarction in more than 90 percent of patients [6]. Within a few seconds of total interruption of coronary blood flow, systolic shortening of ischemic myocardial segments decreases, and after approximately 30 seconds of ischemia, little or no effective work is performed by the ischemic segments [7–9]. Within a few minutes, ischemic regions demonstrate bulging during isovolumic systole and akinesis during the ejection phase [7, 10]. Paradoxical shortening of the ischemic myocardium is observed during isovolumic relaxation and the early diastolic phases.

The degree of functional impairment of the ischemic myocardium is related to the magnitude of the reduction of coronary blood flow. In the presence of preexisting adequate collateral blood flow, the magnitude of reduction of effective myocardial perfusion is less despite complete occlusion of the infarct-related artery. When subtotal occlusion of the infarct-related artery is the anatomic and pathophysiologic mechanism of myocardial infarction, the degree of ischemia is also relatively less and is usually confined to the subendocardium [11]. When functionally collateral vessels are present, the extent of myocardial necrosis and the degree of functional impairment tend to be less [12–15]. The hemodynamic disturbances are likewise less pronounced.

Perfusion may be reestablished shortly after total interruption of blood flow (e.g., within 15 to 20 minutes), and significant recovery of systolic function of the ischemic myocardium may occur, minimizing the hemodynamic disturbances [16–18]. If reperfusion occurs after 60 minutes of ischemia, recovery of ventricular function may require up to 4 weeks [19]. This prolonged impairment in myocardial function despite reestablishment of adequate coronary blood flow has been termed stunned myocardium [20]. The hemodynamic abnormalities resulting from nonfunctioning ischemic myocardium therefore are not immediately corrected by delayed reperfusion, although the function of the stunned myocardium ultimately recovers along with improvement in hemodynamics. Thus the timing of recanalization of the infarct-related artery and reperfusion of the ischemic myocardium following the onset of myocardial infarction is directly related to the severity of the hemodynamic disturbances. Although early reperfusion may avert significant hemodynamic abnormalities, delayed reperfusion may still be associated with marked hemodynamic derangements, requiring aggressive supportive and corrective therapy.

Impaired systolic function is also observed in the relatively nonischemic regions adjacent to the infarcted segments. Functional alterations can occur in the subepicardial regions with milder degrees of myocardial ischemia when subendocardial blood flow declines with little or no reduction of flow in the subepicardium [21–23]. Adjacent nonischemic subendocardial regions may also demonstrate altered function. This phenomenon probably results from mechanical "tethering" of the infarcted and nonischemic zones.

Augmented systolic function of the myocardial segments remote from the area of infarction is frequent at the early phase of infarction [1–3]. Hyperfunction of the nonischemic areas primarily results from increased utilization of the Frank-Starling mechanism, which is due to increased end-diastolic pressure, a hemodynamic consequence of acute myocardial ischemia [8, 10]. Enhanced sympathetic stimulation may also contribute to the hyperfunction of the nonischemic zones [2]. Experimental studies in animals, however, suggest that the "compensatory" increase in shortening of the nonischemic myocardial segments primarily causes stretching of the ischemic region during isovolumic (paradoxical) systole, and there is little or no increase in the ejection phase shortening of the nonischemic zones [10]. If there is no increase in end-diastolic pressure, there is no increased utilization of the Frank-Starling mechanism, and in these circumstances there may be an actual decrease in ejection phase shortening in nonischemic regions [24]. The results of these experimental studies explain the relatively higher ''optimal filling pressure'' in patients with acute myocardial infarction (14 to 18 mm Hg pulmonary capillary wedge pressure). The absence of augmented systolic motion of the ventricular wall opposite the region of the acute infarct is an important risk factor for the development of severe pump failure, cardiogenic shock with its hemodynamic abnormalities, and death [66, 67].

Diastolic Dysfunction in Acute Myocardial Infarction

Regional and global diastolic dysfunction is as frequent as systolic dysfunction in patients with acute myocardial ischemia or infarction. Indeed, diastolic dysfunction and its hemodynamic consequences tend to precede impairment of systolic function.

During acute spontaneous or induced myocardial ischemia, the ischemic region shortens paradoxically during isovolumic relaxation and early diastolic phases, presumably due to elastic recoil of the passively stretched ischemic region or persistent late systolic active shortening [7, 25]. Nonischemic zones may demonstrate early lengthening during the isovolumic relaxation phase; the mechanism and significance of this phenomenon, however, remain unclear. Abnormalities of ventricular relaxation are also reflected in a decrease in the peak rate of left ventricular pressure fall (peak dP/dt) and an increase in the time constant of left ventricular pressure fall during isovolumic relaxation (τ or tau) [26–30].

Alterations in diastolic filling characteristics are frequent consequences of acute myocardial ischemia and infarction. Peak diastolic filling rates decrease during induced myocardial ischemia [31, 32]. In patients with ischemic heart disease, successful reperfusion by coronary angioplasty increases the peak filling rate [33]. The precise mechanism for impaired filling in patients with ischemia or infarction has not been clarified; regional abnormality of diastolic function, incomplete ventricular relaxation, and alteration in myocardial stiffness may be contributory [34]. Increased end-systolic volume and pressure resulting from impaired systolic emptying enhance inflow impedance and impair diastolic filling [25]. Elevated left ventricular diastolic pressure also offers increased resistance to diastolic filling and decreases effective filling time [35].

Left ventricular filling pressures are elevated in many patients, particularly early during the acute phase of myocardial infarction [2, 36–39]. A number of mechanisms appear to contribute to high ventricular diastolic pressure. The left ventricular diastolic pressure-volume relation is shifted upward during induced myocardial ischemia [40–42]. Impaired ventricular relaxation [28, 29], ventricular interaction effects [43], and increased myocardial stiffness [44, 45] might be contributory. Whatever the mechanism, elevated ventricular filling pressure is a common hemodynamic consequence of abnormal diastolic function.

A mild to moderate increase in left ventricular filling pressure may augment cardiac performance because of increased utilization of the Frank-Starling mechanism by the noninfarcted, nonischemic regions. However, an excessive increase in left ventricular filling pressure can produce several deleterious effects. Increased left ventricular diastolic pressure is associated with a passive increase in left atrial and pulmonary venous pressures—the hemodynamic determinant of pulmonary congestion and pulmonary edema. Compromised subendocardial perfusion resulting from decreased transmyocardial pressure gradient may enhance subendocardial ischemia and cause further deterioration of systolic and diastolic function. The therapeutic implications are that when the left ventricular filling pressure is low, it should be increased to the ''optimal range'' to augment stroke volume and cardiac output, if indicated. The left ventricular filling pressure should be lowered when it is excessively high in order to avoid pulmonary congestion and to improve subendocardial perfusion.

Hemodynamic Subsets of Acute Myocardial Infarction

Based on hemodynamic derangements and their clinical manifestations, several subsets can be recognized [29, 46]. The hemodynamic subsets are based on changes in cardiac output and pulmonary capillary wedge pressure following acute myocardial infarction that reflect changes in left ventricular function. Changes in cardiac output are manifested clinically by changes in peripheral organ perfusion, and the level of pulmonary capillary wedge pressure is correlated to pulmonary congestion.

Bedside hemodynamic evaluation was performed in 200 patients with acute myocardial infarction within 72 hours of the onset of symptoms [29, 46]. Based on the initial level of pulmonary capillary wedge pressure and cardiac index, four hemodynamic subsets could be identified (Table 13-1).

In patients in subset I, the pulmonary capillary wedge pressure was 18 mm Hg or less, and the cardiac index was more than 2.2 L/min/m^2. Clinical evidence for pulmonary congestion or tissue hypoperfusion was absent. Hemodynamic disturbances were mild, left ventricular function was not markedly compromised, and the hospital mortality was low, only 3 percent. This hemodynamic profile occurred in approximately 25 percent of patients. No specific therapy was required until a complication supervened. As these patients could be recognized clinically, hemodynamic monitoring was also not indicated.

In patients in subset II, pulmonary capillary wedge pressure was elevated ($\geq$ 18 mm Hg), but the cardiac index remained higher than 2.2 L/min/m^2. Clinically, these patients presented with signs and symptoms of pulmonary congestion without evidence for hypoperfusion. Approximately 25 percent of patients presented with this hemodynamic and clinical profile, and their immediate prognosis appeared to be worse than that of patients in subset I; hospital mortality was 9 percent.

The primary hemodynamic objective of treatment is to decrease pulmonary capillary wedge pressure with morphine, diuretics, and nitrates. If there is prompt relief of pulmonary edema, hemodynamic monitoring is not required in most patients. If the symptoms and signs of pulmonary congestion persist or hypotension and hypoperfusion occur, determination of pulmonary capillary wedge pressure and cardiac output aids in making further therapeutic decisions. Echocardiography-Doppler evaluation is also helpful to exclude silent, mitral regurgitation. Subsequent therapy can be tailored according to the hemodynamic abnormalities: If pulmonary capillary wedge pressure remains high, nitroglycerin and diuretics are continued. When cardiac output is also low or when pulmonary capillary wedge pressure remains elevated, the addition of sodium nitroprusside or phentolamine can produce an increase in cardiac output and further reduction of pulmonary capillary wedge pressure. Alternatively, phosphodiesterase inhibitors (amrinone, milrinone, enoximone) can be used to increase cardiac output and decrease pulmonary capillary wedge pressure. Systemic vasodilators or phosphodiesterase inhibitors, however, should be used with caution if arterial pressure is low.

The hemodynamic profile of patients in subset III was characterized by a low cardiac index ($<$ 2.2 L/min/m^2) and low pulmonary capillary wedge pressure ($\leq$ 18 mm Hg). Thus signs and symptoms of hypoperfusion rather than symptoms of pulmonary congestion were more apparent clinically. This hemodynamic profile was detected in approximately 15 percent of patients. The hospital mortal-

Table 13-1
Subsets of acute myocardial infarction

	Clinical manifestations		Hemodynamic correlates	
Subset	Pulmonary congestion	Hypoperfusion	PCWP (mm Hg)	CI (L/min/m^2)
I	Absent	Absent	$\leq$18	>2.2
II	Present	Absent	$\geq$18	>2.2
III	Absent	Present	$\leq$18	<2.2
IV	Present	Present	$\geq$18	<2.2

PCWP = pulmonary capillary wedge pressure; CI = cardiac index.
Source: Modified from J. S. Forrester et al. Medical therapy of acute myocardial infarction by application of hemodynamic subsets (first two parts). *N. Engl. J. Med.* 295:1361, 1976. Reprinted by permission.

ity, however, was considerably higher, about 23 percent, suggesting that a decline in cardiac output is associated with worse prognosis than when only pulmonary capillary wedge pressure is elevated.

The mechanisms for the hemodynamic profile of patients in subset III are not entirely clear. Relative or absolute hypovolemia associated with decreased left and right ventricular preload can explain the low cardiac output and low ventricular filling pressures. However, the incidence of hypovolemia is low and is unlikely to be the sole or principal mechanism for these hemodynamic abnormalities. Decreased contractile function, increased ventricular outflow resistance, or both may produce a similar hemodynamic profile in patients with markedly reduced preload (e.g., excessive use of diuretics) prior to the onset of infarction. The hemodynamic abnormalities following right ventricular myocardial infarction may also be similar; however, in patients with right ventricular myocardial infarction, there is usually disproportionate elevation of right atrial pressure compared to pulmonary capillary wedge pressure. It is apparent that it is necessary to establish the mechanism of the hemodynamic profile of patients in subset III in order to select appropriate therapy. Concomitant noninvasive assessment of ventricular chamber size (radionuclide ventriculography or echocardiography) along with hemodynamic determinations can potentially clarify the pathophysiologic mechanisms. Decreased right ventricular systolic function with relatively preserved left ventricular function suggests right ventricular failure, indicating right ventricular myocardial infarction in these clinical circumstances. Normal or decreased ventricular chamber size with relatively preserved systolic function indicates abnormal ventricular compliance as a mechanism for the hemodynamic changes. It is, however, appropriate to consider "volume challenge" with fairly rapid administration of intravenous fluids for the differential diagnosis and the selection of appropriate therapy. When cardiac output does not increase appreciably despite a considerable increase in pulmonary capillary wedge pressure (e.g., > 20 mm Hg), it is likely that marked impairment of left ventricular systolic function is the principal cause for the hemodynamic profile of patients in subset III [47]. In patients with true or absolute hypovolemia, a significant increase in stroke volume and cardiac output is expected along with the increase in right atrial and pulmonary capillary wedge pressures. In patients with markedly decreased left ventricular compliance, volume challenge increases left ventricular filling pressure with no substantial increase in left ventricular preload.

The hemodynamic abnormalities in patients in subset IV were characterized by an elevated pulmonary capillary wedge pressure equal to or exceeding 18 mm Hg and a low cardiac index, less than 2.2 L/min/m^2. Clinically, signs and symptoms of pulmonary congestion and hypoperfusion were present. Approximately 35 percent of the patients had this hemodynamic profile, and the hospital mortality was highest in this subset of patients, approximately 51 percent.

Marked impairment of left ventricular systolic function (reduced ejection fraction) is the principal mechanism for these hemodynamic changes. In addition to the decreased cardiac index and high pulmonary capillary wedge pressure, left ventricular stroke work index is reduced, and frequently sinus tachycardia and relative hypotension are observed. In patients with cardiogenic shock, the systolic arterial pressure is 90 mm Hg or less, and the cardiac index may be 1.5 L/min/m^2 or even less. Because of hypotension and low cardiac output, features of hypoperfusion are universally present: decreased urine output (< 20 ml/hr) and renal failure, hepatic dysfunction, pancreatic and gastrointestinal ischemia, cool and clammy skin, peripheral cyanosis, and mental obtundation. Enhanced anaerobic metabolism and metabolic acidosis frequently result and progressively worsen until a prompt increase in cardiac output can be achieved with appropriate therapeutic interventions. The cardiogenic shock syndrome occurs in approximately 10 to 15 percent of patients with acute myocardial infarction, and the immediate hospital mortality remains high, exceeding 80 percent, despite aggressive pharmacotherapy. Severe pump failure with or without clinical features of cardiogenic shock usually results from markedly impaired systolic function of large areas of ventricular myocardium. However, mechanical complications such as acute left ventricular aneurysm, papillary muscle infarction, and ventricular septal rupture may precipitate severe pump failure even in the presence of less extensive myocardial damage.

Prompt supportive therapy, based on the severity of the hemodynamic abnormalities and the hemody-

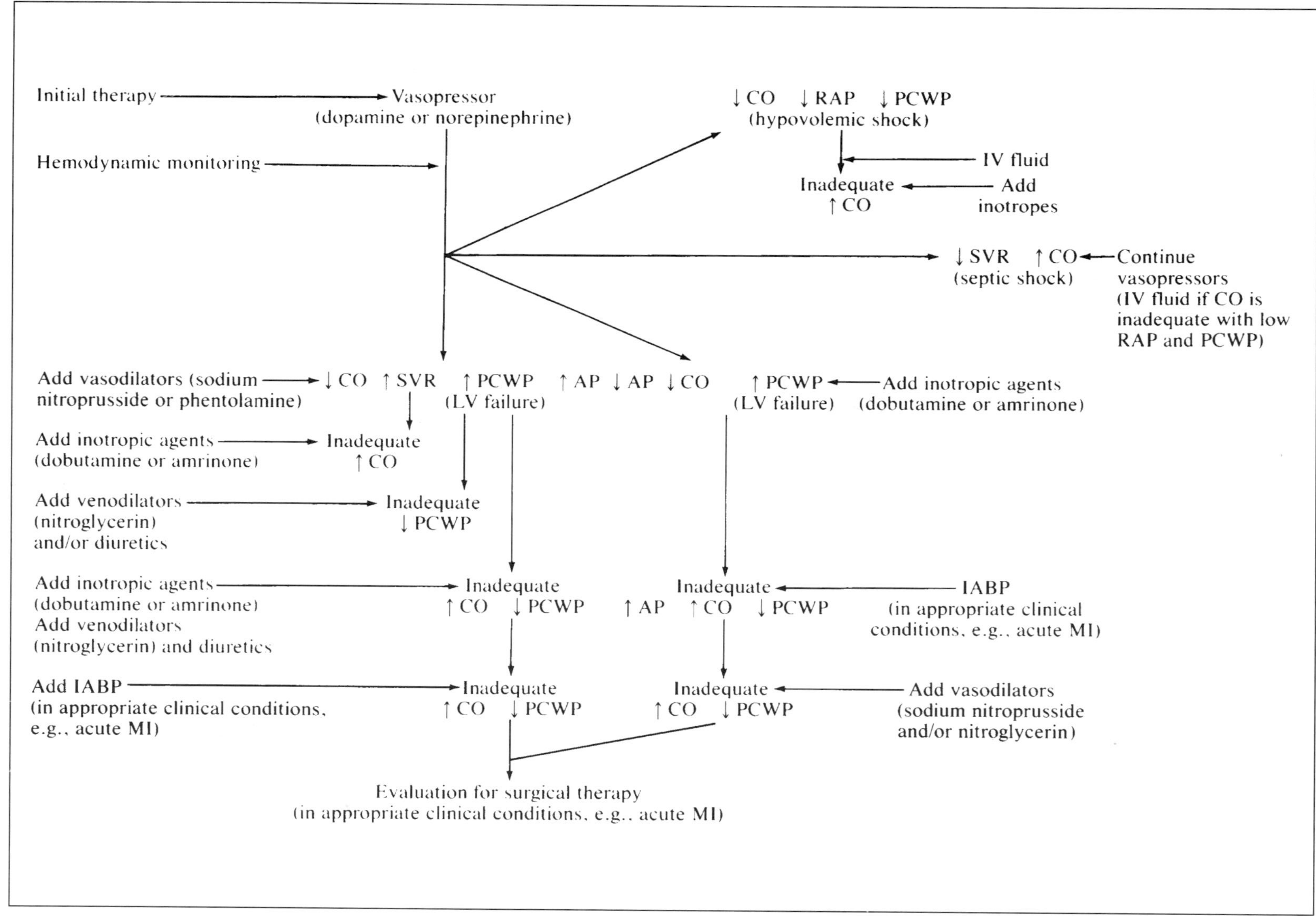
Initial therapy
Vasopressor (dopamine or norepinephrine)
Hemodynamic monitoring
↓CO ↓RAP ↓PCWP (hypovolemic shock)
IV fluid
Inadequate ↑CO
Add inotropes
↓SVR ↑CO (septic shock)
Continue vasopressors (IV fluid if CO is inadequate with low RAP and PCWP)
Add vasodilators (sodium nitroprusside or phentolamine)
↓CO ↑SVR
↑PCWP (LV failure)
↑AP ↓AP ↓CO
↑PCWP (LV failure)
Add inotropic agents (dobutamine or amrinone)
Add inotropic agents (dobutamine or amrinone)
Inadequate ↑CO
Add venodilators (nitroglycerin) and/or diuretics
Inadequate ↓PCWP
Add inotropic agents (dobutamine or amrinone) Add venodilators (nitroglycerin) and diuretics
Inadequate ↑CO ↓PCWP
↑AP
Inadequate ↑CO ↓PCWP
IABP (in appropriate clinical conditions, e.g., acute MI)
Add IABP (in appropriate clinical conditions, e.g., acute MI)
Inadequate ↑CO ↓PCWP
Inadequate ↑CO ↓PCWP
Add vasodilators (sodium nitroprusside and/or nitroglycerin)
Evaluation for surgical therapy (in appropriate clinical conditions, e.g., acute MI)

namic response to therapeutic intervention, is essential. Thus hemodynamic monitoring is indicated in patients in subset IV. Preliminary uncontrolled studies suggested that early recanalization by angioplasty of the infarct-related artery with or without prior administration of thrombolytic agents may improve the prognosis of patients with cardiogenic shock [48, 68]. Although benefits of such a therapeutic approach in the management of cardiogenic shock have not been firmly established, reperfusion therapy with angioplasty should be considered in appropriate patients, as the prognosis with supportive therapy alone remains poor. However, supportive therapy including the use of support devices is required, as hemodynamics and ventricular function do not improve immediately even when adequate recanalization of the infarct-related artery is established promptly [69].

The major objectives of the therapy of severe pump failure with or without the clinical features of cardiogenic shock are to improve cardiac performance, correct hemodynamic abnormalities, maintain viability of ischemic myocardium, and limit the extent of myocardial damage. At present, early reperfusion therapy provides the best chance for limiting infarct size. No conclusive evidence exists to support the routine use of nitroglycerin, nitroprusside, beta blockers, calcium entry–blocking agents, or intra-aortic balloon counterpulsation in patients with significant pump failure (subset IV) to decrease the extent of myocardial injury. Pharmacotherapy and intra-aortic balloon counterpulsation are employed to correct hemodynamic abnormalities and to improve cardiac performance. It is necessary to determine the hemodynamic profile, which should include, at least, arterial pressures, cardiac output, pulmonary capillary wedge pressure, and systemic vascular resistance. Prompt assessment of the hemodynamic response to an intervention is also necessary to decide "when and what" additional therapeutic interventions should be considered. The general outline for the therapy of pump failure complicating acute myocardial infarction based on hemodynamics is summarized in Figure 13-1 [49].

Acute Mitral Regurgitation

Mitral regurgitation can result from ischemia or necrosis of the left ventricular papillary muscles and adjacent left ventricular walls anchoring the papillary muscles, producing papillary muscle dysfunction. Rupture of the tip or trunk of the papillary muscle causes severe mitral regurgitation.

Mild mitral regurgitation is common, occurring in approximately 30 percent of patients, during the acute phase of myocardial infarction. Minor degrees of papillary muscle dysfunction resulting from ischemia of the papillary muscles or of the left ventricular walls contiguous to the papillary muscles is the likely mechanism [50]. It is likely that inefficient contraction of the papillary muscles or contraction along an abnormal axis, shifted inappropriately by dyssynergic motion of the ventricular walls anchoring papillary muscles, produces inadequate coaptation of the mitral leaflets during systole. Mitral regurgitation resulting from mild papillary muscle dysfunction does not impose any significant hemodynamic burden, and no specific hemodynamic derangements are recognized.

Papillary muscle infarction with or without rupture produces severe mitral regurgitation and is a catastrophic complication of acute myocardial infarction. The incidence is approximately 1 percent, and it accounts for about 5 percent of deaths of patients with acute myocardial infarction [51, 52]. More frequently, posteromedial papillary muscle is involved, associated with inferior or inferoposterior

Fig. 13-1
Hypotension may be due to low cardiac output, low systemic vascular resistance, or both. Treatment of hypotension and pump failure is aided by hemodynamic monitoring in critically ill patients. ↑ = increase; ↓ = decrease; CO = cardiac output; SVR = systemic vascular resistance; PCWP = pulmonary capillary wedge pressure; AP = arterial pressure; RAP = right atrial pressure; IABP = intra-aortic balloon counterpulsation; LV = left ventricular; MI = myocardial infarction. (From K. Chatterjee. Bedside hemodynamic monitoring. In W. Parmley and K. Chatterjee, eds., *Cardiology*. Philadelphia: Lippincott, 1988. With permission.)

myocardial infarction due to occlusion of the right or left circumflex coronary artery. The extent of myocardial necrosis is relatively small in approximately 50 percent of patients and not infrequently is associated with single-vessel coronary artery disease.

Hemodynamic diagnosis of severe mitral regurgitation is usually made at the bedside by catheterization of the right side of the heart with balloon flotation catheters [49]. An early giant V wave in the pulmonary capillary wedge pressure tracing usually indicates acute or subacute severe mitral regurgitation. A reflected V wave, when recognized in the pulmonary artery pressure tracing, is pathognomonic of severe acute mitral regurgitation (Fig. 13-2) [49]. Giant V waves, however, may occur in the absence of mitral regurgitation, such as in patients with left-to-right shunt resulting from ventricular septal rupture. Giant V waves in the absence of mitral regurgitation are due to marked accentuation of the normal V wave because of decreased left atrial compliance or a marked increase in the venous return to the left atrium. The onset and peak of the V wave in these circumstances are delayed, in contrast to the "regurgitant wave" of mitral regurgitation, when the V waves occur at the beginning of systole. Thus with careful attention to the details of the changes in the waveforms of pulmonary artery and pulmonary capillary wedge pressure tracings, the diagnosis of mitral regurgitation can be established at the bedside. However, clinical examination and echocardiography-Doppler evaluation are necessary and are valuable for making the correct diagnosis.

The severity of the hemodynamic derangements is related to the degree of mitral regurgitation and ischemia–infarct-related left ventricular dysfunction. In general, papillary muscle infarct produces severe mitral regurgitation and rapidly deteriorating hemodynamics. The forward stroke volume and cardiac output decline, and reflex tachycardia occurs. Systolic blood pressure falls, and the diastolic blood pressure may be maintained owing to marked peripheral vasoconstriction, and thus the pulse pressure is reduced. There is a marked increase in pulmonary venous pressure, an obligatory rise in pulmonary artery pressure, and frequently an increase in right atrial pressure, indicating right ventricular failure. Mitral regurgitation decreases left ventricular systolic impedance, elevating its ejection fraction.

Therapeutic strategies consist of rapid stabilization and early surgical intervention. Early corrective surgery may result in a significant improve-

Fig. 13-2
Diagnosis of mitral regurgitation by bedside hemodynamic monitoring. A reflected V wave in the pulmonary artery pressure tracing and a giant V wave in the pulmonary artery wedge pressure tracing suggest severe acute or subacute mitral regurgitation. (From K. Chatterjee. Bedside hemodynamic monitoring. In W. Parmley and K. Chatterjee, eds., *Cardiology*. Philadelphia: Lippincott, 1988. With permission.)

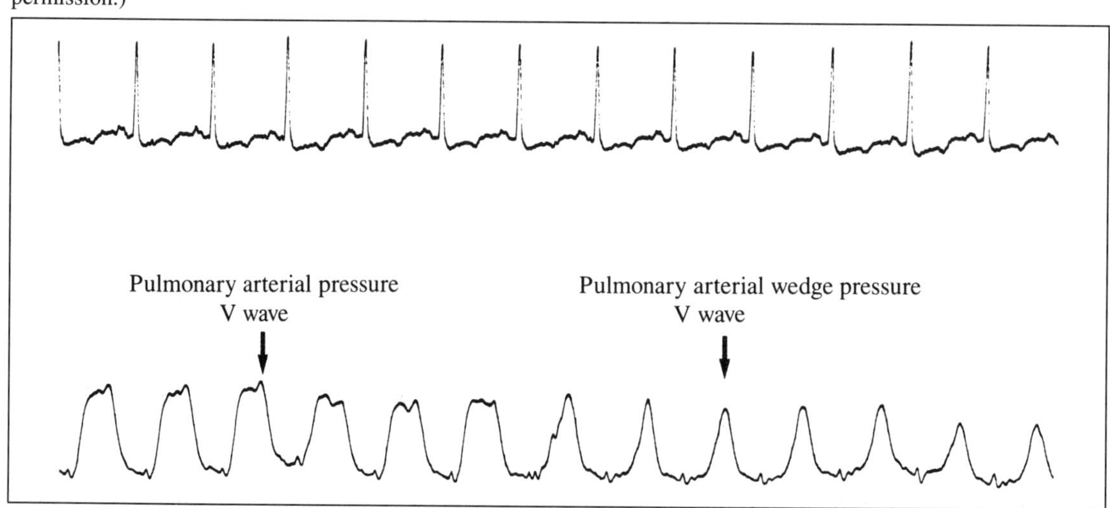

ment in prognosis; 60 to 70 percent of patients may survive this catastrophic complication. With conservative supportive therapy, mortality remains high, about 94 percent within 8 weeks, despite hemodynamic and clinical improvement initially in many patients [51–53].

The objectives of supportive therapy are to decrease regurgitant volume, increase forward stroke volume and cardiac output, and reduce pulmonary venous, pulmonary arterial, and systemic venous pressures. The severity of mitral regurgitation is related not only to the degree of anatomic derangement of the mitral valve apparatus but also to the aortic impedance. With increasing aortic impedance, regurgitant volume increases; with decreased impedance, regurgitant volume declines and forward stroke volume increases. Vasodilators such as sodium nitroprusside and hydralazine decrease systemic vascular resistance, reduce regurgitant volume, and increase forward stroke volume [54, 55]. Along with decreased regurgitant volumes, pulmonary venous pressures fall, and hemodynamics of the right side of the heart improve. In general, with nitroglycerin there is little or no increase in forward stroke volume, although regurgitant volume and pulmonary venous pressures decrease. Thus nitroprusside and hydralazine are preferable to nitroglycerin to correct the hemodynamic abnormalities of severe mitral regurgitation. The addition of inotropic agents such as dobutamine and amrinone may cause a further improvement in hemodynamics. Intra-aortic balloon counterpulsation is associated with decreased left ventricular outflow resistance and an increase in forward stroke volume and cardiac output. Pulmonary venous pressure decreases, presumably owing to reduction of the regurgitant volume, and the arterial diastolic pressure (perfusion pressure) is enhanced owing to diastolic augmentation. In hypotensive patients, intra-aortic balloon counterpulsation should be employed prior to vasodilator therapy. Hemodynamic monitoring is necessary to assess the response to therapy during stabilization of these patients.

Ventricular Septal Rupture

Rupture of the interventricular septum is another catastropic complication of acute myocardial infarction. The incidence is about 0.5 to 2.0 percent and accounts for 1 to 5 percent of all infarct-related deaths [56]. Ventricular septal rupture produces left-to-right shunt and volume overload on the right and left ventricles. Right atrial, pulmonary artery, and pulmonary capillary wedge pressures increase. With increasing left-to-right shunt, systemic output declines with a reflex increase in systemic vascular resistance, which causes a further increase in the magnitude of left-to-right shunt.

The diagnosis can be confirmed at the bedside by demonstrating a step-up in oxygen saturation ($\geq$ 10 percent) from the right atrium to the right ventricle or proximal pulmonary artery. It can also be established by two-dimensional echocardiography, Doppler flow study, or radionuclide studies [57, 58].

The rapidity of hemodynamic deterioration is relatively slower in patients with ventricular septal rupture than in patients with papillary muscle infarction. However, the mortality associated with septal rupture remains high, 24 percent within 24 hours, 46 percent at 1 week, and 67 to 82 percent at 2 months [51–53]. Early aggressive surgical therapy with repair of the ventricular septal defect and, when necessary, coronary artery bypass surgery and aneurysmectomy have been reported to improve the short-term and long-term prognosis [59]. Conservative therapy is thus indicated only to stabilize the patient prior to early corrective surgery. The objectives of supportive therapy are to decrease left-to-right shunt, increase systemic output, and reduce the pulmonary capillary wedge, right atrial, and pulmonary arterial pressures.

The magnitude of the left-to-right shunt in patients with ventricular septal rupture is primarily determined by the ratio of the pulmonary and systemic vascular resistance, as the defect is usually large and offers little resistance to left-to-right shunt. A greater decrease in systemic vascular resistance than in pulmonary vascular resistance is associated with decreased left-to-right shunt and increased systemic output.

Intra-aortic balloon counterpulsation selectively decreases left ventricular outflow resistance without causing any primary change in right ventricular outflow resistance. Thus with intra-aortic balloon counterpulsation, systemic output increases along with decreased left-to-right shunt. Pulmonary and systemic venous pressures also decrease along with augmented arterial diastolic pressure.

Vasodilator drugs can improve hemodynamics, decrease left-to-right shunt, and increase systemic output. However, changes in left-to-right shunt and systemic output due to vasodilators depend on the relative changes in pulmonary and systemic vascular resistance. If the reduction in pulmonary vascular resistance is relatively greater, left-to-right shunt increases. Thus vasodilators with less pronounced effects on the pulmonary vascular bed (e.g., hydralazine) are preferable to vasodilators that cause a substantial decrease in pulmonary vascular resistance (e.g., sodium nitroprusside, nitroglycerin).

It is apparent that hemodynamic monitoring is required during supportive therapy, particularly monitoring of the oxygen saturation changes in right atrial, pulmonary, arterial, and systemic arterial blood.

Right Ventricular Infarction

Predominant right ventricular infarction occurs almost exclusively in patients with inferior or inferoposterior infarction [60, 61], and is associated with worse prognosis in these patients [70]. Total right coronary artery occlusion, proximal to the origins of the right ventricular branches, is the usual anatomic basis for extensive right ventricular infarction, although multivessel coronary artery disease frequently accompanies it. A small right ventricular infarction may produce no hemodynamic abnormalities. A relatively large infarct, however, results in significant hemodynamic derangements and may be associated with decreased systemic output and hypotension. Disproportionate elevation of right atrial pressure compared to pulmonary capillary wedge pressure is the usual finding, and the ratio of the right atrial to the pulmonary capillary wedge pressure exceeds 0.86. In many patients with "low-output state," equalization of right atrial and pulmonary capillary wedge pressures is observed simulating the hemodynamic abnormalities of cardiac tamponade [62]. The equalization of the "diastolic pressure" results from the increased intrapericardial pressure as the stiff pericardium does not stretch quickly enough to compensate for the increased right ventricular volume [63]. In experimental isolated right ventricular infarction in dogs, pericardiectomy prevents equalization of diastolic pressures.

There are multiple hemodynamic mechanisms that contribute to the reduction of systemic output with right ventricular infarction. Decreased right ventricular pump function reduces the venous return to the left ventricle, reducing left ventricular preload. Increased intrapericardial pressure also restricts left ventricular filling. The interventricular septal shift toward the left ventricle also decreases left ventricular diastolic volume. Decreased and incoordinated contraction of the interventricular septum also contributes to the decrease in systemic output.

Right ventricular pump failure results not only from decreased contractility but also from augmented afterload. Right ventricular dilatation is associated with its increased wall stress. Increased left ventricular diastolic pressure resulting from increased intrapericardial pressure causes a passive increase in pulmonary arterial pressure, which also increases right ventricular outflow resistance. There is a further reduction of right ventricular stroke volume, which in turn decreases the left ventricular stroke volume. Impaired right atrial systolic function due to right atrial ischemia or infarction in patients with right ventricular infarction may also contribute to decreased right ventricular stroke volume. Thus a number of interacting hemodynamic mechanisms contribute to decreased left ventricular preload, which is the principal mechanism for decreased systemic output (Table 13-2).

Table 13-2
Mechanisms of decreased systemic output in right ventricular myocardial infarction

1. Decreased RV contractile function → reduced RVSV → decreased LV preload
2. Restricted ventricular filling due to the constraining effect of pericardium
3. Dilated RV with increased wall stress → increased RV afterload → reduced RVSV → decreased LV preload
4. Increased intrapericardial pressure → increased pulmonary venous and pulmonary arterial pressure → increased RV ejection impedance → decreased RVSV → decreased LV preload
5. Interventricular septal shift toward the left ventricle → decreased LV preload

RV = right ventricle; LV = left ventricle; RVSV = right ventricular stroke volume.

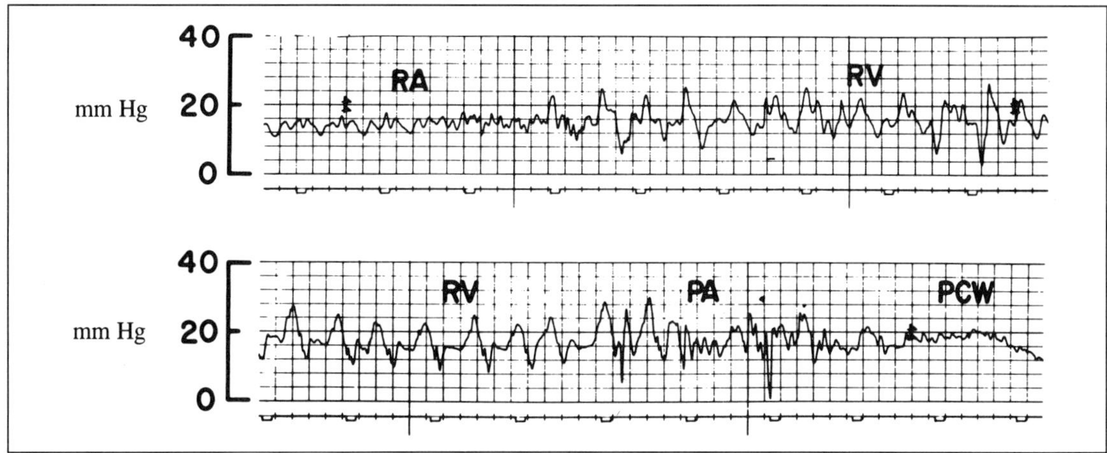

Fig. 13-3
Hemodynamic abnormalities in acute right myocardial infarction include a disproportionate elevation of right atrial (RA) pressure compared to pulmonary capillary wedge (PCW) pressure. In some patients the mean right atrial, right ventricular (RV) diastolic, pulmonary artery (PA) diastolic, and mean PCW pressures are similar. (From K. Chatterjee. Bedside hemodynamic monitoring. In W. Parmley and K. Chatterjee, eds., *Cardiology*. Philadelphia: Lippincott, 1988. With permission.)

Table 13-3
Hemodynamic management of "low-output state" in right ventricular infarction

Low cardiac output, right atrial pressure and pulmonary capillary wedge pressure <15 mm Hg: intravenous fluid → inadequate response → vasodilators if blood pressure is adequate → inadequate response → dobutamine.
Low cardiac output, right atrial pressure and pulmonary capillary wedge pressure >15 mm Hg: dobutamine or nitroprusside → inadequate response → combined dobutamine and nitroprusside.
Low cardiac output, right atrial pressure and pulmonary capillary wedge pressure >15 mm Hg, hypotension: dopamine → inadequate response → add dobutamine → inadequate response but blood pressure is higher → add nitroprusside.
In the presence of left ventricular failure: intraaortic balloon counterpulsation, in addition to vasodilator therapy and inotropic agents, may be required.

Assessment of hemodynamics has direct relevance during the management of a low-output state complicating right ventricular infarction (Fig. 13-3). Although intravenous fluid administration sometimes increases systemic output [64], volume expansion therapy is usually ineffective when the pulmonary capillary wedge and right atrial pressures are already elevated (> 12 to 15 mm Hg). It is feasible that in these circumstances intravenous fluid therapy does not cause a significant increase in left ventricular preload (end-diastolic volume or transmural pressure), although right atrial and pulmonary capillary wedge pressures increase because of increased intrapericardial pressures. Inotropic drugs such as dobutamine and dopamine appear to be more effective than vasodilators or intravenous fluid therapy for increasing systemic output and improving right ventricular pump function. When vasodilators such as sodium nitroprusside and nitroglycerin are used, concomitant intravenous fluid therapy is frequently required to maintain adequate right and left ventricular preload. The therapeutic approach for the treatment of a low-output state complicating right ventricular infarction based on hemodynamic abnormalities is summarized in Table 13-3.

References

1. Corya, B. C., Rasmussen, S., Knoebel, S. B., et al. Echocardiography in acute myocardial infarction. *Am. J. Cardiol.* 36:1, 1975.
2. Rigand, M., Rochar, P., Boschat, J., et al. Regional left ventricular function assessed by contrast angiography in acute myocardial infarction. *Circulation* 60:130, 1979.

3. Stack, R. S., Phillips, H. R., III, Grierson, D. S., et al. Functional improvement of jeopardized myocardium following intracoronary streptokinase infusion in acute myocardial infarction. *J. Clin. Invest.* 72:84, 1983.
4. Viquerat, C. E., Daly, P., Swedberg, K., et al. Endogenous catecholamines in chronic heart failure: Relation to the severity of hemodynamic abnormalities. *Am. J. Med.* 78:455, 1985.
5. Chatterjee, K., and Parmley, W. W. Role of vasodilator therapy in heart failure. *Prog. Cardiovasc. Dis.* 19:301, 1977.
6. DeWood, M. A., Spores, J., Notske, R. N., et al. Prevalence of total coronary occlusion during the early hours of transmural myocardial infarction. *N. Engl. J. Med.* 303:897, 1980.
7. Tennant, R., and Wiggins, C. J. The effect of coronary occlusion on myocardial contraction. *Am. J. Physiol.* 112:351, 1935.
8. Theroux, P., Franklin, D., Ross, J., Jr., et al. Regional myocardial function during acute coronary artery occlusion and its modification by pharmacologic agents in the dog. *Circ. Res.* 35:896, 1974.
9. Tyberg, J. V., Forrester, J. S., Wyatt, H. L., et al. An analysis of segmental ischemic dysfunction utilizing the pressure-length loop. *Circulation* 49:748, 1974.
10. Low, W. Y. W., Chen, Z., Guth, B., et al. Mechanisms of augmented segment shortening in nonischemic areas during acute ischemia of the canine left ventricle. *Circ. Res.* 56:351, 1985.
11. Gallagher, K. P., Osakada, G., Hess, O. M., et al. Subepicardial segmental function during coronary stenosis and the role of myocardial fiber orientation. *Circ. Res.* 50:352, 1982.
12. Williams, D. O., Amsterdam, E. A., Miller, R. R., et al. Functional significance of coronary collateral vessels in patients with acute myocardial infarction: Relation to pump performance, cardiogenic shock and survival. *Am. J. Cardiol.* 37:345, 1976.
13. Nohara, R., Kambara, H., Murakami, T., et al. Collateral function in early acute myocardial infarction. *Am. J. Cardiol.* 52:955, 1983.
14. Bertrand, M. E., Lefebvre, J. M., Laisne, C. L., et al. Coronary arteriography in acute transmural myocardial infarction. *Am. Heart J.* 97:61, 1979.
15. Betriu, A., Castaner, A., Sanz, G. A., et al. Angiographic findings one month after myocardial infarction: A prospective study of 259 survivors. *Circulation* 65:1099, 1982.
16. Theroux, P., Ross, J., Jr., Franklin, D., et al. Regional myocardial function in the conscious dog during acute coronary occlusion and responses to morphine, propranolol, nitroglycerin and lidocaine. *Circulation* 53:302, 1976.
17. Heyndrickx, G. R., Baig, H., Nellens, P., et al. Depression of regional blood flow and wall thickening after brief coronary occlusions. *Am. J. Physiol.* 234:H653, 1978.
18. Heyndrickx, G. R., Millard, R. W., McRitchie, R. J., et al. Regional myocardial functional and electrophysiologic alterations after brief coronary artery occlusion in conscious dogs. *J. Clin. Invest.* 56: 978, 1975.
19. Lanakee, M., Cox, D., Pastrick, T. A., et al. Salvage of myocardial function by coronary artery reperfusion 1, 2, and 3 hours after occlusion in conscious dogs. *Circ. Res.* 53:235, 1983.
20. Braunwald, E., and Kloner, R. A. The stunned myocardium: Prolonged post-ischemic ventricular dysfunction. *Circulation* 66:1146, 1982.
21. Weintraub, W. S., Hastton, S., Agarwal, J. B., et al. The relationship between myocardial blood flow and contraction by myocardial layer in the canine left ventricle during ischemia. *Circ. Res.* 48:430, 1981.
22. Gallagher, K. P., Osakada, G., Hess, O. M., et al. Subepicardial segmental function during coronary stenosis and the role of myocardial fiber orientation. *Circ. Res.* 50:352, 1982.
23. Hattori, S., Weintraub, W. S., Agarwal, J. B., et al. Contrasting ischemic contraction patterns by zone and layer in canine myocardium. *Am. J. Physiol.* 243:H852, 1982.
24. Lew, W. Y. W., and Ban-Hayashi, E. Mechanisms of improving regional and global ventricular function by preload alterations during acute ischemia in the canine left ventricle. *Circulation* 72:1125, 1985.
25. Hess, O. M., Osakada, G., Lavelle, J. F., et al. Left ventricular geometry during partial and complete coronary occlusion in the conscious dog. *Int. J. Cardiol.* 1:387, 1982.
26. Waters, D. D., DaLuz, P., Wyatt, H. L., et al. Early changes in regional and global left ventricular function induced by graded reduction in regional coronary perfusion. *Am. J. Cardiol.* 39:537, 1977.
27. Kumada, T., Karliner, J. S., Pouleur, H., et al. Effects of coronary occlusion on early ventricular diastolic events in conscious dogs. *Am. J. Physiol.* 237: H542, 1979.
28. Mann, T., Goldberg, S., Mudge, G. H., Jr., et al. Factors contributing to altered left ventricular diastolic properties during angina pectoris. *Circulation* 59:14, 1979.
29. Carroll, J. D., Hess, O. M., Hirzel, H. O., et al. Exercise-induced ischemia: The influence of altered relaxation on early diastolic pressures. *Circulation* 67:521, 1983.
30. Sharma, B., Behrens, T. W., Erlein, D., et al. Left ventricular diastolic properties and filling characteristics during spontaneous angina pectoris at rest. *Am. J. Cardiol.* 52:704, 1983.
31. Reduto, L. A., Wickemeyer, W. J., Young, J. B., et al. Left ventricular diastolic performance at rest and during exercise in patients with coronary artery disease: Assessment with first-pass radionuclide angiography. *Circulation* 63:1228, 1981.
32. Poliner, L. R., Farber, S. H., Glaeser, D. H., et al. Alteration of diastolic filling rate during exercise radionuclide angiography: A highly sensitive technique for detection of coronary artery disease. *Circulation* 70:942, 1984.

33. Bonow, R. O., Kent, K. M., Rosing, D. R., et al. Improved left ventricular diastolic filling in patients with coronary artery disease after percutaneous transluminal coronary angioplasty. *Circulation* 66: 1159, 1982.
34. Bonow, R. O., Vitale, D. F., Bacharach, S. L., et al. Asynchronous left ventricular regional function and impaired global diastolic filling in patients with coronary artery disease: Reversal after coronary angioplasty. *Circulation* 71:297, 1985.
35. Weisfeldt, M. L., Armstrong, P., Scully, H. E., et al. Incomplete relaxation between beats after myocardial hypoxia and ischemia. *J. Clin. Invest.* 53:1626, 1974.
36. Hamosh, P., and Cohn J. N. Left ventricular function in acute myocardial infarction. *J. Clin. Invest.* 50:523, 1971.
37. Rackley, C. E., and Russell, R. O., Jr. Left ventricular function in acute myocardial infarction and its clinical significance. *Circulation* 45:231, 1972.
38. Chatterjee, K., Parmley, W. W., Ganz, W., et al. Hemodynamic and metabolic responses to vasodilator therapy in acute myocardial infarction. *Circulation* 48:1183, 1973.
39. Forrester, J. S., Diamond, G., Chatterjee, K., et al. Medical therapy of acute myocardial infarction by application of hemodynamic subsets. *N. Engl. J. Med.* 295:1356(part I), 1404(part II), 1976.
40. Diamond, G., and Forrester, J. S. Effect of coronary artery disease and acute myocardial infarction on left ventricular compliance in man. *Circulation* 45:11, 1972.
41. Barry, W. H., Brooker, J. Z., Alderman, E. L., et al. Changes in diastolic stiffness and tone of the left ventricle during angina pectoris. *Circulation* 49: 255, 1974.
42. Mann, T., Brodie, B. R., Grossmasn, W., et al. Effect of angina on the left ventricular diastolic pressure-volume relationship. *Circulation* 55:761, 1977.
43. Hess, O. M., Osakada, G., Lavelle, J. F., et al. Diastolic myocardial wall stiffness and ventricular relaxation during partial and complete coronary occlusions in the conscious dog. *Circ. Res.* 52:387, 1983.
44. Theroux, P., Ross, J., Jr., Franklin, D., et al. Regional myocardial function in the conscious dog during acute coronary occlusion and responses to morphine, propranolol, nitroglycerin, and lidocaine. *Circulation* 53:302, 1976.
45. Edwards, C. H., II, Rankin, J. S., McHale, P. A., et al. Effects of ischemia on left ventricular regional function in the conscious dog. *Am. J. Physiol.* 240:H413, 1981.
46. Forrester, J. S., Chatterjee, K., and Jobin, G. A new conceptual approach to the therapy of acute myocardial infarction. *Adv. Cardiol.* 15:111, 1975.
47. Crexells, C., Chatterjee, K., Forrester, J. S., et al. Optimal level of left heart filling pressures in acute myocardial infarction. *N. Engl. J. Med.* 289:1263, 1973.
48. Lee, L., Erbel, R., Brown, T. M., et al. Multicenter registry of angioplasty therapy of cardiogenic shock: Initial and longterm survival. *J. Am. Coll. Cardiol.* 17:599, 1991.
49. Chatterjee, K. Bedside hemodynamic monitoring. In W. Parmley and K. Chatterjee (eds.), *Cardiology*. Philadelphia: Lippincott, 1993. Pp. 1–24.
50. Shelburne, J. C., Rubinstein, D., and Gorlin, R. A reappraisal of papillary muscle dysfunction: Correlative clinical and angiographic study. *Am. J. Med.* 46:862, 1969.
51. Nishimura, R. A., Schaff, H. V., Shuh, C., et al. Papillary muscle rupture complicating acute myocardial infarction: Analysis of 17 patients. *Am. J. Cardiol.* 51:373, 1983.
52. Wei, J. Y., Hutchins, G. M., and Bulkley, B. H. Papillary muscle rupture in fatal acute myocardial infarction. *Ann. Intern. Med.* 90:149, 1979.
53. Clements, S. D., Story, W. E., Hurst, J. W., et al. Ruptured papillary muscle, a complication of acute myocardial infarction: Clinical presentation, diagnosis and treatment. *Clin. Cardiol.* 8:93, 1985.
54. Chatterjee, K., Parmley, W. W., Swan, H. J. C., et al. Beneficial effects of vasodilator agents in severe mitral regurgitation due to dysfunction of subvalvular apparatus. *Circulation* 48:684, 1973.
55. Greenberg, B. H., Massie, B. M., Botvinick, E. H., et al. Beneficial effects of hydralazine in severe mitral regurgitation. *Circulation* 58:273, 1978.
56. Fox, A. C., Glassman, E., and Isom, O. W. Surgically remediable complications of myocardial infarction. *Prog. Cardiovasc. Dis.* 21:461, 1979.
57. Fargot, J. C., Borsante, L., Rigaud, M., et al. Two-dimensional echocardiographic visualization of ventricular septal rupture after acute anterior myocardial infarction. *Am. J. Cardiol.* 45:370, 1980.
58. Missri, J. C., Spath, E. A., Stark, S., et al. Ventricular septal rupture detected by two-dimensional echocardiography. *J. Cardiovasc. Ultrasound.* 2:259, 1983.
59. Gray, R. J., Sethna, D., and Matloff, J. M. The role of cardiac surgery in acute myocardial infarction with mechanical complications. *Am. Heart J.* 106: 723, 1983.
60. Shah, P. K., Maddahi, J., Berman, D. S., et al. Scintigraphically detected predominant right ventricular dysfunction in acute myocardial infarction: Clinical, hemodynamic correlates and implications for therapy and prognosis. *J. Am. Coll. Cardiol.* 6:1264, 1985.
61. Isner, J. M., and Roberts, W. C. Right ventricular infarction complicating left ventricular infarction complicating coronary artery disease. *Am. J. Cardiol.* 42:885, 1978.
62. Lorrell, B., Leinbach, R. C., Pohost, G. M., et al. Right ventricular infarction: Clinical diagnosis and differentiation from cardiac tamponade and pericardial constriction. *Am. J. Cardiol.* 43:465, 1979.
63. Goldstein, J. A., Vlahakes, G. J., Verrier, E. D., et al. The role of right ventricular systolic dysfunction and elevated intrapericardial pressure in the genesis

of low output in experimental right ventricular infarction. *Circulation* 65:513, 1982.
64. Goldstein, J. A., Vlahakes, G. J., Verrier, E. D., et al. Volume loading improves low cardiac output in experimental right ventricular infarction. *J. Am. Coll. Cardiol.* 2:270, 1983.
65. Calliff, R. M., and Bengston, J. R. Cardiogenic shock. *N. Engl. J. Med.* 330:1724, 1994.
66. Frid, D. J., Young, S., and Woodlief, L. H., et al. Undercompensation: The role of the non-infarct-related zone in the pathogenesis of cardiogenic shock. *Circulation* 82(Suppl III):III-430, 1990.
67. Grines, C. L., Topol, E. J., Califf, R. M., et al. Prognostic implications and predictors of enhanced regional wall motion of the noninfarct zone after thrombolysis and angioplasty therapy of acute myocardial infarction. *Circulation* 80:245, 1989.
68. Grines, C. L., Brown, K. F., Marco, J., et al. A comparison of immediate angioplasty with thrombolytic therapy for acute myocardial infarction. *N. Engl. J. Med.* 328:673, 1993.
69. Gacioch, G. M., Ellis, S. G., Lee, L., et al. Cardiogenic shock complicating acute myocardial infarction: The use of coronary angioplasty and the integration of the new support devices into patient management. *J. Am. Coll. Cardiol.* 19:647, 1992.
70. Zehender, M., Kasper, W., Kauder, E., et al. Right ventricular infarction as an independent predictor of prognosis after acute inferior myocardial infarction. *N. Engl. J. Med.* 328:981, 1993.

14. Pharmacologic Support of the Failing Circulation in Acute Myocardial Infarction

Jay N. Cohn

Acute myocardial infarction is the most dramatic event that may impair ventricular performance and produce acute circulatory failure. Although the mass of the myocardium infarcted is an important determinant of pump performance and thus plays a critical role in the genesis of circulatory failure [1], a number of other factors may contribute importantly to an overall depression in ventricular pump function and the development of the shock syndrome. They include both cardiac and peripheral factors.

Factors Influencing Ventricular Function

Location of Infarction

The importance of the location of the infarction in the genesis of pump dysfunction is uncertain. Anterior infarcts certainly produce more hemodynamic derangement than inferior infarcts, but this difference may be largely due to the larger mass of anterior wall infarcts. Inferior infarcts often are accompanied by damage to the posterior septum and the right ventricular free wall, resulting in impairment of right ventricular function [2]. The syndrome of right ventricular infarction may precipitate circulatory failure out of proportion to the extent of the left ventricular myocardial damage. When infarcts involve valvular structures, mechanical factors may contribute to the pump dysfunction (see below).

Behavior of Infarcted Myocardium

Infarcts may retain some contractile function because of islands of viable myocardium within the infarcted area protected by collateral flow; infarcts may become akinetic by virtue of the loss of contractile function but with residual stiffness in the area of infarction; or infarcts may become dyskinetic because of systolic bulging in the area of the infarction [3]. The more dyskinetic the infarct area becomes, the more likely it is that it will contribute to systolic pump dysfunction and circulatory failure.

Peri-infarction Ischemia

Even in transmural infarctions it is likely that some tissue in the infarcted zone as well as viable myocardium at the transmural or lateral borders of the infarcted area will remain ischemic because of inadequacy of blood flow. Such ischemia, even if transient, may contribute to profound depression of overall ventricular performance. The time course of recovery of this "stunned myocardium" is controversial [4].

Ventricular Arrhythmias

Premature ventricular depolarizations and runs of ventricular tachycardia are common complications of acute myocardial infarction. Although occasional premature beats have little impact on overall ventricular performance or myocardial energy requirements, frequent ventricular premature beats may have a significant adverse effect on overall myocardial function, both by impairment of systolic emptying during the premature contraction and by an increase in myocardial oxygen consumption generated by the premature beat with no appreciable external mechanical work performed by the ventricle.

Acute Mechanical Defects

Rupture of the septum or ventricular free wall, or ischemia or infarction of the papillary muscles, may precipitate acute hemodynamic stress that may be corrected only by surgical repair of the physical defect. In general, surgical repairs are best postponed for several weeks until healing improves the quality of the tissue to be sutured [5].

Systemic Vasoconstriction

Vasoconstriction places an added burden on the impaired left ventricle by virtue of an increase of aortic impedance and ventricular preload [6]. In the setting of acute myocardial infarction, this vasoconstriction may at least in part be contributed by activation of the sympathetic nervous system or the renin-angiotensin system. Although these systems may be activated to support blood pressure at levels compatible with life, it is likely that some of the neurohormonal response may actually be deleterious to pump function and impair it more severely than would have been the case if systemic vasoconstriction had not been stimulated by the neurohormonal mechanisms.

Sodium and Water Retention

Impaired delivery of sodium to the distal nephron of the kidney may result from both cardiac and neurohormonal changes in the setting of acute myocardial infarction. The resultant sodium retention may contribute to an increase in intravascular volume that produces signs and symptoms of pulmonary and systemic congestion.

Recognition of Circulatory Failure

Some degree of ventricular pump dysfunction accompanies most acute myocardial infarctions [7]. Therefore the challenge to the physician is to recognize when pump function is so severely impaired that pharmacologic or mechanical support for the circulation is necessary. Hemodynamic monitoring is essential for this task because it becomes vital to monitor both the cardiac filling pressure and the stroke volume in order to understand the severity of the pump dysfunction and to assess its response to treatment. Arterial pressure monitoring, preferably with an intra-arterial cannula and transducer, also is essential for guiding therapy.

In the past it was considered prudent to avoid pharmacologic support of the circulation unless the shock syndrome developed with evidence of impaired perfusion to critical vascular beds [8]. The present approach is considerably more aggressive because of the recognition that intelligent use of pharmacologic and mechanical support not only may improve the performance of the ventricle acutely but also may contribute to a long-term benefit [9].

Hemodynamic monitoring of ventricular pump function usually is complemented by monitoring of urine output, blood lactate levels, and arterial blood gases for assessment of the metabolic state [10]. When metabolic acidosis begins to develop, it is clear that aggressive correction of the regional flow deficiency is mandatory. Specific deficiencies in pump function or of organ functional abnormalities may require specific therapeutic approaches.

Ventricular Filling Pressure

Because acute myocardial infarction usually involves the left ventricle, the pulmonary capillary pressure or left ventricular filling pressure generally is increased out of proportion to the right ventricular filling pressure [7]. The exception to this situation occurs in patients in whom the infarction involves significant portions of the free wall of the right ventricle. Under these circumstances, right ventricular filling pressure may be as high or even higher than left ventricular filling pressure, suggesting predominant right ventricular failure [2].

Correction of the elevated left ventricular filling pressure may be important for several reasons: (1) The elevated pulmonary capillary pressure may contribute to pulmonary edema, impairment of oxygenation, and increased work of breathing; (2) elevated diastolic pressure in the left ventricle during diastole may impair subendocardial blood flow owing to the compressive forces of the high ventricular chamber pressure during diastole [11] and thus contribute to aggravation of myocardial ischemia and progressive impairment of pump performance; and (3) a high ventricular diastolic pressure impairs ventricular filling and may contribute to impaired systolic pump performance.

The increase in pulmonary capillary that accompanies acute myocardial infa result from a decrease in compliance ventricle as well as from impairmen emptying. The compliance abnormal with acute ischemia and infarction m the first 48 hours in the hospital, gradual fall in pulmonary capillary patients who are monitored durin Because this reduction of pulmo sure is not necessarily accompa ment in left ventricular ejecti likely that all of the changes i pressure can be accounted f systolic performance.

Reduction of the elevat pressure may be accomp intravascular volume, an increase tricular capacitance, or improvement in pump performance. In general, the latter therapeutic approach is the least effective for acutely reducing the pulmonary capillary pressure [13].

Cardiac Output

A low cardiac output following acute myocardial infarction may be reflected by clinical signs of impaired organ perfusion. Output generally is quantitated by an indicator dilution technique, most commonly using iced dextrose solution injected into the right atrium with a thermistor probe in the pulmonary artery [14]. A low cardiac output also should be reflected in a wide arterial-pulmonary arterial oxygen difference that can be quantitated by blood gas or oximetry measurements.

The goal of therapy should be to increase a depressed cardiac output without unduly burdening the dysfunctional left ventricle. Because increases in heart rate, blood pressure, and contractility demand greater myocardial oxygen consumption [15], the ischemic ventricle may be ill-served by interventions that result in such changes. Similarly, increases in ventricular volume result in a rise in wall stress that demands more oxygen. In contrast, the cost of myocardial fiber shortening in terms of energy consumption is low. Therefore interventions that improve shortening (e.g., a reduction in aortic impedance) without altering contractility or raising blood pressure or ventricular volume would be pre-

The failing circula include diuretics, vasod pic drugs, and vasoconstrictor mic drugs often are employed in th tion, but they are discussed elsewhere.

Diuretics

Administration of furosemide or potent loop diuretics in patients with acute myocardial infarction may result in a considerable diuresis that gradually reduces the elevated pulmonary capillary pressure. Caution is necessary, though, during the first 30 minutes after intravenous administration of drugs such as furosemide because a vasoconstrictor effect may be stimulated by the loop diuretics perhaps by virtue of stimulation of the renin-angiotensin system and the sympathetic nervous system [18]. This early vasoconstrictor effect of furosemide may counterbalance the beneficial volume-depleting effect of the drug and sometimes may even precipitate an acute further rise of pulmonary capillary pressure until the diuresis has become well established.

The major concern with diuretic therapy for acute myocardial infarction is that a reduction in left ventricular preload may result in a further reduction in stroke volume and cardiac output. The risk of such an adverse effect can be minimized by monitoring pulmonary arterial diastolic or wedge

bly
upper
ctively.
many ex-
concomitant
iuretics in the
ion. The vasodi-
venous capacitance
elevated ventricular
mpedance-lowering ef-
cardiac output. Thus di-
asodilators seem to provide
amic and renal profile.

Drugs

rugs are employed in the management ry failure primarily for their systemic effect of reducing the loading conditions eft ventricle. Because some of these drugs xert an effect on the coronary circulation, the nonary vasculature, and certain regional vascu- beds, their actions may be considerably more complicated than their effects on left ventricular loading alone.

The most popular vasodilator agents for intravenous use in circulatory failure are nitroglycerin and sodium nitroprusside. Phentolamine and trimethaphan are no longer used because of potential adverse effects. Phosphodiesterase (PDE) inhibitors exert vasodilator as well as inotropic effects, but they are considered with the inotropic drugs. The converting enzyme inhibitors and hydralazine are vasodilator drugs that are generally taken orally. However, parenteral forms of these compounds are available and may find some use in the management of circulatory failure.

The most striking difference in the circulatory effects of various vasodilator drugs is their relative action on venous capacitance, arterial compliance, arteriolar resistance, and heart rate. The differing effects of some of the vasodilators are depicted in Table 14-1. Increases in venous capacitance lead to redistribution of intravascular volume so that the intrathoracic volume falls, which usually results in decreased cardiac filling pressures. Arterial compliance and arteriolar resistance are the major factors influencing impedance to left ventricular ejection. An increase in compliance or a reduction in resistance allows better left ventricular emptying in patients with left ventricular dysfunction. The result is an increase in cardiac output. The heart rate effects of various vasodilators appear to differ, perhaps because of differing effects on baroreceptors or independent effects on baroreceptor function or sympathetic reflexes. It is also clear that there is considerable individual variation in the heart rate response to vasodilating drugs, perhaps in part because of differences in neurohormonal state or concomitant drug therapy [20].

Nitroglycerin

Nitroglycerin and the other nitrates have a dominant action on venous capacitance and a prominent relaxing effect on the arterial compliance vessels [21]. The net effect of infusion of this drug is a reduction in ventricular filling pressure, a fall in systolic arterial pressure, and a slight increase in cardiac output with only a modest increase in heart rate.

Because nitroglycerin relaxes conduit coronary arteries and coronary collateral vessels, the drug has also been used for acute myocardial infarction

Table 14-1
Hemodynamic response to vasodilators

Vasodilator	Arterial compliance	Arteriolar resistance	Venous capacitance	Reflex response
Nitrates	++	+	++	+
Nitroprusside	++	+++	++	++
Ca^{2+} antagonists	++	++	+	+
Hydralazine	0	+++	0	+++
Angiotensin-converting enzyme inhibitors	+	++	++	0

in an effort to limit infarct size [22–24]. To have such a beneficial effect it may be necessary to begin infusion within the first few hours after the onset of pain.

Nitroglycerin infusion is usually begun at a dose of about 20 μg/min, with gradual increases in the infusion rate until the pulmonary arterial diastolic or wedge pressure has been reduced to the goal pressure, usually about 15 mm Hg. Side effects of headache or nausea limit increments in dosage in some patients. Although there is considerable concern expressed about the development of vascular tolerance during continuous intravenous infusion of nitroglycerin [25], some hemodynamic effect appears to persist [26].

Sodium Nitroprusside

Sodium nitroprusside exerts a venous capacitance effect similar to that of the nitrates, but in the doses used it produces far more potent arteriolar dilation [27]. Therefore impedance is strikingly reduced, and in the patient with left ventricular failure there usually is a prominent increase in cardiac output as well as a fall in right atrial and pulmonary capillary pressures [28]. Although nitroprusside appears to exert a relaxing effect on large arteries, including the conduit coronary arteries, it has not been thought to be as effective as nitroglycerin in increasing coronary collateral flow [29]. Therefore, nitroprusside may not be the drug of choice for improving perfusion of ischemic myocardium.

A controlled double-blind trial of a 48-hour nitroprusside infusion in patients with acute myocardial infarction complicated by an elevated pulmonary wedge pressure confirmed the favorable hemodynamic effects (compared to a placebo infusion) [9]. Furthermore, the study revealed contrasting effects on survival depending on the time of institution of the infusion. Early intervention within the first 8 hours after the onset of infarction appeared to increase mortality, whereas later intervention led to a long-term reduction in mortality. The best explanation for this difference is that the early-intervention group included patients whose elevated pulmonary wedge pressure was not necessarily a manifestation of severe left ventricular systolic dysfunction and would have fallen spontaneously without treatment. Hypotension induced in these patients might have a deleterious effect on the myocardium. In contrast, patients with persistent elevation of pulmonary capillary pressure probably represent a group with more severe systolic dysfunction who benefit from the preload and impedance reduction induced by nitroprusside.

The appropriate clinical implication from this study should be to reserve nitroprusside therapy for patients who manifest clear evidence of severe ventricular systolic dysfunction after acute myocardial infarction. In that group prolonged therapy may have a favorable impact on survival.

Nitroprusside is infused intravenously in increasing doses with a dual aim of reducing elevated ventricular filling pressure and increasing cardiac output and tissue perfusion. Infusions may be initiated at 15 to 20 μg/min, with increases by 20 μg/min increments at 5- to 10-minute intervals until the desired effect is achieved. Rarely is it necessary in patients with acute myocardial infarction to exceed a dose of 200 μg/min. The limiting factor in infusion increments is the fall in arterial pressure. With acute infarction, care must be taken to avoid severe hypotension, which may further aggravate flow deficiency to the ischemic myocardium.

Once a desired hemodynamic response to nitroprusside has been achieved, the effect generally is stable with a constant infusion of the drug. Continuous infusions for 2 to 5 days are usually well tolerated, although a rebound overshoot of arterial and pulmonary capillary pressures may be observed when the drug infusion is withdrawn. During long-term infusion, blood thiocyanate levels should be measured occasionally to be certain that this toxic metabolic product of nitroprusside is not accumulating [30]. Levels below 10 mg/dl are well tolerated.

Calcium Antagonists

The dihydropyridine calcium antagonists exert potent vasodilating effects that may be beneficial in certain clinical situations. These drugs appear to have more profound arterial than venous effects, so that their major action is to reduce impedance; they have only a modest effect on preload [31]. Many of these drugs also have the potential to produce a negative inotropic effect that can directly impair myocardial contractility. An increase in coronary artery caliber in response to these drugs also may have a favorable effect on flow through stenotic coronary arteries [17].

Intravenous infusion of verapamil or diltiazem exerts electrophysiologic and negative inotropic effects that are more prominent than their vasodilator effect [32]. Dihydropyridines exert a potent vasodilator action but their safety in patients with acute myocardial infarction has not been demonstrated.

Other Vasodilators

Hydralazine, a potent arteriolar dilator [33], is available in a parenteral form. However, it probably is not a drug of choice for the acutely ischemic ventricle because it is difficult to titrate accurately, and it could aggravate myocardial ischemia.

The angiotensin-converting enzyme (ACE) inhibitors captopril, enalapril, lisinopril, ramipril, and quinapril have been used in the setting of acute myocardial infarction, but drug titration is difficult because of the steep dose-response effect of these agents [34]. It seems prudent to use directly acting vasodilators for the acute phase of circulatory instability and initiate ACE inhibitor therapy later, if needed, to produce a chronic reduction in preload and aortic impedance. ACE inhibitors are now being used in the early phase of acute infarction for their ability to prevent left ventricular remodeling and reduce long-term mortality. This application of ACE inhibitors should preferably be delayed until the patient is hemodynamically stable.

Phentolamine, an alpha-adrenoceptor antagonist, has been used in the past as an intravenous dilator for acute infarction. The drug, however, tends to produce a prominent reflex tachycardia, and its venous capacitance effects are less prominent than those of nitroprusside [35].

Trimethaphan is a ganglionic blocker that markedly augments venous capacitance and reduces aortic impedance. Unfortunately, however, the severe side effects (orthostatic hypotension and parasympathetic blockade) make it a relatively undesirable vasodilator drug.

Inotropic Drugs

Inotropic drugs are employed in the setting of left ventricular pump failure based on the hypothesis that there is contractile reserve in the myocardium that can be called on to augment ventricular contraction and improve the depressed cardiac performance. It is assumed that the contractility increase induced by these drugs augments myocardial oxygen consumption and thus potentially aggravates a delicate balance between oxygen delivery and consumption in marginally ischemic myocardium. Inotropic agents usually also exert peripheral vascular effects of constriction or dilation. Drugs with potent inotropic actions will be considered here even though they also may function as vasodilators or vasoconstrictors.

Most drugs currently available as potent inotropic agents exert their effect either by stimulating myocardial beta receptors or by increasing cyclic adenosine monophosphate (cAMP) through another mechanism, usually by inhibition of PDE. Digitalis is a less potent inotropic drug whose action to increase contractility is exerted through inhibition of Na^+, K^+-ATPase with a resultant increase in intracellular Ca^{2+}. Because of its relative lack of acute potency, its modest vasoconstrictor effect [36], and its low toxic therapeutic ratio, digitalis is not generally advocated as an agent to increase myocardial contractility in acute unstable circulatory states.

Dobutamine

Dobutamine is a well-tolerated inotropic drug that exerts its effect through activation of myocardial beta-1 adrenoceptors. Because it does not release norepinephrine and has only mild direct vascular effects, the pharmacodynamic response to the drug infusion can be attributed largely to its positive inotropic properties. Furthermore, it produces less chronotropic effect than other beta agonists [37] and therefore appears to be the drug of choice when increases in contractility, without tachycardia or blood pressure effects, are sought.

Dobutamine has a fairly reproducible dose-response effect that usually reaches an optimal effect on cardiac output at a dose of 10 to 15 μg/kg/min [38]. Infusions are generally begun at a dose of 2.5 to 5.0 μg/kg/min and increased gradually until the desired hemodynamic effect is achieved. Tachycardia or ventricular arrhythmia may limit the dosing increments. Because dobutamine as well as other sympathomimetic drugs may produce hypokalemia, serum potassium levels should be monitored during the infusion and potassium administered if necessary.

Dopamine

Dopamine is a beta-1 agonist that exerts peripheral alpha-agonistic vasoconstrictor effects as well as dopamine-mediated vasodilator effects in the renal and splanchnic beds [39]. Although low doses may exhibit predominant vasodilator action, the usual clinical doses tend to raise blood pressure in part by peripheral vasoconstrictor effects. Inotropic properties augment cardiac output, but the increase in output is generally less than with dobutamine because of the increased impedance generated by peripheral vasoconstriction [40]. Tachycardia is a common complication of higher-dose dopamine administration.

When an inotropic effect is desired in a severely hypotensive patient, dopamine is the agent of choice because it probably produces less adverse effects on visceral perfusion than norepinephrine. When a selective increase in renal perfusion is present, low doses of dopamine are occasionally beneficial. However, selective vasodilation usually is a less effective means of improving renal perfusion than the increase in perfusion that accompanies inotropic agent–mediated increases in cardiac output.

Amrinone, Milrinone, and Phosphodiesterase Inhibitors

A variety of chemical compounds that inhibit cardiac PDE have been demonstrated to exert in vitro and in vivo inotropic effects. These cardiac actions, which appear to be largely due to increased myocardial concentration of cAMP, are usually accompanied by vasodilation, also caused by PDE inhibition [41]. The relative cardiac and peripheral vascular effects of these drugs appear to vary from agent to agent and to depend on the dose of the drug employed. During intravenous infusion of these drugs the major side effects relate to ventricular arrhythmias and hypotension.

Because the action of these PDE inhibitors does not depend on intact beta receptors, the drugs have a theoretical advantage in individuals who may have blocked or down-regulated beta receptors. However, beta agonists rarely are ineffective when the dose is titrated upward, and the disadvantage of the PDE inhibitors is that one cannot independently titrate the inotropic and vasodilator properties as can be done with independent infusions of dobutamine and nitroprusside. Nonetheless, amrinone [42] and milrinone [43] exert favorable hemodynamic effects and for severe pump failure may be particularly useful in combination with adrenergic agents [44].

Norepinephrine

During intravenous infusion the neurotransmitter norepinephrine exerts potent beta-1 inotropic and alpha-1 and alpha-2 vasoconstrictor effects. The net effect is a dose-dependent increase in arterial pressure often at the cost of a reduction in visceral perfusion. Norepinephrine should be viewed as emergency therapy for a severely hypotensive patient whose immediate survival is threatened by impaired cerebral or coronary perfusion. More appropriate pharmacologic or mechanical attempts to increase cardiac output should be instituted as soon as the severe hypotension has been moderated.

Epinephrine, Isoproterenol

The catecholamines epinephrine and isoproterenol exert considerable beta-2-agonist properties that increase skeletal blood flow and myocardial contractility via beta-1-stimulating properties. Tachycardia and maldistribution of cardiac output render these drugs less desirable for restoring disturbed hemodynamics during pump failure.

Vasoconstrictors

Drugs that constrict the peripheral vascular bed with little or no positive inotropic effect tend to have an adverse effect on left ventricular performance. Therefore drugs such as angiotensin, methoxamine, phenylephrine, and vasopressin have no place in the management of acute myocardial infarction.

Management of the Patient

The goals of therapy are to improve tissue perfusion; control the elevated ventricular filling pressure; support arterial pressure at a level adequate to maintain renal, cerebral, and coronary perfusion; and minimize the metabolic burden on the myocardium. These goals may be only partially attainable with pharmacologic interventions, but judicious use of the available agents effectively restores hemodynamic stability to most patients with pump failure accompanying acute myocardial infarction.

The cornerstones of therapy are the manipulation of preload and impedance to left ventricular ejection. Arterial pressure represents the integration of these factors and myocardial contractility.

Ventricular Preload

In the past it often was recommended that left ventricular preload be "optimized" by volume manipulations intended to bring pulmonary capillary pressure to about 20 mm Hg, the "peak" of the Frank-Starling curve. In more recent years this approach has been replaced by pharmacologic efforts to reduce pulmonary capillary pressure to the *lowest level compatible with adequate tissue perfusion.* The pulmonary capillary pressure can be reduced by diuretic administration (usually high-dose furosemide, bumetanide, or torsemide) or by intravenous infusion of nitroglycerin or nitroprusside. If these interventions result in a fall in pressure below levels that maintain adequate cardiac output, volume infusion in the form of crystalloid or colloid can restore pulmonary capillary pressure to a more suitable level. It should be recognized, however, that these patients usually are sensitive to volume, and even small amounts may profoundly raise filling pressure.

Right ventricular infarcts that produce predominant right ventricular failure require a different approach to therapy. Under these circumstances high right atrial (or central venous) pressures may be necessary to produce adequate left ventricular filling, and higher volumes of fluid may be required to correct the low cardiac output.

Impedance

The acutely damaged left ventricle functions optimally when impedance to left ventricular emptying is low. Therefore vasodilator drugs should be employed whenever possible to keep impedance at the lowest level compatible with adequate arterial pressure.

In patients with pump failure accompanied by systolic arterial pressure above 120 to 130 mm Hg, vasodilator therapy should be the primary form of therapy. Titration of nitroprusside to lower the filling pressure and improve cardiac output and tissue perfusion is the most effective therapy. In patients with borderline blood pressure nitroprusside may still be the agent of choice, but careful arterial pressure monitoring is mandatory, and the need for concomitant inotropic drug support must be considered. In patients who are already severely hypotensive, vasodilator therapy should be deferred until arterial pressure can be supported by other means.

Use of agents that increase impedance in order to support arterial pressure should be discouraged unless hypotension control is the primary agenda. Vasoconstrictor agents should be employed only if they also exert an inotropic effect. Norepinephrine and dopamine may be used for this purpose.

Contractility

Agents that increase contractility have as their major adverse effects an increase in myocardial oxygen consumption and an increase in arrhythmia risk. Consequently, preload and impedance manipulation should generally be employed when appropriate before attempts to increase contractility are initiated. Dobutamine in a dose of 5 to 15 μg/kg/min is the agent of choice when an inotropic effect is sought.

Regional Perfusion

Failure to stabilize tissue perfusion with the optimal pharmacologic support described above calls for more aggressive measures. The combination of inotropic and vasodilator drugs may exert some favorable effect, but such patients usually have a grim prognosis unless interventional or surgical procedures can be performed. Intra-aortic balloon pumping, ventricular assist devices, emergency revascularization, and correction of structural defects are rational approaches in such patients. Heart transplantation may be the only viable long-term approach if ventricular function is irretrievably impaired.

References

1. Page, D. L., Caulfield, J. B., Kastol, J. A., et al. Myocardial changes associated with cardiogenic shock. *N. Engl. J. Med.* 285:133, 1971.

2. Cohn, J. N., Guiha, N. H., Broder, M. I., and Limas, C. J. Right ventricular infarction: Clinical and hemodynamic features. *Am. J. Cardiol.* 33:209, 1974.
3. Weisse, A. B., Saffa, R. S., Levinson, G. E., et al. Left ventricular function during the early and late stages of scar formation following experimental myocardial infarction. *Am. Heart J.* 79:370, 1970.
4. Braunwald, E., and Kloner, R. The stunned myocardium: Prolonged, postischemic ventricular dysfunction. *Circulation* 66:1146, 1982.
5. Cohn, L. H. Surgical management of mechanical complications of myocardial infarction. *Am. Heart J.* 102:1049, 1981.
6. Cohn, J. N. Vasodilator therapy of myocardial infarction (Editorial). *N. Engl. J. Med.* 290:1433, 1974.
7. Hamosh, P., and Cohn, J. N. Left ventricular function in acute myocardial infarction. *J. Clin. Invest.* 50:523, 1971.
8. Cohn, J. N. Treatment of shock following myocardial infarction. *Calif. Med.* 111:66, 1969.
9. Cohn, J. N., Franciosa, J. A., Francis, G. S., et al. Effect of short-term infusion of sodium nitroprusside on mortality rate in acute myocardial infarction complicated by left ventricular failure. *N. Engl. J. Med.* 306:1129, 1982.
10. Cohn, J. N. Monitoring techniques in shock. *Am. J. Cardiol.* 26:565, 1970.
11. Salisbury, P. F., Cross, E. C., and Rieban, P. A. Acute ischemia of inner layers of ventricular wall. *Am. Heart J.* 66:650, 1963.
12. Franciosa, J. A., Guiha, N. H., Limas, C. J., et al. Arterial pressure as a determinant of left ventricular filling pressure after acute myocardial infarction. *Am. J. Cardiol.* 34:506, 1974.
13. Mikulic, E., Cohn, J. N., and Franciosa, J. A. Comparative hemodynamic effects of inotropic and vasodilator drugs in severe heart failure. *Circulation* 56:528, 1977.
14. Forrester, J. S., Ganz, W., Diamond, G., et al. Thermodilution cardiac output with a single flow-directed catheter. *Am. Heart J.* 83:306, 1978.
15. Sonnenblick, E. H., Ross, J., Jr., and Braunwald, E. Oxygen consumption of the heart: New concepts of its multifactorial determination. *Am. J. Cardiol.* 22:328, 1968.
16. Franciosa, J. A., Notargiacomo, A. V., and Cohn, J. N. Comparative haemodynamic and metabolic effects of vasodilator and inotropic agents in experimental myocardial infarction. *Cardiovasc. Res.* 12: 294, 1978.
17. Cohn, J. N., Bache, R. J., and Schwartz, J. S. Calcium entry blockers in coronary artery disease. In R. P. Rubin, G. B. Weiss, and J. W. Putney (eds.), *Calcium in Biological Systems.* New York: Plenum, 1985. Pp. 471–477.
18. Francis, G. S., Siegel, R. M., Goldsmith, S. R., et al. Acute vasoconstrictor response to intravenous furosemide in patients with chronic congestive heart failure. *Ann. Intern. Med.* 103:1, 1985.
19. Cohn, J. N., and Franciosa, J. A. Vasodilator therapy of cardiac failure. *N. Engl. J. Med.* 297:27, and 254, 1977.
20. Cohn, J. N. Myocardial infarction shock revisited. *Am. Heart J.* 74:1, 1967.
21. Zobel, L. R., Finkelstein, S. M., Carlyle, P. F., and Cohn, J. N. Pressure pulse contour analysis in determining the effect of vasodilator drugs on vascular hemodynamic impedance characteristics in dogs. *Am. Heart J.* 100:81, 1980.
22. Derrida, J. P., Sal, R., and Chiche, P. Favorable effects of prolonged nitroglycerin infusion in patients with acute myocardial infarction. *Am. Heart J.* 96:833, 1978.
23. Bussmann, W. D., Passek, D., Seidel, W., and Kaltenbach, M. Reduction of CK and CK-MB indexes of infarct size by intravenous nitroglycerin. *Circulation* 63:615, 1981.
24. Flaherty, J. T., Becker, L. C., Bulkley, B. H., et al. A randomized prospective trial of intravenous nitroglycerin in patients with acute myocardial infarction. *Circulation* 68:576, 1983.
25. Abrams, J. Nitrate tolerance and dependence. *Am. Heart J.* 99:113, 1980.
26. Leier, C. V., Bambach, D., Thompson, M. J., et al. Central and regional hemodynamic effects of intravenous isosorbide dinitrate, nitroglycerin and nitroprusside in patients with congestive heart failure. *Am. J. Cardiol.* 48:1115, 1981.
27. Cohn, J. N., and Burke, L. P. Diagnosis and treatment —drugs five years later: Nitroprusside. *Ann. Intern. Med.* 91:752, 1979.
28. Franciosa, J. A., Guiha, N. H., Limas, C. J., et al. Improved left ventricular function during nitroprusside infusion in acute myocardial infarction. *Lancet* 1:650, 1972.
29. Chiariello, M., Gold, H. K., Leinbach, R. C., et al. Comparison between the effects of nitroprusside and nitroglycerin on ischemic injury during acute myocardial infarction. *Circulation* 54:766, 1976.
30. McDowall, D. G., Keaney, N. P., Turner, J. M., et al. The toxicity of sodium nitroprusside. *Br. J. Anaesth.* 46:327, 1974.
31. Olivari, M. T., Levine, T. B., and Cohn, J. N. Acute hemodynamic effects of nitrendipine in chronic congestive heart failure. *J. Cardiovasc. Pharmacol.* 6:S1002, 1984.
32. Millard, R. W., Lathrop, D. A., Grupp, G., et al. Differential cardiovascular effects of calcium channel blocking agents. Potential mechanisms. *Am. J. Cardiol.* 49:499, 1982.
33. Franciosa, J. A., Pierpont, G., and Cohn, J. N. Hemodynamic improvement after oral hydralazine in left ventricular failure: A comparison with nitroprusside infusion in 16 patients. *Ann. Intern. Med.* 86:388, 1977.
34. Chaterjee, K., Rouleau, J. L., and Parmley, W. W. Hemodynamic and myocardial metabolic effects of captopril in chronic heart failure. *Br. Heart J.* 47:233, 1982.
35. Richards, D. A., Woodings, E. P., and Pritchard,

B. N. C. Circulatory and alpha-adrenoceptor blocking effects of phentolamine. *Br. J. Clin. Pharmacol.* 5:507, 1978.

36. Cohn, J. N., Tristani, F. E., and Khatri, I. M. Cardiac and peripheral vascular effects of digitalis in clinical cardiogenic shock. *Am. Heart J.* 78:318, 1969.
37. Tuttle, R. R., and Mills, J. Dobutamine: Development of a new catecholamine to selectively increase myocardial contractility. *Circ. Res.* 36:185, 1975.
38. Akhtar, N., Mikulic, E., Cohn, J. N., and Chaudhry, M. H. Hemodynamic effect of dobutamine in patients with severe heart failure. *Am. J. Cardiol.* 36:202, 1975.
39. Goldberg, L. I. Cardiovascular and renal action of dopamine: Potential clinical applications. *Pharmacol. Rev.* 24:1, 1972.
40. Francis, G. S., Sharma, B., and Hodges, M. Comparative hemodynamic effects of dopamine and dobutamine in patients with acute cardiogenic circulatory collapse. *Am. Heart J.* 103:995, 1982.
41. Benotti, J. R., Grossman, W., Braunwald, E., et al. Hemodynamic assessment of amrinone: A new inotropic agent. *N. Engl. J. Med.* 299:373, 1978.
42. Marcus, R. H., Raw, K., Patel, J., et al. Comparison of intravenous amrinone and dobutamine in congestive heart failure due to idiopathic dilated cardiomyopathy. *Am. J. Cardiol.* 66:1107, 1990.
43. Klocke, R. K., Mager, G., Kux, A., et al. Effects of a 24-hour milrinone infusion in patients with severe heart failure and cardiogenic shock as a function of the hemodynamic initial condition. *Am. Heart J.* 121:1965, 1991.
44. Gage, J., Rutman, H., Lucido, D., et al. Additive effects of dobutamine and amrinone on myocardial contractility and ventricular performance in patients with severe heart failure. *Circulation* 74:367, 1986.

15. Mechanical Support of the Failing Circulation in Acute Coronary Insufficiency and Myocardial Infarction

Gordon L. Pierpont

Pathology studies have demonstrated that loss of function of more than 40 percent of the left ventricle leads to almost certain death [1]. If damage to the heart is extensive or large areas of myocardium are rendered functionally inadequate, a point can be reached where the heart cannot maintain adequate circulation even with the most aggressive and judicious use of supportive pharmacologic therapy. When this situation occurs, mechanical assist of left ventricular function may be the only option that can maintain survival.

This chapter reviews various methods of providing mechanical assist to the heart. After the physiologic goals of mechanical support are defined, the spectrum of devices available is placed in clinical perspective. The role of circulatory assist in the treatment of acute coronary insufficiency is emphasized, with only brief mention of applications to other cardiac disorders.

Physiologic Goals of Mechanical Support

There are several desired effects of mechanical support devices aimed at reversing the pathophysiologic changes that occur when acute coronary insufficiency leads to severe left ventricular dysfunction (Table 15-1). The primary goal is to improve coronary blood flow, thereby reversing the precipitating defect of ischemia-induced myocardial dysfunction. This can be achieved by several mechanisms. Because almost all effective coronary perfusion occurs during diastole, increasing systemic aortic pressure during diastole improves coronary perfusion pressure. Concomitant lowering of left ventricular diastolic pressure further augments coronary flow by increasing the transmyocardial perfusion gradient. Hemodynamic benefits of enhanced myocardial perfusion pressure should benefit myocardial regions perfused by both normal and stenosed coronary arteries.

A second major goal of mechanical support is to decrease cardiac work, thereby diminishing myocardial oxygen demand. This can be accomplished by decreasing both afterload and preload, with the beneficial effects of lowering afterload predominating. Decreasing afterload is accomplished by lowering systemic pressure during systole; preload is lowered indirectly by mechanical circulatory support through improved cardiac output. If the heart rate is high or significant cardiac dysrhythmias are present, promoting a slow, stable, physiologic rhythm also can have marked beneficial metabolic consequences.

At the same time that cardiac work is decreased, cardiac output needs to be maintained to improve peripheral perfusion. This requires maintaining adequate systemic perfusion pressure while lowering peripheral vascular resistance, preferably selectively in the most vital organs. A final goal in most patients with severe left ventricular dysfunction is to decrease pulmonary and venous congestion. This is basically synonymous with decreasing diastolic left ventricular filling pressure (preload). As noted already, this can be achieved by improving overall left ventricular performance, and by promoting diuresis through increased blood flow to the kidneys.

It is evident that to achieve these goals requires balancing some seemingly dichotomous interactions of the hemodynamic variables involved, for

Table 15-1
Goals of mechanical support

Improve myocardial perfusion
Increase coronary perfusion pressure
Decrease diastolic wall tension
Decrease myocardial work
Decrease afterload
Decrease preload
Stabilize heart rate
Improve peripheral blood flow
Relieve pulmonary and venous congestion

example, increasing diastolic pressure while lowering systolic pressure, or simultaneously maintaining peripheral perfusion pressure while reducing cardiac afterload. Indirect effects of mechanical support may also be important. If systemic pressure and peripheral perfusion are maintained, the beneficial effects of lowering adrenergic nervous system activity, promoting diuresis, and decreasing activation of the renin-angiotensin system may be achieved. The ultimate usefulness of a mechanical support device will be determined by the extent to which these therapeutic goals are attained with minimal complications, low cost, rapid application, and ease of use.

Noninvasive Devices

External circulatory assist by *mechanical compression of the chest,* either manually or mechanically, falls into the category of cardiac resuscitation rather than cardiac assist. For information on this topic, the reader is referred to Chapter 22.

Rotating tourniquets are of historical interest only. Although recommended well into the 1970s as a method of decreasing pulmonary congestion by diminishing venous return and thereby pooling fluid in the extremities, there was scant scientific support of the efficacy of this procedure. In a systematic study of ten patients with acute congestive heart failure, Bertel and Steiner [2] found no beneficial hemodynamic effects of rotating tourniquets. In view of the rapid and effective decreases in pulmonary capillary wedge pressure obtainable with currently available vasodilators, diuretics, and inotropic agents (see Chapter 14), the devices previously sold to provide rotating tourniquets for treating pulmonary congestion are obsolete.

Military antishock trousers (MAST) compress the abdomen, legs, or both. They are used primarily for hypovolemic shock in out-of-hospital settings and have no role in supporting the circulation during acute cardiac ischemia associated with left ventricular failure or shock. According to one report [3], certain individuals in cardiogenic shock appeared to benefit from the MAST suit, but these patients were concomitantly volume depleted. Rapid volume expansion would be most appropriate in such situations. Most patients in cardiogenic shock already have a high preload. By further increasing the preload and by aggravating dyspnea because of mechanical restraints to thoracic movement, the MAST unit is more likely to be detrimental than beneficial for acute coronary insufficiency associated with left ventricular failure [4].

The concept of supporting the circulation using *synchronized external lower body counterpulsation (ECP)* was promoted in 1963 by Dennis et al. [5]. They were able to lower peak systolic aortic pressure and raise aortic diastolic pressure using an electronically controlled external counterpulsator on the hindquarters of dogs. Further experimental support for this methodology was provided by Soroff et al. [6], who noted a decrease in systolic pressure, as well as an increase in cardiac output, in dogs provided external assist. Silverstein et al. [7] demonstrated that ECP can increase diastolic perfusion pressure and improve coronary flow in experimental myocardial infarction. Their results were supported by Watson et al. [8], who studied dogs with ischemia induced by coronary artery ligation. With ECP, they were able to produce increases in coronary collateral flow to ischemic myocardium equivalent to the increases obtained with the intra-aortic balloon pump (IABP).

According to Wright, clinical application of external cardiac assist was partially responsible for survival in four patients in cardiogenic shock following cardiopulmonary bypass surgery [9]. In 17 patients with acute myocardial infarction, Parmley et al. [10] used ECP in conjunction with nitroprusside to produce hemodynamic effects that were better than those seen with either nitroprusside or external assist alone. ECP also has been used to support the right side of the heart [11, 12]. A patient undergoing ECP is seen in Figure 15-1.

In conjunction with reports by Kern et al. [13] of 14 patients with normal left ventricular function and Beckman et al. [14] of 29 surgical patients, it

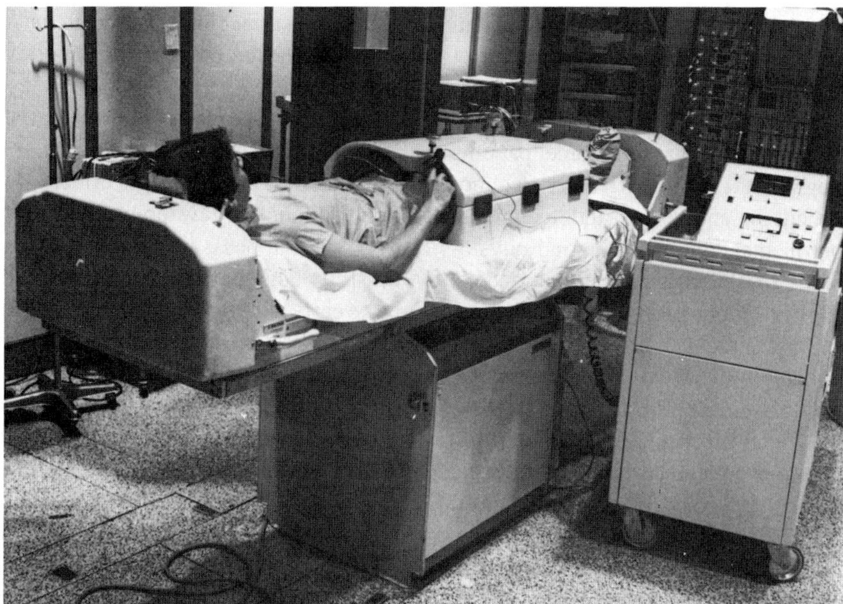

Fig. 15-1
Patient prepared for external counterpulsation of the legs. (From M. I. Kern et al. Effects of pulsed external augmentation of diastolic pressure on coronary and systemic dynamics in patients with coronary artery disease. *Am. Heart J.* 110:728, 1985. With permission.)

is evident that augmentation of systemic diastolic pressure can be achieved in patients using ECP, with variable increases in cardiac output. These studies provided background for a randomized cooperative trial of ECP for acute myocardial infarction that reported improved survival in patients with mild left ventricular failure treated with ECP [15]. Kuhn [16] pointed out some of the limitations of this study, and ECP has not gained clinical acceptance. The Bethesda Conference Task Force V assessment [4] is appropriate in saying that ''routine clinical use cannot be currently justified, and practical issues in addition to efficacy are patient discomfort and equipment cost.''

Invasive Devices

Arterial Counterpulsator

An arterial counterpulsator removes blood from the systemic arterial system to a reservoir chamber during ventricular systole, thereby decreasing ventricular afterload. It then empties back into the systemic circulation during diastole to augment diastolic perfusion pressure and flow to the coronary arteries and periphery. Such a device, described by Clauss et al. in 1961 [17], was used experimentally in dogs. Subsequent studies demonstrated the potential of this type of device to improve hemodynamics in experimental heart failure [18], decrease myocardial oxygen consumption [19–21], increase coronary blood flow [20, 21], and preserve ischemic myocardium [22, 23], perhaps in part by opening dormant coronary collateral channels [24]. Despite continued evaluation of such devices [25, 26], they have not progressed to significant clinical use, perhaps in a large part because of evident superiority of the concomitantly developed IABPs and left ventricular assist devices.

Intra-aortic Balloon Pump

The IABP can be considered the circulatory assist device of choice [4]. Intra-aortic balloon counterpulsation was introduced during the early 1960s by Moulopoulous et al. [27]. It was successfully applied clinically by Kantrowitz et al. in 1967 [28] to two patients with cardiogenic shock complicating acute myocardial infarction, and one of the patients survived to leave the hospital. Early clinical use, often in preterminal patients, frequently met with relatively poor survival rates [28–35]. Nonetheless, it became clear that this technology offered improved chances of survival for some patients with dismal prognosis. It led to progressive technologic improvement in equipment and technique, continued experimental studies evaluating physiologic effects of the IABP in various animal models, and broader clinical application. A collective review by Weber and Janicki in 1974 [36] summarized the early data on the IABP.

Operation of this device is conceptually illustrated in Figure 15-2. A long balloon connected to a controlling pump is positioned in the aorta distal to the great vessels but above the renal arteries. During systole, when blood is being ejected from the left ventricle, the balloon is collapsed so as to interfere minimally with blood flow. By synchronizing with the cardiac cycle, the balloon is inflated during diastole to help force blood rapidly out of the aorta to the periphery and proximally to the heart and head. As the balloon collapses again with the next systole, blood volume in the aorta is lower, allowing easier ejection of blood from the left ventricle.

Over two decades of clinical and research application of the IABP has resulted in a sound understanding of the physiologic effects of this intervention, although a few points remain controversial. The fact that peak diastolic pressure could be successfully augmented in the aorta was demonstrated quite early in both animals [27, 37] and humans [28, 30–32, 38]. The increased peak diastolic pressure is usually associated with a lower end-diastolic aortic pressure. Augmentation of peak diastolic aortic pressure occurs independent of the status of the left ventricle so long as the aortic valve is competent. Additional studies supported these findings and demonstrated that systolic pressure decreases [30, 31, 38, 39] whereas mean aortic pressure changes little [38] or rises slightly [33, 40, 41] during IABP support. These effects of the IABP on aortic pressure are illustrated in Figures 15-3 and 15-4. Cardiac output is improved [30, 31, 33, 35, 38, 40, 42], and pulmonary artery wedge pressure falls [33,

Fig. 15-2
Mechanism of circulatory support by intra-aortic balloon pumping. The balloon is collapsed during systole, allowing minimal interference with normal blood flow. Inflating the balloon during diastole increases the diastolic pressure and enhances flow out of the aorta centrally and peripherally.

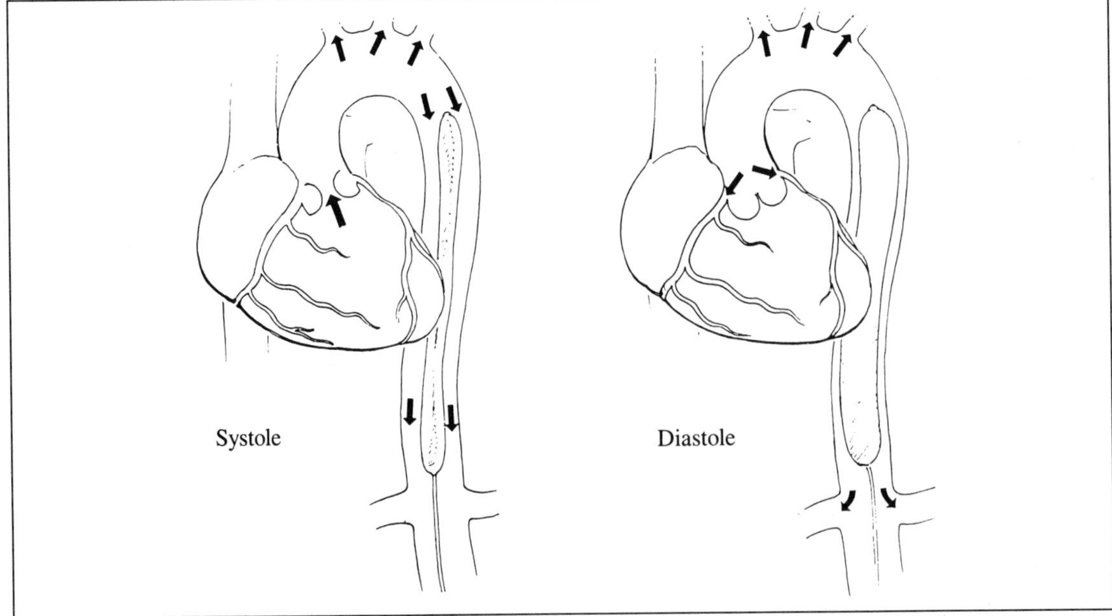

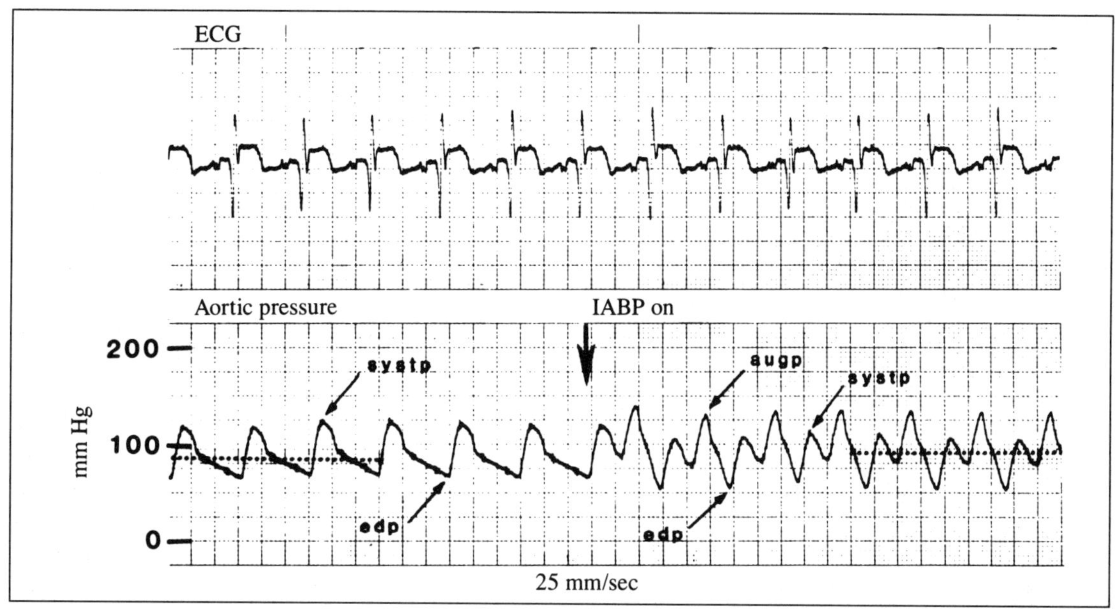

Fig. 15-3
Effect of the intra-aortic balloon pump (IABP) on systemic arterial pressure in a patient requiring postoperative support. With IABP treatment the peak diastolic pressure (ausp) is increased, the end-diastolic pressure (edp) is decreased, the peak systolic pressure (systp) is decreased, and the mean pressure increases only slightly.

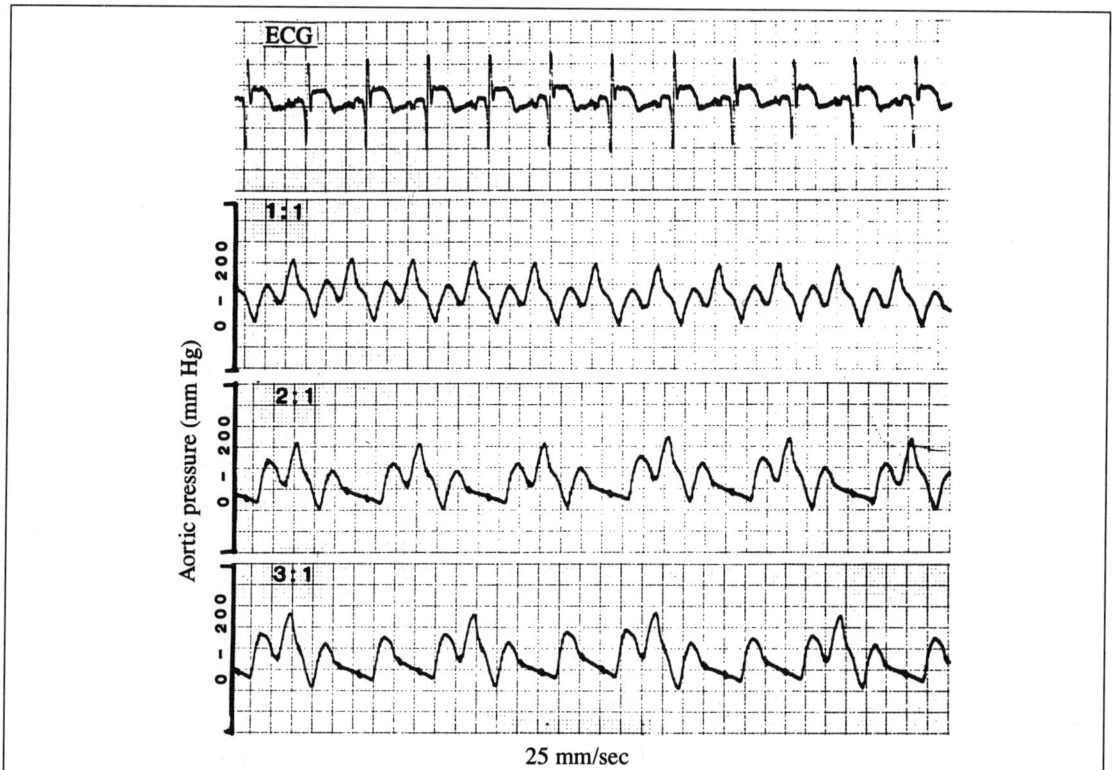

Fig. 15-4
The effects of intra-aortic balloon pumping on systemic pressure are evident as a patient is ''weaned'' from support by progressing from 1:1 augmentation (balloon inflated during every diastole) to 2:1 and then 3:1 augmentation (balloon inflated every third diastole).

35, 42]. Collectively, these hemodynamic changes result in improved values for derived indexes of ventricular performance. For example, the increase in cardiac output is usually greater than the increase in mean aortic pressure such that calculated peripheral vascular resistance is decreased [40, 42]. Ejection fraction [43] and stroke volume index [35] are increased. Secondarily, heart rate is decreased [35, 38–40], and cardiac arrhythmias can sometimes be stabilized. Indeed the IABP has even been used for the specific indication of treating postinfarction ventricular arrhythmias [44, 45].

Whereas the systemic hemodynamic effects of IABP support have been reproducible, changes in myocardial blood flow have been more difficult to predict. Numerous experimental preparations in dogs produced conflicting results. For example, total coronary flow (coronary sinus flow) in dogs with normal hearts was decreased using IABP support in a study by Feola et al. [46] but was essentially unchanged in a study by Talpins et al. [47]. Talpins et al. also found no effect of the IABP on total coronary flow when the dogs were subjected to hemorrhage or sustained left ventricular injury by temporary left ventricular outflow occlusion. Yet following coronary artery ligation, both Talpins et al. [47] and Feola et al. [46] noted improved total coronary flow with the IABP. In right heart bypass preparations studied by Tyberg et al. [48], Powell et al. [49], and McDonnell et al. [50], the IABP during control conditions did not alter coronary blood flow. However, in this preparation coronary blood flow was improved by the IABP at a low cardiac output [48] and low aortic blood pressures [49] but not following coronary artery ligation at normal systemic pressure [50].

Collectively these results would suggest that at least in some situations (but not likely under normal conditions) it may be possible to increase total coronary blood flow by intra-aortic balloon pumping. However, in ischemic heart disease, total coronary blood flow may not be as important as regional flow to ischemic or peri-infarction zones. Flow to areas fed by normal vessels would be of less importance unless left ventricular failure was severe enough to compromise total coronary flow. Using electromagnetic flow meters, several investigators studied flow in uninvolved coronaries with or without ligation of a separate coronary artery [51–54]. Collectively these four studies also suggest that the IABP has little effect on coronary blood flow under normal conditions, but flow can be increased by intra-aortic balloon pumping in normal coronaries after an adjacent coronary is ligated. Weber and Janicki [55] found similar results in calves (i.e., the IABP improved coronary flow only in hypotensive animals).

Additional pertinent experimental data come from studies using alternative methods of measuring regional myocardial blood flow. Direct measurements of retrograde collateral flow distal to a coronary ligation made by Gundel et al. [56] and Feola et al. [57] in dogs demonstrated improved collateral flow during IABP support. These findings were supplemented by Gill et al. [58], who used radioactive microspheres to demonstrate improved coronary blood flow to ischemic myocardium with the IABP; in this study, however, flow to normal myocardium decreased with IABP support. The data of Chen et al. [59] support these findings by demonstrating a positive inotropic effect of the IABP in ischemic myocardium, but not normal myocardium. Shaw et al. [60] also used microspheres in dogs with ligated coronary arteries and found that the IABP increased subendocardial blood flow in peri-infarction areas and normal areas but not in the infarction zone. These results were interpreted as improved collateral flow during IABP support. On the other hand, using $Na^{131}I$ to measure "nutrient blood flow" to myocardium, Saini et al. [61] found that following coronary artery ligation, the IABP increased flow to all zones (i.e., normal, peri-infarction, and central infarction). Finally, in a study of pigs by Gewertz et al. [62], the IABP failed to alter either pressure or flow (by microspheres) distal to a coronary stenosis.

Despite the variability in the data on coronary blood flow, most studies consistently demonstrated that the IABP can decrease myocardial oxygen utilization ($M\dot{V}O_2$) in experimental myocardial ischemia or infarction [49, 50, 62]. It thus remains difficult to assess whether the beneficial effects of the IABP on limiting infarct size [63, 64] or diminishing ischemic injury [65] are primarily due to decreased cardiac workload and MVO_2, or to improved myocardial perfusion.

Data from patients fail to provide a definitive answer to this question. Results of clinical studies measuring total coronary flow using coronary sinus catheterization, like the studies in animals, have been contradictory. Leinbach et al. [66] found the IABP to have a variable effect on coronary flow in patients with acute myocardial infarction, with an overall surprising lack of improvement. Two reports by Mueller et al. [31, 40], on the other hand, suggested that coronary flow increases in most patients during IABP support.

Similarly contradictory data evolved from studies selectively looking at flow in the great cardiac vein (which returns blood from the anterior myocardium) in patients with lesions in the left anterior descending coronary artery. Williams et al. [41] reported a decrease in selective flow from the affected area of myocardium during IABP support and concluded that decreased myocardial work was more important than changes in myocardial perfusion. This was supported by the results of Port et al. [39], who used xenon 133 washout to measure a decrease in coronary blood flow, consistent with decreased myocardial workload, when intra-aortic balloon pumping was instituted. Additionally, the IABP failed to augment distal coronary perfusion pressure during percutaneous transluminal coronary angioplasty in three patients studied by MacDonald et al. [67]. By contrast, Fuchs et al. [68] found that great cardiac vein flow increased proportional to increases in systemic diastolic pressure with the IABP in a similar group of patients. Using intracoronary Doppler flow probes, Kern et al. [69] found that the IABP "unequivocally" augmented proximal coronary blood flow velocity in critically ill patients. However, in another study by the same group [70], flow did not improve beyond a critical stenosis before angioplasty with the IABP, but did after amelioration of the coronary obstruction. Using a similar technique, Ishihara et al. [71] demonstrated an increase in peak coronary blood flow in successfully dilated vessels during IABP support, but no change in mean flow. Whatever the mechanism (increased perfusion or decreased workload), the IABP can improve myocardial lactate metabolism (i.e., increased lactate uptake and/or decreased lactate production [38]) and improve regional wall motion in ischemic but not infarcted areas of the heart [72].

The inconsistencies in the results of these clinical and experimental studies are not surprising when the large number of variables that can alter coronary blood flow are considered. The effect of the IABP on myocardial perfusion will depend on such factors as baseline coronary and regional myocardial blood flow, the level of systemic perfusion pressure and left ventricular end-diastolic pressure, the myocardial workload, the extent to which autoregulatory mechanisms are still intact and functional, the severity of metabolic abnormalities both locally in the myocardium and systemically (e.g., pH, oxygen), the degree of systemic and cardiac adrenergic activation and concentration of circulating neurohormones, the depth and type of anesthesia, the amount of myocardial functional reserve and extent to which pathologic changes in the myocardium are reversible, and the nature of the underlying pathologic process or processes initiating the myocardial dysfunction. Many of these factors were discussed in the reports of the studies just described, including some of the studies using an arterial counterpulsator, and differences in any one or more factors could easily account for variations in the results observed. It is unlikely that any single study could ever be so complete as to allow accurate prediction of the response of an individual patient with coronary insufficiency and left ventricular dysfunction to the IABP. Nonetheless, independent of the mechanisms involved, it is reasonable to make two general statements.

1. The IABP will not likely be of benefit unless there is significant underlying pathology, and the underlying process has some reversible component.
2. The IABP can improve systemic hemodynamics and directly benefit the myocardium in appropriately selected patients.

To properly assess the potential benefits of the IABP, the risks of this intervention must be carefully considered. Numerous reports described myriad complications that can occur with IABP support. Overall complication rates have ranged from 11 to 36 percent [73–101]. These reports concerned 5921 patients who had a total of 1112 complications, for an aggregate rate of 18.8 percent. Differences between the complication rates among the reports can often be explained by factors such as whether investigators differentiated between major and minor complications, whether the series was prospective or retrospective, and the percent of patients in whom extensive necropsy analysis was included. Selection criteria, insertion and maintenance techniques, and the time period over which the data were collected also may be pertinent. To gain a proper perspective, it is therefore instructive to review the incidence of specific complications.

Not all attempts to insert an intra-aortic balloon are successful. Some studies on the complications of IABP support failed to note specifically the number of failed attempts and whether the failures were included in the series. Obviously, complications can occur even when the attempt at IABP support is unsuccessful. In 12 studies that reported the failure rate of attempted IABP support [77, 80, 82–84, 87, 95, 102–106], the failure rate ranged from 5.7 to 21.0 percent, but in most it was approximately 10 percent.

The types of complications that can occur with IABP support are listed in Table 15-2 in relative order of frequency. The incidence of each type of major complication in Table 15-2 is a collective estimate based on the literature cited here.

By far the most common complication of IABP support is leg ischemia [73, 75–78, 82, 83, 91, 95, 98, 101, 107–116]. The leg is the most common site of ischemia because the femoral artery is by far the most common site of insertion for the intra-aortic balloon. Ischemia can be caused by mechanical occlusion of the vessel from the balloon catheter or insertion sheath, by thrombosis, or by emboli that are either thrombotic or atherosclerotic in origin. Ischemia can progress to necrosis requiring surgical intervention, including possible amputation. It can also lead to nerve damage resulting in footdrop or peripheral neuropathies. Residual obstruction can leave the patient who recovers with claudication.

Table 15-2
Complications of IABP treatment

Complication	Incidence (%)
Insertion failure	10
Leg ischemia	10
Mechanical obstruction	
Thromboembolism	
Vascular injury	5
Dissection	
Perforation	
Infection	2
Embolization/thrombosis	1
Hematologic disorder	1
Mechanical failure	1

The reported frequency of leg ischemia with IABP support ranges from a low of 3 percent to as high as 42 percent. However, some series reported ischemia only when subsequent permanent damage occurred; others, if an additional procedure was required; and some, if there was any evidence of ischemia during or following the IABP procedure, even if the ischemia was only transient. Collectively, based on the reports just cited, limb ischemia causing permanent damage or requiring intervention might be expected in 10 percent of patients undergoing treatment with IABP.

Anticoagulation with heparin is usually used to help present thrombosis and embolization. Anticoagulation, of course, presents risks of bleeding, particularly in postoperative patients supported with the IABP. Pericardial tamponade due to anticoagulation has occurred [75], so this consideration is not trivial. Heparin can cause thrombocytopenia, and this may occur in as many as 4.5 percent of IABP-treated patients [117]. The need to maintain pulsation of the balloon to decrease the incidence of thrombosis is well recognized and was clearly demonstrated by Bernstein and Murphy [118]. It is possible that bleeding complications may be higher when the IABP is used subsequent to thrombolytic therapy, but pertinent data are scarce (see below).

Vascular trauma is also reasonably common in patients undergoing IABP support. Trauma to vessels is usually dissection or perforation and can lead to pseudoaneurysm formation, obstruction of branch vessels, bleeding, and hematoma formation. These complications can be expected to occur in approximately 5 percent of patients, as the incidence of vascular trauma ranged from 2.5 to 8.0 percent [77, 100, 103, 112]. Vascular complications may well occur at the time of removal of the intra-aortic balloon [113], and careful attention to the technique of removal is needed [104, 119, 120].

Infection occurs in 1 to 6 percent of patients [73, 77, 82, 88, 103, 112], depending on whether or not local infections are included. Three studies differentiated local infection from sepsis [73, 77, 88]. In these reports the rate of sepsis ranged from 1.0 to 2.3 percent, and that of local infection from 3.0 to 5.7 percent. Unusual infections such as osteomyelitis of the spine [76] and infected arteriovenous fistula [121] also have been reported. Because of the possibility of infection, many programs routinely use prophylactic antibiotics during IABP support.

Embolization or thrombosis of vessels other than the one used for insertion has led to a variety of complications involving multiple organ systems, including splenic infarction [122], spinal cord infarction [123–127], mesenteric [77, 88, 105] or small-bowel [128] infarction, renal artery thrombosis [38, 79], subclavian artery occlusion [129], and even cerebral vascular accident [83, 88]. The overall incidence of any one of these complications is low, but collectively a complication of this type can occur in 1 to 2 percent of patients.

Hematologic disorders, including hemolysis and thrombocytopenia, occur infrequently. Balloon malfunction (e.g., malposition, gas embolus, or balloon damage) also occurs in a small percentage of patients. Several instances of balloon rupture, with or without clot formation and entrapment, have been reported [130–135]. Basically, with the widespread use of the IABP, it is fair to say that almost any complication can potentially occur. For example, McCabe et al. [77] included a case of lymphocele (cystic lymphangioma) formation with lymphedema in their series. In a patient with right ventricular infarction reported by Hasan et al. [136], the IABP reduced left atrial pressure and thereby promoted right-to-left shunting through a valve patent foramen ovale. Finally, IABP support may impact on the patient's psychological status [137], particularly because it most likely is to be used in patients already under severe physical and psychological stress.

Complications are not equally likely to occur in all patients, and several factors have been identified to define patients at higher risk (Table 15-3). Peripheral vascular disease would be expected to be important and has been documented to be so by several authors [82, 88, 96, 101, 115]. Perhaps in part because of the high prevalence of vascular disease, diabetes mellitus is also a risk factor [101, 105, 114, 115]. Similarly, advanced age may be important according to Weintraub et al. [138] and Goldberger et al. [92], although it was not in the series by Gottleib et al. [88]. Sisto et al. [139] used IABP in 25 octogenarians with a reasonable complication rate. Women are more likely to have a complication of IABP treatment than men [86, 88, 93, 114, 115], perhaps because of the generally smaller size of their vessels. The importance of the status of the vasculature was further emphasized when Goldman et al. [82] noted that complications are more likely when insertion of the balloon is difficult. Aortoiliac angiography has been recommended [140] at the time of heart catheterization to assist in assessment of the pertinent vasculature for those patients likely to need IABP treatment. Not surprisingly, patients in shock may be more likely to have a complication than are those with unstable angina but near-normal hemodynamics [82, 88, 109, 138]. Complication rates are higher with emergency IABP use than with elective insertion [97, 141]. Hypertension has been identified as a risk factor [99, 114] but it is not as likely to be important as the other factors just noted.

Early use of the IABP involved surgical techniques for balloon insertion. It was hoped that development of percutaneous techniques [80, 102, 111, 142, 143] would help decrease the incidence of complications. Unfortunately, this did not occur, and several studies documented that the complication rate with percutaneous insertion is equal to or higher than that seen with surgical insertion [83–86, 88, 92–94, 119, 130, 144]. A recent randomized study comparing surgical and percutaneous removal of the IABP suggested that the majority of the balloons inserted percutaneously may be safely removed percutaneously, but surgical removal should be done in patients who have bleeding diathesis or hemorrhagic or ischemic complications, and those who had the balloon inserted surgically [120]. Complication rates increase the longer the balloon is in place [76, 82, 86, 88, 114, 145, 146] and a well-organized program of continuous patient monitoring is necessary to help minimize complications. Even so, the complications of IABP are not trivial, in either incidence or severity, making the decision to use the IABP in an individual patient a major and sometimes difficult option.

Table 15-3
Risk factors for IABP complications

Risk factors
Peripheral vascular disease
Diabetes mellitus
Advanced age
Female gender
Shock
Hypertension
Percutaneous insertion/removal
Duration of use

Clinical experience with the IABP and knowledge of the likely outcome of its application in specific types of patients enhance the decision-making process when considering this intervention. Numerous institutions, encompassing thousands of patients, reported their experience with clinical outcome following IABP treatment. The literature includes a series of specific groups with unstable angina [138, 147–150], myocardial infarction [109, 151–165], postoperative circulatory inadequacy [106, 166–173], or combinations of these and other disorders [72–75, 78, 81, 85, 87, 90, 92, 145, 174–178]. Experience with the IABP in patients undergoing coronary angioplasty is expanding, with the IABP inserted either electively prior to the procedure in high-risk patients [179–183] or during the procedure for patients experiencing reocclusion or acute complications [183, 184]. Use of the IABP has even expanded to patients undergoing noncardiac surgery who are at increased risk because of severe heart disease [185–188]. It becomes clear from an analysis of this collective experience that indications for IABP use cannot be easily listed in a way that will be all-inclusive. Nor is it reasonable to construct a simple decision tree that will guide us directly to the proper decision for every patient who may potentially benefit from IABP, as there are too many important factors to consider. Rather, we must carefully analyze the status of the patient along a spectrum of critical areas, and then weigh the potential risks against the possible benefits of IABP treatment.

IABP therapy is useful in patients with coronary insufficiency only when coronary lesions are extremely critical, left ventricular function is inadequate to maintain peripheral perfusion despite optimal medical support, there are concomitant lesions such as mitral insufficiency or acquired ventricular septal defect causing inadequate cardiac output, or a combination of these situations. Moreover, since IABP therapy is supportive, not curative, the lesions must be potentially reversible. With rare exception this means that the patient with acute coronary insufficiency needs to be a candidate for surgery, angioplasty, or possibly cardiac transplantation in order for the physician to reasonably consider IABP therapy. *The first step in considering use of the IABP therefore is to establish that the patient is a candidate for further invasive procedures.*

Once it is established that a patient with acute coronary insufficiency is a candidate for aggressive, invasive therapy, subsequent management is determined by the severity of the symptoms, extent of myocardial damage (and consequently the degree of hemodynamic compromise), amount of myocardium at risk, nature and severity of coronary obstruction, and presence of complications. The subsequent paragraphs provide a perspective on how IABP therapy is considered as the patient is assessed in each of these categories.

Symptoms of coronary insufficiency can range from not being present at all despite severe ischemia or infarction (silent ischemia), to severe intractable chest pain. Although the IABP has been successfully used to help alleviate pain in patients with unstable angina [138, 147], severe chest pain alone is not sufficient indication for its use. If the patient is hemodynamically stable, the symptoms should be treated aggressively with antianginal medication and then cardiac catheterization [189]. Olinger et al. [190] demonstrated that most patients with unstable angina can be revascularized without IABP therapy. Only when the intractable symptoms are also associated with significant cardiac dysfunction [191] or extremely critical coronary anatomy (see below) is IABP therapy necessary. If such is the case, the IABP can be used as an adjunct to angioplasty or surgery. It must also be realized that if there is ongoing myocardial necrosis, none of the available interventions may completely alleviate pain, and narcotic analgesics are often both necessary and appropriate.

The extent of myocardial damage and consequent degree of circulatory impairment are assessed with a complete hemodynamic profile, as discussed in Chapter 13. *The functional status of the heart as a pump is the most critical factor determining the need for IABP treatment.* Pump function depends not only on the extent of myocardial dysfunction but also on the structural and functional integrity of the heart valves, interventricular septum, and electrical conduction system. Whenever there is clinical evidence of inadequate circulation, IABP support should be considered a potential option. However, it should be instituted only after it is evident that pharmacologic support alone (see Chapter 14) is inadequate.

Assessment of the amount of myocardium at risk, as well as the nature and severity of coronary obstruction, requires cardiac catheterization, often supplemented with data obtained by electrocardiography, echocardiography, nuclear imaging, and serum enzyme analysis. As mentioned previously, the IABP is not likely to be helpful unless a reversible component to the disease is delineated with these studies. In the absence of severe pump failure, the IABP may still be useful when there is a large area of myocardium at risk from a single critical coronary artery stenosis. Such is the case when there is a more than 90 percent stenosis of the left main coronary artery. This lesion carries a poor prognosis [192] and increases the risk of both cardiac catheterization [193] and coronary artery bypass surgery [194]. Perturbations in hemodynamic status that might otherwise be easily tolerated may be fatal with severe left main coronary artery disease. The experience of Cooper et al. [195] further supports use of the IABP in this situation.

Specific mention should be made of studies designed to prove the efficacy of using the IABP in acute myocardial infarction. Two randomized trials failed to detect a difference in mortality or morbidity with IABP therapy in this setting. The study by O'Rourke et al. [152] evaluated the benefit of counterpulsation in limiting infarct size and improving survival in patients with acute myocardial infarction not considered for bypass surgery. Flaherty et al. [164] limited their study to patients in Killip class I or II at the time of entry, a group that would not likely meet the above-mentioned criteria for utilizing the IABP. Thus neither study examined use of the IABP in the type of clinical setting in which we currently consider it most beneficial. In patients with acute myocardial infarction and cardiogenic shock, Waksman et al. [196] found better in-hospital and 1-year survival rates in patients provided IABP support (most of whom subsequently received early revascularization) than in a similar group for whom the IABP was not available. Although this was not a randomized study, it better approximates the usual clinical application of the IABP in acute myocardial infarction. Additional large-scale cooperative randomized trials to test the efficacy of the IABP in patients with acute coronary insufficiency are unlikely to be forthcoming in the future. It would be much too difficult to limit the options available so that all patients are treated similarly, and thus allow a fairly homogeneous group of patients to be randomized to receive IABP support versus conventional therapy. Moreover, "conventional therapy" is not easily defined.

The management of acute coronary insufficiency has advanced dramatically. Interventions such as thrombolytic therapy were not widely used during the time much of the clinical experience with the IABP was obtained. The known risk of bleeding complications from IABP support warrants caution when considering its use in patients receiving thrombolytic therapy. However, use of the IABP is not an absolute contraindication to lytic therapy, and these two interventions have been used together with relative safety [197]. The pressure lumen of the IABP can even be used to infuse the lytic agent [198]. The collective experience of the Thrombolysis and Angioplasty in Acute Myocardial Infarction (TAMI) Study Group suggests that when the IABP is used in high-risk patients with large infarctions, an improvement in global and noninfarct-zone left ventricular function can be attained [199]. However, despite IABP use, such patients can be expected to have a high mortality and in-hospital complication rate.

The basic functional components of the IABP as described earlier in this chapter are fairly consistent, but many technologic aspects of IABP support are continually expanding and improving. Balloons are smaller and easier to insert and, when necessary, can be inserted through the axillary artery [200]. Modifications of the techniques for percutaneous insertion and removal allow physicians to choose a method designed to fit an individual patient's needs. This may include using a sheath with a side hole to maintain limb perfusion [201], no sheath at all [202, 203], or a suprainguinal prosthetic vascular graft [204]. If peripheral vascular disease is present, peripheral angioplasty may allow successful balloon insertion [205]. Modifications of the insertion technique can provide improved patient mobility while under IABP support [206]. "Closed-loop" pump systems can make beat-to-beat adjustments automatically to optimize augmentation [207], and modifications can allow an IABP to act as a pneumatic ventricular device controller [208]. Use of IABP does not preclude application of additional support methods when necessary [209]. The balloon itself can potentially be modified to provide intraventricular and intra-aortic pumping timed to work in concert [210]. Technology independent of the IABP system is also important. Echocardiography, especially transesophageal echocardiography, is being used to help evaluate the physiologic effects of the IABP on ventricular function [211] and coronary flow [212, 213], to diagnose aortic dissection [214], and to guide insertion when aortic dissection is present [215].

Once IABP therapy is instituted, a well-structured program of patient monitoring and system maintenance by a coordinated team of well-trained physicians, nurses, and technicians is necessary to ensure a good outcome and minimize complications. Routine care of patients on IABP therapy includes use of prophylactic antibiotics, heparin anticoagulation to prevent thrombus and embolism, optimization of pump settings, treatment of complications, and careful determination of the appropriate timing and technique of balloon weaning and removal.

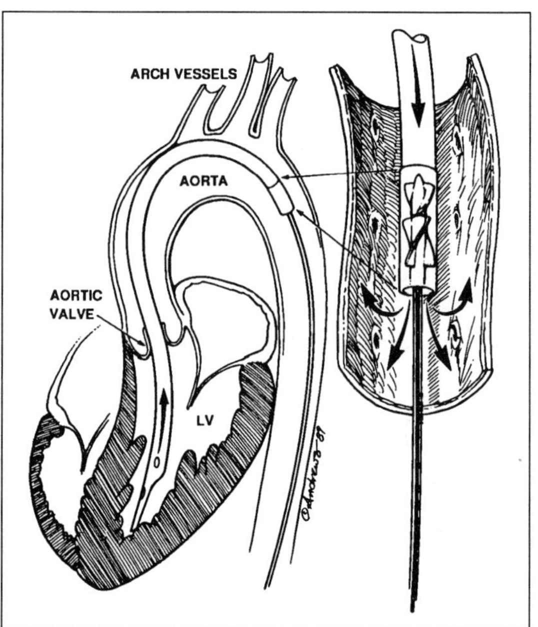

Fig. 15-5
Schematic diagram of the Hemopump intraventricular coaxial flow pump. LV = left ventricle. (Reprinted with permission from the Society of Thoracic Surgeons [*The Annals of Thoracic Surgery,* 1989, vol. 48, page 733].)

Intraventricular Coaxial Flow Pump

A device with potentially the same clinical indications as the IABP provides for left ventricular assist using an intraventricular coaxial flow pump mounted in a catheter positioned retrograde across the aortic valve. The device is manufactured by Johnson and Johnson Interventional Systems (Rancho Cordova, CA) under the trade name Hemopump, and is schematically diagrammed in Figure 15-5 [216]. At the time of this writing, it has not been approved by the Food and Drug Administration for use in the United States, but is available in some countries. The Hemopump turbine produces a continuous flow from the left ventricle to the aorta, thus unloading the failing left ventricle and supporting systemic pressure. Scholz et al. [217] demonstrated improved cardiac output, an increase in mean aortic pressure, and a decrease in myocardial oxygen consumption when Hemopump support was provided to sheep with congestive heart failure induced by high-frequency ventricular pacing. In animals with ventricular fibrillation [218], the Hemopump supported adequate circulation for up to 30 minutes.

The Hemopump could be particularly advantageous in heart failure due to acute ischemia or infarction. Efficient left ventricular unloading with sustained coronary perfusion pressure would provide collateral flow to ischemic zones, and potentially reduce infarct size. In experimental ischemia in dogs, the Hemopump can improve blood flow to ischemic territory [219], as well as nonischemic zones [220], and improve myocardial metabolism as evidenced by decreased myocardial lactate extraction [221]. In a direct comparison to the IABP, Smalling et al. [222] found that compared to control animals, both the Hemopump and the IABP salvaged myocardium when the left anterior descending coronary artery was ligated in 18 dogs, with the Hemopump slightly more beneficial than the IABP. However, Wouters et al. [223] failed to demonstrate any modification of infarct size using the Hemopump in 12 dogs, despite effective global and regional circulatory support. Shiiya et al. [224] suggested that the effects of Hemopump support depend significantly on the severity of myocardial dysfunction, providing a much greater reduction in myocardial oxygen demand when dysfunction is severe. Such findings could help explain some of the discrepancies between studies.

Clinical experience with the Hemopump is somewhat limited, but several reports clearly demonstrated the ability of the pump to improve hemodynamics in patients with failing left ventricular function [225–227]. Cardiac output increases during Hemopump support, while pulmonary wedge pressure decreases. Mean aortic pressure is improved, and heart rate frequently decreases. A preliminary study by Dubois-Rande et al. [228], measuring coronary flow in postangioplasty vessels of five patients, suggested that Hemopump assistance may improve myocardial perfusion, consistent with what has been reported in experimental animals. In addition to use in patients with decompensating left ventricular function, the Hemopump has been used for perioperative support [229], including treatment of heart transplant failure [230], during mechanical resuscitation [231], in conjunction with hemofiltration [232], and during high-risk angioplasty [233–235]. An acceptable quality of life was reported by Baldwin et al. [236] for survivors of Hemopump support.

Potential problems with the Hemopump left ventricular support device include the same type of vascular damage that can occur with the IABP (i.e., thrombosis, perforation, anticoagulation associated bleeding, and embolization). Inability to insert or position the device due to technical or vascular problems can be expected in some patients, and there is always a risk of infection. In addition, the catheter in the ventricle can cause arrhythmias, and there is a theoretical potential for direct damage to the myocardium or valvular apparatus. The catheter inflow orifice can become obstructed by the anterior papillary muscle [237], or the device can be ejected from the left ventricle, both of which can be corrected by repositioning the cannula. Mechanical breakdown is also possible. An interesting problem that can occur with this device is hypoxia due to right-to-left shunting through a patent foramen ovale when left atrial pressure decreases below right atrial pressure [238]. As with any system that exposes blood to moving mechanical mechanisms, hemolysis and thrombocytopenia are of concern. Clinical experience with the Hemopump is still too limited to determine the relative frequency with which these various complications are likely to occur. Additional data are clearly needed to allow a proper assessment of the risk-benefit ratio for this device.

Left Ventricular Assist Devices

Several systems have been devised to provide direct mechanical assist for the failing left ventricle. These devices are often labeled according to the degree of assist provided, whether they are designed to be temporary or permanent, and if they oxygenate the blood as well as circulate it.

Artificial hearts permanently replace the human heart and take over the total burden of maintaining circulation. None of the currently available models can maintain a person for the long term. Although the evolution of artificial hearts continues, they are currently limited to use at selected centers as a "bridge to cardiac transplantation." A detailed discussion of artificial heart technology and of the moral and ethical considerations applicable to the use of artificial hearts is beyond the scope of this treatise.

Cardiopulmonary bypass temporarily provides the body functions of both the heart and the lungs, and is more appropriately presented in textbooks on cardiovascular surgery. However, with current technology, there is not always a clear distinction between a cardiopulmonary bypass system and the more-advanced left ventricular assist devices. When combined with an extracorporeal membrane oxygenator (ECMO), some left ventricular assist systems basically become partial or even total cardiopulmonary bypass systems. This chapter does not discuss the systems designed specifically for open-heart surgery.

Skeletal muscle assistance of the left ventricle has several theoretical advantages. The energy source is intrinsic, running on mitochondrial energy derived from the food we eat, eliminating bulky power packs or lines to external power sources. In addition, when autogenous expendable muscle bundles are used, problems with rejection of foreign tissue or reaction to synthetic materials can be avoided. A potential advantage in ischemic cardiomyopathy is the possibility of neorevascularization from the skeletal muscle to the myocardium, which could help relieve intractable angina [239]. Since 1958, when Kantrowitz and McKinnon [240] first reported use of skeletal muscle to aid the heart, there have been many attempts to refine the technique. Muscle groups used experimentally have included sections of diaphragm, the rectus abdominus, the latissimus dorsi, the pectoralis major, and the quadriceps femoris. The muscles have been wrapped around the heart or aorta, formed into inlay or onlay grafts, fashioned into ventricular structures, or applied to chambers to act as counterpulsation devices or valved conduits. In every configuration it is necessary to have a muscle-stimulating device that also senses cardiac activity and times the muscle contraction appropriately in systole or diastole.

Despite the fact that successful augmentation can be achieved, fatigue continues to be a factor potentially limiting the technique of using skeletal muscle for left ventricular assist. The structure and metabolic functions of skeletal muscle differ from those of cardiac muscle in several important ways. Whereas cardiac muscle is arranged in a syncytium that contracts in unison, skeletal muscle is organized into motor units that are recruited individually. Cardiac action potentials are much longer than skeletal muscle action potentials, thus sustaining contraction throughout all of systole. Myocardium has more than tenfold as many mitochondria as skeletal muscle, and is better suited for sustained aerobic metabolism to produce the high-energy requirements of maintaining circulation. In addition, the contractile and membrane-bound proteins differ in the two types of muscle. Muscle relaxation can also be a problem, and skeletal muscle may impair diastolic relaxation [241].

Chronic low-frequency stimulation can condition skeletal muscle to be more fatigue resistant. Capillary density increases, mitochondria and enzymes of aerobic metabolism increase, and there are alterations in sarcoplasmic reticulum and contractile proteins. These changes result in transformation of "fast-twitch" fibers to the slower contracting and more fatigue-resistant "slow-twitch" fibers. It is possible for conditioning to occur while the muscle is functioning as an assist device, and studies to determine the optimal stimulation protocol continue [242].

Of the several techniques for utilizing skeletal muscle for ventricular assist, *latissimus dorsi cardiomyoplasty* has emerged as the preferred technique for clinical application. Since the first successful clinical application of this procedure by Carpentier and Chachques in 1985 [243], worldwide experience with cardiomyoplasty has rapidly expanded to include hundreds of patients. However, since surgery is needed, followed by time for recovery and weeks of conditioning, this modality has little

Fig. 15-6
A pneumatically powered ventricular assist device is shown before chest closure as it would be used to remove blood from the left atrium and then pump it into the ascending aorta. (From W. S. Pierce et al. Ventricular-assist pumping in patients with cardiogenic shock after cardiac operations. *N. Engl. J. Med.* 305:1606, 1981. With permission.)

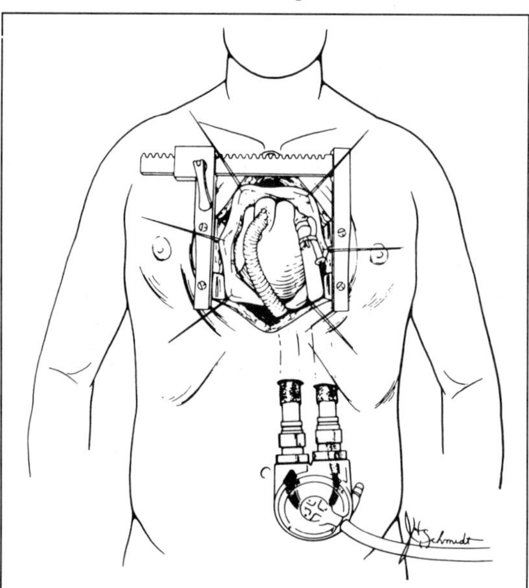

Fig. 15-7
Brushless DC electric motor–driven cam blood pump with Bjork-Shiley inflow and outflow valves (clinical left ventricular assist device). (From W. E. Gaines et al. Development of a long-term electric motor left ventricular assist system. *Heart Transplant* 3:323, 1984. With permission.)

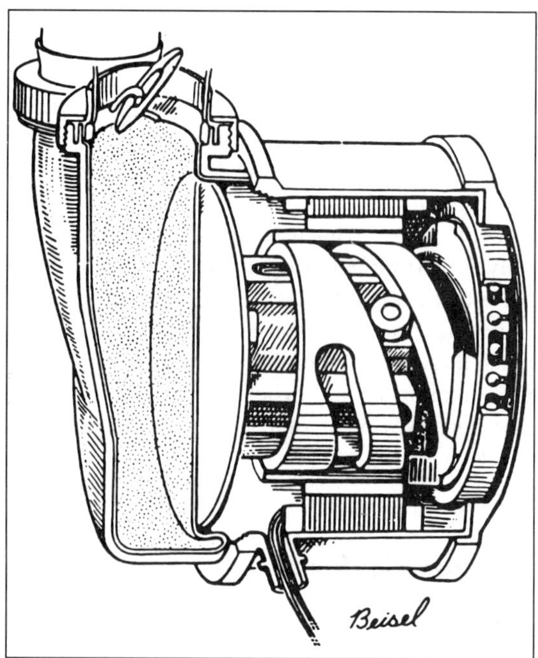

potential for emergency left ventricular support of acutely injured myocardium.

Electrically driven impeller pumps, roller pumps, pneumatic or electrically powered valved chamber pumps, and centrifugal pumps have all seen service as *left ventricular assist devices.* Impeller pumps have generally been limited by problems with thrombosis and hemorrhage. Roller pumps, long used in cardiopulmonary bypass machines, have primarily been used to sustain patients who cannot be weaned from cardiopulmonary bypass following cardiac surgery. They can be used in the short term for cardiogenic shock [244] but are similarly restricted from long-term use because of blood trauma. Thus most left ventricular assist devices currently in clinical use provide either pulsatile flow using chamber pumps or continuous flow using centrifugal pumps.

Chamber pumps consist of a flexible blood-filled chamber inside a rigid housing. The chamber has inlet and outlet valves to ensure unidirectional pulsatile flow as the chamber is intermittently compressed. Usually different function modes can allow pump ejection to be timed to the cardiac cycle, to run independently at set rates, or to begin ejection when complete filling is detected. One such pump, the Pierce-Donnachy [245, 246], developed at Pennsylvania State University, is shown in Figure 15-6. The same group developed a similar pump (Fig. 15-7) with a pusher plate powered by a low-speed, brushless, DC motor [247]. Other pumps of this general type (Figs. 15-8 through 15-11) include an abdominal left ventricular assist device from the Collar Laboratory of the Texas Heart Institute [248], an electromechanical pusher-plate pump [249] developed at Children's Hospital and Harvard Medical School in Massachusetts, a microprocessor-controlled electromagnetic energy converter dual pusher-plate sactype unit from Stanford University [250], and the hydraulic pump used at the Cleveland Clinic [251]. Most chamber pumps are designed for implantation, although some can be used either internally or externally. The ultimate goal of chamber pumps is long-term application in ambulatory patients with a portable power source, often as a bridge to cardiac transplantation. Most of these pumps are ill-suited for emergency use in decompensating patients with acute myocardial ischemia or infarction. The devices illustrated here provide examples of the variety of technologic approaches being applied for cardiac support, but a detailed discussion of the comparative risks and benefits of these and other available units is more appropriately presented in texts on cardiovascular surgery.

Centrifugal pumps constitute the other major class of devices used for left ventricular assist. These pumps move blood by centrifugal force transmitted to the blood from the rotor cones and impeller. A pump of this type, the Biomedicus (Fig. 15-12), is manufactured by Biomedics (Minneapolis, MN) [246, 252–255]. Similar devices include

Fig. 15-8
Single-chambered balloon left ventricular assist device designed for intra-abdominal use with an external pneumatic drive console. (From D. A. Cooley. Staged cardiac transplantation: Report of three cases. *Heart Transplant.* 1:145, 1982. With permission.)

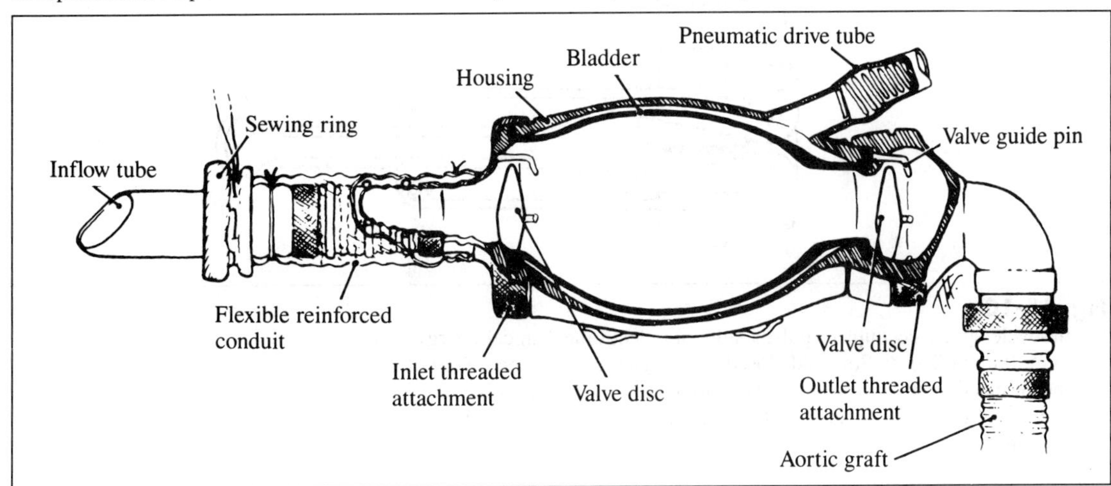

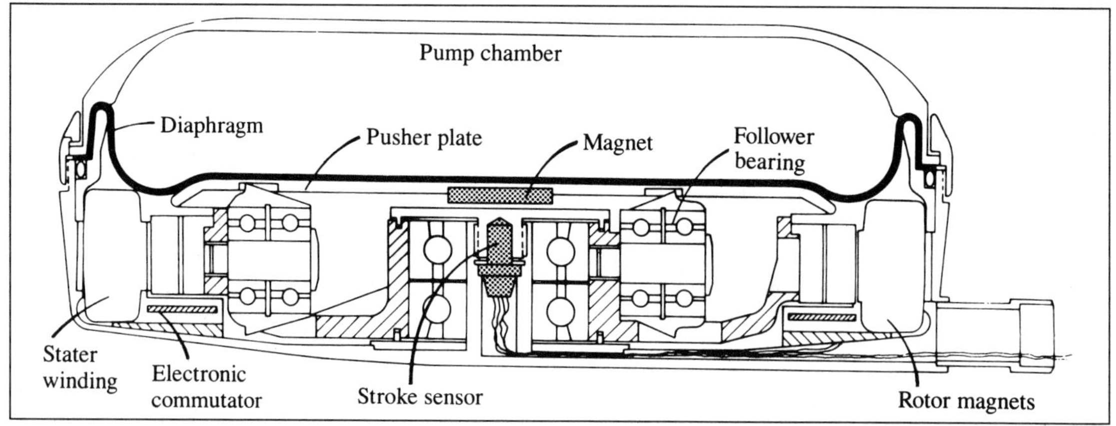

Fig. 15-9
Lateral view of an implantable pusher-plate pump powered by a 50-V low-speed torque motor. (From W. F. Bernhard et al. Investigations with an implantable electrically activated ventricular assist device. *J. Thorac. Cardiovasc. Surg.* 88:11, 1984. With permission.)

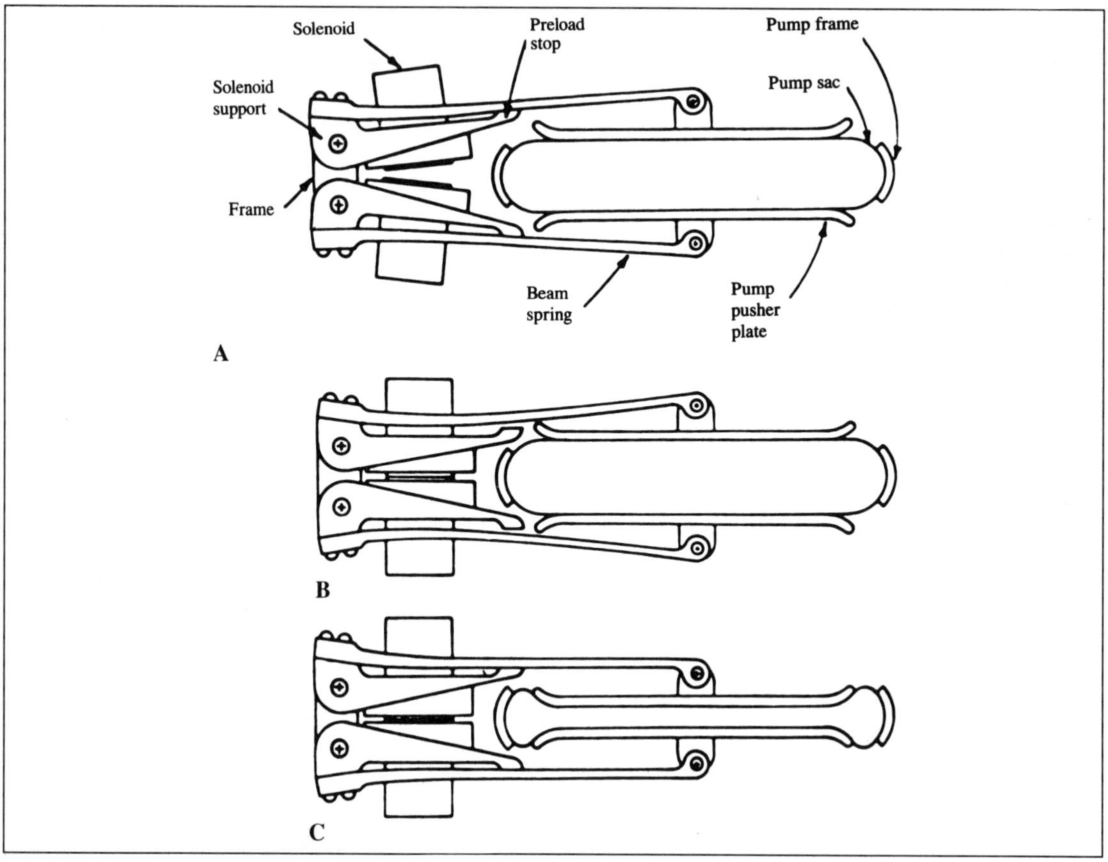

Solenoid
Preload stop
Pump frame
Solenoid support
Pump sac
Frame
Beam spring
Pump pusher plate
A
B
C

Fig. 15-10
Single-cycle spring-decoupled, pulsed solenoid electromechanical energy converter pump. *A*. Pump filled. *B*. Solenoid closed and magnetically latched. Start of ejection stroke. *C*. End of ejection stroke. (From P. M. Portner et al. An alternative in end-stage heart disease: Long-term ventricular assistance. *Heart Transplant.* 3:47, 1983. With permission.)

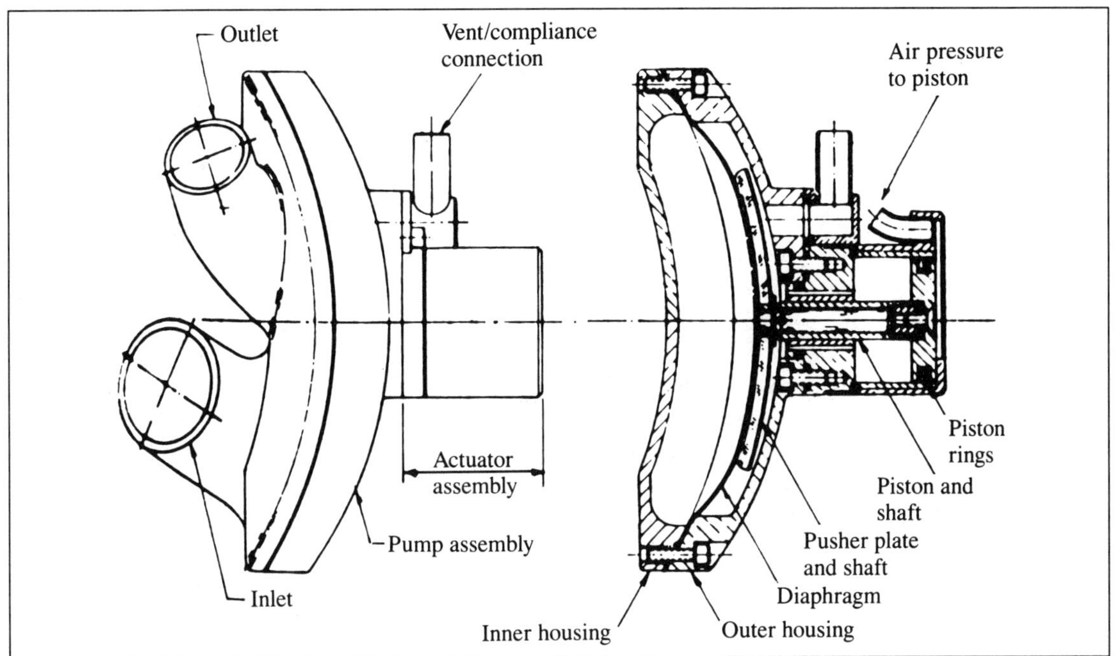

Fig. 15-11
Pneumatically powered pusher-plate left ventricular assist device. (From Y. Nose et al. Experimental results for chronic left ventricular assist and total artificial heart development. *Artif. Organs* 7:55, 1983. With permission.)

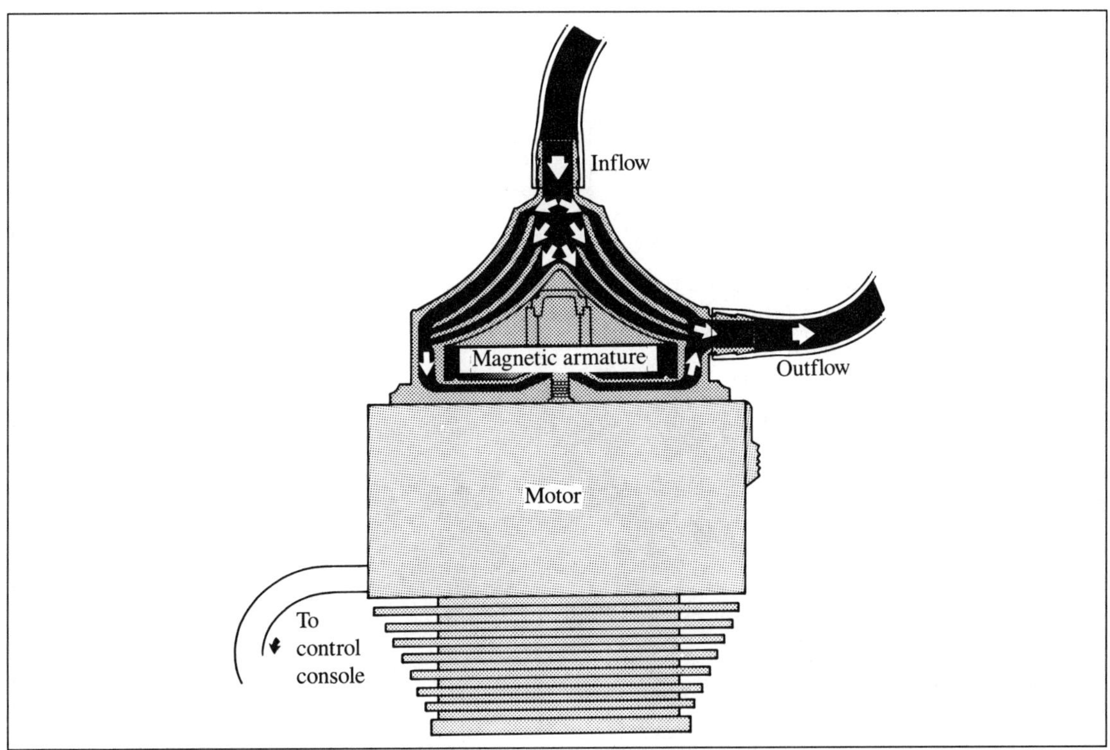

Fig. 15-12
Biomedicus centrifugal blood pump.

the Delphin made by Sarns 3M Health Care (Ann Arbor, MI) [255, 256], and the Lifestream Centrifugal Pump by St. Jude Medical (Little Canada, MN). A seal-less centrifugal pump (Gyro Pump) is under development at Baylor College (Houston, TX) [257]. Although the pulsatile flow of the chamber pumps described here is more physiologic than the continuous flow provided by centrifugal pumps, centrifugal pumps do provide some advantages. Mechanically, these pumps are generally less complex than chamber pumps. Blood trauma is low, as is the propensity for air emboli to develop. In conjunction with an oxygenator and heat exchanger, these pumps can provide cardiopulmonary bypass.

The centrifugal pumps are more restraining than chamber pumps, and currently are not considered for long-term ambulatory support. However, with the development of percutaneous insertion techniques [252, 258], emergency rapid institution of ventricular support for patients with acute decompensation from ischemic heart disease is more feasible. Figure 15-13 illustrates how such a pump can be hooked up for emergency left ventricular support. Percutaneous cannulation of the femoral artery and vein minimizes the time required to initiate support. This allows timely initiation of bypass support for shock from acute myocardial infarction [259, 260], during cardiac arrest [261–263], or more electively for high-risk coronary angioplasty patients [264]. By contrast, Figure 15-14 illustrates use of a pump inserted surgically as might be done for ventricular assist following cardiovascular surgery. This latter method ''unloads'' the ventricle more efficiently, but requires major surgery to initiate its use.

The potential use of left ventricular assist for ischemic heart disease was demonstrated in experiments by Pennock et al. [265] and Grossi et al. [266]. Both groups presented evidence that infarct size in dogs can be decreased using left atrial to

Fig. 15-13
External left ventricular assist device and extracorporeal oxygenator as it may be set up for emergency application using percutaneous arterial and venous access.

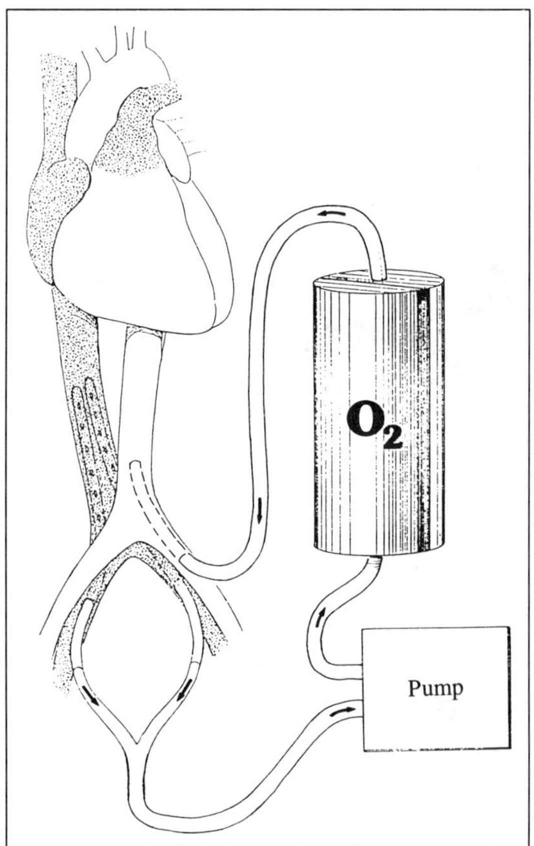

Fig. 15-14
Left ventricular assist device as it would be used to ''unload'' the left ventricle and sustain systemic perfusion. Surgical insertion is required.

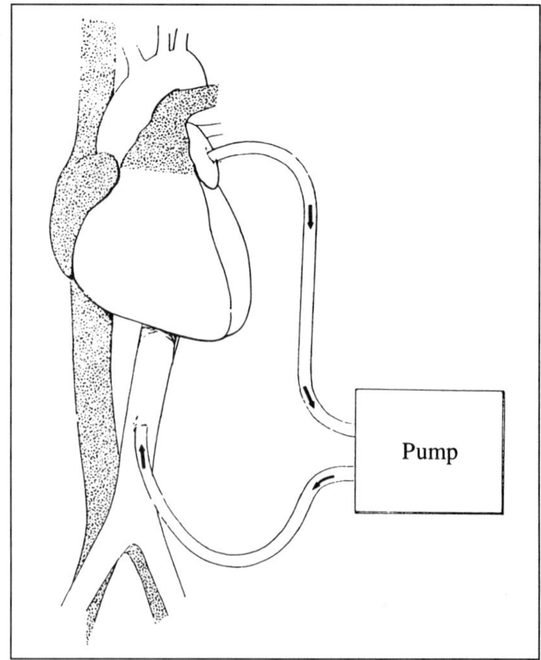

systemic arterial bypass. These findings were supported by Mickleborough et al. [253], who compared circulatory support with a centrifugal pump to that of IABP therapy combined with dopamine in dogs with myocardial depression from temporary ischemic arrest. They found less histologic evidence of necrosis in the dogs supported by left ventricular assist. The survival rate in pigs following coronary artery ligation was higher with the left ventricular assist device than with IABP support in a study by Zobel et al. [267].

Comparisons between the IABP and left ventricular assist device in patients can be made from clinical experience [268], but the unstable status of the critically ill patients who are candidates for these devices makes well-controlled comparative study most difficult. The IABP remains the first mechanical support system to be considered in acute decompensation of ischemic heart disease. Emergency percutaneous bypass may be necessary in patients for whom the IABP is clearly going to be inadequate. Surgical attachment of a left ventricular assist device can be added (or possibly substituted) if the IABP alone is inadequate to support the circulation, or the need for support is anticipated to extend beyond acceptable time limits for percutaneous cannulae to remain in place. The relative role of each of these devices will likely change in the future as both technology and application techniques continue to evolve.

References

1. Page, D. L., Caulfield, J. B., Kastor, J. A., et al. Myocardial changes associated with cardiogenic shock. *N. Engl. J. Med.* 285:133, 1971.
2. Bertel, O., and Steiner, A. Rotating tourniquets do not work in acute congestive heart failure and pulmonary edema. *Lancet* 1:762, 1980.
3. Wayne, M. A. The MAST suit in the treatment of cardiogenic shock. *J. Am. Coll. Emerg. Physicians* 7:107, 1978.
4. Parmley, W. W., Hatcher, C. R., Ewy, G. A., et al. Task Force V: Physical interventions and adjunctive therapy. *Am. J. Cardiol.* 50:409, 1982.
5. Dennis C., Moreno, J. R., Hall, D. P., et al. Studies on external counterpulsation as a potential measure for acute left heart failure. *Trans. Am. Soc. Artif. Int. Organs* 9:186, 1963.
6. Soroff, H. S., Birtwell, W. C., Giron, F., et al. Support of the systemic circulation and left ventricular assist by synchronous pulsation of extramural pressure. *Surg. Forum* 16:148, 1965.
7. Silverstein, D. M., Hamilton, G. W., and Hammermeister, K. E. The effect of external pressure diastolic augmentation on regional myocardial perfusion in experimental myocardial infarction. *Cardiology* 60:329, 1975.
8. Watson, J. T., Platt, M. R., Rogers, D. E., et al. Similarities in coronary flow between external counterpulsation and intra-aortic balloon pumping. *Am. J. Physiol.* 230:1616, 1976.
9. Wright, P. W. External counterpulsation for cardiogenic shock following cardiopulmonary bypass surgery. *Am. Heart J.* 90:231, 1975.
10. Parmley, W. W., Chatterjee, K., Charuzi, Y., and Swan, H. J. C. Hemodynamic effects of noninvasive systolic unloading (nitroprusside) and diastolic augmentation (external counterpulsation) in patients with acute myocardial infarction. *Am. J. Cardiol.* 33:819, 1974.
11. Heck, H. A., and Doty, D. B. Assisted circulation by phasic external lower body compression. *Circulation* 64:II-118, 1981.
12. Milliken, J. C., Laks, H., and George, B. Use of a venous assist device after repair of complex lesions of the right heart. *J. Am. Coll. Cardiol.* 8:922, 1986.
13. Kern, M. J., Henry, R. H., Lembo, N., et al. Effects of pulsed external augmentation of diastolic pressure on coronary and systemic hemodynamics in patients with coronary artery disease. *Am. Heart J.* 110:727, 1985.
14. Beckman, C. B., Dietzman, R. H., Romero, L. H., et al. Hemodynamic evaluation of external counterpulsation in surgical patients. *Surgery* 74:846, 1973.
15. Amsterdam, E. A., Banas, J., Criley, J. M., et al. Clinical assessment of external pressure circulatory assistance in acute myocardial infarction. Report of a cooperative clinical trial. *Am. J. Cardiol.* 45:349, 1980.
16. Kuhn, L. A. External pressure circulatory assistance: No light on the shadow. *Am. J. Cardiol.* 46:1069, 1980.
17. Clauss, R. H., Birtwell, W. C., Albertal, G., et al. Assisted circulation. I. The arterial counterpulsator. *J. Thorac. Cardiovasc. Surg.* 41:447, 1961.
18. Ellis, P. R. ,Lee, C., Wong, S. H., et al. Assisted circulation in treatment of experimental heart failure. *Arch. Surg.* 90:879, 1965.
19. Lefemine, A. A., Low, H. B. C., Cohen, M. L., et al. Assisted circulation. III. The effect of synchronized arterial counterpulsation on myocardial oxygen consumption and coronary flow. *Am. Heart J.* 64:789, 1962.
20. Hirsch, L. J., Lluch, S., and Katz, L. N. Counterpulsation effects of coronary blood flow and cardiac oxygen utilization. *Circ. Res.* 19:1031, 1966.
21. Spotnitz, H. M., Covell, J. W., Ross, J., and Braunwald, E. Left ventricular mechanics and oxygen consumption during arterial counterpulsation. *Am. J. Physiol.* 217:1352, 1969.
22. Goldfarb, D., Friesinger, G. C., Conti, C. R., et al.

Preservation of myocardial viability by diastolic augmentation after ligation of the coronary artery in dogs. *Surgery* 63:320, 1968.

23. Sugg, W. L., Webb, W. R., and Ecker, R. R. Reduction of extent of myocardial infarction by counterpulsation. *Ann. Thorac. Surg.* 7:310, 1969.
24. Jacobey, J. A., Taylor, W. J., Smith, G. T., et al. A new therapeutic approach to acute coronary occlusion. II. Opening dormant coronary collateral channels by counterpulsation. *Am. J. Cardiol.* 11:218, 1963.
25. Nanas, J. N., Mason, J. W., Taenaka, Y., and Olsen, D. B. Comparison of an implanted abdominal aortic counterpulsation device with the intraaortic balloon pump in a heart failure model. *J. Am. Coll. Cardiol.* 7:1028, 1986.
26. Zelano, J. A., Ko, W., Lazzaro, R., et al. Evaluation of an extraaortic counterpulsation device in severe cardiac failure. *Ann. Thorac. Surg.* 53:30, 1992.
27. Moulopoulos, S. D., Topaz, S., and Kolff, W. J. Diastolic balloon pumping (with carbon dioxide) in the aorta—a mechanical assistance to the failing circulation. *Am. Heart J.* 63:669, 1962.
28. Kantrowitz, A., Tjonneland, S., Freed, P. S., et al. Initial clinical experience with intra-aortic balloon pumping in cardiogenic shock. *J.A.M.A.* 203:135, 1968.
29. Kantrowitz, A., Krakauer, J. S., Rosenbaum, A., et al. Phase-shift balloon pumping in medically refractory cardiogenic shock. *Arch. Surg.* 99:739, 1969.
30. Buckley, M. J., Leinbach, R. C., Kastor, J. A., et al. Hemodynamic evaluation of intra-aortic balloon pumping in man. *Circulation* 41, 42:II-130, 1970.
31. Mueller, H., Ayres, S. M., Conklin, E. F., et al. The effects of intra-aortic counterpulsation on cardiac performance and metabolism in shock associated with acute myocardial infarction. *J. Clin. Invest.* 50:1885, 1971.
32. Bregman, D., and Goetz, R. H. Clinical experience with a new cardiac assist device. The dual-chambered intra-aortic balloon assist. *J. Thorac. Cardiovasc. Surg.* 62:577, 1971.
33. Dunkman, W. B., Leinbach, R. C., Buckley, M. J., et al. Clinical and hemodynamic results of intra-aortic balloon pumping and surgery for cardiogenic shock. *Circulation* 46:465, 1972.
34. Leinbach, R. C., Gold, H. K. Dinsmore, R. E., et al. The role of angiography in cardiogenic shock. *Circulation* 47:III-95, 1973.
35. Dilley, R. B., Ross, J., Jr., and Bernstein, E. F. Serial hemodynamics during intra-aortic balloon counterpulsation for cardiogenic shock. *Circulation* 47, 48:III-99, 1973.
36. Weber, K. T., and Janicki, J. S. Intra-aortic balloon counterpulsation. A review of physiological principles, clinical results, and device safety. *Ann. Thorac. Surg.* 17:602, 1974.
37. Urschel, C. W., Eber, L., Forrester, J., et al. Alteration of mechanical performance of the ventricle by intra-aortic balloon counterpulsation. *Am. J. Cardiol.* 25:546, 1970.
38. Scheidt, S., Wilner, G., Mueller, H., et al. Intra-aortic balloon counterpulsation in cardiogenic shock. Report of a cooperative clinical trial. *N. Engl. J. Med.* 288:979, 1973.
39. Port, S. C., Patel, S., and Schmidt, D. H. Effects of intra-aortic balloon counterpulsation on myocardial blood flow in patients with severe coronary artery disease. *J. Am. Coll. Cardiol.* 3:1367, 1984.
40. Mueller, H., Ayres, S. M., Giannelli, S., Jr., et al. Effect of isoproterenol, l-norepinephrine, and intra-aortic counterpulsation on hemodynamics and myocardial metabolism in shock following acute myocardial infarction. *Circulation* 45:335, 1972.
41. Williams, D. O., Korr, K. S., Gewirtz, H., and Most, A. S. The effect of intra-aortic balloon counterpulsation on regional myocardial blood flow and oxygen consumption in the presence of coronary artery stenosis in patients with unstable angina. *Circulation* 66:593, 1982.
42. Ehrich, D. A., Biddle, T. L., Kronenberg, M. W., and Yu, P. N. The hemodynamic response to intra-aortic balloon counterpulsation in patients with cardiogenic shock complicating acute myocardial infarction. *Am. Heart J.* 93:274, 1977.
43. Steele, P., Pappas, G., Vogel, R., et al. Isosorbide dinitrate and intra-aortic balloon pumping in preinfarctional angina. *Chest* 69:712, 1976.
44. Mundth, E. D., Buckley, M. J., DeSanctis, R. W., et al. Surgical treatment of ventricular irritability. *J. Thorac. Cardiovasc. Surg.* 66:943, 1973.
45. Hanson, E. C., Levine, F. H., Kay, H. R., et al. Control of postinfarction ventricular irritability with the intra-aortic balloon pump. *Circulation* 62:I-130, 1980.
46. Feola, M., Adachi, M., Akers, W. W., et al. Intra-aortic balloon pumping in the experimental animal. *Am. J. Cardiol.* 27:129, 1971.
47. Talpins, N. L., Kripke, D. C., and Goetz, R. H. Counterpulsation and intra-aortic balloon pumping in cardiogenic shock. *Arch. Surg.* 97:991, 1968.
48. Tyberg, J. V., Keon, W. J., Sonnenblick, E. H., and Urschel, C. W. Effectiveness of intra-aortic balloon counterpulsation in the experimental low output state. *Am. Heart J.* 80:89, 1970.
49. Powell, W. J., Jr., Daggett, W. M., Magro, A. E., et al. Effects of intra-aortic balloon counterpulsation on cardiac performance, oxygen consumption, and coronary blood flow in dogs. *Circ. Res.* 26:753, 1970.
50. McDonnell, M. A., Kralios, A. C., Tsagaris, T. J., and Kuida, H. Comparative effect of counterpulsation and bypass on left ventricular myocardial oxygen consumption and dynamics before and after coronary occlusion. *Am. Heart J.* 97:78, 1979.
51. Brown, B. G., Goldfarb, D., Topaz, S. R., and Gott, V. L. Diastolic augmentation by intra-aortic balloon. Circulatory hemodynamics and treatment of severe, acute left ventricular failure in dogs. *J. Thorac. Cardiovasc. Surg.* 53:789, 1967.
52. Yahr, W. Z., Butner, A. N., Krakauer, J. S., et al. Cardiogenic shock: Dynamics of coronary blood

flow with intra-aortic phase-shift balloon pumping. *Surg. Forum* 19:142, 1968.
53. Corday, E., Swan, H. J. C., Lang, T., et al. Physiologic principles in the application of circulatory assist for the failing heart. Intra-aortic balloon circulatory assist and venoarterial phased partial bypass. *Am. J. Cardiol.* 26:595, 1970.
54. Chatterjee, S., and Rosensweig, J. Evaluation of intra-aortic balloon counterpulsation. *J. Thorac. Cardiovasc. Surg.* 61:405, 1971.
55. Weber, K. T., and Janicki, J. S. Coronary collateral flow and intra-aortic balloon counterpulsation. *Trans. Am. Soc. Artif. Int. Organs* 19:395, 1973.
56. Gundel, W. D., Brown, B. G., and Gott, V. L. Coronary collateral flow studies during variable aortic root pressure waveforms. *J. Appl. Physiol.* 29:579, 1970.
57. Feola, M., Haiderer, O., and Kennedy, J. H. Intra-aortic balloon pumping (IABP) at different levels of experimental acute left ventricular failure. *Chest* 59:68, 1971.
58. Gill, C. C., Wechsler, A. S., Newman, G. E., and Oldham, H. N., Jr. Augmentation and redistribution of myocardial blood flow during acute ischemia by intra-aortic balloon pumping. *Ann. Thorac. Surg.* 16:445, 1973.
59. Chen, J., Jiang, Y. S., Fang, F. Z., et al. The effect of IABP on ventricular contractility of the normal and ischemic canine heart assessed in situ by T-Emax. *Adv. Exp. Med. Biol.* 248:517, 1989.
60. Shaw, J., Taylor, D. R., and Pitt, B. Effects of intra-aortic balloon counterpulsation on regional coronary blood flow in experimental myocardial infarction. *Am. J. Cardiol.* 34:552, 1974.
61. Saini, V. K., Hood, W. B., Jr., Hechtman, H. B., and Berger, R. L. Nutrient myocardial blood flow in experimental myocardial ischemia. Effects of intra-aortic balloon counterpulsation and coronary reperfusion. *Circulation* 52:1086, 1975.
62. Gewirtz, H., Ohley, W., Williams, D. O., et al. Effect of intra-aortic balloon counterpulsation on regional myocardial blood flow and oxygen consumption in the presence of coronary artery stenosis: Observations in an awake animal model. *Am. J. Cardiol.* 50:829, 1982.
63. Nachlas, M. M., and Siedband, M. P. The influence of diastolic augmentation on infarct size following coronary artery ligation. *J. Thorac. Cardiovasc. Surg.* 53:698, 1967.
64. Roberts, A. J., Alonso, D. R., Combes, J. R., et al. Role of delayed intra-aortic balloon pumping in treatment of experimental myocardial infarction. *Am. J. Cardiol.* 41:1202, 1978.
65. Maroko, P. R., Bernstein, E. F., Libby, P., et al. Effects of intra-aortic balloon counterpulsation on the severity of myocardial ischemic injury following acute coronary occlusion. Counterpulsation and myocardial injury. *Circulation* 40:1150, 1972.
66. Leinbach, R. C., Buckley, M. J., Austen, W. G., et al. Effects of intra-aortic balloon pumping on coronary flow and metabolism in man. *Circulation* 43(Suppl I):I-77, 1971.
67. MacDonald, R. G., Hill, J. A., and Feldman, R. L. Failure of intra-aortic balloon counterpulsation to augment distal coronary perfusion pressure during percutaneous transluminal coronary angioplasty. *Am. J. Cardiol.* 59:359, 1987.
68. Fuchs, R. M., Brin, K. P., Brinker, J. A., et al. Augmentation of regional coronary blood flow by intra-aortic balloon counterpulsation in patients with unstable angina. *Circulation* 68:117, 1983.
69. Kern, M. J., Aguirre, F. V., Tatineni, S., et al. Enhanced coronary blood flow velocity during intraaortic balloon counterpulsation in critically ill patients. *J. Am. Coll. Cardiol.* 21:359, 1993.
70. Kern, M. J., Aguirre, F., Bach, R., et al. Augmentation of coronary blood flow by intra-aortic balloon pumping in patients after coronary angioplasty. *Circulation* 87:500, 1993.
71. Ishihara, M., Sato, H., Tateishi, H., et al. Effects of intraaortic balloon pumping on coronary hemodynamics after coronary angioplasty in patients with acute myocardial infarction. *Am. Heart J.* 124:1133, 1992.
72. Nichols, A. B., Pohost, G. M., Gold, H. K., et al. Left ventricular function during intra-aortic balloon pumping assessed by multigated cardiac blood pool imaging. *Circulation* 58(Suppl I):I-176, 1978.
73. Beckman, C. B., Geha, A. S., Hammond, G. L., and Baue, A. E. Results and complications of intra-aortic balloon counterpulsation. *Ann. Thorac. Surg.* 24:550, 1977.
74. Curtis, J. J., Barnhorst, D. A., Pluth, J. R., et al. Intra-aortic balloon assist. Initial Mayo Clinic experience and current concepts. *Mayo Clin. Proc.* 52:723, 1977.
75. Lefemine, A. A., Kosowsky, B., Madoff, I., et al. Results and complications of intra-aortic balloon pumping in surgical and medical patients. *Am. J. Cardiol.* 40:416, 1977.
76. Pace, P. D., Tilney, N. L., Lesch, M., and Couch, N. P. Peripheral arterial complications of intra-aortic balloon counterpulsation. *Surgery* 82:685, 1977.
77. McCabe, J. C., Abel, R. M., Subramanian, V. A., and Gay, W. A. Complications of intra-aortic balloon insertion and counterpulsation. *Circulation* 57:769, 1978.
78. McEnany, M. T., Kay, H. R., Buckley, M. J., et al. Clinical experience with intra-aortic balloon pump support in 728 patients. *Circulation* 58:I-124, 1978.
79. Isner, J. M., Cohen, S. R., Virmani, R., et al. Complications of the intra-aortic balloon counterpulsation device: Clinical and morphologic observations in 45 necropsy patients. *Am. J. Cardiol.* 45:260, 1980.
80. Subramanian, V. A., Goldstein, J. E., Sos, T. A., et al. Preliminary clinical experience with percutaneous intra-aortic balloon pumping. *Circulation* 62(Suppl I):I-123, 1980.
81. Singh, J. B., Connelly, P., Kocot, S., et al. Intra-

aortic balloon counterpulsation in a community hospital. *Chest* 79:58, 1981.

82. Goldman, B. S., Hill, T. J., Rosenthal, G. A., et al. Complications associated with use of the intra-aortic balloon pump. *Can. J. Surg.* 25:153, 1982.
83. Hauser, A. M., Gordon, S., Gangadharan, V., et al. Percutaneous intra-aortic balloon counterpulsation. Clinical effectiveness and hazards. *Chest* 82:422, 1982.
84. Alcan, K. E., Stertzer, S. H., Wallsh, E., et al. Comparison of wire-guided percutaneous insertion and conventional surgical insertion of intra-aortic balloon pumps in 151 patients. *Am. J. Med.* 75: 24, 1983.
85. Pennington, D. G., Swartz, M., Codd, J. E., et al. Intra-aortic balloon pumping in cardiac surgical patients: A nine-year experience. *Ann. Thorac. Surg.* 36:125, 1983.
86. Shahian, D. M., Neptune, W. B., Ellis, F. H., and Maggs, P. R. Intra-aortic balloon pump morbidity: A comparative analysis of risk factors between percutaneous and surgical techniques. *Ann. Thorac. Surg.* 36:644, 1983.
87. Weintraub, R. M., and Thurer, R. L. The intra-aortic balloon pump—a ten-year experience. *Heart Transplant.* 3:8, 1983.
88. Gottlieb, S. O., Brinker, J. A., Borkon, A. M., et al. Identification of patients at high risk for complications of intra-aortic balloon counterpulsation: A multivariate risk factor analysis. *Am. J. Cardiol.* 53:1135, 1984.
89. LoCicero, J., Hartz, R. S., Sanders, J. H., Jr., et al. Interhospital transport of patients with ongoing intra-aortic balloon pumping. *Am. J. Cardiol.* 56:59, 1985.
90. Vigneswaran, W. T., Reece, I. J., and Davidson, K. G. Intra-aortic balloon pumping: Seven years' experience. *Thorax* 40:858, 1985.
91. Corral, C. H., and Vaughn, C. C. Intra-aortic balloon counterpulsation: An eleven-year review and analysis of determinants of survival. *Texas Heart Inst. J.* 13:39, 1986.
92. Goldberger, M., Tabak, S. W., and Shah, P. K. Clinical experience with intra-aortic balloon counterpulsation in 112 consecutive patients. *Am. Heart J.* 111:497, 1986.
93. Sanfelippo, P. M., Baker, N. H., Ewy, H. G., et al. Experience with intra-aortic balloon counterpulsation. *Ann. Thorac. Surg.* 41:36, 1986.
94. Goldberg, M. J., Rubenfire, M., Kantrowitz, A., et al. Intra-aortic balloon pump insertion: A randomized study comparing percutaneous and surgical techniques. *J. Am. Coll. Cardiol.* 9:515, 1987.
95. Alpert, J., Parsonnet, V., Goldenkranz, R. J., et al. Limb ischemia during intra-aortic balloon pumping: Indication for femorofemoral crossover graft. *J. Thorac. Cardiovasc. Surg.* 79:729, 1980.
96. Kvilekval, K. H., Mason, R. A., Newton, G. B., et al. Complications of percutaneous intra-aortic balloon pump use in patients with peripheral vascular disease. *Arch. Surg.* 126:621, 1991.
97. Yuen, J. C. Percutaneous intra-aortic balloon pump: Emphasis on complications. *South. Med. J.* 84:956, 1991.
98. Mackenzie, D. J., Wagner, W. H., Kulber, D. A., et al. Vascular complications of the intra-aortic balloon pump. *Am. J. Surg.* 164:517, 1992.
99. Alvarez, J. M., Gates, R., Rowe, D., and Brady, P. W. Complications from intra-aortic balloon counterpulsation: A review of 303 cardiac surgical patients. *Eur. J. Cardiothorac. Surg.* 6:530, 1992.
100. Naunheim, K. S., Swartz, M. T., Pennington, D. G., et al. Intraaortic balloon pumping in patients requiring cardiac operations: Risk analysis and long-term follow-up. *J. Thorac. Cardiovasc. Surg.* 104:1654, 1992.
101. Eltchaninoff, H., Dimas, A. P., and Whitlow, P. L. Complications associated with percutaneous placement and use of intraaortic balloon counterpulsation. *Am. J. Cardiol.* 71:328, 1993.
102. Bregman, D., Nichols, A. B., Weiss, M. B., et al. Percutaneous intra-aortic balloon insertion. *Am. J. Cardiol.* 46:261, 1980.
103. Harvey, J. C., Goldstein, J. E., McCabe, J. C., et al. Complications of percutaneous intra-aortic balloon pumping. *Circulation* 64:II-114, 1981.
104. Vignola, P. A., Swaye, P. S., and Gosselin, A. J. Guidelines for effective and safe percutaneous intra-aortic balloon pump insertion and removal. *Am. J. Cardiol.* 48:660, 1981.
105. Martin, R. S., Moncure, A. C., Buckley, M. J., et al. Complications of percutaneous intra-aortic balloon insertion. *J. Thorac. Cardiovasc. Surg.* 85:186, 1983.
106. Downing, T. P., Miller, D. C., Stofer, R., and Shumway, N. E. Use of the intra-aortic balloon pump after valve replacement. Predictive indices, correlative parameters, and patient survival. *J. Thorac. Cardiovasc. Surg.* 92:210, 1986.
107. Honet, J. C., Wajszczuk, W. J., Rubenfire, M., et al. Neurological abnormalities in the leg(s) after use of intra-aortic balloon pump: Report of six cases. *Arch. Phys. Med. Rehabil.* 56:346, 1975.
108. Alpert, J., Bhaktan, E. K., Gielchinsky, I., et al. Vascular complications of intra-aortic balloon pumping. *Arch. Surg.* 111:1190, 1976.
109. O'Rourke, M. F., Sammel, N., and Chang, V. P. Arterial counterpulsation in severe refractory heart failure complicating acute myocardial infarction. *Br. Heart J.* 41:308, 1979.
110. Sutorius, D. J., Majeski, J. A., and Miller, S. F. Vascular complications as a result of intra-aortic balloon pumping. *Am. Surg.* 45:512, 1979.
111. Grayzel, J. Clinical evaluation of the percor percutaneous intra-aortic balloon: Cooperative study of 722 cases. *Circulation* 66:I-223, 1982.
112. Perler, B. A., McCabe, C. J., Abbott, W. M., and Buckley, M. J. Vascular complications of intra-aortic balloon counterpulsation. *Arch. Surg.* 118:957, 1983.
113. Todd, G. J., Bregman, D., Voorhees, A. B., and Reemtsma, K. Vascular complications associated

with percutaneous intra-aortic balloon pumping. *Arch. Surg.* 118:963, 1983.

114. Kantrowitz, A., Wasfie, T., Freed, P. S., et al. Intra-aortic balloon pumping 1967 through 1982: Analysis of complications in 733 patients. *Am. J. Cardiol.* 57:976, 1986.
115. Alderman, J. D., Gabliani, G. I., McCabe, C. H., et al. Incidence and management of limb ischemia with percutaneous wire-guided intra-aortic balloon catheters. *J. Am. Coll. Cardiol.* 9:524, 1987.
116. Funk, M., Gleason, J., and Foell, D. Lower limb ischemia related to use of the intraaortic balloon pump. *Heart Lung* 18:542, 1989.
117. Walls, J. T., Boley, T. M., Curtis, J. J., and Silver, D. Heparin induced thrombocytopenia in patients undergoing intra-aortic balloon pumping after open heart surgery. *ASAIO J.* 38:M574, 1992.
118. Bernstein, E. F., and Murphy, A. E., Jr. The importance of pulsation in preventing thrombosis from intra-aortic balloons. *J. Thorac. Cardiovasc. Surg.* 62:950, 1971.
119. Cutler, B. S., Okike, N., and Vander Salm, T. J. Surgical versus percutaneous removal of the intra-aortic balloon. *J. Thorac. Cardiovasc. Surg.* 86:907, 1983.
120. Rohrer, M. J., Sullivan, C. A., McLaughlin, D. J., and Cutler, B. S. A prospective randomized study comparing surgical and percutaneous removal of intraaortic balloon pump. *J. Thorac. Cardiovasc. Surg.* 103:569, 1992.
121. Archie, J. P., Jr., and Mann, J. T. Infected femoral arteriovenous fistula after percutaneous insertion of an intra-aortic balloon. *South. Med. J.* 82:778, 1989.
122. Busch, H. M., Jr., Cogbill, T. H., and Gundersen, A. E. Splenic infarction: Complication of intra-aortic balloon counterpulsation. *Am. Heart J.* 109: 383, 1985.
123. Tyras, D. H., and Willman, V. L. Paraplegia following intra-aortic balloon assistance. *Ann. Thorac. Surg.* 25:164, 1978.
124. Rose, D. M., Jacobowitz, I. J., Acinapura, A. J., and Cunningham, J. N. Paraplegia following percutaneous insertion of an intra-aortic balloon. *J. Thorac. Cardiovasc. Surg.* 87:788, 1984.
125. Harris, R. E., Reimer, K. A., Crain, B. J., et al. Spinal cord infarction following intra-aortic balloon support. *Ann. Thorac. Surg.* 42:206, 1986.
126. Riggle, K. P., and Oddi, M. A. Spinal cord necrosis and paraplegia as complications of the intra-aortic balloon. *Critical Care Med.* 17:475, 1989.
127. Orr, E., McKittrick, J., D'Agostino, R., et al. Paraplegia following intra-aortic balloon support. Report of a case. *J. Cardiovasc. Surg.* 30:1013, 1989.
128. Jarmolowski, C. R., and Poirier, R. L. Small bowel infarction complicating intra-aortic balloon counterpulsation via the ascending aorta. *J. Thorac. Cardiovasc. Surg.* 79:735, 1980.
129. O'Rourke, M. F., and Shepherd, K. M. Protection of the aortic arch and subclavian artery during intra-aortic balloon pumping. *J. Thorac. Cardiovasc. Surg.* 65:543, 1973.
130. Milgalter, E., Mosseri, M., Uretzky, G., and Romanoff, H. Intra-aortic balloon entrapment: A complication of balloon perforation. *Ann. Thorac. Surg.* 42:697, 1986.
131. Brodell, G. K., Tuzcu, E. M., Weiss, S. J., and Simpfendorfer, C. Intra-aortic balloon-pump rupture and entrapment. *Cleve. Clin. J. Med.* 56:740, 1989.
132. Millham, F. H., Hudson, H. M., Woodson, J., and Menzoian, J. O. Intraaortic balloon pump entrapment. *Ann. Vasc. Surg.* 5:381, 1991.
133. Nishizawa, J., Konishi, Y., Matsumoto, M., and Yuasa, S. Intraaortic balloon entrapment: A case report and a review of the literature. *Jpn. Circ. J.* 55:563, 1991.
134. Shafei, H., Webb, G., and Lennox, S. C. Entrapping of the clotted intra-aortic balloon in the descending aorta. *Eur. J. Cardiothorac. Surg.* 5:165, 1991.
135. Sutter, F. P., Joyce, D. H., Bailey, B. M., et al. Events associated with rupture of intra-aortic balloon counterpulsation devices. *ASAIO Trans.* 37: 38, 1991.
136. Hasan, R. I., Deiranyia, A. K., and Yonan, N. A. Effect of intra-aortic balloon counterpulsation on right-left shunt following right ventricular infarction. *Int. J. Cardiol.* 33:439, 1991.
137. Patacky, M. G., Garvin, B. J., and Schwirian, P. M. Intra-aortic balloon pumping and stress in the coronary care unit. *Heart Lung* 14:142, 1985.
138. Weintraub, R. M., Voukydis, P. C., Aroesty, J. M., et al. Treatment of preinfarction angina with intra-aortic balloon counterpulsation and surgery. *Am. J. Cardiol.* 34:809, 1974.
139. Sisto, D. A., Hoffman, D. M., Fernandes, S., and Frater, R. W. Is use of the intraaortic balloon pump in octogenarians justified? *Ann. Thorac. Surg.* 54: 507, 1992.
140. Bahn, C. H., Vitikainen, K. J., Anderson, C. L., and Whitney, R. B. Vascular evaluation for balloon pumping. *Ann. Thorac. Surg.* 27:474, 1979.
141. Funk, M., Ford, C. F., Foell, D. W., et al. Frequency of long-term lower limb ischemia associated with intraaortic balloon pump use. *Am. J. Cardiol.* 70:1195, 1992.
142. Wolfson, S., Karsh, D. L., Langou, R. A., et al. Modification of intra-aortic balloon catheter to permit introduction by cardiac catheterization techniques. *Am. J. Cardiol.* 41:733, 1978.
143. Leinbach, R. C., Goldstein, J., Gold, H. K., et al. Percutaneous wire-guided balloon pumping. *Am. J. Cardiol.* 49:1707, 1982.
144. Miller, J. S., Dodson, T. F., Salam, A. A., and Smith, R. B. Vascular complications following intra-aortic balloon pump insertion. *Am. Surg.* 58: 232, 1992.
145. Macoviak, J., Stephenson, L. W., Edmunds, L. H., Jr., et al. The intra-aortic balloon pump: An analysis of five years' experience. *Ann. Thorac. Surg.* 29: 451, 1980.
146. Lazar, J. M., Ziady, G. M., Dummer, S. J., et al. Outcome and complications of prolonged intraaor-

tic balloon counterpulsation in cardiac patients. *Am. J. Cardiol.* 69:955, 1992.
147. Gold, H. K., Leinbach, R. C., Buckley, M. J., et al. Refractory angina pectoris: Follow-up after intra-aortic balloon pumping and surgery. *Circulation* 54:III-41, 1976.
148. Scully, H. E., Gunstensen, J., Williams, W. G., et al. Surgical management of complicated acute coronary insufficiency. *Surgery* 80:437, 1976.
149. Langou, R. A., Geha, A. S., Hammond, G. L., and Cohen, L. S. Surgical approach for patients with unstable angina pectoris: Role of the response to initial medical therapy and intra-aortic balloon pumping in perioperative complications after aortocoronary bypass grafting. *Am. J. Cardiol.* 42:629, 1978.
150. Weintraub, R. M., Aroesty, J. M., Paulin, S., et al. Medically refractory unstable angina pectoris. I. Long-term follow-up of patients undergoing intra-aortic balloon counterpulsation and operation. *Am. J. Cardiol.* 43:877, 1979.
151. O'Rourke, M. F., Chang, V. P., Windsor, H. M., et al. Acute severe cardiac failure complicating myocardial infarction. Experience with 100 patients referred for consideration of mechanical left ventricular assistance. *Br. Heart J.* 37:169, 1975.
152. O'Rourke, M. F., Norris, R. M., Campbell, T. J., et al. Randomized controlled trial of intra-aortic balloon counterpulsation in early myocardial infarction with acute heart failure. *Am. J. Cardiol.* 47:815, 1981.
153. Mundth, E. D., Buckley, M. J., Gold, H. K., et al. Intra-aortic balloon pumping and emergency coronary arterial revascularization for acute myocardial infarction with impending extension. *Ann. Thorac. Surg.* 16:435, 1973.
154. Baron, D. W., and O'Rourke, M. F. Long-term results of arterial counterpulsation in acute severe cardiac failure complicating myocardial infarction. *Br. Heart J.* 38:285, 1976.
155. Bardet, J., Rigaud, M., Kahn, J. C., et al. Treatment of post-myocardial infarction angina by intra-aortic balloon pumping and emergency revascularization. *J. Thorac. Cardiovasc. Surg.* 74:299, 1977.
156. Hagemeijer, F., Laird, J. D., Haalebos, M. M. P., and Hugenholtz, P. G. Effectiveness of intra-aortic balloon pumping without cardiac surgery for patients with severe heart failure secondary to a recent myocardial infarction. *Am. J. Cardiol.* 40:951, 1977.
157. Johnson, S. A., Scanlon, P. J., Loeb, H. S., et al. Treatment of cardiogenic shock in myocardial infarction by intra-aortic balloon counterpulsation and surgery. *Am. J. Med.* 62:687, 1977.
158. Leinbach, R. C., Gold, H. K., Harper, R. W., et al. Early intra-aorta balloon pumping for anterior myocardial infarction without shock. *Circulation* 58:204, 1978.
159. Levine, F. H., Gold, H. K., Leinbach, R. C., et al. Management of acute myocardial ischemia with intra-aortic balloon pumping and coronary bypass surgery. *Circulation* 58:I-69, 1978.
160. Levine, F. H., Gold, H. K., Leinbach, R. C., et al. Safe early revascularization for continuing ischemia after acute myocardial infarction. *Circulation* 60:I-5, 1979.
161. DeWood, M. A., Notske, R. N., Hensley, G. R., et al. Intra-aortic balloon counterpulsation with and without reperfusion for myocardial infarction shock. *Circulation* 61:1105, 1980.
162. Lorente, P., Gourgon, R., Beaufils, P., et al. Multivariate statistical evaluation of intra-aortic counterpulsation in pump failure complicating acute myocardial infarction. *Am. J. Cardiol.* 46:124, 1980.
163. Pierri, M. K., Zema, M., Kligfield, P., et al. Exercise tolerance in late survivors of balloon pumping and surgery for cardiogenic shock. *Circulation* 62:I-138, 1980.
164. Flaherty, J. T., Becker, L. C., Weiss, J. L., et al. Results of a randomized prospective trial of intra-aortic balloon counterpulsation and intravenous nitroglycerin in patients with acute myocardial infarction. *J. Am. Coll. Cardiol.* 6:434, 1985.
165. Laks, H., Rosenkranz, E., and Buckberg, G. D. Surgical treatment of cardiogenic shock after myocardial infarction. *Circulation* 74:III-11, 1986.
166. Buckley, M. J., Craver, J. M., Gold, H. K., et al. Intra-aortic balloon pump assist for cardiogenic shock after cardiopulmonary bypass. *Circulation* 47:III-90, 1973.
167. Bregman, D., Parodi, E. N., Edie, R. N., et al. Intraoperative unidirectional intra-aortic balloon pumping in the management of left ventricular power failure. *J. Thorac. Cardiovasc. Surg.* 70:1010, 1975.
168. Bolooki, H., Williams, W., Thurer, R. J., et al. Clinical and hemodynamic criteria for use of the intra-aortic balloon pump in patients requiring cardiac surgery. *J. Thorac. Cardiovasc. Surg.* 72:756, 1976.
169. Scanlon, P. J., O'Connell, J., Johnson, S. A., et al. Balloon counterpulsation following surgery for ischemic heart disease. *Circulation* 54:III-90, 1976.
170. Stewart, S., Biddle, T., and DeWeese, J. Support of the myocardium with intra-aortic balloon counterpulsation following cardiopulmonary bypass. *J. Thorac. Cardiovasc. Surg.* 72:109, 1976.
171. McGee, M. G., Zillgitt, S. L., Trono, R., et al. Retrospective analyses of the need for mechanical circulatory support (intra-aortic balloon pump/abdominal left ventricular assist device or partial artificial heart) after cardiopulmonary bypass. A 44 month study of 14,168 patients. *Am. J. Cardiol.* 46:135, 1980.
172. Sturm, J. T., McGee, M. G., Fuhrman, T. M., et al. Treatment of postoperative low output syndrome with intra-aortic balloon pumping: Experience with 419 patients. *Am. J. Cardiol.* 45:1033, 1980.
173. Downing, T. P., Miller, D. C., Stinson, E. B., et al. Therapeutic efficacy of intra-aortic balloon pump counterpulsation. Analysis with concurrent "control" subjects. *Circulation* 64:II-108, 1981.

174. Foster, E. D., Subramanian, V. A., Vito, L., et al. Response to intra-aortic balloon pumping. *Am. J. Surg.* 129:464, 1975.
175. Willerson, J. T., Curry, G. C., Watson, J. T., et al. Intra-aortic balloon counterpulsation in patients in cardiogenic shock, medically refractory left ventricular failure and/or recurrent ventricular tachycardia. *Am. J. Med.* 58:183, 1975.
176. Johnson, M. D., Holub, D. A., Winston, D. S., et al. Retrospective analysis of 286 patients requiring circulatory support with the intra-aortic balloon pump. *Cardiovasc. Dis.* 4:428, 1977.
177. Frazier, O. H., Painvin, G. A., Urrutia, C. O., et al. Medical circulatory support: Clinical experience at the Texas Heart Institute. *Heart Transplant.* 2:299, 1983.
178. Folland, E. D., Kemper, A. J., Khuri, S. F., et al. Intra-aortic balloon counterpulsation as a temporary support measure in decompensated critical aortic stenosis. *J. Am. Coll. Cardiol.* 5:711, 1985.
179. Kahn, J. K., Rutherford, B. D., McConahay, D. R., et al. Supported "high risk" coronary angioplasty using intraaortic balloon pump counterpulsation. *J. Am. Coll. Cardiol.* 15:1151, 1990.
180. Morrison, D. A. Percutaneous transluminal coronary angioplasty for rest angina pectoris requiring intravenous nitroglycerin and intraaortic balloon counterpulsation. *Am. J. Cardiol.* 66:168, 1990.
181. Kreidieh, I., Davies, D. W., Lim, R., et al. High-risk coronary angioplasty with elective intra-aortic balloon pump support. *Int. J. Cardiol.* 35:147, 1992.
182. Alcan, K. E., Stertzer, S. H., Wallsh, E., et al. The role of intra-aortic balloon counterpulsation in patients undergoing percutaneous transluminal coronary angioplasty. *Am. Heart J.* 105:527, 1983.
183. Ishihara, M., Sato, H., Tateishi, H., et al. Intraaortic balloon pumping as the postangioplasty strategy in acute myocardial infarction. *Am. Heart J.* 122: 385, 1991.
184. Suneja, R., and Hodgson, J. M. Use of intraaortic balloon counterpulsation for treatment of recurrent acute closure after coronary angioplasty. *Am. Heart J.* 125:530, 1993.
185. Grotz, R. L., and Yeston, N. S. Intra-aortic balloon counterpulsation in high-risk cardiac patients undergoing noncardiac surgery. *Surgery* 106:1, 1989.
186. Georgen, R. F., Dietrick, J. A., Pifarre, R., et al. Placement of intra-aortic balloon pump allows definitive biliary surgery in patients with severe cardiac disease. *Surgery* 106:808, 1989.
187. Siu, S. C., Kowalchuk, G. J., Welty, F. K., et al. Intra-aortic balloon counterpulsation support in the high-risk cardiac patient undergoing urgent noncardiac surgery. *Chest* 99:1342, 1991.
188. Georgeson, S., Coombs, A. T., and Eckman, M. H. Prophylactic use of the intra-aortic balloon pump in high-risk cardiac patients undergoing noncardiac surgery: A decision analytic view. *Am. J. Med.* 92:665, 1992.
189. Bristow, J. D., Burchell, H. B., Campbell, R. W., et al. Report of the ad hoc committee on the indications for coronary arteriography. *Circulation* 55: 969A, 1977.
190. Olinger, G. N., Bonchek, L. I., Keelan, M. H., Jr., et al. Unstable angina: The case for operation. *Am. J. Cardiol.* 42:634, 1978.
191. Brundage, B. H., Ullyot, D. J., Winokur, S., et al. The role of aortic balloon pumping in postinfarction angina. A different perspective. *Circulation* 62:I-119, 1980.
192. Takaro, T., Hultgren, H. N., Lipton, M. J., et al., participants in the VA study group. The VA cooperative randomized study of surgery for coronary arterial occlusive disease. II. Subgroup with significant left main lesions. *Circulation* 54:III-107, 1976.
193. Davis, K., Kennedy, J. W., Kemp, H. G., Jr., et al. Complications of coronary arteriography from the collaborative study of coronary artery surgery (CASS). *Circulation* 59:1105, 1979.
194. Kennedy, J. W., Kaiser, G. C., Fisher, L. D., et al. Multivariate discriminant analysis of the clinical and angiographic predictors of operative mortality from the Collaborative Study in Coronary Artery Surgery (CASS). *J. Thorac. Cardiovasc. Surg.* 80: 876, 1980.
195. Cooper, G. N., Jr., Singh, A. K., Christian, F. C., et al. Preoperative intra-aortic balloon support in surgery for left main coronary stenosis. *Ann. Surg.* 185:242, 1977.
196. Waksman, R., Weiss, A. T., Gotsman, M. S., and Hasin, Y. Intra-aortic balloon counterpulsation improves survival in cardiogenic shock complicating acute myocardial infarction. *Eur. Heart J.* 14:71, 1993.
197. Goodwin, M., Hartmann, J., McKeever, L., et al. Safety of intraaortic balloon counterpulsation in patients with acute myocardial infarction receiving streptokinase intravenously. *Am. J. Cardiol.* 64:937, 1989.
198. Cooper, G., Timms, J., Nashef, S. A., and Smith, G. H. Streptokinase through the pressure lumen of the intraaortic balloon. *J. Thorac. Cardiovasc. Surg.* 101:748, 1991.
199. Ohman, E. M., Califf, R. M., George, B. S., et al. The use of intraaortic balloon pumping as an adjunct to reperfusion therapy in acute myocardial infarction. *Am. Heart J.* 121:895, 1991.
200. McBride, L. R., Miller, L. W., Naunheim, K. S., and Pennington, D. G. Axillary artery insertion of an intraaortic balloon pump. *Ann. Thorac. Surg.* 48:874, 1989.
201. Satoh, H., Kobayashi, T., Hiraishi, T., et al. New side-holed sheath for intraaortic balloon pumping to maintain limb perfusion. *Ann. Thorac. Surg.* 54: 794, 1992.
202. Nash, I. S., Lorell, B. H., Fishman, R. F., et al. A new technique for sheathless percutaneous intraaortic balloon catheter insertion. *Cathet. Cardiovasc. Diagn.* 23:57, 1991.

203. Phillips, S. J., Tannenbaum, M., Zeff, R. H., et al. Sheathless insertion of the percutaneous intraaortic balloon pump: An alternate method. *Ann. Thorac. Surg.* 53:162, 1992.
204. LaMuraglia, G. M., Valahakes, G. J., Moncure, A. C., et al. The safety of intraaortic balloon pump catheter insertion through suprainguinal prosthetic vascular bypass grafts. *J. Vasc. Surg.* 13:830, 1991.
205. Lewis, B. E., Sumida, C., Hwang, M. H., and Loeb, H. S. New approach to management of intraaortic balloon pumps in patients with peripheral vascular disease: Case reports of four patients requiring urgent IABP insertion. *Cathet. Cardiovasc. Diagn.* 26:295, 1992.
206. Phillips, S. J., Kreamer, R., Kongatahworn, C., et al. Permanent left ventricular assistance for outpatients. *Texas Heart Inst. J.* 16:275, 1989.
207. Kantrowitz, A., Freed, P. S., Cardona, R. R., et al. Initial clinical trial of a closed loop, fully automatic intra-aortic balloon pump. *ASAIO J.* 38:M617, 1992.
208. Macrae, D. J., Glenville, B., McCarthy, T., et al. Use of an intraaortic balloon pump as a pneumatic ventricular assist device controller. *Ann. Thorac. Surg.* 47:752, 1989.
209. Phillips, S. J., Zeff, R. H., Kongtahworn, C., et al. Benefits of combined balloon pumping and percutaneous cardiopulmonary bypass. *Ann. Thorac. Surg.* 54:908, 1992.
210. Moulopoulos, S. D., Stamatelopoulos, S. F., Zacopoulos, N. A., et al. Intraventricular plus intra-aortic balloon pumping during intractable cardiac arrest. *Circulation* 80:III-167, 1989.
211. Shimamoto, H., Kawazoe, K., Kito, Y., et al. Effects of intraaortic balloon pumping on mitral flow dynamics in patients with coronary artery bypass operations. *Am. Heart J.* 123:1229, 1992.
212. Kyo, S., Matsumura, M., Takamoto, S., and Omoto, R. Transesophageal color Doppler echocardiography during mechanical assist circulation. *ASAIO Trans.* 35:722, 1989.
213. Katz, E. S., Tunic, P. A., and Kronzon, I. Observations of coronary flow augmentation and balloon function during intraaortic balloon counterpulsation using transesophageal echocardiography. *Am. J. Cardiol.* 69:1635, 1992.
214. Jacobs, L. E., Fraifeld, M., Kotler, M. N., and Ioli, A. W. Aortic dissection following intraaortic balloon insertion: Recognition by transesophageal echocardiography. *Am. Heart J.* 124:536, 1992.
215. Nakatani, S., Beppu, S., Tanaka, N., et al. Application of abdominal and transesophageal echocardiography as a guide for insertion of intraaortic balloon pump in aortic dissection. *Am. J. Cardiol.* 64:1082, 1989.
216. Duncan, J. M., Frazier, O. H., Radovancevic, B., and Velebit, V. Implantation techniques for the Hemopump. *Ann. Thorac. Surg.* 48:733, 1989.
217. Scholz, K. H., Hering, P., Schröder, T., et al. Protective effects of the Hemopump left ventricular assist device in experimental cardiogenic shock. *Eur. J. Cardiothorac. Surg.* 6:209, 1992.
218. Schröder, T., Hering, J. P., Uhlig, P., et al. Efficiency of the left ventricle assist device Hemopump in cardiac fibrillation. *Br. J. Anaesth.* 68:536, 1992.
219. Merhige, M. E., Smalling, R. W., Cassidy, D., et al. Effect of the Hemopump left ventricular assist device on regional myocardial perfusion and function: Reduction of ischemia during coronary occlusion. *Circulation* 80:III-158, 1989.
220. Shiiya, N., Zelinsky, R., Deleuze, P. H., and Loisance, D. Y. Effects of Hemopump support on left ventricular unloading and coronary blood flow. *ASAIO Trans.* 37:M361, 1991.
221. Hering, J. P., Schröder, T., Uhlig, P., et al. Myocardial support and protection during regional myocardial ischemia using the Hemopump assist device. *Thorac. Cardiovasc. Surg.* 39:257, 1991.
222. Smalling, R. W., Cassidy, D. B., Barrett, R., et al. Improved regional myocardial blood flow, left ventricular unloading, and infarct salvage using an axial-flow, transvalvular left ventricular assist device: A comparison with intra-aortic counterpulsation and reperfusion alone in a canine infarct model. *Circulation* 85:1152, 1992.
223. Wouters, P. F., Sukehiro, S., Möllhoff, T., et al. Left ventricular assistance using a catheter-mounted coaxial flow pump (Hemopump) in a canine model of regional myocardial ischaemia. *Eur. Heart J.* 14:567, 1993.
224. Shiiya, N., Zelinsky, R., Deleuze, P. H., and Loisance, D. Y. Changes in hemodynamics and coronary blood flow during left ventricular assistance with the Hemopump. *Ann. Thorac. Surg.* 53:1074, 1992.
225. Phillips, S. J., Barker, L., Balentine, B., et al. Hemopump support for the failing heart. *ASAIO Trans.* 36:M629, 1990.
226. Deeb, G. M., Bolling, S. F., Nicklas, J., et al. Clinical experience with the Nimbus pump. *ASAIO Trans.* 36:M632, 1990.
227. Wampler, R. K., Frazier, O. H., Lansing, A. M., et al. Treatment of cardiogenic shock with the Hemopump left ventricular assist device. *Ann. Thorac. Surg.* 52:506, 1991.
228. Dubois-Rande, J. L., Deleuze, P., Zelinsky, R., et al. Coronary hemodynamics during Hemopump left-intraventricular assistance. *Int. J. Artif. Organs* 15: 234, 1992.
229. Burnett, C. M., Vega, J. D., Radovancevic, B., et al. Improved survival after Hemopump insertion in patients experiencing postcardiotomy cardiogenic shock during cardiopulmonary bypass. *ASAIO Trans.* 36:M-626, 1990.
230. Duncan, J. M., Baldwin, R. T., and Frazier, O. H. Preoperative and postoperative Hemopump support for patients undergoing orthotopic heart transplantation. *Ann. Thorac. Surg.* 53:349, 1992.
231. Scholz, K. H., Tebbe, U., Chemnitius, M., et al. Transfemoral placement of the left ventricular assist

device ''Hemopump'' during mechanical resuscitation. *Thorac. Cardiovasc. Surg.* 38:69, 1990.

232. Duncan, J. M., Burnett, C. M., Vega, J. D., et al. Rapid placement of the Hemopump and hemofiltration cannula. *Ann. Thorac. Surg.* 50:667, 1990.
233. Loisance, D., Dubois-Rande, J. L., Deleuze, P. H., et al. Prophylactic intraventricular pumping in high-risk coronary angioplasty. *Lancet* 335:438, 1990.
234. Lincoff, M. A., Poma, J. J., Bates, E. R., et al. Successful coronary angioplasty in two patients with cardiogenic shock using the Nimbus Hemopump support device. *Am. Heart J.* 120:970, 1990.
235. Gacioch, G. M., Ellis, S. G., Lee, L., et al. Cardiogenic shock complicating acute myocardial infarction: The use of coronary angioplasty and the integration of the new support devices into patient management. *J. Am. Coll. Cardiol.* 19:647, 1992.
236. Baldwin, R. T., Radovancevic, B., Duncan, J. M., et al. Quality of life in long-term survivors of the Hemopump left ventricular assist device. *ASAIO Trans.* 37:M422, 1991.
237. Baldwin, R. T., Radovancevic, B., Duncan, J. M., et al. Management of patients supported on the Hemopump cardiac assist system. *Texas Heart Inst. J.* 19:81, 1992.
238. Baldwin, R. T., Duncan, J. M., Frazier, O. H., and Wilansky, S. Patent foramen ovale: A cause of hypoxemia in patients on left ventricular support. *Ann. Thorac. Surg.* 52:865, 1991.
239. Mannion, J. D., Buckman, P. D., Mango, M. G., and Dimeo, F. Collateral blood flow from skeletal muscle to normal myocardium. *J. Surg. Res.* 53:578, 1992.
240. Kantrowitz, A., and McKinnon, W. M. P. The experimental use of the diaphragm as an auxiliary myocardium. *Surg. Forum* 9:266, 1958.
241. Corin, W. J., George, D. T., Sink, J. D., and Santamore, W. P. Dynamic cardiomyoplasty acutely impairs left ventricular diastolic function. *J. Thorac. Cardiovasc. Surg.* 104:1662, 1992.
242. Soberman, M. S., Wornom, I. L., Justicz, A. G., et al. Latissimus dorsi dynamic cardiomyoplasty of the right ventricle: Potential for use as a partial myocardial substitute. *J. Thorac. Cardiovasc. Surg.* 99:817, 1990.
243. Carpentier, A., and Chachques, J. C. Myocardial substitution with a stimulated skeletal muscle: First successful clinical case. *Lancet* 6:1267, 1985.
244. Rose, D. M., Connolly, M., Cunningham, J. N., Jr., and Spencer, F. C. Technique and results with a roller pump left and right heart assist device. *Ann. Thorac. Surg.* 47:124, 1989.
245. Pierce, W. S., Parr, G. V. S., Myers, J. L., et al. Ventricular-assist pumping in patients with cardiogenic shock after cardiac operations. *N. Engl. J. Med.* 305:1606, 1981.
246. Pennington, D. G., Codd, J. E., Merjavy, J. P., et al. The expanded use of ventricular bypass systems for severe cardiac failure and as a bridge to cardiac transplantation. *Heart Transplant.* 3:38, 1983.
247. Gaines, W. E., Rosenberg, G., Pennock, J. L., and Pierce, W. S. Development of a long-term electric motor left ventricular assist system. *Heart Transplant.* 3:323, 1984.
248. Cooley, D. A. Staged cardiac transplantation: Report of three cases. *Heart Transplant.* 1:145, 1982.
249. Bernhard, W. F., Gernes, D. G., Clay, W. C., et al. Investigations with an implantable, electrically actuated ventricular assist device. *J. Thorac. Cardiovasc. Surg.* 88:11, 1984.
250. Portner, P. M., Oyer, P. E., Jassawalla, J. S., et al. An alternative in end-stage heart disease: Long-term ventricular assistance. *Heart Transplant.* 3:47, 1983.
251. Nose, Y., Jacobs, G., Kiraly, R. J., et al. Experimental results for chronic left ventricular assist and total artificial heart development. *Artif. Organs* 7:55, 1983.
252. Phillips, S. J., Ballentine, B., Slonine, D., et al. Percutaneous initiation of cardiopulmonary bypass. *Ann. Thorac. Surg.* 36:223, 1983.
253. Mickleborough, L. L., Rebeyka, I., Wilson, G. J., et al. Comparison of left ventricular assist and intraaortic balloon counterpulsation during early reperfusion after ischemic arrest of the heart. *J. Thorac. Cardiovasc. Surg.* 93:597, 1987.
254. Bolman, R. M., Cox, J. L., Marshall, W., et al. Circulatory support with a centrifugal pump as a bridge to cardiac transplantation. *Ann. Thorac. Surg.* 47:108, 1989.
255. Noon, G. P., Sekela, M. E., Glueck, J., et al. Comparison of Sarns and Biomedicus pumps. *ASAIO Trans.* 36:M616, 1990.
256. Joyce, L. D., Kiser, J. C., Eales, F., et al. Experience with the Sarns centrifugal pump as a ventricular assist device. *ASAIO Trans.* 36:M619, 1990.
257. Minato, N., Sakuma, I., Sasaki, T., et al. A seal-less centrifugal pump (Baylor Gyro Pump) for application to long-term circulatory support. *Artif. Organs* 17:36, 1993.
258. Pennington, D. G., Merjavy, J. P., Codd, J. E., et al. Extracorporeal membrane oxygenation for patients with cardiogenic shock. *Circulation* 70:I-130, 1984.
259. Shawl, F. A., Domanski, M. J., Hernandez, T. J., and Punja, S. Emergency percutaneous cardiopulmonary bypass support in cardiogenic shock from acute myocardial infarction. *Am. J. Cardiol.* 64:967, 1989.
260. Nahhas, A. T., Mooney, J. F., Gobel, F. L., et al. The use of emergency percutaneous cardiopulmonary support and coronary angioplasty as a bridge to surgery in a patient with acute ischemic papillary muscle rupture and circulatory collapse. *J. Invasive Cardiol.* 5:138, 1993.
261. O'Neill, P., Menendez, T., Hust, R., et al. Prolonged ventricular fibrillation-salvage using a new percutaneous cardiopulmonary support system. *Am. J. Cardiol.* 64:545, 1989.
262. Sugimoto, J. T., Baird, E., and Bruner, C. Percuta-

neous cardiopulmonary support in cardiac arrest. *ASAIO Trans.* 37:M282, 1991.

263. Mooney, M. R., Arom, K. N., Joyce, L. D., et al. Emergency cardiopulmonary bypass support in patients with cardiac arrest. *J. Thorac. Cardiovasc. Surg.* 101:450, 1991.
264. Vogel, R. A., Shawl, F., Tommaso, C., et al. Initial report of the National Registry of Elective Cardiopulmonary Bypass Supported Coronary Angioplasty. *J. Am. Coll. Cardiol.* 15:23, 1990.
265. Pennock, J. L., Pierce, W. S., and Waldhausen, J. A. Quantitative evaluation of left ventricular bypass in reducing myocardial ischemia. *Surgery* 79: 523,1976.
266. Grossi, E. A., Krieger, K. H., Cunningham, J. N., Jr., et al. Time course of effective interventional left heart assist for limitation of evolving myocardial infarction. *J. Thorac. Cardiovasc. Surg.* 91:624, 1986.
267. Zobel, G., Dacar, D., Kuttnig, M., et al. Mechanical support of the left ventricle in ischemia induced left ventricular failure: An experimental study. *Int. J. Artif. Organs* 15:114, 1992.
268. Nawa, S., Yamada, M., and Teramoto, S. Evaluation of conventional circulatory assist devices: Intraaortic balloon pumping, venoarterial bypass, and extracorporeal membrane oxygenation. *Chest* 95:261, 1989.

16. Pump Failure, Shock, and Cardiac Rupture in Acute Myocardial Infarction

Prediman K. Shah and Gary S. Francis

Nearly one million patients are hospitalized in the United States each year with a diagnosis of acute myocardial infarction, and the early course (the first 2 to 4 weeks) of this disease is associated with a 5 to 15 percent mortality. Pump failure secondary to extensive myocardial loss is the leading cause of in-hospital mortality as well as a major determinant of postdischarge morbidity and mortality [1, 2]. Recent data from the Worcester Heart Attack Registry concerning more than 4700 patients demonstrate that the overall incidence of cardiogenic shock has not declined over the past 14 years, averaging around 7.5 percent [73]. Similarly the overall mortality has not changed appreciably during this period, ranging from 65 to 80 percent despite the use of pharmacologic agents and intra-aortic balloon counterpulsation [73]. In this chapter we discuss the pathogenesis, clinical presentation, and contemporary management of this important and potentially lethal complication of acute myocardial infarction.

Pathogenesis of Acute Myocardial Infarction

Coronary Artery Occlusion

That coronary thrombosis is the culprit of evolving acute myocardial infarction in nearly all patients has now been amply confirmed by in vivo angiographic studies, careful autopsy studies, and recovery of a coronary thrombus from the artery of infarction in patients undergoing emergency coronary artery bypass surgery [3–5]. Thus the previous controversy regarding the primary versus the secondary nature of coronary thrombosis has now been laid to rest, and the primary role of coronary thrombosis in the pathogenesis of acute myocardial infarction is firmly established [4, 5].

Fissuring of an atherosclerotic plaque with subsequent exposure of the subintimal lipid-rich matrix to circulating platelets appears to initiate the process of platelet-rich thrombus formation, with additional fibrin accretion resulting from locally generated thrombin through a tissue factor–mediated pathway [75]. Coronary thrombus is totally occlusive in about 80 percent of patients studied within the early hours of evolving transmural myocardial infarction, whereas in about 20 percent of patients coronary thrombus results in subtotal or intermittent occlusion.

Wave-Front Progression of Myocardial Necrosis

The dynamic and temporal dependence of myocardial necrosis following coronary artery occlusion has been demonstrated. After acute coronary occlusion in experimental animals, necrosis begins within 15 to 20 minutes near the subendocardium within the myocardial area at risk, and progresses toward the epicardium in a wave front of cell death such that it involves about 70 to 80 percent of the risk area by 6 hours [6]. When coronary occlusion is subtotal rather than total or when there are well-developed collaterals to the area at risk, the progression of myocardial necrosis may proceed more slowly and to a smaller transmural extent.

In humans, studies of myocardial perfusion, viability, and recovery of function following reperfusion suggest that the pattern and time sequence of myocardial necrosis may be similar to that in dogs and primates, with nearly complete necrosis of the

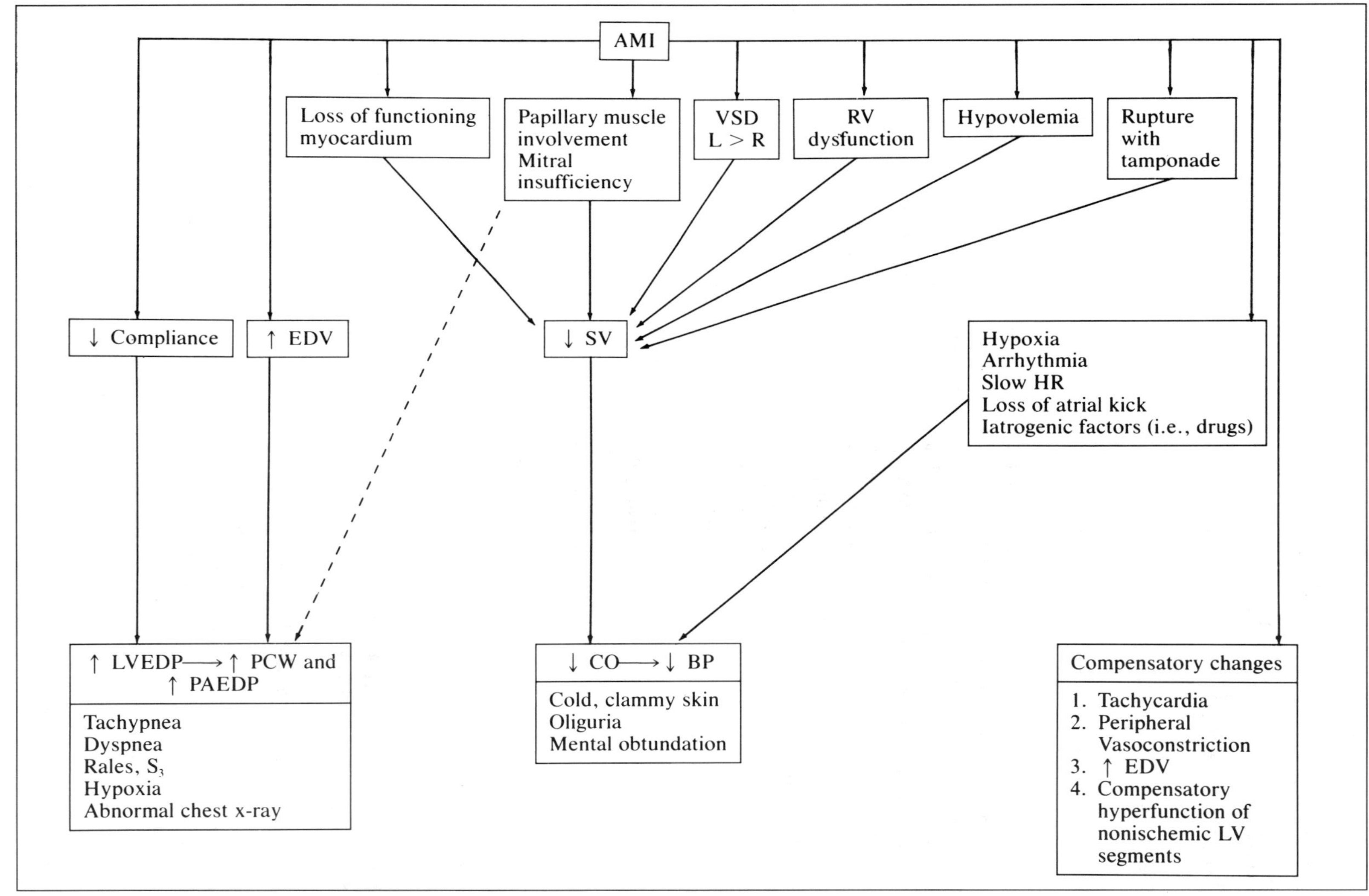
AMI
Loss of functioning myocardium
Papillary muscle involvement
Mitral insufficiency
VSD
L > R
RV dysfunction
Hypovolemia
Rupture with tamponade
↓ Compliance
↑ EDV
↓ SV
Hypoxia
Arrhythmia
Slow HR
Loss of atrial kick
Iatrogenic factors (i.e., drugs)
↑ LVEDP⟶↑ PCW and ↑ PAEDP
Tachypnea
Dyspnea
Rales, S_3
Hypoxia
Abnormal chest x-ray
↓ CO⟶↓ BP
Cold, clammy skin
Oliguria
Mental obtundation
Compensatory changes
1. Tachycardia
2. Peripheral Vasoconstriction
3. ↑ EDV
4. Compensatory hyperfunction of nonischemic LV segments

area at risk within 3 to 6 hours of persistent and total occlusion of the coronary artery, although in individual patients the time required for transmural spread of necrosis may vary as a function of the magnitude of residual flow (antegrade, collateral derived, or both) and myocardial oxygen demand. Recent clinical studies suggested that collateral-mediated perfusion can be accurately detected by echo-contrast studies (even in the absence of angiographically visible collaterals) in myocardial segments supplied by totally occluded arteries and that such hibernating myocardium may remain viable for days and weeks [76]. The recognition of time-dependent evolution of necrosis provides a brief ''window of opportunity'' during which interventions can be applied to abort the transmural speed of necrosis and to limit the eventual size of the infarction.

Pump Failure

The clinical syndrome of pump failure in acute myocardial infarction (Fig. 16-1) results from one or more of the following consequences of acute myocardial infarction:

1. Regional contractile dysfunction of the left or right ventricle (or both). Contractile dysfunction results from hypofunction of the ischemic and necrotic segments, persistent postischemic dysfunction (stunned myocardium), as well as the tethering effects of akinetic segments on nonischemic segments.
2. Regional and global diastolic dysfunction.
3. Infarct expansion and ventricular remodeling.
4. Mechanical complications such as mitral regurgitation, interventricular septal rupture, and cardiac free-wall rupture.

Additional factors contributing to the pump failure syndrome include sustained or recurrent supraventricular or ventricular arrhythmias, persistent severe bradyarrhythmias including complete heart block, use of potent negative inotropic drugs, relative or absolute hypovolemia, electrolyte disturbances, acid-base disequilibrium, and abnormalities of pulmonary gas exchange.

Contractile Dysfunction

Severe reduction or total cessation of coronary blood flow, the proximate cause of acute myocardial infarction, results in abnormalities of regional contractile function ranging from hypokinesis (reduction in the extent of shortening), to akinesis (loss of contraction), to dyskinesis (systolic expansion) [7] (Fig. 16-2). The extent of myocardium involved, as well as the type of regional contractile dysfunction, determines the ultimate change in global left ventricular volumes and ejection fraction (see Fig. 16-2). Without compensatory mechanisms, progressive abnormalities of regional contractile function result in an increased end-systolic volume with a consequent decrease in stroke volume and ejection fraction. Similarly, an increasing extent of myocardium involved in contractile dysfunction leads to a progressively larger end-systolic volume and a lower stroke volume and ejection fraction. Reduction in stroke volume, in turn, leads to a reduction in cardiac output. When contractile dysfunction involves 10 percent of the left ventricular perimeter, the left ventricular ejection fraction declines with a minimal decrease in stroke volume, whereas fatal cardiogenic shock is usually associated with involvement of 30 to 40 percent or more. Clinical evidence of heart failure is generally observed when contractile dysfunction involves 25 to 40 percent of the left ventricular perimeter.

Fig. 16-1
Pathogenesis of pump failure following acute myocardial infarction (AMI). VSD = ventricular septal defect; HR = heart rate; RV = right ventricular; SV = stroke volume; CO = cardiac output; BP = blood pressure; EDV = end-diastolic volume; PCW = pulmonary capillary wedge pressure; LVEDP = left ventricular end-diastolic pressure; PAEDP = pulmonary arterial end-diastolic pressure; LV = left ventricular. (From P. K. Shah. Complications of acute myocardial infarction. In W. Parmley and K. Chatterjee, eds., *Cardiology*. Philadelphia: Lippincott, 1987.)

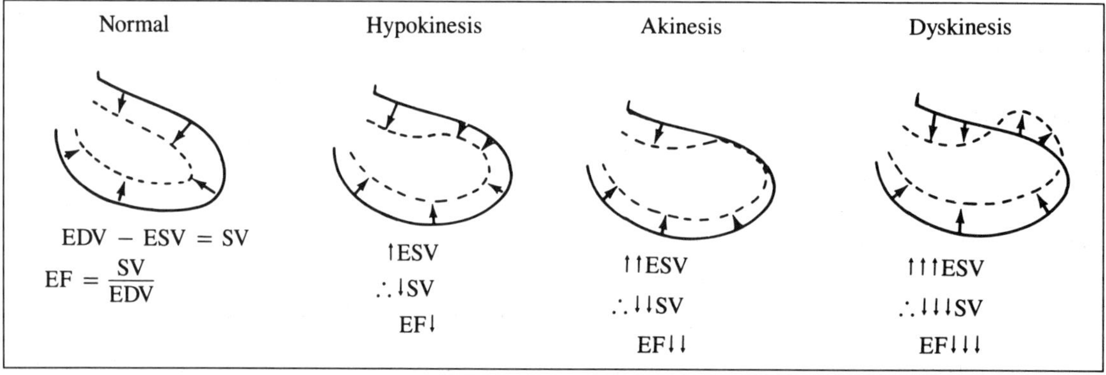

Fig. 16-2
Patterns of left ventricular regional contractile dysfunction and their influence on end-diastolic volume (EDV), end-systolic volume (ESV), stroke volume (SV), and ejection fraction (EF). Note the progressive declines in EF with increasing ESV consequent to increasing gradation of contractile dysfunction. (From P. K. Shah. Complications of acute myocardial infarction. In W. Parmley and K. Chatterjee, eds., *Cardiology*. Philadelphia: Lippincott, 1987.)

Compensatory Mechanisms

Several compensatory mechanisms are activated to minimize the hemodynamic consequences of contractile dysfunction in acute myocardial infarction.

1. Increased sympathoadrenal activity with increased circulating catecholamines helps to increase the heart rate, systemic vascular resistance, and inotropic state of the residual myocardium. Sympathoadrenal stimulation, however, may also increase the risk of arrhythmias, exacerbate myocardial ischemia by increasing myocardial oxygen consumption, and increase left ventricular afterload by producing systemic vasoconstriction.
2. Left ventricular dilatation allows the heart to utilize the Frank-Starling mechanism to minimize declines in stroke volume in the setting of a depressed ejection fraction. Left ventricular dilatation, however, may produce deleterious consequences by (a) increasing wall tension and myocardial oxygen demand, (b) leading to pulmonary venous congestion because of associated increases in left ventricular end-diastolic pressure, and (c) leading to mitral annulus dilatation, papillary muscle dysfunction and consequent mitral regurgitation.
3. Normally perfused remote myocardial segments may overwork to reduce the end-systolic volume, preserve the global ejection fraction, and minimize decreases in stroke volume. Such compensatory hyperfunctioning of remote myocardium may not be possible if remote myocardial segments become ischemic when their blood supply is jeopardized.

Diastolic Dysfunction

Diastolic function is frequently abnormal with acute myocardial infarction as reflected by changes in the ventricular diastolic pressure-volume relation or compliance. Because pulmonary capillary wedge pressure closely approximates the left ventricular mean diastolic pressure in the absence of mitral valve disease, an elevated left ventricular diastolic pressure also raises the pulmonary capillary wedge pressure. Left ventricular end-diastolic pressure may increase owing to an increased end-diastolic volume, reduce compliance, or both (Fig. 16-3). Infarct expansion appears to be an important contributor to left ventricular dilatation with acute myocardial infarction. Infarct expansion results from stretching, lengthening, and thinning of the myocardial segments with transmural necrosis, usually affecting the apical segment, which in return results in ventricular remodeling and dilatation [8, 9]. Disruption of the connective tissue framework and myofibrillar slippage may be responsible for infarct expansion.

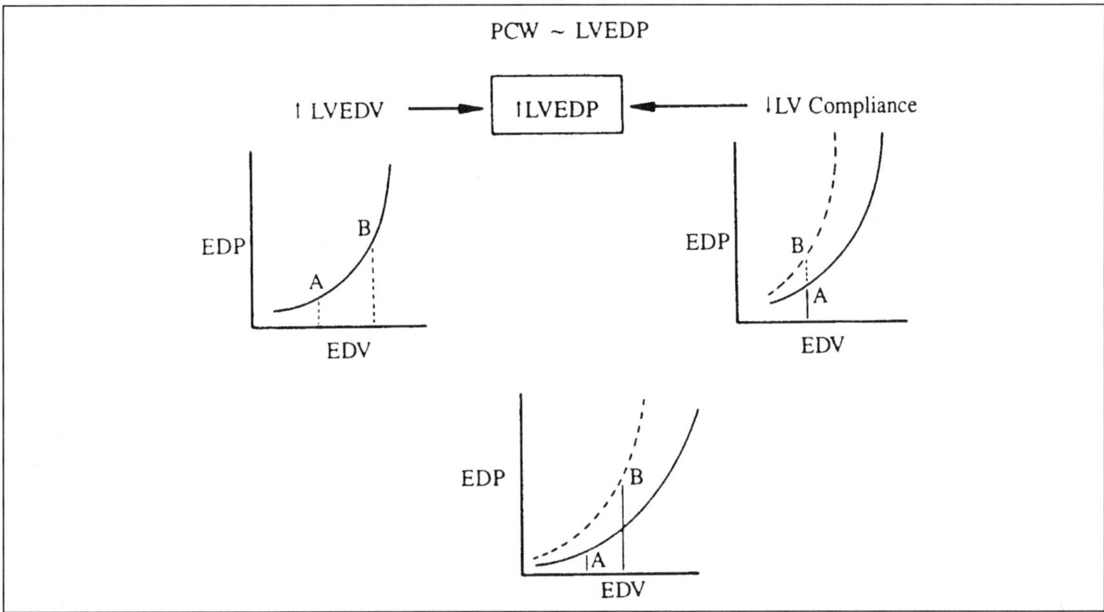

Fig. 16-3
Two mechanisms contributing to elevation of left ventricular (LV) end-diastolic pressure (EDP)—and consequently elevation of the pulmonary capillary wedge pressure (PCW)—are illustrated on the pressure-volume plots. *Left.* Elevation of EDP secondary to an increase in end-diastolic volume (EDV), as the patient moves from A to B. *Right.* Leftward and upward displacement of the pressure-volume curve with an increase in EDP without a change in EDV, reflecting reduced compliance, as the patient moves from A to B. *Bottom.* Composite of increased EDV and reduced compliance, as the patient moves from A to B. Note that mitral regurgitation can raise the PCW by directly increasing the left atrial pressure, without involving any of these mechanisms. (From P. K. Shah. Complications of acute myocardial infarction. In W. Parmley and K. Chatterjee, eds., *Cardiology.* Philadelphia: Lippincott, 1987.)

Alteration in left ventricular diastolic compliance occurs frequently in acute myocardial infarction and may be detectable even with infarction of a limited extent. Although in some instances overall compliance appears to be increased in the early phase of acute myocardial infarction, most studies suggested that the overall compliance is generally reduced, probably reflecting alterations in viscoelastic properties of the ischemic and necrotic tissue due to cellular and interstitial edema during the acute phase and healing with fibrosis during the subacute and chronic phases [10–12]. Right ventricular dilatation and dysfunction accompanying ischemia or infarction of the right ventricle may produce a leftward bulging of the interventricular septum into the left ventricle as well as an increase in intrapericardial pressures, contributing to abnormalities of diastolic function of the left ventricle [13].

Severity of Pump Failure and Prognosis

The importance of ventricular function as the chief determinant of short-term as well as long-term survival following acute myocardial infarction has been well established [1, 13–17]. Infarct size, in turn, is a major determinant of ventricular function, although alterations in compliance, contractile function of noninfarcted remote myocardium, and mechanical disruption of infarcted structures may modify this relation. Investigators have attempted to characterize the severity of ventricular dysfunction and pump failure using clinical, invasive, hemodynamic, and noninvasive techniques, not only to assist in prognostic assessment but also to provide rational guidelines for therapeutic interventions [15–18].

Clinical Subsets

In 1967 Killip and Kimbal [15] characterized patients with acute myocardial infarction into four classes based on physical findings on admission: class I—no signs of left ventricular failure; class II—S_3 gallop and/or pulmonary congestion limited to basal lung segments; class III—acute pulmonary edema; and class IV—shock syndrome (Table 16-1). Subsequently, Forrester and colleagues stratified patients with acute myocardial infarction into four subsets: subset I—no evidence of pulmonary congestion or systemic hypoperfusion; subset II—evidence of pulmonary congestion without evidence of systemic hypoperfusion; subset III—evidence of systemic hypoperfusion without evidence of pulmonary congestion; and subset IV—evidence of pulmonary congestion and systemic hypoperfusion [16, 17].

More recently, patients with acute myocardial infarction also have been characterized into prognostic subsets based on left and right ventricular ejection fractions determined by radionuclide ventriculography (Fig. 16-4) [18]. Such categorization is particularly relevant in patients who do not have clinical signs of severe pump failure on admission. The severity of ventricular dysfunction determined by more objective invasive or noninvasive means often shows considerable overlap between various clinical classes and subsets of patients. Such discrepancies arise because patients exhibit clinical "phase lags" as pulmonary congestion develops or resolves, when symptoms and signs secondary to coexistent chronic obstructive lung disease are mistakenly interpreted as pulmonary congestion, or when patients pass from one subset to another with or without therapy or due to confounding effects of changes in ventricular compliance or loading conditions that occur with mechanical complications such as mitral regurgitation and cardiac rupture.

Hemodynamic Assessment of Pump Dysfunction

Introduction of the balloon-flotation pulmonary artery thermodilution catheter by Swan, Ganz, and

Table 16-1
Clinical and hemodynamic subsets in acute myocardial infarction (AMI)

Subset	Clinical features	Approximate % of patients with AMI	Hospital mortality (%)
Killip class			
I	No signs of CHF	40–50	6
II	S_3 gallop, bibasilar rales	30–40	17
III	Acute pulmonary edema	10–15	38
IV	Cardiogenic shock	5–10	81
Cedars-Sinai clinical subsets			
I	No pulmonary congestion or tissue hypoperfusion	25	1
II	Pulmonary congestion only	25	11
III	Tissue hypoperfusion only	15	18
IV	Pulmonary congestion and tissue hypoperfusion	35	60
Cedars-Sinai hemodynamic subsets	Hemodynamic features		
I	PCW $\leq$18; CI $>$2.2	25	3
II	PCW $>$18; CI $>$2.2	25	9
III	PCW $\leq$18; CI $\leq$2.2	15	23
IV	PCW $>$18; CI $\leq$2.2	35	51

CHF = congestive heart failure; PCW = pulmonary capillary wedge pressure (mm Hg); CI = cardiac index (L/min/m^2).
Source: From P. K. Shah. Complications of acute myocardial infarction. In W. Parmley and K. Chatterjee, eds., *Cardiology.* Philadelphia: Lippincott, 1987.

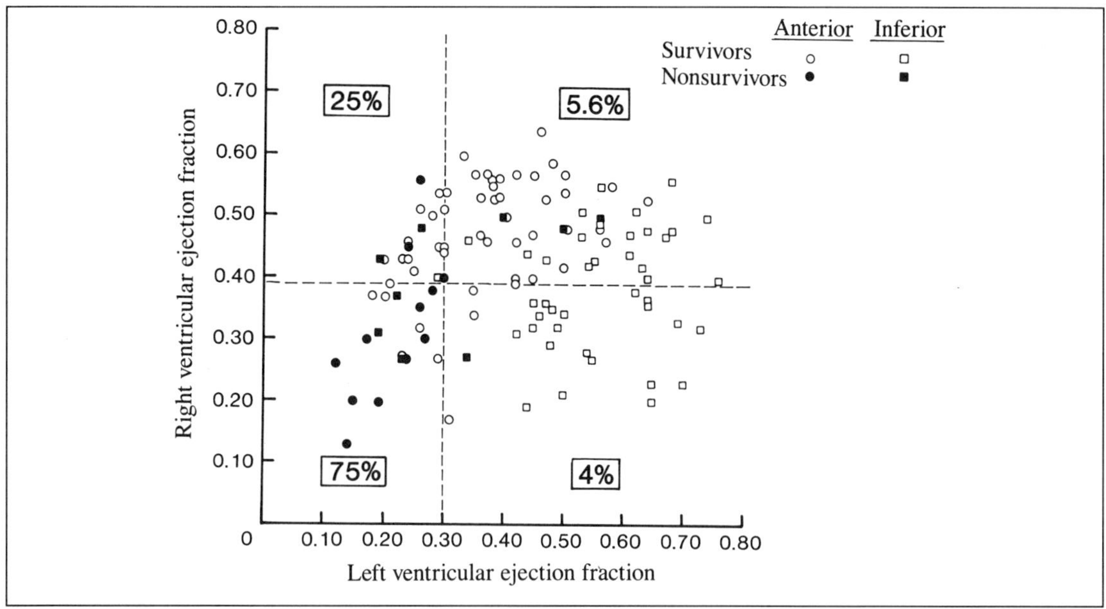

Fig. 16-4
Relation of mortality to left and right ventricular ejection fractions during acute myocardial infarction in 112 Killip class I patients. Note that mortality is high when the left ventricular ejection fraction is below 0.30 and right ventricular ejection fraction is lower than 0.38, whereas mortality is low in the presence of a left ventricular ejection fraction above 0.30 regardless of the right ventricular ejection fraction.

colleagues during the early 1970s made it feasible to objectively assess left ventricular function in acute myocardial infarction [19]. Based on invasive hemodynamic evaluation of pulmonary capillary wedge pressure and cardiac index in 200 patients with acute myocardial infarction, Forrester and associates described four subsets of patients (see Table 16-1) [16, 17]. This stratification was suggested for predicting mortality, and it also can be used as a guide for selecting appropriate therapy.

In acutely ill patients with myocardial infarction, clinical evidence of pulmonary congestion is often present when the pulmonary capillary wedge pressure is 18 to 20 mm Hg or higher, whereas evidence of systemic hypoperfusion is frequently present when the cardiac index is less than 2.0 to 2.2 L/min/m^2. However, in 20 to 30 percent of patients, discrepancies between clinical findings and hemodynamic variables may be found for reasons described earlier.

Role of Hemodynamic Monitoring

There is little evidence to support the practice of routine hemodynamic monitoring in patients with a clinically uncomplicated acute myocardial infarction. Such patients can be well assessed by careful and meticulous clinical observation, which takes into account the overall appearance of the patient, heart rate and rhythm, systemic blood pressure, careful repeated cardiac examination for gallops or murmurs, careful pulmonary auscultation for rales, assessment of pulmonary vasculature on chest radiography, and assessment of the adequacy of vital organ perfusion (i.e., urine output, mental status).

On the other hand, hemodynamic monitoring may be useful in selected subsets of patients with hemodynamic complications following an acute myocardial infarction, in order to (1) clarify the role of hypovolemia, left ventricular failure, valvular regurgitation, septal rupture, right ventricular infarction, and cardiac tamponade in producing a state of hypotension, low-output syndrome, or pulmonary congestion and edema; and (2) assist in the selection of appropriate therapeutic interventions and follow the response to the intervention (Table 16-2). Thus hemodynamic monitoring should be considered only in patients with acute myocardial infarction who demonstrate clinical evidence of se-

Table 16-2
Invasive hemodynamic monitoring of acute myocardial infarction

Uses
1. Clarifying role of hypovolemia, left ventricular failure, mitral regurgitation, interventricular septal rupture, right ventricular infarction, and cardiac tamponade in the genesis of pump failure.
2. Selection of appropriate therapy for pump failure, i.e., inotropes, vasodilators, volume
3. Rapid assessment of response to therapy
4. Prognostic assessment (see Table 16-1)

Indications
1. Persistent low-output state, hypotension, or shock
2. Recurrent or refractory pulmonary congestion or edema
3. Appearance of a a new systolic murmur
4. During the use of intravenous vasoactive drugs or intra-aortic balloon counterpulsation
5. Unexplained persistent sinus tachycardia

Source: From P. K. Shah. Complications of acute myocardial infarction. In W. Parmley and K. Chatterjee, eds., *Cardiology*. Philadelphia: Lippincott, 1987.

vere low-output state, persistent hypotension and shock unrelated to correctable bradycardia, persistent unexplained sinus tachycardia, or appearance of a new systolic murmur.

In recent years, noninvasive studies such as two-dimensional echocardiography, color flow and Doppler echocardiography, and radionuclide scintigraphy have proved to be extremely useful for fully characterizing abnormalities of regional and global left and right ventricular function and detection of complications of myocardial infarction (Table 16-3). Thus in contemporary practice, invasive monitoring for diagnosing complications of acute myocardial infarction has been largely supplanted by Doppler echocardiography and scintigraphic studies, with hemodynamic monitoring assuming a secondary role in selected patients.

Subsets of Pump Failure

It is useful to categorize patients with pump failure following acute myocardial infarction into subsets that are clinically meaningful and that provide guidelines for appropriate diagnostic and therapeutic strategies (Table 16-4).

Pulmonary Congestion Without a Low-Output State

Some degree of pulmonary congestion (pulmonary capillary wedge pressure of 18 to 25 mmHg) is common in patients with acute myocardial infarction. The increased pulmonary capillary wedge pressure results from an elevated left ventricular end-diastolic pressure due to decreased diastolic compliance, increased end-diastolic volume, or both, although it may also be due to mitral regurgitation. The patient may be asymptomatic or may complain of dyspnea and orthopnea. Findings on physical examination may include tachypnea, bibasilar pulmonary rales, and mild to moderate hypoxemia, and there may be radiologic evidence of mild to moderate pulmonary venous congestion.

Therapy in such patients is aimed at ensuring adequate arterial oxygenation and relieving pulmonary venous congestion. These goals can usually be accomplished by supplemental oxygen and judicious use of small doses of intravenous diuretics. Reduction of left ventricular filling pressure not only relieves pulmonary congestion but also may reduce left ventricular volume, wall tension, and myocardial oxygen demand while facilitating subendocardial coronary perfusion. Measurements of venous capacitance in patients with acute myocardial infarction have suggested that the diuretic effect of intravenous furosemide may be preceded by a venodilator action, contributing to its preload-reducing effect [20], although a transient vasoconstrictor effect preceding a diuretic effect has been noted in patients with chronic congestive heart failure [21]. Excessive diuresis should be avoided to prevent electrolyte depletion (notably hypokalemia) and hypotension secondary to hypovolemia.

Vasodilators such as nitrates or sodium nitroprusside may also be used, particularly when pulmonary congestion is accompanied by evidence of mitral regurgitation or systemic hypertension. Vasodilators produce their beneficial effects in pulmonary congestion by producing (1) venodilation, (2) improved ventricular compliance directly or by unloading the right ventricle, (3) decreased ventricular afterload through arteriolar dilator effects resulting in improvement in left ventricular function, and (4) reduction in mitral regurgitation or the degree of left-to-right shunt across a ventricular septal rupture. Nitrates, such as sublingual isosorbide dinitrate (in doses of 2.5 to 10.0 mg) every 3 to 4

Table 16-3
Role of noninvasive techniques for assessing complications of acute myocardial infarction with pump dysfunction

Technique	Useful for diagnosis
Echocardiography	Papillary muscle rupture Ventricular septal rupture Pseudoaneurysm True aneurysm and mural thrombus Infarct expansion Right ventricular infarction Pericardial effusion and tamponade
Doppler echocardiography	Acute mitral regurgitation Ventricular septal rupture
Radionuclide techniques	
Radionuclide ventriculography	Ventriculopenic state Right ventricular infarction Ventricular septal rupture (first-pass method) Pseudoaneurysm and true aneurysm Mural thrombus Subacute cardiac rupture with intrapericardial bleeding
Rest and redistribution thallium 201 scintigraphy	Differentiation of ischemia and viable tissue from infarcted myocardium
Technetium 99m pyrophosphate scintigraphy	Diagnosis of right ventricular infarction

Source: From P. K. Shah. Complications of acute myocardial infarction. In W. Parmley and K. Chatterjee, eds., *Cardiology*. Philadelphia: Lippincott, 1987.

Table 16-4
Categories of pump dysfunction in acute myocardial infarction

Clinical category	Pathophysiologic basis	Equivalent clinical subsets: Killip	Equivalent clinical subsets: Cedars-Sinai	Equivalent Cedars-Sinai hemodynamic subset
Subclinical	Compensated ventricular dysfunction or normal or near-normal ventricular function	I	I	I
Clinically overt				
Pulmonary congestion	Systolic and/or diastolic LV dysfunction Mitral regurgitation Ventricular septal rupture	II	II	II
Acute pulmonary edema	As above but more severe	III	II	II
Low-output state, hypotension, and shock				
With pulmonary congestion and edema				
Ventriculopenic state	Severe systolic and diastolic LV dysfunction	IV	IV	IV
Mechanical lesions	Acute mitral regurgitation Septal rupture	IV	IV	IV
Without pulmonary congestion or edema	Hypovolemia Dominant RV dysfunction Cardiac rupture Cardiac tamponade Electromechanical dissociation Severe bradyarrhythmias	IV	III	III

LV = left ventricular; RV = right ventricular.
Source: From P. K. Shah. Complications of acute myocardial infarction. In W. Parmley and K. Chatterjee, eds., *Cardiology*. Philadelphia: Lippincott, 1987.

hours or 2% nitroglycerin ointment (0.5 to 1.0 inch) applied cutaneously every 6 to 8 hours may provide mild to moderate vasodilator effects. Although hemodynamic monitoring is not generally necessary in patients with pulmonary congestion and adequate perfusion, objective documentation of effects of vasodilators, if they are used, may be appropriate when clinical assessment of efficacy is ambiguous. Continuous exposure to nitrates may lead to tolerance, and nitrate therapy should be used in such a way as to allow a 6- to 12-hour nitrate-free interval during each 24-hour period of therapy.

Acute Pulmonary Edema Without a Low-Output State

Acute pulmonary edema without shock is characterized by severe, dramatic manifestations of acute pulmonary congestion, that is, severe respiratory distress, sometimes accompanied by expectoration of pink, frothy sputum and frequently accompanied by increased heart rate, cool, clammy, diaphoretic skin, and elevated blood pressure indicative of a reactive sympathoadrenal response. Pulmonary edema may be precipitated by (1) extensive left ventricular contractile failure due to massive acute myocardial infarction or cumulative effects of old and new myocardial infarction; (2) primary decrease of diastolic function with only modest systolic contractile dysfunction (stiff heart); (3) acute, persistent, or intermittent mitral regurgitation resulting from papillary muscle dysfunction or rupture; or (4) profound global myocardial ischemia in association with a relatively small or modest degree of myocardial necrosis (ischemic paralysis).

Patients with pulmonary edema usually exhibit severe hypoxemia and may demonstrate respiratory alkalosis or metabolic acidosis depending on the degree and duration of the problem. Physical examination generally reveals tachypnea, cyanosis, tachycardia, elevated blood pressure, cool and moist skin, and extensive bilateral pulmonary rales, occasionally accompanied by wheezing (cardiac asthma) or even diminished breath sounds due to poor respiratory efforts. Acute pulmonary edema in myocardial infarction is invariably due to a rapid, marked elevation of pulmonary capillary wedge pressure (> 25 mm Hg), although in some patients decreased capillary colloid oncotic pressure has been thought to play a contributory role. A hypo-oncotic state has been implicated when pulmonary edema is precipitated by rapid infusion of crystalloid solution that results in dilution of serum proteins and a fall in intravascular oncotic pressure. Acute pulmonary edema complicating myocardial infarction is associated with a 30 to 50 percent mortality.

The salient principles of therapy for acute pulmonary edema involve general supportive therapy consisting of maintenance of adequate gas exchange, maintenance of a stable rhythm and blood pressure, and rapid reduction of pulmonary capillary wedge pressure. However, it should be emphasized that when pulmonary edema complicates an evolving acute myocardial infarction, primary attention should be paid to achieving rapid reperfusion with thrombolytic therapy or percutaneous transluminal coronary angioplasty (PTCA). This issue is discussed in more detail later in this chapter.

Maintenance of Adequate Gas Exchange. Maintenance of adequate gas exchange requires immediate analysis of arterial blood gases and administration of high concentrations (50 to 100%) of oxygen via a face mask. Use of continuous positive airway pressure may be helpful in maintaining adequate gas exchange in severely hypoxic cases, often eliminating the need for intubation. Endotracheal intubation should be considered when patients are moribund, are unable to maintain an arterial oxygen pressure of at least 60 mm Hg with a face mask, or develop a rising carbon dioxide pressure or falling arterial pH. Following endotracheal intubation, mechanical ventilation may need to be supplemented with positive end-expiratory pressure (PEEP) to maintain adequate systemic oxygenation and allow the use of relatively safer concentrations of oxygen (i.e., fraction of inspiratory oxygen < 60 percent). PEEP should be used judiciously to avoid lung barotrauma and to minimize declines in cardiac output secondary to reduced left ventricular preload and increased right ventricular afterload. Hemodynamic and arterial blood gas monitoring is useful for determining the effects of PEEP on tissue oxygen delivery (a product of cardiac output and arterial oxygen content) and for selecting optimal amounts of PEEP.

Rapid Decrease in Pulmonary Capillary Wedge Pressure. Nitrates are extremely useful for rapidly lowering an elevated pulmonary capillary wedge pressure in the presence of acute pulmonary edema [22, 23]. Nitrates produce a pharmacologic phlebotomy by their peripheral venodilator effects, shifting blood away from the intrathoracic compartment to the extrathoracic compartment, thereby rapidly lowering pulmonary venous and capillary pressures. A direct vasodilator effect of nitrates on pulmonary vasculature may contribute in some patients to unloading of the right ventricle, resulting in improved left ventricular compliance. Improvement in left ventricular function resulting from a reduction in afterload and improved function of ischemic segments, as well as a decrease or elimination of mitral regurgitation consequent to reduction of afterload, may be additional important acute effects of nitrates. The effects of nitrates may be supplemented by small intravenous doses of morphine sulfate, which helps calm the agitated patient and contributes to venodilator and arteriolar dilator actions.

Diuretics, especially intravenous furosemide, are frequently used as the primary treatment; however, their effect is slower and their use should generally be considered as secondary and adjunctive to nitrates. In severely hypertensive patients or in those with significant mitral regurgitation, continuous infusion of sodium nitroprusside may also be useful. Acute digitalization, intermittent positive-pressure ventilation, and routine use of aminophylline are generally not beneficial for acute pulmonary edema. In some patients, use of rotating tourniquets or phlebotomy is recommended, but in our experience it is rarely necessary. The role of inotropic-vasopressor therapy and intra-aortic balloon pumping for acute pulmonary edema in selected patients is discussed later in this chapter.

While emergency supportive therapy of acute pulmonary edema is being implemented, patients should be assessed for the presence of (1) intermittent or persistent severe mitral regurgitation, (2) ventricular septal rupture, and (3) ongoing or intermittent ischemia. Recognition of these complications is important, as mechanical intervention (revascularization, repair, or both) would be highly desirable for such patients.

Shock

Shock can be defined as a clinical syndrome characterized by evidence of acute, severe, prolonged tissue hypoperfusion, usually associated with a low arterial blood pressure (< 90 mm Hg systolic) and a markedly reduced cardiac output. In addition to hypotension and tachycardia, patients generally have cool, clammy skin, diaphoresis, mental obtundation, and oliguria. Depending on the dominant pathophysiologic event precipitating shock, additional clinical findings also may be present. Similarly, hemodynamic findings of shock may also vary depending on the pathophysiologic state resulting in the shock syndrome. Shock syndrome can be considered under two main categories: shock with pulmonary congestion or edema, and shock without pulmonary congestion or edema.

Shock Syndrome with Pulmonary Congestion or Edema

Shock syndrome with associated pulmonary congestion or edema may result from extensive left ventricular dysfunction (ventriculopenic state) or mechanical complications, that is, acute mitral regurgitation or ventricular septal rupture or a combination of the two.

Ventriculopenic Shock

Ventriculopenic shock syndrome occurs in 5 to 15 percent of patients with acute myocardial infarction. Despite a subjective impression that in recent years the incidence of cardiogenic shock may have declined, data from the Worcester Heart Attack Registry in fact show no substantive decrease in the incidence of cardiogenic shock over the past 14 years [73]. Shock generally results from severe left ventricular contractile dysfunction due to (1) extensive acute myocardial infarction; (2) acute myocardial infarction of less severe nature in patients with prior loss of myocardial function from old infarction; and (3) less commonly, large areas of ischemic nonfunctioning but viable myocardium along with only modest areas of myocardial infarction (ischemic paralysis). It may be the predominant mechanism of shock that occurs within the first hours of onset of acute myocardial infarction. Aggressive strategies aimed at reperfusion during early evolving myocardial infarction may be most useful for salvaging ischemic but viable myocardium in this subset of patients with cardiogenic shock.

Several pathology studies indicated that patients succumbing to this type of shock invariably demonstrate a cumulative involvement of at least 30 to 40 percent of the total left ventricular mass [24, 25]. In addition, patients frequently demonstrate marginal extension of recent areas of necrosis and focal necrotic areas remote from the major location of recent infarction. Profound impairment of ventricular function perpetuates ischemia and necrosis secondary to hypotension and the coronary artery underperfusion. This vicious cycle is responsible for the progressive nature of myocardial damage found in this syndrome, reflected by stuttering and progressive elevation of plasma levels of myocardium-specific enzymes [26]. Nearly 70 percent of patients succumbing to this type of shock demonstrate extensive, severe multivessel coronary obstructive disease with a high prevalence of left anterior descending coronary artery involvement [27]. It has been suggested that early thinning, lengthening, and stretching of transmurally necrotic myocardium (infarct expansion) may contribute to acute ventricular dilatation and precipitation of pump failure in patients with acute myocardial infarction [8, 28, 29].

Severe hypoperfusion of various body organs due to low cardiac output and hypotension results in impairment of organ function, for example, renal failure, hepatic dysfunction, pancreatic and gastrointestinal ischemia, enhanced anaerobic metabolism, and lactic acidosis. Pulmonary congestion and edema produce hypoxemia, atelectasis, and in rare cases, acute respiratory distress syndrome. Supraventricular and ventricular arrhythmias are common, and complications such as systemic or pulmonary sepsis, renal failure, and gastrointestinal hemorrhage further contribute to the poor overall outlook of the patient. The overall incidence of shock increases with increasing prevalence of risk factors such as advancing age, diabetes mellitus, and prior myocardial damage [73, 74]. While cardiogenic shock may supervene soon after the onset of acute myocardial infarction in patients who present with shock on admission, shock develops in as many as 25 to 30 percent of patients 2 to 5 days after admission. This delayed appearance of shock may be related to factors such as infarct expansion with progressive functional deterioration as well as to infarct extension or development of mechanical complications.

Patients in shock are generally cool and clammy with peripheral cyanosis, oliguria, and impaired mental status [30]. The systolic blood pressure is generally less than 90 mm Hg, or 60 mm Hg below the previous basal level, and the pulse is rapid with a narrow pulse pressure. Lactic acidosis may be present in advanced cases. Indirect cuff pressures may be 10 to 20 mm Hg lower in the presence of intense peripheral vasoconstriction, arguing in favor of direct intra-arterial measurements. Some patients have recurrent episodes of ischemic cardiac pain, whereas other remain moribund. Depending on the severity of the pulmonary congestion, patients demonstrate varying degrees of respiratory distress, hypoxemia, and hyperpnea. Cerebral underperfusion and use of narcotic analgesics, particularly in elderly patients, may result in Cheyne-Stokes respirations. Other clinical features of organ dysfunction may also be evidence as the shock syndrome progresses. Cardiac examination generally demonstrates diminished intensity of heart sounds, atrial or ventricular gallop (or both), pericardial friction rub, and dyskinetic apical impulse; the pulmonary examination reveals rales of varying distribution.

Hemodynamic findings demonstrate a low arterial pressure, severely depressed cardiac and stroke work indexes, and elevated pulmonary arterial and capillary wedge pressures. Systemic vascular resistance and arteriovenous oxygen differences are also increased. The left ventricle is generally dilated with severe and extensive regional contractile dysfunction, and the global ejection fraction is frequently less than 30 percent.

The prognosis of this type of "cardiogenic shock" is poor, with 80 to 100 percent in-hospital mortality, which has not appreciably changed in the past 10 to 15 years [73]. The small number of hospital survivors often live with continued heart failure and dysrhythmias, and they are faced with a low probability of long-term survival. Prognosis appears to be more favorable in relatively young patients, in those with single-vessel coronary disease, and in that subgroup of patients in whom early reperfusion with or without subsequent coronary artery revascularization salvages substantial amounts of jeopardized nonfunctioning but viable myocardium [31–34, 77–87].

Treatment Strategies

The main goals of management of ventriculopenic cardiogenic shock are (1) to improve ventricular performance and cardiac output, maintain adequate systemic arterial pressure to sustain perfusion to vital organs, reduce pulmonary congestion, and maintain adequate gas exchange (general supportive therapy); and (2) to limit the degree of myocardial damage, preserve the viability and maintain or improve the function of ischemic myocardium, minimize ongoing ventricular remodeling, and correct mechanical abnormalities.

General Supportive Measures

General supportive measures are essential and include relief of pain and discomfort with judicious use of small doses of analgesics such as morphine, maintenance of adequate oxygenation and ventilation (which requires endotracheal intubation in some patients), prompt correction of electrolyte and acid-base abnormalities, control of fever, treatment of nausea and vomiting, control of cardiac dysrhythmias, and maintenance of an adequate heart rate with atrioventricular synchrony. An ischemic ventricle is more susceptible to negative inotropic effects of drugs, particularly the antiarrhythmic agents, which are frequently misused in such patients. The need for such drugs and their dosage must be carefully reviewed and monitored, to avoid deleterious consequences.

Specific Therapeutic Modalities

Until a few years ago specific therapy for "cardiogenic shock" not only required careful clinical assessment but also virtually mandated the use of bedside hemodynamic monitoring using a Swan-Ganz thermodilution catheter as well as an indwelling intra-arterial cannula. Such invasive monitoring has been useful for excluding the presence of other complications that could produce pump failure or shock, that is, mitral regurgitation, septal or free-wall rupture, hypovolemia, and right ventricular infarction (Table 16-5). Moreover, it has helped in the selection of specific drugs and other therapeutic interventions, as well as in monitoring the response to such therapy. Refinements in noninvasive techniques such as two-dimensional echocardiography, color-flow Doppler techniques, and radionuclide scintigraphy have made it possible to expand and refine the information obtained by clinical means. In most modern cardiac intensive care units, bedside assessment of critically ill patients can now be made expeditiously with a combination of clinical and noninvasive techniques that considerably facilitate diagnosis and treatment.

Specific therapeutic interventions used in patients with shock are pharmacologic agents (inotropic and vasopressor drugs, vasodilators, diuretics), mechanical circulatory assist devices (intra-aortic balloon pumping, left heart assist device, percutaneous cardiopulmonary bypass, intraventricular coaxial flow pumps [Hemopump]), reperfusion (thrombolysis, percutaneous transluminal angioplasty, coronary artery bypass graft surgery), and surgery for the correction of mechanical complications (Table 16-6). Prior to the era of aggressive reperfusion, most of the therapeutic efforts were directed at improving the hemodynamic state of the patient by pharmacologic or mechanical manipulation of loading conditions and the inotropic state of the myocardium [17]. While such essentially palliative therapy is still an important adjunct in the management of these critically ill patients, the realization that such therapy alone seldom achieves a significant reduction in acute or long-term mortality has directed attention to reperfusion as the most important primary therapeutic intervention for severe pump failure complicating acute myocardial infarction.

Early Reperfusion and Revascularization. Because ventriculopenic shock results from large areas of nonfunctioning left ventricular myocardium, a consequence of ischemia and necrosis, early restoration of myocardial blood flow during the evolutionary phase of myocardial infarction, before extensive myocardial loss has been completed and when substantial amounts of nonfunctioning myocardium are still viable, is emerging as the most rational and effective therapy for curtailing the high mortality and morbidity associated with cardiogenic shock [34, 78, 79, 84, 85, 86, 87]. Early reperfusion can interrupt the necrotic wave front by relieving ischemia of jeopardized myocardium; restore its contractile function immediately or over time; render reperfused, salvaged but nonfunctioning myocardium more responsive to inotropic agents; limit the eventual degree of necrosis; preserve or improve ventricular function and topography; and dramatically improve the outlook in these patients. Because of the high baseline mortality associated with cardiogenic shock in patients treated with supportive and pharmacologic approaches alone, randomized trials of reperfusion have not been conducted in this specific subset of patients and it is highly unlikely that such trials will be conducted in the future. However, several

Table 16-5
Low-output state and shock following acute myocardial infarction

Underlying abnormality	Recognition			Guide to management
	Clinical	Hemodynamic	Others	
Ventriculopenic shock	Shock syndrome Rales, S_3 Abnormal chest x-ray	Elevated PCW Depressed CI High SVR Low BP	Markedly depressed LVEF (i.e., ≤0.30)	Inotropes-pressors to maintain systolic BP ~90 mm Hg and CI of >2 L/m^2 Vasodilators added to keep PCW 12–15 mm Hg IABP if no response to above + General supportive care Consider acute reperfusion with PTCA and/or thrombolysis
Acute severe mitral regurgitation	Shock syndrome Rales, S_3, abnormal x-ray Holosystolic murmur; occasionally murmur not heard or soft and brief	Elevated PCW with tall V waves Depressed CI High SVR Low BP	LVEF may be normal, elevated, or variably depressed depending on extent of necrosis of LV Echo shows flail leaflet Doppler shows regurgitation	Vasodilators + inotropes to maintain systolic BP ~90, PCW 12–15 mm Hg, and CI >2 L/m^2 IABP followed by early catheterization and surgery + General supportive care
Acute VSD	Shock syndrome Rales, S_3 Holosystolic murmur with precordial thrill in 50%	O_2 stepup from RA to RV or PA Thermodilution curve shows evidence of L→R shunt	First-pass radionuclide study shows L→R shunt LV and RVEF are variable as in mitral regurgitation and depend on extent of necrosis 2D echo visualizes defect Shunt seen on Doppler	Same as above + General supportive care

Hypovolemia	Shock syndrome Lungs and x-rays do not show signs of LV failure (but in some patients may show persistent signs of LV failure if hypovolemia is superimposed on a patient with prior LV failure, generally from overdiuresis) Orthostatic ↑ in HR and/or ↓ in BP	PCW generally $<$12–15 mm Hg CI depressed SVR may be high BP may be low Some patients with this profile have RV infarction		If patient has clinical evidence for hypoperfusion, then rapid but careful volume expansion until PCW is ~15 mm Hg but no higher than 18 mm Hg
Predominant acute right ventricular infarction	Shock syndrome in a patient with inferior infarction JVD or HJR in 70% of cases Lungs and x-rays generally clear with minimal or no signs of LV failure Occasionally pulsus paradoxus and Kussmaul sign Rarely severe hypoxia from R→L shunt across a PFO	RA pressure $\geq$PCW Reduced PA and RV pulse pressure Depressed CI 30% may have normal RA pressure (Volume challenge may bring out occult findings)	Dilated RV with ↓ RVEF ($<$0.39) LVEF generally $>$0.45 Some patients have severely depressed LV and such patients should be categorized differently	Increase volume if PCW $<$15 mm Hg PCW is ~15 mm Hg If no improvement, add inotropic agent and/or vasodilator depending on BP

PCW = pulmonary capillary wedge pressure; CI = cardiac index; SVR = systemic vascular resistance; BP = blood pressure; LVEF = left ventricular ejection fraction; IABP = intra-aortic balloon pumping, PTCA = percutaneous transluminal coronary angioplasty; LV = left ventricle; VSD = ventricular septal defect; RA = right atrium; RV = right ventricle; PA = pulmonary artery; L→R = left to right; RVEF = right ventricular ejection fraction; 2D = two-dimensional; HR = heart rate; JVD = jugular venous distention; HJR = hepatojugular reflux; PFO = patent foramen ovale.

Source: From P. K. Shah. Complications of acute myocardial infarction. In W. Parmley and K. Chatterjee, eds., *Cardiology*. Philadelphia: Lippincott, 1987.

Table 16-6
Beneficial and adverse effects of therapeutic interventions for postinfarction pump dysfunction

Intervention	Potential effects	
	Beneficial	Adverse
↑ Heart rate	May ↑ depressed CO and BP if HR is slow	↑ MVO_2 and possible increase in ischemia, loss of atrial contribution if ventricular pacing is performed
Diuretics	Decrease PCW, improve pulmonary congestion	Hypovolemia, low CO and BP, azotemia, hypokalemia
Volume loading	May ↑ depressed CO and BP in presence of hypovolemia or RV infarction	↑ MVO_2 by increasing preload, and possible ↑ in ischemia, pulmonary edema if PCW is not carefully monitored
Inotropic agents Digitalis Dopamine Norepinephrine Dobutamine	May ↑ depressed CO and BP in presence of LV failure	May ↑ MVO_2 by ↑ HR (dopamine, dobutamine, norepinephrine), ↑ contractility (all agents), ↑ SVR (norepinephrine, digitalis, dopamine), may worsen LV failure and produce tissue hypoperfusion if SVR increased markedly or tachyarrhythmias occur
Vasodilators Nitroprusside Nitroglycerin	May decrease elevated PCW and SVR, reduce MR, L→R shunt, and elevate depressed CO	May ↑ BP and compromise myocardial and other organ perfusion; may produce hypoxia; may produce toxic effects
IABP	Similar to above with maintenance and/or augmentation of diastolic coronary perfusion pressure	Complications related to IABP insertion and stay in the vascular compartment, i.e., vascular insufficiency, infection
Early reperfusion (thrombolysis, anticoagulants, PTCA)	May stop ischemia, limit infarction, improve LV function, restore inotropic responsiveness, prevent ischemia-related arrhythmias, reverse conduction abnormalities, prevent mural thrombus formation	Bleeding complication, hypotension, allergy, etc. (with thrombolytic anticoagulant drugs)

CO = cardiac output; BP = blood pressure; HR = heart rate; LV = left ventricular; RV = right ventricular; PCW = pulmonary capillary wedge pressure; SVR = systemic vascular resistance; MR = mitral regurgitation; L→R = left to right; MVO_2 = myocardial O_2 demand; HR = heart rate; IABP = intra-aortic balloon pumping; PTCA = percutaneous transluminal angioplasty.

retrospective and observational series, using historical control subjects clearly showed that early, successful and sustained reperfusion, whether achieved with PTCA, coronary artery bypass surgery, or both, is associated with significantly better short- and long-term survival rates (40 to 60 percent) than is conventional therapy or failed reperfusion [31–34, 78–87]. In this regard it is worthwhile noting that thrombolytic therapy alone, in sharp contrast to PTCA or coronary artery bypass surgery, has had little impact on survival in patients with cardiogenic shock [82, 88] (Table 16-7). Although reversal of cardiogenic shock and improvement in survival may occur following successful reperfusion with thrombolytic therapy, the overall failure of thrombolysis alone to achieve a significant mortality reduction in reported series may well be due to reduced delivery of the lytic agent associated with markedly reduced cardiac output and arterial pressure and suboptimal adjunctive antithrombotic therapy [31, 83, 89]. The experience at William Beaumont Hospital suggests that the overall survival rate for patients with cardiogenic shock treated with pharmacologic therapy alone is 10 percent, which is sharply lower than the survival rates associated with the use of thrombolytic therapy (23 percent), PTCA (55 percent), and coronary artery bypass surgery (57 percent). The data from a multicenter registry compiled by Lee et al. [34] documented a 59 percent in-hospital survival rate among 69 patients with cardiogenic shock after an acute myocardial infarction who were treated with coronary bal-

Table 16-7
Effects of reperfusion on mortality in patients with postinfarction cardiogenic shock

Intervention	% Mortality
Medical therapy (conventional)	70–80
Thrombolytic therapy	65–70
PTCA	40–50
Successful PTCA	*20–30*
CABG	30–40

PTCA = percutaneous transluminal coronary angioplasty; CABG = coronary artery bypass grafting.
Source: Data compiled from a composite review of published data and personal observations.

loon angioplasty. When angioplasty was successful, the short-term survival rate was 69 percent, compared to a 20 percent survival rate when angioplasty failed to accomplish reperfusion. At a mean of 32 months' follow-up, 55 percent of successfully reperfused patients were alive, compared to only 20 percent of those in whom angioplasty had failed [34]. In another study involving 53 patients, the survival rate was 40 percent among patients who were successfully reperfused with angioplasty, thrombolytic therapy, or both within 6 hours after the onset of symptoms, whereas nonreperfused patients had only a 19 percent survival rate [77].

The potential value of myocardial revascularization in the absence of mechanical complications of rupture or acute aneurysm depends largely on the existence of ischemic but viable myocardium. After stabilization of the patient with general supportive, specific pharmacologic, and in many, balloon counterpulsation therapy, prompt cardiac catheterization is recommended to define the presence and feasibility of cardiac surgery. Survival rates of 50 to 75 percent may be accomplished with this approach in properly selected patients, especially when bypass surgery is performed within 12 to 24 hours after shock develops [80, 81]. Cardiac surgery also improves the overall survival rate of patients with cardiogenic shock resulting from a potentially lethal mechanical complication (i.e., severe mitral regurgitation or ventricular septal or subacute free-wall rupture) [35, 80, 81].

Thus based on experience gained in the past few years, the contemporary approach to the management of cardiogenic shock consists of an aggressive strategy aimed at achieving rapid and sustained reperfusion using PTCA as the primary modality supplemented by general supportive measures, vasoactive and inotropic agents, and mechanical circulatory assist devices (such as the intra-aortic balloon pumping, heart bypass, assist devices, and Hemopump). Cardiac surgery is reversed for patients unsuitable for PTCA, for patients in whom PTCA failed, and for patients with cardiac rupture where surgical repair is imperative. For selected patients unsuitable for coronary bypass surgery or those with refractory shock and dependence on circulatory assist devices, cardiac transplantation may be yet another option.

Supportive Pharmacologic Therapy. In many patients, *inotropic and vasopressor agents*—cardiac glycosides, sympathomimetic agents, and nonsympathomimetic inotropic agents—are necessary to maintain peripheral tissue perfusion by improving cardiac output and maintaining an adequate systemic blood pressure (usually in the range of at least 90 to 100 mm Hg systolic).

Cardiac glycosides are relatively ineffective or only marginally effective in patients with severe pump failure following acute myocardial infarction. Ischemic myocardium appears to be more susceptible to the arrhythmogenic effects of digitalis, and the coronary and peripheral vasoconstrictor effects of rapid intravenous administration of digitalis have produced deleterious consequences [36]. However, digitalis may be indicated for atrial arrhythmias (i.e., fibrillation, flutter) complicating myocardial infarction and pump failure.

Sympathomimetic drugs are the most commonly used inotropic-vasopressor drugs for cardiogenic shock (Table 16-8). Dopamine and dobutamine are the most frequently used agents, whereas norepinephrine is used infrequently.

Dopamine exerts its cardiovascular effects by directly stimulating dopaminergic-specific receptors as well as releasing endogenous norepinephrine from sympathetic nerve endings [37, 38]. At low doses (2 to 5 μg/kg/min) in most patients, stroke volume and cardiac output increase. Renal blood flow is also increased, with redistribution toward the inner one-third of the renal cortex, an effect mediated by interaction with dopaminergic-specific receptors. At this low dose, chronotropic and peripheral vasoconstrictor effects are minimal, and deleterious effects on myocardial ischemia are not generally observed. With increasing doses, there is

Table 16-8
Guidelines for use of intravenous catecholamines and vasodilators in pump failure following myocardial infarction

Catecholamines
- Begin with a low dose and titrate every 10–15 minutes to a therapeutic endpoint without provoking unacceptable adverse effects.
  - *Dopamine:* Begin with 1–3 μg/kg/min and increase as needed to increase blood pressure.
  - *Dobutamine:* Begin with 2–5 μg/kg/min and increase as needed to improve cardiac output; dobutamine is not effective as sole therapy to increase blood pressure and should be used only when BP has been adequately restored.
  - *Norepinephrine:* Begin with 1–3 μg/min and increase by 0.5–2.0 μg increments. Preferably use in combination with alpha blocker, i.e., phentolamine.
- Use acidic solutions as diluents.
- Observe for adverse effects.
  - Sinus tachycardia (rarely bradycardia may occur with norepinephrine-induced hypertension)
  - Accelerated AV conduction and increased ventricular response in supraventricular arrhythmias
  - Atrial and ventricular premature beats and tachyarrhythmias
  - Worsening or provocation of ischemia or ventricular dysfunction
  - Tissue hypoperfusion from excessive vasoconstriction; necrosis (from extravascular extravasation) from dopamine or norepinephrine
- Nausea and vomiting

Vasodilators
- Begin with low doses and titrate every 10–15 minutes to a therapeutic endpoint without provoking adverse effects.
  - *Sodium nitroprusside:* Begin with 10–20 μg/min and increase by 10–20 μg/min increments.
  - *Intravenous nitroglycerin:* Begin with 10–20 μg/min and increase by 10–20 μ/min increments.
  - *Intravenous phentolamine:* Begin with 0.5 mg/min and increase by 0.25 mg/min increments.
  - Use freshly prepared solutions of nitroprusside (<6–8 hours old) and shield the reservoir from light.
- Preferably use nonabsorbent plastic tubings when giving intravenous nitroglycerin to avoid adherence of nitroglycerin to plastic tubing.
- Observe for adverse effects.
  - Flushing, headaches, hypotension
  - Reflex tachycardia; rarely reflex bradycardia
  - Worsening or precipitation of ischemia due to excessive hypotension and tachycardia and, possibly, maldistribution of coronary nutrient flow
  - Arterial desaturation from intrapulmonary shunting
  - Methemoglobinemia (nitroglycerin and nitroprusside)
  - Thiocyanate and cyanide intoxication (nitroprusside)
  - Precipitation of increased intracranial and intraocular pressures (nitrates)
  - Ethanol intoxication during prolonged high-dose infusions of intravenous nitroglycerin containing ethanol as a vehicle

Miscellanous
- Infuse these potent drugs through free-flowing non-posture-dependent large-bore intravenous, preferably central, lines using well-calibrated constant-infusion pumps.
- Avoid abrupt cessation of infusion (unless serious adverse effects occur); preferably, wean gradually.
- Avoid flushing infusion lines through which catecholamines or vasodilators are infusing without first clearing the infusion line by withdrawing blood through it.
- If cardiac outputs are being performed using a Swan-Ganz catheter, avoid infusing drugs through the right atrial port of the Swan-Ganz catheter.

BP = blood pressure; AV = atrioventricular.
Source: From P. K. Shah. Complications of acute myocardial infarction. In W. Parmley and K. Chatterjee, eds., *Cardiology.* Philadelphia: Lippincott, 1987.

a dose-dependent increase in chronotropic arrhythmogenic and alpha-adrenergic receptor–mediated vasoconstrictor and vasopressor effects that may result in decreased tissue perfusion and increased pulmonary arterial and left ventricular filling pressures secondary to elevated afterload. At large doses (>15 to 20 μg/kg/min), inotropic, chronotropic, and vasopressor effects may provoke or exacerbate myocardial ischemia.

The dose of dopamine infusion for "cardiogenic shock" requires careful individual titration beginning with a low dose (2 to 5 μg/kg/min). The object of therapy is to improve cardiac output, increase renal and other organ perfusion, and maintain a systolic blood pressure of 90 to 100 mm Hg without permitting excessive increases in heart rate (>110 to 115 bpm), arrhythmias, or excessive peripheral vasoconstriction to occur. Because of marked individual variations in dose response, it is crucial to use the lowest dose that produces optimal hemodynamic and clinical improvement with the fewest adverse effects. Adverse effects include sinus tachycardia; atrial and ventricular arrhythmias; excessive peripheral vasoconstriction and compromise of tissue blood flow; precipitation or worsening of myocardial ischemia; gangrene at the infusion site, especially when extravascular extravasation occurs; nausea and vomiting; and increased heart rate in the presence of supraventricular arrhythmias resulting from facilitation of atrioventricular conduction.

Dobutamine, a synthetic catecholamine, differs from dopamine in that it has predominantly beta-adrenergic agonist actions (accounting for its positive inotropic and chronotropic effects) with only minimal alpha-adrenergic agonist effects (accounting for its lack of appreciable vasoconstrictor effects even at large doses) [39]. Furthermore, dobutamine does not release endogenous norepinephrine and has no direct renal vasodilator effects. Dobutamine produces dose-dependent increases in stroke volume and cardiac output, and a modest reduction in pulmonary capillary wedge pressure. Excessive increases in heart rate are uncommon at infusion rates under 15 to 20 μg/kg/min, and vasoconstriction does not occur.

Because dobutamine tends to produce equivalent increases in cardiac output but with lesser increments in heart rate, a lower risk of arrhythmias, no vasoconstrictor effects, and a more consistent reduction in left ventricular filling pressures than dopamine, it is generally preferred as a starting drug. However, lack of direct renal vasodilator effects and only a modest pressor effect compared to dopamine make dobutamine less desirable when arterial pressure is low (i.e., < 80 mm Hg). The optimal use of dobutamine for cardiogenic shock requires that guidelines similar to those for dopamine be followed.

Norepinephrine produces potent arteriolar and venous constrictor effects through stimulation of alpha-adrenergic receptors. It has relatively modest, beta-1-adrenergic receptor–mediated myocardial inotropic and chronotropic effects. The peripheral vasoconstrictor effects of norepinephrine make it a potent pressor agent with much fewer overall positive chronotropic or arrhythmogenic effects compared to dopamine or dobutamine. Although such effects may temporarily maintain adequate arterial pressure in severely hypotensive patients, little increase or an actual decrease in cardiac output and compromise of peripheral organ blood flow may result in later deterioration [40]. However, in patients with cardiogenic shock with a low systemic arterial pressure (70 mm Hg) and a normal or reduced systemic vascular resistance in whom pressor doses of dopamine produce serious adverse effects (tachyarrhythmias), small doses of norepinephrine may be used to maintain systemic arterial pressure around 90 mm Hg systolic, with improvement in cardiac output in some patients. Use of norepinephrine combined with an alpha-adrenergic blocking drug (e.g., phentolamine) or direct vasodilators (e.g., nitroglycerin or sodium nitroprusside) is preferred, as such therapy minimizes peripheral vasoconstrictor effects and helps unmask the positive inotropic effects of norepinephrine [41]. As with dopamine and dobutamine, norepinephrine is generally begun at a low dose (1 to 4 μg/min) and increased to an optimal clinical and hemodynamic effect before excessive peripheral vasoconstriction or arrhythmias occur. Adverse effects are mostly related to excessive vasoconstriction and compromise of organ blood flow, worsening of ventricular function due to increased afterload, tissue necrosis and sloughing if extravascular extravasation occurs, increased heart rate, and cardiac arrhythmias. In some patients, an excessive increase in blood pressure may produce reflex slowing of the heart rate.

A number of new *nonsympathomimetic inotropic agents* with vasodilator effects (amrinone, milrinone, enoximone) that inhibit the breakdown of cyclic adenosine monophosphate by blocking phosphodiesterase, thereby increasing cytosolic calcium, have been investigated in recent years with regard to the management of acute and chronic heart failure. While these agents have proved to be of limited use in the long-term management of chronic heart failure, they have been useful in the short-term management of acute pump failure, in a manner analogous to that of drugs such as dobutamine. Limited experience in postinfarction patients with acute pump failure suggests that these agents, by themselves or in combination with other inotropic drugs, may be of short-term value to patients unresponsive to routine pharmacotherapy.

The rationale for using *vasodilators* in patients with shock is predicated on their ability to (1) reduce ventricular afterload by dilating the systemic arteriolar bed and (2) reduce ventricular preload by dilating the peripheral venous capacitance bed. Reduction in ventricular afterload results in decreased outflow impedance to left ventricular ejection, thereby increasing forward stroke volume and cardiac output. In the presence of mitral regurgitation and ventricular septal rupture, decreased impedance to ejection into the aorta reduces the degree of regurgitation and left-to-right shunt while increasing forward output into the aorta. Preload reduction contributes to the reduction of ventricular filling pressures, thereby reducing pulmonary capillary wedge, pulmonary arterial, and right atrial pressures. Although favorably influencing ventricular function, the afterload and preload reducing effects also tend to decrease myocardial oxygen demand and may favor subendocardial perfusion during diastole. Vasodilators may also influence the left ventricular diastolic pressure-volume relation, shifting it down and to the right owing to right ventricular unloading and reduction in the degree of pericardial restraint.

The use of vasodilators in this clinical setting is limited by their potential to produce excessive hypotension. Blood flow through coronary arteries with severe flow-limiting stenosis is highly dependent on perfusion pressure because of loss of autoregulatory reserve. Thus vasodilator-induced hypotension provokes a reflex tachycardia. Hypotension may also compromise perfusion to other organs (i.e., brain, kidney, splanchnic bed). Excessive reduction of left ventricular filling pressures or use of vasodilators in patients with low or normal filling pressures predisposes to hypotension and tachycardia. Because of these considerations, caution is necessary when using vasodilators in critically ill patients with a precarious hemodynamic state.

The effects of vasodilator therapy on the outcome of patients with cardiogenic shock have never been examined in properly controlled studies. Chatterjee and colleagues [42] reported an apparent improvement in short-term survival of close to 50 percent in a small group of patients who had severe pump failure complicating acute myocardial infarction and were treated with vasodilators; the 1-year survival rate, however, was 20 percent, and most survivors continued to have severe heart failure [42].

Currently the most commonly used vasodilators in patients with severe heart failure and shock are intravenous sodium nitroprusside and nitrates. Intravenous agents are preferred because they have a rapid onset of action (1 to 2 minutes) and a short half-life (2 to 4 minutes), and their effects rapidly dissipate within 10 to 15 minutes after cessation of the infusion.

Sodium nitroprusside infusion has a prompt peripheral vasodilator effect on both arterial and venous circulations. It produces hemodynamic and short-term clinical improvement in patients with severe heart failure with or without shock accompanying acute myocardial infarction [43]. The beneficial effects tend to be greater in patients with a markedly elevated pulmonary capillary wedge pressure and in those with mitral regurgitation or septal rupture. Therapy is generally begun with a low dose (10 to 20 μg/min) followed by rapid increases every 15 to 20 minutes, without permitting systolic arterial pressure to drop below 90 mm Hg (see Table 16-8). In many patients with cardiogenic shock, vasodilator therapy alone may produce unacceptable degrees of arterial hypotension unless combined with an inotropic drug (dopamine or dobutamine) or intra-aortic balloon counterpulsation.

Adverse effects of nitroprusside therapy include excessive hypotension with reflex tachycardia, potential for worsening of myocardial ischemia, accumulation of thiocyanate (particularly in the presence of renal insufficiency and prolonged infusions) with thiocyanate toxicity, accumulation of cyanide and cyanide toxicity, worsening of arterial hypoxemia due to an increasing intrapulmonary ventilation-perfusion mismatch, and rarely, methemoglobinemia and vitamin B_{12} deficiency. Limiting the dose and duration of therapy, frequent monitoring of serum thiocyanate levels to avoid exceeding levels of 6 mg/dl, and prophylactic use of the cyanide chelating agent hydroxycobalamin have been recommended to avoid cyanide intoxication [44]. Thiocyanate and cyanide toxicity are rarely observed.

Intravenous *nitroglycerin* is a rapidly acting vasodilator that tends to reduce the pulmonary capillary wedge pressure with more variable increases in stroke volume and cardiac output in patients with severe left ventricular failure [45]. These differential effects have been attributed to preferential venodilation, particularly at lower doses, but significant arteriolar dilation is also observed with increasing doses. Nitroglycerin may have a more favorable effect on the distribution of coronary blood flow to ischemic myocardium than nitroprusside, but there have been no careful comparative studies in patients with cardiogenic shock to confirm or refute the superiority of one agent over the other.

The adverse effects of nitroglycerin, like those of nitroprusside, include hypotension with reflex tachycardia, headaches due to cerebral vasodilation and possibly increased intracranial pressure, increasing intraocular pressure in patients with glaucoma, methemoglobinemia, Wernicke's encephalopathy, and ethanol intoxication (ethanol is the vehicle for many intravenous nitroglycerin preparations). Hypotension and paradoxical profound bradycardia are rare but generally respond to atropine administration and cessation of nitroglycerin therapy [46]. As with nitroprusside therapy, the use of intravenous nitroglycerin for cardiogenic shock frequently requires concomitant use of an inotropic drug (dopamine or dobutamine) or intra-aortic balloon counterpulsation to maintain or elevate a low systemic arterial pressure.

Phentolamine was one of the earliest agents to be used as a vasodilator. It is a nonselective alpha-adrenergic blocking agent with direct, smooth muscle relaxant effects and mild direct, inotropic and chronotropic effects. In comparison to nitroprusside and nitroglycerin, phentolamine produces a relatively greater increase in heart rate (and cardiac output) and a lesser decrease in filling pressures; it is considerably more expensive. Phentolamine is mainly used to minimize the vasoconstrictor effects of norepinephrine infusion and the deleterious effects of extravascular extravasation of norepinephrine or dopamine.

Combinations of vasodilator and sympathomimetic agents may be used to treat patients in cardiogenic shock. Afterload- and preload-reducing effects of vasodilators improve cardiac output and lower ventricular filling pressures, but systemic arterial hypotension remains a potential drawback. Inotropic drugs may improve ventricular function and cardiac output, but it may have inconsistent effects on ventricular filling pressures and potentially deleterious excessive peripheral vasoconstrictor effects. Thus by using lower doses of more than one agent, combined therapy may offset each other's adverse effects while augmenting overall ventricular function. Vasodilators frequently used for this purpose include alpha-adrenergic blockers such as phentolamine and direct vasodilators such as nitroglycerin and sodium nitroprusside. The principal advantage of adding a vasodilator to dopamine or dobutamine is that increments in cardiac output are achieved at much lower left ventricular filling pressures and systemic vascular resistance. Combined use of dopamine and dobutamine has also been suggested for the treatment of cardiogenic shock as a means of achieving a better acute hemodynamic response at lower doses.

Mechanical Circulatory Assist Devices. Intra-aortic balloon counterpulsation (see Chapter 15) is a mechanical circulatory assist device commonly used for the management of shock syndrome. The development of a percutaneous insertion technique has made it easier to initiate balloon counterpulsation, although rarely insertion through a surgical femoral arteriotomy is needed. Intra-aortic balloon pumping reduces left ventricular oxygen demand by its afterload-reducing effect while the increased diastolic aortic pressure helps to maintain or improve coronary perfusion pressure and subendocardial blood flow. The combined systolic unloading and diastolic augmentation tend to reduce myocardial ischemia, left ventricular filling pressures, mitral regurgitation, and left-to-right shunt across a ventricular septal rupture, whereas the forward stroke volume and cardiac output tend to increase. Electrocardiographic synchronization is used to begin balloon inflation at the time of aortic valve closure to produce diastolic pressure augmentation and to initiate deflation just prior to the onset of systole, thereby causing systolic unloading (Fig. 16-5). Hemodynamic effects of balloon counterpulsation may be further augmented by concomitant use of vasodilator or inotropic drugs.

Although patients with cardiogenic shock frequently demonstrate temporary clinical and hemodynamic improvement during intra-aortic balloon pumping, short- and long-term mortality rates remain high unless intra-aortic balloon pumping is used for short-term stabilization of the patient; it should be used in preparation for salvage of jeopardized nonfunctioning (but still viable) ischemic myocardium with coronary revascularization or for correction of severe mechanical complications (i.e.,

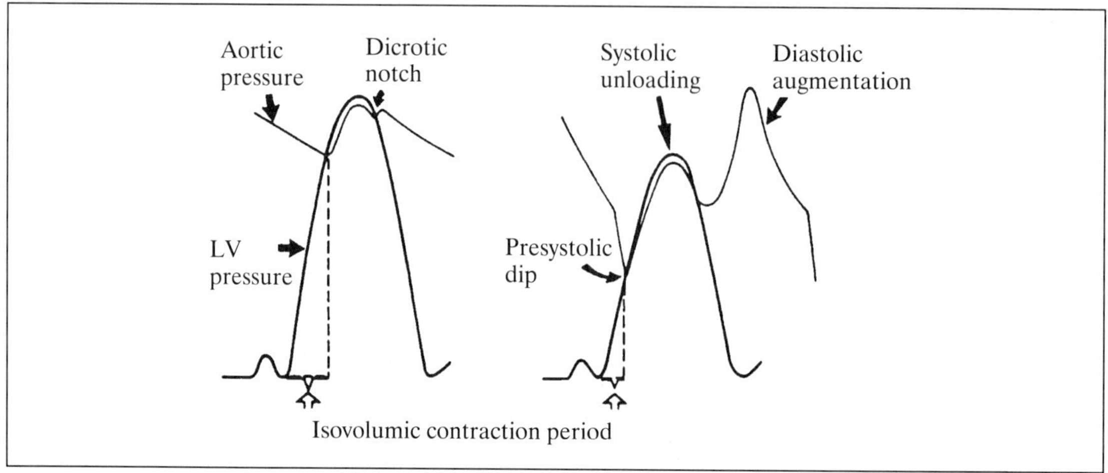

Fig. 16-5
Principle of intra-aortic balloon counterpulsation. Initiation of balloon inflation is timed to the arterial dicrotic notch producing diastolic augmentation in arterial pressure, whereas deflation of the balloon prior to the next ventricular systole contributes to systolic unloading. LV = left ventricle. (From P. K. Shah. Complications of acute myocardial infarction. In W. Parmley and K. Chatterjee, eds., *Cardiology*. Philadelphia: Lippincott, 1987.)

mitral regurgitation and ventricular septal rupture). The patients least likely to benefit from intra-aortic balloon pumping are those with multiple previous infarctions, those with large areas of myocardial scarring with massive irreversible necrosis, and those with late and advanced stages of cardiogenic shock; elderly patients with peripheral vascular disease who are most at risk of morbidity from insertion of the device also belong in this group [47, 48]. For patients with evidence of large areas of ischemic but viable myocardium or in whom there are mechanical complications (both amenable to definitive surgical therapy), balloon counterpulsation begun within a few hours after development of shock offers the best prospect of benefit when subsequent definitive surgical intervention is planned [35, 49, 50, 80, 81].

From a pragmatic standpoint, balloon counterpulsation should be considered for relatively young patients who are free of severe aortoiliac disease or aortic regurgitation, who have developed cardiogenic shock after their first infarction, and who have failed to improve with a trial of pharmacologic therapy given for 30 to 60 minutes. Every attempt should be made to determine the presence of surgically remediable lesions as described earlier using noninvasive and invasive techniques. Early cardiac catheterization, usually within 48 to 96 hours after the onset of balloon counterpulsation, should be performed and surgical intervention instituted for suitable patients. Patients who are unsuitable for surgery or in whom surgery must be delayed because of intercurrent complications should undergo weaning from balloon counterpulsation after a stabilization period of 2 to 4 days. The prognosis in such patients is generally unfavorable.

Complications occur in up to 30 percent of patients subjected to intra-aortic balloon counterpulsation and tend to be more frequent with the use of percutaneous methods [47, 48]. The complications are mostly vascular (i.e., vascular compromise of extremities and abdominal viscera, damage to femoral artery, aortic dissection) but also include infection, hemolysis, thrombocytopenia, gas leak, and embolism. In our experience, complications are particularly likely in older individuals (> 70 years), especially older women, and in those with aortoiliac vascular disease [47]. We generally recommend the use of small-caliber balloon catheters for the elderly and for women whose native vessels tend to be smaller.

In addition to intra-aortic balloon pumping, other methods of providing circulatory assistance in patients with severe pump failure or shock in preparation for definitive surgery (bypass, correction of mechanical defects, transplantation) include the use of percutaneous cardiopulmonary bypass, left-heart assist device, and the Nimbus Hemopump device [90–92]. Although the comparative usefulness of these newer devices remains to be clearly defined, preliminary results from limited experience are encouraging [90, 91].

Shock Syndrome Without Pulmonary Congestion or Pulmonary Edema

A clinical syndrome of a low-output hypotensive state following myocardial infarction may occur without signs of left ventricular failure. Such a clinical syndrome may result from bradyarrhythmias, hypovolemia, right ventricular infarction, and superimposed complications such as pulmonary embolism and sepsis.

Invasive hemodynamic studies of acute myocardial infarction demonstrated that in some patients with shock, the left ventricular filling pressure is normal, low, or only minimally elevated; and in some of these patients the clinical and hemodynamic state may improve with rapid volume loading. The precise reasons for this hypovolemic state are not clear, but overdiuresis, excessive use of vasodilators, possible reflexly mediated inappropriate peripheral vasodilation, and in some patients diaphoresis and vomiting resulting in dehydration may contribute to volume depletion. These patients can be recognized when a low-output state or shock is associated with collapsed neck veins without signs of pulmonary congestion on physical examination and chest radiographs and without an S_3 gallop. In other patients the diagnosis can be made with certainty only using invasive hemodynamic monitoring. The hemodynamic profile of these patients is typified by the Cedars-Sinai subset III, that is, a cardiac index of 2.2 or less with a pulmonary capillary wedge pressure of, at most, 18 mm Hg but usually considerably lower. It is also important to recognize that some patients with predominant right ventricular dysfunction complicating an acute inferior infarction may have a similar hemodynamic profile.

The treatment of hypovolemic shock requires rapid volume infusion using aliquots of 50 to 100 ml of fluid (colloid or crystalloid) under close clinical and hemodynamic observation until the pulmonary capillary wedge pressure is elevated to a maximum of 15 to 18 mm Hg. Further volume infusion may precipitate pulmonary congestion or edema and should be avoided. In some patients, particularly those receiving crystalloid infusions, pulmonary congestion and edema may even occur at lower pulmonary wedge pressures, possibly owing to a reduction in intracapillary oncotic pressure resulting from dilutional hypoalbuminemia. Thus careful clinical assessment in addition to hemodynamic monitoring is essential while volume loading is under way. In some patients, pump function fails to improve despite restoration of the pulmonary capillary wedge pressure to seemingly adequate levels. Such patients generally have severely reduced left ventricular systolic function with the ventricle operating along a flat Starling curve. Alternatively, volume loading may elevate the pulmonary capillary wedge pressure without a real increase in left ventricular preload or end-diastolic volume when left ventricular compliance is abnormal.

Right Ventricular Infarction

Ischemia and infarction of the right ventricle may occur in as many as 30 to 40 percent of patients with acute inferior or posterior myocardial infarction and rarely with anterior infarction [51, 52]. Associated infarction of the posterior part of the interventricular septum and variable degrees of inferoposterior left ventricular infarction are common, as these territories share a common blood supply from the right coronary artery [51]. Right ventricular dysfunction due to ischemia or infarction is clinically silent in many patients, but in 30 to 40 percent of patients it is associated with a low-output, hypotensive syndrome often simulating true cardiogenic shock. Diagnosis of hemodynamically significant predominant right ventricular dysfunction (Fig. 16-6) should be considered in any patient with acute inferior or posterior myocardial infarction complicated by a low-output or hypotensive syndrome; it is especially considered when accompanied by elevated jugular venous pressure or increased jugular venous pressure during inspiration (Kussmaul's sign) or during abdominal compression (abdominojugular reflux) with little evidence of pulmonary congestion. In about 30 percent

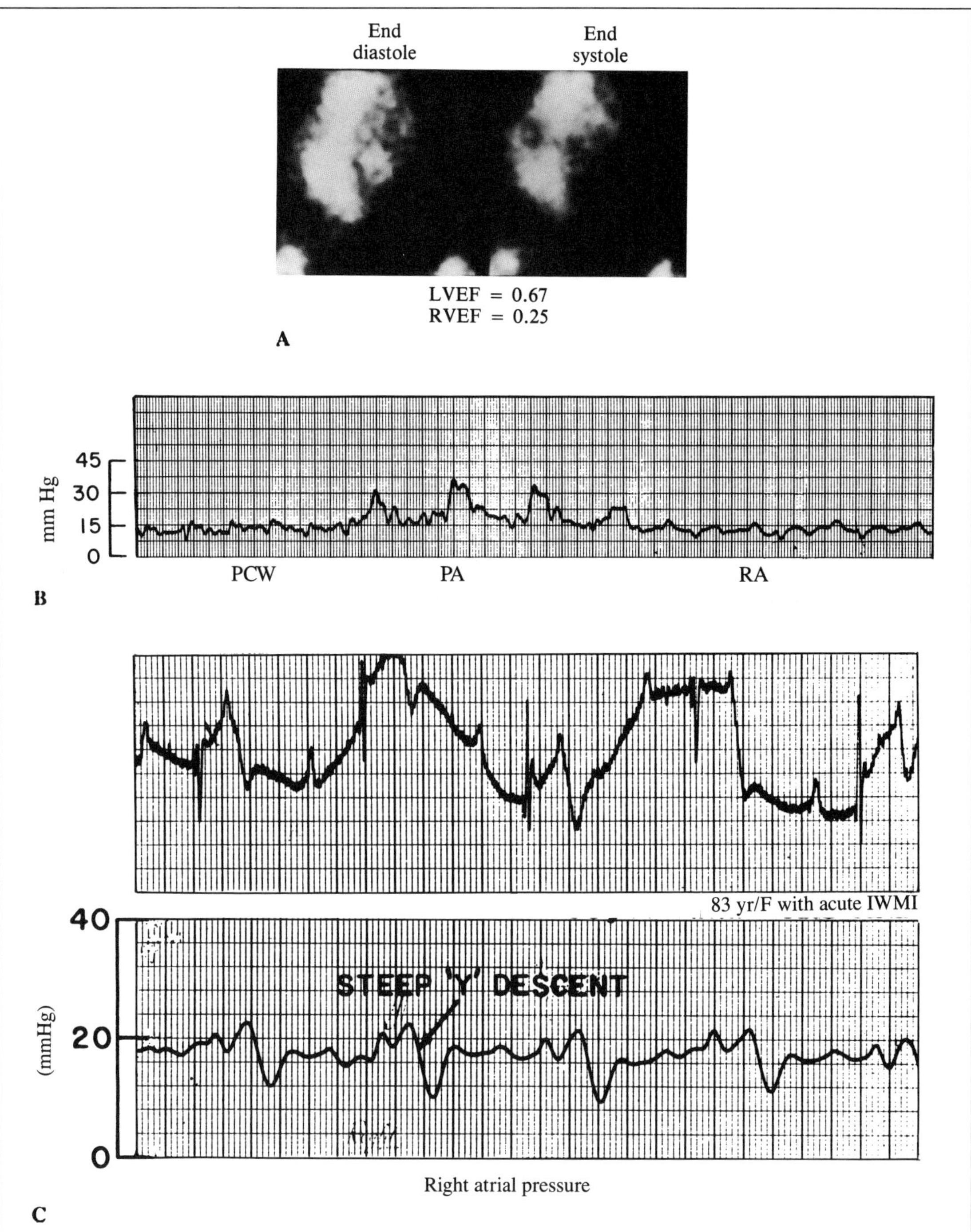

Fig. 16-6
A. Radionuclide ventriculogram in a 45-degree left anterior oblique projection demonstrating predominant right ventricular dysfunction in a patient with acute inferior infarction. LV = left ventricle; RV = right ventricle; EF = ejection fraction. *B.* Hemodynamic findings of equalization of right atrial (RA) and pulmonary capillary wedge (PCW) pressures in a patient with postinfarction predominant right ventricular dysfunction. PA = pulmonary artery. *C.* Abnormal right atrial pressure waveform showing a steep y descent in a patient with postinfarction predominant right ventricular dysfunction. (From P. K. Shah. Complications of acute myocardial infarction. In W. Parmley and K. Chatterjee, eds., *Cardiology.* Philadelphia: Lippincott, 1987.)

of patients, however, the jugular venous pressure may be within normal limits on initial assessment. Rarely, a murmur of tricuspid regurgitation secondary to right ventricular papillary muscle dysfunction may be heard. The presence of pulsus paradoxus in some patients with right ventricular infarction may lead to an erroneous diagnosis of a cardiac tamponade [53].

The electrocardiogram, in addition to the changes of acute inferior infarction, frequently shows ST segment elevation in right-sided precordial leads (V_{3R} or V_{4R}) or, less commonly, over V_1-V_5. The ST segment elevation in lead III often exceeds that in lead II and there is disproportionately less ST depression in V_2 compared to the ST elevation in aVF [93]. Precordial ST elevations from right ventricular infarction may create confusing electrocardiographic patterns simulating concomitant left anterior descending coronary occlusion [54].

A wide spectrum of hemodynamic abnormalities may be observed, with elevated right atrial and right ventricular end-diastolic pressures equal to or above the pulmonary capillary wedge pressure, which may be low, normal, or only modestly elevated. Other hemodynamic findings may include a steep right atrial y descent (see Fig. 16-6C) with a paradoxical increase in the right atrial pressure during inspiration (Kussmaul's sign), a dip and plateau during diastole in the right ventricular pressure tracing, pulmonary arterial and right ventricular pulsus alternans, and diminished pulse pressures in the right ventricle and pulmonary artery. Many of these hemodynamic findings overlap with those of cardiac tamponade, constrictive pericarditis, or restrictive myocardial disease [53]. In nearly 30 percent of patients, however, abnormalities of right atrial pressure are not evident initially but appear only later in the course of illness or following volume infusion. Severe arterial desaturation secondary to a right-to-left shunt through a stretched patent foramen ovale has rarely been observed [55].

Echocardiography and radionuclide ventriculography demonstrate disproportionate right ventricular dilation, dyssynergy, and a depressed ejection fraction (< 0.39) compared to the left ventricle, which generally demonstrates an ejection fraction of 0.45 or more. Technetium 99m pyrophosphate imaging may show uptake in the right ventricle. However, severe left ventricular global and regional dysfunctions coexist in some patients with right ventricular infarction, and such patients with severe biventricular dysfunction may behave differently from patients with predominant right ventricular dysfunction [18].

The low-output hypotensive syndrome results predominantly from reduced left ventricular filling and low left ventricular end-diastolic volume [52]. However, bradyarrhythmias, which are frequently observed with this syndrome (particularly when associated with loss of appropriately timed atrial contraction), may aggravate or even precipitate the low-output syndrome. The reduction in left ventricular volume results from reduced right ventricular systolic function with a consequent decrease in pulmonary blood flow and left ventricular inflow, as well as an increase in intrapericardial pressure secondary to right ventricular dilation, producing in effect a tamponade of the left ventricle [52, 53, 56]. In addition, diastolic septal bulge into the left ventricle (reverse Bernheim's effect) may contribute to decreased left ventricular volume. In some patients an increase in circulating atrial natriuretic factor, resulting from right atrial distention, may contribute to the hypotensive state.

It is important to recognize that timely reperfusion with either thrombolytic therapy or PTCA can rapidly reverse the low-output hypotensive state accompanying right ventricular infarction and thus should be considered in all patients without any contraindications. It is also important to recognize that in such patients volume infusion alone is rarely successful in improving the hemodynamic or clinical state and that concomitant use of inotropic or vasoactive drug therapy is necessary to stabilize most patients [52]. Such pharmacologic therapy should be considered as a supplement to reperfusion therapy. For patients with hemodynamically compromising bradyarrhythmias, treatment with atropine or the use of atrioventricular sequential pacing should be considered as additional supportive therapy. Although some studies have suggested that electrocardiographic signs of right ventricular infarction portend an adverse prognosis for patients with acute inferior infarction [94], the overall survival rate is generally favorable in this subset of patients provided there is no concomitant severe left ventricular dysfunction or a mechanical complication [18, 52]. Furthermore spontaneous improvement in right ventricular function over time is a frequent occurrence [52]. However, when severe left ventricular dysfunction (hemodynamic evidence of which may remain masked) coexists or if papillary muscle, free-wall, or ventricular septal rupture occurs, the outlook becomes grave [18, 52]. Rarely, tricuspid valve replacement is necessary to treat shock and severe tricuspid regurgitation, and closure of patent foramen ovale is necessary for refractory right-to-left shunt and life-threatening hypoxemia.

Mechanical Complications

Mechanical complications following myocardial infarction include acute mitral regurgitation (papillary muscle dysfunction and rupture) or septal or free-wall rupture. Cardiac rupture contributes to 15 to 30 percent of all deaths related to acute myocardial infarction. Papillary muscle rupture accounts for 5 percent of all cardiac ruptures; ventricular septal rupture, for 10 percent; and free-wall rupture, for 85 percent.

Acute Mitral Regurgitation

Acute mitral regurgitation following myocardial infarction can result from (1) ischemia or necrosis of the left ventricular papillary muscles and the contiguous portion of the left ventricular wall from where the papillary muscles originate (papillary muscle dysfunction); (2) rupture of the tip or, less commonly, the trunk of papillary muscle; and (3) rarely, rupture of the chordae tendineae.

Papillary Muscle Dysfunction

An intricate balance of geometry and function of components of the mitral valve complex is necessary for normal competent function of the mitral valve, failure of which can result in varying degrees of malfunction and regurgitation. The mitral valve complex consists of the annulus, mitral leaflets (anterior and posterior), papillary muscles (anterolateral and posteromedial), 120 chordae tendineae, the left ventricular wall where the two papillary muscles are attached, and the left atrial wall. The posteromedial papillary muscle receives blood supply predominantly from the posterior descending branch of the angiographically dominant coronary artery (commonly the right [90 percent] but occasionally the left [10 percent] circumflex) with few twigs from the nondominant artery. The anterolateral papillary muscle receives its blood supply from the left anterior descending coronary artery or its diagonal branches and from the marginal termination of the left circumflex coronary artery. The anterolateral papillary muscle originates from the midportion of the anterolateral left ventricular wall and receives chordal attachment from both mitral leaflets. The bulkier posteromedial papillary muscle originates from the junction of the lower or middle one-third of the ventricular wall, and it receives chordal attachment from the medial one-half of both mitral leaflets. The high propensity of papillary muscle for ischemia and infarction in coronary disease is related partly to its disadvantaged blood supply from inconstant and tenuous sources and its innermost cardiac location at the terminus of cardiac arterial circulation; it is also subject to exiguous perfusion and a relatively high degree of tension development during systole. Its attendant high metabolic oxygen cost is similar to that of subendocardial myocardium. Ischemia, infarction, or rupture of the posteromedial papillary muscle is five to ten times more common than that of anterolateral papillary muscle, possibly because of its more tenuous blood supply, which comes predominantly from a single artery.

Papillary muscle ischemia or infarction is rarely sufficient to result in severe mitral regurgitation unless there is associated deranged contractile function of the left ventricular myocardium [57]. It is likely that in many patients, mitral regurgitation resulting from papillary muscle dysfunction occurs when papillary muscle contraction fails to occur or occurs along an abnormal axis, shifted inappropriately by coexistent ventricular dilatation and dyssynergy, resulting in an inability of the mitral leaflets to coapt appropriately during systole.

Recognition of papillary muscle dysfunction complicating acute myocardial infarction is based on the appearance of intermittent or persistent mitral regurgitation. Mitral regurgitation is suspected in patients with a new systolic apical murmur of variable intensity, duration, pitch, and radiation who demonstrate disproportionately large V waves on pulmonary capillary wedge pressure tracings or severe mitral regurgitation on left ventricular angiography. However, the systolic murmur may be ephemeral and lingering, soft or loud, high- or low-pitched, holosystolic or midsystolic, or even completely absent despite severe mitral regurgitation [58, 59]. Depending on the concomitant severity of left ventricular dysfunction and the degree of acute mitral regurgitation, the patient may develop clinical manifestations of persistent or intermittent pulmonary congestion, pulmonary edema, hypotension, or shock.

Recognition of severe mitral regurgitation, persistent or intermittent, requires a high index of clinical suspicion. Advances in echocardiography and Doppler techniques have made it possible to detect mitral regurgitation and assess its severity at the bedside. Such patients should be subjected to prompt cardiac catheterization followed by surgery that may include mitral valve repair or replacement as well as coronary artery bypass.

In preparation for cardiac catheterization and surgery, the condition of a severely symptomatic patient may require stabilization using pharmacologic support (intravenous vasodilators and inotropic agents) and mechanical circulatory assistance (intra-aortic balloon pumping). A report of three patients with acute myocardial infarction complicated by mitral regurgitation and pulmonary edema or shock who were treated successfully with coronary angioplasty is provocative, as prompt resolution of hemodynamic instability and resolution of mitral regurgitation were documented [60].

Papillary Muscle Rupture

Rupture of the left ventricular papillary muscle, a serious complication of acute myocardial infarction, occurs in approximately 1 percent of patients and accounts for up to 5 percent of infarcts resulting in death [61, 62, 95]. Papillary muscle rupture tends to occur 2 to 7 days after infarction, but up to 20 percent of ruptures may occur within 24 hours after the onset of infarction. Most of the ruptures involve the posteromedial papillary muscle, a complication of inferior or posterior infarction resulting from occlusive disease of the circumflex or the right coronary artery for reasons described earlier. The degree of left ventricular myocardial necrosis is variable, with nearly 50 percent of patients demonstrating relatively small or subendocardial infarction [62]. Likewise, the extent of coronary artery disease is variable, with nearly 50 percent of patients having single-vessel disease [61]. The most frequent form of papillary muscle rupture involves one of the smaller heads of the papillary muscle, whereas rupture of the main trunk of the papillary muscle is less common and generally incompatible with more than brief survival [61].

The clinical presentation of papillary muscle rupture is dominated by the sudden development of severe pulmonary congestion and pulmonary edema, with many patients rapidly progressing to shock. A loud holosystolic apical murmur with widespread radiation may be detected. However, the systolic murmur may be brief (owing to rapid equilibration of left atrial and left ventricular pressures during late systole), nondescript, or even completely absent (silent mitral regurgitation) in some patients. The severe respiratory distress and adventitious pulmonary sounds caused by pulmonary edema may make it difficult to hear a murmur even when it is present. A palpable thrill is distinctly rare with papillary muscle rupture. The electrocardiogram often shows evidence of inferior or posterior infarction, which in many cases may be limited to seemingly minor ST-T changes, a deceptively benign appearance despite the catastrophic clinical deterioration. The chest radiograph shows pulmonary congestion or edema, which may be preferentially distributed to upper lung lobes, particularly on the right side, simulating pulmonary infiltrates. This preferential location may be the outcome of the mitral regurgitant jet being directed toward the orifice of the right upper lobe pulmonary veins. The left ventricular ejection fraction may be normal or supernormal because of the relatively limited degree of myocardial necrosis coupled with the unloading effect of severe mitral regurgitation, or depressed when infarction is extensive. However, the right ventricular ejection fraction may be depressed owing to associated acute pulmonary arterial hypertension or coexistent right ventricular infarction.

The diagnosis can be made noninvasively in the presence of the appropriate clinical context. Echocardiography may show a flail mitral leaflet as well as hyperdynamic left ventricular wall motion. When a Doppler flow study is performed, the presence and severity of mitral regurgitation can be gauged at the bedside. Even when a characteristic mitral valve echo of papillary muscle rupture is not

Table 16-9
Papillary muscle rupture with acute mitral regurgitation versus ventricular septal rupture

Papillary muscle rupture with acute mitral regurgitation	Ventricular septal rupture
Characteristics	
Occurs in 1% of all infarcts	Occurs in 1–2% of all infarcts
Peak incidence 3–5 days after infarct	Peak incidence 3–5 days after infarct
More frequent in inferoposterior infarcts (posterior papillary more frequently involved)	Equally frequent in anterior and inferior infarcts
Murmur usually loud and holosystolic but may be soft and nonholosystolic or completely absent	Murmur loud and holosystolic with widespread radiation
Palpable precordial thrill, rarely	Palpable precordial thrill in 50%
Diagnostic techniques	
Two-dimensional echocardiography: flail or prolapsing leaflet	Visualization of defect in septum (with or without contrast echocardiography)
Doppler: systolic regurgitant jet into left atrium	Detection of transseptal left-to-right shunt
Radionuclide ventriculography: normal, increased, or reduced LV ejection fraction with abnormal stroke/count ratio	Normal, increased, or reduced LV ejection fraction with abnormal stroke/count ratio; left-to-right shunt on a first-pass study
Pulmonary artery catheterization	
Prominent V waves on PCW tracing, reflected V waves on PA tracing	Oxygen saturation in RV and PA shows a step-up compared to RA (PA>RA by ≥10% saturation)
LV angiography: mitral regurgitation visualized	Ventricular septal defect visualized

LV = left ventricular; PCW = pulmonary capillary wedge pressure; PA = pulmonary artery; RV = right ventricular; RA = right atrium.

observed on echocardiography, hyperdynamic left ventricular wall motion in a postinfarction patient with pulmonary edema and shock suggests the diagnosis. Hemodynamic evaluation usually shows elevated pulmonary capillary wedge pressure with tall V waves, which are sometimes reflected in the pulmonary arterial tracing as well. Papillary muscle rupture can be differentiated from ventricular septal rupture by several features (Table 16-9).

Patients with papillary muscle rupture experience 50 percent mortality within 24 hours and 94 percent mortality within 8 weeks [61–63]. Although some patients appear to stabilize and improve with supportive medical therapy, such improvement is transitory and is usually followed by deterioration. Early surgical correction by valve replacement or repair can salvage up to 60 to 70 percent of patients. The catastrophic clinical course, the frequent evidence of relatively limited extent of myocardial necrosis and obstructive coronary artery disease, and a better outcome with surgery provide an impetus and rationale for early recognition of and early surgery for papillary muscle rupture [61, 62]. In preparation for urgent cardiac catheterization and subsequent surgery, patients frequently require intra-aortic balloon pumping and additional diuretic, vasodilator, or inotropic therapy for temporary stabilization. Papillary muscle rupture is one of the few causes of pulmonary edema or shock complicating myocardial infarction whereby aggressive and early surgical correction can result in improved short- and long-term survival rates compared to the natural history of this complication when untreated.

Ventricular Septal Rupture

Rupture of the interventricular septum is a catastrophic and serious complication of acute myocardial infarction that occurs in 0.5 to 2.0 percent of infarction patients and is responsible for 1 to 5 percent of all infarct-related deaths [64]. Septal rupture occurs with both anterior and inferior or posterior infarction and is associated with infarction of the interventricular septum as well as a variable extent of the left or right ventricular myocardium. Although multivessel obstructive coronary artery disease is common, septal rupture may complicate single-vessel disease. Rupture of the septum may occur as early as within the first 24 hours after the onset of infarction or as late as 2 weeks hence; however, most often it occurs 3 to 7 days after infarction. Rupture of the septum results in a left-to-right interventricular shunt, producing right ventricular volume overload, increased pulmonary blood flow, and reduced systemic blood flow. Reduction in systemic blood flow results in a low-output hypotensive syndrome that rapidly progresses to shock. The left ventricular ejection fraction is usually normal or supernormal but may be variably depressed depending on the magnitude of the ventricular infarction. The unloading effect of the left-to-right shunt may result in a higher left ventricular ejection fraction relative to the extent of myocardial necrosis. The right ventricular ejection fraction may be depressed secondary to right ventricular volume overload and increased pulmonary arterial pressure, particularly in patients with concomitant ischemic damage or infarction of the right ventricle.

Ventricular septal rupture is associated with the development of a new, harsh, loud holosystolic precordial murmur with widespread radiation. It is accompanied by a palpable thrill in about 50 percent of patients. Clinically, the patient may have recurrence of chest pain and dyspnea followed by signs and symptoms of a low-output state, hypotension, or shock. Right ventricular volume overload secondary to the shunt, concomitant right ventricular ischemic damage, and tricuspid regurgitation may produce signs of systemic venous congestion out of proportion to those of pulmonary venous congestion. The diagnosis can be confirmed rapidly at the bedside using two-dimensional echocardiography, which demonstrates the site and approximate size of the septal rupture [65, 66]. The diagnosis can be further refined by using echo-bubble contrast or Doppler and color-flow imaging [96, 97]. First-pass radionuclide ventriculography may also demonstrate an intracardiac left-to-right shunt. Bedside catheterization of the right side of the heart is useful for confirming the diagnosis and permits an approximate calculation of the degree of left-to-right shunt. An increase in oxygen saturation (> 10 percent) from the right atrium to the right ventricle or proximal pulmonary artery in the appropriate clinical setting is virtually diagnostic of ventricular septal rupture.

The clinical course of septal rupture is ominous, with a 24 percent mortality within 24 hours, 46 percent mortality at 1 week, 67 to 82 percent mortality at 2 months, and only a 5 to 7 percent survival rate at 1 year [35, 64]. Conservative medical therapy of septal rupture is generally ineffective. Afterload reduction by vasodilators may decrease left ventricular systolic pressure and reduce the degree of left-to-right shunt, but more pulmonary than systemic vasodilation could actually increase the shunt. Severe systemic hypotension frequently precludes the aggressive use of vasodilators. Inotropic and vasopressor drug therapy may be necessary to sustain arterial blood pressure, but it could produce tachyarrhythmias, systemic vasoconstriction with increasing left-to-right shunt, and myocardial ischemia. Transient stabilization can be achieved with intra-aortic balloon counterpulsation alone or in conjunction with vasodilator and inotropic drug therapy, but such stabilization is often temporary and should be used only in preparation for urgent cardiac catheterization to confirm the diagnosis, define the coronary anatomy, or determine mitral valve competence and left ventricular function.

Stabilization should be followed by prompt cardiac surgery involving repair of the defect and, when necessary, coronary bypass surgery and aneurysmectomy. Such an approach results in a 48 to 75 percent short-term survival rate [35]. Follow-up over 17 to 91 months has shown a late mortality of 5 to 14 percent in some series [35]. Cardiogenic shock, right ventricular infarction, and evidence of end-organ failure (pulmonary, renal) appear to portend a higher perioperative mortality [58]. The results of surgery appear more favorable for anteriorly located septal ruptures compared to posteriorly located defects, possibly because of technical problems encountered during repair of posteriorly located defects, coexistent mitral regurgitation, and ischemic right ventricular dysfunction.

Free-Wall Rupture

Free-wall rupture contributes to 8 to 24 percent of deaths related to acute myocardial infarction and occurs in 1.5 to 8.0 percent of all patients with acute myocardial infarcts [67]. The peak incidence of rupture appears to be around the second to eighth day after infarction, although about 30 percent of ruptures occur within 24 hours after the onset of infarction. Rupture occurs through an area of transmural necrosis and expansion; the infarct-related coronary artery is invariably totally occluded with a thrombus, and the collateral circulation is sparse or absent [67, 68]. In addition to transmural necrosis being a prerequisite, cardiac rupture is probably facilitated by quantitative or qualitative alterations in the connective tissue matrix such as breakdown of collagen or its cross-links that can result from ischemia or plasmin-induced activation of latent interstitial collagenases [98, 99]. In fact, the pressure required to rupture a normal porcine heart is dramatically reduced when collagenase is infused into the coronary circulation and collagen breakdown is produced (H. Anderson, personal communication, 1992).

The rupture occurs mainly in the left ventricle. Free-wall rupture may occur with anterior or inferior infarcts. Rarely, right ventricular rupture occurs as a complication of right ventricular infarction. Free-wall rupture occurs most frequently after a first infarction, with lateral infarction, during and after the seventh decade of life, in women, and in those with a history of systemic hypertension or hypertension complicating acute myocardial infarction [68]. Early ambulation, short-term use of anti-inflammatory drugs (steroids, indomethacin), and anticoagulants have been implicated in predisposing to cardiac rupture, although firm evidence is lacking.

Early thrombolytic-anticoagulant therapy initiated before transmural infarction is complete does not appear to increase the risk of cardiac rupture [100, 101]. Early reperfusion therapy may in fact halt transmural spread of myocardial infarction and thereby reduce the risk of free-wall rupture by preserving a viable shell of epicardial tissue. This theory is supported by published data on the incidence of cardiac rupture among patients receiving thrombolytic therapy when compared to conventionally treated patients with acute myocardial infarction [101]. It is possible, however, that thrombolytic-anticoagulant therapy, when administered after completion of transmural necrosis and occurrence of pericarditis, may actually increase the risk of cardiac rupture or hemopericardium. This conclusion is supported by a recent meta-analysis of published literature which suggests that the odds ratio for rupture exceeds unity when the time from the onset of infarction to the initiation of thrombolytic therapy exceeds 10 to 12 hours [100]. Cardiac rupture may also account, at least in part, for the excess mortality that results from thrombolytic therapy in the first day of treatment [102].

Free-wall rupture generally presents as a catastrophic clinical syndrome characterized by sudden severe and often tearing pain that is rapidly followed by hypotension, jugular venous distention, and electromechanical dissociation. Frequently there is a vagally mediated junctional or sinus bradycardia associated with the hypotension. In some patients this clinical scenario may be preceded or accompanied by intense agitation and mental confusion, whereas in other patients intermittent chest pain, simulating postinfarction angina or infarct extension, may precede the full-blown catastrophic syndrome. The electrocardiogram may remain unchanged or demonstrate more ST segment elevation (simulating infarct extension), failure of the expected T-wave inversion, or reversal of an inverted T wave to an upright position. In most such patients, death from hemopericardium and tamponade ensues rapidly, and few patients with this presentation can be salvaged by anything short of heroic measures (i.e., immediate pericardiocentesis, emergency thoracotomy, and surgical repair).

A more subacute form of free-wall rupture with progressively increasing signs of cardiac tamponade over hours or days occurs in some patients. Only a high index of suspicion can lead to proper investigation, diagnosis, and appropriate surgery [69]. It is important to recognize this subacute form of rupture, since nearly 30 percent of all ruptures follow this pattern and timely diagnosis and surgery can lead to gratifying long-term results [35, 69, 103, 104]. In a consecutive study of 1247 patients with acute myocardial infarction, Lopez-Sendon and colleagues [103] confirmed the diagnosis of subacute rupture in 33 (2.6 percent) patients. The combination of hypotension with echocardiographic evidence of a pericardial effusion larger than 5 mm, intrapericardial echoes, and right atrial/ventricular compression (indicative of tamponade) correctly identified 87.9 percent of patients with rupture, with only 9.4 percent false-positive diagnoses [103]. Of the 33 patients with subacute cardiac rupture, 25 (76 percent) survived surgical repair and 16 (48.5 percent) were alive at a median follow-up of 2.5 years [103]. In another large series involving a consecutive cohort of 2608 patients with acute myocardial infarction, Pollak and coworkers [104] described 24 (0.92 percent) patients with subacute cardiac rupture, in 15 of whom the correct clinical diagnosis had been missed. A high clinical index of suspicion coupled with early use of echocardiography and in selected patients, radionuclide ventriculography offers the best approach for a timely diagnosis and subsequent surgery [103–106]. Although experimental studies suggested that volume loading and inotropic support with dobutamine may improve the hemodynamic state in the canine model of hemopericardium from rupture, surgical repair is the only hope for survival in patients with subacute cardiac rupture [107].

Rarely, free-wall rupture of the left ventricle leads to the formation of a pseudoaneurysm, which is a consequence of containment of the resulting hemopericardium by circumferential adhesions between the pericardium and epicardium (Fig. 16-7). Most pseudoaneurysms reported in the literature, however, resulted from complications of cardiac surgery, chest trauma, and bacterial endocarditis [70]. In one retrospective review, a pseudoaneurysm was detected in 0.5 percent of 1050 patients referred for cardiac catheterization [71]. The pseudoaneurysm frequently contains a thrombus and communicates with the body of the left ventricle through a narrow isthmus. It may remain small or enlarge progressively, eventually becoming larger than the main left ventricle in some patients. In contrast to a true aneurysm, the walls of the pseudoaneurysm are composed of pericardium and adhesions and are devoid of myocardial tissue and coronary arteries. Pseudoaneurysm may remain clinically silent and be discovered only during routine investigation. In some patients it leads to progressively worsening congestive heart failure, recurrent ventricular arrhythmias, cardiomegaly with an abnormal bulge on the cardiac border, and persistent elevation of the ST segment overlying an area of infarction on the electrocardiogram, thereby simulating a true aneurysm. Systolic and diastolic murmurs, presumably related to back-and-forth movement of blood across the narrow isthmus of the aneurysm, may rarely occur, simulating valvular heart disease [72]. The pseudoaneurysm is prone to free rupture with an invariably fatal outcome (although long-term survival is possible), whereas such a complication is rare with chronic true aneurysm [70]. Two-dimensional echocardiography, radionuclide ventriculography or invasive left ventriculography, cine-computed tomography, and magnetic resonance imaging can be used to make a diagnosis of pseudoaneurysm. Surgical resection is strongly recommended in symptomatic as well as asymptomatic patients, irrespective of the size of the pseudoaneurysm, to prevent a catastrophic outcome from rupture.

Rarely an intramural rupture of an infarct with an overlying thin shell of myocardium (pseudo-

Fig. 16-7
Differences between a pseudoaneurysm and a true aneurysm. (From P. K. Shah. Complications of acute myocardial infarction. In W. Parmley and K. Chatterjee, eds., *Cardiology*. Philadelphia: Lippincott, 1987.)

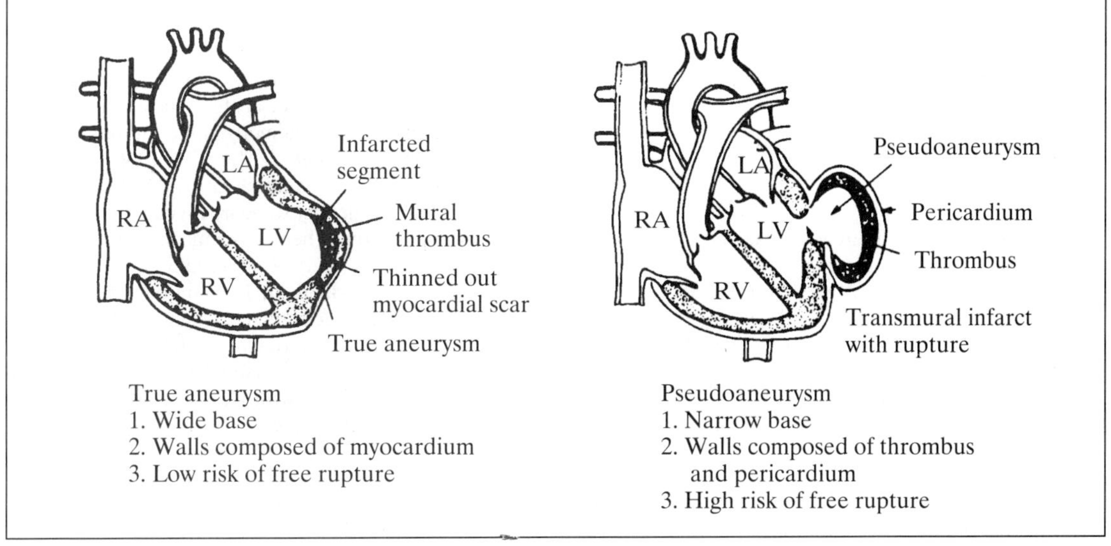

pseudoaneurysm) may also occur, simulating a pseudoaneurysm on imaging tests. These variants are probably best managed with surgical repair.

Future Perspectives

Pump failure and cardiogenic shock, whether resulting from severe contractile dysfunction or mechanical complications, remain the primary causes of mortality following acute myocardial infarction. It is clear that after the development of shock, aggressive interventional approaches using PTCA and cardiac surgery, can significantly improve survival but regrettably the mortality still remains prohibitively high (40 to 50 percent). These statistics may further improve with further refinements in reperfusion strategies [108, 109]. It is, however, clear that the best approach to further improving the survival of patients with acute myocardial infarction is to prevent the development of shock by reducing myocardial infarct size and serious ventricular dysfunction (with early rapid and sustained reperfusion). Recent data from the TAPS study suggest that the incidence of cardiogenic shock may be reduced with relatively rapid administration of tissue plasminogen activator followed by therapeutic levels of intravenous heparin [110]. Furthermore, preventing progressive functional and topographic deterioration following large myocardial infarction, with prophylactic use of nitrates and angiotensin-converting inhibitors, may further reduce the incidence of severe pump failure [111–113]. This is particularly relevant since cardiogenic shock may not be present on admission but may develop 2 to 3 days later in 25 to 30 percent of all patients [73, 114].

References

1. Multicenter Post Infarction Research Group. Risk stratification and survival after myocardial infarction. *N. Engl. J. Med.* 309:331, 1983.
2. May, G. S., Furberg, C. D., Eberlein, K. A., et al. Secondary prevention after myocardial infarction: A review of short term acute phase trials. *Prog. Cardiovasc. Dis.* 25:335, 1983.
3. Herrick, J. B. Clinical features of sudden obstruction of the coronary arteries. *J.A.M.A.* 59:2015, 1912.
4. Roberts, W. C. Coronary arteries in fatal acute myocardial infarction. *Circulation* 45:215, 1972.
5. DeWood, M. A., Spores, J., Notske, R., et al. Prevalence of total coronary occlusion during the early hours of transmural myocardial infarction. *N. Engl. J. Med.* 303:897, 1981.
6. Reimer, K. A., Lowe, J. E., Rasmussen, M. D., et al. The wave-front phenomenon of ischemic cell death. *Circulation* 56:786, 1977.
7. Herman, M. V., Heinle, R. A., Klein, M. D., et al. Localized disorders in myocardial contraction. *N. Engl. J. Med.* 227:222, 1967.
8. Eaton, L. W., and Bulkley, B. H. Expansion of acute myocardial infarction: Its relationship to infarct morphology in a canine model. *Circ. Res.* 49:80, 1981.
9. Erlebacher, J. A., Weiss, J. L., Eaton, L. W., et al. Late effects of acute infarct dilation on heart size: A two dimensional echocardiographic study. *Am. J. Cardiol.* 49:1120, 1982.
10. Bertrand, M., Rousseau, M. D., LaBlanche, J. M., et al. Cineangiographic assessment of left ventricular function in the acute phase of transmural myocardial infarction. *Am. J. Cardiol.* 43:472, 1979.
11. Bardet, J., Rocha, P., Rigaud, M., et al. Left ventricular compliance in acute myocardial infarction in man. *Cardiovasc. Res.* 11:122, 1977.
12. Swan, H. J. C., Forrester, J. S., Diamond, G., et al. Hemodynamic spectrum of myocardial infarction and cardiogenic shock. *Circulation* 45:1097, 1972.
13. Shah, P. K., Pichler, M., Berman, D. S., et al. Left ventricular ejection fraction determined by radionuclide ventriculography in early stages of first transmural myocardial infarction: Relation to short term prognosis. *Am. J. Cardiol.* 45:542, 1980.
14. Bigger, J. T., Fleiss, J. L., Kleiger, R., et al. The relationship among ventricular arrhythmias, left ventricular dysfunction, and mortality in the 2 years after myocardial infarction. *Circulation* 69:250, 1984.
15. Killip, T., and Kimbal, J. T. Treatment of myocardial infarction in a coronary care unit: A two year experience with 250 patients. *Am. J. Cardiol.* 20:457, 1967.
16. Forrester, J. S., Diamond, G. A., Chatterjee, K., et al. Medical therapy of acute myocardial infarction by application of hemodynamic subsets (first of two parts). *N. Engl. J. Med.* 295:1356, 1976.
17. Forrester, J. S., Diamond, G. A., Chatterjee, K., et al. Medical therapy of acute myocardial infarction by application of hemodynamic subsets (second of two parts). *N. Engl. J. Med.* 295:1404, 1976.
18. Shah, P. K., Maddahi, J., Staniloff, H. M., et al. The variable spectrum and prognostic implications of left and right ventricular ejection fractions determined early in the course of acute myocardial infarction associated with clinical evidence of no or mild heart failure. *Am. J. Cardiol.* 58:387, 1986.
19. Swan, H. J. C., Ganz, W., Forrester, J., et al. Catheterization of the heart in man with use of flow-directed balloon-tipped catheter. *N. Engl. J. Med.* 283:447, 1970.

20. Dikshit, K., Vyden, J. K., Forrester, J. S., et al. Renal and extrarenal hemodynamic effects of furosemide in congestive heart failure after acute myocardial infarction. *N. Engl. J. Med.* 288:1087, 1973.
21. Francis, G. S., Siegel, R. M., Goldsmith, S. R., et al. Acute vasoconstrictor response to intravenous furosemide in patients with chronic congestive heart failure. *Ann. Intern. Med.* 103:1, 1985.
22. Bussman, W. D., and Kaltenbach, M. Sublingual nitroglycerin in the treatment of left ventricular failure and pulmonary edema. *Eur. J. Cardiol.* 4:327, 1976.
23. Shah, P. K. Buccal nitroglycerin ointment in acute cardiac pulmonary edema. *Ann. Intern. Med.* 103: 153, 1985.
24. Page, D. L., Caulfield, J. B., Kastor, J. A., et al. Myocardial changes associated with cardiogenic shock. *N. Engl. J. Med.* 285:133, 1971.
25. Alonso, D. R., Scheidt, S., Post, M., et al. Pathophysiology of cardiogenic shock: Quantification of myocardial necrosis: Clinical, pathologic and electrocardiographic correlation. *Circulation* 48:588, 1973.
26. Gutovitz, A. L., Sobel, B. E., and Roberts, R. Progressive nature of myocardial injury in selected patients with cardiogenic shock. *Am. J. Cardiol.* 41:469, 1978.
27. Wackers, F. J., Lie, K. I., and Becker, A. E. Coronary artery disease in patients dying from cardiogenic shock or congestive heart failure in the setting of acute myocardial infarction. *Br. Heart J.* 38: 906, 1976.
28. Eaton, L. W., Weiss, J. L., Bulkley, B. H., et al. Regional cardiac dilatation after acute myocardial infarction: Recognition by 2-D echocardiography *N. Engl. J. Med.* 300:57, 1979.
29. Meizlish, J. L., Berger, H. J., Plankey, M., et al. Functional left ventricular aneurysm formation after acute anterior transmural myocardial infarction: Incidence, natural history and prognostic implications. *N. Engl. J. Med.* 311:1001, 1984.
30. Doherty, N. E., Ades, A., Shah, P. K., et al. Hypothermia as a consequence of acute myocardial infarction. Reversal with intra-aortic balloon counterpulsation. *Ann. Intern. Med.* 101:863, 1984.
31. Lew, A. S., Weiss, A. T., Shah, P. K., et al. Extensive myocardial salvage and reversal of cardiogenic shock after reperfusion of the left main coronary artery by intravenous streptokinase. *Am. J. Cardiol.* 54:450, 1984.
32. Mathey, D. G., Kuck, K. H., Tishner, V., et al. Nonsurgical coronary artery recanalization in acute transmural myocardial infarction. *Circulation* 63: 489, 1981.
33. Meyer, J., Merx, W., Dorr, R., et al. Successful treatment of acute myocardial infarction shock by combined percutaneous transluminal coronary artery recanalization and angioplasty. *Am. Heart J.* 103:132, 1982.
34. Lee, L., Erbel, R., Brown, T. M., et al. Multicenter registry of angioplasty therapy of cardiogenic shock: Initial and long-term survival. *J. Am. Coll. Cardiol.* 17:599, 1991.
35. Gray, R. J., Sethna, D., and Matloff, J. M. The role of cardiac surgery in acute myocardial infarction with mechanical complications. *Am. Heart J.* 106: 723, 1983.
36. Cohn, J. N., Tristani, F. E., and Khatri, I. M. Cardiac peripheral vascular effects of digitalis in clinical cardiogenic shock. *Am. Heart J.* 78:318, 1969.
37. Goldberg, L. O. Cardiovascular and renal actions of dopamine. I. Potential clinical applications. *Pharmcol. Rev.* 21:1, 1972.
38. Mueller, H. S., Evans, R., and Ayres, S. M. Effects of dopamine on hemodynamics and myocardial metabolism in shock following acute myocardial infarction in man. *Circulation* 57:361, 1978.
39. Sonnenblick, E. H., Frishman, W. H., and Lejemtel, T. H. Dobutamine: A new synthetic cardioactive sympathetic amine. *N. Engl. J. Med.* 300:17, 1979.
40. Mueller, H., Ayres, S., Giarinelli, S., Jr., et al. Effect of isoproternol, I-norepinephrine and intraaortic counterpulsation on hemodynamics and myocardial metabolism in shock following myocardial infarction. *Circulation* 55:325, 1972.
41. Gray, R. J., Shah, P. K., Singh, B. N., et al. Low cardiac-output states following open heart surgery: Comparative hemodynamic effects of dobutamine, dopamine and norepinephrine plus phentolamine. *Chest* 80:16, 1981.
42. Chatterjee, K., Swan, H. J. C., Kaushik, V. S., et al. Effects of vasodilator therapy for severe pump failure in acute myocardial infarction on short term and late prognosis. *Circulation* 53:797, 1976.
43. Franciosa, J. B., Buiha, N. M., Limas, C. J., et al. Improved left ventricular function during nitroprusside infusion in acute myocardial infarction. *Lancet* 1:650, 1972.
44. Cottrell, J. E., Casthely, P., Brodie, J. D., et al. Prevention of nitroprusside induced cyanide toxicity with hydroxycobalamin. *N. Engl. J. Med.* 298:809, 1978.
45. Jaffe, A. S., and Roberts, R. The use of intravenous nitroglycerin in cardiovascular disease. *Pharmacotherapy* 2:273, 1983.
46. Nemerowski, M., and Shah, P. K. Syndrome of severe bradycardia and hypotension following sublingual nitroglycerin administration. *Cardiology* 67: 180, 1981.
47. Goldberger, M., Tabak, S. W., and Shah, P. K. Clinical experience with intra-aortic balloon counterpulsation in 112 consecutive patients. *Am. Heart J.* 111:497, 1986.
48. Isner, J. M., Cohen, S. R., Vermani, R., et al. Complications of intra-aortic balloon counterpulsation device, clinical and morphological observations in 45 necropsy patients. *Am. J. Cardiol.* 45:260, 1980.
49. Dewood, M. A,. Notske, R. N., Hensley, G. R., et al. Intra-aortic balloon counterpulsation with or

without reperfusion for myocardial infarction shock *Circulation* 61:1105, 1980.
50. Leinbach, R. C., and Gold, H. K. Intra-aortic balloon pumping: Use in treatment of cardiogenic shock and acute myocardial ischemia. In J. S. Karliner and G. Gregoratos (eds.), *Coronary Care.* New York: Churchill Livingstone, 1981.
51. Isner, J. M., and Roberts, W. C. Right ventricular infarction complicating left ventricular infarction complicating coronary artery disease. *Am. J. Cardiol.* 42:885, 1978.
52. Shah, P. K., Maddahi, J., Berman, D. S., et al. Scintigraphically detected predominant right ventricular dysfunction in acute myocardial infarction: Clinical, hemodynamic correlates and implications for therapy and prognosis. *J. Am. Coll. Cardiol.* 6:1264, 1985.
53. Lorrell, B., Leinbach, R. C., Pohost, G. M., et al. Right ventricular infarction: Clinical diagnosis and differentiation from cardiac tamponade and pericardial constriction. *Am. J. Cardiol.* 43:465, 1979.
54. Gest, I. L.,Shah, P. K., Rodriguez, L., et al. ST elevations in leads V_1 to V_5 may be caused by right coronary occlusion and acute right ventricular infarction. *Am. J. Cardiol.* 53:991, 1984.
55. Morris, A. L., and Donen, N. Hypoxia and intracardiac right to left shunt complicating inferior myocardial infarction with right ventricular extension. *Ann. Intern. Med.* 138:1405, 1978.
56. Goldstein, J. H., Blahaker, G. J., Verriez, E. D., et al. The role of right ventricular systolic dysfunction and elevated intrapericardial pressure in the genesis of low cardiac output in experimental right ventricular infarction. *Circulation* 65:513, 1981.
57. Shelburne, J. C., Rubinstein, D., and Gorlin, R. A reappraisal of papillary muscle dysfunction: Correlative clinical and angiographic study. *Am. J. Med.* 46:862, 1969.
58. Heikkila, J. Mitral incompetence complicating acute myocardial infarction. *Acta Med. Scand.* 176: 287, 1967.
59. Forrester, J. S., Diamond, G., Freedman, S., et al. Silent mitral insufficiency in acute myocardial infarction. *Circulation* 44:877, 1971.
60. Heuser, R. R., Maddoux, G. L., Gross, J. E., et al. Coronary angioplasty for acute mitral regurgitation due to myocardial infarction. *Ann. Intern. Med.* 107:852, 1987.
61. Nishimura, R. A., Schaff, H. V., Shuh, C., et al. Papillary muscle rupture complicating acute myocardial infarction: Analysis of 17 patients. *Am. J. Cardiol.* 51:373, 1983.
62. Wei, J. Y., Hutchins, G. M., and Bulkley, B. H. Papillary muscle rupture in fatal acute myocardial infarction. *Ann. Intern. Med.* 90:149, 1979.
63. Clements, S. D., Story, W. E., Hurst, J. W., et al. Ruptured papillary muscle, a complication of acute myocardial infarction: Clinical presentation, diagnosis and treatment. *Clin. Cardiol.* 8:93, 1985.
64. Fox, A. C., Glassman, E., and Isom, O. W. Surgically remediable complications of myocardial infarction. *Prog. Cardiovasc. Dis.* 21:461, 1979.
65. Farcot, J. C., Borsante, L., Rigaud, M., et al. Two dimensional echocardiographic visualization of ventricular septal rupture after acute anterior myocardial infarction. *Am. J. Cardiol.* 45:370, 1980.
66. Richards, K. L., Hoekenga, D. E., Leach, J. K., et al. Doppler cardiographic diagnosis of interventricular septal rupture. *Chest* 76:101, 1979.
67. Rasmussen, S., Leth, A., Kjoller, E., et al. Cardiac rupture in acute myocardial infarction: A review of 72 consecutive cases. *Acta Med. Scand.* 205:11, 1979.
68. Bates, R. J., Beutler, S., Resnekov, L., et al. Cardiac rupture—challenge in diagnosis and management. *Am. J. Cardiol.* 40:1231, 1977.
69. O'Rourke, M. F. Subacute heart rupture following myocardial infarction—clinical features of a correctable condition. *Lancet* 2:124, 1973.
70. Knowlton, A. A., Grauer, J., Plehn, J. F., et al. Ventricular pseudoaneurysm: A rare but ominous condition. *Cardiovasc. Rev. Rep.* 6:508, 1985.
71. Catherwood, E., Mintz, G. S., Kotler, M. N., et al. Two dimensional echocardiographic recognition of left ventricular pseudoaneurysm. *Circulation* 62: 294, 1980.
72. Lopez-Martinez, J. I. Pulsatory phenomena in pseudoaneurysm of the heart. *Am. J. Cardiol.* 15:422, 1965.
73. Goldberg, R. J., Gore, J. M., Alpert, J. S., et al. Cardiogenic shock resulting from acute myocardial infarction: A fourteen year community wide perspective. *N. Engl. J. Med.* 325:1117, 1991.
74. Hands, M. E., Rutherford, J. D., Muller, J. E., et al. The in-hospital development of cardiogenic shock after myocardial infarction: Incidence, predictors of occurrence, outcome and prognostic factors. *J. Am. Coll. Cardiol.* 14:40, 1989.
75. Shah, P. K., and Forrester, J. Pathophysiology of acute coronary syndromes. *Am. J. Cardiol.* 68:16c, 1991.
76. Sabia, P. J., Powers, E. R., Ragosta, M., et al. An association between collateral blood flow and myocardial viability in patients with recent myocardial infarction. *N. Engl. J. Med.* 327:1825, 1992.
77. Ramos, R. G., et al. The effect of coronary reperfusion on the survival of patients with cardiogenic shock due to acute myocardial infarction (Abstract). *J. Am. Coll. Cardiol.* 9:233A, 1987.
78. Bengtson, J. R., Kaplan, A. J., Pieper, K. S., et al. Prognosis in cardiogenic shock after acute myocardial infarction in the interventional era. *J. Am. Coll. Cardiol.* 20:1482, 1992.
79. O'Neill, W. W. Angioplasty therapy of cardiogenic shock: Are randomized trials necessary? *J. Am. Coll. Cardiol.* 19:915, 1992.
80. Dewood, M. A., Notske, R. N., Hensley, G. R., et al. Intra-aortic balloon counterpulsation with or without reperfusion for myocardial infarction shock. *Circulation* 61:1105, 1980.

81. Moosvi, A. R., Khaja, F., Villanueva, L., et al. Early revascularization improves survival in cardiogenic shock complicating acute myocardial infarction. *J. Am. Coll. Cardiol.* 19:907, 1992.
82. Bates, E. R., and Topol, E. J. Limitations of thrombolytic therapy for acute myocardial infarction complicated by congestive heart failure and cardiogenic shock. *J. Am. Coll. Cardiol.* 18:1077, 1991.
83. Becker, R. C. Hemodynamic, mechanical, and metabolic determinants of thrombolytic efficacy: A theoretical framework for assessing the limitations of thrombolysis in patients with cardiogenic shock. *Am. Heart J.* 125:919, 1993.
84. Hibbard, M. D., Holmes, D. R., Jr., Bailey, K. R., et al. Percutaneous transluminal coronary angioplasty in patients with cardiogenic shock. *J. Am. Coll. Cardiol.* 19:639, 1992.
85. Ellis, S. G., O'Neill, W. W., Bates, E. R., et al. Implications for triage from survival and left ventricular function recovery analyses in 500 patients treated with coronary angioplasty for acute myocardial infarction. *J. Am. Coll. Cardiol.* 13:1251, 1989.
86. Eckman, M. H., Wong, J. B., Salem, D. N., and Pauker, S. G. Direct angioplasty for acute myocardial infarction. A review of outcomes in clinical subsets. *Ann. Intern. Med.* 117:667, 1992.
87. Klein, L. W. Optimal therapy of cardiogenic shock: The emerging role of coronary angioplasty. *J. Am. Coll. Cardiol.* 19:654, 1992.
88. Mueller, H. S., Cohen, L. S., Braunwald, E., et al. Predictors of early morbidity and mortality after thrombolytic therapy of acute myocardial infarction. Analysis of patient subgroups in the Thrombolysis in Myocardial Infarction (TIMI) Trial Phase II. *Circulation* 85:1254, 1992.
89. Prewitt, R. M., Gu, S., Garber, P. J., and Ducas, J. Marked systemic hypotension depresses coronary thrombolysis induced by intracoronary administration of recombinant tissue plasminogen activator. *J. Am. Coll. Cardiol.,* in press.
90. Overlie, P. A. Emergency use of portable cardiopulmonary bypass. *Cathet. Cardiovasc. Diagn.* 20:27, 1990.
91. Mooney, M. R., Mooney, J. F., Van Tassel, R. A., et al. The Nimbus Hemopump: A new left ventricular assist device that combines myocardial protection with circulatory support. *J. Invasive Cardiol.* 2: 169, 1990.
92. Moritz, A., and Wolner, E. Circulatory support with shock due to acute myocardial infarction. *Ann. Thorac. Surg.* 55:238, 1993.
93. Shah, P. K. New insights into the electrocardiogram of acute myocardial infarction. In B. Gersh and S. Rahimtoola (eds.), *Acute Myocardial Infarction.* New York: Elsevier, 1990.
94. Zehender, M., Kasper, W., Kauder, E., et al. Right ventricular infarction as an independent predictor of prognosis after acute inferior myocardial infarction. *N. Engl. J. Med.* 328:981, 1993.
95. Lavie, C. J., and Gersh, B. J. Mechanical and electrical complications of acute myocardial infarction. *Mayo Clin. Proc.* 65:709, 1990.
96. Maurer, G., Czer, L. S. C., Shah, P. K., and Chaux, A. Assessment by Doppler color flow mapping of ventricular septal defect after acute myocardial infarction. *Am. J. Cardiol.* 64:668, 1989.
97. Smyllie, J. H., Sutherland, G. R., Geuskens, R., et al. Doppler color flow mapping in the diagnosis of ventricular septal rupture and acute mitral regurgitation after acute myocardial infarction. *J. Am. Coll. Cardiol.* 15:1449, 1990.
98. Takahishi, S., Barry, A. C., and Factor, S. M. Collagen degradation in ischemic rat hearts. *Biochem. J.* 265:233, 1990.
99. Peuhkurinen, K. J., Risteli, L., Melkko, J. T., et al. Thrombolytic therapy with streptokinase stimulates collagen breakdown. *Circulation* 83:1969, 1991.
100. Honan, M. B., Harrell, F. E., Reimer, K. A., et al. Cardiac rupture, mortality and the timing of thrombolytic therapy: A meta-analysis. *J. Am. Coll. Cardiol.* 16:359, 1990.
101. Nakamura, F., Minamino, T., Highashino, Y., et al. Cardiac free wall rupture in acute myocardial infarction: Ameliorative effect of coronary reperfusion. *Clin. Cardiol.* 15:244, 1992.
102. ISIS-3: A randomized comparison of streptokinase vs tissue plasminogen activator vs anistreplase and of aspirin plus heparin vs aspirin alone among 41,299 cases of suspected acute myocardial infarction. *Lancet* 339:753, 1992.
103. Lopez-Sendon, J., Gonzalez, A., De Sa, E. L., et al. Diagnosis of subacute ventricular rupture after acute myocardial infarction: Sensitivity and specificity of clinical, hemodynamic and echocardiographic criteria. *J. Am. Coll. Cardiol.* 19:1145, 1992.
104. Pollak, H., Diez, W., Spiel, R., et al. Early diagnosis of subacute free wall rupture complicating acute myocardial infarction. *Eur. Heart J.* 14:640, 1993.
105. Bateman, T. M., Czer, L. S. C., Gray, R. J., et al. Detection of occult pericardial hemorrhage early after open-heart surgery using technetium-99m red blood cell radionuclide ventriculography. *Am. Heart J.* 108:1198, 1984.
106. Leor, J., Hod, H., Kaplinsky, E., et al. Pseudoakinesis: A radionuclide ventriculography sign for subacute heart rupture and tamponade early after acute myocardial infarction. *Am. Heart J.* 118: 612, 1988.
107. Hoit, B. D., Gabel, M., and Fowler, N. O. Hemodynamic efficacy of rapid saline infusion and dobutamine versus saline infusion alone in a model of cardiac rupture. *J. Am. Coll. Cardiol.* 16:1745, 1990.
108. Beyersdorf, F., Sarai, K., Maul, F. D., et al. Immediate functional benefits after controlled reperfusion during surgical revascularization for acute coronary occlusion. *J. Thorac. Cardiovasc. Surg.* 102:856, 1991.
109. Beyersdorf, F., and Buckberg, G. D. Myocardial

protection in patients with acute myocardial infarction and cardiogenic shock. *Semin. Thorac. Cardiovasc. Surg.* 5:151, 1993.

110. Neuhaus, K. L., Von Essen, R., Tebbe, U., et al. Improved thrombolysis in acute myocardial infarction with front-loaded administration of alteplase. Results of the rt-PA APSAC Patency Study (TAPS). *J. Am. Coll. Cardiol.* 19:885, 1992.
111. Jugdutt, B. I. Intravenous nitroglycerin unloading in acute myocardial infarction. *Am. J. Cardiol.* 18:52D, 1991.
112. Pfeffer, M., Lamas, G. A., Vaughn, D. E., et al. Effect of captopril on progressive ventricular dilation after anterior myocardial infarction. *N. Engl. J. Med.* 319:80, 1988.
113. Pfeffer, M. A., Braunwald, E., Moye, L. A., et al. Effect of captopril on mortality and morbidity in patients with left ventricular dysfunction after myocardial infarction. *N. Engl. J. Med.* 327:669, 1992.
114. Leor, J., Goldbourt, U., Reicher-Reiss, H., et al. Cardiogenic shock complicating acute myocardial infarction in patients without heart failure on admission. *Am. J. Med.* 94:265, 1993.

17. Left Ventricular Remodeling Following Acute Myocardial Infarction

Edward J. Brown, Jr., and Marc A. Pfeffer

Advances in the treatment of acute myocardial infarction have resulted in a decline in both morbidity and mortality over the past 30 years. Establishment of coronary care units with prompt use of cardiac defibrillators to interrupt life-threatening arrhythmias produced the initial decrease in mortality. An understanding of the determinants of myocardial oxygen demand has resulted in hemodynamic monitoring and therapies designed to reduce the size of the myocardial infarct, and the implementation of pharmacologic and direct measures to acutely restore coronary blood flow has resulted in further improvements in survival for patients with acute myocardial infarctions. Survivors of the acute phase of myocardial infarctions also have benefited from the use of beta-blocking drugs that reduce death and recurrent myocardial infarction, and the use of coronary angioplasty and surgery for revascularization. Further long-term improvements in survival now appear possible with aggressive control of risk factors, with the potential that significant regression or stabilization of atherosclerotic lesions in coronary arteries may become a clinical reality.

Despite improved survival, left ventricular dysfunction continues to be a problem for survivors of acute myocardial infarctions, and congestive heart failure leads to death and disability for many survivors of acute myocardial infarctions. Until recently, efforts to prevent left ventricular dysfunction have focused on reduction of infarct size and prevention of recurrent myocardial infarctions. Efforts to reduce infarct size are effective but must be instituted within a few hours after the onset of acute infarction.

During the past 15 years an understanding of left ventricular remodeling has provided physicians with additional opportunities to prevent further deterioration in left ventricular function in survivors of acute myocardial infarctions [1]. Left ventricular remodeling refers to an enlargement of the cardiac chamber provoked by alterations in both infarcted and noninfarcted myocardium that can lead to a progressive deterioration in left ventricular function and increased mortality and morbidity for survivors of acute myocardial infarctions. Therapies to prevent or attenuate left ventricular remodeling in both the early and the late phases of acute myocardial infarction can improve left ventricular function and long-term clinical outcome (Tables 17-1, 17-2).

Left Ventricular Remodeling: Early Postinfarction Phase

Following coronary artery occlusion, necrotic myocardium is malleable, and remodeling can result in infarct expansion, a thinning and dilation of infarcted myocardium [2]. Infarct expansion can occur over a period of days, but gradually necrotic tissue is replaced with collagen that renders the infarct resistant to further changes in shape. Infarct expansion occurs most commonly after large transmural infarctions, particularly those involving the anteroapical region of the heart. Infarct expansion has been associated with a higher incidence of congestive heart failure, aneurysm formation, cardiac rupture, and increased mortality. Perhaps the most easily overlooked problem associated with infarct expansion is the increase in left ventricular volume that accompanies the expansion of an infarct. Large infarcts that expand can result in left ventricular

Table 17-1
Early postinfarction left ventricular (LV) remodeling

- A. Promote early LV remodeling
  1. Anti-inflammatory agents
     - a. Glucocorticoids
     - b. Ibuprofen
     - c. Indomethacin
  2. Hypertension
  3. Transmural infarction
  4. Anteroapical infarct location
  5. ? Exercise
- B. Prevent or attenutate early LV remodeling
  1. Coronary artery reperfusion
  2. ? Angiotensin-converting enzyme inhibitors
  3. Nitrates

Table 17-2
Late postinfarction left ventricular (LV) remodeling

- A. Promote late LV remodeling
  1. Extensive myocardial damage
  2. ? Exercise
- B. Prevent or attenuate late LV remodeling
  1. Angiotensin-converting enzyme inhibitors
  2. Milrinone (experimental infarctions)

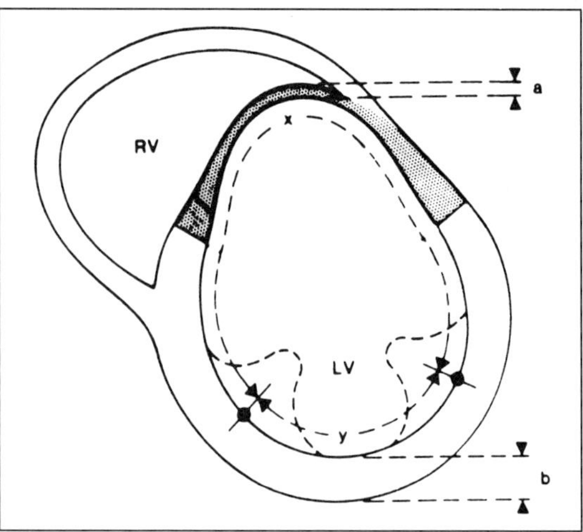

Fig. 17-1
Diagram of two-dimensional cross-sectional echocardiographic view of the left ventricle at the midpapillary muscle level. This view is used to identify the presence and extent of infarct expansion, which is a thinning and dilation of the infarct. The extent of infarct thinning (a) is expressed as a percent of the noninfarcted wall thickness (b). The extent of infarct dilation (x) is expressed as a percent of the noninfarcted segment length (y). The papillary muscles are used to separate the infarcted segment (x) and the noninfarcted segment (y). (From B. I. Jugdutt and B. L. Michorowski. *Clin. Cardiol.* 10:641, 1987. With permission.)

volumes that are 25 to 40 percent larger than volumes associated with similar-sized infarcts that do not expand [3]. Increased left ventricular volume increases wall stress and myocardial oxygen consumption, and can lead to subsequent congestive heart failure, angina, and death.

The premortem clinical diagnosis of infarct expansion can be made by noninvasive (two-dimensional echocardiography or magnetic resonance imaging) or left ventricular angiographic demonstration of left ventricular distortion due to elongation and thinning of the noncontractile infarcted segment in the absence of enzyme evidence of further myocardial necrosis [4]. This is to be distinguished from further distortion of the infarcted myocardium due to extension of the infarct. As shown in Figure 17-1, a short-axis two-dimensional echocardiogram at the papillary muscle level is used to determine anterior and posterior segments. Expansion is considered present when the length of the segment containing the infarct exceeds the length in normal subjects [5].

Pathophysiologic Observations

Histologic examination of expanded infarcts has revealed that thinning of the infarcted region is a consequence of slippage between muscle bundles, resulting in a reduction in the number of myocytes across the infarcted region [6]. During the course of healing, connective tissue cells enter the myocyte compartment and connect disrupted myocyte fibers, providing resistance to further stretching.

Anti-inflammatory Agents

Although the mechanism of infarct expansion is not well understood, several clinically important observations have been made. Some anti-inflammatory agents promote infarct expansion [7]. In experimental rat and dog myocardial infarctions, glucocorticoids, indomethacin, and ibuprofen promoted infarct expansion. Chronic administration of these agents is not necessary, and even a single day of treatment at the time of the acute infarction can result in expanded infarcts when hearts are examined several days to weeks later. Retrospective analyses of patients who died due to myocardial rupture after infarction demonstrated an association between rupture and treatment with anti-inflammatory agents [8, 9]. The relatively common past practice to use indomethacin and glucocorticoids to treat postinfarction pericarditis (Dressler's syndrome) may have inadvertently contributed to the process of infarct expansion. For unexplained reasons, other agents with anti-inflammatory properties have no effect on infarct shape. Heparin, aspirin, and superoxide dismutase are three agents with anti-inflammatory properties that do not promote infarct expansion. A report by Jugdutt and Basualdo [10] highlighted the clinical importance of these experimental findings. Patients receiving either indomethacin or ibuprofen during an acute myocardial infarction had a greater degree of infarct expansion than did a similar group of patients not receiving these agents. The patients treated with indomethacin had a higher incidence of aneurysm formation and congestive heart failure during the follow-up. Although more definitive randomized trials have not been performed, agents that interfere with scar formation and wound healing should be avoided in the early phase of acute myocardial infarction.

Nitrates

In a small randomized trial of nitroglycerin versus placebo, intravenous nitroglycerin was administered within 2 hours after an acute myocardial infarction and continued for 48 hours [11]. Echocardiography was used to measure infarct expansion at baseline, and then 3 and 10 days after infarction. Titrated nitroglycerin therapy limited the expansion of both anterior and inferior infarcts. In another clinical trial, intravenous nitroglycerin plus intra-aortic balloon counterpulsation or pumping (IABP) was compared to conventional therapy during the acute phase of myocardial infarctions [12]. Patients treated with nitroglycerin and IABP had less infarct expansion than did patients treated conventionally. Although judicious use of nitroglycerin was associated with less infarct expansion in the above-mentioned trials, two large prospective trials [13, 14] failed to demonstrate any beneficial effect on survival in a broad population with acute myocardial infarction. The Gruppo Italiano per lo Studio della Sopravvivenza nell'Infarto Miocardico (GISSI-3) trial compared placebo to nitrate therapy in patients with acute myocardial infarctions [13]. Patients in the treated group received a 24-hour infusion of nitroglycerin started within the first 24 hours after myocardial infarction followed by a 12-hr/day transdermal nitrate treatment for 6 weeks. Nitrate therapy had no effect on survival or on left ventricular function assessed 6 weeks after myocardial infarction. The ISIS-4 trial also failed to demonstrate a survival benefit when nitrate therapy was started in the early postinfarction period [14]. While it is possible that benefits on infarct remodeling do not manifest as improved survival as early as 6 weeks after myocardial infarction, the results of this large trial suggest that routine nitrate therapy is not necessary for asymptomatic patients in the early postinfarction period.

Exercise

Exercise will transiently increase wall stress and can produce eccentric ventricular hypertrophy with a proportional increase in both mass and volume in rats with normal hearts. In studies of recently infarcted rats, exercise altered infarct healing and caused infarct thinning [15, 16]. One other study, however, found no adverse effects of postinfarct exercise on infarct remodeling [17]. Although there has been a trend toward shorter hospital stays for patients with acute myocardial infarctions, it would still seem prudent to restrict activities, especially in patients with large transmural myocardial infarctions, for the first few postinfarction weeks until the infarct is healed and resistant to remodeling.

Thrombolytic Therapy

Coronary artery reperfusion performed early after the onset of coronary occlusion will reduce infarct size and improve regional and global left ventricular function. However, the 18 to 47 percent reductions in mortality observed in patients randomized to receive thrombolytic therapy seem too large to be explained by the modest improvements in global ejection fraction that have been associated with the use of thrombolytic therapy. Restoration of coronary blood flow early enough to salvage ischemic myocardium will also reduce the extent of infarct expansion. Reperfusion too late to salvage myocytes still has a favorable effect by continuing to modify infarct expansion [18]. Touchstone et al. [19] demonstrated an increased risk of infarct expansion in patients in whom thrombolytic therapy was unsuccessful and infarct regions were supplied by totally occluded coronary arteries. Using quantitative ventriculography, two studies demonstrated that patients receiving thrombolytic therapy had smaller ventricular volumes than did comparable patients with acute infarcts not receiving thrombolytic therapy [20, 21]. A cohort in the GISSI trial followed by echocardiographic assessment of ventricular volumes demonstrated that thrombolytic therapy was associated with reduced ventricular volume both before discharge and 6 months after myocardial infarction [22]. Some of the benefits of reperfusion on survival, particularly when reperfusion is accomplished more than 6 hours after the onset of acute myocardial infarction, may be attributed to a reduction in ventricular remodeling.

Reperfusion early enough after infarction to decrease infarct size salvages a rim of epicardium and reduces the fraction of the infarct that is transmural. The viable subepicardium may act as a buttress to support underlying necrotic myocardium and prevent infarct expansion. The mechanism by which reperfusion too late to decrease infarct size reduces infarct expansion is unclear. Perhaps the restored blood flow acts as a scaffolding to support the necrotic infarct, thereby preventing infarct expansion. Another possibility supported by recent experimental evidence suggests that even late reperfusion salvages islets of subepicardial myocytes. Although insufficient in number to decrease the measurement of overall infarct size, the islets of viable cells may buttress the underlying necrotic myocardium and prevent infarct expansion [23].

Hypertension

Hypertension induced by methoxamine 1 to 5 hours after experimental canine myocardial infarction has occurred has a long-term adverse effect by promoting infarct expansion [24]. In experimental rat myocardial infarctions, chronic hypertension produced by aortic banding also increases the extent of infarct expansion [25]. In patients, higher arterial pressure was associated with a greater risk of infarct expansion [26]. The observation that prevention of hypertension during the acute infarction period is associated with clinical benefits [27] may in part be related to prevention of infarct expansion.

Angiotensin-Converting Enzyme Inhibitors

The effect of angiotensin-converting enzyme (ACE) inhibitor therapy on infarct expansion is not clear. However, because hypertension promotes infarct expansion, it is likely that the hypotensive effects of ACE inhibitor therapy will have a beneficial effect on infarct remodeling when it is administered during the acute postinfarction period. Sharpe et al. [28] demonstrated that captopril started orally 24 to 48 hours after acute infarction prevented left ventricular dilation over a 3-month follow-up period. The beneficial effect on ventricular dilation appeared to be greater than benefits from ACE inhibitor therapy started more than 1 week after acute infarction. A large randomized trial demonstrated that early postinfarction captopril treatment improves survival [14]. Whether early ACE therapy improves clinical outcome by decreasing infarct expansion remains unknown.

Left Ventricular Remodeling: Late Postinfarction Phase

Compensatory Postinfarction Left Ventricular Dilation

Loss of functioning myocardium as the result of acute infarction results in a decline in global ejection fraction and cardiac performance. Compensatory mechanisms are activated to maintain stroke volume as ejection fraction declines. Acute left ventricular distention activates the Frank-Starling mechanism, which together with increased adrenergic activity increases heart rate and contractility, and serves to maintain cardiac performance. However, this distention, or enlargement of the cavity as a consequence of increased filling pressure, also augments the wall stress. This increase in wall stress provides the stimulus for myocyte hypertrophy, which serves to return wall stress levels to normal, thereby reducing the stimulus for further left ventricular enlargement. In some instances the initial loss of myocardium can initiate an adequate compensation with minimal chamber enlargement and concomitant fiber hypertrophy.

Pathologic Postinfarction Left Ventricular Dilation

Although left ventricular hypertrophy can often offset the increase in wall stress following acute infarctions, ventricular dilation with large insults may exceed the potential to increase left ventricular mass. When hypertrophy is inadequate to compensate for the loss of myocytes, the increased wall stress continues to stimulate further left ventricular dilation that goes beyond that necessary to maintain stroke volume [29]. A vicious cycle is thereby created in which left ventricular dilation progressively increases wall stress, which opposes contraction and stimulates even further increases in left ventricular cavity size. The balance between cavity dilation and maintenance of cardiac function is upset and progressive left ventricular dilation becomes a pathologic process.

Histologic healing of a myocardial infarction in humans occurs in 8 to 10 weeks. By this time, the infarcted area becomes more resistant to further deformation. However, global left ventricular remodeling continues, and changes in noninfarcted myocardium can cause progressive left ventricular dilation and further deterioration in left ventricular function. Data from the Framingham Study demonstrate that the incidence of clinically apparent congestive heart failure increases with time after a myocardial infarction [30]. While 5 percent of acute infarct survivors developed congestive heart failure in the first year after infarction, this number increased to 22 percent by 10 years after infarction. Although in some patients congestive heart failure may have been due to recurrent infarctions and further loss of viable myocardium, left ventricular remodeling was probably an important contributor to the increasing incidence of late congestive heart failure.

In experimentally induced myocardial infarctions, the extent of left ventricular enlargement was related not only to infarct size, but also to the duration of time after the infarction [31]. Measurements of pressure-volume relationships showed that for similar end-diastolic pressures, left ventricular volume progressively increased over time (Fig. 17-2). This late volume increase was not due to left ventricular distention, but rather to structural changes in both viable as well as infarcted areas of myocardium.

Similar progressive increases in volume have been recorded in patients with the use of echocardiography, radionuclide ventriculography, or angiography to measure serial changes in left ventricular volume. Progressive volume increases to 20 to 40 percent were recorded after 1 year in patients who had large myocardial infarctions that resulted in depressed left ventricular ejection fractions. Techniques for measuring left ventricular volumes are not readily available in clinical practice, and it is understandable that such large increases in left ventricular volume were often undetected in the past. Unless specifically examined for, progressive left ventricular dilation can go unrecognized until associated with a deteriorating clinical status.

Ventricular Enlargement and Prognosis

Roentgenographic evidence of cardiac enlargement after a myocardial infarction is associated with reduced survival. Kostuk et al. [32] reported a threefold increase in mortality (24 versus 8 percent) for survivors of myocardial infarction developing cardiac enlargement as compared to those maintaining a normal silhouette. At almost 1 year of follow-up, 32 percent of the patients with an enlarged heart, but only 2 percent of the patients with a normal-sized heart manifested New York Heart Association class III symptoms of either congestive heart failure or angina. Studies using left ventriculography, which is a more sensitive means of detecting left ventricular enlargement, observed that increases in left ventricular volume predict a poor prognosis, even when the overall heart size appears normal on plain chest roentgenography [33, 34].

Modification of Left Ventricular Enlargement

A likely explanation for the progressive increase in left ventricular volume is that the initial loss of functioning myocardium during the infarction increases wall stress. Wall stress stimulates further

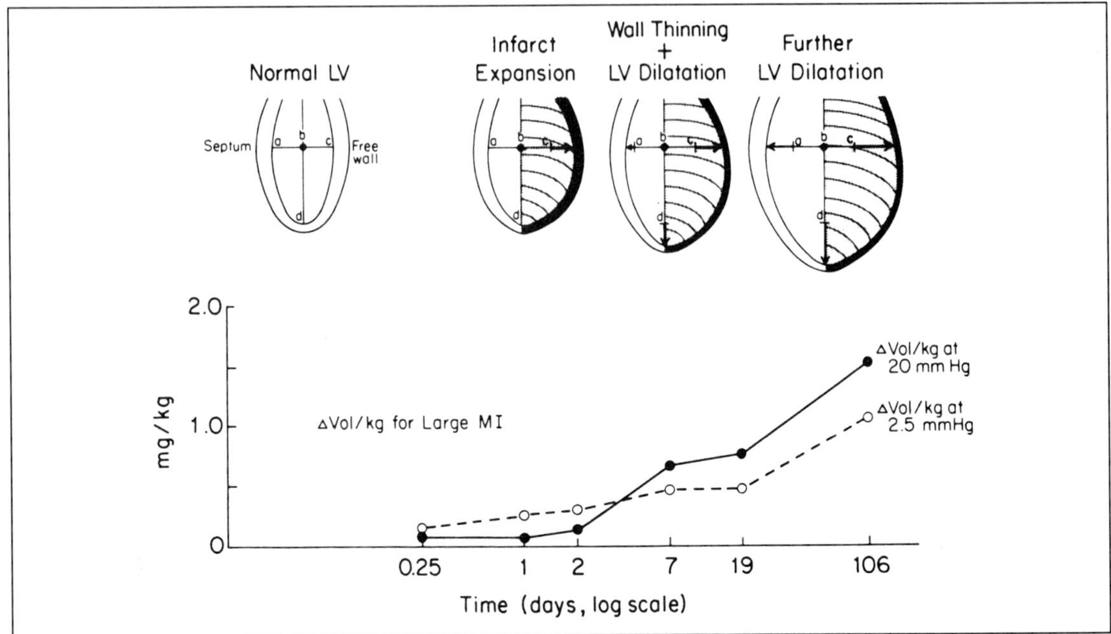

Fig. 17-2
Schematic representing left ventricular remodeling during the early postinfarction phase and during the late postinfarction phase following an experimental rat myocardial infarction. During the first few days after infarction, the infarcted area (*darkly shaded*) thins and expands, resulting in an increase in left ventricular volume. Healing of the infarct into a collagenized scar restricts further change in infarct shape. Over the following weeks to months, further increases in left ventricular volume occur as the result of structural changes in the noninfarcted myocardium. (From J. M. Pfeffer. *Am. J. Cardiol.* 68:17D, 1991. With permission.)

increases in left ventricular volume, which result in yet further increases in wall stress. This hypothesis was tested in rats undergoing myocardial infarction by left coronary artery ligation [31]. Wall stress was reduced by administering captopril, an agent that reduces wall stress by decreasing both preload and afterload. After 3 months of treatment, left ventricular volume in the captopril-treated rats was smaller than volumes in nontreated rats.

The observations concerning the benefits of ACE inhibitor therapy in rats have been extended to patients. Left ventricular volume was measured after myocardial infarction and again 1 year later in patients with moderate-sized to large infarctions [35]. In patients treated with captopril beginning 12 to 31 days after infarction, left ventricular volume remained unchanged for the 1-year follow-up period, while patients in a placebo control group experienced a 23 percent increase in left ventricular volume.

The clinical importance of these mechanistic observations was tested in the Survival and Ventricular Enlargement (SAVE) study [36]. More than 2000 patients with acute myocardial infarctions and left ventricular ejection fractions of at least 40 percent were randomly assigned to receive either captopril or placebo 3 to 16 days after myocardial infarction. At the end of a 3$^1/_2$-year follow-up period, captopril-treated patients experienced reduced mortality, and fewer developed congestive heart failure. The reduction in mortality and morbidity that accompanied captopril therapy was additive to the benefits of beta blockers, aspirin, and thrombolytic therapy. An echocardiographic substudy demonstrated an association between an adverse clinical outcome and progressive left ventricular dilation [37]. An increase in left ventricular volume was a strong predictor of cardiovascular mortality and adverse cardiovascular events. An attenuation in ventricular enlargement in patients treated with captopril was associated with a decrease in adverse clinical events. This new use of therapy with captopril provides further opportunity to improve the outcome for selected patients with acute myocardial infarctions.

Remodeling of noninfarcted myocardium resulting in progressive left ventricular dilation may not be confined to patients with recent myocardial infarctions. The Studies of Left Ventricular Dysfunction (SOLVD) randomized patients with depressed left ventricular function (left ventricular ejection fraction ≤ 35 percent) of all causes to receive enalapril or placebo [38]. Although 30 percent of the patients in this trial had left ventricular dysfunction due to causes other than coronary artery disease, and none had a recent myocardial infarction, a substudy of quantitative radionuclide ventriculography to measure changes in left ventricular volume demonstrated a time-related increase in ventricular volume in the placebo group, while patients treated with enalapril had no such increase [39]. Thus, progressive left ventricular dilation should be viewed as a chronic modifiable process that is not only confined to patients with recent myocardial infarctions.

Exercise may have an adverse effect on remodeling of noninfarcted myocardium in some patients. Jugdutt et al. [40] demonstrated that exercise started 15 weeks after infarction and continued for 12 weeks in patients with large anterior Q-wave infarctions had an adverse effect. Exercised patients had echocardiographic evidence of deterioration in ventricular function and further deterioration of the infarct region topography with an increase in the extent of infarct expansion and infarct thinning. While these results need to be confirmed in a larger group of patients, they do raise a cautionary note that although exercise after infarction is generally well tolerated, the potential to adversely affect ventricular function exists, particularly in patients with extensive infarctions.

References

1. Pfeffer, M. A., and Braunwald, E. Ventricular remodeling after myocardial infarction. Experimental observations and clinical implications. *Circulation* 81:1161, 1990.
2. Hutchins, G. M., and Bulkley, B. H. Infarct expansion versus extension: Two different complications of acute myocardial infarction. *Am. J. Cardiol.* 41: 1127, 1978.
3. Brown, E. J., Jr., Swinford, R. D., Gadde, P., and Lillis, O. Acute effects of delayed reperfusion on infarct shape and left ventricular volume. A potential mechanism of additional benefits from thrombolytic therapy. *J. Am. Coll. Cardiol.* 17:1641, 1991.
4. Eaton, L. W., Weiss, J. L., Bulkley, B. H., et al. Regional cardiac dilatation after acute myocardial infarction. *N. Engl. J. Med.* 300:57, 1979.
5. Weiss, J. L., Bulkley, B. H., Hutchins, G. R., and Mason, S. J. Two-dimensional echocardiographic recognition of myocardial injury in man: Comparison with post mortem studies. *Circulation* 63:401, 1981.
6. Weisman, H. F., Bush, D. E., Mannisi, J. A., et al. Cellular mechanisms in myocardial infarct expansion. *Circulation* 78:186, 1988.
7. Hammerman, H., Schoen, F. J., Braunwald, E., and Kloner, R. A. Drug-induced expansion of infarct: Morphologic and functional correlations. *Circulation* 69:611, 1984.
8. Bowden, W. E., and Sadaniantz, A. Ventricular septal rupture during ibuprofen therapy for pericarditis after acute myocardial infarction. *Am. J. Cardiol.* 55:1631, 1985.
9. Silverman, H. S., and Pfeffer, M. A. Relation between use of antiinflammatory agents and left ventricular free wall rupture during acute myocardial infarction. *Am. J. Cardiol.* 59:303, 1987.
10. Jugdutt, B. I., and Basualdo, C. A. Myocardial infarct expansion during indomethacin or ibuprofen therapy for symptomatic postinfarction pericarditis: Influence of other pharmacologic agents during remodeling. *Can. J. Cardiol.* 5:211, 1989.
11. Jugdutt, B. I., and Warnica, J. W. Intravenous nitroglycerin therapy to limit myocardial infarct size, expansion and complications: Effect of timing, dosage, and infarct location. *Circulation* 78:906, 1988.
12. Flahrty, J. T., Becker, L. C., Weiss, J. L., et al. Results of a randomized prospective trial of intraaortic balloon counterpulsation and intravenous nitroglycerin in patients with acute myocardial infarction. *J. Am. Coll. Cardiol.* 6:434, 1985.
13. Gruppo Italiano per lo Studio della Sopravvivenza nell'Infarto Miocardico. GISSI-3: Effects of lisinopril and transdermal glyceryl trinitrate singly and together on 6-week mortality and ventricular function after acute myocardial infarction. *Lancet* 343: 1115, 1994.
14. Collins, R., on behalf of the ISIS-4 Collaborative Group. Captopril, oral mononitrate and magnesium in acute myocardial infarction. Presented at the American Heart Association 66th Scientific Sessions, November 8–11, 1993. Atlanta, GA.
15. Kloner, R. A., and Kloner, J. A. The effects of early exercise on myocardial infarct scar formation. *Am. Heart J.* 106:1009, 1983.

16. Hammerman, H., Schoen, F. J., and Kloner, R. A. Short-term exercise has a prolonged effect on scar formation after experimental acute myocardial infarction. *J. Am. Coll. Cardiol.* 7:979, 1983.
17. Hochman, J. S., and Healy, B. Effect of exercise on acute myocardial infarction in rats. *J. Am. Coll. Cardiol.* 7:126, 1986.
18. Hochman, J. S., and Choo, H. Limitation of myocardial infarct expansion by reperfusion independent of myocardial salvage. *Circulation* 75:299, 1987.
19. Touchstone, D. A., Beller, G. A., Nygaard, T. W., et al. Effects of successful intravenous reperfusion therapy on regional myocardial function and geometry in humans. A tomographic assessment using two-dimensional echocardiography. *J. Am. Coll. Cardiol.* 13:1506, 1989.
20. Hirai, T., Fujita, M., Nakajima, H., et al. Importance of collateral circulation for prevention of left ventricular aneurysm formation in acute myocardial infarction. *Circulation* 79:791, 1989.
21. Jeremy, R. W., Hackworthy, R. A., Bautovich, G., et al. Infarct artery perfusion and changes in left ventricular volume in the month after acute myocardial infarction. *J. Am. Coll. Cardiol.* 9:989, 1987.
22. Marino, P., Zanolla, L., Zardini, P., on behalf of GISSI. Effect of streptokinase on left ventricular modeling and function after myocardial infarction: The GISSI (Gruppo Italiano per lo Studio della Streptochinaisi nell'Infarto Miocardico) Trial. *J. Am. Coll. Cardiol.* 14:1149, 1989.
23. Alhaddad, I. A., Hakim, I., Garno, J. L., et al. Benefits of late coronary artery reperfusion on infarct expansion evolve as a wave-front over time. *J. Am. Coll. Cardiol.* 21:301A, 1993.
24. Hammerman, H., Kloner, R. A., Alker, K. J., et al. Effects of transient increased afterload during experimentally induced acute myocardial infarction in dogs. *Am. J. Cardiol.* 55:566, 1985.
25. Nolan, S. E., Mannisi, J. A., Bush, D. E., et al. Increased afterload aggravates infarct expansion after acute myocardial infarction. *J. Am. Coll. Cardiol.* 12:1318, 1988.
26. Pierard, L. A., Albert, A., Gillis, F., et al. Hemodynamic profile of patients with acute myocardial infarction at risk of infarct expansion. *Am. J. Cardiol.* 60:5, 1987.
27. Shell, W. E., and Sobel, B. E. Protection of jeopardized ischemic myocardium by reduction of ventricular afterload. *N. Engl. J. Med.* 291:481, 1974.
28. Sharpe, D. N., Smith, H., Murphy, J., et al. Early prevention of left ventricular dysfunction following myocardial infarction with angiotensin converting enzyme inhibition. *Lancet* 337:872, 1991.
29. Ross, J., Jr. Afterload mismatch and preload reserve: A conceptual framework for the analysis of ventricular function. *Prog. Cardiovasc. Dis.* 18:255, 1976.
30. Kamel, W. B., Sorlie, P., and McNamara, P. M. Prognosis after initial myocardial infarction: The Framingham Study. *Am. J. Cardiol.* 44:53, 1979.
31. Pfeffer, J. M., Pfeffer, J. M., and Braunwald, E. Influence of chronic captopril therapy on the infarcted left ventricle of the rat. *Cir. Res.* 57:84, 1985.
32. Kostuk, W. J., Kazamias, T. M., Gander, M. P., et al. Left ventricular size after acute myocardial infarction: Serial changes and their prognostic significance. *Circulation* 47:1174, 1973.
33. White, H. D., Norris, R. M., Brown, M. A., et al. Left ventricular end-diastolic volume as the major determinant of survival after recovery from myocardial infarction. *Circulation* 76:44, 1987.
34. Hammermeister, K. E., DeRouen, T. A., and Dodge, H. T. Variables predictive of survival in patients with coronary disease: Selection by univariate and multivariate analyses from the clinical, electrocardiographic, exercise, arteriographic, and quantitative angiographic evaluations. *Circulation* 59:421, 1979.
35. Pfeffer, M. A., Lamus, G. A., Vaughan, D. E., et al. Effect of captopril on progressive ventricular dilatation after anterior myocardial infarction. *N. Engl. J. Med.* 319:80, 1988.
36. Pfeffer, M. A., Braunwald, E., Moye, L. A., et al. Effect of captopril on mortality and morbidity in patients with left ventricular dysfunction after myocardial infarction. *N. Engl. J. Med.* 327:669, 1992.
37. St. John Sutton, M., Pfeffer, M. A., Plappert, T., et al., for the SAVE Investigators. Quantitative two-dimensional echocardiographic measurements are major predictors of adverse cardiovascular events after acute myocardial infarction. The protective effects of captopril. *Circulation* 89:68, 1994.
38. The SOLVD Investigators. Effect of angiotensin converting enzyme inhibition with enalapril on survival in patients with reduced left ventricular ejection fraction and congestive heart failure: Results of the Treatment Trial of the Studies of Left Ventricular Dysfunction (SOLVD): A randomized double blind trial. *N. Engl. J. Med.* 325:293, 1991.
39. Konstam, M. A., Rousseau, M. F., Kronenberg, M. W., et al. for the SOLVD Investigators. Effects of the angiotensin converting enzyme inhibitor enalapril on the long-term progression of left ventricular dysfunction in patients with heart failure. *Circulation* 86:431, 1992.
40. Jugdutt, B. I., Michowski, B. L., and Kappagoda, C. T. Exercise training after anterior Q wave myocardial infarction: Importance of regional left ventricular function and topography. *J. Am. Coll. Cardiol.* 12:362, 1988.

18. Pericardial Complications of Myocardial Infarction

David H. Spodick

The pericardium, the nearest neighbor of the heart, participates directly or indirectly in many cardiac lesions and cardiac responses to physiologic, pharmacologic, and metabolic challenges [1] (Table 18-1). These are due in part to the immediate proximity of the pericardial sac, by direct anatomic involvement or by pericardial constraint of the heart [2]. The latter, a function of the parietal pericardium, begins to proceed after anything more than minimal cardiac dilation or individual chamber enlargement due to injury or to circulatory volume overload [3]. Thus there is an increasingly recognized pericardial role in ventricular failure, acute valvular regurgitation, and rapid chamber enlargement, as, for example, acute right ventricular myocardial infarction [4]. These entities sometimes raise problems in the differential diagnosis from primarily pericardial disease.

The pericardial tissue responses to all the foregoing include irritative, inflammatory, transudative, and immunopathic reactions [40] and healing, that is, pericardial scarring [5], individually and in combinations. It must be emphasized, first, as with most disease, data obtained at necropsy differ from clinical and laboratory (e.g., imaging) results obtained during life, and second, that the differences are exaggerated as these types of data are temporarily separated.

Acute Fibrinous "Pericarditis" (*Pericarditis Epistenocardiaca*)

Forty percent of patients who die during acute myocardial infarction show fibrinous exudation into the pericardial sac [6]. Although this response is classically known as epistenocardiac pericarditis [7], it appears to be irritative rather than inflammatory, as no separate leukocytic response necessarily accompanies it—hence the term "pericarditis" [8]. An important datum here is that every patient with fresh infarct-associated pericarditis [9] has an *anatomically* transmural infarct [6]. ("Anatomically" is stressed here because the electrocardiogram is incapable of detecting infarct transmurality with certainty [10].) Thus although transmural infarction need not be a homogeneously necrotic block of tissue, at least the apex of the infarcted "pyramid" must extend into the epicardial muscle layers and involve the visceral pericardium to account for the production of fibrin at that point, which is also the site of any future pericardial scarring or adhesion. Smaller amounts of fibrinous exudate remain localized, whereas larger amounts are spread throughout the pericardial cavity by the action of the heart. Heart size appears to be unrelated to the occurrence of epistenocardiac pericarditis [11].

Clinical Characteristics

Epistenocardiac pericarditis appears most often to be clinically silent—without subjective or objective manifestations. Pain is probably the most frequent manifestation, but unfortunately can be firmly ascribed to pericardial involvement only if a pericardial rub is discovered [9]. However, the characteristics of the pain are such that the inference of pericardial involvement can be strong. The most common pain is precordial or substernal and is pleuritic, increased by breathing, body movement, and usually recumbency, all of which tend to distinguish it from renewed ischemic pain.

The only pain quasi-pathognomonic of pericardial injury is that which is perceived in one (usually

Table 18-1
Pericardial complications of myocardial infarction

Fibrinous "pericarditis" (*pericarditis epistenocardiaca*)
Intrapericardial bleeding
Pericardial effusion
Noncompressing
Acute: transudative or exudative
Chronic
Compressing: cardiac tamponade
Recurrent acute pericarditis (postmyocardial infarction syndrome)
Clinically "dry"
Effusive
Constrictive
Pericardial scarring
Epistenocardiac adhesions
Constrictive pericarditis
Effusive-constrictive pericarditis
Pseudoaneurysm

the left) or both *trapezius ridges,* either in association with chest pain or by itself [7]. It is important to have the patient point to the area of involvement because he or she (or the physician) usually describes it as "shoulder" pain. Shoulder pain also occurs with pericarditis, which indeed can have all the areas of reference and radiation of anginal pain [7]; anginal pain, however, is not referred to the trapezius ridge.

On a scale of one to ten, the pain of epistenocardiac pericarditis is commonly rated between one and five, though occasionally it can be as much as ten; such cases may represent an early Dressler's syndrome (post–myocardial infarction); in some patients it is more distressing than the pain of their myocardial infarction. The mildest pain may not evoke spontaneous complaints from the patient and may be transient, though often fluctuating in presence and intensity. Persistence for more than 2 to 3 days is unusual. It is important to distinguish it from extending or renewed infarction, as pericardial involvement does not appear to worsen the in-hospital prognosis.

Because of the rarity of characteristic electrocardiographic changes (see below), virtually the only objective manifestation of pericardial involvement in acute myocardial infarction is the appearance of a pericardial rub. More than perhaps most other types of pericarditis, the rub here not only fluctuates rapidly but is especially likely to be evanescent and therefore largely undiscovered. Indeed, its discovery is strongly linked to the frequency of auscultation, not only because of transience but also because many patients with possible or probable pericardial pain do not appear to have rubs, whereas occasional pain-free patients have them. This situation is responsible for the wide discrepancy in the proportion of patients with acute myocardial infarction reported to have pericarditis: roughly between 6 and 30 percent [9]. In a large series of consecutive patients with acute myocardial infarction in which patients with pericarditis were carefully compared with either the other patients with infarcts as a control group or selected control patients, the incidence of infarction-associated pericarditis ranged from 6.3 to 10.1 percent [12].

Pericardial rubs are an early phenomenon, most appearing within the first 4 days after admission, with more than one-half of them on day 1 or day 2 [9]. In the absence of the postmyocardial infarction syndrome of recurrent pericarditis (never a secure exclusion), rubs may first appear as late as the twelfth day and, exceptionally, may disappear only to reappear from the first to the third week after onset.

Pericardial rubs may be typical, that is, three-component [13], in patients with sinus rhythm; but often they are biphasic, and some are confined to atrial or more often, ventricular systole. In each case, differentiation from a murmur is essential, although usually easy, unless a murmur coexists with a rub. Rubs, like pain, are likely to vary more with posture and respiration than most murmurs associated with infarction, and they nearly always sound "more superficial," as if they are just under the diaphragm of the stethoscope (which is preferred for auscultation because nearly every rub is comprised of high-frequency vibrations).

The most important differential diagnoses are from papillary muscle dysfunction, which may be perceived as a murmur anywhere from the apex to the left lower sternal border, ventricular septal perforation (which may be heard in the same areas), and tricuspid regurgitation (detected at the right lower sternal border). The pericardial lesion is distinguished from these entities (again, so long as they do not coexist) by the absence of expected hemodynamic abnormalities and of characteristic pharmacologic and physiologic responses to challenges such as respiratory and postural maneuvers as well as administration of nitrates. Echocardiographic Doppler study usually detects any of these entities; significantly increased pericardial fluid more often reflects cardiac failure than pericardial irritation.

Electrocardiography

Although there is some evidence that special techniques can show somewhat increased total ST segment elevation (Σ ST) in patients with infarct-associated pericarditis, the electrocardiogram is of virtually no help, probably because the pericardial involvement is local and because there is not usually an element of primarily pericardial inflammation. Thus the quasi-diagnostic stage I electrocardiographic changes of pericarditis [7, 14] were found in only 1 of 31 consecutively diagnosed patients [9]. Experience shows that in these rare cases the J points are displaced from the baseline in accordance with the criteria for stage I ST changes, obliterating any preexisting ST depressions, reciprocal or otherwise, but usually not interfering with any T-wave evolution of the infarct that has already commenced. In contrast to the approximately 43 percent of atypical electrocardiograms in patients with acute pericarditis of mixed causes [15], the rarity of this finding among patients with acute myocardial infarction raises strong questions of an intercurrent true pericarditis of other etiology, myopericarditis masquerading from the outset as myocardial infarction [16], or any very early "postmyocardial infarction" syndrome.

Other Characteristics

Careful observations failed to show any increase in the incidence of arrhythmias in patients with pericarditis of myocardial infarction [9, 12], which is not surprising because even generalized, truly inflammatory pericarditis does not by itself provoke arrhythmias [17] and because pericardial involvement is strictly localized to the ventricular infarct itself [6]. This is of additional interest because most patients with pericarditis have Q-wave infarcts [9, 12], and an increased number of patients are in Killip classes II, III, and IV [9]. Yet in prospectively observed series the in-hospital mortality of patients with pericarditis versus patients without pericarditis is no different [9, 12]. Predictably, the postdischarge mortality is increased, as expected for patients categorized in higher Killip classes. Finally, it is not surprising that pericardial rubs are discovered approximately equally among anterior and inferior infarcts, as the exudate is free to slosh throughout the pericardial sac. The sporadic identification of a more generalized pericardial involvement may well be related to the unusually early appearance of the postmyocardial infarction (Dressler's) syndrome (see below), which could also be a cause of the rare stage I electrocardiographic changes. Finally, in company with most forms of pericardial disease [15] there is a male-female ratio of about 4:1, far in excess of the male dominance (< 2:1) among coronary care unit patients with acute myocardial infarction [9].

Treatment for infarct-associated pericarditis is primarily for relief of pain. Nonsteroidal anti-inflammatory drugs (NSAIDs), usually aspirin or ibuprofen, are preferred. Indomethacin should be avoided because it has deleterious effects on coronary flow in humans and animals and increases the size of experimental infarcts. (Ibuprofen appears to increase coronary flow and reduce infarct size, although the ultimate effects on infarct healing, which is impaired by corticosteroids, are uncertain as are the effects of aspirin, which has been the first choice.) In occasional patients with severe pain, narcotics are indicated.

Intrapericardial Bleeding

Although many, if not most, forms of pericardial inflammation are accompanied by some escape of red blood cells into the pericardial cavity, this entity is associated with either direct injury of the pericardium by the inciting agent or disease or the capillary-rich granulation tissue that appears with early healing [7]. With infarction-associated pericardial involvement, this problem should be minimal to absent because of the common absence of true inflammation and the restriction of the lesion to the smallest part of any transmural infarct, that is, its epicardial apex. (An unusually early postmyocardial infarction syndrome could be an exception owing to presumably widespread pericardial involvement.) Thus the source of any significant intrapericardial bleeding could be a smaller or larger myocardial perforation (rupture) into the sac [18–20]. This explanation, of course, raises the question as to the effect of antithrombotic—including anticoagulant, "antiplatelet," and thrombolytic—therapy, which would either promote hemorrhage or impede its cessation [41]. Overall experience indicates that any of these treatments, even after recognition of pericarditis, does not usually produce catastrophic bleeding (including patients who were put in a thrombolytic state by treatment when acute pericarditis was mistaken for acute myocardial infarction). Evidence, on the other hand, exists for individuals given anticoagulants and thrombolytics with significant pericardial bleeding, that is, hemopericardium, sometimes causing cardiac tamponade that was not always recognized before death. The problem of mistaken diagnosis has been exacerbated by erroneous computer-generated electrocardiographic interpretations, typically "anterolateral infarction" instead of "acute pericarditis." Some of the older reports of hemopericardium come from an era when anticoagulant control was not at the present standards, and indeed the target level of anticoagulation was higher than the currently accepted levels [20]. Moreover, adverse experience now is more with heparin than coumarin derivatives. Finally, the major cause of frank hemopericardium appears to be ventricular rupture.

The danger of hemopericardium from anticoagulant therapy appears to be remote in patients with infarct-associated pericardial lesions, particularly with appropriate, careful control of the level of anticoagulation and of thrombolysis, and therefore these forms of therapy should be applied if there is an appropriate indication. Of course, it is prudent on such occasions to increase further the already high level of patient observation following the appearance or persistence of pericardial rubs or effusion (see below), particularly when they appear later than the first week after the onset of infarction. Cardiac tamponade (also discussed under Pericardial Effusion) is a major, though rare, emergency with or without an underlying infarct and indeed may be difficult to diagnose from other consequences of infarction. Because of these possibilities, echocardiographic Doppler studies should be performed as often as appropriate questions arise.

Pericardial Effusion

Despite the 40 percent incidence of pericarditis in necropsied patients with infarct-associated pericardial involvement [6], only about 18 percent were found to have excess pericardial fluid content (although despite a careful necropsy-clinical correlation it was unclear how many of them were the same patients [11]). Clinical experience and laboratory evaluation (principally by echocardiography) indicate that very different individuals may be involved because pericardial effusion can be inflammatory or irritative (an exudate) or noninflammatory (a transudate). An exudative effusion could be further complicated by intrapericardial bleeding of the types mentioned above. Transudates accumulate because of either metabolic abnormalities, including fluid and electrolyte imbalances, or high intracapillary pressures due to heart failure or venous and lymphatic obstruction. Such transudates are probably much more common and are usually small.

Careful echocardiography of consecutive patients with acute myocardial infarction by Galve et al. [21] and Pierard et al. [22] detected 28 and 26 percent, respectively, with pericardial effusion and compared them with acute myocardial infarction patients who did not develop pericardial effusions. In both reports there were no significant differences for the following factors: sex, initial acute infarction, Q-wave versus non-Q-wave infarction, in-hospital mortality, and major supraventricular arrhythmias. In both studies pericardial effusion was more often associated with anterior infarction and with heart failure. In Galve et al.'s study [21] there was no difference in peak creatine kinase MB (CK-MB); in Pierard et al.'s study [22] peak CK was higher with pericardial effusion, as was peak lactate dehydrogenase. In the latter study late mortality (15 days to 1 year) was higher in those with pericardial effusion, whereas in Galve et al.'s study the 6-month mortality was no different. Moreover, Galve et al. found no difference among those requiring resuscitation maneuvers, cardioversion, or both and no statistical difference for atrioventricular block, ventricular arrhythmias, and non-Q-wave infarction [21]. Pierard et al. found no difference among those with lateral infarcts and no difference between the groups for heparin therapy, but patients with pericardial effusion had a higher average Killip class, more ventricular arrhythmias, and much more aneurysm formation with their first acute infarction, along with an equally heavy preponderance of wall motion abnormalities [22]. These careful reports clearly supersede earlier investigations utilizing only M-mode echograms.

Finally, pericardial effusion may rarely be localized in patients with acute infarction [23] and is probably related to new or preexisting pericardial adhesions. Series such as that of Wunderink [24] can be discounted because they involved M-mode studies and especially because the echocardiographic incidence (5.6 percent) is equivalent to the prevalence of posterior echo-free spaces (5 percent) found in the Framingham Study for individuals of the same age and sex [25] and for the same control group by Galve et al. [21]—which by itself can be accounted for by pericardial fat [26]. (Several differences between the carefully studied series of Galve et al. [21] and Pierard et al. [22] may be ascribed largely to group differences and perhaps in part to study protocol.)

It is important that the presence of excess pericardial fluid does not correlate with the presence of pericardial rubs or inflammatory signs but rather with the clinical extent of the infarction, cardiac dilation, and particularly aneurysm formation (an expected feature of anterior infarctions especially). It also correlates with both heart failure and admission Killip class, as well as late mortality [21, 22]. The absence of correlation with heparin therapy is also significant. Indeed, there were no differences in the incidence of pericardial effusion in patients at either full- or low-dose heparin and no case with severe effusion or tamponade [21].

Pericardial effusion is thus common during acute myocardial infarction and is usually small, although slowly reabsorbed. It is probably rarely, if ever, related to a fibrinous pericardial reaction to localized injury but rather to heart failure with the attendant hemodynamic and fluid-electrolyte effects that can produce effusions in other serous cavities as well. It is not clear if aneurysm formation produces irritative effects of its own. The poor late prognosis probably reflects only the larger zone of acute damage and generally poor prognosis for patients with myocardial infarction who have developed congestive heart failure.

Occasional patients show persistence (i.e., poor reabsorption) of pericardial fluid, which may be related to persistent cardiac failure and attendant fluid-electrolyte abnormalities. It has been shown that even a small amount of fluid has detectable physiologic, if not pathologic, effects [27]. This finding suggests its corollary—that rapid cardiac dilation in the presence of otherwise clinically insignificant amounts of fluid may raise the pressure in the pericardial sac to some level of cardiac compression (tamponade).

Cardiac Tamponade

Following acute myocardial infarction, cardiac tamponade is virtually always due to bleeding into the pericardial sac with or without concomitant pericardial effusion. Any demonstrable association with anticoagulant and antithrombotic therapy is not clear (see above), but that situation is rare, as is atrial rupture [28], whereas ventricular rupture is a relatively common mode of death during early infarction because it causes overwhelming cardiac tamponade and acute constriction by massive clotting, usually before treatment is available; it has the characteristic sign of electromechanical dissociation. Rupture may be preceded by a somewhat lesser degree of tamponade, resembling (and extremely difficult to differentiate from) cardiogenic shock. Especially because of extremely low blood pressures, the characteristic sign, pulsus paradoxus, may be imperceptible (and does not occur in many hypertrophied hearts). Because bedside pressure curves and portable radiographs may be difficult to interpret, the situation calls for emergency echocardiography. In patients with either a minute myocardial perforation or myocardial hemorrhage of other cause, an increase in cardiopericardial silhouette with pulsus paradoxus, particularly with clear lung fields, should prompt a hemodynamic study (for diastolic pressure equilibration and amputation of the y descent in venous and atrial curves); emergency echocardiography is also desirable.

There is but one effective treatment for cardiac tamponade: evacuation of the pericardial contents. Little proof exists that the medical measures to support the hemodynamic state or augment intravascular fluid volume (which is dangerous in some patients with heart disease) have more than evanescent, temporizing effects on cardiac tamponade. Therefore needle pericardiocentesis [42], subxiphoid surgical drainage (which can be done under local anesthesia if necessary), or thoracoscopic drainage [43] should be instituted as soon as there is a firm diagnosis or on reasonable suspicion if the patient's condition is deteriorating rapidly. Needless to say, should bloody fluid be encountered, all anticoagulant and antithrombotic therapy should be discontinued.

Postmyocardial Infarction (Dressler's) Syndrome

Between 1 week and 2 months after an acute myocardial infarction (occasionally earlier [29, 30] and rarely later) patients may develop constitutional symptoms such as malaise and fever along with pericardial and pleuritic pain (sometimes severe and nearly always more intense than that of epistenocardiac pericarditis). Also present are leukocytosis, rapid erythrocyte sedimentation rate, sinus tachycardia, and sometimes pulmonary infiltrates and effusion. The latter are seen on chest films, and at the bedside pericardial and pleural rubs are frequent.

Examination of the patient may also reveal signs of the acute infarction if it is an early postmyocardial infarction syndrome. Indeed, this immunopathic syndrome can appear almost simultaneously with the clinical onset of infarction. This is explained by infarctions that remain asymptomatic for variable periods [10, 16] after actual onset. (Many infarcts, of course, appear to have been totally asymptomatic.)

The new syndrome may be disconcerting, particularly in patients recovering from a painless or minimally symptomatic infarction. The rub is more likely to be loud and to have two or three components than is the usual rub of infarct pericarditis. The pain is virtually always much greater than that of epistenocardiac pericarditis. Cardiac tamponade is rare [31], although it is probably always indicative of a generalized pericarditis, in contrast to the infarct lesion, which is localized. Individual attacks are also more protracted, even with therapy, and may last as long as 6 weeks.

Chest films usually show some increase in the cardiopericardial silhouette. Pleural effusion may be bilateral, but as with other forms of pericarditis, it is usually on the left, irrespective of whether there is pericardial effusion [32]. There are no cardiac enzyme changes unless there is also extension of the infarct. Echocardiography should show any pericardial effusion as well as the expected wall motion and other changes due to infarction. The electrocardiogram is sometimes unchanged, although J-ST changes may occur and are more often typical of pericarditis (i.e., stage I) than the customary absence of diagnostic electrocardiographic changes in epistenocardiac pericarditis [30]. PR segments may or may not be depressed.

Recurrences are common and may go on indefinitely after the index attack, although 2 years is a common cutoff point. Recurrence is thus one of the characteristics that point to an immunopathic basis for the postmyocardial infarction syndrome, that is, an immune response to products of myocardial damage, including antimyocardial antibodies [33], like the postmyocardial and pericardial injury syndromes. The other characteristics pointing to an immune basis include the time interval from the tissue damage, frequent evidence of generalized pericardial involvement as well as systemic signs and symptoms, and response to anti-inflammatory treatment. On the other hand, the question has been raised of activation of a latent virus [34] producing what is clinically idiopathic or viral pericarditis complicating or succeeding infarction. This situation is more likely in patients with a lesion confined to the pericardium; although these forms of pericarditis recur, one rarely sees associated lesions.

The incidence of postmyocardial infarction syndrome appears to be declining; in Dressler's hospital there were no cases among 229 consecutive patients [35]. Elsewhere three cases were found among 779 patients [36]. It is unclear why this syndrome may be disappearing. Perhaps there is some element in the management of infarct patients—for example, no longer is there prolonged strict bed rest, and the anticoagulant dicumarol is not used—but this remains speculative.

Differential diagnosis includes epistenocardiac pericarditis, usually distinguished by the differences noted previously, its early onset in nearly every patient, and a much milder course. Recurrent or extending acute infarction should be recognizable by enzyme increases, and its pain should be different. Cardiac tamponade is rare [31] but may mimic right ventricular infarction by producing increased jugular venous pressure with essentially clear lungs and pulsus paradoxus [3]. Moreover, a pericardial rub was found in 11 of 12 patients with right ventricular infarction [4]. The differential diagnosis should be made by pulmonary artery catheterization for the characteristic features of right ventricular infarction (a right ventricular pressure curve resembling pericardial constriction and right atrial pressure equal to or greater than left atrial pressure versus left ventricular infarction with left atrial pressure exceeding right atrial pressure); right precordial leads may show ST elevation but without stage I electrocardiographic changes of pericarditis (unless they coexist); pericardial effusion is usually absent by echocardiography. Differentiation from pulmonary embolism is important [44], as anticoagulants are needed for that condition but are relatively, if not absolutely, contraindicated by the presence of postmyocardial infarction syndrome. Exclusion of pericarditis by bedside and laboratory techniques is the most dependable differential approach. Should the picture resemble pneumonia, appropriate sputum and blood cultures (negative in patients with postmyocardial infarction syndrome), as well as careful radiography, are needed.

Patients who had been discharged should be readmitted to the hospital for their initial episode of postmyocardial infarction syndrome because of the remote possibility of cardiac tamponade and especially for the differential diagnosis of the conditions already noted. For subsequent recurrent episodes, admission is not needed so long as they are recognizable and so long as the patient is not seriously uncomfortable or threatened by any of the changes.

Treatment is primarily with nonsteroidal anti-inflammatory agents, including aspirin as tolerated. Perhaps the first drug to use is ibuprofen because it has the widest dose range and the lowest side effect profile (except for salicylates). Indomethacin should be avoided because, at least in experimental animals, it reduces coronary flow, raises blood pressure, and increases infarct size. If nonsteroidal agents are of no avail after trying several, corticosteroid therapy may be attempted. It is likely to work but may predispose to recurrences and, in some patients, to steroid side effects and dependence. Standard doses of prednisone (e.g., 60 mg/day in divided doses) may be given until symptoms and signs have decreased (usually rapidly). This agent should be tapered over approximately 2 weeks while introducing a nonsteroidal agent, which can then be tapered after the last dose of prednisone.

Pericardial Scarring

Adhesions and scarring of the pericardium, usually minor and localized, are the rule after epistenocardiac pericarditis [5]. They are localized to the area of the infarct and are of little or no clinical significance. Rare patients develop constrictive pericarditis [37] or effusive-constrictive pericarditis [38]. It is so uncommon as to raise a question of intercurrent infectious pericarditis or postmyocardial infarction syndrome masquerading as epistenocardiac pericarditis, as postmyocardial infarction syndrome rarely does proceed to constriction.

Pseudoaneurysm

Occasionally, ventricular rupture is minor and not fatal, occurring in such a form and at such a tempo that the pericardium contains the bleeding. Thus an aneurysmal bulge that may resemble a true ventricular aneurysm is formed [45]. However, the wall is formed by pericardium, usually with a narrow neck connecting the aneurysm cavity to the ventricular cavity, in contrast to a true ventricular aneurysm, which has a wide communication with the ventricle and a wall of myocardium in various states of damage and fibrosis [39]. Because pseudoaneurysms are more likely to rupture than aneurysms, the diagnosis should lead to surgical intervention whenever possible. Echocardiography with Doppler flow studies of the aneurysm's neck are most efficient for graphic diagnosis.

References

1. Spodick, D. H. The normal and diseased pericardium: Current concepts of pericardial physiology, diagnosis and treatment. *J. Am. Coll. Cardiol.* 1:240, 1983.
2. Spodick, D. H. Threshold of pericardial constraint: The pericardial reserve volume and auxiliary pericardial functions. *J. Am. Coll. Cardiol.* 6:296, 1985.
3. Applegate, R. J., Johnston, W. E., Vinten-Johansen, J., et al. Restraining effect of intact pericardium dur-

ing acute volume loading. *Am. J. Physiol.* 262: H1725, 1992.
4. Lorell, B., Leinbach, R. C., Pohost, G. M., et al. Right ventricular infarction: Clinical diagnosis and differentiation from cardiac tamponade and pericardial constriction. *Am. J. Cardiol.* 43:465, 1979.
5. Spodick, D. H. *Chronic and Constrictive Pericarditis.* New York: Grune & Stratton, 1964.
6. Erhardt, L. R. Clinical and pathological observations in different types of acute myocardial infarction: A study of 84 patients deceased after treatment in a coronary care unit. *Acta Med. Scand. Suppl.* 560: 1, 1974.
7. Spodick, D. H. *Acute Pericarditis.* New York: Grune & Stratton, 1959.
8. Roberts, W. C., and Spray, T. L. Pericardial heart disease: A study of its causes, consequences, and morphologic features. In D. H. Spodick (ed.), *Pericardial Diseases.* Philadelphia: Davis, 1976. Pp. 11–65.
9. Krainin, F. M., Flessas, A. P., and Spodick, D. H. Infarction-associated pericarditis: Rarity of diagnostic electrocardiogram. *N. Engl. J. Med.* 311:1211, 1984.
10. Spodick, D. H. Q-wave infarction versus ST-infarction: nonspecificity of ECG criteria for differentiating transmural and nontransmural lesions. *Am. J. Cardiol.* 51:913, 1983.
11. Roeske, W. R., Savage, R. M., O'Rourke, R. A., and Bloor, C. M. Clinicopathologic correlations in patients after myocardial infarction. *Circulation* 63:36, 1981.
12. Lichstein, E., Liu, H. M., and Gupta, P. Fundamentals of clinical cardiology: Pericarditis complicating acute myocardial infarction: Incidence of complications and significance of electrocardiogram on admission. *Am. Heart J.* 87:246, 1974.
13. Spodick, D. H. The pericardial rub: A prospective, multiple observer investigation of pericardial friction in 100 patients. *Am. J. Cardiol.* 35:357, 1975.
14. Spodick, D. H. The electrocardiogram in acute pericarditis: Distributions of morphologic and axial changes by stages. *Am. J. Cardiol.* 33:470, 1974.
15. Bruce, M. A., and Spodick, D. H. Atypical electrocardiogram in acute pericarditis: Characteristics and prevalence. *J. Electrocardiol.* 13:61, 1980.
16. Spodick, D. H. Infection and infarction: Acute viral (and other) infection in the onset, pathogenesis and mimicry of acute myocardial infarction. *Am. J. Med.* 81:661, 1986.
17. Spodick, D. H. Frequency of arrhythmias in acute pericarditis determined by Holter monitoring. *Am. J. Cardiol.* 53:843, 1984.
18. Miller, R. L. Hemopericardium with use of oral anticoagulant therapy. *J.A.M.A.* 209:1362, 1969.
19. Anderson, M. W., Christensen, N. A., and Edwards, J. E. Hemopericardium complicating myocardial infarction in the absence of cardiac rupture. *Arch. Intern. Med.* 90:634, 1952.
20. Goldstein, R., and Wolff, L. Hemorrhagic pericarditis in acute myocardial infarction treated with bishydroxycoumarin. *J.A.M.A.* 146:616, 1951.
21. Galve, E., Garcia-Del-Castillo, H., Evangelista, A., et al. Pericardial effusion in the course of myocardial infarction: Incidence, natural history, and clinical relevance. *Circulation* 73:294, 1986.
22. Pierard, L. A., Albert, A., Henrard, L., et al. Incidence and significance of pericardial effusion in acute myocardial infarction as determined by two-dimensional echocardiography. *J. Am. Coll. Cardiol.* 8:517, 1986.
23. Gore, J. M., Haffagee, C. I., Love, J. C., and Dalen, J. E. Isolated right ventricular tamponade after pericarditis from acute myocardial infarction. *Am. J. Cardiol.* 53:372, 1984.
24. Wunderink, R. G. Incidence of pericardial effusion in acute myocardial infarctions. *Chest* 85:494, 1984.
25. Savage, D. D., Garrison, R. J., Anderson, B. F., et al. Prevalence and correlates of posterior extra echocardiographic spaces in a free-living population based sample (the Framingham Study). *Am. J. Cardiol.* 51:1207, 1983.
26. Rifkin, R. D., Isner, J. M., Carter, B. L., and Bankoff, M. S. Combined posteroanterior subepicardial fat simulating the echocardiographic diagnosis of pericardial effusion. *J. Am. Coll. Cardiol.* 3:1333, 1984.
27. Spodick, D. H., Paladino, D., and Flessas, A. P. Respiratory effects on systolic time intervals during pericardial effusion. *Am. J. Cardiol.* 51:1033, 1983.
28. Bishop, L. H., Jr., Estes, E. H., Jr., and McIntosh, H. D. The electrocardiogram as a safeguard in pericardiocentesis. *J.A.M.A.* 162:264, 1956.
29. Khan, A. H. The postcardiac injury syndromes. *Clin. Cardiol.* 15:67, 1992.
30. Berman, J., Haffagee, C. I., and Alpert, J. S. Therapy of symptomatic pericarditis after myocardial infarction: Retrospective and prospective studies of aspirin, indomethacin, prednisone, and spontaneous resolution. *Am. Heart J.* 101:750, 1981.
31. Tew, F. T., Mantle, J. A., Russell, R. O., and Rackley, C. E. Cardiac tamponade with nonhemorrhagic pericardial fluid complicating Dressler's syndrome. *Chest* 72:93, 1977.
32. Weiss, J. M., and Spodick, D. H. Association of left pleural effusion with pericardial disease. *N. Engl. J. Med.* 308:696, 1983.
33. Fowler, N. O. Autoimmune heart disease. *Circulation* 44:159, 1971.
34. Burch, G. E., and Colcolough, H. L. Postcardiotomy and postinfarction syndrome—a theory. *Am. Heart J.* 80:290, 1970.
35. Lichstein, E., Arsura, E., Hollander, G., et al. Current incidence of postmyocardial infarction (Dressler's) syndrome. *Am. J. Cardiol.* 50:1269, 1982.
36. Thadani, U., Chopra, M. P., Aber, C. P., et al. Pericarditis after acute myocardial infarction. *B.M.J.* 2: 135, 1971.
37. Haiat, R. Post-myocardial infarction constrictive pericarditis (Letter). *Am. Heart J.* 101:358, 1981.
38. Friedman, B. J., and Segal, B. L. Chronic effusive

pericarditis associated with healed myocardial infarction: Report of a case. *Dis. Chest* 49:217, 1966.
39. Wang, R., DeSantola, J. R., Reichek, N., and Edie, R. An unusual case of postoperative pseudoaneurysm of the left ventricle: Doppler echocardiographic findings. *J. Am. Coll. Cardiol.* 8:699, 1986.
40. Maisch, B. Myocarditis and pericarditis: Old questions and new answers. *Herz* 17:65, 1992.
41. Eriksen, U. H., Molgaard, H., Ingerslev, J., and Nielsen, T. T. Fatal haemostatic complications due to thrombolytic therapy in patients falsely diagnosed as acute myocardial infarction. *Eur. Heart J.* 13: 840, 1992.
42. Wall, T. C., Campbell, P. T., O'Connor, C. M., et al. Diagnosis and management (by subxiphoid pericardiotomy) of large pericardial effusions causing cardiac tamponade. *Am. J. Cardiol.* 69:1075, 1992.
43. Millaire, A., Wurtz, A., de Groote, P., et al. Malignant pericardial effusions: Usefulness of pericardioscopy. *Am. Heart J.* 124:1030, 1992.
44. Belenkie, I., Dani, R., Smith, E. R., and Tyberg, J. V. The importance of pericardial constraint in experimental pulmonary embolism and volume loading. *Am. Heart J.* 123:733, 1992.
45. Brack, M., Asinger, R. W., Sharkey, S. W., et al. Two-dimensional echocardiographic characteristics of pericardial hematoma secondary to left ventricular free wall rupture complicating acute myocardial infarction. *Am. J. Cardiol.* 68:961, 1991.

19. Diastolic Abnormalities of Acute Myocardial Infarction

J. A. Bianco

The Observation

In 1970 Hood and colleagues [1] first demonstrated that left ventricular (LV) relaxation, distensibility, stiffness, or compliance, as measured post mortem by pressure-volume or pressure-segment length curves, was reduced in canine acute myocardial infarction during the 3- to 5-day postinfarct period. This observation is diagrammed in Figure 19-1. The practical implications of this observation are that patients with acute myocardial infarction (1) can have LV diastolic failure (e.g., dyspnea), even if systolic function is normal, and (2) can be pushed into pulmonary edema by volume loading when the preload is medically increased [2]. One is also tempted to relate this observation with the process of LV remodeling, as will be described.

Pathophysiologic Concepts

Diastole [3] consists of (1) an initial and rapid filling phase that occurs during the completion of active myocardial relaxation, (2) a phase of slow passive filling (i.e., diastasis), and (3) the phase of atrial contraction (i.e., the atrial systolic kick). During tachycardia the duration of diastasis is greatly curtailed.

The phases of diastole are shown in Figure 19-2. Note that a noninvasive study of diastole can be performed with the Doppler echocardiographic method [4] or by multigated radionuclide cineangiography [3] depending on institutional expertise. During the initial rapid phase of diastole, the maximal relaxation rate or peak filling rate (PFR) is calculated. It is a useful parameter of ventricular diastolic function. The normal range for the radionuclide-determined PFR is 3.15 ± 0.5 L/sec. Bonow, Bacharach, and Green at the National Institutes of Health and Pollack and Bianco in Boston [3] determined that more than 90 percent of patients with a history of myocardial infarction and 50 to 75 percent of patients with coronary artery disease without a history of infarction have subnormal PFR values. In recent work, the radionuclide diastolic function was the gold standard against which ultrafast computed tomography was compared [5].

The Doppler equivalent of the PFR is the peak of the E wave, while the second peak (the A wave) is obviously related to the radionuclide atrial kick wave. In a noncompliant ventricle the peak of the A wave increases at the expense of the peak of the E wave.

Over 75 percent of LV filling occurs during the initial rapid phase. This phase is related to the decay of the calcium transient, which is due to the reuptake of Ca^{2+} into the sarcoplasmic reticulum mediated by the sarcoplasmic reticulum calcium adenosinetriphosphatase (ATPase) and the extrusion of calcium by the sodium-calcium exchange [6].

Determinants of Diastolic Function

It is widely accepted in classic hemodynamic investigations [7] that reduced LV distensibility or compliance implies the need for a higher LV distensibility or compliance at any given LV end-diastolic volume, as shown in Figure 19-1, for acute cardiac infarction where fibrosis replaces cardiac tissue. LV diastolic function is, however, modified by a variety of variables other than diastolic compliance, which should be considered when assessing LV diastolic function in a given patient:

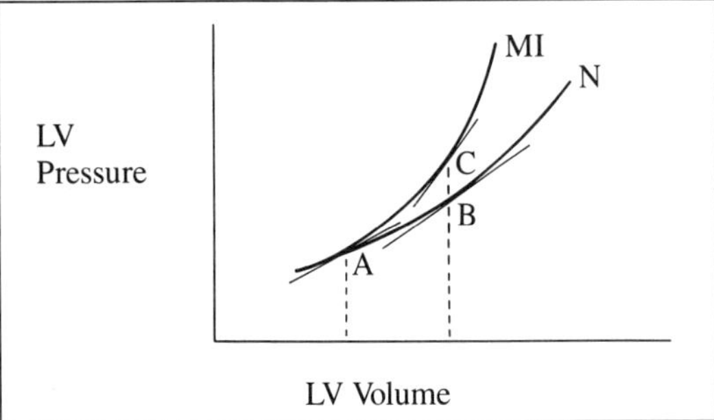

Fig. 19-1
Left ventricular (LV) pressure is plotted against the LV volume, according to observations obtained in the excised, emptied LV. Fluid was slowly infused to the LV while the LV pressure was being recorded continuously. N is the normal curve. The stiffness or distensibility of the LV in the noninfarcted heart is given by the tangents to the curve at points A and B. MI is the LV curve of a heart with acute myocardial infarction in the healing phase. At low volumes (A), the stiffness of both the normal and the infarcted LV is similar. However, at larger volumes (B), the infarcted heart (C) develops more pressure. This indicates that the infarcted heart has reduced diastolic compliance when compared to the normal heart. (Adapted from D. Gibson. Ventricular Function. In R. H. Anderson, F. J. MacCartney, E. A. Shinebourne, and M. Tynan, eds., *Pediatric Cardiology* [vol. 1]. New York: Churchill Livingstone, 1987. P. 174.)

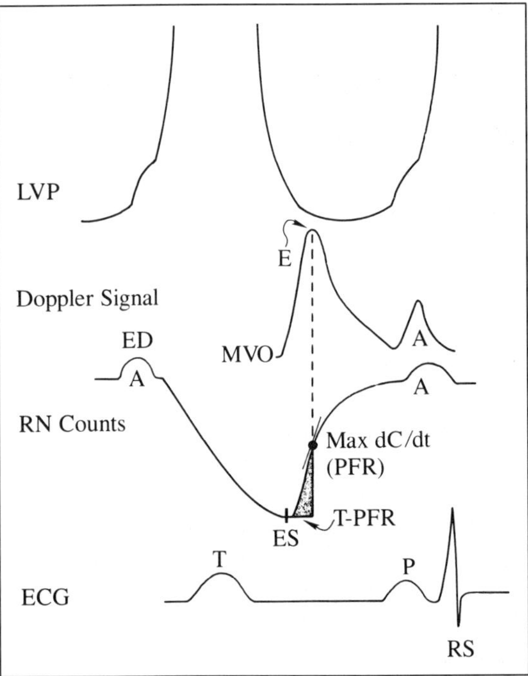

Fig. 19-2
Relation between left ventricular (LV) filling parameters and hemodynamics. The figure is structured to portray four physiologic recordings. *Top to bottom:* Bottom part of LV pressure (LVP) tracing, Doppler signal, radionuclide (RN) counts as a function of time, and electrocardiogram (ECG).

The LVP tracing is shown as a reference to highlight the diastolic phase of the cardiac cycle. With the Doppler signal, transmitral flow occurs mainly as early diastolic (E) and late diastolic (A = atrial contraction–related) components. The areas under the velocity signals reflect the amount of diastolic inflow.

The radionuclide time-activity curve is closely equivalent to the Doppler signal. It is expressed as counts (C) as a function of time, that is, C(t). The maximum rate of filling, dC/dt_{max} = PFR, defines the maximal derivative of early rapid diastolic filling, which corresponds to the peak of the velocity signal on the Doppler recording (E). The second flow signal in the radioisotopic C(t) curve is the atrial kick (A), which corresponds to the A signal on the Doppler signal. The time interval between end-systole (ES) and PFR is designated as time to peak filling rate (T-PFR). The shaded area under the diastolic time-activity curve corresponds to the maximal fraction of diastolic filling.

1. Pericardium. LV distensibility is less in the presence of the pericardium than in its absence [7].
2. Right ventricular diastolic function. In patients with right ventricular infarction, right and left ventricular pressures may be increased.
3. Aging. Aging prolongs the isovolumetric relaxation period and increases the atrial contribution to LV filling (in the aged, fractional early diastolic filling decreases from 80 percent to 50 percent).
4. Level of LV atrial pressure, preload, positive inotropic agents, LV ejection fraction, and heart rate. These factors singly or in combination have a direct relation with early diastolic filling [7–9].
5. Peripheral arterial vasoconstriction. This has a reciprocal relation with early diastolic filling. Peripheral vasodilators may improve diastolic function by this mechanism.

Effects of Myocardial Infarction on Diastolic Function

Before acutely necrotic cardiac tissue is replaced by fibrosis, LV diastolic distensibility may *actually* improve (increase) for a few days and this is thought to minimize a rise in filling pressure [10].

Many investigations have been designed to evaluate the changes in LV volumes associated with a previous myocardial infarction. McKay et al. [11] used LV angiography and echocardiography on admission and 2 weeks after thrombolytic therapy in 30 patients presenting with acute myocardial infarction. At 2 weeks after thrombolysis, there was an increase in LV end-diastolic and end-systolic volumes. The increase in LV volume correlated directly with the percentage of the LV that was akinetic or dyskinetic on initial catheterization. The postinfarct increase in LV volume was by far more common in patients with anterior infarcts and could have been related to an increase in LV pressure.

Lamas and Pfeffer [12] determined the relationship between LV volumes and magnitude of wall motion abnormalities in the chronic (i.e., at least 8 weeks) post–myocardial infarction period. These investigators studied 55 patients with left anterior descending coronary artery disease. Marked increases in end-diastolic and end-systolic volumes were observed across groups of increasing wall motion abnormality. The increases in LV diastolic volumes were not associated with increases in LV end-systolic pressure.

Seals et al. [13] studied 54 patients with a first acute myocardial infarction, using radionuclide angiography and plasma creatine kinase MB activity. Substantial LV dilation was documented within the initial 24 hours of acute infarction. Again, patients with anterior infarcts had the larger increases in LV end-diastolic and end-systolic volumes. The noted LV diastolic dysfunction (with lower peak diastolic filling rates) was the rule even in patients with preserved LV function. This finding was in agreement with the frequent observation of elevated LV filling pressure during the acute infarction. Finally, the authors noted that on day 10 after acute infarction, the end-diastolic volume was increased further.

Despite the findings in the above-mentioned investigations, the role of LV enlargement after infarction is unclear.

Gaudron et al. [14] studied 39 patients with small and 37 with large myocardial infarctions from 4 days and 4 weeks to 6 months after infarction before and during supine exercise. In patients with large infarctions, end-diastolic volume indexes increased at a constant wedge pressure. LV dilation within 4 weeks of infarction was considered to be compensatory since stroke volume in these patients increased during exercise. After 4 weeks, the dilation was noncompensatory since the stroke volume augmentation during exercise was lost.

Rumberger et al. [15] investigated 18 patients with acute infarction, at the time of hospital discharge and 6 weeks, 6 months, and 1 year after the infarction occurred. Patients with anterior infarcts demonstrated a progressive increase in LV end-diastolic volume from the time of hospital discharge to 1 year after the infarct was diagnosed. This was accompanied by a decrease in LV mass.

Loss of Left Ventricular Compliance

Acute myocardial infarction produces a shift in the pressure-volume characteristics of the LV. This is known as reduced LV diastolic compliance. As a consequence of this phenomenon there is increased resistance to LV filling. At rest and during exercise, the loss of LV compliance can result in exercise intolerance and symptoms of LV failure. Further, systolic dysfunction need not exist even when diastolic dysfunction is present [16]. Optimization of preload by volume loading can worsen the pressure-volume characteristics of the LV and precipitate an onset of pulmonary edema. During the first year after acute myocardial infarction there is a progressive increase in LV end-diastolic volume. This is thought to be associated with the phenomenon of *ventricular remodeling*.

Therapeutic Principles

Five recent publications discuss concepts related to therapy of diastolic dysfunction in patients who have had a myocardial infarction [2, 7, 15, 17, 18].

After acute infarction, fluids should be administered but should be done so *cautiously* to avoid pulmonary edema, and tachycardia should be avoided to maintain ventricular filling.

Determination and interpretation of the amount and the speed of initial and late diastolic filling by echocardiography, Doppler studies, or alternatively radionuclide cineangiography should be correlated to factors such as age, ejection fraction, heart rate, preload, left atrial pressure, synchronicity of ventricular activation, peripheral vascular resistance, and pericardial restraint [3, 4, 7–9, 18]. Increases in heart rate worsen the diastolic function of the infarcted heart.

The detrimental effects of increased LV volumes from remodeling can be prevented by using angiotensin-converting enzyme inhibitors or nitroglycerin [17, 18]. After a myocardial infarction results in reduced ejection fraction, angiotensin-converting enzyme inhibitors should be used.

Pipilis et al. [19] studied 81 patients within 36 hours after the onset of symptoms of suspected myocardial infarction and randomized them to receive oral captopril, isosorbide mononitrate, or matching placebo for 1 month. Captopril increased stroke volume. Both captopril and isosorbide mononitrate reduced systemic vascular resistance.

The rationale for ameliorating the effects of diastolic failure after acute myocardial infarction is to prevent upward and leftward shifts of the pressure-volume curve representing the LV. The recent introduction of the concept of remodeling has emphasized the usefulness of drugs such as angiotensin-converting enzyme inhibitors [18, 19] for patients with diastolic dysfunction.

Calcium channel blockers may be beneficial drugs to improve impaired systolic relaxation, which is the initial event in diastolic dysfunction [18]. More clinical studies are needed to define their proper role in relation to the stage of ventricular dysfunction.

References

1. Hood, W. B., Jr., Bianco, J. A., Kumar, R., and Whiting, R. B. Experimental myocardial infarction. IV. Reduction of left ventricular compliance in the healing phase. *J. Clin. Invest.* 49:1316, 1970.
2. Francis, G. S., and Archer, S. L. Diagnosis and management of acute congestive heart failure in the intensive care unit. *J. Intens. Care Med.* 4:84, 1989.
3. Harizi, R. C., Bianco, J. A., and Alpert, J. S. Diastolic function of the heart in clinical cardiology. *Arch. Intern. Med.* 148:99, 1988.
4. Labovitz, A. J., and Pearson, A. C. Evaluation of left ventricular diastolic function: Clinical relevance and recent Doppler echocardiographic insights. *Am. Heart J.* 114:836, 1987.
5. Rumberger, J. A. Use of ultrafast computed tomography to assess early diastolic filling in man. In W. Stanford and J. A. Rumberger (eds.), *Ultrafast Computed Tomography in Cardiac Imaging: Principles and Practice.* Mount Kisko, NY: Futura, 1992. Pp. 161–175.
6. Barry, W. H., and Bridge, J. H. B. Intracellular calcium homeostasis in cardiac myocytes. *Circulation* 87:1806, 1993.
7. Lorell, B. H. Significance of diastolic dysfunction of the heart. *Annu. Rev. Med.* 42:411, 1991.
8. Ishida, Y., Meisner, J. S., Tsujioka, K., et al. Left ventricular filling dynamics: Influence of left ventricular relaxation and left atrial pressure. *Circulation* 74:187, 1986.
9. Bianco, J. A., Filiberti, A. W., Baker, S. P., et al. Ejection fraction and heart rate correlate with diastolic peak filling rate at rest and during exercise. *Chest* 88:107, 1985.
10. Forrester, J. S., Diamond, G., Parmley, W. W., and Swann, H. J. C. Early increase in LV compliance after myocardial infarction. *J. Clin. Invest.* 51:598, 1972.
11. McKay, R. G., Pfeffer, M. A., Pasternak, R. C., et al. Left ventricular remodeling after myocardial infarction: A corollary to infarct expansion. *Circulation* 74:693, 1986.
12. Lamas, G. A., and Pfeffer, M. A. Increased left ventricular volume following myocardial infarction in man. *Am. Heart J.* 111:30, 1986.
13. Seals, A. A., Pratt, C. M., Mahmarian, J. J., et al. Relation of left ventricular dilatation during acute myocardial infarction to systolic performance, diastolic dysfunction, infarct size and location. *Am. J. Cardiol.* 61:224, 1988.
14. Gaudron, P., Eilles, C., Ertl, G., and Kochsiek, K. Adaptation to cardiac dysfunction after myocardial infarction. *Circulation* 87(Suppl IV):IV-83, 1993.
15. Rumberger, J. A., Behrenbeck, T., Breen, J. R., et al. Nonparallel changes in global left ventricular chamber volume and muscle mass during the first year after transmural myocardial infarction in humans. *J. Am. Coll. Cardiol.* 21:673, 1993.
16. Doughherty, A. H., Nacarelli, G. V., Gray, E. L., et al. Congestive heart failure with normal systolic function. *Am. J. Cardiol.* 54:778, 1984.
17. In M. D. Cheitlin, M. Sokolow, and M. D. McIlroy (eds.), *Clinical Cardiology.* Norwalk, CT: Appleton & Lange, 1993. Pp. 204–205.

18. Brutsaert, D. L., Sys, S. U., and Gillebert, T. C. Diastolic failure: Pathophysiology and therapeutic implications. *J. Am. Coll. Cardiol.* 22:318, 1993.

19. Pipilis, A., Flather, M., Collins, R., et al. Hemodynamic effects of captopril and isosorbide mononitrate started early in acute myocardial infarction: A randomized placebo-controlled study. *J. Am. Coll. Cardiol.* 21:73, 1993.

V. Miscellaneous Complications of Acute Myocardial Infarction

20. Unstable Angina Pectoris

Gary S. Francis

There is no general agreement about the precise definition of unstable angina. The condition is said to present when there is recurrent rest angina that is more prolonged, intense, and more frequent than usual. There are often ST-T changes observed on the electrocardiogram (ECG) during pain and no significant rise in serum enzyme levels. It may be defined as the new onset of angina pectoris or previously "stable" angina that is now brought on by minimal activity. Unstable angina may also be a change from previously predictable, exertional angina to rest angina.

Although most patients with acute myocardial infarction have a prodrome of discomfort (60 to 70 percent) (see Chapter 5), only 7 to 22 percent of patients with unstable angina go on to develop acute myocardial infarction [1–3]. On the other hand, the 1-year mortality is high following the onset of unstable angina [4] and can approach 20 percent [3]. Patients with unstable angina whose symptoms do not promptly respond to medical therapy (< 48 hours) are a particularly high-risk group [5], as are patients who develop frequent episodes of ECG changes without chest pain (silent ischemia) [6].

Pathophysiology

There are now compelling angiographic [7–13], angioscopic [14], and autopsy [15, 16] data to indicate that unstable angina is due to a change in the coronary endothelial surface. For reasons that are still unclear, an atherosclerotic plaque ruptures, platelets are activated, and thrombus formation ensues. Vasospasm, progression of underlying disease, and an increased myocardial demand for oxygen under certain conditions can also play some role. The pathogenesis of unstable angina has been extensively discussed in several reviews [17–22] as well as in Chapter 1.

It is now recognized that plaque disruption is the major underlying event that seems to precede most acute coronary syndromes [15, 20, 23]. It is often superimposed on the progression of underlying coronary stenosis [24]. Complex arteriographic lesions including eccentric stenosis, scalloping, and overhanging edges are observed angiographically and at autopsy in patients with unstable angina [7, 25]. A plaque may rupture within a relatively minor preexisting lesion. Thrombosis may be intermittent in unstable angina, in contrast to a Q-wave or non-Q-wave infarction in which the thrombosis may be more firmly fixed. Aggregated platelets may contribute to local vasoconstriction by releasing thromboxane [26]. Fibrinopeptide A, a sensitive marker of in vivo thrombin generation, is increased in patients with unstable angina [27], as is the concentration of fibrin and fibrinogen-related antigens [28]. Taken together, these observations strongly support a role for endothelial change (plaque fissure/rupture, platelet adhesion and activation, vasoconstriction, thrombosis, spontaneous lysis) in the pathogenesis of unstable angina.

Diagnosis

The diagnosis of unstable angina depends on the definition and is therefore subjective. A characteristic history accompanied by ECG changes during pain is conventionally used to make the diagnosis. Enzymes are usually not increased, although some investigators have allowed the presence of a "slight enzyme leak." We have stressed the importance of obtaining a 12-lead ECG *during pain* to confirm the diagnosis; we also accept for diagnosis a change from a previous ECG in the absence of enzyme changes. This strategy, however, does not take into account that more than 90 percent of ECG changes are asymptomatic in the setting of unstable angina

Table 20-1
Subset classification of unstable angina

New-onset angina or "de novo" angina—the first manifestation of angina pectoris
Crescendo angina—a distinctive increase in the number, severity, or duration of angina episodes in a patient with previous angina or "de novo" angina
Acute coronary insufficiency—prolonged chest pain, 20 or 30 min or more in duration, usually occurring at rest, incompletely relieved by nitroglycerin
Early postinfarction angina—recurrent chest pain between 24–48 hr after acute myocardial infarction
Postangioplasty angina—angina occurring within 6 mo after the procedure
Post–bypass surgery angina—angina following bypass surgery; it usually has a worse prognosis
Prinzmetal's variant angina—angina at rest associated with transient ST segment elevation

when calibrated amplitude-modulated Holter monitoring recordings are used [6].

Unstable angina is a broad term that encompasses many variations (Table 20-1). Clinical judgment is always necessary when making the diagnosis, and no simple algorithm will suffice. In its current use, the terminology implies an active coronary process, and intervention is therefore clearly justified.

Management

Medical Management

Most if not all patients should be admitted to the coronary care or intensive care unit, where appropriate surveillance and intensive nursing care are available. Although invasive monitoring is usually not necessary, it should be available if the patient becomes hemodynamically unstable. Providing supplemental oxygen by nasal prongs and sedation with benzodiazepam is standard care. Pharmacologic therapy for unstable angina has improved substantially, and our experience is that roughly 80 percent of patients respond to medical treatment. Urgent cardiac catheterization is reserved for a subset of patients who continue to have angina despite aggressive medical therapy (Table 20-2).

Intravenous nitroglycerin is used for nearly all patients because it is easier to titrate than oral nitrates and may offer additional benefit [29, 30]. The dose is highly variable, but 10 to 200 μg/min usually relieves or prevents angina.

Aspirin has been extensively studied in patients with unstable angina, where it has proved to be exceptionally beneficial [31, 32]. In the Veterans Administration Cooperative Study [31] 1266 men were treated with aspirin or placebo for 12 weeks following admission to the hospital for unstable angina. The authors observed a 51 percent reduction in mortality and acute myocardial infarction in the aspirin group ($p < .0005$). The Canadian Multicenter Trial [32] randomized 555 patients with unstable angina to receive aspirin, sulfinpyrazone, both drugs, or placebo; the investigators then followed these patients for up to 2 years. The incidence of cardiac death or nonfatal myocardial infarction was reduced by 51 percent in patients treated with aspirin ($p = .008$), once again establishing the utility of aspirin for the treatment of unstable angina. Taken together, these two well-controlled studies offer strong support for the role of platelet activation in the syndrome of unstable angina.

Combining heparin and aspirin has the distinct advantage of providing anticoagulant and antiplatelet activity. Intravenous heparin appears to significantly reduce progression to transmural infarction when compared to atenolol in patients with unstable angina [33]. The Risk of Myocardial Infarction and Death (RISC) trial demonstrated that the combination of aspirin (low dose, 75 mg) and intravenous heparin reduced the risk of infarction by 75 percent [75]. However, in a study from the Montreal Heart Institute, the combination of aspirin and heparin added no benefit compared to heparin alone [76]. It now seems clear that abrupt discontinuation of intravenous heparin can cause reactivation of unstable angina [76]. Therefore, patients should be taking aspirin for several days (3 to 4 days) before heparin is stopped. One can make a case to gradually taper heparin in patients with unstable angina [77]. New antithrombins such as hirudin and related peptides may result in more complete and safer control of unstable angina [78]. Although still controversial, the combined use of oral aspirin (324 mg/day) and intravenous heparin is recommended for the treatment of unstable angina (see Table 20-2).

In one small, controlled study, intravenous heparin significantly reduced progression to transmural infarction when compared to atenolol in patients with unstable angina [33]. Although not systematically studied, a small dose of aspirin (325 mg/day or less) used with full-dose heparin may prevent progression to infarction while minimizing bleeding complications. It has been our strategy to use both low-dose aspirin and full-dose heparin in patients with unstable angina unless contraindicated.

Numerous studies have demonstrated improved control of rest angina by adding calcium channel blockers to nitrates or beta blockers. One well-controlled study demonstrated that adding nifedipine to nitrates and propranolol significantly reduced sudden death, myocardial infarction, or persistent angina requiring surgery [34]. Similar controlled studies demonstrated the usefulness of verapamil in patients with unstable angina [35, 36]. The precise reasons whereby calcium channel blockers improve unstable angina are not clear, but multiple mechanisms are likely operative. Coronary blood flow may improve, spasm may be prevented, and verapamil and diltiazem are well known to reduce the heart rate. Moreover, all three commonly used calcium channel blockers (nifedipine, verapamil, and diltiazem) are known to have some antiplatelet activity [37].

The use of beta blockers for unstable angina is more controversial. Although they were introduced during the early 1970s as treatment for unstable angina [4], only one controlled trial demonstrated their usefulness [38]. Another controlled trial failed to show the effectiveness of propranolol [39], and some experts questioned the drug's use for unstable angina [40]. It appears that benefit is best derived when propranolol is combined with nifedipine [38].

Our own experience with beta blockers for treating unstable angina is that they are generally beneficial. In fact, the ultrashort-acting agent esmolol may help to control severe angina when used in selected patients who are refractory to more conventional therapy.

Invasive Supportive Measures

Some patients continue to have rest angina despite maximal medical therapy. Intra-aortic balloon counterpulsation (IABC) has been demonstrated to control refractory symptoms [41]. However, there is a substantial risk when using IABC, especially in older patients, women, diabetics, and those with severe peripheral vascular disease [42]. Patients who remain refractory to medical therapy are likely to undergo urgent cardiac catheterization and possibly angioplasty or surgery. The IABC device now serves primarily as a temporary support system prior to urgent catheterization, angioplasty, or surgery (see Chapter 15).

Coronary sinus retroperfusion is a technique that allows delivery of arterial blood and medications to the coronary veins during diastole. Venous drainage occurs during systole through a synchronized coronary sinus balloon catheter and pump system. Animal studies have documented beneficial effects with coronary sinus retroperfusion [43–45], and preliminary experience in patients appears promising [46]. More experience is necessary with this device and with the newer catheter-based systems, including laser, intracoronary stents, and atherectomy techniques, before their role in unstable angina is secured.

Thrombolytic Therapy

The well-recognized role of intracoronary thrombus in unstable angina has generated much interest in thrombolytic therapy for this syndrome. Intravenous [47] and intracoronary [48, 49] streptokinase has been used with expected success. Gold and colleagues [50, 51] have used recombinant tissue-type plasminogen activator (rt-PA) in patients with unstable angina. In a placebo-controlled trial, rt-PA in doses of 1.75 mg/kg intravenously over 12 hours was given at a rate of 0.75 mg/kg over 1 hour and 0.5 mg/kg over 11 hours; it ameliorated angina in 11 of 12 patients, whereas placebo was effective in only 6 of 11 patients. Oozing at puncture sites was not observed in patients treated with placebo but occurred in 8 of 12 patients treated with rt-PA. In 3 patients rt-PA was terminated before the 12-hour infusion was completed because of bleeding complications. Subsequent coronary arteriography demonstrated subocclusive thrombus in 8 of 11 patients receiving placebo but in none of the patients treated with rt-PA. The third Thrombolysis in Myocardial Infarction (TIMI III) trial showed no advantage for rt-PA in patients with unstable angina, but only a small number of patients demonstrated thrombus in this study [79]. It is still possible that a small subset of patients with unstable angina and thrombus formation may benefit from thrombo-

Table 20-2
Treatment of unstable angina

Drug category	Clinical condition	When to avoid[a]	Dose
Aspirin[b]	Unstable angina	Hypersensitivity Active bleeding Severe bleeding risk	324 mg (160–324) daily
Heparin	Unstable angina in high-risk category	Active bleeding History of heparin-induced thrombocytopenia Severe bleeding risk Recent stroke	80 units/kg intravenous bolus Constant intravenous infusion at 18 units/kg/hr Titrated to maintain activated partial thromboplastin time between 1.5–2.5 times control
Nitrates	Symptoms are not fully relieved with three sublingual nitroglycerin tablets and initiation of beta-blocker therapy	Hypotension	5–10 μg/min by continuous infusion Titrated up to 75–100 μg/min until relief of symptoms or limiting side effects (headache or hypotension with a systolic blood pressure < 90 mm Hg or more than 30% below starting mean arterial pressure levels if significant hypertension is present) Topical, oral, or buccal nitrates are acceptable alternatives for patients without ongoing or refractory symptoms
Beta blockers[c]	Unstable angina	PR ECG segment > 0.24 sec Second- or third-degree atrioventricular (AV) block Heart rate < 60 bpm Blood pressure < 90 mm Hg Shock Left ventricular failure with congestive heart failure Severe reactive airway disease	**Metoprolol** 5-mg increments by slow (over 1–2 min) intravenous administration Repeated every 5 min for a total initial dose of 15 mg Followed in 1–2 hr by 25–50 mg by mouth every 6 hr If a very conservative regimen is desired, initial doses can be reduced to 1–2 mg **Propranolol** 0.5–1.0-mg intravenous dose Followed in 1–2 hr by 40–80 mg by mouth every 6–8 hr **Esmolol** Starting maintenance dose of 0.1 mg/kg/min intravenously Titration in increments of 0.05 mg/kg/min every 10–15 min as tolerated by blood pressure until the desired therapeutic response has been obtained, limiting symptoms develop, or a dose of 0.20 mg/kg/min is reached

			Optional loading dose of 0.5 mg/kg may be given by slow intravenous administration (2–5 min) for more rapid onset of action **Atenolol** 5-mg intravenous dose Followed 5 min later by a second 5-mg intravenous dose and then 50–100 mg orally every day initiated 1–2 hr after the intravenous dose
Calcium channel blockers	Patients already on adequate doses of nitrates and beta blockers or patients unable to tolerate adequate doses of one or both of these agents or patients with variant angina	Pulmonary edema Evidence of left ventricular dysfunction	Dependent on specific agent
Morphine sulfate	Patients whose symptoms are not relieved after three serial sublingual nitroglycerin tablets or whose symptoms recur with adequate anti-ischemic therapy	Hypotension Respiratory depression Confusion Obtundation	2–5-mg intravenous dose May be repeated every 5–30 min as needed to relieve symptoms and maintain patient comfort

[a]Allergy or prior intolerance contraindication for all categories of drugs listed in this chart.

[b]Patients unable to take aspirin because of a history of hypersensitivity or major gastrointestinal intolerance should be started on ticlopidine 250 mg twice a day, as a substitute.

[c]Choice of the specific agent is not as important as ensuring that appropriate candidates receive this therapy. If there are concerns about patient intolerance due to existing pulmonary disease, especially asthma, left ventricular dysfunction, or risk of hypotension or severe bradycardia, initial selection should favor a short-acting agent, such as propranolol or metoprolol or the ultrashort-acting agent esmolol. Mild wheezing or a history of chronic obstructive pulmonary disease should prompt a trial of a short-acting agent at a reduced dose (e.g., 2.5 mg of intravenous metopolol, 12.5 mg of oral metoprolol, or 25 μg/kg/min of esmolol as initial doses) rather than complete avoidance of beta-blocker therapy.

Note: Some of the recommendations in this guide suggest the use of agents for purposes or in doses other than those specified by the Food and Drug Administration (FDA). Such recommendations are made after consideration of concerns regarding nonapproved indications, where such recommendations are based on more recent clinical trials or expert consensus.

Source: Adapted from E. Braunwald, D. B. Mark, R. H. Jones, et al. *Unstable Angina: Diagnosis and Management.* Clinical practice guideline number 10. AHCPR Publication No. 94-0602. Rockville, MD: Agency for Health Care Policy and Research and the National Heart, Lung, and Blood Institute, Public Health Service, U.S. Department of Health and Human Services, March 1994.

lytic therapy, but it cannot be recommended as routine therapy.

Interventional Management

The timing and even the necessity of coronary arteriography for patients with unstable angina have been controversial and even somewhat cyclical. The early 1970s was an era of emergency arteriography and surgery [52, 53], soon followed by a general consensus that if patients can be medically controlled, arteriography and catheterization can be delayed [54, 55]. This change was in part predicated on the large National Cooperative Study Group report on unstable angina, which concluded that patients with unstable angina can be managed acutely with intensive medical therapy, followed by elective surgery performed if the patient fails to respond to medical therapy [56]. In this study 36 percent of medically treated patients crossed over to surgery because of refractory symptoms during follow-up. The Veterans Administration Cooperative Study on Unstable Angina [57] found a similar survival rate at 2 years' follow-up in patients treated medically or surgically, but once again 34 percent of patients assigned to receive chronic medical therapy became refractory with recurrent symptoms and crossed over to surgery. Interestingly, the Veterans Administration study found that patients with a modestly low ejection fraction (30 to 59 percent) demonstrated significantly greater improvement in survival when treated surgically [57]. This improvement in survival in surgically treated patients with unstable angina who showed some reduction in ejection fraction is similar to observations made in patients with stable angina [58, 59].

It is probably fair to say that many centers, at least until recently, treated most patients with unstable angina medically in the coronary care unit, performed coronary arteriography electively within 2 to 3 days when patients were pain free, and operated on a substantial proportion of patients depending on the individual circumstances. Indeed, when performed in an elective manner in a stable, quiescent patient, coronary bypass surgery has proved to be a safe, effective treatment for medically refractory or medically responsive unstable angina pectoris. Our approach is to obtain coronary arteriography data early in the patient's hospital course because knowledge of the anatomy helps the physician make judgments regarding therapy and sometimes helps to avoid later emergency catheterization in patients who subsequently become unstable.

Percutaneous transluminal coronary angioplasty (PTCA) has more recently been used to treat patients with unstable angina [60, 61] and those with evolving acute myocardial infarction [62–64] (see Chapter 23). Reports of angioplasty in patients with unstable angina have generally been favorable [65–73], with primary success rates of 61 to 93 percent and complication rates of 2.0 to 12.5 percent.

Coronary angioplasty when performed in patients with unstable angina is associated with more frequent complications [80], with the risk approximating 10 percent for combined myocardial infarction, urgent surgery, and death. Higher complication rates are related to the presence of an intracoronary thrombus [80]. PTCA is preferably performed as a semielective procedure after initial medical stabilization. Coronary artery bypass surgery may be the preferred choice when there is multivessel disease. When three-vessel disease coexists with left ventricular dysfunction, patients will benefit more from surgery.

There has been interest in "culprit lesion angioplasty," in which PTCA is performed on a single lesion in patients with unstable angina and multivessel disease [81]. The culprit lesion is identified by observing ECG changes during ischemia or by regional thallium redistribution. Angiography, exercise-induced wall motion abnormalities during exercise gated blood pool scan, dipyridamole thallium perfusion scintigraphy, and positron emission tomography can also be used to identify culprit lesions. The good symptomatic response to culprit lesion angioplasty in patients with unstable angina suggests that the single-site dilation strategy should be the rule unless there is a substantial amount of myocardium in jeopardy from other lesions.

The past few years have witnessed a remarkable transition in therapeutic approaches to the acutely ischemic myocardium. Reduction in myocardial oxygen demand, a strategy shown to be beneficial in the laboratory setting for reducing infarct size, has not proved to reduce infarct size in patients [74]. Instead, a realization that unstable angina may be caused by a reversible change in the endothelial surface of the coronary artery has emerged. This new concept of how stable coronary disease becomes unstable is still incompletely understood, but it has nevertheless fostered new approaches to therapy.

Antiplatelet drugs, usually in the form of low-dose aspirin, are now routinely given to patients unless there is a contraindication. A strong case can also be made for administering intravenous heparin to patients with unstable angina. Beta-adrenergic blocking drugs may be useful in selected patients with unstable angina who have excessive myocardial oxygen demands. Intravenous nitroglycerin followed by long-acting oral nitrates are time-proved remedies for unstable angina. Calcium channel–blocking agents may be useful. If nifedipine is used, it should be combined with a beta blocker. Lytic therapy with streptokinase or tPA might be considered, but experience with these agents to date is primarily in patients with evolving acute transmural (Q-wave) infarction and not unstable angina.

Early cardiac catheterization is usually indicated in patients once they respond to treatment and have stabilized. Patients who fail to stabilize should have urgent cardiac catheterization with consideration toward angioplasty of the culprit lesion. Rarely, IABC and emergency catheterization are necessary. Operative therapy is preferred for many patients, especially those with multivessel disease and modest left ventricular dysfunction.

References

1. Fulton, M., Lutz, W., Donald, R. W., et al. Natural history of unstable angina. *Lancet* 1:860, 1972.
2. Gazes, P. C., Mobley, E. M., Jr., Faris, H. M., Jr., et al. Preinfarction (stable) angina—a prospective study: Ten year follow-up prognostic significance of eletrocardiographic changes. *Circulation* 48:331, 1973.
3. Mulcahy, R., Awahdi, A. H. L., de Buitleor, M., et al. Natural history and prognosis of unstable angina. *Am. Heart J.* 109:753, 1985.
4. Fischl, S. J., Herman, M. V., and Gorlin, R. The intermediate coronary syndrome: Clinical angiographic and therapeutic aspects. *N. Engl. J. Med.* 288:1193, 1973.
5. Roberts, K. B., Califf, R., Harrell, F. E., Jr., et al. The prognosis for patients with new-onset angina who have undergone cardiac catheterization. *Circulation* 68:970, 1983.
6. Gottleib, S. O., Weisfeldt, M. L., Ouyang, P., et al. Silent ischemia as a marker for early unfavorable outcomes in patients with unstable angina. *N. Engl. J. Med.* 314:1214, 1986.
7. Ambrose, J. A., Winters, S. L., Stern, A., et al. Angiographic morphology and the pathogenesis of unstable angina. *J. Am. Coll. Cardiol.* 5:609, 1985.
8. Alpert, J. S. Coronary vasomotion, coronary thrombosis, myocardial infarction and the camel's back (Editorial). *J. Am. Coll. Cardiol.* 5:617, 1985.
9. Bresnahan, D. R., Davis, J. L., Holmes, D. R., Jr., et al. Angiographic occurrence and clinical correlates of intraluminal coronary artery thrombus: Role of unstable angina. *J. Am. Coll. Cardiol.* 6:285, 1985.
10. Ambrose, J. A., Winters, S. L., Arora, R. R., et al. Angiographic evolution of coronary artery morphology in unstable angina. *J. Am. Coll. Cardiol.* 7:472, 1986.
11. Gotoh, K., Minamino, T., Katoh, O., et al. The role of intracoronary thrombus in unstable angina: Angiographic assessment and thrombolytic therapy during ongoing anginal attacks. *Circulation* 77:526 1988.
12. Wilson, R. F., Holida, M. D., and White, C. W. Quantitative angiographic morphology of coronary stenoses leading to myocardial infarction or unstable angina. *Circulation* 73:286, 1986.
13. Ambrose, J. A., and Hjemdalh-Monsen, C. E. Arteriographic anatomy and mechanisms of myocardial ischemia in unstable angina (Editorial). *J. Am. Coll. Cardiol.* 9:1397, 1987.
14. Sherman, C. T., Litvack, F., Grundfest, W., et al. Coronary angioscopy in patients with unstable angina pectoris. *N. Engl. J. Med.* 315:913, 1986.
15. Falk, E. Unstable angina with fatal outcome: Dynamic coronary thrombosis leading to infarction and/or sudden death. *Circulation* 71:699, 1985.
16. Davies, M. J., Thomas, A. C., Knapman, P. A., et al. Intramyocardial platelet aggregation in patients with unstable angina suffering sudden ischemic cardiac death. *Circulation* 73:418, 1986.
17. Epstein, S. E., and Palmeri, S. T. Mechanisms contributing to precipitation of unstable angina and acute myocardial infarction: Implications regarding therapy. *Am. J. Cardiol.* 54:1245, 1984.
18. Fuster V., and Chesebro, J. W. Mechanism of unstable angina. *N. Engl. J. Med.* 315:1023, 1986.
19. Willerson, J. T., Hillis, L. D., Winniford, M., et al. Speculation regarding mechanisms responsible for acute ischemic heart disease syndromes (Editorial). *J. Am. Coll. Cardiol.* 8:245, 1986.
20. Gorlin, R., Fuster, V., and Ambrose, J. A. Anatomic-physiologic links between acute coronary syndromes (Editorial). *Circulation* 74:6, 1986.
21. Forrester, J. S., Litvack, F., and Grundfest, W. A perspective of coronary disease seen through the arteries of living man. *Circulation* 75:505, 1987.
22. Fuster, V., Badiman, L., Cohen, M., et al. Insights into the pathogenesis of acute ischemic syndromes. *Circulation* 77:1213, 1988.
23. Davies, M. J., and Thomas, A. C. Plaque fissuring: The cause of acute myocardial infarction, sudden

ischemic death, and crescendo angina. *Br. Heart J.* 53:363, 1985.
24. Moise, A., Théroux, P., Taymans, Y., et al. Unstable angina and progression of coronary atherosclerosis. *N. Engl. J. Med.* 309:685, 1983.
25. Levin, D. C., and Fallon, J. T. Significance of the angiographic morphology of localized coronary stenosis: Histopathological correlates. *Circulation* 66:316, 1982.
26. Fitzgerald, D. J., Roy, L., Catella, F., et al. Platelet activation in unstable coronary disease. *N. Engl. J. Med.* 315:983, 1986.
27. Théroux, P., Latour, J-G., Léger-Gauthier, C., et al. Fibrinopeptide A and platelet factor levels in unstable angina pectoris. *Circulation* 75:156, 1987.
28. Kruskal, J. B., Commerford, P. J., Franks, J. J., et al. Fibrin and fibrinogen-related antigens in patients with stable and unstable coronary artery disease. *N. Engl. J. Med.* 317:1361, 1987.
29. Kaplan, K., Davison, R., Parker, M., et al. Intravenous nitroglycerin for the treatment of angina at rest unresponsive to standard nitrate therapy. *Am. J. Cardiol.* 51:694, 1983.
30. Curfman, G. D., Heinsimer, J. A., Lozner, E. C., et al. Intravenous nitroglycerin in the treatment of spontaneous angina pectoris. *Circulation* 67:276, 1983.
31. Lewis, H. D., Jr., Davis, J. W., Archibald, D. G., et al. Protective effects of aspirin against acute myocardial infarction and death in men with unstable angina. *N. Engl. J. Med.* 309:396, 1983.
32. Cairns, J. A., Gent, M., Singer, J., et al. Aspirin, sulfinpyrazone, or both in unstable angina: Results of a Canadian multicenter trial. *N. Engl. J. Med.* 313:1369, 1985.
33. Telford, A. M., and Wilson, C. Trial of heparin versus atenolol in prevention of myocardial infarction in intermediate coronary syndrome. *Lancet* 1:1225, 1981.
34. Gerstenblith, G., Ouyang, P., Achuff, S. C., et al. Nifedipine in unstable angina: A double-blind, randomized trial. *N. Engl. J. Med.* 306:885, 1982.
35. Mehta, J., Pepine, C. J., Day, M., et al. Short-term efficacy of oral verapamil in rest angina—a double-blind, placebo-controlled trial in CCU patients. *Am. J. Med.* 71:977, 1981.
36. Parodi, O., Maseri, A., and Simonetti, I. Management of unstable angina at rest by verapamil: A double-blind, cross-over study in the coronary care unit. *Br. Heart J.* 41:167, 1979.
37. Johnson, G. J., Leis, L. A., and Francis, G. S. The calcium channel blockers, nifedipine and verapamil, have different effects on alpha$_2$ adrenergic receptors and thromboxane-induced aggregation of human platelets. *Circulation* 73:847, 1986.
38. Gottlieb, S. O., Weisfeldt, M. L., Ouyang, P., et al. Effect of the addition of propranolol to therapy with nifedipine for unstable angina pectoris: A randomized, double-blind, placebo-controlled trial. *Circulation* 73:331, 1986.
39. Parodi, O., Simonetti, I., Michelassi, C., et al. Comparison of verapamil and propranolol therapy for angina pectoris at rest: A randomized, multiple-crossover, controlled trial in the coronary care unit. *Am. J. Cardiol.* 57:899, 1986.
40. Singh, B. H., and Nademanee, K. Beta-adrenergic blockade in unstable angina pectoris. *Am. J. Cardiol.* 57:992, 1986.
41. Gold, H. K., Leinbach, R. C., Sanders, C. A., et al. Intraaortic balloon pumping for control of recurrent myocardial ischemia. *Circulation* 47:1197, 1973.
42. Alderman, J. D., Gablioni, G. I., McCabe, C. H., et al. Incidence and management of limb ischemia with percutaneous wire-guided intraaortic balloon catheters. *J. Am. Coll. Cardiol.* 9:524, 1987.
43. Meerbaum, S., Lang, T., Osher, J. V., et al. Diastolic retroperfusion of acutely ischemic myocardium. *Am. J. Cardiol.* 37:588, 1976.
44. Drury, J. K., Yamazaki, S., Fishbein, M. C., et al. Synchronized diastolic coronary venous retroperfusion: Results of a pre-clinical safety and efficacy study. *J. Am. Coll. Cardiol.* 6:328, 1985.
45. Chang, B-L., Drury, J. K., Meerbaum, S., et al. Enhanced myocardial washout and retrograde blood delivery with synchronized retroperfusion during acute myocardial ischemia. *J. Am. Coll. Cardiol.* 9:1091, 1987.
46. Gore, J. M., Weiner, B. H., Benotti, J. R., et al. Preliminary experience with synchronized coronary sinus retroperfusion in humans. *Circulation* 74:381, 1986.
47. Lawrence, J. R., Shephard, J. T., Bone, I., et al. Fibrinolytic therapy in unstable angina: A controlled clinical trial. *Thromb. Res.* 17:767, 1980.
48. Vetrovec, G. W., Leinbach, R. C., Gold, H. K., et al. Intracoronary thrombolysis in syndromes of unstable ischemia: Angiographic and clinical results. *Am. Heart J.* 104:946, 1982.
49. Shapiro, E. P., Brinker, J. A., Gottleib, S. O., et al. Intracoronary thrombolysis 3 to 13 days after acute myocardial infarction for postinfarction angina pectoris. *Am. J. Cardiol.* 55:1453, 1985.
50. Gold, H. K., Johns, J. A., Leinbach, R. C., et al. A randomized, blinded, placebo-controlled trial of recombinant human tissue-type plasminogen activator in patients with unstable angina pectoris. *Circulation* 75:1192, 1987.
51. Gold, H. K., Johns, J. A., Leinbach, R. C., et al. Thrombolytic therapy for unstable angina pectoris: Rationale and results. *J. Am. Coll. Cardiol.* 10: 91B, 1987.
52. Bonchek, L. I., Rahimtoola, S. H., Anderson, R. B., et al. Late results following emergency saphenous vein bypass grafting for unstable angina. *Circulation* 50:972, 1974.
53. Matloff, J. M., Sustaita, H., Chatterjee, K., et al. The rationale for surgery in preinfarction angina. *J. Thorac. Cardiovasc. Surg.* 69:73, 1975.
54. Golding, L. A. R., Loop, F. D., Sheldon, W. C., et al. Emergency revascularization for unstable angina. *Circulation* 58:1163, 1978.
55. Cohn, L. H., Alpert, J., Koster, J. K., et al. Changing

indications for the surgical treatment of unstable angina. *Arch. Surg.* 113:1312, 1978.
56. Russell, R. O., Jr., Moraski, R. E., Kouchoukos, N., et al. Unstable angina pectoris: National Cooperative Study Group to compare surgical and medical therapy. *Am. J. Cardiol.* 42:839, 1978.
57. Luchi, R. J., Scott, S. M., Deupree, R. H., et al. Comparison of medical and surgical treatment for unstable angina pectoris. *N. Engl. J. Med.* 316: 977, 1987.
58. Passamani, E., Davis, K. B., Gillespie, M. J., et al. A randomized trial of coronary artery bypass surgery: Survival of patients with a low ejection fraction. *N. Engl. J. Med.* 312:1665, 1985.
59. Veterans Administration Coronary Artery Bypass Surgery Cooperative Study Group. Eleven-year survival in Veterans Administration randomized trial of coronary bypass surgery for stable angina. *N. Engl. J. Med.* 311:1333, 1984.
60. Meltzer, R. S., van den Brand, M., Serruys, P. W., et al. Sequential intracoronary streptokinase and transluminal angioplasty in unstable angina with evolving myocardial infarction. *Am. Heart J.* 104: 1109, 1982.
61. De Feyter, P. J., Serruys, P. W., van den Brand, M., et al. Emergency coronary angioplasty in refractory unstable angina. *N. Engl. J. Med.* 313:342, 1985.
62. Goldberg, S., Urban, P. L., Greenspon, A., et al. Combination therapy for evolving myocardial infarction: Intracoronary thrombolysis and percutaneous transluminal angioplasty. *Am. J. Med.* 72:994, 1982.
63. Myer, J., Merx, W., Schmitz, H., et al. Percutaneous transluminal coronary angioplasty immediately after intracoronary streptolysis of transmural myocardial infarction. *Circulation* 66:905, 1982.
64. Yasuno, M., Saito, Y., Ishida, M., et al. Effects of percutaneous transluminal coronary angioplasty: Intracoronary thrombolysis with urokinase in acute myocardial infarction. *Am. J. Cardiol.* 53:1217, 1984.
65. Williams, D. O., Riley, R. S., Singh, A. K., et al. Evaluation of the role of coronary angioplasty in patients with unstable angina pectoris. *Am. Heart J.* 102:1, 1981.
66. Meyer, J., Schmitz, H., Erbel, R., et al. Treatment of unstable angina pectoris with percutaneous transluminal coronary angioplasty (PTCA). *Cathet. Cardiovasc. Diagn.* 7:361, 1981.
67. Erbel, R., Moyer, J., Schmitz, H., et al. Percutaneous transluminal coronary angioplasty in patients with unstable angina. *Postgrad. Med. J.* 59(Suppl 3):22, 1983.
68. Faxon, D. P., Detre, K. M., McCabe, C. H., et al. Role of percutaneous transluminal coronary angioplasty in the treatment of unstable angina: Report from the National Heart, Lung and Blood Institute percutaneous transluminal coronary angioplasty and coronary artery surgery study registries. *Am. J. Cardiol.* 53: 131C, 1984.
69. Quigley, P. J., Erwin, J., Maurer, B. J., et al. Percutaneous transluminal coronary angioplasty in unstable angina: Comparison with stable angina. *Br. Heart J.* 55:227, 1986.
70. Timmis, A. D., Griffen, B., Crick, J. C. P., et al. Early percutaneous transluminal coronary angioplasty in the management of unstable angina. *Int. J. Cardiol.* 14:25, 1987.
71. De Feyter, P. J., Serruys, P. W., Soward, A., et al. Coronary angioplasty for early postinfarction unstable angina. *Circulation* 74:1365, 1986.
72. Gottlieb, S. O., Walford, G. D., Ouyang, P., et al. Initial and late results of coronary angioplasty for early postinfarction unstable angina. *Cathet. Cardiovasc. Diagn.* 13:93, 1987.
73. Safian, R. D., Snyder, L. D., Snyder, B. A., et al. Usefulness of percutaneous transluminal coronary angioplasty for unstable angina pectoris after non-Q-wave acute myocardial infarction. *Am. J. Cardiol.* 59:263, 1987.
74. Roberts, R., Croft, C., Gold, H. K., et al. Effect of propranolol on myocardial infarct size in a randomized blinded multicenter trial. *N. Engl. J. Med.* 311:218, 1984.
75. The RISC Group. Risk of myocardial infarction and death during treatment with low dose aspirin and intravenous heparin in men with unstable coronary disease. *Lancet* 336:827, 1990.
76. Théroux, P., Waters, D., Lam, J., et al. Reactivation of unstable angina following discontinuation of heparin. *N. Engl. J. Med.* 327:141, 1992.
77. Conti, R. Heparin after unstable angina, myocardial infarction and coronary angioplasty: When and how should the drug be stopped? (Editorial). *Clin. Cardiol.* 15:793, 1992.
78. Markwardt, F., Kaiser, B., and Novak, G. Studies on antithrombotic effects of recombinant hirudin. *Thromb. Res.* 54:377, 1989.
79. TIMI III. Presented at the Nov. 1994 American Heart Association meeting by E. Braunwald.
80. deFeyter, P. J., Suryapranata, H., Serruys, P. W., et al. Coronary angioplasty for unstable angina: Immediate and late results in 200 consecutive patients with identification of risk factors for unfavorable early and late outcome. *J. Am. Coll. Cardiol.* 12:324, 1988.
81. Théroux, P., and Lidón, R-M. Unstable angina: Pathogenesis, diagnosis, and treatment. *Curr. Probl. Cardiol.* 18:157, 1993.

21. Pulmonary Embolism and Systemic Embolism in Patients with Acute Myocardial Infarction

James E. Dalen

The incidence of venous thromboembolism (VTE) in patients with acute myocardial infarction has decreased dramatically. The primary factors predisposing to VTE in patients with acute myocardial infarction are immobility and congestive heart failure. In the past patients with acute myocardial infarction were kept at bed rest for weeks, whereas at the present time patients with uncomplicated myocardial infarction rarely remain in bed for more than a few days and the total hospital stay is usually less than a week. The clinical incidence of pulmonary embolism in patients with uncomplicated myocardial infarction is approximately 1 to 8 percent [1].

VTE is most likely to occur in myocardial infarction patients who are at prolonged bed rest due to complications, particularly those associated with congestive heart failure. The myocardial infarction patients who are at greatest risk are those who have additional risk factors for VTE (Table 21-1). A history of VTE is an important risk factor.

Prevention of Venous Thromboembolism

In patients with an uncomplicated myocardial infarction who do not have additional risk factors for VTE, low-dose heparin (5000 units subcutaneously every 12 hours) and early mobilization are adequate to prevent VTE [2]. The risks of low-dose heparin are minimal. It is our policy to begin low-dose heparin in all patients who are admitted with suspected acute myocardial infarction. When the infarction is excluded and the patient is ambulatory, heparin is discontinued. If the diagnosis of myocardial infarction is confirmed, we continue low-dose heparin until the patient is out of the coronary care unit and is ambulating actively.

In patients with myocardial infarction complicated by congestive heart failure or prolonged bed rest, and in those with additional risk factors for VTE (see Table 21-1), low-dose heparin is inadequate to prevent VTE. In this circumstance, intravenous heparin is indicated. After a 5000-unit bolus, intravenous heparin at a rate of 1000 units/hr is begun. The hourly dose is adjusted to prolong the partial thromboplastin time (PTT) to 1.5 to 2.0 times the control value. Heparin should be continued until the patient is ambulatory.

If heparin is contraindicated, external compression devices can effectively prevent deep vein thrombosis [3]. They should be utilized until the patient is ambulatory. In patients at very high risk (e.g., a patient with recent VTE whose myocardial infarction is complicated and in whom heparin is contraindicated), it may be appropriate to place a filter in the inferior vena cava [4].

Detection of Deep Vein Thrombosis

Pulmonary embolism nearly always originates as venous thrombosis in the lower extremities. Unfortunately, this process is usually clinically silent. The most specific sign of proximal deep vein thrombosis is unilateral leg swelling; however, this finding is not sensitive in that it occurs in only a few patients with deep vein thrombosis.

The most useful diagnostic test for deep vein thrombosis is impedance plethysmography, which is noninvasive and is easily performed at the bedside [5]. A unilaterally positive result is essentially

Table 21-1
Risk factors for venous thromboembolism in patients with acute myocardial infarction

Prolonged bed rest, especially when due to congestive heart failure
History of venous thromboembolism
Cancer
Advanced age
Obesity

diagnostic of proximal deep vein thrombosis, and this finding is sufficient to begin full-dose heparin therapy [6]. Bilaterally normal findings on impedance plethysmography essentially exclude proximal deep vein thrombosis. Duplex ultrasound is equally sensitive and specific for proximal deep vein thrombosis [7].

If proximal deep vein thrombosis is documented by impedance plethysmography or venography, full-dose intravenous heparin is indicated to prevent pulmonary embolism. If heparin is contraindicated, an inferior vena cava filter should be placed.

Detection of Pulmonary Embolism

If deep vein thrombosis is not prevented, and if it is not detected and treated, pulmonary embolism may occur and cause one of three syndromes: acute cor pulmonale, pulmonary infarction, or acute unexplained dyspnea.

Acute Cor Pulmonale

Acute cor pulmonale due to massive pulmonary embolism obstructing more than 60 percent of the pulmonary circulation is the most dramatic but the least frequent manifestation of acute pulmonary embolism. When more than 60 percent of the pulmonary circulation is acutely obstructed by emboli, the right ventricle dilates and fails. The central venous pressure increases and the stroke volume and cardiac output decrease, with resultant hypotension, syncope, or cardiac arrest [8].

The principal symptoms of acute cor pulmonale are dyspnea, anxiety, and possible syncope. On physical examination, one notes tachypnea (> 20/min), tachycardia, and hypotension in most patients. The signs of acute right ventricular failure include distended neck veins, an S_3 gallop, and a parasternal heave. The lungs are usually clear. The most important diagnostic tests are the electrocardiogram (ECG), which demonstrates a new S_1 Q_3 T_3 pattern or new incomplete right bundle branch block in most patients [9]. Arterial blood gas analysis demonstrates significant hypoxemia, hypocapnia, and respiratory alkalosis. The diagnosis may be confirmed by a ventilation-perfusion (V/Q) lung scan or pulmonary angiography.

Pulmonary Infarction

Pulmonary infarction occurs when pulmonary embolism causes complete obstruction of a distal branch of the pulmonary circulation [10]. Because patients with pulmonary infarction have submassive pulmonary embolism, there are no signs or symptoms of acute cor pulmonale. The dominant symptom of pulmonary infarction is pleuritic chest pain, which may be accompanied by dyspnea, cough, and hemoptysis. The pleuritic pain may be confused with the pain of pericarditis, or it may be attributed to a pulmonary infection.

On physical examination the principal findings are in the lungs, and may include rales, wheezes, or a pleural friction rub. In addition to tachypnea, tachycardia may be present. The cardiac examination remains unchanged.

The ECG is of little benefit other than helping to exclude pericarditis. The chest radiograph is usually abnormal, demonstrating an infiltrate (which is rarely wedge shaped) or a small unilateral pleural effusion [9].

Arterial blood gas analysis may demonstrate hypoxemia, or the oxygen pressure may remain in the low-normal range, as a small portion of the pulmonary circulation is compromised. Hypocapnia and respiratory alkalosis are usually present.

Because the principal differential diagnosis is pulmonary infection, viral or bacterial, the white blood cell count, temperature, and sputum analysis are important. The diagnosis can usually be determined by V/Q scan and impedance plethysmography. If the lung scan is nonspecific and impedance plethysmography or duplex ultrasound results are bilaterally normal, pulmonary embolism is unlikely [11]. If the findings are inconclusive, a selective pulmonary angiogram to evaluate the findings of the perfusion scan may be indicated.

Acute, Unexplained Dyspnea

If pulmonary embolism is submassive, and if pulmonary infarction does not occur, the only symptoms may be dyspnea and possibly anxiety. Pulmonary embolism is often overlooked in this setting. The physical examination is unchanged except for tachypnea and possibly tachycardia. The ECG and chest radiograph are unchanged. The dyspnea is often attributed to left ventricular failure secondary to acute myocardial infarction. Examination of the lungs and a chest radiograph help to exclude left ventricular failure. If a pulmonary artery catheter is in place, the wedge pressure is normal in the absence of left ventricular failure, but the pulmonary artery pressure is elevated owing to precapillary pulmonary hypertension secondary to the pulmonary embolism [12]. Measurement of arterial blood gases is helpful in this setting. If dyspnea is due to acute pulmonary embolism, the arterial oxygen tension (breathing room air) demonstrates obvious hypoxemia. A V/Q or duplex ultrasound scan and impedance plethysmography should lead to the correct diagnosis.

Treatment of Acute Pulmonary Embolism

The cornerstone of treatment for acute pulmonary embolism in patients with acute myocardial infarction is heparin given by intravenous infusion at a rate sufficient to prolong the PTT to 1.5 to 2.0 times control values. Heparin should be continued for 5 to 7 days [13]. Studies are currently under way to determine whether a shorter course of heparin is sufficient.

Warfarin should be begun early in the treatment course, perhaps on day 1 or 2 of heparin therapy. The dose of warfarin should be adjusted to prolong the prothrombin time to an international normalized ratio (INR) of 2.0 to 3.0 [14]. The duration of warfarin therapy depends on the factors that predispose to VTE. If these factors are ongoing (e.g., a patient immobilized by severe congestive heart failure), warfarin therapy should be continued indefinitely. In patients in whom the predisposition to VTE is chronic, inferior vena caval interruption with a filter may be considered. Anticoagulant therapy with heparin followed by warfarin is effective in patients with pulmonary embolism uncomplicated by hypotension. The major threat to life in these patients is recurrent, potentially lethal episodes of pulmonary embolism.

In patients with massive pulmonary embolism complicated by acute cor pulmonale and hypotension, prophylactic therapy with anticoagulation may be insufficient. In this circumstance, definitive therapy may be indicated. Pulmonary embolectomy is rarely, if ever, feasible in patients with acute myocardial infarction. However, in some centers transvenous pulmonary embolectomy may be feasible [15].

As an alternative to embolectomy in patients with massive pulmonary embolism complicated by shock, fibrinolytic therapy may be appropriate. The most extensive experience is with urokinase and streptokinase. Treatment with these agents has been shown to increase the early resolution rate of pulmonary embolism, but they have not been shown to decrease the mortality associated with acute pulmonary embolism [16]. The primary complication of fibrinolytic therapy is bleeding, especially from the sites of arterial or venous procedures. Preliminary reports indicate that treatment of pulmonary embolism with tissue plasminogen activator (t-PA) may be more effective than treatment with urokinase and streptokinase [17]. However, further studies are required to determine the efficacy and the hemorrhagic complication rate of t-PA.

It should be stressed that only a few patients with pulmonary embolism require definitive therapy with embolectomy of fibrinolytic agents. Most of these patients do well if further episodes are prevented with appropriate prophylactic therapy.

Systemic Embolism

Systemic emboli in patients with acute myocardial infarction may arise from two sources: the left ventricle and the left atrium. Left atrial thrombi leading to systemic embolism may occur in patients with atrial fibrillation [18] or other arrhythmias characterized by a lack of effective atrial contraction [19] and in patients with coexistent mitral valve disease [20].

The most common source of systemic embolism in patients with acute myocardial infarction is left ventricular thrombi. It is clear from studies utilizing two-dimensional echocardiography that left ventricular thrombi are most frequently associated with transmural anterior wall infarction, where the incidence of thrombi may be as high as 30 to 40 percent [21]. The incidence in patients with inferior wall infarction is much lower. It should be noted that two-dimensional echocardiography fails to detect up to 20 percent of left ventricular thrombi [22] and that only a few left ventricular thrombi result in systemic embolism.

The exact incidence of systemic embolism in patients with acute myocardial infarction is uncertain because many systemic emboli are not detected clinically. In postmortem studies the incidence was 5 percent [23]. Most (70 percent) systemic emboli result in cerebral embolism. Embolic stroke occurs in approximately 3 percent of patients with acute myocardial infarction [24].

Prevention of Systemic Embolism

At least three clinical trials have demonstrated that full-dose heparin followed by oral anticoagulants decreases the incidence of stroke in patients with acute myocardial infarction [25–27]. In these three studies, the incidence of stroke was decreased from 2 to 3 percent in control patients to approximately 1 percent in patients who were anticoagulated. Given the hemorrhagic complications of anticoagulant therapy, full-dose anticoagulation is not appropriate in all patients with acute myocardial infarction.

The high incidence of left ventricular thrombi in patients with transmural anterior myocardial infarction indicates that they are the acute myocardial infarction patients at greatest risk of systemic embolism. Several small case-control studies have shown that anticoagulation decreases the incidence of left ventricular thrombi in patients with transmural anterior myocardial infarction as detected by two-dimensional echocardiography [28, 29]. To date, no large randomized trial has demonstrated that anticoagulation decreases the incidence of systemic embolism in patients with transmural anterior myocardial infarction.

Given the available incomplete data, the ACCP National Conference on Antithrombotic Therapy [30] recommended that in the absence of contraindications, patients with transmural anterior myocardial infarction should receive full-dose anticoagulation. They recommended heparin sufficient to prolong the PTT to 1.5 to 2.0 times control, followed by low-intensity warfarin therapy (prothrombin time prolonged to an INR of 2.0 to 3.0) for 3 months.

It must be noted that there is no evidence that low-dose heparin, aspirin, or other platelet-active agents decrease the incidence of systemic embolism in patients with acute myocardial infarction.

Treatment of Systemic Embolism

The treatment of systemic embolism in patients with acute myocardial infarction depends on the site of the embolism. Emboli to the upper or lower extremities may be removed by the use of the Fogarty catheter [31], with follow-up anticoagulation with heparin and warfarin to prevent recurrent embolism. When emboli affect the viscera, thrombolytic therapy may be appropriate in addition to anticoagulation.

Treatment of the most common form of systemic embolism—cerebral embolism—is somewhat controversial. Some clinicians are reluctant to anticoagulate because of the fear of brain hemorrhage due to hemorrhagic transformation of a bland infarct. The Cerebral Embolism Study Group addressed this problem, utilizing serial computed tomography (CT) scans [32]. They found that the incidence of hemorrhagic transformation was greatest in patients with large infarcts and in those in whom anticoagulation was initiated less than 12 hours after the onset of symptoms [32]. The recommendation of the ACCP/Task Force on Antithrombotic Therapy [33] was that nonhypertensive patients with small to moderate-sized embolic strokes should have a CT scan 48 hours or more after stroke onset. If the CT scan documents the absence of spontaneous hemorrhage and there are no contraindications, intravenous heparin treatment sufficient to prolong the PTT to 1.5 to 2.0 times control should be initiated. Heparin therapy should be followed by warfarin therapy at a dose that prolongs the prothrombin time to an INR of 2.0 to 3.0. Warfarin therapy should be continued for 3 months.

References

1. Salzman, E. W., and Hirsch, J. Prevention of venous thromboembolism. In R. W. Colman et al. (eds.), *Hemostasis and Thrombosis: Basic Principles and Clinical Practice* (2nd ed.) Philadelphia: Lippincott, 1987.
2. Hull, R. D., and Hirsch, J. Preventing venous thromboembolism. *J. Cardiovasc. Med.* 9:63, 1984.
3. Moser, G., Krahenbuhl, B., Barroussel, R., et al. Mechanical versus pharmacologic prevention of deep venous thrombosis. *Surgery* 152:448, 1981.
4. Kanter, B., and Moser, K. M. The Greenfield vena cava filter. *Chest* 93:170, 1988.
5. Wheeler, H. B. Diagnosis of deep vein thrombosis. *Am. J. Surg.* 150:7, 1985.
6. Hull, R. D., Hirsch, J., Carter, C. J., et al. Diagnostic efficacy of impedance plethysmography for clinically suspected deep-vein thrombosis. *Ann. Intern. Med.* 102:21, 1985.
7. Polak, J. F. Doppler ultrasound of the deep leg veins. *Chest* 99:1655, 1991.
8. Thames, M. D., Alpert, J. S., and Dalen, J. E. Syncope in patients with pulmonary embolism. *J.A.M.A.* 238:2509, 1977.
9. Szucs, M., Jr., Brooks, H. L., Johnson, L. W., et al. Diagnostic sensitivity of laboratory findings in acute pulmonary embolism. *Ann. Intern. Med.* 74:161, 1971.
10. Dalen, J. E., Haffajee, C. I., Alpert, J. S., et al. Pulmonary embolism, pulmonary hemorrhage, pulmonary infarction. *N. Engl. J. Med.* 296:1431, 1977.
11. Dalen, J. E. When can treatment be withheld in the treatment of patients with suspected pulmonary embolism? *Arch. Intern. Med.* 153:1415, 1993.
12. Dalen, J. E., Dexter, L., Ockene, I. S., and Carlson, J. Precapillary pulmonary hypertension: Its relationship to pulmonary venous hypertension. *Trans. Am. Clin. Climatol. Assoc.* 86:207, 1974.
13. Hyers, T. M., Hull, R. D., and Weg, J. G. Antithrombotic therapy for venous thromboembolic disease *Chest* 102:4085, 1992.
14. Hyers, T. M., Hull, R. D., and Weg, J. G. Antithrombotic therapy for venous thromboembolic disease. *Chest* 102:408S, 1992.
15. Greenfield, L. J., and Zocco, J. J. Intraluminal management of acute massive pulmonary thromboembolism. *J. Thorac. Cardiovasc. Surg.* 77:402, 1979.
16. Dalen, J. E. The case against fibrinolytic therapy. *J. Cardiovasc. Med.* 5:799, 1980.
17. Goldhaber, S. Z., Markis, J. E., Meyerovitz, M. F., et al. Acute pulmonary embolism treated with tissue plasminogen activator. *Lancet* 1:886, 1986.
18. Abbott, W. M., Maloney, R. D., McCabe, C. C., et al. Arterial embolism: A 44 year perspective. *Am. J. Surg.* 1243:460, 1982.
19. Fairfax, A. J., Lambert, C. D., and Leatham, A. Systemic embolism in chronic sinoatrial disorder. *N. Engl. J. Med.* 295:190, 1976.
20. Coulshed, N., Epstein, E. J., McKendrick, C. S., et al. Systemic embolism in mitral valve disease. *Br. Heart J.* 32:26, 1970.
21. Asinger, R. W., Mikell, F. L., Elsperger, J., et al. Incidence of left ventricular thrombosis after acute transmural myocardial infarction. *N. Engl. J. Med.* 305:297, 1981.
22. Ezekowitz, M. D., Wilson, D. A., Smith, E. O., et al. Comparison of indium-111 platelet scintigraphy and two-dimensional echocardiography in the diagnosis of left ventricular thrombi. *N. Engl. J. Med.* 306:1509, 1982.
23. Hilden, T., Iversen, K., Raaschou, F., et al. Anticoagulants in acute myocardial infarction. *Lancet* 2:327, 1961.
24. Drapkin, A., and Merskey, C. Anticoagulant therapy after acute myocardial infarction: Relation of therapeutic benefit to patient's age, sex and severity of infarction. *J.A.M.A.* 222:541, 1972.
25. United States Veterans Administration: Long-term anticoagulant therapy after myocardial infarction. *J.A.M.A.* 193:157, 1965.
26. Second Report of the Working Party on Anticoagulant Therapy in Coronary Thrombosis to the Medical Research Council: An assessment of long-term anticoagulant administration after cardiac infarction. *B.M.J.* 2:837, 1964.
27. Veterans Administration Cooperative Trial on Anticoagulation. Anticoagulants in acute myocardial infarction: Results of a cooperative clinical trial. *J.A.M.A.* 225:724, 1973.
28. Weinreich, D. J., Burke, J. F., and Pauletto, F. J. Left ventricular mural thrombi complicating acute myocardial infarction: Long-term follow-up with serial echocardiography. *Ann. Intern. Med.* 100:789, 1984.
29. Keating, E. C., Gross, S. A., Schlamowitz, R. A., et al. Mural thrombi in myocardial infarctions: Prospective evaluation of two-dimensional echocardiography. *Am. J. Med.* 74:989, 1983.
30. Cairns, J. A., Hirsh, J., Lewis, H. D., et al. Antithrombotic agents in coronary artery disease. *Chest* 102: 456S, 1992.
31. Sheiner, N. M., Zeltzer, J., and MacIntosh, E. Arterial embolectomy in the modern era. *Can. J. Surg.* 25:373, 1982.
32. Cerebral Embolism Study Group: Cardioembolic stroke, early anticoagulation, and brain hemorrhage. *Arch. Intern. Med.* 147:636, 1987.
33. Sherman, D. G., Dyken, M. L., Fisher, M., et al. Antithrombotic therapy for cerebrovascular disorders. *Chest* 102:529S, 1992.

22. Cardiopulmonary Resuscitation in Patients with Acute Myocardial Infarction

Karl B. Kern and Gordon A. Ewy

Cardiopulmonary resuscitation (CPR) is intended to revive individuals who have experienced an unexpected cardiac arrest [1–3]. Thus not all patients with myocardial infarction are candidates for resuscitation. Although clinical death occurs when the patient's heart stops beating, cellular metabolism continues for a limited period of time. Unless effective CPR is promptly instituted, cellular ischemia and death quickly follow. The probability of successful CPR depends on the duration of the arrest prior to initiating therapy, the age of the patient, the presence of associated illnesses, and the degree of cardiac damage sustained prior to the cessation of circulation [4–6]. Early recognition is an essential initial step. For this reason, all patients with acute or suspected myocardial infarctions should be monitored electrocardiographically.

Defibrillation is the most important single event of successful resuscitation. Accordingly, the guidelines for CPR and emergency cardiac care have been changed and now emphasize early defibrillation capability including the use of automatic external defibrillators [7].

In the intensive care setting, respiratory arrest can precede cardiac arrest, but prompt assisted ventilation prevents the problem. Because this sequence is rare in the patient with acute myocardial infarction, respiratory arrest is not addressed.

Cardiac Arrest Associated with Acute Myocardial Infarction

Cardiac arrest is a known complication of acute myocardial infarction. Goldberg and colleagues [127] showed that approximately 20 percent of patients having an acute myocardial infarction will experience cardiac arrest. Typically about half of these cardiac arrests occur within the first 48 hours after the onset of the myocardial infarction. It is in the emergent treatment of cardiac arrest that coronary care units have had their greatest impact in decreasing acute myocardial infarction mortality. The Worcester Heart Attack Study identified several characteristics of patients who had cardiac arrest with an acute myocardial infarction [127]. Large Q-wave infarctions were significantly more likely to be complicated with sudden cardiac death than were small or non-Q-wave infarctions [127]. Other investigators [128] found that anterior infarctions are more often associated with cardiac arrest than are inferior or lateral wall infarcts. In-hospital mortality is higher in patients having cardiac arrest but long-term survival rates are similar between acute myocardial infarction patients with and those without initial cardiac arrest [127].

Though sudden cardiac death related to coronary artery disease and acute myocardial infarction is the most prevalent cause of death in America today, prompt and appropriate out-of-hospital and in-hospital treatment of cardiac arrest can prevent a large number of these deaths [7].

Mechanism of Blood Flow with External Chest Compression

In 1960 Kouwenhouven and associates [1] described a noninvasive technique for CPR. Over the ensuing two decades there was little change in what was known as conventional or standard CPR. By the mid-1970s, one of the few remaining questions concerning CPR was the rate at which external chest compression should be applied. In 1977

Taylor [8] and others [9] indicated that over a range of 40 to 80 compressions per minute the *duration* of chest compression was more important than the *rate* of chest compression. At 50 percent chest compression and 50 percent relaxation, duty cycle at a rate of 60 compressions per minute was thought to be optimal [7]. However, work from Duke University indicated that a faster chest compression rate produces better blood flow during closed-chest CPR [10, 11]. Some of these data were available at the time of the 1985 National Conference on CPR [129]. Consequently, this information played a role in the recommendations for a chest compression rate of 80 to 100 per minute [129].

Physiologists and physicians have assumed that external chest compression in the arrested patient created artificial circulation by compressing the heart in much the same manner as open-chest internal cardiac massage. It was assumed that during sternal compression there was cardiac compression and that blood moved from the left ventricle into the aorta as closure of the mitral valve prevented retrograde blood flow. This widely held concept was challenged during the late 1970s by Weisfeldt and associates [12–16]. These physicians believed that this concept was inconsistent with a number of observations. The first was that when sternal compression was performed in a patient with a flail chest no radial arterial blood pressure was recorded until the remainder of the chest was bound to prevent paradoxical expansion [12, 14]. The second clinical observation was that patients with chronic obstructive lung disease and a marked increase in anterior-posterior chest diameter and a relatively small heart could be resuscitated by sternal compression [12, 14]. The third observation was that during conventional CPR the compression cycle that followed ventilation often resulted in increased blood pressure and blood flow [12, 14]. Weisfeldt's group extended these observations by maintaining airway pressure with a bag-mask device and noted that this method also increased radial artery pressure during external chest compression [12]. These findings suggested that forward blood flow was related to an increase in intrathoracic pressure. This theory was supported by the studies of Criley and associates [17] on "cough CPR" (see below).

Another important observation was the rediscovery that the pressures in the aorta and right atrium were often similar during external sternal compression. This observation was reported by Weale and Rothwell-Jackson in 1962 [18] but received little attention. Weisfeldt and associates [12, 14] found that during chest compression not only were the central venous and aortic pressures similar but also the pressures in all cardiac chambers as well as in all the intrathoracic structures were nearly equal. In a fluid-filled system with a resistance, there must be a pressure gradient across the resistance to allow fluid to flow. When the heart is pumping normally, there is a large pressure gradient between the aorta and the central veins and right atrium. The lack of a gradient during external chest compression in their arrested subjects suggested to these investigators that the heart was not functioning as a pump [12, 14]. They concluded that the entire thorax was the "pump" during CPR.

In contrast to the similar pressures inside the thorax, Weisfeldt and associates [14] found a significant pressure difference between the extrathoracic carotid artery and jugular veins. This pressure gradient was thought to be sufficient to produce cerebral blood flow. The reason for the pressure difference between the intrathoracic and extrathoracic veins was initially not clear [14]. At the same time, Criley and coworkers [17] demonstrated that jugular venous valves were operative during coughing. This observation led to a renewed appreciation of the internal jugular valves that were well described by early anatomists [19]. Figure 22-1 illustrates how the thorax, in conjunction with these jugular venous valves, acts as a "pump."

Early two-dimensional echocardiographic studies during CPR in humans showed that the mitral valve did not close and that the left ventricular internal diameter was little changed [20, 21]. These findings supported the observation that in some patients increased intrathoracic pressure and not cardiac compression accounted for the forward blood flow during external chest compression.

Cardiac compression does occur in humans [12]. In a few of the patients studied by the Johns Hopkins group, simultaneous central venous pressures were lower than arterial pressures during external chest compression, indicating cardiac compression [12]. It is of interest that in patients in whom cardiac compression is present the arterial pressure generated is generally higher than that found in patients without cardiac compression [9]. Weisfeldt and associates [12] emphasized that "in these patients in

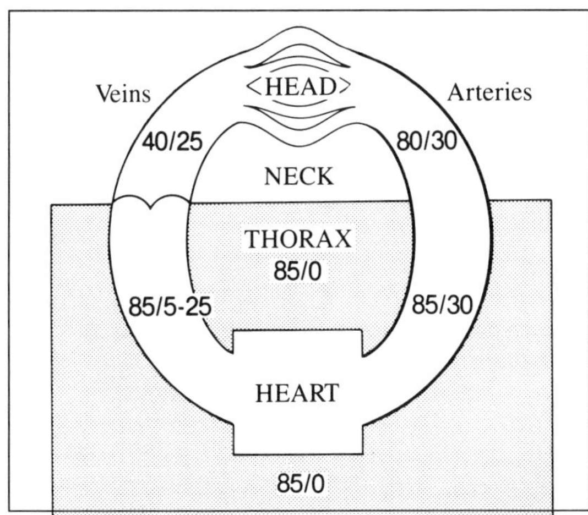

Fig. 22-1
Thoracic "pump" wherein pressures produced in the thorax are equally transmitted to an intrathoracic vascular structure. Note the reflection of that transmitted pressure by the extrathoracic venous jugular valve, which allows a pressure gradient across the central nervous system vascular bed resulting in antegrade flow to the head.

whom direct cardiac compression can be applied effectively, a particularly attractive feature of the maneuver is that the aortic diastolic pressure seems to rise significantly more than it does when the blood is moved solely by manipulating intrathoracic pressure; this means coronary perfusion is probably improved. For this reason, we strongly recommend that chest compression be included in any new CPR system designed to take advantage of the potentially useful effects of manipulating generalized intrathoracic pressure." The importance of this statement has been underscored by more recent studies (see below).

If in most patients blood flow during external chest compression depends on increased intrathoracic pressure, the question that logically follows is if altering techniques of conventional CPR could enhance blood flow during external chest compression. Accordingly, Weisfeldt and associates [14] at Johns Hopkins explored two basic strategies: direct increases in intrathoracic pressure and abdominal binding. Although increased intrathoracic pressure could be obtained by clamping the endotracheal tube during chest compression, the initial increase in pressure and flow dissipated rapidly, undoubtedly because venous return is inhibited by the continuous high intrathoracic pressure [12]. These investigators [14] then reported that maintaining inflated lungs during external chest compression resulted in a significant increase in arterial pressure and carotid flow when compared to conventional CPR (Table 22-1). These results were confirmed by other investigators using simultaneous high-pressure ventilation and chest compression in large [22] but not small [22, 23] dogs. In small dogs, true cardiac compression evidently occurs with relatively good blood pressure and flow, and the addition of simultaneous high-pressure ventilation does not appear to improve these hemodynamics [22]. In large animals, where cardiac compression plays a small role, the addition of simultaneous ventilation improves peripheral circulation [22].

The second approach to augment blood flow during CPR was abdominal binding (see Table 22-1). Redding [24] was the first to show that abdominal binding during CPR improves survival as well as hemodynamics. However, further investigation of this technique was interrupted by studies that reported a high incidence of liver laceration secondary to abdominal binding [25]. Studies that applied abdominal binding during CPR using military antishock trousers (MAST) also revealed a high incidence of liver laceration and exsanguination [26]. The technique advocated by the group at Johns Hopkins utilized a device similar to an enlarged blood pressure cuff that distributes pressure over the abdomen in a broader fashion. They then reported the use of such a device in humans [16].

The ultimate utility of simultaneous high-pressure ventilation or abdominal binding would be determined by whether these interventions resulted in an increase in survival. In an effort to answer

Table 22-1
Effects of maintaining lungs inflated and binding the abdomen during chest compression

Treatment	Aortic systolic blood pressure (mm Hg)	Carotid flow (ml/min)
Chest compression plus	27	9
lungs inflated	58	29
Chest compression plus	29	15
abdominal binding	58	32

Source: After M. T. Rudikoff, W. L. Maughan, M. Effron et al. Mechanisms of blood flow during cardiopulmonary resuscitation. *Circulation* 61:345, 1980.

this question, an experimental form of CPR that utilized high-pressure (60 torr) ventilation, chest compression with a broad flat surface, and abdominal binding (60 torr) was compared to standard CPR in our laboratory. Standard or experimental CPR was performed during ventricular fibrillation [27]. Five of the six animals that underwent standard CPR had a return of blood pressure and survived, whereas none of the six animals that underwent simultaneous high-pressure ventilation, diffuse chest compression, and abdominal pressure had a return of blood pressure following defibrillation, and none could be resuscitated despite intensive efforts [27]. Nevertheless, a National Heart, Lung, and Blood Institute (NHLBI)–funded study in humans was performed in Dade County, Florida. The mortality was higher in patients randomized to receive simultaneous chest compression and ventilation [28]. The hemodynamic reasons for the deleterious effect of simultaneous chest compression and ventilation are discussed below.

In contrast to the "thoracic pump" mechanism of blood flow during CPR, Rankin and associates were convinced from their clinical experience that faster chest compression rates were more effective and that cardiac compression was the mechanism of blood flow during CPR. Maier, Rankin, and associates [10, 11] studied the effects of varying the manual compression rate, force, and duration in large dogs. They reported that the relative contributions of the thoracic pump and direct cardiac compression mechanisms to blood flow varied with the method of CPR being performed [10, 11]. Direct cardiac compression seemed to be more significant during high-impulse (increased frequency) CPR, and the thoracic pump mechanism was predominant during low-momentum compression techniques. Echocardiographic studies by Deshmukh and associates [29, 30] in anesthetized minipigs demonstrated cardiac valve motion and a change in left ventricular dimensions during the early phases of closed-chest CPR, adding further support for direct cardiac compression as a mechanism of blood flow during CPR.

As with most disagreements, there is probably truth on both sides. It is our conclusion that the mechanism of blood flow during closed-chest compression is a spectrum varying from a purely thoracic pump mechanism (cough or vest CPR) on one end of the spectrum and cardiac compression (open-chest CPR) on the other; with still others, for example, standard, mechanical thumper, or high-impulse CPR, there are varying combinations of thoracic pump and cardiac pump depending on the anatomic attributes of the subject and the duration of CPR. This conclusion is based on the following observations. Patients in sinus rhythm and subjects in cardiac arrest undergoing open-chest cardiac compression display a large difference between the aortic and right atrial systolic pressures. In contrast, there appears to be little or no systolic pressure difference between the aorta and right atrium in those subjects in whom blood moves by the thoracic pump mechanism during CPR. Because of this observation we evaluated the absolute difference between aortic and right atrial systolic pressure (which we called the systolic pressure gradient, or SPG) in 63 adult mongrel dogs undergoing five methods of CPR [31]. After 3 minutes of "down time," during which no CPR was performed, the animals were ventilated and one of five methods of CPR was initiated. Systolic pressure gradients were measured at 1, 7, and 17 minutes of CPR. The systolic pressure gradient was greatest during open-chest cardiac massage (true cardiac compression), intermediate with external mechanical (thumper) and standard CPR, and lowest with CPR performed with a combined thoracic and abdominal vest apparatus (predominantly thoracic pump) [31]. The findings are shown in Figure 22-2.

It was also noted that the 24-hour survival rate was greatest in the groups treated with cardiac compression and least in those treated with the thoracic pump mechanism (see Fig. 22-2) [31]. This latter observation is of interest in light of the report by Deshmukh and associates concerning a two-dimensional echocardiographic study of eight minipigs [29, 30]. The aortic and mitral valves demonstrated appropriate systolic and diastolic behavior for the first 5 minutes in all animals but for 12 minutes in the three minipigs successfully resuscitated [29, 30].

We concluded that the mechanism of blood flow during closed-chest CPR varies according to *technique;* it is greatest with the open-chest technique (see below) and high-impulse CPR and lowest with vest CPR. The mechanism also varies with *duration* of CPR, with cardiac compression being the mechanism early and thoracic pump later. The fact is that the patients reported by the Johns Hopkins group

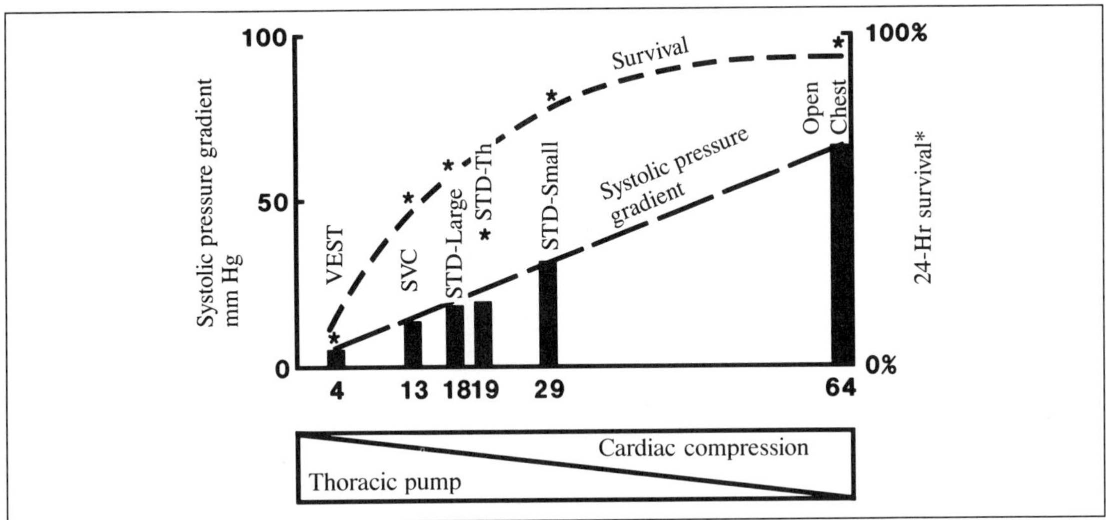

Fig. 22-2
Systolic pressure gradient as a potential indicator of the mechanism of cardiopulmonary resuscitation (CPR)–generated blood flow. Of note is the relation between increased survival and CPR blood flow resulting from cardiac compression. SVC = simultaneous ventilation and compression CPR; STD = standard CPR; Th = thumper CPR.

were studied only after the house staff had ''given up'' and turned the patient over to the CPR research team, who then had to instrument the patients prior to their studies. The average *systolic* arterial pressure generated by these investigators with standard CPR was less than 30 mm Hg (see Table 22-1). Thus by the time these measurements were made, the thoracic pump mechanism was predominant. The third determinant of blood flow during closed-chest CPR is the *anatomic makeup* of the subject. Patients with narrow anterior-posterior chest diameters and a large heart have more cardiac compression than does the emphysematous patient with a large anterior-posterior chest diameter and a small heart.

Recent transesophageal echocardiography studies during CPR in humans at the Mayo Clinic [130] indicated that cardiac compression, especially right ventricular compression, is the mechanism of blood flow during CPR in humans. In summary, the mechanism of blood flow during closed-chest CPR depends on the anatomy and pathology of the patient, the duration of CPR, and the technique used. We recommend a compression rate of at least 100 per minute with a 50 percent compression/50 percent relaxation ratio.

Since cardiac compression is often the major mechanism of blood flow in humans, and since a fixed stroke volume is moved forward with each compression, a rapid compression rate is essential. We showed that audioguidance is often necessary for the would-be rescuer to maintain an optimal rate of near 100 chest compressions per minute [131].

Cough Resuscitation

Criley and associates [32, 33] introduced cough CPR, which is accomplished by having the patient with recent-onset asystole or ventricular fibrillation cough forcefully every 1 to 2 seconds. The obvious disadvantage of this technique is that it must be initiated before the patient loses consciousness. Forceful cough results in an abrupt increase in intrathoracic pressures, which can result in striking aortic systolic pressures (Fig. 22-3). By employing cough CPR in the cardiac catheterization laboratory, Criley and coworkers [32, 33] had patients sustain consciousness for 24 and 39 seconds after the onset of ventricular fibrillation. Cough CPR has several advantages: It enables laboratory personnel to turn their full attention to preparing for and using the defibrillator rather than performing cardiac massage; it can be performed by a patient in any position and on any surface, including the lateral position of the angiographic cradle; and finally, not

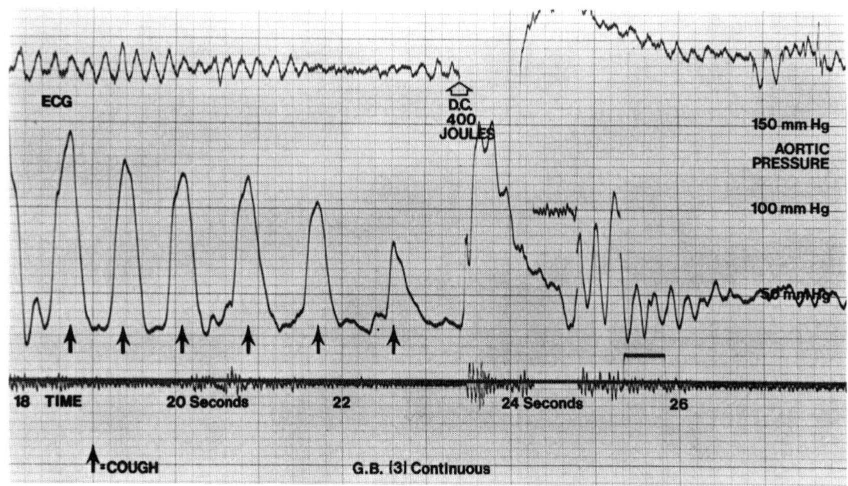

Fig. 22-3
Marked aortic pressure spikes seen with simple rhythmic coughing during ventricular fibrillation. Aortic peak pressure ranges from 80 to 145 mm Hg. No compressions of any type were performed during this tracing. (From G. A. Ewy and R. Bressler, eds., *Cardiovascular Drugs and Management of Heart Disease.* New York: Raven Press, 1982. P. 365.)

only are the hazards of fracture avoided, but also ventilation occurs spontaneously [32, 33]. The potential for using cough CPR in areas other than the cardiac catheterization laboratory needs further exploration. A recent case report suggested the use of cough CPR as a less traumatic resuscitation technique in arresting patients with acute myocardial infarction, thereby not eliminating the later use of thrombolytic agents [132]. Cough has been used not only for resuscitation but also for termination of ventricular tachycardia [34].

Open-Chest Cardiac Massage

Open-chest cardiac massage sounds primitive in the present era but may well be indicated in selected situations. Conventional CPR, which produces only 6 to 30 percent of normal blood flow, cannot sustain tissue viability—it only slows the process of dying. The question is whether open-chest cardiac massage provides sufficient increase in blood flow over standard noninvasive resuscitation methods to justify its use.

There have been few published studies in humans comparing closed- and open-chest CPR. Del Guercio and associates [35] recorded hemodynamics of patients undergoing CPR with closed-chest compression and repeated these measurements with open-chest cardiac massage. The cardiac output and circulation times were significantly improved by the open-chest technique. However, this study was criticized because the green dye dilution techniques used are inaccurate at low flow states [36].

There are indications for open-chest cardiac massage in clinical medicine. Patients with cardiac arrest and major chest trauma or penetrating chest wounds should be treated with open-chest massage once they arrive at the hospital. Patients undergoing thoracic surgery should also undergo open-chest massage should they arrest. The major question concerns the use of open-chest massage when standard closed-chest compression is not effective. This issue is further complicated by another major deficit in the field of CPR, namely the inability to determine the effectiveness of closed-chest compression. If an arterial pulse is not perceptible, one can be sure that external chest compression alone is inadequate. If a pulse is palpable, the question remains whether this pulse is only a transmitted pressure wave or is a true arterial pulse. Even if it is a true arterial pulse, if the diastolic pressure is not adequate the subject is not likely to survive.

If a pulse cannot be generated after a reasonable trial of external chest compression, the patient may be hypovolemic or have cardiac tamponade—conditions that are difficult to diagnose during cardiac arrest. Likewise, the patient might simply be inadequately perfused with closed-chest compression CPR. How long should efforts with ineffective closed-chest compression persist before more drastic therapy such as open-chest cardiac massage be instituted? In an experimental model of cardiac arrest, we found open-chest massage effective when instituted after 15 minutes of ineffective closed-chest resuscitation [37]. However, when internal massage was delayed for 20 minutes of closed-chest efforts, successful resuscitation with open-chest massage was less likely, and when 25 minutes elapsed before open-chest cardiac compressions were performed, none of the experimental subjects could be resuscitated. It appears that though open-chest massage can effectively produce excellent myocardial perfusion pressures, if a lengthy period of poor myocardial perfusion precedes the use of internal resuscitation techniques, no improvement in resuscitation outcome results.

Open-chest cardiac massage has clearly been shown to improve hemodynamics, cardiac output, and short-term resuscitation success. However, the long-term effects of internal resuscitation, with its inherent morbidity, were less clear. Could open-chest cardiac massage, when instituted after 15 minutes of closed-chest compressions, improve long-term survival as well as initial resuscitation outcome? In an experiment designed to evaluate this question, we found that open-chest massage begun after 15 minutes of ventricular fibrillation and closed-chest compression was strikingly superior for producing 7-day survival compared to continued closed-chest efforts [38] (Fig. 22-4).

Geehr and associates [39]performed a limited trial of open-chest cardiac massage in victims of out-of-hospital cardiac arrest. They found no difference in open-chest massage versus continued closed-chest compressions in 50 patients. Both groups had three initial resuscitated survivors, but no patient lived long term [39]. Careful evaluation of the details of this study revealed that all patients had a minimum of 20 to 30 minutes of cardiac arrest and closed-chest compression prior to randomization to continue closed-chest efforts versus open-chest massage. Hence their results were similar to the findings of our experimental work showing that open-chest cardiac massage does not improve survival when instituted after a lengthy period of closed-chest efforts. In both experimental models and limited clinical trials it appears that open-chest cardiac massage is unlikely to improve survival from cardiac arrest when used only as a last ditch effort. Nonetheless, it is also apparent that with proper timing, open-chest cardiac massage is clearly the superior resuscitation technique at present.

Fig. 22-4
Open-chest cardiac massage (*closed bars*) improves initial resuscitation results, 24-hour survival, and 7-day survival when instituted after 15 minutes of standard closed-chest compression CPR (*hatched bars*) and failed external defibrillation.

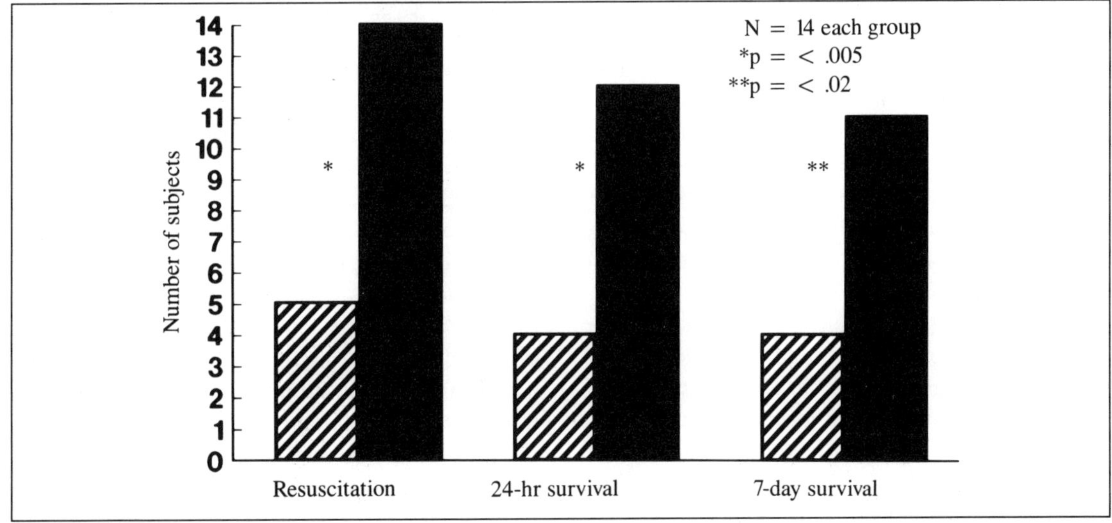

Open-Chest Cardiac Massage During Acute Myocardial Infarction

Open-chest massage is one resuscitation technique that has been experimentally evaluated in the setting of myocardial infarction and cardiac arrest. Weiser and associates [40] studied the hemodynamic effects of closed- and open-chest cardiac resuscitation in both normal dogs and those with myocardial infarction. Experimental myocardial infarctions were attempted by injecting plastic microspheres into the ascending aorta and allowing random entry into the coronary circulation, though no documentation of actual infarction was provided. The authors commented on the superiority of open-chest massage for producing higher aortic pressures and cardiac outputs, but no analysis compared the effect of the bead-induced myocardial infarction on hemodynamics, cardiac output, or outcome.

Cardiopulmonary Resuscitation in Subjects with Chronic Ischemia

A study of external versus internal cardiac massage in normal and chronically ischemic dogs was reported in 1980 by Byrne and associates [41]. These investigators measured myocardial blood flow using radioactive microspheres in normal animals and in those with complete circumflex coronary artery occlusions produced by a surgically placed aneroid constrictor. Myocardium supplied by the occluded circumflex artery, presumably then perfused by canine epicardial collaterals, had significantly less blood flow than any other area during external cardiac massage. The authors speculated that similar hypoperfused areas of myocardium are likely to exist in many patients who developed cardiac arrest and that such areas may be more adequately perfused by internal massage. No data were given concerning the relation of CPR-produced intravascular pressures, the amount of blood flow to the normal and ischemic myocardium, or the success of the resuscitation effort.

We adapted a nonsurgical method for the production of a coronary stenosis in closed-chest animals for CPR research. The model, originally described by Gewirtz and Most [42], involves percutaneous transcatheter placement of a plastic cylinder in a coronary artery of the pig. We modified this procedure for the production of a discrete anterior myocardial infarction by occluding the midportion of the left anterior descending coronary artery. We found that allowing thrombotic occlusion of the stenosis in the mid left anterior coronary artery resulted in an anteroseptal infarction involving 28 ± 3 percent of the left ventricle [43]. Subsequently, we produced both discrete patent stenoses and complete coronary occlusions in the pig through the judicious use of anticoagulation therapy.

We applied this model of coronary obstructive disease in preliminary studies of coronary blood flow during CPR. Swine were studied with nonradioactive, colored microspheres for regional blood flow during normal sinus rhythm and ventricular fibrillation treated with external CPR [44, 133]. All animals had one or more Teflon cylinders successfully placed in the left anterior coronary artery during the study. An advantage of this method for creating an "abnormal" heart model for CPR research is avoidance of a thoracotomy. External chest compressions can be performed without concern for nonphysiologic changes within the thorax or chest wall.

We found that prior to coronary manipulations left ventricular myocardial blood flow was 124 ± 56 ml/min/100 gm during sinus rhythm. These data correspond well to published levels of myocardial blood flow in pigs [45–51]. Comparisons of left ventricular blood flow during sinus rhythm showed no difference between the anterior and lateral locations or between blood flows to the epicardium and endocardium.

Blood flow to the left ventricular anterior wall supplied by the left anterior descending coronary artery was studied above and below the location of the experimentally placed intracoronary cylinder. Preliminary data showed that in pigs in which the cylinder is occluded no distal left anterior descending flow occurred. Hence regardless of the coronary perfusion pressure generated by CPR, no blood flow occurred to the myocardium below the level of the obstruction [44]. This initial finding, if confirmed, is important to understanding the distribution of CPR-produced blood flow during acute myocardial infarctions complicated by cardiac arrest. Evidence indicates that most myocardial infarctions indeed result from acute thrombotic occlusions [52]. Hence if a person arrests during an acute coronary occlusion and myocardial infarction, CPR does not produce the same regional myocardial blood flow as in patients without such coronary disease.

The most important finding is that CPR performed in an arrest victim with a left anterior descending coronary artery stenosis produces markedly different regional myocardial blood flows above and below that lesion [133]. We found that for any given coronary perfusion pressure, blood flow below a patent stenosis was only one-half of that above the coronary lesion. The consequences of diminished myocardial blood flow in the presence of coronary stenosis and occlusion are of obvious importance, as greater CPR-produced perfusion pressure may be needed to produce enough blood flow for successful resuscitation.

A better understanding of the effect of coronary lesions and thrombotic occlusions on CPR-generated myocardial blood flow has renewed interest in optimizing myocardial perfusion pressure during resuscitation efforts. Recently, using intracoronary Doppler flow measurements during external CPR, we showed that the hope of antegrade coronary blood flow during the compression phase of CPR was not realized [134]. In spite of positive systolic coronary perfusion pressure gradients with some techniques of CPR, no appreciable forward flow occurred in the large epicardial coronary arteries. Further work is needed on improving myocardial perfusion during CPR in those with coronary artery lesions.

Drug Therapy During Cardiac Arrest

Proper drug therapy generally increases the effectiveness of CPR. The objectives of drug therapy during cardiac arrest are, first, to increase peripheral vascular constriction and, second, to minimize the adverse effects of metabolic acidosis.

The value of epinephrine in cardiac resuscitation has long been known. Because the drug has both inotropic and chronotropic (beta-adrenergic) effects on the beating heart and also produces peripheral vasoconstriction (alpha-adrenergic effects), there has been confusion regarding which of these effects is the most important to restarting an arrested heart. As early as 1906, Crile and Dolley [53] noted the importance of securing an adequate aortic diastolic perfusion pressure during cardiac resuscitation. They stated that it usually was not possible to achieve an adequate aortic diastolic pressure via cardiac massage without the addition of epinephrine. Since that time, it has been repeatedly demonstrated that the value of epinephrine does not lie in its direct action on the heart. Instead, epinephrine increases peripheral vascular resistance, transiently decreasing perfusion of most of the body and, in the process, increasing aortic diastolic pressure [54, 55]. The increased peripheral vascular constriction increases aortic diastolic blood pressure, which improves the coronary perfusion pressure. Because coronary artery blood flow occurs during diastole in either the spontaneously beating or arrested heart, the result is increased coronary blood flow.

The now classic studies of Redding and Pearson [56], in which asphyxial cardiac arrest was produced, are worth emphasizing. Standard CPR and drug administration resulted in survival of all of ten animals that received epinephrine, none of ten animals that received isoproterenol, and nine of ten animals that received methoxamine [56]. In a similar study of cardiac arrest produced by ventricular fibrillation, one of ten animals survived without drugs, nine of ten with epinephrine, and ten of ten with phenylephrine. In a reexamination of this phenomenon, it was found that alpha-adrenergic blockade administered with epinephrine prevented resuscitation in animals with cardiac arrest. Resuscitation of animals with beta-adrenergic blocking drugs administered with epinephrine was uniformly successful [57]. Table 22-2 summarizes these data.

Table 22-2
Successful drug therapy for cardiac arrest

Cardiac arrest	Survival
Asphyxial arrest	
Epinephrine	10/10
Isoproterenol	0/10
Methoxamine	9/10
Ventricular fibrillation arrest	
Epinephrine	9/10
Phenylephrine	10/10
Saline	1/10
Epinephrine	10/10
Phenylephrine plus propranolol	10/10
Isoproterenol plus phenoxybenzamine	3/11

Drugs that have their principal effect by cardiac stimulation, such as isoproterenol, dobutamine, and calcium salts, may be useful for supporting the circulation after the heart has restarted but have not been shown to be helpful during the period of cardiac arrest. Drugs that do not have epinephrine's cardiac stimulating effect but are potent peripheral vasoconstrictors, such as phenylephrine, methoxamine, and dopamine, are as effective as epinephrine during CPR [54–60]. However, because none of these medications has been shown to be superior to epinephrine, epinephrine remains the drug of choice. There should be no delay in using an appropriate dose of epinephrine during resuscitation from either cardiac standstill or ventricular fibrillation. Because the useful action of the drug is on the peripheral circulation, intracardiac injection has no advantage over intravenous injection. In fact, when an endotracheal tube is in place and intravenous access is not available, drugs may be diluted and administered via the endotracheal tube (see below). Intracardiac injections, although relatively safe [60], should be reserved for the rare situation where intravenous and endotracheal routes are not available.

One of the major areas of interest addressed by the recent American Heart Association's guidelines for CPR and emergency cardiac care was the optimal dose of epinephrine in the treatment of cardiac arrest [7]. Enthusiastic support for using higher doses than previously recommended came from experimental animal data suggesting that milligram-per-kilogram doses equivalent to a 10-mg bolus in humans resulted in marked improvements in perfusion pressure and myocardial blood flow [135]. Case reports of individuals responding to high doses of epinephrine following no response to standard doses also contributed to the enthusiasm. Four separate randomized, prospective clinical trials of standard-dose epinephrine versus high-dose epinephrine have now been completed [136–139]. All failed to show a survival advantage for high-dose epinephrine. Therefore, only a minor change was made in the recommended guidelines, namely increasing the frequency with which epinephrine should be given to every 3 minutes during the resuscitation effort, but not changing the initial dose of an intravenous 1-mg bolus [7]. There is new emphasis that individual physicians in charge of the resuscitation effort may opt to try other dosing schemes, particularly if no response is seen with the usual dose. Caution in using high-dose epinephrine is still warranted. Work from our experimental laboratory at the University of Arizona shows that high-dose epinephrine may not only fail to improve survival, but also in some cases may result in increased refractory ventricular arrhythmias, myocardial dysfunction, and ultimately increased early death following resuscitation [140]. This may be especially true in patients with acute myocardial infarction who have cardiac arrest.

Two drugs, sodium bicarbonate and calcium chloride, are often used in excess during CPR. In the absence of adequate tissue perfusion, anaerobic metabolism results in the production of lactic acid and other metabolites that cause metabolic acidosis. Following the widespread adoption of CPR, there were many advocates of the early use of sodium bicarbonate to correct the acidosis on the assumption that it would promote early restoration of cardiac function. For several years it was common to observe the administration of large amounts of sodium bicarbonate while drugs of established value were neglected. This attitude was based on observations that the administration of bicarbonate to the animals before the induction of cardiac arrest made the animals easier to resuscitate, that acidotic animals had a diminished response to catecholamines, and that calves made hypotensive by infusion of hydrochloric acid could be restored by infusion of sodium bicarbonate [61–63].

Subsequent investigation showed that sodium bicarbonate alone given during CPR did not promote return of cardiac contractility [64]. In fact, accurate correction of metabolic acidosis was not feasible until cardiac resuscitation had been successful and improved tissue perfusion mobilized acid metabolites sequestered in the tissues. Administration of bicarbonate did not potentiate the effect of suboptimal doses of epinephrine, whereas 1 mg of epinephrine was found to be effective even in the presence of severe metabolic acidosis [64]. Other experiments demonstrated that the susceptibility of the heart to the development of ventricular fibrillation was increased in the presence of metabolic acidosis, and that it could be corrected by administration of bicarbonate. However, respiratory acidosis or alkalosis had no such effect [65]. Hyperosmolar states considered incompatible with life were found in a series of patients given bicarbonate during resuscitation efforts. The hyperosmolar state was attributed directly to the injection of hypertonic sodium bicarbonate [66, 67]. Sodium bicarbonate infusion results in a significant rise in arterial carbon dioxide tension that parallels the rise in pH [68].

These facts indicate that caution should be used in the administration of sodium bicarbonate. Observations by Bishop and Weisfeldt [68] indicated that cardiac arrest can be managed for a "considerable period of time" by adequate ventilation in patients not previously acidotic. Animals fibrillated and immediately begun on CPR with adequate ventilation become progressively alkalotic during the first 5 minutes. After 20 minutes of standard CPR, metabolic acidosis is present. Thus if a patient develops primary ventricular fibrillation, sodium bicarbonate is probably not needed unless CPR is excessively long. In this situation, the need for sodium bicarbonate should be determined by blood gas analysis. In some patients, cardiac arrest is secondary to acidosis. In these patients, sodium bicarbonate at 1 mg/kg should be administered initially with subsequent doses based on blood gas determinations. If blood gases are not available, one-half of the initial dose can be given empirically every 10 to 15 minutes during arrest [2].

The second drug that is probably used in excess during cardiac arrest is calcium. Calcium ions have long been known to increase the force of myocardial contraction [69–71]. Because of their integral role in myocardial excitation-contraction coupling, calcium ions have been postulated to be useful during profound cardiovascular collapse when accompanied by electrical mechanical dissociation, and for restoring electrical rhythm in some instances of electrical standstill. Not only are there few experimental data to support this postulate [56, 72], but also intravenous injections in the quantities usually given result in potentially dangerous high serum calcium levels in the arrested patient [73, 74]. After 5 mg of 10% calcium chloride administration as an intravenous bolus to arrested victims, serum calcium levels were found to vary from 12.9 to 18.2 ml/dl [74]. The mean serum calcium level was 15.3 ml/dl at 5 minutes and 11.2 ml/dl at 10 minutes. Calcium has the potential of being particularly dangerous in patients receiving digitalis.

Calcium may be needed in a rare patient, as in a cardiac arrest victim who has had considerable blood loss and citrated blood replacement or the hyperkalemic patient who arrests. The near routine use of calcium chloride in victims of cardiac arrest and during asystole or idioventricular rhythm has little support in the medical literature and is no longer recommended [7].

Endotracheal Administration of Drugs

Epinephrine is rapidly absorbed when given via the endotracheal tube (Table 22-3); epinephrine peak blood levels occur within 15 seconds, but the effects last much longer than with intravenous administration [75–78]. Because metabolism of the drug is the same following intravenous or endotracheal administration, the endotracheal route must provide a depot for continued delayed release [75–79]. Other drugs that have been shown to be well absorbed via the endotracheal route are atropine and lidocaine for dysrhythmias, naloxone for morphine overdose, and diazepam for therapy of status epilepticus [80] (see Table 22-3).

All endotracheally administered drugs have a two to five times longer duration of action than when given by the intravenous route [81, 82]. Repeated doses by the endotracheal route should be administered with this extended period in mind. The volume of endotracheal drug should not be excessive.

Sterile normal saline is probably the diluent of choice for endotracheal drug administration because this solution should result in less deleterious effects than distilled water. However, Redding et al. [75] showed that endotracheal epinephrine has a faster effect when diluted in distilled water than when diluted in saline. Endotracheal drugs should be administered deep into the lungs, preferably with a catheter as long as the endotracheal tube. Forceful

Table 22-3
Endotracheal administration of cardiac arrest drugs

Acceptable	Not acceptable
Epinephrine	Calcium
Atropine	Norepinephrine
Lidocaine	
Naloxone	
Diazepam	

administration with nebulization of the solution enhances its absorption. Its delivery should be followed by a short period of hyperventilation (about five inflations with a breathing bag).

Because absorption is nearly complete, drugs administered endotracheally have the same toxicity as those administered intravenously. Drugs that should not be administered via the endotracheal tube are calcium chloride and norepinephrine. Sodium bicarbonate has not been studied but will probably not be practical if for no other reason than because of the large volume of fluid necessary for an effective dose.

The endotracheal route of administration of drugs may be especially valuable in the prehospital CPR setting where paramedics have the skills for endotracheal intubation but where field conditions or patient factors might preclude efficient intravenous access.

Bradydysrhythmias During Cardiac Arrest

Asystole and idioventricular rhythm are the dominant bradydysrhythmias seen during cardiac arrest and resuscitation. Occasional asystole or a "flat line" on the electrocardiogram is actually fine ventricular fibrillation masquerading as asystole [141]. A reorientation of the electrocardiographic leads will reveal this "variant," allowing for its appropriate treatment. During cardiac arrest these disorders of impulse formation and conduction are almost invariably the result of myocardial ischemia and do not respond to pacing. Even when pacing results in electrical depolarization of the myocardium, there is seldom an associated myocardial contraction. Thus during CPR one must resist the temptation to focus only on the electrocardiogram. The therapy of choice is to improve myocardial perfusion by appropriate CPR techniques and drugs. Pacing is seldom indicated.

On rare occasions, sinus arrest, profound sinus bradycardia, and advanced heart block with long periods of ventricular asystole occur because of isolated conduction defects. In these patients, emergency pacing is indicated. In such acute emergencies, temporizing measures may be necessary before pacing can be initiated. These temporizing measures include cough CPR, rhythmic chest thumps, standard CPR, and intravenous drugs.

Cough CPR may be effective if initiated before the patient loses consciousness. A sharp blow to the precordium (chest thump) may initiate cardiac contraction. Continued rhythmic chest thumps are indicated only if each blow produces a palpable pulse or the series maintains consciousness [83].

If the patient is unconscious and chest thumps are ineffective, standard external chest compression and assisted ventilation should be initiated while an intravenous access is being obtained. Drugs that might be beneficial in patients with severe bradycardia or recent-onset asystole include anticholinergic drugs such as atropine and beta-adrenergic stimulants such as isoproterenol. Some patients who have sustained trauma or have an acute illness may develop a marked vasovagal reaction that results in profound bradycardia or asystole. In these patients, intravenous atropine at 0.5 to 1.0 mg or even more may be effective. The potential for adverse reactions to a single dose of atropine in the setting of asystole or severe bradycardia is so minimal that its use is to be encouraged. Isoproterenol infusion may also be helpful in patients with high-grade heart block or severe symptomatic bradycardia, but as noted (see Drug Therapy During Cardiac Arrest) isoproterenol is contraindicated in the patient with true cardiac arrest. In such patients, epinephrine is the drug of choice.

There are three basic approaches to pacing: transvenous, transthoracic, and external. External pacing is the oldest and simplest technique and is another temporizing approach to stabilizing patients with profound bradydysrhythmias [84]. The major virtue of external pacing is its ease of application. Zoll and coworkers [85] modified the external electrodes and the pacing waveform to effect external cardiac pacing without excessive pain or skeletal-muscle stimulation. This device is now available for clinical use [86].

Ventricular Fibrillation

Cardiac arrest may result from a variety of dysrhythmias including ventricular fibrillation, ventricular tachycardia, ventricular asystole, electromechanical dissociation, and high-grade heart block. Ventricular fibrillation, the most common cause of cardiac arrest, almost invariably requires defibrillation for definitive therapy. Ventricular tachycardia may respond to pharmacologic therapy but frequently requires electrical intervention. The remaining ventricular dysrhythmias often require some form of electrical intervention as definitive or adjunctive therapy. Fifty to seventy percent of the annual deaths from coronary artery disease occur suddenly and are the result of ventricular fibrillation [87]. Fortunately, primary ventricular fibrillation is usually responsive to immediate defibrillation [88]. Patients with witnessed, exertion-related cardiac arrest in well-established cardiac rehabilitation units have been reported to respond uniformly to prompt defibrillation [89]. Similarly, nearly 40 percent of patients treated for out-of-hospital cardiac arrest are discharged alive following prompt application of CPR and early defibrillation [90, 91]. Because rapidity of delivery of defibrillation continues to be the major determinant in survival from cardiac arrest secondary to ventricular fibrillation, therapy that can be administered by bystanders or emergency medical technicians trained in defibrillation is assuming increasing importance [92–94].

A sharp blow to the chest with the fist 8 to 12 inches above the precordium, the chest thump, is effective in only 2 percent of patients with ventricular fibrillation [95] but has the distinct advantages of ready availability and ease and speed of application. These features have resulted in the recommendation that the chest thump be the initial therapy for witnessed unmonitored cardiac arrest [7].

Recommended Management

1. In a witnessed arrest due to ventricular fibrillation the initial step is prompt defibrillation, providing a defibrillator is available.
2. If a defibrillator is not available, initiate external sternal compression and assisted ventilation (basic cardiac life support [BCLS]) and call for defibrillation equipment and assistance. If the patient is monitored and has ventricular fibrillation or has witnessed nonasphyxial unmonitored collapse, give a precordial thump.
3. The following steps should be followed while interrupting chest compressions for as brief a time as possible.
   a. Apply conductive, low-resistance interface to metal defibrillator paddles or apply self-adhesive electrodes.
   b. Place electrode paddles so that the delivered current traverses the left ventricle.
   c. Select the appropriate energy level (joules) and charge the defibrillator capacitor. In adults the initial attempt at defibrillation is made using approximately 200 joules of delivered energy. If defibrillation is successful at 200 joules but the patient later has recurrent ventricular fibrillation, higher energies are not necessary for subsequent shocks.
   d. If the first shock is unsuccessful, the second shock is 200 to 300 joules.
   e. If unsuccessful, a third shock of up to 360 joules is administered as soon as possible.
   f. If the patient does not defibrillate following the third shock, look for factors producing high impedance.
   g. Administer epinephrine, continue chest compression and assisted ventilation, and administer an additional one or two shocks at 360 joules. Follow American Heart Association recommendations for advanced cardiac life support (ACLS).
4. After delivery of electrical current, the electrocardiogram and arterial pulse are assessed to determine the effectiveness of therapy.

Successful defibrillation of patients in ventricular fibrillation depends on many factors, including the duration of the ventricular fibrillation, the environment and condition of the myocardium, and whether an adequate electrical current traverses a critical mass of the ventricles [96, 97]. Current delivery through the ventricles depends on the energy delivered from the defibrillator, the resistance (impedance) between the defibrillator capacitor and the heart, and the electrode size and position.

Energy Requirements for Defibrillation

The amount of energy desirable for direct-current external defibrillation is controversial [98]. It is clear that a defibrillation threshold exists; that is, shocks of inadequate strength do not defibrillate [99–103]. Yet excessively strong defibrillation shocks are known to produce dysrhythmias and myocardial damage [99]. Animals varying markedly in size require a wide range of energy for defibrillation [99]. However, observations in human adults indicate that body weight is not a major determinant of the energy levels necessary for defibrillation [103–106]. It is now generally agreed that although there is a relation between body size and the energy needed for defibrillation (infants and small children require less energy than large adults) over the range of weights in most adults, size does not appear to be a clinically important variable [107].

Previous ACLS guidelines advised that "the initial attempt at defibrillation should be made using 200 to 300 joules of delivered energy" [2]. Since this recommendation was made, two clinical studies [108, 109] suggested that an initial shock energy of no more than 200 joules should be used. In a prospective out-of-hospital study, Weaver and colleagues [108] compared the effects of low- and high-energy shocks in 249 patients with ventricular fibrillation. Low-energy shocks (two 175-joule shocks; if ineffective, an additional 320-joule shock) were compared on alternate days with high-energy shocks (three 320-joule shocks). Defibrillation rates were virtually identical with either shock energy, as was the proportion of patients resuscitated and subsequently discharged from the hospital [108]. Kerber and associates [109] conducted a prospective in-hospital study of 183 patients who received direct-current shocks for ventricular fibrillation. Patients received initial shocks of either 200 joules or 300 to 400 joules. This study also showed no difference in the first-shock or cumulative success rates of these two energy levels. Neither study therefore showed any benefit from initial shocks above 200 joules. Moreover, using a lower energy may be safer. Weaver and associates [108] found a higher incidence of atrioventricular block in patients receiving 320-joule shocks compared to the lower-energy shocks; it was particularly evident in patients who received several shocks at the higher energy level.

The appropriate energy level for the second shock is still somewhat controversial. The previous ACLS guidelines suggested that the initial and second shock should be of similar energies [2]. This recommendation was based on three points. First, defibrillation appears to be a probability function; that is, at any given energy there is a specific probability that defibrillation can be achieved [110]. Thus if the first shock fails, there is a possibility that a second shock of the same energy will succeed. The rationale for a second shock is that transthoracic impedance declines with repeated shocks [111, 112]. Such a decline results in greater current flow for any given energy, and this increase in current flow should improve the chances of achieving defibrillation with a second shock using the same energy. However, Kerber and associates [113] showed that although the transthoracic impedance in humans does fall with repeated shocks, the change is modest. They concluded that a greater and more predictable increase in current flow occurs if the shock energy is raised. Another argument against increasing the energy for the second shock is the result of a study by Weaver and coworkers [108]. Because of the conflicting evidence, the present recommendation for the strength of the second shock remains at 200 to 300 joules [2]. Should the first two shocks fail to defibrillate, a third shock not to exceed 360 joules should be delivered immediately. This method is another change incorporated in the 1986 guidelines for ACLS [2].

Because defibrillation success is significantly decreased by a delay of minutes, the present guidelines suggest three consecutive shocks [2, 114]. Again, because early defibrillation is so important, the guidelines are written so that it is acceptable to deliver three successive 200-joule shocks (the maximum output of the presently available automatic external defibrillators is less than 360 joules).

For recurrent ventricular fibrillation, it may not be necessary to increase the defibrillation energy on successive shocks. If ventricular fibrillation recurs frequently, it may be desirable to reduce the energy of subsequent defibrillatory shocks. This approach has the theoretical advantage of minimizing electrical injury to the heart. Appropriate external chest compression and assisted ventilation should be performed until a defibrillator is available and between shocks while the defibrillator capacitor is charging, *except* with automatic or semiautomatic external defibrillators. These devices require a period of time for diagnosis and capacitor charging. During this time, external chest compression interferes with the diagnostic process and delays or aborts discharge. Therefore because the most important aspect of survival in out-of-hospital fibrillation is prompt defibrillation, a period of up to 1.5 minutes for diagnosing and delivering three shocks by automatic or semiautomatic external defibrillators without chest compression is, by consensus, acceptable [115].

Transthoracic Resistance

Defibrillation is accomplished by passage through the heart of an electrical current of sufficient energy to depolarize a critical mass of the myocardium. Although the operator selects the energy (joules), it is the current flow (amperes) that is responsible for defibrillation. Current flow is determined by the shock strength and the transthoracic resistance (impedance). Many of the factors determining transthoracic impedance to direct-current defibrillator discharge are known. They include the energy level [116], electrode size [117–120], interface between the skin and the electrode [119, 121, 122], number and time interval of previous shocks [111, 112], phase of ventilation [123], distance between electrodes [113], and paddle electrode pressure [113]. Human transthoracic impedance to cardioversion or defibrillator shock ranges between 14 and 143 ohms [124]. If the impedance is high, low-energy shocks fail to defibrillate [125]. Factors affecting transthoracic impedance are less important at high-energy defibrillations. However, if all three defibrillation attempts fail, one should evaluate factors that may contribute to a high transthoracic impedance or resistance to defibrillation. These factors include pneumothorax, inadequate electrode chest wall interface, inadequate electrode position or skin contact, excessive distance between electrodes, and inadequate electrode pressure.

Electrode Position

Because defibrillation depends on an adequate current traversing the myocardium, *paddle electrode placement* is critical. The electrodes should be placed in a position that maximizes current flow through the ventricular myocardium. There are two accepted locations for paddle placement. The standard placement is one electrode with its edge just to the right of the upper sternum and below the clavicle, with the other paddle placed to the left of the nipple with the center of the electrode in the mid-axillary line. An alternative approach is to place one paddle anteriorly over the left precordium and the other posteriorly behind the heart. The paddle should be applied to the chest wall with firm pressure (about 25 lb).

On occasion, external cardioversion of defibrillation is necessary in patients with a permanent pacemaker. The external defibrillation electrodes should not be placed too near (not closer than 5 inches) the subcutaneous pacemaker generator, as defibrillation shocks may cause pacemaker malfunction by raising the pacing threshold [126]. It has been suggested that patients with permanent pacemakers who have been defibrillated or cardioverted should have the pacing thresholds checked at frequent intervals for 6 weeks after the shock [126].

Thrombolytic Therapy in Acute Myocardial Infarction Patients Requiring Cardiopulmonary Resuscitation

CPR has been considered a contraindication for the subsequent administration of a thrombolytic agent in patients having an acute myocardial infarction [142]. With the survival advantages of such lytic therapy now well documented, this issue is both important and timely. Tenaglia and coworkers [128] reviewed the incidence and results of cardiac arrest in patients enrolled in the first three Thrombolysis in Acute Myocardial Infarction (TAMI) trials. By exclusion criteria no patient with more than 10 minutes of CPR was enrolled in the TAMI studies. Included were 59 patients who had cardiac arrest and received less than 10 minutes of CPR. The mean duration of CPR was only 1 minute, but among these patients no bleeding complications were attributed to the use of thrombolysis after CPR. Still the 1990 recommendation from the joint American College of Cardiology/American Heart Association task force on guidelines for the early management of acute myocardial infarction included as ''absolute contraindications'' to thrombolytic therapy ''prolonged or traumatic cardiopulmonary resuscitation'' [143]. Neches and colleagues [144] reported a case of successful and uncomplicated thrombolysis after 13 minutes of CPR. They concluded that thrombolytic therapy should be used in acute myocardial infarction victims and should not be excluded because of the duration of resuscitation. Scholz [145] also reported on 43 patients who received thrombolytic drugs within 24 hours of CPR. They could not identify any bleeding complications directly attributable to cardiocompressions from CPR.

It seems reasonable to consider all acute myocardial infarction patients requiring CPR for thrombolytic therapy unless there is obvious trauma and injury resulting from the resuscitation.

References

1. Kouwenhoven, W. B., Jude, J. R., and Knickerbocker, G. C. Closed chest cardiac massage. *J.A.M.A.* 137:1064, 1960.
2. Standards and guidelines for cardiopulmonary resuscitation (CPR) and emergency cardiac care (ECC). *J.A.M.A.* 244:453, 1980.
3. McIntyre, K. M., and Lewis, A. J. *Textbook of Advanced Cardiac Support.* Dallas: American Heart Association, 1981.
4. Cole, S. L., and Corday, E. Four minute limit for cardiac resuscitation. *J.A.M.A.* 161:1454, 1956.
5. Cobb, L. A., Baum, R. S., Alvarez, J., et al. Resuscitation from out-of-hospital ventricular fibrillation. *Circulation* 51, 52(Suppl 3):223, 1975.
6. Eisenberg, M. S., Bergner, L., and Hallstrom, A. Cardiac resuscitation in the community: Importance of rapid provision and implications of program planning. *J.A.M.A.* 241:1905, 1979.
7. Emergency Cardiac Care Committee and Subcommittees, American Heart Association. Guidelines for cardiopulmonary resuscitation and emergency cardiac care, I: Introduction. *J.A.M.A.* 268:2172, 1992.
8. Taylor, G. J., Tucker, W. M., Green, H. L., et al. Importance of prolonged compression duration during cardiopulmonary resuscitation in man. *N. Engl. J. Med.* 296:1515, 1977.
9. Fitzgerald, K. R., Babbs, C. F., Frissors, H. A., et al. Cardiac output during cardiopulmonary resuscitation at various compression rates and durations. *Am. J. Physiol.* (*Heart Circ.*) 10:H442, 1981.
10. Maier, G. W., Tyson, G. S., Olsen, C. O., et al. The physiology of external cardiac massage: High impulse cardiopulmonary resuscitation. *Circulation* 70:86, 1984.
11. Maier, G. W., Tyson, G. S., Olsen, C. O., et al. Optimal techniques of external cardiac massage. *Surg. Forum* 33:282, 1982.
12. Weisfeldt, M. I., Chandra, N., Tsitlik, J. E., et al. New attempts to improve blood flow during CPR. In J. Schluger and A. F. Lyon (eds.), *CPR and Emergency Cardiac Care. Looking to the Future.* New York: EM Books, 1980. Pp. 29–45.
13. Chandra, N., Rudikoss, M., Tsitlik, J., et al. Augmentation of carotid flow during cardiopulmonary resuscitation (CPR) in the dog by simultaneous compression and ventilation with high airway pressure. *Am. J. Cardiol.* 43:422, 1979.
14. Rudikoff, M. T., Maughan, W. L., Effron, M., et al. Mechanisms of blood flow during cardiopulmonary resuscitation. *Circulation* 61:345, 1980.
15. Chandra, N., Rudikoff, M., and Weisfeldt, M. L. Simultaneous chest compression and ventilation at high airway pressure during cardiopulmonary resuscitation. *Lancet* 1:175, 1980.
16. Chandra, N., Snyder, L. D., and Weisfeldt, M. L. Abdominal binding during cardiopulmonary resuscitation in man. *J.A.M.A.* 246:351, 1981.
17. Niemann, J. T., Garner, D., Rosborough, D. S., et al. The mechanism of blood flow in closed chest cardiopulmonary resuscitation (Abstract). *Circulation* 59(Suppl II):74, 1979.
18. Weale, F. E., and Rothwell-Jackson, R. L. The efficiency of cardiac massage. *Lancet* 1:1990, 1962.
19. Weathersby, H. T. The valves of the axillary, subclavian, and internal jugular vein (Abstract). *Anat. Rec.* 124:379, 1956.
20. Werner, J. A., Greene, H. L., Janko, C., et al. Visualization of cardiac valve motion in man during external chest compression using two-dimensional echocardiography: Implications regarding the mechanism of blood flow. *Circulation* 63:1417, 1981.
21. Rich, S., Wix, H. L., and Shapiro, E. Two-dimensional echocardiography resuscitation in man. *Am. J. Cardiol.* 47:398, 1981.
22. Babbs, C. F., Tacker, W. A., Paris, R. J., et al. Cardiopulmonary resuscitation with simultaneous compression and ventilation at high airway pressure in four animal models. In *Abstracts of the Fourth Purdue Conference on Cardiac Defibrillation and Cardiopulmonary Resuscitation.* Purdue University, September 15–17, 1981. P. 5.
23. Redding, J. S., Haynes, R. R., and Thomas, J. D. ''Old'' and ''new'' CPR manually performed in dogs. *Crit. Care Med.* 9:386, 1981.
24. Redding, J. S. Abdominal compression in cardiopulmonary resuscitation. *Anesth. Anagl.* 50:668, 1971.
25. Harris, L. C., Kirimli, B., and Safar, P. Augmentation of artificial circulation during cardiopulmonary resuscitation. *Anesthesia* 28:730, 1967.
26. Alifimoff, J. K., Barnett, W. M., Safar, P., et al. Comparisons of standard cardiopulmonary resuscitation, new CPR, abdominal restraint—augmented CPR and open-chested CPR. In *Abstracts of the Fourth Purdue Conference on Cardiac Defibrillation and Cardiopulmonary Resuscitation.* Purdue University, September 15–17, 1981. P. 2.
27. Sanders, A., Ewy, G. A., Alferness, C., et al. Failure of one method of simultaneous chest compression, ventilation, and abdominal binding during cardiopulmonary resuscitation. *Crit. Care Med.* 10:509, 1982.
28. Krischer, J. P., Fine, E. G., Weisfeldt, M. L., et al. Comparison of prehospital conventional and simultaneous compression-ventilation cardiopulmonary resuscitation. *Crit. Care Med.* 17:1263, 1989.
29. Deshmukh, H. G., Weil, M. H., Gudipati, C. V., et al. Blood flow during CPR is maintained by direct cardiac compression (Abstract). *Clin. Res.* 34:88A, 1986.
30. Deshmukh, H. G., Weil, M. H., Rackow, E. C., et al. Echocardiographic observations during cardiopulmonary resuscitation: A preliminary report. *Crit. Care Med.* 13:904, 1985.
31. Raessler, K. L., Kern, K. B., Sanders, A. B., et al. Aortic and right atrial systolic pressures as an

indicator of the mechanism of blood flow during CPR. *Am. Heart J.* 115:1021, 1988.
32. Criley, J. M., Blaufuss, A. H., and Kissel, G. L. Cough-induced cardiac compression. *J.A.M.A.* 236: 1246, 1976.
33. Criley, J. M. Cough CPR. In J. Schluger and A. F. Lyon (eds.), *CPR and Emergency Cardiac Care: Looking to the Future.* New York: EM Books, 1980. P. 47.
34. Wei, J. Y., Greene, H. L., and Weisfeldt, M. L. Cough facilitated conversion of ventricular tachycardia. *Am. J. Cardiol.* 45:174, 1980.
35. Del Guercio, L. R. M., Feins, N. R., Cohn, J. D., et al. Comparison of blood flow during external and internal cardiac massage in man. *Circulation* 31, 32(Suppl 1):171, 1965.
36. Jacobson, S. Current status of open chest procedures. In J. Schluger and A. F. Lyon (eds.), *CPR and Emergency Cardiac Care: Looking to the Future.* New York: EM Books, 1980. P. 127.
37. Sanders, A. B., Kern, K. B., Atlas, M., et al. Importance of the duration of inadequate coronary perfusion pressure on resuscitation from cardiac arrest. *J. Am. Coll. Cardiol.* 6:113, 1986.
38. Kern, K. B., Sanders, A. B., Badylak, S. F., et al. Long-term survival with open chest cardiac massage after ineffective closed chest compression in a canine preparation. *Circulation* 75:498, 1987.
39. Geehr, E. C., Lewis, F. R., and Auerbach, P. S. Failure of open heart massage to improve survival after pre-hospital non-traumatic cardiac arrest. *N. Engl. J. Med.* 314:1189, 1986.
40. Weiser, F. M., Adler, L. N., and Kuhn, L. A. Hemodynamic effects of closed and open chest cardiac resuscitation in normal dogs and those with acute myocardial infarction. *Am. J. Cardiol.* 10:555, 1962.
41. Byrne, D., Pass, H. I., Neely, W. A., et al. External versus internal cardiac massage in normal and chronically ischemic dogs. *Am. Surg.* 46:657, 1980.
42. Gewirtz, H., and Most, A. S. Production of a critical coronary stenosis in closed chest laboratory animals. *Am. J. Cardiol.* 47:589, 1981.
43. Lancaster, L. D., Kern, K. B., Morrison, D., et al. Right ventricular dysfunction during acute anteroseptal myocardial infarction in pigs (Abstract). *Clin. Res.* 35:179A, 1987.
44. Kern, K. B., Lancaster, L. D., Goldman, S., et al. The effect of coronary artery lesions on the relationship between coronary perfusion pressure and myocardial blood flow during cardiopulmonary resuscitation. *Am. Heart J.* 120:324, 1990.
45. White, F. C., Roth, D. M., and Bloor, C. M. The pig as model for myocardial ischemia and exercise. *Lab. Anim. Sci.* 36:351, 1986.
46. Bellamy, R. F., DeGuzman, L. R., and Pedersen, D. C. Coronary blood flow during cardiopulmonary resuscitation in swine. *Circulation* 69:174, 1984.
47. Guth, B. D., White, F. C., Gallagher, K. P., and Bloor, C. M. Decreased systolic wall thickening in myocardium adjacent to ischemic zones in conscious swine during brief coronary artery occlusion. *Am. Heart J.* 107:458, 1984.
48. Fedor, J. M., McIntosh, D. M., Rembert, J. C., and Greenfield, J., Jr. Coronary and transmural myocardial blood flow responses in awake domestic pigs. *Am. J. Physiol.* 255:H435, 1978.
49. Tranquilli, W. J., Manohar, M., Parks, C. M., et al. Systemic and regional blood flow distribution in unanesthetized swine and swine anesthetized with halothane and nitrous oxide, halothane, or enflurane. *Anesthesiology* 56:369, 1982.
50. Manohar, M., and Parks, C. M. Porcine systemic and regional organ flow during 1.0 and 1.5 minimum alveolar concentrations of sevoflurane anesthesia without and with 50 percent nitrous oxide. *J. Pharmacol. Exp. Ther.* 231:640, 1984.
51. Brown, C. G. Regional blood flow measurements during cardiopulmonary resuscitation following prolonged ventricular fibrillation in a swine model. *Resuscitation* 16:107, 1988.
52. DeWood, M. A., Spores, J., Motske, R., et al. Prevalence of total occlusion during the early hours of transmural myocardial infarction. *N. Engl. J. Med.* 303:897, 1980.
53. Crile, G., and Dolley, D. H. Experimental research into resuscitation of dogs killed by anesthetics and asphyxia. *J. Exp. Med.* 8:713, 1906.
54. Pearson, J. W., and Redding, J. S. Epinephrine in cardiac resuscitation. *Am. Heart J.* 66:210, 1963.
55. Pearson, J. W., and Redding, J. S. Influence of peripheral vascular tone on cardiac resuscitation. *Anesth. Analg.* 46:253, 1967.
56. Redding, J. S., and Pearson, J. W. Evaluation of drugs for cardiac resuscitation. *Anesthesiology* 24: 203, 1963.
57. Yakaitis, R. W., Otto, C. W., and Blitt, C. D. Relative importance of alpha- and beta-adrenergic receptors during resuscitation. *Crit. Care Med.* 7: 293, 1979.
58. Otto, C. W., Yakaitis, R. W., and Blitt, C. D. Mechanism of action of epinephrine in resuscitation from asphyxial arrest. *Crit. Care Med.* 9:364, 1981.
59. Otto, C. W., Yakaitis, R. W., Redding, J. S., et al. Comparison of dopamine, dobutamine, and epinephrine in CPR. *Crit. Care Med.* 9:366, 1981.
60. Davison, R., Barresi, V., Parker, M., et al. Intracardiac injections during cardiopulmonary resuscitation: A low-risk procedure. *J.A.M.A.* 244:1110, 1980.
61. Ledingham, I. M. A., and Norman, J. N. Acid-base studies in experimental circulatory arrest. *Lancet* 2:967, 1962.
62. Thrower, W. B., Darby, T. D., and Aldinger, E. E. Acid-base derangements and myocardial contractibility. *Arch. Surg.* 82:56, 1961.
63. Stewart, J. S. S. Management of cardiac arrest. *Lancet* 1:106, 1964.
64. Redding, J. S., and Pearson, J. W. Metabolic acido-

sis: A factor in cardiac resuscitation. *South. Med. J.* 60:926, 1967.
65. Gerst, P. H., Fleming, W. H., and Malm, J. R. Increased susceptibility of the heart to ventricular fibrillation during metabolic acidosis. *Circ. Res.* 19:63, 1966.
66. Mattar, J. A., Weil, M. H., Shubin, H., et al. Cardiac arrest in the critically ill. II. Hyperosmolar states following cardiac arrest. *Am. J. Med.* 56:162, 1974.
67. Cohn, J. D., and Del Guercio, L. R. M. Cardiorespiratory analysis of cardiac arrest and resuscitation. *Surg. Gynecol. Obstet.* 123:1066, 1966.
68. Bishop, R. L., and Weisfeldt, M. L. Sodium bicarbonate administration during cardiac arrest: Effect on arterial pH, PCO_2, and osmolality. *J.A.M.A.* 235:506, 1976.
69. Niedergerke, R. The rate of action of calcium ions on the contraction of the heart. *J. Physiol. (Lond.)* 138:506, 1957.
70. Weber, A., Herz, R., and Reiss, I. Role of calcium in contraction and relaxation of muscle. *Fed. Proc.* 28:896, 1964.
71. Borle, A. B. Calcium metabolism of the cellular level. *Fed. Proc.* 32:1944, 1973.
72. White, B. C., Petinga, T. J., Hoehner, P. J., et al. Incidence, etiology and outcome of pulseless idioventricular rhythm treated with dexamethasone during advanced CPR. *J. Am. Coll. Emerg. Physicians* 8:188, 1979.
73. Carlon, G. C., Howland, W. S., Kahn, R. C., et al. Calcium chloride administration in normocalcemic critically ill patients. *Crit. Care Med.* 8:209, 1980.
74. Dembo, D. H. Calcium in advanced life support. *Crit. Care Med.* 9:358, 1981.
75. Redding, J. S., Asuncion, J. S., and Pearson, J. W. Effective routes of drug administration during cardiac arrest. *Anesth. Analg.* 46:253, 1967.
76. Roberts, J. R., Greenberg, M. I., Kanub, M. A., et al. Blood levels following intravenous and endotracheal epinephrine administration. *J. Am. Coll. Emerg. Physicians* 8:53, 1979.
77. Roberts, J. R., Greenberg, M. I., and Baskin, S. I. Endotracheal epinephrine in cardiorespiratory collapse. *J. Am. Coll. Emerg. Physicians* 8:515, 1979.
78. Greenberg, M. I., Roberts, J. R., and Baskin, S. I. Endotracheal naloxone reversal of morphine-induced respiratory depression in rabbits. *Ann. Emerg. Med.* 9:289, 1980.
79. Greenberg, M. I., Roberts, J. R., and Krusz, J. C. Endotracheal epinephrine in a canine anaphylactic shock model. *J. Am. Coll. Emerg. Physicians* 8:500, 1979.
80. Greenberg, M. I. Endotracheal medication in cardiac emergencies. In *Abstracts of the Fourth Purdue Conference on Cardiac Defibrillation and Cardiopulmonary Resuscitation.* Purdue University, September 15–17, 1981. P. 9.
81. Roberts, J. R., Greenberg, M. I., Knaub, M., et al. Comparison of the pharmacological effects of epinephrine administered by the intravenous and endotracheal routes. *J. Am. Coll. Emerg. Physicians* 7:260, 1978.
82. Elam, J. O. The interpulmonary route for CPR drugs. In P. Safar and J. O. Elam (eds.), *Advances in Cardiopulmonary Resuscitation.* New York: Springer-Verlag, 1977.
83. Zoll, P. M., Belgard, A. H., Weintraub, M. J., and Frank, H. A. External mechanical cardiac stimulation. *N. Engl. J. Med.* 294:1274, 1976.
84. Zoll, P. M. Resuscitation of the heart in ventricular standstill by external electrical stimulation. *N. Engl. J. Med.* 247:768, 1952.
85. Zoll, R. H., Zoll, P. M., and Belgard, A. H. Noninvasive cardiac stimulation. In *Abstracts of the Fourth Purdue Conference on Cardiac Defibrillation and Cardiopulmonary Resuscitation.* Purdue University, September 15–17, 1981. P. 20.
86. Zoll, P. M., Zoll, R. H., Falk, R. H., et al. External noninvasive temporary cardiac pacing: Clinical trial. *Circulation* 71:937, 1985.
87. Julian, D. G. Toward preventing coronary death from ventricular fibrillation. *Circulation* 54:360, 1976.
88. Eisenberg, M. S., Copass, M. K., Hallstrom, A. P., et al. Treatment of out-of-hospital cardiac arrests with rapid defibrillation by emergency medical technicians. *N. Engl. J. Med.* 302:1379, 1980.
89. Hossck, K. F., and Hartwig, R. Cardiac arrest associated with supervised cardiac rehabilitation. *J. Cardiac Rehabil.* 2:402, 1982.
90. Cobb, L. A., and Hallstrom, A. P. Community-based cardiopulmonary resuscitation: What have we learned? *Ann. N.Y. Acad. Sci.* 382:330, 1982.
91. Eisenberg, M. S., Bergner, L., and Hallstrom, A. P. Cardiac resuscitation in the community: Importance of rapid provision and implications for program planning. *J.A.M.A.* 241:1905, 1979.
92. Stults, K. R., Brown, D. D., Schug, V. L., and Bean, J. A. Pre-hospital defibrillation performed by emergency medical technicians in rural communities. *N. Engl. J. Med.* 310:219, 1984.
93. Rozkovec, A., Crossley, J., Walesby, R., et al. Safety and effectiveness of a portable external automatic defibrillator-pacemaker. *Clin. Cardiol.* 6:527, 1983.
94. Weaver, W. D., Copass, M. K., Cobb, L. A., et al. A new, compact, automatic external defibrillator designed for layperson use (Abstract). *J. Am. Coll. Cardiol.* 5:457, 1985.
95. Caldwell, G., Millor, G., Quinn, E., et al. Simple mechanical method of cardioversion: Defense of the precordial thump and cough version. *B.M.J.* 291:627, 1985.
96. Garrey, W. E. The nature of fibrillatory contractions of the heart and its relation to tissue mass and form. *Am. J. Physiol.* 33:397, 1914.
97. Zipes, D. P., Fisher, J., King, R. M., et al. Termination of ventricular fibrillation in dogs by depolarizing a critical amount of myocardium. *Am. J. Cardiol.* 36:37, 1975.

98. Ewy, G. A., and Tacker, W. A., Jr. Transchest electrical ventricular defibrillation. *Am. Heart J.* 91:403, 1976.
99. Geddes, L. A., Tacker, W. A., Rosborough, J. P., et al. Electrical dose for ventricular defibrillation of large and small animals using precordial electrodes. *J. Clin. Invest.* 53:310, 1974.
100. Gutgesell, H. P., Tacker, W. A., Geddes, L. A., et al. Energy dose for defibrillation in children. *Pediatrics* 58:898, 1976.
101. Dahl, C. F., Ewy, G. A., Warner, E. D., et al. Myocardial necrosis from direct current countershock. *Circulation* 50:956, 1974.
102. Warner, E. D., Dahl, C., and Ewy, G. A. Myocardial injury from transthoracic defibrillator countershock. *Arch. Pathol.* 99:55, 1975.
103. Pantridge, J. R., Adgey, A. A. J., Webb, S. W., et al. Electrical requirements for ventricular defibrillation. *B.M.J.* 2:313, 1975.
104. Adgey, A. A. Electrical energy requirements for ventricular defibrillation. *Br. Heart J.* 40:1197, 1978.
105. Crampton, J. A., Crampton, R. S., Sipes, J. N., et al. Energy levels and patient weight in ventricular defibrillation. *J.A.M.A.* 242:1380, 1984.
106. Gascho, J. A., Crampton, R. S., Cherwek, M. L., et al. Determinants of ventricular defibrillation in adults. *Circulation* 60:231, 1979.
107. Lown, B., Crampton, R. S., DeSilva, R. A., and Gascho, J. The energy for ventricular fibrillation—too little or too much? *N. Engl. J. Med.* 298:1252, 1978.
108. Weaver, W. D., Cobb, L. A., Copass, M. K., and Hallstrom, A. P. Ventricular defibrillation—a comparative trial using 175 J and 320 J shocks. *N. Engl. J. Med.* 307:1101, 1982.
109. Kerber, R. E., Jensen, S. R., Gascho, J. A., et al. Determinants of defibrillation: Prospective analysis of 183 patients. *Am. J. Cardiol.* 52:739, 1985.
110. Tacker, W. A., and Geddes, L. A. *Electrical Defibrillation.* Boca Raton, FL: CRC Press, 1980. P. 141.
111. Geddes, L. A., Tacker, W. A., Cabler, D. P., et al. Decrease in transthoracic resistance during successive ventricular defibrillation trials. *Med. Instrum.* 9:179, 1975.
112. Dahl, C. F., Ewy, G. A., Ewy, M. D., and Thomas, E. D. Transthoracic impedance to direct current discharge: Effect of repeated countershocks. *Med. Instrum.* 10:151, 1976.
113. Kerber, R. E., Grayzel, J., Hoyt, R., et al. Transthoracic resistance of human defibrillation: Influence of body weight, chest size, serial shocks, paddle size and paddle contact pressure. *Circulation* 63:676, 1981.
114. Yakaitis, R. W., Ewy, G. A., Oho, C. W., et al. Influence of time and therapy on ventricular defibrillation in dogs. *Crit. Care Med.* 8:157, 1980.
115. Ewy, G. A. Electrical therapy for cardiovascular emergencies. *Circulation* 74(Suppl IV):111, 1986.
116. Ewy, G. A., Ewy, M. D., Nuttall, A. J., and Nuttall, A. W. Canine transthoracic resistance. *J. Appl. Physiol.* 32:91, 1972.
117. Thomas, E. D., Ewy, G. A., Dahl, C. F., and Ewy, M. D. Effectiveness of direct current defibrillation; Role of paddle electrode size. *Am. Heart J.* 93: 463, 1977.
118. Patel, A. S., and Galysh, F. T. Experimental studies to design safe external pediatric paddles for DC defibrillation. *IEEE Trans. Biomed. Eng.* 19:228, 1972.
119. Connell, P. N., Ewy, G. A., Dahl, C. F., et al. Transthoracic impedance to defibrillation discharge: Effect of electrode size and electrode chest wall interface. *J. Electrocardiol.* 6:313, 1973.
120. Ewy, G. A., and Horan, W. J. Effectiveness of direct current defibrillations. II. Role of paddle electrode size. *Am. Heart J.* 93:674, 1977.
121. Ewy, G. A., Horan, W. J., and Ewy, M. D. Disposable defibrillator electrodes. *Heart Lung* 6:127, 1977.
122. Ewy, G. A., and Taren, D. Comparison of paddle electrode pastes used for defibrillation. *Heart Lung* 6:847, 1977.
123. Ewy, G. A., Hellman, D. A., McClung, S., et al. Influence of ventilation phase on transthoracic impedance and defibrillation effectiveness. *Crit. Care Med.* 3:164, 1980.
124. Ewy, G. A., Ewy, M. K., and Silverman, J. Determinants of human transthoracic resistance to direct current discharge. *Circulation* 46(Suppl II):II-150, 1972.
125. Kerber, R. E., Kouba, C., Martins, J., et al. Advanced prediction of transthoracic impedance in human defibrillation and cardioversion: Importance of impedance in determining the success of low energy shocks. *Circulation* 70:303, 1984.
126. Levine, P. A., Barold, S. S., Fletcher, R. D., and Talbot, P. Adverse acute and chronic effects of electrical defibrillation and cardioversion on implanted unipolar cardiac pacing systems. *J. Am. Coll. Cardiol.* 1:1413, 1983.
127. Goldberg, R. J., Gore, J. M., Haffajee, C. I., et al. Outcome after cardiac arrest during myocardial infarction. *Am. J. Cardiol.* 59:251, 1987.
128. Tenaglia, A. N., Califf, R. M., Candela, R. J., et al. Thrombolytic therapy in patients requiring cardiopulmonary resuscitation. *Am. J. Cardiol.* 68: 1015, 1991.
129. Standards and guidelines for cardiopulmonary resuscitation (CPR) and emergency cardiac care (ECC). *J.A.M.A.* 255:2905, 1986.
130. Higano, S. T., Oh, J. K., Ewy, G. A., et al. The mechanism of blood flow during closed chest cardiac massage in humans: Transesophageal echocardiographic observations. *Mayo Clin. Proc.* 65:1432, 1990.
131. Kern, K. B., Sanders, A. B., Raife, J., et al. A study of chest compression rates during cardiopulmonary

resuscitation in humans. *Arch. Intern. Med.* 152:145, 1992.

132. Rieser, M. J. The use of cough-CPR in patients with acute myocardial infarction. *J. Emerg. Med.* 10:291, 1992.
133. Kern, K. B., and Ewy, G. A. Minimal coronary stenoses and left ventricular blood flow during cardiopulmonary resuscitation. *Ann. Emerg. Med.* 21:1066, 1992.
134. Kern, K. B., Hilwig, R., and Ewy, G. A. Retrograde coronary blood flow during cardiopulmonary resuscitation in swine: An intra-coronary Doppler evaluation. *Am. Heart J.,* 128:490, 1994.
135. Brown, C. G., Werman, H. A., Davis, E. A., et al. The effects of graded doses of epinephrine on regional myocardial blood flow during cardiopulmonary resuscitation in swine. *Circulation* 75:491, 1987.
136. Lindner, K. H., Ahnefeld, F. W., and Prengel, A. W. Comparison of standard and high-dose adrenaline in the resuscitation of asystole and electromechanical dissociation. *Acta Anaesthesiol. Scand.* 35:253, 1991.
137. Stiell, I. G., Hebert, P. C., Weitzman, B. N., et al. High-dose epinephrine in adult cardiac arrest. *N. Engl. J. Med.* 327:1045, 1992.
138. Brown, C. G., Martin, D. R., Pepe, P. E., et al. A comparison of standard-dose and high-dose epinephrine in cardiac arrest outside the hospital. *N. Engl. J. Med.* 327:1051, 1992.
139. Callaham, M., Madsen, C. D., Barton, C. W., et al. A randomized clinical trial of high-dose epinephrine and norepinephrine vs standard-dose epinephrine in prehospital cardiac arrest. *J.A.M.A.* 268: 2667, 1992.
140. Berg, R. A., Otto, C. W., Kern, K. B., et al. High dose epinephrine results in greater early mortality following resuscitation from prolonged cardiac arrest in pigs. *Crit. Care Med.* 22:282, 1994.
141. Ewy, G. A., Dahl, C. F., Zimmerman, M., et al. Ventricular fibrillation masquerading as ventricular standstill. *Crit. Care Med.* 9:841, 1981.
142. Sherry, S., Bell, W. R., Duckert, F. H., et al. Thrombolytic therapy in thrombosis: A National Institutes of Health Consensus Development Conference. *Ann. Intern. Med.* 93:141, 1980.
143. Subcommittee to Develop Guidelines for the Early Management of Patients with Acute Myocardial Infarction. Guidelines for the early management of patients with acute myocardial infarction: A report of the American College of Cardiology/American Heart Association Task Force on Assessment of Diagnostic and Therapeutic Cardiovascular Procedures. *J. Am. Coll. Cardiol.* 16:249, 1990.
144. Neches, R. B., Goldfarb, A. M., and Saviano, G. J. Thrombolytic therapy in acute myocardial infarction following prolonged cardiopulmonary resuscitation. *Clin. Cardiol.* 14:616, 1991.
145. Scholz, K. H., Tebbe, U., Herrman, C., et al. Frequency of complications of cardiopulmonary resuscitation after thrombolysis during acute myocardial infarction. *Am. J. Cardiol.* 69:724, 1992.

VI.
Special Procedures in Acute Myocardial Infarction

23. Coronary Arteriography in Acute Ischemic Syndromes

Marcus A. DeWood

Until the past few years, there has been a general reluctance to subject patients to coronary arteriography during acute ischemic syndromes. Arteriography was usually limited to patients with chronic stable angina pectoris. However, increasing experience demonstrated that coronary arteriography could be used to define the nature and extent of coronary obstruction in acute ischemic syndromes, including their most profound expression, acute myocardial infarction (AMI) [1–4]. Because standard investigational techniques involved in animal models and autopsy studies frequently do not mimic the clinical situation, interest shifted to the pathophysiology of AMI in patients; therapies directed toward thrombolysis, restoration of myocardial perfusion, and limitation of the extent of AMI have evolved.

Coronary vasculature in the various acute ischemic syndromes is different and probably reflects a spectrum of acute manifestations of chronic coronary disease. Thus, precise categorization of arteriographic findings is difficult (1) because of the variability in the biology of the coronary lesion for each type of coronary event, and (2) because arteriographic features differ over time [1, 5].

Clinically, the manifestation of Q-wave (transmural) infarction is similar from patient to patient. It is known that coronary thrombosis occurs frequently [6], but the interaction between underlying atherosclerotic plaque, coronary arterial spasm, and platelet aggregates is variable and the contribution of each is not well defined. In contrast, non-Q-wave (nontransmural or subendocardial) myocardial infarction (MI) presents a confusing and variable clinical picture [5, 7] associated with less frequent coronary thrombosis and coronary occlusion.

Supported in part by the Deaconess Medical Center Foundation, the Sacred Heart Medical Center Foundation, the Max Baer Heart Fund of the Fraternal Order of Eagles, and the Spokane Heart Research Foundation.

Finally, the status of the coronary tree soon after sudden cardiac death associated with MI is mostly unknown, and the mechanisms of the associated ventricular arrhythmias are largely undefined. In AMI, ventricular tachycardia, fibrillation, or both may occur secondary to complete coronary occlusion or may be associated with reperfusion rhythm disturbances. Arrhythmias associated with coronary occlusion are usually termed *ischemic arrhythmias,* whereas the category associated with antegrade blood flow is termed *reperfusion arrhythmias.* The mechanisms of each differ significantly and have been defined in the laboratory [8–12].

The patient who undergoes sudden cardiac death is usually perceived as unstable, and the clinician is reluctant to perform arteriography or thrombolytic therapy soon after cardiopulmonary arrest or resuscitation, especially if the patient's cerebral status is not immediately clear. Therefore, little prospective investigation has been done in this area, and the nature and extent of coronary obstruction following sudden death have been undetermined.

The goal of this chapter is to present the angiographic findings for early stages of Q-wave myocardial infarction as well as those associated with non-Q-wave infarction. Some of the complications associated with arteriography during bouts of each type of acute ischemic syndrome are explored. Data regarding the angiographic findings in patients evaluated soon after sudden cardiac death are also discussed.

Q-Wave (Transmural) Myocardial Infarction

Early Q-wave MI is defined as chest pain in conjunction with persistent ST segment elevation on the electrocardiogram with evolution of pathologic Q waves and typical cardiac enzyme elevations.

Despite reticence to perform arteriography during early acute infarction, multiple clinical studies [1, 6, 13–16] have demonstrated that the prevalence of total coronary occlusion is high in the first few hours after the onset of symptoms of Q-wave MI. Results reported from most centers also suggest that coronary thrombosis is present in the involved coronary artery in approximately 80 percent of cases seen early. Coronary arteriography for acute myocardial infarction has been performed in our community since 1970, and we conducted a 10-year retrospective study [6] to define the arteriographic findings with and without coronary thrombosis during Q-wave myocardial infarction.

Patient Population

During the 10-year period from 1971 to 1981, 517 patients underwent coronary arteriography and left ventriculography within 24 hours of symptom onset of Q-wave MI. The overall average age for the study group was 54 years (range 32 to 76 years). Seventy-nine percent were male. Seventy-two patients (13.9 percent) had suffered previous MI.

Because earlier data [1] demonstrated that the prevalence of total coronary occlusion in Q-wave MI changed over time, the 517 patients were divided into three time-related subsets. The subsets reflected the time interval from symptom onset to performance of coronary arteriography. The study also attempted to define the frequency of total coronary occlusion and to investigate the prevalence of coronary thrombosis in each patient group. The population characteristics of each subset are presented in Table 23-1. The clinical classification of each group is described according to average age, gender, area of infarction defined by the electrocardiogram on study entry, and clinical class [17]. As Table 23-1 demonstrates, 368 patients underwent coronary arteriography within 0 to 6 hours of symptom onset, and 85 patients and 64 patients underwent investigation in the 6- to 12-hour and the 12- to 24-hour periods, respectively. Anterior wall infarction included anterior, anteroseptal, and lateral infarcts. Inferior infarction included inferior, inferoposterior, and inferolateral infarction, that is, infarcts likely caused by occlusion of the right or circumflex system.

Arteriographic Features of Coronary Thrombosis

The angiographic features that best define ''fresh'' intracoronary thrombus include (1) staining of intraluminal material at the distal end of the column of injected contrast agent (Figs. 23-1 and 23-2), (2) local retention of the contrast agent in the involved coronary artery (Figs. 23-1B and 23-2B), and (3) an intracoronary filling defect usually seen best in patients with subtotal coronary obstruction (Fig. 23-3).

Table 23-1
Clinical characteristics of subsets on study entry

Characteristics	At 0–6 hours	At 6–12 hours	At 12–24 hours
No. of patients	368	85	64
Age (yr)	52.5±7.2	53.7±8.2	55.1±8.2
Sex (% male)	79.4	82.3	76.8
Area of infarction by ECG			
Anterior	199 (51.9%)	46 (54.1%)	32 (50.0%)
Inferior	177 (48.1%)	39 (45.8%)	32 (50.0%)
Clinical class*			
I	227 (61.7%)	47 (55.3%)	39 (61.0%)
II	99 (26.9%)	23 (27.0%)	15 (23.4%)
III	18 (4.9%)	4 (4.7%)	2 (3.2%)
IV	24 (6.5%)	11 (12.9%)	8 (12.5%)

Values are mean ± SD.
*Criteria of Killip and Kimball [17].

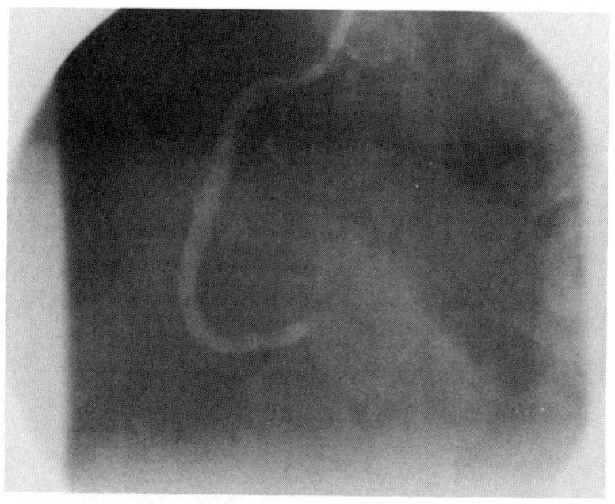

A

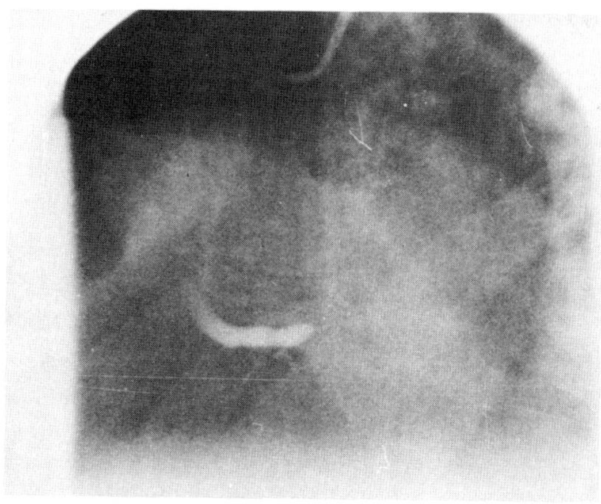

B

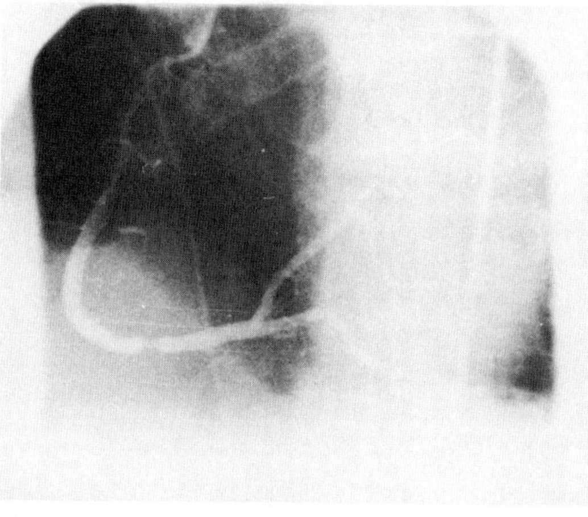

C

Fig. 23-1
A. Total coronary occlusion of the right coronary artery in a patient seen within 3 hours of acute myocardial infarction. *B.* Retention of dye in the involved vessel. *C.* After intracoronary streptokinase perfusion of the distal right coronary artery. (From M. A. DeWood et al. Coronary arteriographic findings in acute transmural myocardial infarction. *Circulation* 68[Suppl I]:I-39, 1983. By permission of the American Heart Association, Inc.)

Results of Arteriographic Studies

Prevalence of Coronary Thrombosis

In the *overall* population, angiographic features suggestive of coronary thrombosis were observed in 73 percent (379 of 517). Of the patients evaluated within 6 hours of symptom onset, one or more angiographic features consistent with thrombus were present in 80 percent (294 of 368), whereas the frequency of coronary thrombosis fell to 59 percent (50 of 85) and 54 percent (35 of 64) in the 6- to 12-hour and 12- to 24-hour groups, respectively. The decline in the frequency of coronary thrombosis on angiography showed a statistically significant trend (Fig. 23-4).

Prevalence of Total Coronary Occlusion

Eighty-one percent of the patients in the overall population (419 of 517) demonstrated total coronary occlusion. As with coronary thrombosis, the frequency of total coronary occlusion declined over time. The patient group evaluated within 6 hours of symptom onset demonstrated an 85 percent (320 of 368) frequency of complete coronary occlusion. The frequency fell to 68 percent (58 of 85) in the 6- to 12-hour group and to 64 percent (41 of 64) in the 12- to 24-hour group. This trend was statistically significant (Fig. 23-5).

As Figure 23-5 demonstrates, the decline in arteriographic features favoring coronary thrombus parallels the fall in the prevalence of total coronary

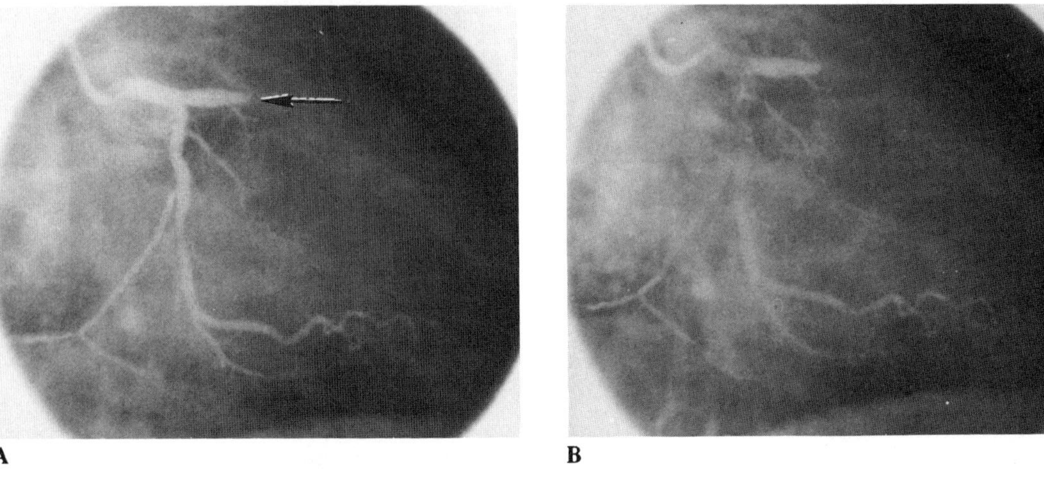

A B

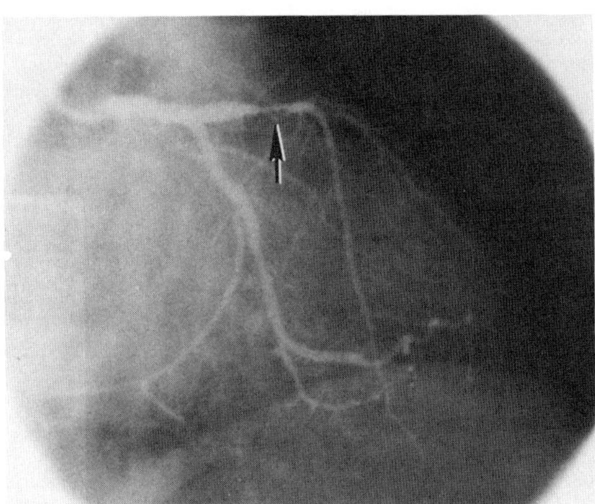

C

Fig. 23-2
A. Complete occlusion of the left anterior descending coronary artery (*arrow*). *B.* Retention of dye with staining of the intraluminal material in the same vessel while contrast is disappearing from the circumflex system. *C.* Restoration of blood flow to the left anterior descending artery after guidewire recanalization. Thrombus is noted (*arrow*) after reinjection of the vessel. (From M. A. DeWood et al. Coronary arteriographic findings in acute transmural myocardial infarction. *Circulation* 68[Suppl I]:I-39, 1983. By permission of the American Heart Association, Inc.)

occlusion over time. However, the frequencies of total coronary occlusion and of coronary thrombosis are slightly different even though most patients with thrombus are completely occluded. The difference between occlusion and thrombosis (approximately 10 percent) was systematic and suggests that the two phenomena differ somewhat in some patients. Other factors that may affect the coronary tree at the point of occlusion and coronary thrombus may not be present in these patients. For example, rupture of a softened plaque with progressive occlusion of the coronary lumen (Fig. 23-6), coronary spasm (Fig. 23-7), or gradual reduction of blood flow due to multiple stenoses (Fig. 23-8) may cause MI. The angiographic findings detailed in Figure 23-9 suggest that the pathophysiology of MI in a selected group may not involve coronary thrombus even though complete occlusion is usual. This difference between prevalence of occlusion and thrombus may partly explain failure of thrombolytic agents to restore antegrade blood flow in selected patients [13–16].

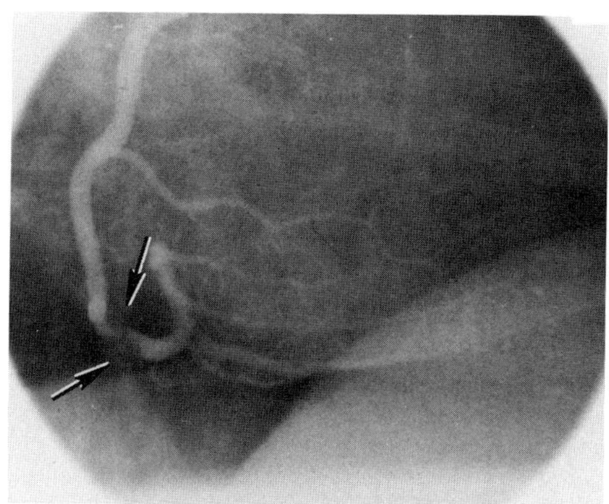

Fig. 23-3
Subtotal occlusion of the right coronary artery demonstrating an intraluminal filling defect (*arrows*). Thrombus was recovered at surgery. (From M. A. DeWood et al. Coronary arteriographic findings in acute transmural myocardial infarction. *Circulation* 68[Suppl I]:I-39, 1983. By permission of the American Heart Association, Inc.)

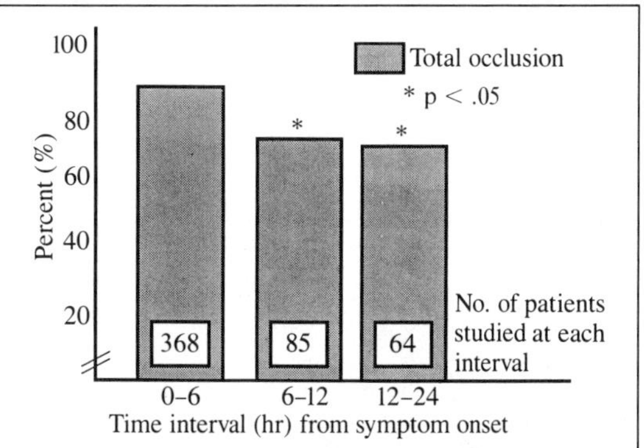

Fig. 23-5
Frequency of total occlusion in patient groups evaluated during time intervals over 24 hours after the onset of symptoms in Q-wave myocardial infarction. There is less complete occlusion in the 6- to 12-hour and the 12- to 24-hour groups than in the patients studied from 0 to 6 hours. (From M. A. DeWood et al. Coronary arteriographic findings in acute transmural myocardial infarction. *Circulation* 68[Suppl I]:I-39, 1983. By permission of the American Heart Association, Inc.)

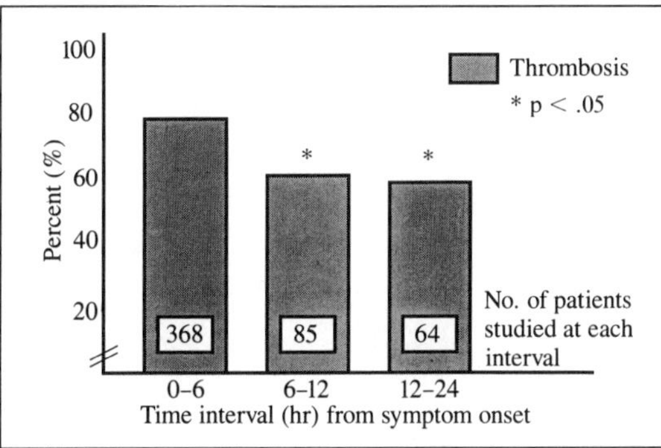

Fig. 23-4
Frequency of coronary thrombosis detected by coronary arteriography in patients evaluated during discrete time intervals after symptom onset. There was a significant decrease ($p < .05$) in the prevalence of coronary thrombosis that paralleled the decrease in total coronary occlusion. (From M. A. DeWood et al. Coronary arteriographic findings in acute transmural myocardial infarction. *Circulation* 68[Suppl I]:I-39, 1983. By permission of the American Heart Association, Inc.)

Correlation of Surgical and Pathologic Findings

To assess the accuracy of coronary arteriography in determining the presence or absence of coronary thrombus, the surgical findings in 96 patients who underwent emergency bypass surgery for Q-wave MI were reviewed. This procedure has been described elsewhere [1]. Briefly, at surgery a Fogarty catheter was passed into the infarct-related coronary vessel in an attempt to retrieve thrombus. Of the 96 patients, there were 71 in the 0- to 6-hour group, 14 in the 6- to 12-hour group, and 11 in the 12- to 24-hour group. Before surgery, the coronary obstruction observed during arteriography was graded as positive or negative for the presence of thrombus depending on criteria agreed on prospectively. Seventy-three of the 96 patients (76 percent) had angiographic features of thrombus and clot was recovered from the infarct-related coronary artery in 65 patients (89 percent). These thrombi were situated at or near a critical stenosis. In contrast, coronary thrombus was incorrectly judged to be present in eight patients with features of coronary thrombosis (11% false-positive rate). Spontaneous thrombolysis may have occurred in the interval between arteriography and surgery. This interval was usually 1 hour or less.

It is noteworthy that a 26 percent false-negative rate was observed, because even though thrombus was judged absent, thrombus was recovered in 6 of 23 cases (see Fig. 23-6). This finding suggests

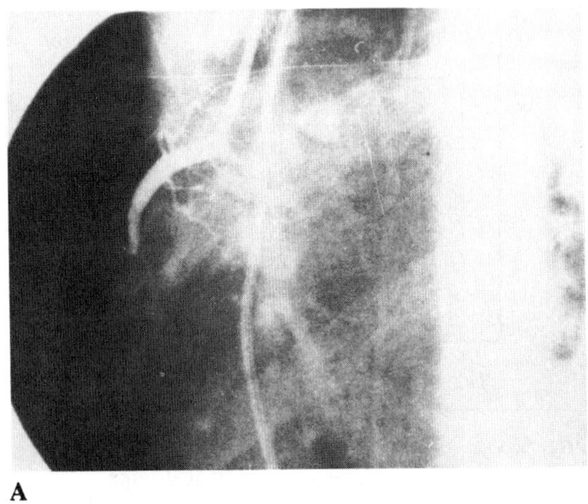

A

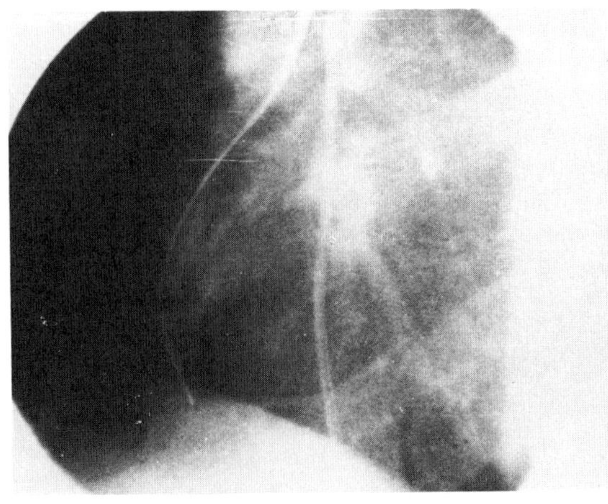

B

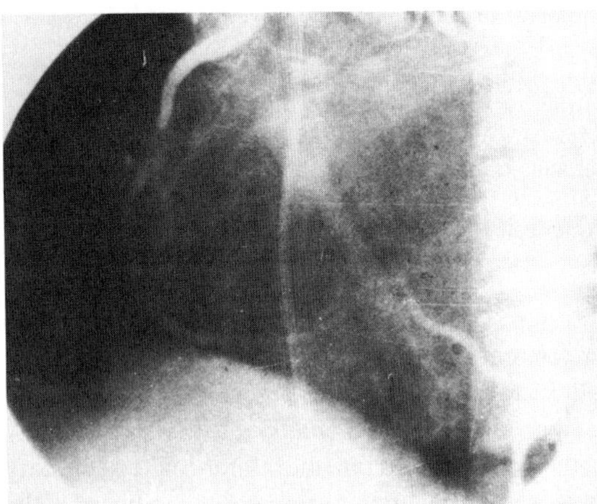

C

Fig. 23-6
A. Abrupt cutoff of forward flow in the right coronary artery with retention of dye. There was no staining, however. *B.* Passage of a guidewire through the lumen of the right coronary artery demonstrates that reperfusion of the distal vessel is possible. *C.* Perfusion of the distal right coronary artery is present. Beyond the previous occlusion, a channel through the thrombus has been generated by the guidewire. (From M. A. DeWood et al. Coronary arteriographic findings in acute transmural myocardial infarction. *Circulation* 68[Suppl I]:I-39, 1983. By permission of the American Heart Association, Inc.)

that in selected patients the presence of thrombus is not detected by the resolution of the coronary angiogram. Nevertheless, coronary arteriography appears to be very sensitive in the detection of coronary thrombus during the early hours of Q-wave infarction.

Complications Associated with Coronary Arteriography

Of the 517 patients, 51 (10 percent) had major complications during the arteriographic procedure. Most (44 of 51) complications were due to ventricular fibrillation. Overall, this represented an 8.5 percent (44 of 517) prevalence of ventricular fibrillation. None of these instances was fatal. More than half of the 44 patients with complications had experienced recurrent bouts of paired or multiple premature ventricular contractions, ventricular tachycardia, or fibrillation prior to the procedure. Other complications included intramyocardial injection of contrast agent, which occurred twice (0.4 percent), and plaque raised in a vessel not involved with the acute infarct in two other patients (0.4 percent).

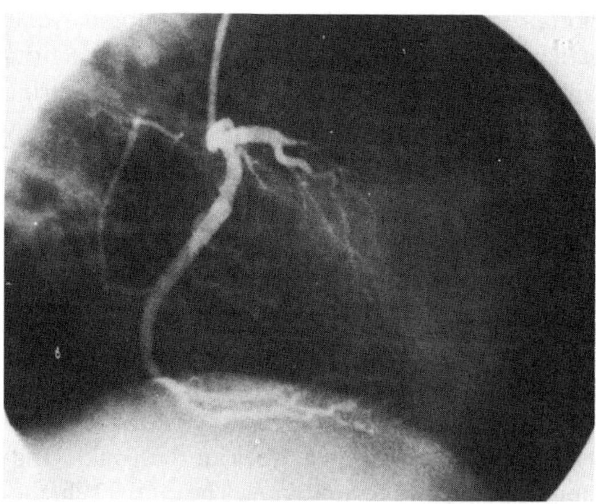

A

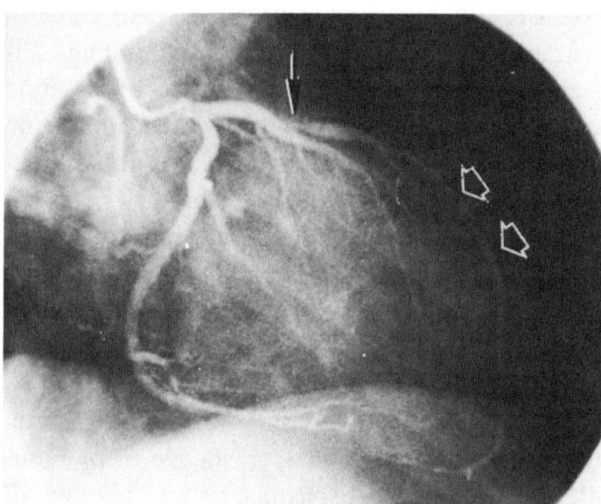

B

Fig. 23-7
A. Right anterior oblique projection of the left anterior descending coronary artery showing "beaking" appearance. *B.* After injection of intracoronary nitroglycerin, the distal left anterior descending coronary artery is injected as resolution of coronary spasm has occurred. (From M. A. DeWood et al. Coronary arteriographic findings in acute transmural myocardial infarction. *Circulation* 68[Suppl I]: I-39, 1983. By permission of the American Heart Association, Inc.)

Four patients (0.7 percent) did not survive the procedure. Three of these had been suffering from cardiogenic shock prior to the procedure. Hypotension was occasionally observed; however, no deaths occurred secondary to hypotension associated with cardiac catheterization. Thus, with an experienced operator, cardiac catheterization during early acute Q-wave MI is relatively safe and is associated with low morbidity and mortality.

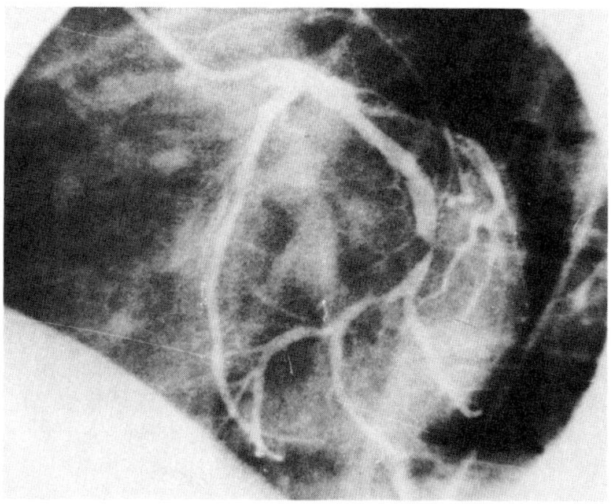

Fig. 23-8
Multiple severe stenosis of the circumflex vessels causative of Q-wave myocardial infarction. Several stenoses were observed in multiple eccentric lesions. No thrombus was seen. (From M. A. DeWood et al. Coronary arteriographic findings in acute transmural myocardial infarction. *Circulation* 68 [Suppl I]:I-39, 1983. By permission of the American Heart Association, Inc.)

Non-Q-Wave (Nontransmural) Myocardial Infarction

Although early Q-wave MI is usually diagnosed by ST segment elevation with evolution of pathologic Q waves on the electrocardiogram, non-Q-wave MI is not associated with a distinctive electrocardiographic marker. Frequently, these patients present with chest pain, elevation of cardiac enzymes, and nondiagnostic ST and T-wave abnormalities, but they do not develop Q waves.

The clinical distinction between Q-wave and non-Q-wave MI relies heavily on electrocardiographic criteria, but autopsy studies have shown that these criteria are relatively nonspecific [18–22]. Furthermore, patients with ST and T-wave abnormalities on the electrocardiogram but with only minor abnormalities of cardiac enzymes have been perceived as having unstable angina pectoris or other less important forms of coronary disease.

Because of this perception, few prospective clinical studies aimed at defining the arteriographic features associated with non-Q-wave infarction have been performed in the past. Because the arteriographic features of Q-wave infarction have been well defined, however, investigation of the acute ischemic syndromes has recently shifted to non-Q-

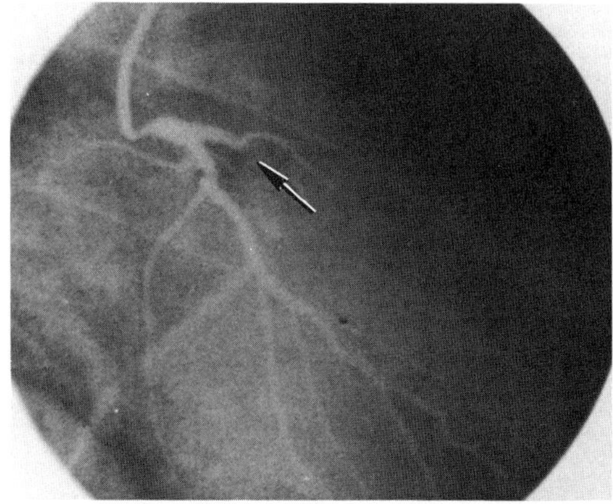

A

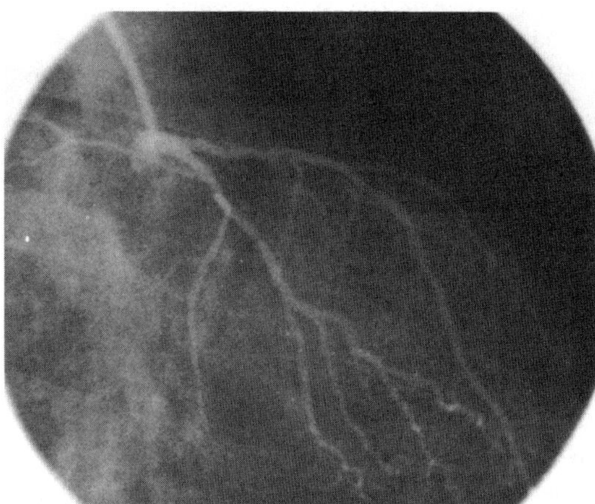

B

Fig. 23-9
A. Total occlusion of the left anterior descending coronary artery in the right anterior oblique projection. There was no staining or retention of dye on the left anterior descending vessel. Contrast agent perfused the circumflex system, which is well defined. *B.* Successful reperfusion of the distal left anterior descending coronary artery after thrombolytic therapy. There was a minor irregularity noted. (From M. A. DeWood et al. Coronary arteriographic findings in acute transmural myocardial infarction. *Circulation* 68[Suppl I]I-39, 1983. By permission of the American Heart Association, Inc.)

wave myocardial infarction. This is especially so because the clinical behavior of non-Q-wave infarction indicates that the initial mortality is lower, but most reports indicate the overall mortality equals or surpasses mortality associated with Q-wave infarction in long-term observations [23–27]. Therefore, one could assume that high long-term mortality reflects unstable pathophysiologic events in the coronary arteries. Our study analyzed angiography over a 10-year period in patients suffering early non-Q-wave infarction. The goals of the study were (1) to define the frequency of complete coronary occlusion within 1 week of non-Q-wave MI and (2) to correlate the arteriographic and clinical findings associated with non-Q-wave MI.

Patient Population

From 1974 through 1984, 341 patients underwent left heart studies within 1 week of the peak symptoms of non-Q-wave infarction. The clinical characteristics of the patients are summarized in Table 23-2. Because earlier studies with Q-wave MI demonstrated that coronary arteriographic findings differed with the duration from symptom onset to performance of arteriography, the total population with non-Q-wave MI was divided into three time-related groups.

One group (192 patients) underwent left heart catheterization within 24 hours of peak symptoms, another group (94 patients) underwent evaluation within the 24- to 72-hour period, and a third group (55 patients) underwent left heart catheterization 3 to 7 days after peak symptoms. Table 23-2 demonstrates that the age, gender, incidence of previous MI, creatinine kinase characteristics, number of vessels diseased, and the area of infarction seen by electrocardiogram were similar among the three groups. Similar to the Q-wave MI group, anterior infarction included patients with anterior, anteroseptal, anterolateral, and lateral infarctions, whereas inferior wall infarction encompassed inferior, inferoposterior, posterior, and inferolateral infarctions.

Results of Arteriographic Studies

Prevalence of Coronary Occlusion

In contrast to the Q-wave MI group (see Fig. 23-4, only 32 percent (107 of 341) of the entire population demonstrated complete coronary occlusion. Figure 23-10 shows that total coronary occlusion occurred in 26 percent (49 of 192) of the 0- to 24-hour group, 37 percent (35 of 94) of the 24- to 72-hour group, and 42 percent (23 of 55) of the 3- to 7-day group ($p < .05$). Thus, a significant increase in the frequency of complete coronary oc-

Table 23-2
Clinical characteristics of the three subsets of patients on entry into the study*

	Time after peak symptoms		
Characteristic	<24 hours	24–72 hours	72 hours–7 days
No. of patients	192	94	55
Age (yr), mean ± SD	59±10	59±9	60±9
Men (No. and % of total)	166 (86%)	83 (88%)	45 (82%)
Previous MI (No.)	42 (22%)	28 (30%)	10 (18%)
Mean initial CK (IU)	200	198	218
Mean peak CK (IU)	547	465	358
No. of diseased vessels			
1	53 (28%)	25 (27%)	11 (20%)
2	77 (40%)	28 (30%)	21 (38%)
3 or more	62 (32%)	41 (44%)	23 (42%)
Area of infarct by ECG			
Anterior	96 (50%)	51 (54%)	32 (58%)
Inferior	45 (23%)	26 (28%)	11 (20%)
Indeterminate	28 (15%)	7 (7%)	5 (9%)
Both	23 (12%)	10 (11%)	7 (13%)

*The three groups did not differ significantly in any of the characteristics on entry into the study. MI = myocardial infarction; CK = total creatinine kinase activity (>90 IU = abnormal); ECG = electrocardiogram.

clusion in the infarct-related vessel was observed over time.

Importantly, in the same groups, stenosis of 90 to 99 percent (i.e., subtotal occlusion) occurred in 34 percent (65 of 192), 26 percent (24 of 94), and 18 percent (10 of 55), respectively ($p < .05$). As shown in Figure 23-10, stenosis of 70 to 90 percent occurred in similar proportions across the patient populations studied. Stenosis of less than 70 percent was seen in 3 percent, 1 percent, and 0 percent in the three groups, respectively. Thus, a clear trend toward higher prevalence of total coronary occlusion occurred over time with a decline in the frequency of subtotal occlusion.

Prevalence of Collaterals

Figure 23-10 also shows the prevalence of collaterals beyond the infarct-related vessel. Collateralization occurred almost universally with patients who had complete coronary occlusion and in 32 percent of the entire population (107 of 341). When complete coronary occlusion was present (Fig. 23-11), usually the distal vessel was completely opacified by collaterals from a noninfarct-related vessel. As shown in Figure 23-10, collateral vessels occurred in 27 percent (52 of 192) in the 0- to 24-hour group, 34 percent (32 of 94) in the 24- to 72-hour group, and 42 percent (23 of 55) of the patients in the 3- to 7-day group ($p < .05$). Thus, there was a parallel increase in visible collateral vessels associated with the increase in total coronary occlusion among the three groups over time.

Prevalence of Coronary Thrombus

In contrast to the prevalence of coronary thrombus in Q-wave MI (see Fig. 23-4), non-Q-wave MI occasionally demonstrated intraluminal filling defects consistent with intracoronary thrombus. Because these defects were rarely associated with complete coronary occlusion, there was neither local retention of contrast agent nor staining of intraluminal material (see Figs. 23-12 and 23-13). More recent studies using intraoperative angioscopy have confirmed that intraluminal filling defects observed by angiographic methods are microthrombi [28].

Complications Associated with Coronary Arteriography

Although the rate of complications was 10 percent in the Q-wave MI group, the study observed a much lower rate of 2 percent (8 of 341) in patients with non-Q-wave MI. Major complications included ventricular fibrillation (N = 3), allergic dye response (N = 1), and severe hypotension (N = 3) that required extensive volume expansion and

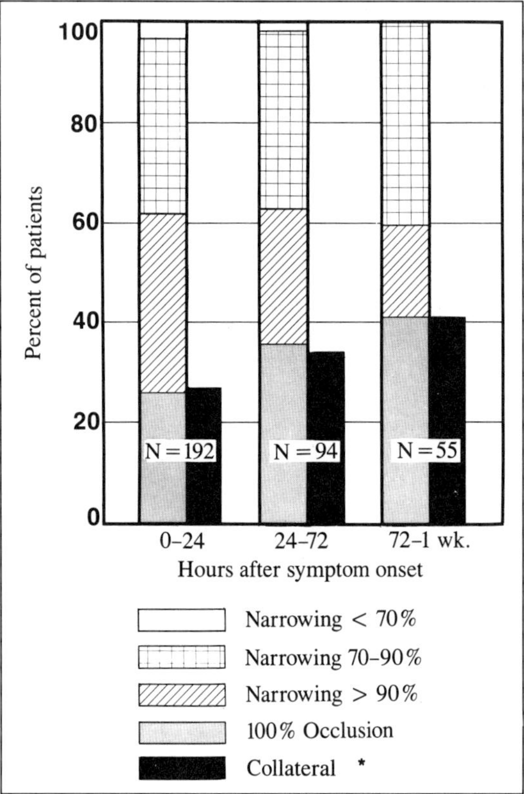

Fig. 23-10
Extent of occlusion in the three groups suffering non-Q-wave myocardial infarction. Percentage of stenosis applies to the infarct-related vessel. There was a significant increase in the frequency of coronary occlusion with time in the three groups and an inverse decrease (90 percent or more) in the percentage of patients with stenosis. There is no significant change in patients with 70 to 90 percent narrowing. (From M. A. DeWood et al. Coronary angiographic findings soon after non-Q-wave myocardial infarction. *N. Engl. J. Med.* 315:417, 1986. With permission.)

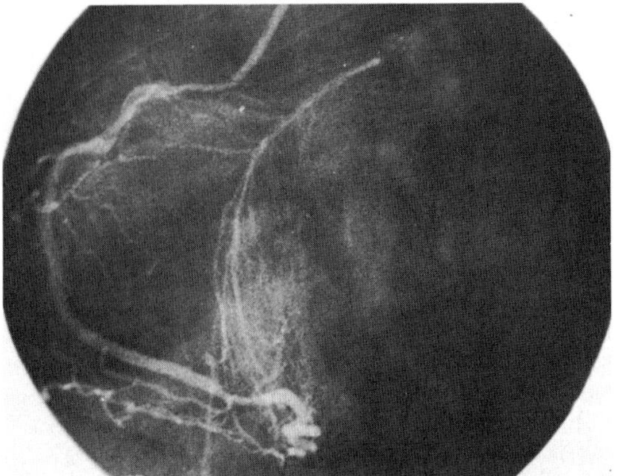

Fig. 23-11
Complete filling of the left anterior descending coronary artery in a patient with an anterior non-Q-wave myocardial infarction. The right coronary artery completely fills the distal left anterior descending coronary artery.

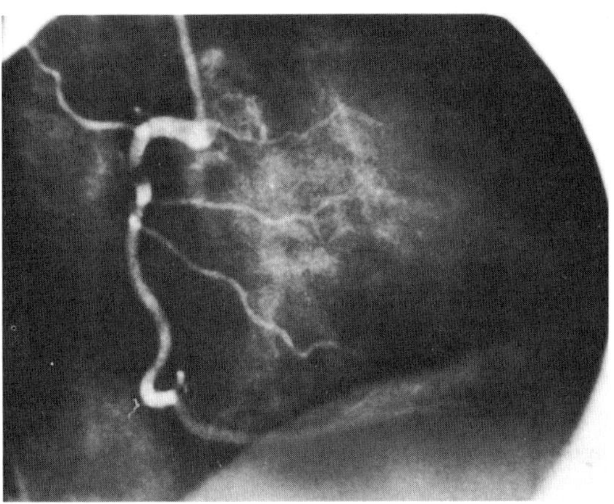

Fig. 23-12
Subtotal occlusion with a large thrombus in the right coronary artery causative of non-Q-wave inferior wall myocardial necrosis.

vasopressor therapy. In addition, one patient needed transvenous pacing. No deaths were attributable to cardiac catheterization.

Myocardial Infarction with and Without Sudden Death

The mechanisms of ventricular rhythm disturbances in cardiac death are generally unknown. Ventricular tachycardia or fibrillation may be secondary to complete coronary occlusion or it may be due to reperfusion rhythm disorders. Arrhythmias associated with complete coronary occlusion are usually termed *ischemic arrhythmias;* others are designated as *reperfusion arrhythmias.* The mechanisms for each differ in the experimental setting [8–12, 29–34].

Laboratory investigation with animals [35] indicated that coronary blood flow is phasic. In the laboratory, a 70 percent reduction in luminal diameter of coronary arteries was generated by placement of a snare, resulting in periodic and phasic decreases in coronary blood flow in more than half of the animals. Usually there was a gradual decrease in flow followed by a return to control levels. How-

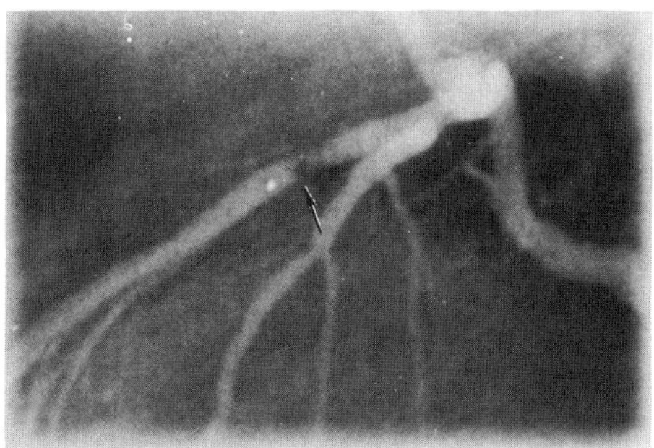

Fig. 23-13
Small thrombus in the left anterior descending coronary artery in the lateral projection vessel in a patient soon after symptom onset of non-Q-wave myocardial infarction. The patient has recurrent bouts of severe ischemia and required coronary bypass surgery. Thrombus was retrieved at surgery.

ever, some animals spontaneously occluded, which resulted in ventricular fibrillation and sudden cardiac death. Equally as important, abrupt *restoration* of blood flow may also result in ventricular fibrillation. The duration of preceding ischemia has been shown to influence the incidence of malignant arrhythmias associated with reperfusion [34]. Of note, the cyclic changes in coronary blood flow can be inhibited by antiplatelet agents, suggesting that thrombus formation at the site of the narrowing is a factor in some instances.

In patients, little is known about the status of the coronary arteries after sudden death except for pathologic data. These data usually demonstrate that almost all cases of sudden cardiac death are accompanied by some abnormality, although none is pathognomonic of sudden death. Some studies have shown microthrombi; others [36] describe platelet aggregates in the microcirculation of young patients who had no other abnormalities of the coronary arteries.

In patients successfully resuscitated after sudden cardiac death, coronary arteriography suggests extensive and diffuse coronary atherosclerosis, but only 20 percent of these patients evolve Q waves consistent with MI [37]. Thus, study of patients without evolution of Q waves results in two groups of patients: (1) those who have primary electrocardiographic disturbances but no evidence of acute myocardial necrosis, and (2) those with non-Q-wave infarction. Although cardiac enzyme studies confirm MI in 40 percent of patients who undergo successful resuscitation [37], most do not undergo coronary angiography until several weeks after the acute event. Arteriographic findings associated with disturbances soon after the onset of MI are poorly described and little is known about whether coronary thrombus or platelet aggregates are partially responsible for either ischemic or reperfusion rhythm disturbances.

Accordingly, we performed a series of studies. The goals of our investigations were (1) to define the prevalence of coronary occlusion in patients with sudden cardiac death associated with Q-wave MI, (2) to determine whether coronary anatomy is different from that in patients who sustain Q-wave MI but not sudden cardiac death, and (3) to determine whether most rhythm disturbances are caused by ischemic arrhythmias or reperfusion rhythm disturbances.

The clinical characteristics, coronary arteriographic features, and left ventriculographic findings in 78 patients with documented ventricular fibrillation, tachycardia, or asystole leading to sudden cardiac death after the symptoms of MI were investigated [38] (Table 23-3). In each case sudden death was witnessed and rhythm disturbances were docu-

Table 23-3
Overall group characteristics

Characteristics	Nonsudden death	Sudden death
No. of patients	78	78
Age (± SD)	54±10	54±10
Gender (% male)	78	75
Area of myocardial infarction		
Anterior	39	39
Inferior	39	39
Previous myocardial infarction	12/78 (15%)	11/78 (14%)
No. vessels diseased		
1	36/78 (46%)	35/78 (45%)
2	28/78 (36%)	32/78 (41%)
3 or more	14/78 (18%)	11/78 (14%)
Global EF	51±10	47±13*
LVFP (mm Hg)	21±9	20±9
A_0 (mm Hg)	101±15	98±18

EF = ejection fraction; LVFP = left ventricular filling pressure, A_0 = mean aortic pressure.
*Number of patients was 71.

mented by a cardiac monitor, either by paramedics in the field or by hospital personnel.

The sudden cardiac death group was compared to the nonsudden cardiac death group. Both groups were diagnosed with AMI and underwent left heart catheterization, left ventriculography, and coronary arteriography within 6 hours of the onset of infarction symptoms. The groups were matched for age, area of infarction (determined by the electrocardiogram), and the vessels believed to be responsible for the infarct. Other variables included number of vessels diseased, prevalence of complete coronary occlusion, incidence of previous MI, left ventricular filling pressure, central aortic blood pressure, and left ventricular function (estimated by global ejection fraction determinations).

The patient in Figure 23-14 presented to the emergency room with chest discomfort. He experienced ventricular fibrillation following ventricular tachycardia. When the patient became pulseless,

Fig. 23-14
Supraventricular arrhythmia with acute inferior wall myocardial infarction. The arrhythmia deteriorates into ventricular tachycardia and fibrillation. Electrical countershock is applied, and normal sinus rhythm resumes. Note the significant ST segment elevation in lead II.

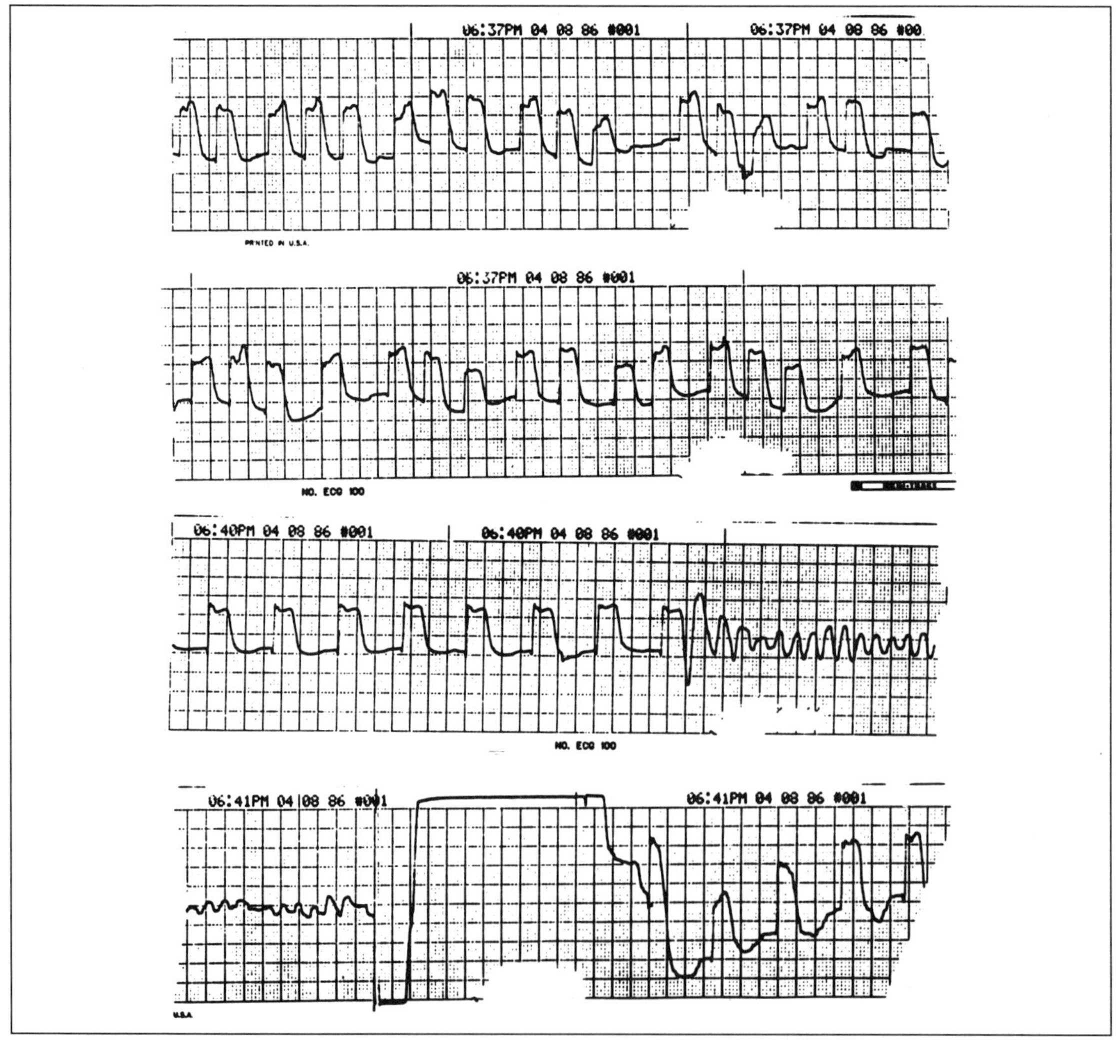

he was defibrillated. Regular rhythm and blood pressure were immediately restored. Coronary arteriography was performed within the hour of this instance of sudden death. The results are demonstrated in Figure 23-15. Intracoronary retention of the contrast agent suggested evidence of coronary thrombus.

There was a significant difference in the prevalence of coronary occlusion between groups. The study suggests that total coronary occlusion is frequent in sudden cardiac death associated with MI and supports the concept that most rhythm disturbances are due to ischemic arrhythmias. Within this group, however, there is an unexpected but significant lower frequency of complete coronary occlusion as compared to a matched group not sustaining sudden death in this clinical situation; it may be that sudden cardiac death is secondary to spontaneous thrombolysis and reperfusion rhythm disturbances. Further investigation to define the frequency of each type of arrhythmia and its clinical significance is needed.

Fig. 23-15
A. Left anterior oblique projection of the right coronary artery, which was causative of the Q-wave myocardial infarction in a sudden death patient (characterized in Fig. 23-14). *B.* Staining of the thrombus in the right coronary artery is seen in the same patient. *C.* The patient underwent coronary angioplasty and was discharged uneventfully in 3 days. The floppy guidewire is seen in the distal right coronary artery. Good perfusion of the distal vasculature was observed.

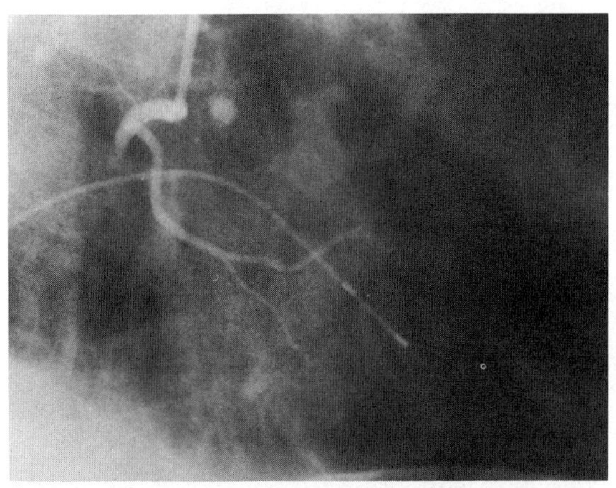
A

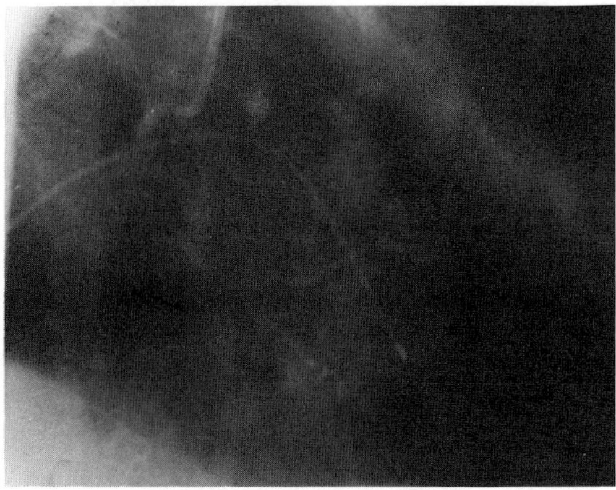
B

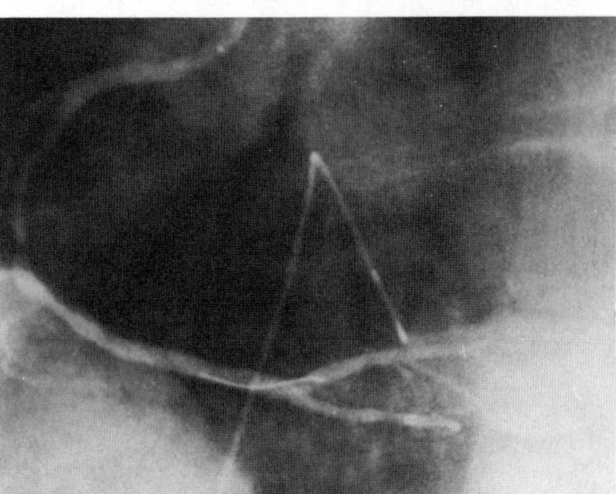
C

Coronary Arteriography for Acute Myocardial Infarction—When Is It Applicable?

Although early data [1, 5] demonstrate that coronary arteriography in AMI is safe, the question of when it should be performed remains.

Non-Q-Wave Myocardial Infarction

Two studies of acute non-Q-wave MI [5, 7] have demonstrated that whether arteriography is performed acutely [5] or delayed [7] there is no increase in mortality or morbidity. This applies if a patient's coronary anatomy is known to be relatively "safe" and only a small amount of myocardial tissue is in jeopardy. On the other hand, in patients with previous MI, it may be better to perform early arteriography to define the coronary tree, with an eye toward revascularization. Temporizing with heparin and antiplatelet agents also may be a safe option in the early hours [5] or 1 to 2 weeks [7] after non-Q-wave MI.

Q-Wave Myocardial Infarction

Most studies have demonstrated that inferior wall or inferoposterior wall MI is associated with approximately 4 to 5 percent mortality regardless of whether urgent revascularization is performed. Since knowing whether early revascularization is successful depends on an arteriogram, arteriography in these patients can usually be deferred unless the patient becomes unstable or has obvious biventricular infarction.

In the case of anterior infarcts, the case seems different. Patients who present within 12 hours of symptom onset should probably undergo arteriography with anticipation of interventions because hospital mortality data and 10-to-13-year follow-up data have demonstrated that revascularization performed within 12 hours lowers mortality and decreases morbidity. The effects of revascularization and the need for acute coronary arteriography in patients with anterior Q-wave MIs presenting more than 12 hours from symptom onset is unknown. This will be tested in an upcoming study in this and two other centers.

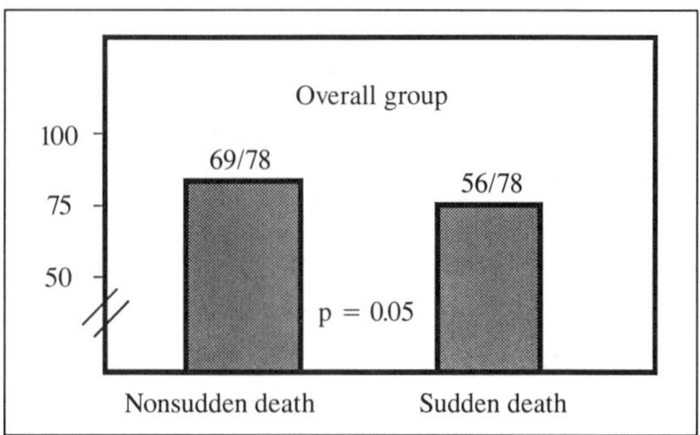

Fig. 23-16
Frequency of coronary occlusion in sudden death versus nonsudden death patients suffering Q-wave myocardial infarction. There was significantly less coronary occlusion in patients who suffered sudden cardiac death following myocardial infarction than in patients who did not.

Coronary thrombosis is the final common pathway converting chronic coronary disease to acute ischemia in the presence of Q-wave MI. Coronary thrombosis occurs in approximately 80 percent of patients with chronic coronary disease within 6 hours of symptom onset. This finding has been confirmed with multiple studies. There is less certainty when dealing with non-Q-wave MI because few systematic prospective studies have been done. However, certain features are suggestive of coronary thrombus with this syndrome.

Coronary arteriographic findings in sudden death patients are currently an area of investigation. Among many patients who evolve AMI, coronary thrombus is present, as is total coronary occlusion with thrombosis. However, there is less coronary occlusion than in patients who have no ventricular fibrillation or tachycardia (Fig. 23-16). In selective cases this finding may indicate spontaneous thrombolysis.

References

1. DeWood, M. A., Spores, J., Notske, R., et al. Prevalence of total coronary occlusion during the early hours of transmural myocardial infarction. *N. Engl. J. Med.* 303:897, 1980.
2. Oliva, P. B., and Breckenridge, J. C. Arteriographic evidence of coronary arterial spasm in acute myocardial infarction. *Circulation* 56:366, 1977.
3. Neill, W. A., Wharton, T. P., Jr., Fluri-Lundeen, J., et al. Acute coronary insufficiency—coronary occlu-

sion after intermittent ischemic attacks. *N. Engl. J. Med.* 302:1157, 1980.

4. Alison, H. W., Russell, R. O., Jr., Mantle, J. A., et al. Coronary anatomy and arteriography in patients with unstable angina pectoris. *Am. J. Cardiol.* 41:204, 1978.
5. DeWood, M. A., Stifter, W. F., Simpson, C. S., et al. Coronary angiographic findings soon after non-Q-wave myocardial infarction. *N. Engl. J. Med.* 315:417, 1986.
6. DeWood, M. A., Spores, J., Hensley, G. R., et al. Coronary arteriographic findings in acute transmural myocardial infarction. *Circulation* 68(Suppl I):1–39, 1983.
7. Gibson, R. S., Beller, G. A., Gheorghiade, M., et al. The prevalence and clinical significance of residual myocardial ischemia 2 weeks after uncomplicated non-Q-wave infarction: A prospective natural history study. *Circulation* 73:1186, 1986.
8. Axelrod, P. J., Verrier, R. L., and Lown, B. Vulnerability to ventricular fibrillation during acute coronary arterial occlusion and release. *Am. J. Cardiol.* 36:776, 1975.
9. Corbalan, D., Verrier, R. L., and Lown, B. Differing mechanisms for ventricular vulnerability during coronary artery occlusion and release. *Am. Heart J.* 92:223, 1976.
10. Levite, R., Banka, V. S., and Helfant, R. H. Electrophysiologic effects of coronary occlusion and reperfusion, observation of dispersion of refractoriness and ventricular automaticity. *Circulation* 52:760, 1975.
11. Ramanathan, K. B., Bodenheimer, M. M., Banka, V. S., et al. Electrophysiological effects of partial coronary occlusion and reperfusion. *Am. J. Cardiol.* 40:50, 1977.
12. Battle, W. E., Naimi, S., Avitall, B., et al. Distinction time course of ventricular vulnerability of fibrillation during and after release of coronary ligation. *Am. J. Cardiol.* 34:42, 1974.
13. Raisner, A. E., Tortoledo, F. A., Verani, M. S., et al. Intracoronary thrombolytic therapy in acute myocardial infarction: A prospective, randomized, controlled trial. *Am. J. Cardiol.* 55:301, 1985.
14. Stadius, M. L., Maynard, C., Fritz, J. K., et al. Coronary anatomy and left ventricular function in the first 12 hours of acute myocardial infarction: The Western Washington randomized intracoronary streptokinase trial. *Circulation* 72:292, 1985.
15. Simoons, M. L., Serruys, P. W., Van den Brand, M., et al. Improved survival after early thrombolysis in acute myocardial infarction: A randomized trial by the Interuniversity Cardiology Institute in The Netherlands. *Lancet* 2:578, 1985.
16. Rentrop, K. P., Feit, F., Blanke, H., et al. Effects of intracoronary streptokinase and intracoronary nitroglycerin infusion on coronary angiographic patterns and mortality in patients with acute myocardial infarction. *N. Engl. J. Med.* 311:1457, 1984.
17. Killip, T., III, and Kimball, J. T. Treatment of myocardial infarction in a coronary care unit: A two year experience with 250 patients. *Am. J. Cardiol.* 20:457, 1967.
18. Abbott, J. A., and Scheinman, M. M. Nondiagnostic electrocardiogram in patients with acute myocardial infarction: Clinical and anatomic correlations. *Am. J. Med.* 55:608, 1973.
19. Sullivan, W., Voldaver, Z., Tuna, N., et al. Correlation of electrocardiographic and pathologic findings in healed myocardial infarction. *Am. J. Cardiol.* 42:724, 1978.
20. Savage, R. M., Wagner, G. S., Ideker, R. E., et al. Correlation of postmortem anatomic findings with electrocardiographic changes in patients with myocardial infarction: Retrospective study of patients with typical anterior and posterior infarcts. *Circulation* 55:279, 1977.
21. Cook, R. W., Edwards, J. E., and Pruitt, R. D. Electrocardiographic changes in acute subendocardial infarction. I. Large subendocardial and large nontransmural infarcts. *Circulation* 18:603, 1958.
22. Horan, L. G., Flowers, N. C., and Johnson, J. C. Significance of the diagnostic Q-wave of myocardial infarction. *Circulation* 43:428, 1971.
23. Thanavaro, S., Krone, R. J., Kleiger, R. E., et al. Inhospital prognosis of patients with first nontransmural and transmural infarctions. *Circulation* 61:29, 1980.
24. Fabricius-Bjerre, N., Munkvad, M., and Knudsen, J. B. Subendocardial and transmural myocardial infarction: A five year survival study. *Am. J. Med.* 66:986, 1979.
25. Szklo, M., Goldberg, R., Kennedy, H. L., and Tonascia, J. A. Survival of patients with nontransmural myocardial infarction: A population-based study. *Am. J. Cardiol.* 42:648, 1978.
26. Cannom, D. S., Kevy, W., and Cohen, L. S. The short- and long-term prognosis of patients with transmural myocardial infarction. *Am. J. Med.* 61: 452, 1976.
27. Hutter, A. M., Jr., DeSanctis, R. W., Flynn, T., and Yeatman, L. A. Nontransmural myocardial infarction: A comparison of hospital and late clinical course of patients with that of matched patients with transmural anterior and transmural inferior myocardial infarction. *Am. J. Cardiol.* 48:595, 1981.
28. Sherman, C. T., Litvack, F., Grundfest, W., et al. Coronary angioscopy in patients with unstable angina pectoris. *N. Engl. J. Med.* 315:913, 1986.
29. Penkoske, P. A., Sobel, B. E., and Corr, P. B. Disparate electrophysiological alterations accompanying dysrhythmia due to coronary occlusion and reperfusion in the cat. *Circulation* 58:1023, 1978.
30. Murdock, D. K., Loeb, J. M., Euler, D. E., et al. Electrophysiology of coronary reperfusion, a mechanism for reperfusion arrhythmias. *Circulation* 61:175, 1980.
31. Kaplinsky, E., Ogawa, S., Michelson, E. L., et al. Instantaneous and delayed ventricular arrhythmias after reperfusion of acutely ischemic myocardium:

Evidence for multiple mechanisms. *Circulation* 63:333, 1981.
32. Sewell, W. H., Koth, D. R., and Huggins, C. E. Ventricular fibrillation in dogs after sudden return of flow to the coronary artery. *Surgery* 38:1050, 1955.
33. Scherlag, B. J., El-Sherif, N., Hope, R., et al. Characterization and location of ventricular arrhythmias resulting from myocardial ischemia and infarction. *Circ. Res.* 33:372, 1974.
34. Balke, C. W., Kaplinsky, E., Michelson, E. L., et al. Reperfusion tachyarrhythmias: Correlation with antecedent coronary artery occlusion tachyarrhythmias and duration of myocardial ischemia. *Am. Heart J.* 101:449, 1981.
35. Folts, J. D., Gallagher, K., and Rowe, G. G. Blood flow reductions in stenosed canine coronary arteries: Vasospasm or platelet aggregation. *Circulation* 65: 248, 1982.
36. Frink, R. J., Trowbridge, J. O., and Rooney, P. A., Jr. Nonobstructive coronary thrombosis in sudden cardiac death. *Am. J. Cardiol.* 42:48, 1978.
37. Cobb, L. A., Werner, J. A., and Trobaugh, G. B. Sudden cardiac death. 1. A decade's experience with out-of-hospital resuscitation. *Mod. Concepts Cardiovasc. Dis.* 49:31, 1980.
38. DeWood, M. A., Spores, J., Notske, R. N., et al. Coronary artery occlusion determined early after sudden cardiac death due to myocardial infarction. *J. Am. Coll. Cardiol.* 5:401, 1985.

24. Percutaneous Transluminal Coronary Angioplasty in Acute Myocardial Infarction

Bertram Pitt and Gary S. Francis

Thrombolytic therapy with intravenous streptokinase, recombinant tissue plasminogen activator (rt-PA), and anisoylated plasminogen streptokinase activator complex (APSAC) has been shown to improve ventricular function and survival in patients with acute myocardial infarction. The GISSI-I trial [1], demonstrating a marked reduction in mortality in patients seen within the first few hours of onset of symptoms of infarction, marked the beginning of the modern "reperfusion era." The ISIS-2 trial [2] extended these observations and demonstrated a significant reduction in mortality in patients receiving aspirin, streptokinase, or combination of aspirin and streptokinase seen within 24 hours from onset of symptoms. Similar reductions in mortality have been seen with rt-PA [3] and APSAC [4], at least within the early hours of acute infarction.

Despite the beneficial effects of intravenous thrombolytic agents, animal and clinical data suggest that intravenous thrombolysis alone may not provide optimal results. For example, Tomada [5] compared the effects of coronary artery thrombotic occlusion without intervention, coronary occlusion with thrombolysis, and coronary occlusion with percutaneous transluminal coronary angioplasty (PTCA) in an animal model. He found that the animals who underwent PTCA had a significantly smaller infarct size/area at risk than the animals treated with thrombolysis alone. Studies at the University of Michigan by Grines et al. [6] in patients with acute myocardial infarction undergoing reperfusion show that patients with more than a 50 percent residual stenosis of their infarct-related artery had a significantly increased incidence of postinfarction angina, exercise-induced ischemia prior to hospital discharge, and mortality compared to patients with less than 50 percent stenosis. These observations in animals and man suggest that a residual stenosis of the infarct-related artery may limit the beneficial effects of reperfusion. The residual stenosis of the infarct-related artery after reperfusion with thrombolytic agents is in part due to the underlying atherosclerotic lesion that led to the acute thrombosis and in part to partially lysed thrombus.

Although currently available intravenous agents may achieve reperfusion in 60 to 75 percent of patients [7–9], this reperfusion may not be optimal, at least during the first few hours of thrombolysis. Serial angiographic studies in patients receiving intravenous streptokinase in the Western Washington trial [10] have shown that clot lysis is not complete at 90 minutes and may not be complete for several days. Studies at the University of Michigan by Nicklas et al. [11] have shown that restoration of coronary blood flow after thrombolysis is suboptimal. The failure to completely restore flow after thrombolysis is likely due to the residual stenosis of the infarct-related artery and active vasoconstriction due to continued platelet deposition on to the unlysed residual thrombus, with release of thromboxane A_2 and serotonin as well as other vasoconstrictive agents.

In an attempt to achieve more complete reperfusion, PTCA of patients with acute myocardial infarction was first attempted by Meyer et al. in West Germany [12] and Hartzler et al. in the United States [13]. Hartzler et al. [14] have performed more than 400 direct PTCAs without concomitant thrombolytic therapy in patients with acute myocardial infarction. They have achieved a greater than

90 percent primary success rate with a relatively low in-hospital mortality and excellent long-term follow-up.

The only random trial of direct PTCA without thrombolytic agents to date was performed by O'Neill et al. at the University of Michigan and William Beaumont Hospital [15]. In this study patients with acute myocardial infarction seen within the first 6 hours of onset of symptoms of infarction were randomized to a strategy of PTCA without prior thrombolytic therapy or to thrombolytic therapy alone with intracoronary streptokinase. Approximately 85 percent of patients were successfully reperfused with either PTCA or intracoronary streptokinase. Although the reperfusion rates were similar, the patients randomized to PTCA had significantly less residual stenosis of the infarct-related artery, better improvement in global and regional left ventricular function, less postinfarction angina, less exercise-induced ischemia on prehospital discharge submaximal thallium 201 stress testing, and a tendency toward less reocclusion. Bleeding rates, however, as evidenced by the need for blood transfusion, were similar in the two groups. Although it was postulated that an advantage of direct PTCA might be a reduction in bleeding compared to that seen with thrombolytic agents, it is likely that the concomitant use of intravenous heparin negated this potential advantage. The number of patients in this trial was unfortunately too small to give any insight into the relative effect of these two strategies on survival. Although relatively small (56 patients), this trial provided encouragement for the use of direct (primary) PTCA.

We remain enthusiastic about the potential of direct PTCA, but it is obvious that this strategy is unlikely to be broadly applicable. The advantages of direct PTCA include a high success rate of reperfusion (85–95 percent), a low incidence of residual stenosis of the infarct-related artery, significantly better global and regional left ventricular function, less postinfarction angina, and less exercise-induced ischemia prior to hospital discharge compared to patients receiving thrombolysis alone. A major disadvantage of this strategy, however, is the time necessary to get the patient to the cardiac catheterization laboratory and to perform PTCA compared to the administration of an intravenous thrombolytic agent alone. Second, most patients with acute myocardial infarction are seen in community hospitals without facilities for acute angiography or PTCA. Even in institutions with adequate facilities for PTCA, adoption of a strategy of direct PTCA would result in performance of PTCA in individuals who might not need it if they have received intravenous thrombolytic therapy. Approximately 15 percent of patients who receive an intravenous thrombolytic agent are shown to have a less than 50 percent residual stenosis of their infarct-related artery on follow-up coronary angiography prior to hospital discharge. If seen within the early hours of infarction, these patients may have a more than 50 percent residual stenosis of their infarct-related artery, which might lyse over time and may not be hemodynamically significant (*minimal lesion syndrome*).

Two important reports published in 1993 have confirmed that immediate angioplasty is safe in the setting of acute myocardial infarction and may be preferable in selected patients. However, Gibbons et al. reported that immediate angioplasty does not clearly result in greater myocardial salvage than administration of thrombolytic agent followed by conservative treatment [16]. Grines et al., reporting for the Primary Angioplasty in Myocardial Infarction (PAMI) study group, compared t-PA with immediate PTCA and demonstrated that immediate PTCA reduced the combined occurrence of nonfatal reinfarction or death and was associated with a lower rate of intracranial hemorrhage, although left ventricular systolic function was similar in the two groups at six weeks [17]. It is now generally believed that direct angioplasty has an overall mortality similar to that of thrombolytic therapy [18]. Patients who may benefit more from immediate angioplasty include those with uncontrolled hypertension, recent major surgery, cerebral vascular accident, prolonged cardiopulmonary resuscitation, or bleeding diathesis. Also, patients with cardiogenic shock or very severe left ventricular dysfunction are better managed by immediate PTCA.

In about 10 percent of patients who undergo angioplasty of acute thrombotic coronary artery lesion, the large clot burden may result in markedly reduced coronary blood flow due to intense microvascular constriction [19]. Such microvascular constriction, probably caused by release of potent vasoconstrictors from the clot, may partly explain the failure of emergency angioplasty to reduce infarct size in acute myocardial infarction.

The strategy of immediate angioplasty for acute myocardial infarction continues to have limited application because of severely restricted accessibility of the procedure. When the procedure can be performed promptly (within 1 hour of arriving at the hospital) and expertly, it may be preferred for selected high-risk patients. For most patients with evolving acute Q-wave infarction, intravenous thrombolytic therapy continues to be the best approach.

References

1. Gruppo Italiano per lo Studio della Streptochinasi Nell'Infarto Miocardio (GISSI). Effectiveness of intravenous thrombolytic treatment in acute myocardial infarction. *Lancet* 1:397, 1986.
2. ISIS-2 Collaborative Group. Randomized trial of intravenous streptokinase, oral aspirin, both or neither among 17187 cases of suspected acute myocardial infarction: ISIS-2. *Lancet* 2:349, 1988.
3. Wilcox, R. G., Olsson, C. G., Skene, A. M., et al. Trial of tissue plasminogen activator for mortality reduction in acute myocardial infarction: Anglo-Scandinavian Study of Early Thrombolysis (ASSET). *Lancet* 2:525, 1988.
4. AIMS Trial Study Group. Effect of intravenous APSAC on mortality after acute myocardial infarction: Preliminary report of a placebo-controlled clinical trial. *Lancet* 1:545, 1988.
5. Tomada, H. Experimental study on myocardial salvage by coronary thrombolysis and mechanical recanalization. *Am. Heart J.* 116:687, 1988.
6. Grines, C. L., Topol, E. J., Bates, E. R., et al. Infarct vessel status after intravenous tissue plasminogen activator and acute coronary angioplasty: Prediction of clinical outcome. *Am. Heart J.* 115:1, 1988.
7. Chesebro, J. H., Knatterud, G., Roberts, R., et al. Thrombolysis in Myocardial Infarction (TIMI) Trial, Phase I: A comparison between intravenous tissue plasminogen activator and intravenous streptokinase. *Circulation* 76:142, 1987.
8. Verstraete, M., Brower, R. W., Collen, D., et al. Double-blind randomised trial of intravenous tissue-type plasminogen activator versus placebo in acute myocardial infarction. *Lancet* 2:965, 1985.
9. Topol, E. J., Califf, R. M., George, B. S., et al. A randomized trial of immediate versus delayed elective angioplasty after intravenous tissue plasminogen activator in acute myocardial infarction. *N. Engl. J. Med.* 317:581, 1987.
10. Stadius, M. L., Maynard, C., Fitz, J. K., et al. Coronary anatomy and left ventricular function in the first 12 hours of acute myocardial infarction: The Western Washington Randomized Intracoronary Streptokinase Trial. *Circulation* 72:292, 1985.
11. Nicklas, J. M., Diltz, E. A., O'Neill, W. W., et al. Quantitative measurement of coronary flow during medical revascularization (thrombolysis or angioplasty) in patients with acute infarction. *J. Am. Coll. Cardiol.* 10:284, 1987.
12. Meyer, J., Merx, W., Schmitz, H., et al. Percutaneous transluminal coronary angioplasty after streptolysis of transmural myocardial infarction. *Circulation* 66:905, 1982.
13. Hartzler, G. O., Rutherford, B. D., McConahay, D. R., et al. Percutaneous transluminal coronary angioplasty with and without thrombolytic therapy for treatment of acute myocardial infarction. *Am. Heart J.* 106:965, 1987.
14. Giorgi, L. V., Rutherford, B. D., Hartzler, G. O., et al. Direct PTCA for acute myocardial infarction in patients commonly excluded from thrombolytic trials. *Circulation* 78 (Suppl II):377, 1988.
15. O'Neill, W., Timmis, G., Bourdillon, P., et al. A prospective randomized clinical trial of intracoronary streptokinase versus coronary angioplasty therapy of acute myocardial infarction. *N. Engl. J. Med.* 314:812, 1986.
16. Gibbons, R. J., Holmes, D. R., Reeder, G. S., et al. Immediate angioplasty compared with the administration of a thrombolytic agent followed by conservative treatment for myocardial infarction. *N. Engl. J. Med.* 328:685, 1993.
17. Grines, C. L., Browne, K. F., Marco, J., et al. A comparison of immediate angioplasty with thrombolytic therapy for acute myocardial infarction. *N. Engl. J. Med.* 328:673, 1993.
18. Eckman, M. H., Wong, J. B., Salem, D. N., et al. Direct angioplasty for acute myocardial infarction. A review of outcomes in clinical subsets. *Ann. Int. Med.* 117:667, 1992.
19. Wilson, R. F., Laxson, D. D., Lesser, J. R., et al. Intense microvascular constriction after angioplasty of acute thrombotic coronary arterial lesions. *Lancet* 1:807, 1989.

25. Streptokinase in Acute Myocardial Infarction

Prediman K. Shah, Doron Zahger, and William Ganz

Thrombolytic therapy for acute myocardial infarction (AMI) dates to the 1960s and 1970s, when several large randomized studies assessed the value of intravenous thrombolytic therapy for AMI with inconclusive or negative results [1]. These results, together with a growing belief that thrombosis may not be the primary mechanism for acute coronary artery occlusion and AMI [2], led to the abandonment of thrombolytic therapy. However, better understanding of the pathophysiologic basis for AMI caused renewed interest in reperfusion therapy for AMI in the late 1970s. It became clear that the reason earlier thrombolytic trials had been negative or inconclusive was perhaps the failure of researchers to appreciate the importance of timely therapy, variable dose regimens, and criteria for inclusion.

Early approaches to reperfusion included emergency coronary artery bypass surgery (CABG) [3, 4], but logistic constraints and lack of suitability for widespread application were serious limitations; thus, the need for nonsurgical reperfusion became obvious. The modern era of thrombolytic therapy began when intracoronary administration of thrombolytic agents demonstrated effective coronary recanalization and myocardial reperfusion [5–8]. Animal work and subsequent clinical studies showed that timely reperfusion of the ischemic myocardium reduces infarct size, and thereby improves residual ventricular function and survival. Furthermore, clinical studies repeatedly demonstrated that the earlier reperfusion is achieved, the larger the potential benefit.

Rationale for Thrombolytic Therapy

The experimental and clinical studies of the 1970s and early 1980s greatly enhanced our understanding of the pathophysiology of AMI, confirming the seminal observations of Herrick [9]. It is now clear that the main initiating event of an acute ischemic syndrome such as AMI is rupture of the fibrous cap of an atherosclerotic plaque, often involving a mild, or angiographically insignificant, stenosis [10, 11]; the mechanisms involved are incompletely understood but circumferential shear stress, products of macrophages, the lipid content of the plaque, and the thickness of the collagen cap all seem to be important [11]. When the lipid-rich core of the plaque is exposed to circulating blood, there is rapid platelet recruitment, aggregation and thrombus formation, followed by thrombin-mediated fibrin accretion, leading to abrupt arterial obstruction and myocardial infarction. The extent of necrosis following acute coronary occlusion depends on the extent of myocardium at risk and on the residual blood supply to the ischemic territory as determined by (1) the degree, duration, and persistence of vascular obstruction (thrombus may be occlusive or permit some flow, and there often are spontaneous cycles of thrombolysis and occlusion [12]; and (2) the extent of collateral flow to the ischemic myocardium.

Once severe ischemia has lasted for about 20 minutes, myocardial necrosis ensues, affecting the subendocardium first and then proceeding in a time-dependent wave front to reach the epicardium about 4 to 6 hours later [13, 14]. Restoration of blood flow before necrosis is transmural arrests the progression of necrosis and salvages the still viable but ischemic myocardium that would otherwise proceed to necrosis [13, 14]. This fact, together with the realization that total thrombotic occlusion is central in the pathophysiology of AMI [15], leads to the conclusion that timely thrombolysis may achieve reperfusion of the ischemic myocardial territory, arrest the progression of necrosis, and reduce infarct size.

Process of Thrombolysis

Plasmin is the enzyme responsible for fibrin digestion. It is a nonspecific serine protease that circulates as the inactive proenzyme precursor plasminogen. Plasminogen is a 90-kilodalton (kD) glycoprotein containing 20 percent carbohydrate and composed of a single polypeptide chain of 791 amino acids that is synthesized by the liver [16]. The plasminogen content of plasma is approximately 180 mg/L and its half-life is 2.2 days. The native form of plasminogen, Glu-plasminogen, has glutamic acid in the *N*-terminus position. Another form of plasminogen, which has different biologic properties, is Lys-plasminogen. This molecule has amino-terminal lysine and arises when plasmin cleaves off a 77 amino acid residue from the amino-terminal portion of Glu-plasminogen [17]. Plasmin degrades fibrin (thrombolysis) as well as fibrinogen, clotting factors V, VIII, and XII and some hormones [18]. As a result of plasmin's action on fibrin and fibrinogen, fibrin(ogen) degradation products are detected in plasma. Of these, D-dimers are a marker of degradation of cross-linked fibrin, i.e., clot dissolution.

Fibrinolysis can be inhibited by two main endogenous proteins: alpha$_2$-antiplasmin, which degrades circulating plasmin, and plasminogen-activator inhibitor-1 (PAI-1). Levels of PAI-1 have been found to be elevated in diabetic patients and in survivors of myocardial infarction, raising the possibility that impaired endogenous fibrinolysis may contribute to the risk of AMI [19–21].

The conversion of plasminogen to plasmin can be achieved by endogenous (intrinsic and extrinsic) and exogenous activators and can occur with both fibrin-associated and free plasminogen. The intrinsic activators, which include factor XII kallikrein and kinins, circulate in plasma in a precursor state; the extrinsic plasminogen activators are of tissue or cellular origin (kidney and endothelial cells) and appear to be locally released and to act locally. The exogenous activators are those used for the pharmacologic activation of plasminogen to plasmin. Currently, there are four groups of pharmacologic activators of plasmin: (1) streptokinase (SK) and its related agents, (2) urokinase and its related agents, (3) tissue plasminogen activator (t-PA), and (4) staphylokinase. This chapter focuses primarily on the use of SK as a thrombolytic agent in AMI.

Pharmacology of Streptokinase

Mechanism of Action

SK is an extracellular protein product of hemolytic streptococci [22]. It is composed of a single polypeptide chain with a molecular weight of 47 to 50 kD. SK is not an enzyme; it cannot cleave peptide bonds, has no esterase or amidase activities against synthetic substrates, and is not inhibited by any inhibitors specific for proteolytic enzymes [23]. Reddy and Markus discovered how this nonenzymatic protein catalyzes the enzyme reaction required for plasminogen activation [24] (Table 25-1).

SK rapidly forms a 1:1 stoichiometric complex with plasminogen (either Glu-plasminogen or Lys-plasminogen) (reaction 1). The noncovalent association of these two inactive proteins exposes an active site so that the new complex has enzyme and amidase activities [25, 26]. Plasminogen (both circulating and fibrin-bound) is the only known natural substrate for this enzyme; Lys-plasminogen is activated at a higher rate (sixfold) than native Glu-plasminogen [27]. Activated plasminogen then catalyzes the conversion of plasminogen to plasmin (reaction 2). Although the SK–plasminogen complex can be prepared by mixing stoichiometric amounts of the two components, its existence is short-lived as it is continuously transformed autocatalytically into the SK–plasmin complex; this conversion is completed within 5 minutes at room temperature [24] (reaction 3). Acylated/anisoylated plasminogen SK activator complex (APSAC) (see below) is prepared by blocking the active site with acyl or anisoyl groups, respectively [28]. The plasminogen activator activity of the SK–plasminogen complex is two- to threefold greater than that of the SK–plasmin complex [29].

Table 25-1
Mechanism of action of streptokinase

Reaction sequence	Reaction
1. Plasminogen + SK	SK–plasminogen complex
2. Plasminogen + SK–plasminogen	plasmin
3. SK–plasminogen + SK–plasminogen	SK–plasmin
4. Plasminogen + SK–plasmin	plasmin

SK = streptokinase.

The SK–plasmin complex is the relatively stable form of the enzyme formed by the reaction between SK and plasminogen; it can also be formed by direct reaction of SK with plasmin. Formation of the SK–plasmin complex involves cleavage of two peptide bonds in the plasminogen molecule (Arg 560-Val 561 and Lys 77-Lys 78) giving rise to the two-chain structure of plasmin. The SK molecule undergoes proteolytic cleavages as well and becomes less active as a result [23]. The SK–plasmin complex activates both Glu- and Lys-plasminogens to give Lys-plasmin. The enzyme properties of the SK–plasmin complex are similar to those of plasmin, but its catalytic efficiency is approximately twofold higher. Furthermore, while the interaction of alpha$_2$-antiplasmin with plasmin is practically instantaneous, a 2×10^7-fold reduction is seen in its interaction with the SK–plasmin complex [30–32]. The difference in the reaction of the physiological inhibitor has important consequences for the in vivo activity of SK. Because of the inability of alpha$_2$-antiplasmin to inhibit the SK–plasmin complex, plasminogen activation in the circulation proceeds until both plasminogen and the inhibitor are depleted.

Both the SK–plasminogen and SK–plasmin complexes are plasminogen activators (reaction 4), but the former is two- to threefold more active than the latter [29]. However, SK–plasmin shows higher activity (2.5-fold) toward Lys-plasminogen as the substrate compared to Glu-plasminogen. Thus, if plasmin generated in the circulation during SK thrombolysis is not inactivated rapidly, the cascade of reactions amplifies the rate of plasminogen activation to plasmin. An important consequence of complex formation between SK and plasminogen is that SK consumes an equimolar amount of plasminogen for activator formation and thus decreases the amount of substrate plasminogen available for conversion to plasmin.

In man, both circulating and thrombus-bound plasminogen is converted to plasmin, but the latter is more important in thrombolysis [32–34]. Most circulating plasmin is either rapidly inactivated by antiplasmins and cleared from the circulation [35], or it hydrolyses circulating fibrinogen and other clotting factors, producing the lytic state characterized by hypofibrinogenemia, elevated serum fibrin(ogen) degradation products such as D-dimers, a shortened euglobulin lysis time, and prolonged thrombin and partial thromboplastin times [36–38]. These hemostatic changes are dose-dependent and contribute to the bleeding tendency produced by SK. The half-life of SK is approximately 20 minutes, whereas that of the plasminogen activator complex is about 80 minutes. The systemic lytic effects last even longer and plasma fibrinogen is depressed for 24 to 72 hours with recovery to levels of above 100 mg/dl (minimum for adequate hemostasis) within about 24 hours [39]. The SK–plasmin complex, immune from the action of alpha$_2$-antiplasmin, binds to fibrin via the kringle structure on plasmin [40] and degrades it.

Clot lysis by SK is dependent on the time delay from onset of thrombosis to treatment. Experimental studies have shown that older thrombi are more resistant to lysis [41, 42], probably because they tend to be larger, have a lower plasminogen content due to retraction, and have a higher degree of fibrin cross-linking than fresher thrombi [43, 44]. Older thrombi are therefore more resistant to lysis and require a longer exposure to increased amounts of thrombolytic agents to be lysed than do smaller and fresher thrombi [45]. Consistent with these observations, several clinical studies found that the delay between onset of infarction and treatment was a determinant of both the rate of successful reperfusion and the time required to achieve it [42, 46–49], probably reflecting the fact that the interval between onset of symptoms and treatment is related to the thrombus age. Anderson and colleagues [50] reported reperfusion rates of 85 percent or more in patients who were admitted within 4 hours of the onset of chest pain, whereas the rate of successful reperfusion was 60 to 70 percent in studies that delayed treatment for more than 6 hours after the onset of chest pain [51–55].

Species Specificity

Plasminogens from various mammalian species vary in their interaction with SK [23] and can be divided into three groups.

1. Plasminogens that can be activated with a small amount of SK (human and monkey)
2. Plasminogens that require large amounts of SK (dog and rabbit)
3. Plasminogens that are resistant to activation by SK (cow, sheep, pig, rat, mouse)

The mechanism of plasminogen activation by SK involves several steps, and any block in these steps affects the activation process. For example, cow, sheep, and mouse plasminogens do not form the respective SK–plasminogen complexes, and no activation can take place. In the dog and rabbit, high concentrations of SK are needed for complete activation because the added SK is rapidly degraded. When native SK of 47 kD was added to dog plasminogen, the final product of the reaction was a SK–dog plasmin complex in which the SK was found to be degraded to a fragment of approximately 25 kD [56]. Moreover, the SK–dog plasmin complex had no plasminogen activator activity. Alpha$_2$-antiplasmin inhibited the SK–dog plasmin complex completely but had no effect on the SK–human plasmin complex [57]. Lack of activator activity in the SK–dog plasmin complex and its rapid inhibition by alpha$_2$-antiplasmin explains why SK does not achieve efficient thrombolysis in the dog. Although rabbit plasminogen requires a large excess of SK for in vitro activation, significant thrombolysis is achieved in vivo with low doses of SK due to enhancement of activation by rabbit fibrin [58]. In cats, SK infusion results in depletion of plasminogen and fibrinogen in the circulation, similar to changes seen in humans [59].

Interactions of Streptokinase with the Clotting System and with Platelets

A complex interaction exists between the fibrinolytic system and platelets [60]. Platelets have been found to possess both fibrinolytic and antifibrinolytic properties, whereas thrombolytic agents have been shown to decrease as well as to enhance platelet aggregation. Platelets contain both t-PA and urokinase-type plasminogen activator, although the function of these platelet factors is unclear [61, 62]. Platelets can also bind plasminogen [63]; this can be facilitated by the presence of thrombospondin, a plasminogen-binding protein, on the surface of activated platelets [64]. Thus, platelets can localize fibrinolysis to their vicinity, which may explain their potentiating effects on t-PA-induced plasminogen activation [65]. Platelets also contain two antifibrinolytic substances: plasminogen-activator inhibitor-1 [66] and alpha$_2$-antiplasmin [67]. The net effect of these opposing forces is unclear, and may differ according to circumstances. A dominant antifibrinolytic activity may explain why platelet-rich thrombi are relatively resistant to thrombolysis [68] and why antiplatelet agents are synergistic with thrombolytic agents [69].

In a similar fashion, contradictory observations have been made regarding the effect of thrombolytic therapy on platelet activation [70–73]. SK-induced platelet aggregation may be facilitated by thrombin, which is also induced by SK (see below). Other studies have found, however, that plasmin inhibits platelet function [72] as do fibrin(ogen) degradation products, probably by binding to fibrinogen and its platelet receptor, and thus blocking further aggregation [74].

The net effect of these seemingly conflicting interactions has not yet been elucidated and may vary with different agents, with conjunctive anticoagulation, and with time after treatment. Platelet aggregation has been shown to increase immediately after t-PA infusion in the rabbit, decrease below baseline by 180 minutes and return to baseline at 240 minutes [75]. The clinical benefit of platelet inhibition in conjunction with thrombolysis, however, is clear [69, 76].

Evidence has also accumulated to suggest paradoxical thrombin action and fibrin generation during thrombolysis, mainly through the finding of elevated levels of fibrinopeptide A, a marker of fibrin generation, after in vitro or in vivo thrombolysis [77, 78]. Persistently elevated fibrinopeptide A has also been shown to be associated with early reocclusion, and to be suppressed by adequate anticoagulation [79, 80]. SK has also been shown to induce a state of relative resistance to heparin, which may be explained by ongoing fibrin generation [81]. Thrombin is a potent platelet aggregator; this characteristic may contribute to the proaggregatory effect of SK. The hypercoagulable state induced by thrombolysis may facilitate thrombotic reocclusion or predispose to failure of lysis or to slow lysis [82].

The plasminogen activator activity of SK is enhanced by fibrinogen, fibrin, and fibrinogen fragment D. Fibrinogen was found to stimulate the rate of complex formation between SK and plasminogen as well as the activator activity of the complex [83]. Fibrin stimulates Glu-plasminogen activation to a higher extent (6.5-fold) than fibrinogen (2-fold).

Anticoagulation with heparin or hirudin has been shown in vitro to enhance thrombolysis [84, 85]. Clinically, the role of heparin is not as clear (see "adjunctive therapy" below).

Antigenicity of Streptokinase

Because exposure to streptococcus is ubiquitous in man, an amnestic immunologic response usually follows administration of SK and the titer of circulating anti-SK antibodies substantially increases [86]. This response is variable, but neutralizing antibodies usually appear within about 5 days. They later decline during the first year and reach a plateau level that persists for at least four years, at which time about 50 percent of patients still have neutralizing antibodies to a therapeutic dose of SK [87–90]. Preexisting, naturally occurring antibodies may impair the clinical response to SK thrombolysis [91]. Thus, it seems prudent that patients with known antibodies should receive an alternative agent and that SK, or an SK-containing thrombolytic agent such as anistreplase, should not be used within at least one year, and possibly indefinitely, after previous administration because the time required for determination of the antistreptococcal titer makes it impractical as an aid to early decision-making as AMI evolves. Not all researchers concur, however, that SK thrombolysis may be impaired by preexisting, natural antibodies [92].

Notwithstanding the inhibitory role of antistreptokinase antibodies, allergy following SK is a rare problem in clinical practice. In the Second International Study of Infarct Survival (ISIS-2) mild allergic reactions were observed in 4.4 percent of treated patients and 0.9 percent of controls; this incidence was not reduced in the 22 percent of patients who received steroids [69]. Anaphylaxis was very rare. Allergic reactions to SK are not associated with a worse outcome of treatment [93].

Anistreplase

New forms of SK have been developed by molecular engineering technologies that covalently bind SK–plasminogen activator complex to compounds such as acyl or anisoyl groups, which render the complex inactive. The new product, acylated plasminogen SK activator complex (APSAC), also called anistreplase, becomes a functional plasminogen activator only after removal of the acyl group exposes the active site on the complex [94, 95]. Because deacylation proceeds much more rapidly in the presence of fibrin than in the circulation, APSAC is relatively inert after intravenous injection until it reaches the thrombus interface. However, slow deacylation does occur in the circulation, and the ultimate systemic effects of APSAC are usually similar to those of SK [96]. One advantage of APSAC over SK is that it may be given as a bolus [96] because the systemic activation of plasmin is slow and the drug is less likely than SK to cause hypotension when given rapidly [97]. Otherwise, the thrombolytic and antigenic effects of APSAC are similar to those of SK, as is the clinical outcome [98].

Dosage and Administration of Streptokinase

Intracoronary Streptokinase

In studies of intracoronary SK, the dosage, infusion rate, and technique of infusion varied, but in general a loading dose of 10,000 to 20,000 units of SK was followed by a constant infusion of 2000 to 4000 IU/min until coronary artery patency was restored and for another 30 to 60 minutes to completely lyse the clot. The total dose varied from less than 100,000 units to more than 500,000 units and was usually greater than 250,000 units. Pooled data suggest that administration of larger doses of SK or a subselective infusion result in a higher reperfusion rate, whereas intracoronary nitroglycerin or perforation of the thrombus with a guidewire were of no added benefit and only rarely achieved reperfusion [13, 99]. Despite the encouraging results of intracoronary thrombolysis, it is now used rarely because of the simplicity and widespread applicability of intravenous thrombolysis.

Intravenous Streptokinase

Intravenous thrombolysis proved to be an effective and widely applicable means of achieving reperfusion and is usually the way thrombolysis is currently used as primary treatment for AMI. The rate at which any thrombolytic agent affects clot lysis and reperfusion is in part a function of its plasma concentration [35, 100, 101]; therefore, intravenous studies have used higher doses at faster infusion rates than the intracoronary studies used. A direct relation has been found between dosage and reperfusion rates [49, 53, 102]. In our experience, about 30 percent of the patients treated with 750,000 units received an inadequate dose and required a second dose to achieve reperfusion [103]. Although these patients tended to be heavy (> 75 kg) or had a high titer of anti-SK antibodies, they could not be rapidly recognized before treatment. Therefore, as the larger dose did not cause an increased incidence of bleeding, we currently recommend a routine intravenous SK dose of 1.5 million units. Six and others randomized 189 patients to receive 200,000, 750,000, 1,500,000 or 3,000,000 units of SK [104]. Angiographically determined patency at 2.8 hours was significantly better with the highest dose as compared to the other doses examined. If this observation is confirmed, and bleeding is not found to be substantially increased, a higher dose of SK may prove superior. Reperfusion by intravenous or intracoronary SK is achieved more rapidly by fast infusion rates (Fig. 25-1); slow administration may be relatively ineffective [49]. On the other hand, rapid infusion of SK may cause sudden and sometimes severe hypotension [105] (see Fig. 25-1).

Fig. 25-1
Reciprocal effects of the rate of infusion of streptokinase on the time interval to reperfusion (*bottom*) and the fall in systolic blood pressure (*top*). Slow infusion rates of streptokinase have a small effect on blood pressure but achieve reperfusion slowly, whereas rapid infusion rates of streptokinase achieve prompt reperfusion but may cause considerable hypotension.

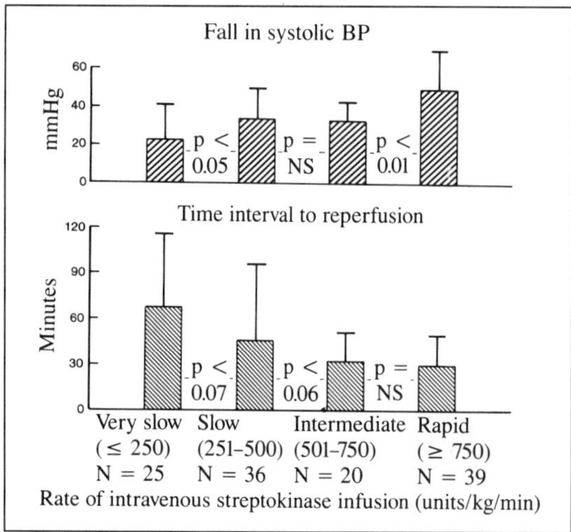

Effects of Streptokinase in Evolving Acute Myocardial Infarction

Coronary Recanalization

Angiography has generally been regarded as the gold standard for assessment of success or failure of reperfusion (Fig. 25-2). It is important to realize, though, that angiographic "patency" is not the equivalent of successful treatment; patency determined at any time after thrombolysis may reflect spontaneous reperfusion before treatment or an ar-

Fig. 25-2
Serial selective right coronary angiograms from a patient with inferior acute myocardial infarction showing (*A*) complete proximal occlusion and (*B*) restoration of patency following intracoronary streptokinase.

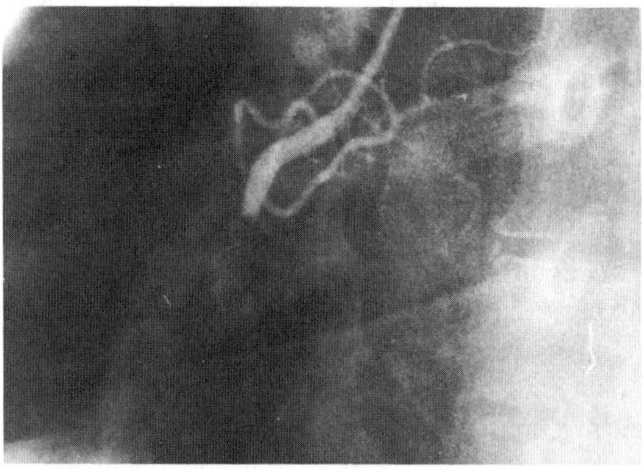

A

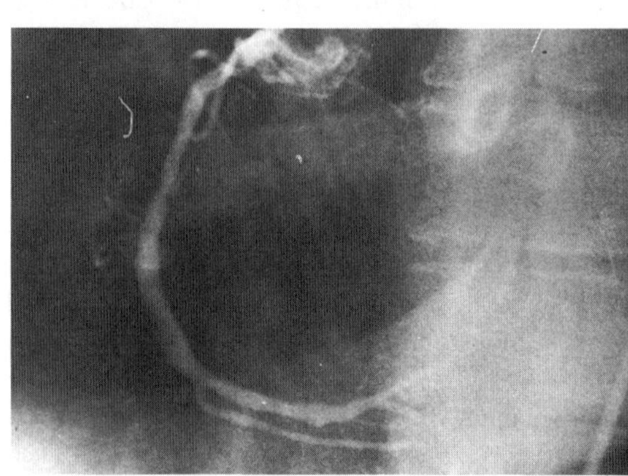

B

tery that was never totally occluded. Therefore, a stricter measure of the success of treatment is "reperfusion" or "recanalization," which implies an angiographically occluded artery before treatment. The first angiographic sign of reperfusion is often the establishment of a sluggish flow of contrast through the thrombus. In both experimental and clinical studies, the lumen and coronary flow generally increase as thrombolysis continues, although frequently a cyclic pattern of reperfusion and reocclusion precedes definitive recanalization [4, 106]. In our experience, once reperfusion is evident, the artery remains open if thrombolytic therapy is continued, even when patency is initially intermittent. Neither nitroglycerin nor calcium channel blocking drugs have proved effective in accelerating complete reperfusion.

The following four-point scoring code was proposed by the investigators of the Thrombolysis in Myocardial Infarction (TIMI-I) group to grade the antegrade flow in an infarct-related artery [107]:

TIMI 0 = no antegrade perfusion
TIMI 1 = contrast penetrates beyond the occlusive thrombus but does not fill the entire distal artery
TIMI 2 = the entire distal artery fills sluggishly at a rate much slower than that in the normal coronary arteries
TIMI 3 = normal, brisk antegrade perfusion

Although TIMI flow grades 0 to 1 and 2 to 3 were considered in past trials to reflect failed or successful reperfusion, respectively, it has recently become clear that TIMI flow grade 2 is insufficient and is associated with worse outcome as compared to TIMI flow grade 3 [108–111]. In the recently completed Global Utilization of Streptokinase and t-PA for Occluded Coronary Arteries (GUSTO-1) angiographic study [111], TIMI flow grades of 0 to 1, 2, and 3 were associated with a mortality of 9 percent, 7.9 percent, and 4.3 percent, respectively. Therefore, TIMI flow grades 0 and 1 represent failed reperfusion, and TIMI flow grades 2 and 3 signify incomplete and complete reperfusion, respectively. Patients with failed or incomplete reperfusion should be considered for alternative methods of recanalization (e.g., rescue angioplasty).

Because of the dynamic nature of coronary obstruction during thrombolysis, coronary patency at any particular time point is merely a "snapshot" of a changing process; to fully appreciate the effect of treatment one would have to know the time course of reperfusion; this can be inferred from studies that have examined patency at different time points (Table 25-2).

Most studies of intracoronary thrombolytic therapy for AMI have used SK, but similar results were reported with other agents [112, 113]. In these studies, reperfusion occurred in 60 to 79 percent of completely occluded infarct-related arteries, which is probably an underestimation of the ultimate reperfusion rate because few studies observed patients for longer than 90 minutes. The reperfusion rate averaged about 75 percent for 1453 patients enrolled in three large registries of intracoronary SK [47, 48, 114] with a mean time interval from commencement of SK to reperfusion of about 40 minutes for successfully treated patients.

Intravenous SK achieves reperfusion rates that are comparable to those obtained by the intracoronary route [51–54, 102, 115]. When examined within 3 to 4 hours after symptom onset, 80 to 85 percent of patients have total occlusion of the infarct-related artery [7, 50, 97, 116]. In the absence of reperfusion therapy, the prevalence of total occlusion slowly declines with time, due to spontaneous reperfusion, and at 10 to 21 days after infarction, 45 to 78 percent of patients have patent infarct-related arteries [117, 118]. One hour after initiation of SK, patients in the Pro-Urokinase in Myocardial Infarction (PRIMI) trial [119] had a patency of 48 percent. Most studies have studied coronary patency 90 minutes after initiation of thrombolysis and have reported it as 45 to 64 percent [116, 119–122]. At 2 to 3 hours, patency is

Table 25-2
Coronary patency at various time points after streptokinase thrombolysis*

Time	Patency (%)
Pretreatment	15–20
1 hr	48–52
90 min	43–64
2–3 hr	60–73
24 hr	75–88
⩾3 days	70–90

*Patency was usually defined as incomplete + complete reperfusion. See text for references.

60 to 84 percent [104, 123, 124] and it rises to over 85 percent at 24 hours [119, 122]. When examined later, usually predischarge, patients have coronary patency of 70 to 80 percent [118, 125].

Various studies have performed coronary angiography at different time points; most of them did not have pretreatment angiograms and were therefore examining patency, not reperfusion. Reported patency rates with intravenous SK have varied widely, from as low as 10 to 30 percent [54, 55] to more than 90 percent [126].

In the GUSTO-1 angiographic substudy [111], patency was assessed at 90 and 180 minutes, again at 24 hours, and 5 to 7 days after treatment, allowing appreciation of the time course of reperfusion. In the 120 patients randomized to intravenous SK combined with intravenous heparin, complete reperfusion was achieved in 32 percent and 43 percent of patients at 90 and 180 minutes, respectively. Partial or complete reperfusion (TIMI flow grade 2 or 3), which is the traditionally defined patency, was obtained in 61 percent, 76 percent, and 86 percent of cases at 90 minutes, 180 minutes, and 5 to 7 days, respectively.

Thus, after thrombolysis, reperfusion progresses over a few hours. Patency increases from about 45 to 60 percent at 90 minutes to 70 to 80 percent at three hours, and 80 to 90 percent a few days later.

Effects on Left Ventricular Function

Early reperfusion results in a reduction in the extent of myocardial necrosis as assessed by electrocardiographic [50, 127–129], enzymatic [130–132], scintigraphic [130, 132–138], functional [50,139–144], and metabolic [145, 146] criteria (Fig. 25-3). When assessing the impact of reperfusion on ventricular function, it is important to distinguish between global ventricular function and regional function in the reperfused zone [147]. Because global ventricular function reflects the additive contributions of both the nonischemic and ischemic zones of the myocardium, its recovery may be an insensitive index of myocardial salvage. This is especially true if, before reperfusion, the hypofunction of the ischemic zone was compensated by hyperkinesia in the nonischemic myocardium which, after functional recovery of the salvaged myocardium, subsequently regresses to normal function and thereby neutralizes any measurable gain in global function. This phenomenon may also explain why improvement in global function after reperfusion is more apparent in patients with extensive initial involvement [148, 149], in whom the nonischemic zone is relatively small, and the impact of the early compensatory hyperkinesis and its subsequent regression is relatively minor. Furthermore, because contractile dysfunction of the salvaged and viable myocardium (stunning) may continue for up to several weeks after reperfusion [150], an improvement in ventricular function may not be apparent during the patient's hospital stay [151]. This reflects the time required for the recovery of severely damaged myocardium. It is important to note, however, that this viable but stunned myocardium is responsive to inotropic stimulation immediately after reperfusion [152–154], which may explain why hemodynamically compromised patients who are initially refrac-

Fig. 25-3

Electrocardiographic (*A*), thallium-201 scintigraphic (*B*), and radionuclide ventricular functional (*C*) evidence of myocardial salvage following reperfusion of the left main coronary artery by intravenous streptokinase. *A.* Serial 12-lead electrocardiograms demonstrating rapid resolution of marked anterior ST segment elevations and right bundle branch block without evolution of pathologic Q waves. *B.* Serial thallium-201 scintigrams showing an extensive perfusion defect involving the anterior (Ant), apical (Ap), septal (Sept), and posterolateral (Pl) walls of the left ventricle on day 1. Only posterolateral and apical perfusion defects are present by day 10, with marked improvement of anterior and septal isotope uptake. *C.* Serial technetium 99m radionuclide wall motion studies in the left anterior oblique 45-degree projection showing a dilated and poorly functioning left ventricle with regional ventricular septal, inferoapical, and posterolateral wall motion abnormalities on day 1 that significantly improved by day 10. (From A. S. Lew et al. Extensive myocardial salvage and reversal of cardiogenic shock following reperfusion of the left main coronary artery by intravenous streptokinase. *Am. J. Cardiol.* 54:451, 1984. With permission.)

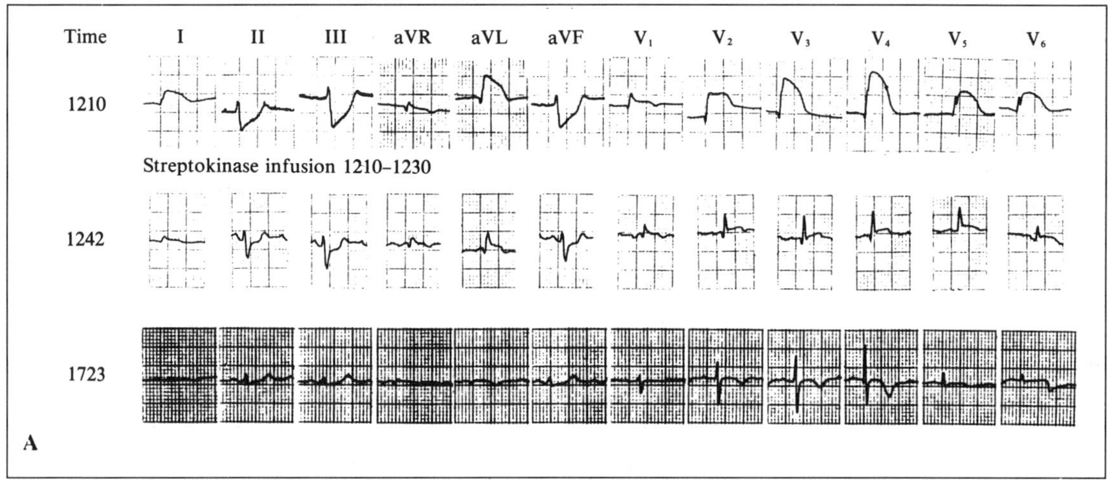
Time
I
II
III
aVR
aVL
aVF
V1
V2
V3
V4
V5
V6
1210
Streptokinase infusion 1210–1230
1242
1723
A

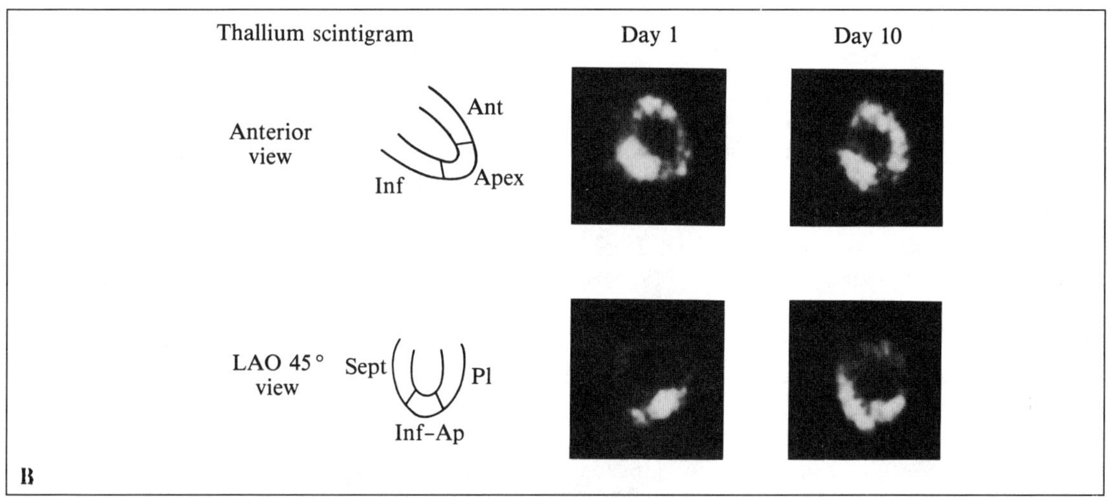
Thallium scintigram
Day 1
Day 10
Anterior view
Ant
Inf
Apex
LAO 45° view
Sept
Pl
Inf–Ap
B

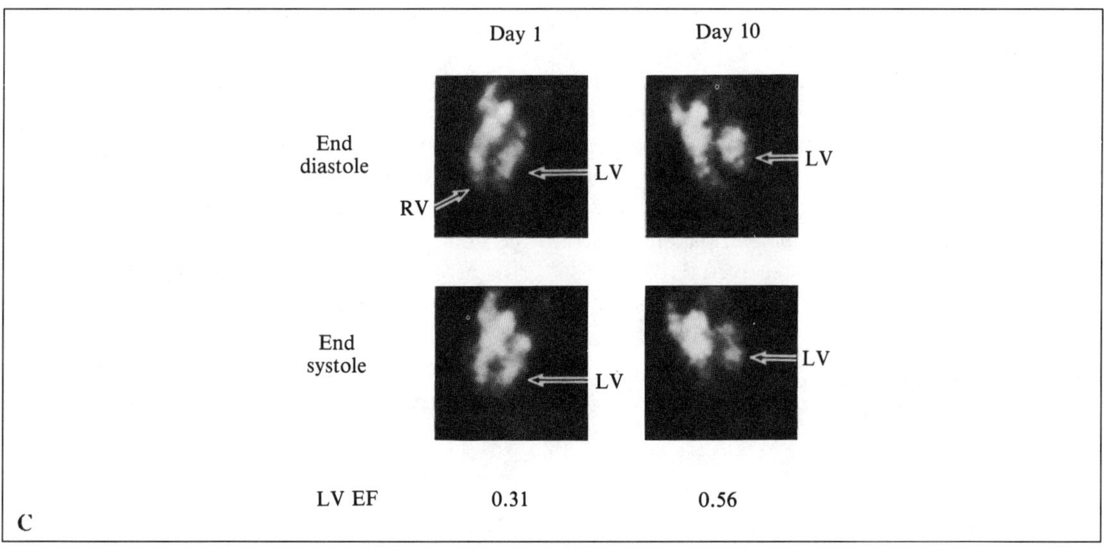
Day 1
Day 10
End diastole
RV
LV
LV
End systole
LV
LV
LV EF
0.31
0.56
C

tory to inotropic agents frequently become responsive to them after reperfusion. This property has important implications for the effective management of patients with cardiac failure or cardiogenic shock.

Because left ventricular (LV) function is a key prognostic marker in survivors of myocardial infarction [155], and myocardial salvage is the assumed mechanism of the benefit of thrombolysis, and since ventricular function is an easily measured continuous variable, multiple studies have tested the outcome of thrombolysis by measuring residual ventricular function as a surrogate measure of survival. Intracoronary SK improved ventricular function in two randomized, placebo-controlled studies [50, 140]. Other studies failed to confirm these observations [156, 157], but small sample sizes or long time delays to treatment may have obscured the effect of treatment. Significantly, the Western Washington intracoronary study [156] found a reduction in mortality but no improvement in ventricular function (see below). Intravenous thrombolysis has been shown to improve residual ventricular function as compared to control by about 2 to 7 percent in a number of randomized trials [117, 118, 158, 159]. Improved ventricular systolic function has also been reported in patients who received treatment late or in whom early reperfusion failed, especially in well-collateralized infarcts [160, 161]. In addition, thrombolytic therapy is associated with less ventricular dilatation and remodeling [162].

Of note, in most studies before the GUSTO-1 trial, either ventricular function or survival, but not both, were significantly improved by thrombolysis [163]. In GUSTO-1 LV function (ejection fraction) was significantly higher in survivors than in nonsurvivors. The difficulties inherent in using global ventricular function as a surrogate measure for survival, missing value in patients who died, and possibly missing poor ventricular function in patients who would have died had they not received thrombolysis, may explain the discrepancy in earlier trials.

Effects on Mortality and Mechanisms of Mortality Reduction

Short-Term Benefit

Two controlled studies of intracoronary SK were able to show improved survival with treatment [156, 164]. A trend toward reduced mortality with intravenous SK was also observed in the Intravenous Streptokinase in Acute Myocardial Infarction (ISAM) and Western Washington studies [118, 158].

The full potential of thrombolysis was widely recognized, however, with the results of two landmark studies of intravenous SK. Gruppo Italiano per lo Studio della Streptokinasi nell'Infarto Miocardico (GISSI-I) was conducted in 176 intensive care units in Italy and randomized 11,806 patients to SK (1.5 million units over 1 hour) or conventional treatment [165]. Hospital mortality was reduced by SK from 13 percent to 10.7 percent, an 18 percent difference that was highly significant. The benefit of treatment diminished with the delay from symptoms to initiation of treatment. ISIS-2, conducted in Europe, Australia, New Zealand, and North America, randomized 17,187 patients with suspected AMI to receive SK (by GISSI protocol) or placebo [69]. In addition, each patient was randomized to receive either enteric-coated aspirin, 160 mg/day, or placebo, thus creating four treatment arms. SK reduced 5-week mortality from 12 percent to 9.2 percent, a 25 percent reduction that was highly significant. Aspirin alone was almost equally effective. The combination of SK and aspirin was additive: patients who received both agents had a 42 percent lower mortality as compared to those who received neither (8 percent versus 13.2 percent). Benefit was highest for patients treated early, but patients treated up to 24 hours after symptom onset had lower mortality. Aspirin reduced the incidence of reinfarction; its beneficial effect was not dependent on the time delay to treatment. Both studies reported an increased mortality with SK during the first 24 hours of treatment, a trend that was later reversed. This early hazard of thrombolytic therapy was mainly attributed to an increased risk of rupture in patients receiving therapy late in the course of evolving AMI and to an increased risk of death from cardiogenic shock during the first day after treatment. A much smaller study from New Zealand confirmed a reduction of mortality and improved ventricular function by SK in patients with a first myocardial infarction (MI) [117].

Long-Term Results

The benefit of thrombolysis is conferred during the hospital phase and maintained thereafter. A number of studies found that the salutary effects of thrombolysis are sustained for at least 1 year. In GISSI-I and ISIS-2 [69, 166] 1-year mortality was reduced by SK by 9.5 percent and 20 percent, respectively. Five-year follow-up of 618 patients from the Western Washington intracoronary and intravenous studies suggests that after this period there is no longer a benefit to patients who were randomized to SK. There was a trend towards improved long-term survival in patients with anterior infarcts [167]. Similar follow-up of 533 patients studied by the Interuniversity Cardiology Institute of the Netherlands found that the benefit of thrombolysis was maintained for up to 5 years; survival after thrombolysis and conventional treatment was 81 percent and 71 percent, respectively. Following thrombolysis there were more cases of reinfarction and coronary intervention [168].

The main mechanism for the mortality reduction achieved by SK is believed to be reduced infarct size and preserved LV function, brought about by timely restoration of blood flow to the ischemic territory. The beneficial effect of a patent infarct artery with brisk flow on LV function and survival was suggested by the Western Washington intracoronary trial and recently confirmed in GUSTO-1 [111]. Thrombolytic therapy has also been associated with better infarct healing and less remodeling and aneurysm formation [169], lower frequency of mural thrombosis [170] and a reduced incidence of ventricular late potentials and inducible ventricular tachycardia [171, 172].

Even when reperfusion does not influence short-term prognosis, it may improve the patient's chance of surviving a subsequent infarction. Physiologic considerations indicate that, in the event that another coronary artery becomes acutely occluded, any patent coronary artery may be a source of collateral perfusion, which reduces the severity of myocardial ischemia and the rapidity of its progression to necrosis [173]. These collaterals may therefore facilitate greater myocardial salvage by reperfusion of the second infarction [174].

Effects of Time Delay to Treatment

As the time-dependency of necrosis in AMI would imply, myocardial salvage is heavily dependent on the time delay to initiation of reperfusion therapy, although in some patients ischemic myocardium supplied by a totally occluded infarct-related artery may remain viable for days to weeks when adequate collateral-mediated perfusion is present [175]. In many instances, this collateral perfusion may be demonstrated by contrast echocardiography but not be visible by angiography [175]. In addition to the time-dependency of myocardial salvage, older clots are probably more difficult to lyse [45]. Patency [111], residual ventricular function [142], and survival [111, 165] have all been shown to be inversely correlated to the time between onset of symptoms and treatment. Treatment initiated within the first hour is associated with particularly good results [69, 176]. In Gruppo Italiano per lo Studio della Streptokinasi nell'Infarto Miocardico II (GISSI-2) [177], the combined endpoint of mortality and severe ventricular damage was observed in 18 percent, 21.5 percent, and 25.1 percent of patients treated within 1, 3, and over 3 hours, respectively. In GUSTO-1 [111] there was a clear gradient of mortality according to the time delay to treatment: 5.4 percent in patients treated within 2 hours, as opposed to 8.3 percent in those treated after more than 6 hours.

Data from ISIS-2 [69] and other studies suggest that late thrombolysis, while still reducing overall mortality, is associated with an increased risk of cardiac rupture [178]. The causes for this association have not been investigated; a possible reason is that subacute rupture may already have taken place in some patients who present many hours after the onset of symptoms (explaining their prolonged pain), and fatal tamponade may then be facilitated by thrombolysis. Other mechanisms may include breakdown of collagen matrix due to plasmin-induced activation of latent interstitial collagenase.

Complications of Streptokinase

An understanding of the risks of thrombolytic therapy is essential for its safe utilization (Table 25-3).

Table 25-3
Major complications of streptokinase thrombolysis

Complication	Streptokinase (% of patients)	Control (% of patients)
Major bleeding	0.6–1	0.2
Intracranial bleeding	0.2–0.5	0.15
Stroke	0.7–1	0.7–1

Bleeding

Hemorrhagic complications are the primary cause of significant morbidity and mortality attributable to thrombolytic therapy [39, 47, 48, 69, 114, 179]. Bleeding results from either (1) lysis of hemostatic thrombi at the site of previous trauma or tissue injury or (2) prevention of adequate clot formation by the hypocoagulable state resulting from fibrinogen depletion, release of degradation products, and the conjunctive use of antiplatelet and anticoagulant drugs. In large series, noncerebral bleeding was reported in 4 to 6 percent of patients, and transfusions were required in about 1 percent [98, 177, 180]. Risk of bleeding increases with age [98, 177, 180] and appears to be higher in women [181], in patients who have invasive procedures [182], and with the conjunctive use of heparin [98, 177, 180]. However, as thrombolysis still reduces infarct size and mortality in such patients, these characteristics do not contraindicate its use but call for closer monitoring.

The most common site of severe bleeding is the puncture site in the femoral artery used for coronary angiography. The factors that predispose to bleeding from this site include repeated attempts at vascular access, puncture of the posterior wall of the femoral artery, and inadequate attention to post-procedure hemostasis, which, after thrombolytic therapy, may require prolonged groin pressure or clamping for up to 4 to 6 hours. Repeated venipuncture is another common cause of minor (or sometimes severe) bleeding. Whenever possible, vascular access lines are maintained until there is recovery of depleted coagulation factors (approximately 24 hours) and until the dissipation of fibrinolytic effects (about 12 to 24 hours for SK or urokinase but less than 1 hour for rt-PA). When a patient who has received thrombolysis requires catheterization of a central vein for hemodynamic monitoring or pacing, the femoral approach or antecubital cutdown should be utilized instead of attempts at jugular or subclavian vein cannulation.

A guide to the management of bleeding complications is presented in Table 25-4. The use of topical thrombin and cryoprecipitate can assist in hemostasis [183], but, as with all blood products, their use should be restricted to refractory bleeding. It is of note that, even for severe bleeding, antifibrinolytic agents such as epsilonaminocaproic acid are usually not indicated if bleeding occurs after the fibrinolytic effects of the drug have dissipated [184]. For early and severe bleeding, currently available antifibrinolytic agents may be useful but should be considered a second-line approach because they are only partially effective and the bleeding is more likely to respond to withdrawal of anticoagulant therapy and repletion of coagulation factors. In the future, monoclonal antibodies that specifically inhibit the circulating plasminogen activators may provide a tool for controlling severe hemorrhage.

Table 25-4
Management of hemorrhagic complications

Minor complications
1. Secure local hemostasis; apply pressure dressings; apply topical thrombin powder or topical cryoprecipitate/thrombin glue.*
2. Discontinue anticoagulation if bleeding cannot be controlled.

Moderate complications
1. As above.
2. Discontinue anticoagulation.
3. Reverse anticoagulation if bleeding not controlled; give protamine sulfate for heparin or fresh frozen plasma for coumadin.

Severe complications
1–3. As above.
4. If fibrinogen <100 mg/dl, administer 5–10 units of cryoprecipitate.
5. Transfuse blood as required.
6. Consider epsilonaminocaproic acid.*
7. Consider surgical control of bleeding site.

*See Complications section in text.

Cardiopulmonary resuscitation, unless prolonged or traumatic, should not preclude the use of thrombolysis, particularly in high-risk patients. Spontaneous hemorrhagic tamponade has been reported following thrombolysis and can be managed conservatively by pericardiocentesis [185]. This complication should be differentiated from myocardial rupture with subsequent hemopericardium, which calls for immediate surgery.

Stroke

The most dreaded complication of thrombolytic therapy is intracranial hemorrhage, which fortunately occurs infrequently with SK, with an overall incidence of about 0.2 to 0.5 percent [69, 111, 186].

In GISSI-2 and the associated international study, the risk of intracranial hemorrhage was increased in women and in patients with a diastolic blood pressure over 110 mm Hg at entry but not by older age, history of hypertension, elevated systolic blood pressure at entry, or diabetes [186]. Severe diastolic hypertension may thus pose an increased risk of intracranial bleeding from thrombolytic therapy. A recent (6 months) nonhemorrhagic stroke or any previous intracranial hemorrhage should be an absolute contraindication for thrombolysis.

While the risk of intracranial bleeding is increased by thrombolysis, the overall risk of stroke is not, reflecting a decreased rate of ischemic and embolic strokes with treatment [69, 165]. The risk of any stroke is about 1 percent; it increases with age, anterior infarction, a higher Killip class, diastolic hypertension on entry, and female sex, but not with body mass index, a history of hypertension, diabetes, or smoking [186].

Hypotension

SK may cause hypotension through multiple mechanisms, including bradykinin release and complement activation [105]. The excess hypotension attributed to SK in the ISIS-2 study was 7.9 percent [69]. SK-associated hypotension is best managed with slowing or stopping the infusion, leg raising, and intravenous fluids. Pressors are rarely necessary. When hypotension has resolved, the infusion can usually be resumed without recurrence [105]. This direct effect of SK should be differentiated from the hypotension and bradycardia that occasionally follow reperfusion of the right coronary artery (through the Bezold-Jarisch reflex) and may require administration of atropine, fluids, or vasopressors.

Peripheral Embolization

Thrombolytic therapy has generally been considered to be contraindicated in the presence of a known or strongly suspected chronic left heart thrombus and in patients with infective endocarditis because of the potential for systemic embolization. Fresh mural LV thrombi in the setting of AMI have been effectively lysed by thrombolytic therapy with a low risk of embolization [187]. However, since embolization from such thrombi has been reported after thrombolysis [188], alternative means of reperfusion should be considered in patients with known mural thrombi.

Hepatocellular Disturbance

A mild, reversible hepatocellular disturbance has been associated with SK, but not with t-PA, thrombolysis. No sequelae have been seen [189].

Cholesterol Embolism Syndrome

The syndrome of cholesterol embolism has been described in a few cases following SK thrombolysis [190]. The mechanism probably involves dislodgment and peripheral embolization of cholesterol that contains mural clots in the aorta.

Risk of Reocclusion and Reinfarction

Following successful thrombolysis, a significant residual stenosis of the infarct-related artery and an unlysed mural thrombus usually remain (Fig. 25-4), predisposing to thrombotic reocclusion. Reocclusion occurs most frequently within the first 72 hours and may remain clinically silent in nearly half the patients [191]. Reinfarction has been reported in 2.8 to 4 percent of patients receiving SK [69, 158, 165]; in ISIS-2, aspirin reduced this risk from 4 percent to 2 percent [69]. The right coronary artery appears to be more prone to reocclusion, as are arteries with incomplete reperfusion [191] (see Fig. 25-4). Reocclusion has been associated with biochemical signs of ongoing thrombin-mediated procoagulant activity [80] and, particularly in the case of t-PA, with inadequate concurrent anticoagulation [192] or transient failure of heparinization. Strict heparin anticoagulation may not be as critical in the presence of aspirin.

The risk of reocclusion is not limited to the hospital phase. Recent data from the Antithrombotics in the Prevention of Reocclusion in Coronary Thrombolysis (APRICOT) trial indicate that 30 percent of infarct-related arteries that are patent early after thrombolysis are found occluded when studied 3 months later. Only a small minority of these patients have clinical reinfarction [193]. Although

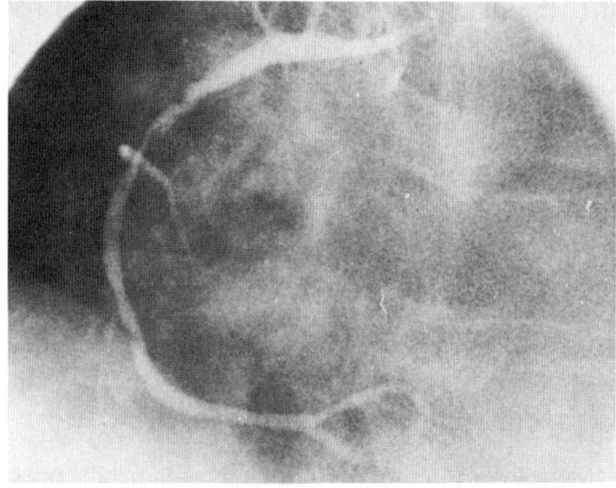

A

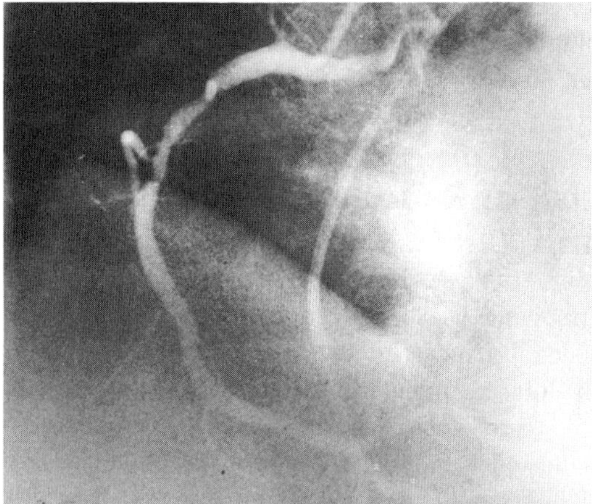

B

Fig. 25-4
Serial selective right coronary angiograms from a patient with inferior acute myocardial infarction at (*A*) 2 hours and (*B*) 24 hours after treatment with intravenous tissue plasminogen activator. Note the early postreperfusion tight residual stenosis of the right coronary artery proximal to the right ventricular branch with a superimposed intraluminal thrombus (*A*) that has markedly improved by 24 hours following additional intravenous rt-PA and anticoagulation with heparin (*B*).

reocclusion may be clinically silent, it often leads to a distinctly worse outcome with reduced regional and global ventricular function and an increased risk of heart failure and death [191, 194].

The risk of recurrent ischemia and reinfarction can be decreased by aspirin and by intravenous metoprolol given immediately [195]. In GUSTO-1 [111] intravenous heparin reduced the risk of reocclusion from 7.7 percent (with subcutaneous heparin) to 5.8 percent. These adjunctive measures are further discussed below.

The treatment of reinfarction following initially successful thrombolysis is aimed at rapid re-establishment of sustained coronary patency. When the clinical presentation is similar to the patient's original one, that is, with chest pain and ST segment elevation in the same leads, complete thrombotic reocclusion is likely. The available therapeutic options are repeat thrombolysis and emergency ("rescue") coronary angioplasty. Barbash and colleagues administered t-PA to 52 patients who had acute reocclusion [196]. Resolution of symptoms was achieved in 85 percent of patients; in 44 percent of them no further intervention was necessary. The risk of bleeding was not excessive. Due to its antigenicity, SK should not be readministered, and alternative agents should be chosen. Since no objective data exist to compare readministration of thrombolytics to mechanical revascularization in this context, the decision should be individualized according to the patient's characteristics and the availability of a coronary intervention team.

Comparison of Streptokinase with Other Agents

Besides SK, the main thrombolytic agents currently in use are t-PA, anistreplase (APSAC), and urokinase. Table 25-5 provides a comparative profile of these agents. As shown first in TIMI-I [116], t-PA achieves coronary recanalization faster than SK. In that study, 90-minute patency was 62 percent with t-PA but 31 percent with SK. Patency with t-PA was improved further by "front-loaded" (i.e., rapid) administration [197]. Following these observations, large clinical trials were launched to compare the various thrombolytic agents. GISSI-2 and its associated international study [177, 180] randomized over 20,000 patients by a 2 × 2 factorial design to either SK or t-PA and to either subcutaneous heparin or no heparin. ISIS-3 [98] was similarly designed but an arm of anistreplase was added and over 41,000 patients were randomized. In both studies, aspirin was given routinely to all patients. The results of these "mega-trials" were similar. When combined, mortality was identical (10 percent) with t-PA or with SK and mortality with anistreplase was also not statistically different. There was a

Table 25-5
Clinical comparison of intravenous thrombolytic agents

	Streptokinase (% of patients)	Alteplase (t-PA) (% of patients)	Anistreplase (APSAC) (% of patients)	Urokinase (% of patients)
Hypotension	11.8	7.1	12.5	10.7
Intracranial bleeding	0.24	0.66	0.55	
90-minute patency	43–74	52–77 (81–91*)	55–100	53–66
2–3 hour patency	60–73	65–80	72–77	65–82
24-hour patency	75–88	78–85 (85–92*)	68–93	65–82
Reinfarction	4	2–6	3.5	7–13 reocclusion
Increased ventricular function	+	+	+	+
↑ Survival	18–25	26–51	34–50	
Cost/dose	$407	$2600	$2061	$4140
Dose	1.5 million U/1 hr	1.25 mg/kg, up to 100 mg/ 90 min	30-U bolus/ 5 min	3 million U/1 hr

+ = yes, ↑ = improved; APSAC = acylated/anisoylated plasminogen streptokinase activator complex; t-PA = tissue plasminogen activator.
*Results with "front-loaded" (rapid) t-PA.

significant excess of hemorrhagic strokes with t-PA as compared to SK (0.66 percent versus 0.24 percent, respectively) and the risk of any stroke was also increased (1.35 percent with t-PA versus 1 percent with SK). Patients allocated to t-PA had a lower reinfarction rate. An important shortcoming of these large trials was their utilization of subcutaneous rather than intravenous heparin, which could have limited the effectiveness of t-PA more than that of SK.

The GUSTO-1 trial [111] randomized 41,021 patients into four treatment arms: front-loaded t-PA, SK with subcutaneous heparin, SK with intravenous heparin, and a combination of SK and t-PA. t-PA was always administered with intravenous heparin. Table 25-6 summarizes some of the results of this trial. Preliminary results indicate that 30-day mortality was 6.3 percent for t-PA, 7.2 percent for SK with subcutaneous heparin, and 7.4 percent for SK with intravenous heparin. When the excess strokes associated with t-PA were taken into account, there was a net benefit of nine lives saved per 1000 patients treated with t-PA as compared to SK. As expected, patency of the infarct-related artery at 90 minutes was higher with t-PA than with SK with intravenous heparin (complete reperfusion achieved in 54 percent and 32 percent, respectively), but this difference disappeared by 180 minutes (42 percent versus 43 percent, respectively). These initial results seem to confirm the hypothesis, previously questioned by results of GISSI-2 and ISIS-3, that more rapid coronary recanalization does indeed translate into improved myocardial salvage and reduced mortality. The difference between t-PA and SK, while statistically significant, was, however, very small (Table 25-7). Furthermore, in patients treated after 4 hours and those over age 75, there was no significant difference in mortality between t-PA-treated and SK-treated patients. Thus, for these subsets of patients, the less expensive drug SK may be appropriate.

Role of Adjunctive Therapies

Antiplatelets: Aspirin

Since ISIS-2 demonstrated the marked synergistic effect aspirin has with SK, it has become routine clinical practice to administer aspirin in conjunction with thrombolysis [69, 198]. To facilitate rapid onset of action, a loading dose of 325 mg is recommended on admission, after which the dose may be reduced to 80 mg/day and continued indefinitely.

Table 25-6
Comparison of SK to t-PA from GUSTO-1 trial results*

	SK with SC heparin	SK with IV heparin	t-PA	t-PA with SK	p pooled value of SK vs. t-PA
No. of patients	9841	10,410	10,396	10,374	
Previous AMI	16	17	17	16	
Time to treatment (hr)	2.7	2.8	2.8	2.8	
24-hr mortality	2.8	2.9	2.3	2.8	0.005
30-day mortality	7.2	7.4	6.3	7	0.001
30-day mortality or nonfatal stroke	7.9	8.2	7.2	7.9	0.006
Cardiogenic shock	6.9	6.3	5.1	6.1	<0.001
Reinfarction	3.4	4	4	4	NS
Recurrent ischemia	19.9	19.6	19	18.8	NS
Total stroke	1.22	1.4	1.55	1.64	0.09
Hemorrhagic stroke	0.49	0.54	0.72	0.94	0.03
Moderate or severe bleeding	5.8	6.3	5.4	6.1	0.04

AMI = acute myocardial infarction; IV = intravenous; NS = not significant; SC = subcutaneous; SK = streptokinase; t-PA = tissue plasminogen activator.
*All values are percentages, unless otherwise indicated.

Table 25-7
Analysis of mortality comparing SK to t-PA from GUSTO-1 trial subgroup results

	SK (% mortality)	t-PA (% mortality)	Significance (p)
Age ≤75 yr	5.5	4.4	<0.001
Age >75 yr	20.6	19.3	NS
Death or nonfatal stroke, age ≤75 yr	6	5	0.001
Death or nonfatal stroke, age >75 yr	21.5	20.2	0.38
Treatment within 0–2 hrs	5.4	4.3	
Treatment within 2–4 hr	6.7	5.5	
Treatment within 4–6 hr	9.3	8.9	
Treatment beyond 6 hr	8.3	10.4	

NS = not significant; SK = streptokinase; t-PA = tissue plasminogen activator.

The antiplatelet effect of aspirin may contribute to maintenance of coronary patency by blocking ongoing platelet aggregation and rethrombosis.

Anticoagulants: Heparin

Experimental evidence suggests that pretreatment with a bolus of heparin may potentiate the efficacy of thrombolysis by inhibiting ongoing fibrin incorporation by the thrombus [84]. There is also considerable clinical evidence that although heparin does not improve acute recanalization, it does enhance late (> 18 hours) coronary patency [199]; this is especially true when agents that have little systemic effect, such as t-PA, are used. Fibrinogen depletion and production of fibrin split products may have a favorable effect on ultimate patency. There is, however, little data on the effect of heparin on SK thrombolysis. One small randomized trial found that high-dose heparin, when started prior to SK, was associated with more rapid recanalization as compared to placebo [200]. In two large randomized controlled trials [98, 180] involving over 60,000 patients, there was either no benefit or only a temporary benefit on reinfarction rate, mortality rate, or both when subcutaneous heparin was added to aspirin and thrombolytic therapy, regardless of whether heparin was initiated within 4 hours [98] or 12 hours [180] of the onset of thrombolytic therapy. In the GISSI-2 trial [177], the incidence of death and severe LV damage was similar (22.7 percent with heparin versus 22.9 percent without heparin) as was the rate of reinfarction and recurrent ischemia. In the international t-PA versus SK trial [180] there was again no difference in mortality with heparin (8.5 percent) compared to no heparin (8.9 percent). In the ISIS-3 trial, in which t-PA, SK, and APSAC were compared, patients were also randomized to subcutaneous high-dose heparin or no heparin [98]. Most patients received aspirin; 80 percent of patients allocated to heparin, as well as 17 percent of patients not allocated to it, actually received heparin. Once again there was no difference in the 5-week mortality (10.3 percent with heparin versus 10.6 percent without it) or reinfarction, although during the 7 days of heparin use there was a slight favorable trend toward lower mortality (7.4 percent versus 7.9 percent; $p = .06$) and reinfarction rates (3.2 percent versus 3.5 percent; $p = .09$) with heparin. In GUSTO-1 [111], intravenous heparin was directly compared to subcutaneous heparin as an adjunct to SK thrombolysis. Preliminary data from this trial suggest that 30-day mortality is actually somewhat higher in patients randomized to intravenous, as compared to subcutaneous, heparin following SK (7.4 percent versus 7.2 percent, respectively). The reocclusion rate was lower with intravenous heparin (5.6 percent versus 7.7 percent with subcutaneous heparin) but this benefit was offset by a higher rate of severe bleeding (0.5 percent versus 0.3 percent).

It may be concluded that subcutaneous heparin should not be used routinely following SK thrombolysis; the value of intravenous heparin is questionable, and final judgment will have to be deferred until full results of GUSTO-1 are available. Heparin remains important for those patients at high risk for systemic or pulmonary embolization, i.e., those with heart failure, large anterior infarcts, prolonged bed rest, or atrial fibrillation. It is emphasized that intravenous heparin should be routinely used in conjunction with t-PA, as well as in patients receiving SK who cannot receive aspirin.

If the decision is made to use intravenous heparin, a bolus loading dose of 5000 units should be given, followed by a continuous drip of 10 IU/kg/h; one should aim to maintain the activated partial thromboplastin time (APTT) at about 70 to 80 seconds. Because individual responses are highly variable, frequent monitoring of the APTT is critical until its level is stable. For several hours after the bolus, anticoagulation can usually be maintained with about 10 IU/kg/hr; but as the effects of the bolus dissipate (4 to 6 hours) and as clotting factors recover and fibrin(ogen) degradation products are cleared from the circulation, the heparin requirements usually increase to about 12 to 15 IU/kg/hr. Heparin requirements after thrombolysis are increased; with the standard dose regimen, 52 percent of all patients and 62 percent of patients weighing less than 80 kg have an APTT below 60 seconds at 24 hours. Patients who weigh over 80 kg, males, and younger patients require larger doses [201]. Because reperfusion may be delayed, heparin should not be withheld on the basis of presumed failure and should not be interrupted prior to angiography, percutaneous transluminal coronary angioplasty (PTCA), or CABG (Table 25-8). When thrombolysis has failed, prolonged anticoagulation may facilitate delayed spontaneous recanalization.

Table 25-8
Anticoagulation*

1. Pretreatment bolus of heparin, 5000 U, IV.
2. Posttreatment heparin infusion at 10–15 U/kg/hr, IV. Do not reduce heparin dose in the first 24 hours on the basis of APTT alone; thereafter adjust heparin dose to maintain the APTT at 60–80 seconds.
3. Heparin requirements may increase during initial 24–48 hours.
4. Heparin is not discontinued prior to coronary angiography, PTCA, or CABG.
5. Heparin is discontinued at 24–72 hours if the course is uncomplicated.

APTT = activated partial thromboplastin time; CABG = coronary artery bypass surgery; IV = intravenous; PTCA = percutaneous transluminal coronary angioplasty.
*The additive benefit of intravenous heparin in patients receiving aspirin in conjunction with streptokinase is unproven (see text).

New Antiplatelet and Antithrombotic Agents

Despite the use of heparin and aspirin, thrombolytic therapy is associated with a failure rate of 15 to 25 percent and a reocclusion rate of 5 to 10 percent [82]. Furthermore, reperfusion with SK is slow, taking an average of 72 minutes [82]. These problems may stem from the paradoxic prothrombotic state that occurs during lytic therapy [82]. Therefore, the search for more effective lytic agents and antithrombotic drugs continues.

Newer antiplatelet agents, some of which antagonize the platelet IIb/IIIA receptor, are being studied as adjuncts to thrombolysis and encouraging preliminary results are available [76].

Unlike heparin, new direct antithrombins such as hirudin, hirulog, and other synthetic agents that effectively inhibit circulating as well as vessel-wall and clot-bound thrombin, are not inhibited by endogenous inhibitors and appear to be significantly more effective as adjuncts to thrombolysis, both in the experimental models [202] and in preliminary clinical trials. Despite this, the risk of bleeding complications appears to be less with these agents than with heparin [203]. Current clinical studies (TIMI-9, GUSTO-2) will fully define the role of these new agents and establish their efficacy and risk-benefit profiles in various acute ischemic syndromes.

Practical Considerations in the Use of Streptokinase in Acute Myocardial Infarction

Patient Suitability and Strategies to Minimize Delay of Treatment

The salutary effects of SK on infarct size and mortality in evolving Q-wave AMI are observed regardless of gender, age, or infarct location and in patients with left bundle branch block (Table 25-9) [69, 117, 165, 204]. In general, the earlier the therapy is initiated and the higher the mortality risk

Table 25-9
Indications and contraindications for thrombolysis

Indications
- AMI manifested by appropriate symptoms and/or ST segment elevation of ≥0.1 mV in at least two electrocardiographically contiguous leads or a left bundle branch block, up to 12 hours after symptom onset. Patients with symptoms compatible with an AMI and precordial ST segment depression with upright T waves may be considered for inclusion as well, as such ST depression may be a mirror image of posterior ST segment elevation.

Contraindications
- Absolute
  1. Active bleeding or serious internal bleeding within preceding 3 months
  2. Known bleeding tendency
  3. Intracranial neoplasm or AV malformation; recent (3–6 months) serious head or spinal trauma surgery
  4. Any history of cerebral hemorrhage; history of nonhemorrhagic stroke in the preceding 6 months
  5. Proliferative diabetic retinopathy
  6. Pericarditis
  7. Aortic dissection or known aortic aneurysm
  8. Recent noncompressible vascular puncture
  9. Pregnancy
  10. Infective endocarditis
- Relative
  1. Uncontrolled hypertension (diastolic pressure >110 mm Hg)
  2. Active peptic disease
  3. Advanced liver or renal disease
  4. Recent major surgery or organ biopsy (within preceding 2–6 weeks)
  5. Prolonged and traumatic CPR
  6. Disseminated cancer
  7. Known or strongly suspected chronic left heart thrombus
  8. Previous administration of streptokinase or anistreplase within 5 days to 4 years (choose alternative agent)

AMI = acute myocardial infarctions; AV = atrioventricular; CPR = cardiopulmonary resuscitation.

associated with the evolving infarct, the larger the potential benefit [69, 165]. Therefore, patients treated within 1 hour of the onset of symptoms and those with anterior MI, left bundle branch block, or higher Killip class (except for patients in cardiogenic shock) derive more benefit from treatment. Similarly, while advanced age was previously considered a contraindication to thrombolysis, the absolute benefit from treatment in the elderly (> 70 years) is actually even larger than in younger patients because of higher baseline mortality. In ISIS-2, thrombolysis in conjunction with aspirin reduced mortality among patients 80 years of age or older from 37 to 20 percent. In an analysis of available data, Krumholz et al. recently showed that thrombolysis is beneficial and cost effective in patients 75 years of age or older [205].

Patients with isolated ST segment depression (except when reflecting a posterior infarction) or a normal electrocardiogram do not appear to benefit from thrombolysis; thrombolysis has generally been less successful in cardiogenic shock [48, 165], probably because the low-flow state may not only facilitate further thrombosis but may also limit the delivery of lytic agent to the thrombus [206].

Because all patients in whom an AMI is still evolving may benefit from limitation of the extent of necrosis by reperfusion, there are three considerations for patient selection from intravenous thrombolytic therapy: (1) the presence of reversibly ischemic myocardium; (2) the risk of complications, primarily hemorrhagic, from the thrombolytic and anticoagulant therapy, and (3) the availability and relative suitability of alternative methods of reperfusion, such as primary coronary angioplasty.

The clinical assessment of reversibility is based on an estimate of the stage of evolution of the infarction and is clinically best gauged by consideration of the duration of chest pain, its persistence or intermittence, and the acuteness of the electrocardiographic changes. Experimental and clinical data indicate that while early treatment achieves the best results [131, 141, 142, 165], thrombolysis may still produce a worthwhile benefit as late as 12 to 24 hours after onset of symptoms [69], especially in those in whom chest pain, acute electrocardiographic changes, or both suggest ongoing ischemia; often these cases involve a "stuttering" pattern of infarction with cyclic occlusion–reperfusion reflected by intermittent pain and electrocardiographic changes. In the Thrombolysis and Angioplasty in Myocardial Infarction (TAMI-6) trial, patients who arrived 6 to 24 hours after the onset of symptoms were randomized to receive t-PA or placebo. No difference in ventricular function was observed but at 6 months there was significantly less ventricular dilatation in the t-PA group [207]. Gil et al. recently reported that thrombolysis given 6 to 24 hours after onset of symptoms improves ventricular function at 1 month as compared to placebo [208]. Preliminary results from the large Late Assessment of Thrombolytic Efficiency (LATE) study [209], which randomized t-PA or placebo to 5700 patients arriving 6 to 24 hours after thrombolysis, suggest a mortality benefit when patients are treated within 12 hours (but not later) after onset of symptoms. Ventricular function was not improved.

Therefore, we currently recommend thrombolysis within 12 hours after onset of infarction for patients with symptoms, ST segment elevation, or both. However, in a patient with persistent chest pain and ST segment elevation, no arbitrary time limit should preclude thrombolysis, provided alternative diagnoses (especially myocardial rupture and pericarditis) have been excluded. A fully evolved electrocardiographic pattern of infarction probably precludes a significant myocardial salvage from reperfusion; whether thrombolysis at this stage may still benefit the patient through other mechanisms (see below) is controversial.

The critical importance of early initiation of treatment has special implications for the organization of emergency services. AMI is a true medical emergency and every effort should be made to start thrombolytic therapy without delay. Treatment should begin as soon as the diagnosis is made and contraindications and other criteria for exclusion have been considered, whether it be in the office, the patient's home, or the emergency department. Prehospital thrombolysis has been shown to be feasible and safe with proper organization [210, 211]; it may shorten the time to initiation of treatment by more than an hour [212, 213] and results in reduced infarct size as compared to hospital thrombolysis [142]. The European Myocardial Infarction Project (EMIP) trial [213] randomized 5469 patients to either prehospital or hospital thrombolysis. There was a 13 percent reduction in mortality ($p = .08$) and a 16 percent reduction in cardiac mortality (p = .049). Prehospital thrombolysis was associated with an increased risk of ventricular fibrillation and hypotension.

Contraindications to Treatment

Table 25-9 lists indications, as well as absolute and relative contraindications, to thrombolysis. Contraindications are defined to minimize the risks of the previously mentioned potential complications of SK. A relative contraindication should prompt the physician to carefully weigh the threat posed by the evolving infarction against the risk of treatment. Immediate coronary angioplasty, where readily available; should be considered for such patients.

Protocol for Administration of Streptokinase

We currently recommend a standard dose of 1.5 million units of SK over about 1 hour for intravenous administration. In our experience, limiting the rate of infusion of SK to about 400 to 500 IU/kg/min together with frequent monitoring of the blood pressure (e.g., every 1 to 2 minutes using a Dinamap) can minimize this risk. For hemodynamically compromised patients and those with baseline hypotension, slower infusion rates of SK (about 200–250 IU/kg/min) may be in order. Table 25-10 contains our recommended protocol for intravenous thrombolysis.

Nonangiographic Recognition of Reperfusion

The main advantage of the intravenous route of thrombolytic therapy is that it does not require pretreatment coronary angiography and therefore can be initiated earlier. Implicit in this approach is the need for nonangiographic recognition of the endpoint of treatment, i.e., reperfusion.

Table 25-10
Protocol for intravenous thrombolysis

1. When a patient presents with suggestive symptoms, obtain an ECG as soon as possible and another immediately before starting lytic therapy.
2. Consider inclusion criteria and contraindications for thrombolysis and rule out other causes of chest pain, e.g., aortic dissection, pericarditis.
3. Insert two large bore antecubital intravenous lines.
4. Dilute 1,500,000 units of SK in 50 ml of saline or dextrose in water; administer over 1 hour using an infusion pump.
5. Unless contraindicated, administer enteric-coated aspirin, 325 mg, followed by a maintenance dose of 80 mg/day. (If patient is already taking aspirin, continue with 80 mg/day).
6. Consider intravenous heparin. If desired, give bolus loading dose of 3000 units and start a drip of 10 U/kg/hr. Check the APTT at baseline and at 6-hour intervals until stable; adjust the infusion after the first 24 hours to maintain the APTT at 60 to 80 seconds. Do not decrease the dose during the first 24 hours regardless of the APTT, unless there is excessive bleeding. (The role of heparin with SK remains controversial).
7. Consider intravenous metoprolol. If desired, give three doses of 5 mg each over 15 minutes, while monitoring blood pressure and heart rate.
8. Monitor the patient closely for changes in chest pain, blood pressure, cardiac rate, and rhythm. Instruct the patient to report any significant change in symptoms.
9. To recognize reperfusion, evaluate patient's symptoms at 5- to 10-minute intervals and assess changes in ST segment elevation in a lead with distinct or maximum pretreatment ST elevation.
10. Reperfusion is signaled by
    a) Rapid decrease in ST segment elevation along with
    b) Decrease in chest pain.
11. Other manifestations of reperfusion may be
    a) Sudden bradycardia with hypotension (Bezold-Jarisch reflex), mostly with infarctions related to the right coronary artery.
    b) Appearance of AIVR at a regular rate.
    c) Disappearance of AV or intraventricular block or ischemic atrial fibrillation if present prior to initiation of therapy.

AIVR = accelerated idioventricular rhythm; APTT = activated partial thromboplastin time; AV = atrioventricular; ECG = electrocardiogram; SK = streptokinase.

Bedside Signs of Reperfusion

Clinical Evidence of Termination of Ischemia

Termination of myocardial ischemia typically results in rapid abatement of chest pain, which is closely accompanied by resolution of ST segment elevation (Fig. 25-5). Relief of chest pain following reperfusion is readily apparent to both the patient and the physician, even after treatment with narcotic analgesics. The patient usually reports a feeling of well-being and also appears well, becoming more conversive and attentive to the environment. Hemodynamic abnormalities, such as hypotension or pulmonary congestion, may rapidly resolve. There is usually rapid resolution of the electrocardiographic manifestations of ischemia, i.e., ST segment elevation [128, 129, 214, 215] (and, occasionally, arrhythmias and conduction abnormalities) followed by rapid evolution of the signs of infarction commensurate with the extent of necrosis that had evolved prior to reperfusion [126, 216, 217]. Frequently, the abatement of chest pain is preceded by a period of fluctuating pain and a cyclic pattern of oscillating ST segment consistent with the intermittency of patency observed angiographically. Paradoxically, many patients manifest a sudden but transient worsening of both chest pain and ST segment elevation at the moment of reperfusion [218, 219] (Fig. 25-6); the pathogenesis of these findings is not known. Patients who have sustained no or minimal necrosis may not develop pathologic Q waves. Nonangiographic, bedside recognition of reperfusion requires close clinical monitoring of the patient. Reperfusion is accompanied by a rapid, progressive decrease of pain intensity within about 30 minutes of the onset of its abatement [217]. Resolution of ST segment elevation is assessed by continuous monitoring of the ST segment in the lead which best reflects the ST segment elevation. We define resolution of ST segment elevation as its progressive decrease within 40 minutes to less than 50 percent of its maximally elevated value. This rapid resolution of chest pain and ST segment elevation represents TIMI grade 3 reperfusion [217].

When recent atrioventricular or intraventricular conduction block is present at the outset, it often disappears shortly after reperfusion [220]. On the other hand, vagally mediated sinus bradycardia may transiently appear at the time of reperfusion in some patients with occlusion of the right coronary artery; it is associated with hypotension, nausea, and vomiting. This reaction is probably due to triggering of the Bezold-Jarisch reflex by reperfusion of the inferior and posterior wall of the left ventricle [221, 222] and responds readily to intravenous atropine. If no clinical signs of reperfusion are evident 2 to 3 hours after initiation of treatment, failure of reperfusion is likely and alternative measures should be considered, particularly when hemodynamic compromise is evident.

Ventricular Arrhythmias

Ventricular arrhythmias that occur at the time of reperfusion or shortly thereafter (reperfusion arrhythmias) have been reported in about 50 percent of patients with proved reperfusion [223–225]. Although experimental studies indicate that the electrophysiologic basis of accelerated idioventricular rhythm (AIVR) is probably an increase of automaticity [226, 227], in clinical practice almost any ventricular arrhythmia may accompany reperfusion. The most common reperfusion arrhythmias are AIVR (see Fig. 25-5B) and ventricular ectopic beats that occur late during diastole and appear either as isolated ectopic or fusion beats or as part of a bigeminal or trigeminal pattern [223, 225]. Although AIVR occurs at the time of reperfusion in only about 50 percent of patients, Holter monitor studies indicate that about 90 percent of patients have self-terminating runs of AIVR at about 70 to 90 beats per minute during the 12 hours following reperfusion [223] (Fig. 25-7). This relative slowness of the AIVR may delay its appearance until the sinus rate slows and may explain why some patients manifest only delayed AIVR. Although reperfusion arrhythmias are generally transient and benign and, therefore, do not usually require any treatment, sustained or rapid ventricular tachycardia occasionally occurs and responds to the usual antiarrhythmic agents. Ventricular fibrillation is a rare arrhythmia following intravenous thrombolysis, but it may become more frequent with earlier reperfusion [213]. The overall incidence of ventricular fibrillation is, in fact, reduced by thrombolysis [165].

Abrupt Rise in Plasma Markers of Myocardial Necrosis

Reperfusion is immediately followed by a marked increase in serum levels of creatine kinase

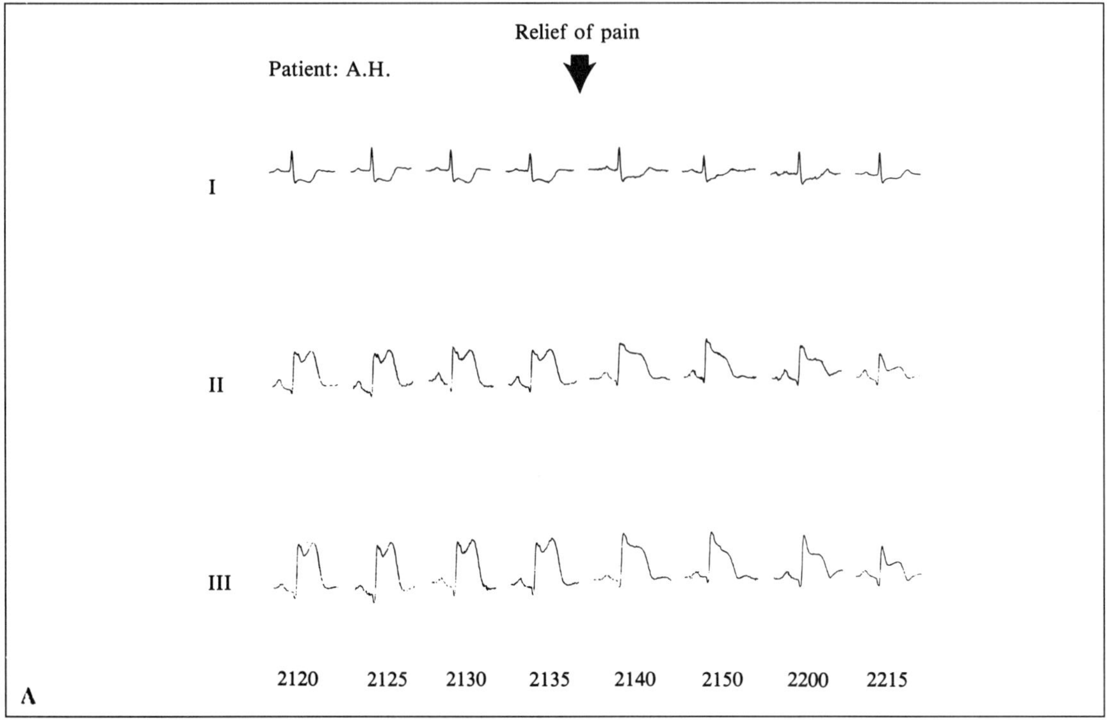

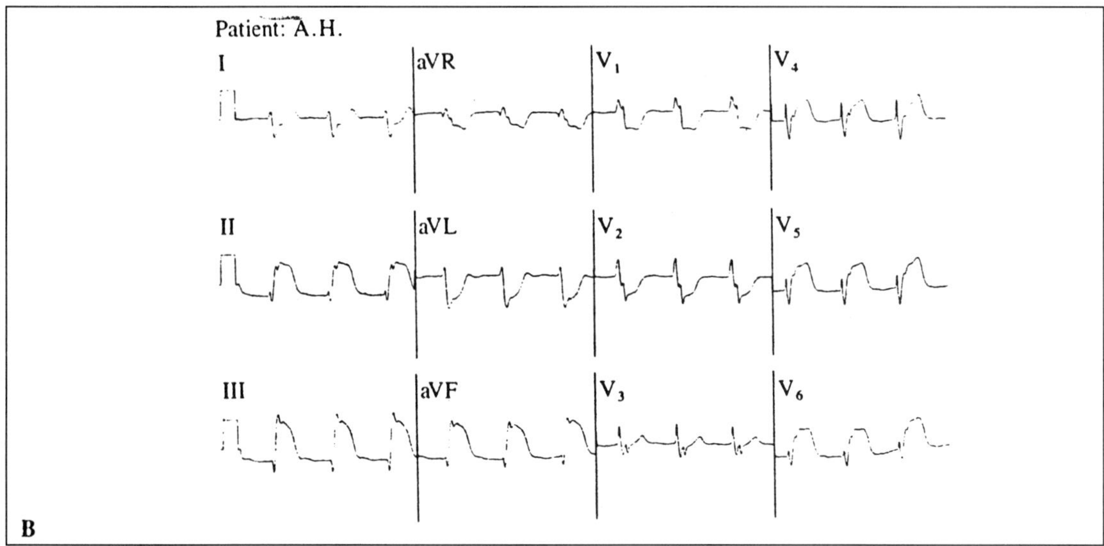

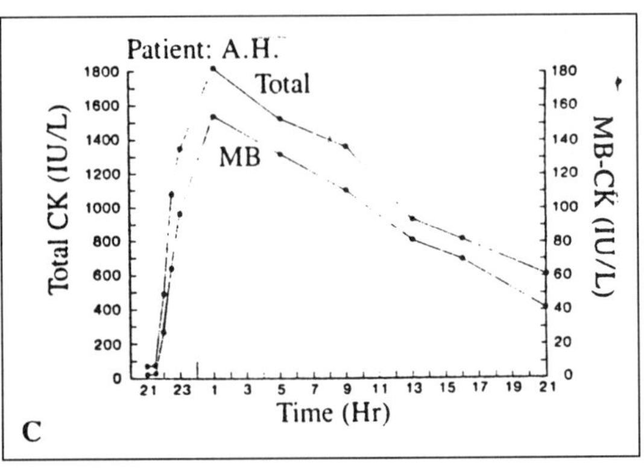

Fig. 25-5
Simultaneous appearance of the nonangiographic signs of reperfusion in a patient with inferior acute myocardial infarction who received intravenous streptokinase commencing at 2120. Note (*A*) the onset of resolution of chest pain and ST segment elevation between 2135 and 2140; (*B*) the occurrence of accelerated idioventricular rhythm at 2142; and (*C*) the onset of an abrupt rise in plasma creatine kinase between 2130 and 2200 followed by early peaking of the time–activity curve within 4 hours of the commencement of its rise.

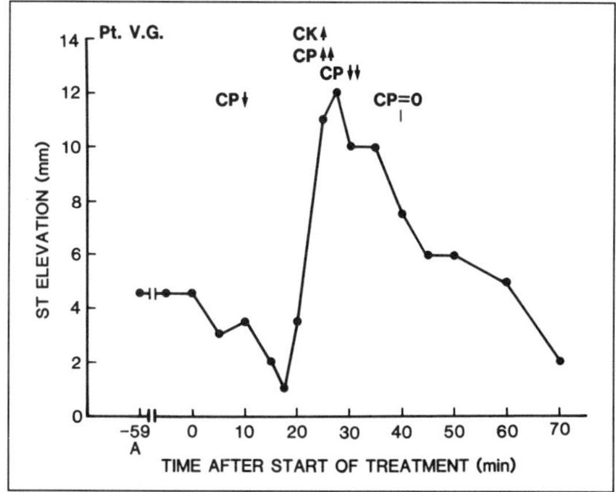

Fig. 25-6
A paradoxical worsening in ST segment elevation in a patient receiving thrombolytic therapy just minutes before the onset of final resolution of chest pain and ST segment elevation. Changes in chest pain (CP) paralleled changes in ST segment elevation, with complete relief (CP=0) occurring in 15 minutes. The plasma creatine kinase activity (CK) increased abruptly, coincident with the onset of progressive resolution of chest pain and ST segment elevation. (From P. K. Shah et al. Angiographic validation of bedside markers of reperfusion. *J. Am. Coll. Cardiol.* 21:55, 1993. With permission.)

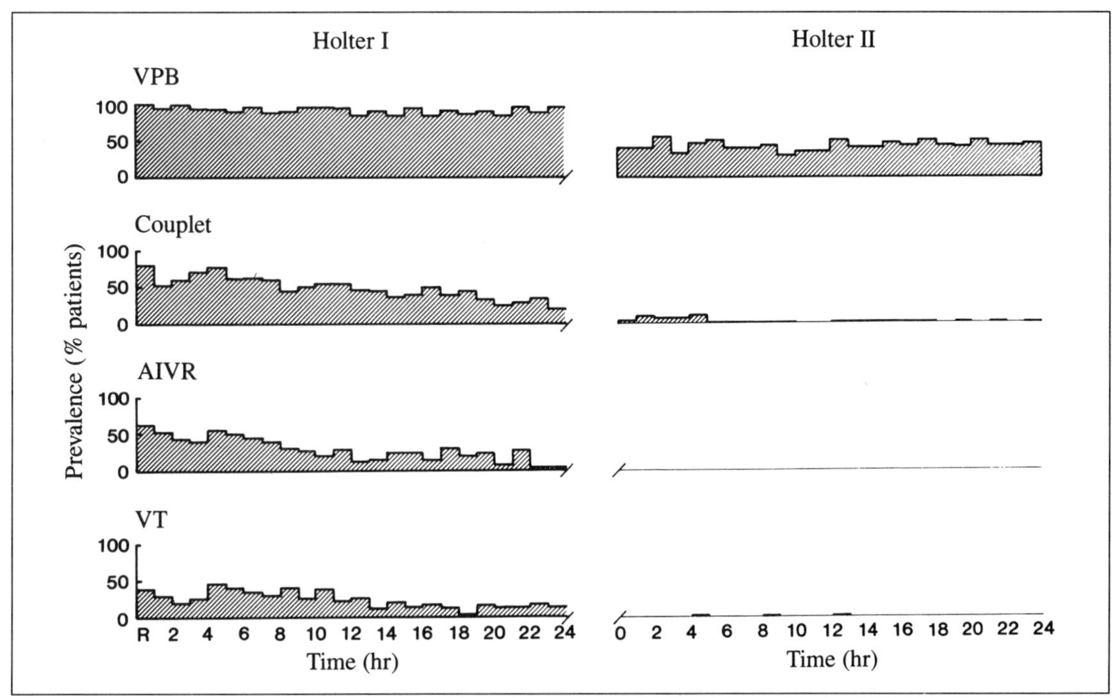

Fig. 25-7
Time course of the prevalence of ventricular arrhythmias during the first 24 hours after reperfusion with intravenous streptokinase. R = hour during which reperfusion occurred; VPB = ventricular premature beat; AIVR = accelerated idioventricular rhythm; VT = ventricular tachycardia. (From B. Cercek et al. Time course and characteristics of ventricular arrhythmias following reperfusion in acute myocardial infarction. *Am. J. Cardiol.* 60:214, 1987. With permission.)

(CK) and other cardiac enzymes, reflecting brisk washout of these proteins into the circulation by the abrupt and marked increase in blood flow to the ischemic myocardium that occurs with reperfusion [228, 229]. Such rapid enzyme washout has also been reported for beta-hydroxydehydrogenase [230], myoglobin [231, 232], and isoforms of CK [233, 234]. The smaller the molecule, the earlier its release from damaged myocardial cells and the earlier the observed serum peak. Usually, the CK time–activity curve peaks earlier with reperfusion (see Fig. 25-5C) than with nonreperfused infarctions [235]. Reperfusion also results in a more complete washout of CK from the myocardium, such that the peak serum CK activity as well as the total amount of CK released are considerably higher following reperfusion than for an equivalent-sized, nonreperfused infarction [236]. Estimation of infarct size from the CK time–activity curve is thus different in reperfused than in nonreperfused infarcts, but the direct relation between infarct size and CK release still holds. CK release is less in patients who have well-developed collaterals [237], implying more gradual washout via collateral circulation, reduced infarct size, or both. The onset of the rise in CK may be identified by sampling blood at 30-minute intervals until reperfusion is clinically evident. An abrupt rise in serum CK is temporally related to the bedside signs of reperfusion. In clinical practice, it may be sufficient to obtain one total CK level on admission, a second one during drug infusion, and another when resolution of chest pain and ST segment elevation suggest reperfusion. A markedly increased CK level obtained at the time of clinical reperfusion is confirmatory. Early peaking of the CK curve is also confirmatory [238] but not essential for the diagnosis of reperfusion; the peak value is helpful in estimating infarct size. If reperfusion fails, CK can be measured at 6-hour intervals until it peaks, to estimate infarct size. The other aforementioned markers of myocardial necrosis have also been shown to be useful in this setting and may permit earlier identification of reperfusion [231, 232, 234]. It is important to remember that because of the time required for CK and other enzyme levels to be determined, this approach is not

Fig. 25-8
Time course of ST segment elevation in lead V3 along with the creatine kinase (CK) time–activity curve during thrombolytic therapy. The close temporal relation of an abrupt increase (↑) in plasma CK activity to the onset of the final rapid and progressive decrease (↓) in ST segment elevation and chest pain (CP) as well as the appearance of accelerated idioventricular rhythm (AIVR) is shown. The marked transient worsening of the ST segment elevation just before the onset of final resolution is also seen. (From P. K. Shah et al. Angiographic validation of bedside markers of reperfusion. *J. Am. Coll. Cardiol.* 21:55, 1993. With permission.)

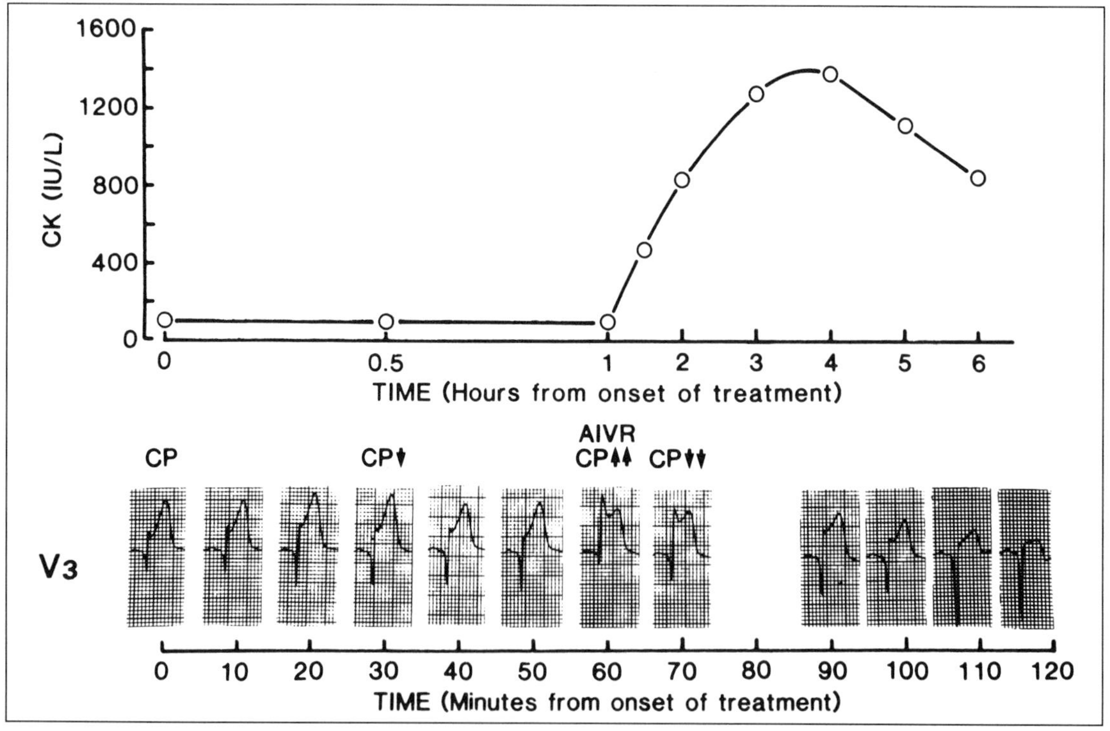

suitable for immediate, on-line assessment of reperfusion during thrombolytic therapy. This situation may change with introduction of advanced technologies for rapid, bedside measurements of enzyme levels [239].

In our experience, the simultaneous occurrence of (1) sudden relief of chest pain, (2) rapid resolution of ST segment elevation, and, possibly, (3) abrupt CK washout reliably indicates complete coronary artery reperfusion in patients undergoing thrombolysis [217, 240] (Fig. 25-8).

Future Directions for Thrombolytic Therapy

In patients with evolving AMI thrombolytic therapy can lyse coronary artery thrombus, restore antegrade coronary blood flow, salvage jeopardized myocardium, preserve myocardial function, and improve survival. Despite the dramatic advances in the use of thrombolytic therapy in AMI, several potential limitations still remain:

1. Only 20 to 30 percent of patients with AMI actually receive lytic therapy in the U.S., even though 50 to 60 percent are probably eligible.
2. Lytic therapy fails in 10 to 15 percent of cases and is followed by reocclusion in 5 to 10 percent, both associated with sharply increased morbidity and mortality.
3. Lytic therapy is slow in producing reperfusion (average of 72 minutes with SK), thereby limiting myocardial salvage.
4. Lytic therapy is being initiated with undue delay from the time of onset of symptoms.
5. Bleeding, especially cerebral bleeding, remains a vexing problem.

There is a pressing need to enlarge the proportion of AMI patients who are given thrombolysis. The clinical impact of reperfusion is critically dependent on how early it is achieved. Future innovative protocols that permit earlier initiation of treatment in the patient's home, in the office, or in the ambulance, together with the introduction of safer, more effective agents and adjunctive antithrombotic agents that can achieve more rapid, sustained thrombolysis, should further enhance the potential benefits of thrombolytic therapy.

References

1. Stampfer, M. J., Goldhaber, S. Z., Yusuf, S., et al. Effect of intravenous streptokinase on acute myocardial infarction: Pooled results from randomized trials. *N. Engl. J. Med.* 307:1180, 1982.
2. Roberts, W. C., and Buja, L. M. The frequency and significance of coronary arterial thrombi and other observations in fatal acute myocardial infarction: A study of 107 necropsy patients. *Am. J. Med.* 52: 425, 1972.
3. Phillips, S. J., Kongtahworn, C., Skinner, J. R., et al. Emergency coronary artery reperfusion; a choice therapy for evolving myocardial infarction: Results in 339 patients. *J. Thorac. Cardiovasc. Surg.* 86: 679, 1983.
4. DeWood, M. A., Spores, J., Berg, R., et al. Acute myocardial infarction: A decade of experience with surgical reperfusion in 701 patients. *Circulation* 68(Suppl. II):8, 1983.
5. Rentrop, P., Blanke, H., Karsch, K. R., et al. Selective intracoronary thrombolysis in acute myocardial infarction and unstable angina pectoris. *Circulation* 63:307, 1981.
6. Ganz, W., Buchbinder, N., Marcus, H., et al. Intracoronary thrombolysis in evolving myocardial infarction. *Am. Heart J.* 101:4, 1981.
7. Ganz, W., Geft, I., Maddahi, J., et al. Nonsurgical reperfusion in evolving myocardial infarction. *J. Am. Coll. Cardiol.* 1:1247, 1983.
8. Mathey, D. G., Kuck, K. H., Tilsner, V., et al. Nonsurgical coronary artery recanalization in acute transmural myocardial infarction. *Circulation* 63: 489, 1981.
9. Herrick, J. B. Clinical features of sudden obstruction of the coronary arteries. *J.A.M.A.* 59:2015, 1912.
10. Ambrose, J. A., Winters, S. L., Arora, R. R., et al. Coronary angiographic morphology in myocardial infarction: A link between the pathogenesis of unstable angina and myocardial infarction. *J. Am. Coll. Cardiol.* 6:1233, 1985.
11. Fuster, V., Badimon, L., Badimon, J. J., et al. The pathogenesis of coronary artery disease and the acute coronary syndromes (2 parts). *N. Engl. J. Med.* 326:242, 310, 1992.
12. Hackett, D., Davies, G., Cheirchia, S., et al. Intermittent coronary occlusion in acute myocardial infarction. *N. Engl. J. Med.* 317:1055, 1987.
13. Reimer, K. A., Lowe, J. E., Rasmussen, M. M., et al. The wave-front phenomenon of ischemic cell death. I. Myocardial infarct size vs. duration of coronary occlusion in dogs. *Circulation* 56:786, 1977.
14. Reimer, K. A., and Jennings, R. B. The wave-front phenomenon of myocardial ischemic cell death. II. Transmural progression of necrosis within the framework of ischemic bed size. *Lab. Invest.* 40: 633, 1979.

15. DeWood, M. A., Spores, J., Notske, R., et al. Prevalence of total coronary occlusion during the early hours of transmural myocardial infarction. *N. Engl. J. Med.* 303:897, 1981.
16. Sottrup-Sensen, L., Clueys, H., Zasdel, M., et al. The primary structure of human plasminogen: Isolation of two lysine binding fragments and one miniplasminogen (MW 38,000) by clastase-catalyzed-specific limited proteolysis. In J. F. Davidson, R. M. Rowan, M. M. Samama, et al. (eds.), *Progress in Chemical Fibrinolysis and Thrombolysis* (Vol. 3). New York: Raven Press, 1978. Pp. 191–209.
17. Claeys, H., Molla, A., and Verstraetc, M. Conversion of NH terminal glutamic acid to NH terminal lysine human plasminogen by plasmin. *Thromb. Res.* 3:515, 1973.
18. Sherry, S., Alkjaersig, N., and Fletcher, A. P. Fibrinolysis and fibrinolytic activity in man. *Physiol. Rev.* 39:343, 1959.
19. Keber, I., and Keber, D. Increased plasminogen activator inhibitor activity in survivors of myocardial infarction is associated with metabolic risk factors of atherosclerosis. *Haemostasis* 22:187, 1992.
20. Hamsten, A., de Faire, U., Walldius, G., et al. Plasminogen activator inhibitor in plasma: Risk factor for recurrent myocardial infarction. *Lancet* 2 (8549):3, 1987.
21. Gray, R. P., Yudkin, J. S., and Patterson, D. L. Plasminogen activator inhibitor: A risk factor for myocardial infarction in diabetic patients. *Br. Heart J.* 69:228, 1993.
22. Tillet, W. S., Edwards, L. B., and Garner, R. L. Fibrinolytic activity of hemolytic streptococci: The development of resistance to fibrinolysis following acute hemolytic streptococcus infections. *J. Clin. Invest.* 13:47, 1934.
23. Reddy, K. N. N. Streptokinase—biochemistry and clinical application. *Enzyme* 40:79, 1988.
24. Reddy, K. N. N., and Markus, G. Mechanism of activation of human plasminogen by streptokinase: Presence of an active center in the streptokinase-plasminogen complex. *J. Biol. Chem.* 247:1683, 1972.
25. Claeson, G., Aureli, L., Karisson, G., et al. Substrate structure and activity relationships. In J. F. Davidson, R. M. Rowan, M. M. Samama, et al. (eds.), *Progress in Chemical Fibrinolysis and Thrombolysis* (Vol. 3). New York: Raven Press, 1978. Pp. 299–304.
26. Robbins, K. C., Summaria, L., and Wohl, R. C. Human plasmin. *Methods Enzymol.* 80:379, 1981.
27. Wohl, R. C., Arzadon, L., Summaria, L., et al. Kinetics of activation of human plasminogen by different activation species at pH 7.4 and 37°C. *J. Biol. Chem.* 255:2005, 1980.
28. Smith, R. A. G., Dupe, R. J., English, P. D., et al. Fibrinolysis with acyl-enzymes: A new approach to thrombolytic therapy. *Nature* 290:505, 1981.
29. Reddy, K. N. N., and Markus, G. Esterase activities in the zymogen moiety of the streptokinase-plasminogen complex. *J. Biol. Chem.* 249:4851, 1974.
30. Cederholm-Williams, S. A., De Cock, F., Lijnen, R., et al. Kinetics of the reaction between streptokinase, plasmin and alpha-antiplasmin. *Eur. J. Biochem.* 100:125, 1979.
31. Wilman, B. On the reaction of plasmin or plasmin-streptokinase complex with aprotinin or alpha-antiplasmin. *Thromb. Res.* 17:143, 1980.
32. Fletcher, A. P., Alkjaersign, N., and Sherry, S. The maintenance of a sustained thrombolytic state in man. I. Induction and effects. *J. Clin. Invest.* 38: 1096, 1959.
33. Fletcher, A. P., Sherry, S., Alkjaersig, N., et al. The maintenance of a sustained thrombolytic state in man. II. Clinical observations on patients with myocardial infarction and other thromboembolic disorders. *J. Clin. Invest.* 38:1111, 1959.
34. Alkjaersig, N., Fletcher, A. P., and Sherry, S. The mechanism of clot dissolution by plasmin. *J. Clin. Invest.* 38:1086, 1959.
35. Spotti, F., and Holzknecht, F. The influence of inhibitors of plasmin and plasminogen activation on the streptokinase-induced fibrinolytic state. *Thromb. Diath. Haemorrh.* 24:101, 1970.
36. Alkjaersig, N., Fletcher, A. P., and Sherry, S. Pathogenesis of the coagulation defect developing during pathological plasma proteolytic (fibrinolytic) states. I. The significance of fibrinogen proteolysis and circulating fibrinogen breakdown products. *J. Clin. Invest.* 41:896, 1962.
37. Alkjaersig, N., Fletcher, A. P., and Sherry, S. Pathogenesis of the coagulation defect developing during pathological plasma proteolytic (fibrinolytic) states. II. The significance of mechanism and consequences of defective fibrin polymerization. *J. Clin. Invest.* 41:917, 1962.
38. Lew, A. S., Berberian, L., Cercek, B., et al. Elevated serum D dimer: A degradation product of cross-linked fibrin (XDP) after intravenous streptokinase during acute myocardial infarction. *J. Am. Coll. Cardiol.* 7:1320, 1986.
39. Timmis, G. C., Gangadharan, V., Ramos, R. G., et al. Hemorrhage and the products of fibrinogen digestion after intracoronary administration of streptokinase. *Circulation* 69:1146, 1984.
40. Cederholm-Williams, S. A. The binding of plasmin-streptokinase complex to fibrin monomer-Sepharose. *Thromb. Res.* 17:573, 1980.
41. Karsch, K. R., Hofmann, M., Rentrop, K. P., et al. Thrombolysis in acute experimental myocardial infarction. *J. Am. Coll. Cardiol.* 1:427, 1983.
42. Rutsch, W., Schartl, M., Mathey, D., et al. Percutaneous transluminal coronary recanalization: Procedure, results, and acute complications. *Am. Heart J.* 102:1178, 1981.
43. Gottlob R., Blumel, G., Piza, F., et al. Studies on thrombolysis with streptokinase. II. The influence of changes due to age in thrombi and whole blood clots. *Thromb. Diath. Haemorrh.* 19:516, 1968.

44. McDonagh, J. Structure and function of factor XIII. In R. W. Colman, J. Hirsch, V. J. Marder, et al. (eds.), *Hemostasis and Thrombosis: Basic Principles and Clinical Practice.* (2nd ed.). Philadelphia: Lippincott, 1987. Pp. 289–300.
45. Kanamasa, K., Watanabe, I., Cercek, B., et al. Selective decrease in lysis of old thrombi after rapid administration of tissue-type plasminogen activator. *J. Am. Coll. Cardiol.* 14:1359, 1989.
46. Lee, G., Amsterdam, E. A., Low, R. I., et al. Coronary thrombolysis by intravenous streptokinase in clinical acute myocardial infarction. *Am. Heart J.* 102(4):783, 1981.
47. Weinstein, J. Treatment of myocardial infarction with intracoronary streptokinase: Efficacy and safety data from 209 United States cases in the Hochst-Roussel registry. *Am. Heart J.* 104:894, 1982.
48. Kennedy, J. W., Gensini, G. G., Timmis, G. C., et al. Acute myocardial infarction treated with intracoronary streptokinase: A report of the Society for Cardiac Angiography. *Am. J. Cardiol.* 55:871, 1985.
49. Lew, A. S., Laramee, P., Cercek, B., et al. The effects of the rate of intravenous infusion of streptokinase and the duration of symptoms on the time interval to reperfusion in acute myocardial infarction. *Circulation* 72:1053, 1985.
50. Anderson, J. I., Marshall, H. W., Askins, J. C., et al. A randomized trial of intravenous and intracoronary streptokinase in patients with acute myocardial infarction. *Circulation* 70:606, 1984.
51. Taylor, G. J., Mikell, F. L., Moses, H. W., et al. Intravenous versus intracoronary streptokinase therapy for acute myocardial infarction in community hospitals. *Am. J. Cardiol.* 54:256, 1984.
52. Valentine, R. P., Pitts, D. E., Brooks-Brunn, J. A., et al. Intravenous versus intracoronary streptokinase in acute myocardial infarction. *Am. J. Cardiol.* 55:309, 1985.
53. Alderman, E. L., Jutzy, K. R., Berte, L. E., et al. Randomized comparison of intravenous versus intracoronary streptokinase for acute myocardial infarction. *Am. J. Cardiol.* 54:14, 1984.
54. Rogers, W. J., Mantle, J. A., Hood, W. P., et al. Prospective randomized trial of intravenous and intracoronary streptokinase in acute myocardial infarction. *Circulation* 68:1051, 1983.
55. Hillis, L. D., Borer, J., Braunwald, E., et al. High dose intravenous streptokinase for acute myocardial infarction: Preliminary results of multicenter trial. *J. Am. Coll. Cardiol.* 6:957, 1985.
56. Reddy, K. N. N. Kinetics of active center formation in dog plasminogen by streptokinase and activity of a modified streptokinase. *J. Biol. Chem.* 251: 6626, 1976.
57. Reddy, K. N. N., Cercek, B., Lew, A. S., et al. Interaction of SK-human plasmin, SK-dog plasmin complexes with alpha-antiplasmin and alpha-macroglobulin. *Thromb. Res.* 41:671, 1986.
58. English, P. D., Smith, R. A. G., Dupe, R. J., et al. The thrombolytic activity of streptokinase in the rabbit. *Thromb. Haemost.* 46:525, 1981.
59. Einarsson, M., Mattso, C., and Nilsson, S. Effect on haemostasis of intravenous injection of alpha-antiplasmin in cats treated with streptokinase. *Thromb. Res.* 30:205, 1983.
60. Coller, B. S. Platelets and thrombolytic therapy. *N. Engl. J. Med.* 322:33, 1990.
61. Jeanneau, C., and Sultan, Y. Tissue plasminogen activator in human megakaryocytes and platelets: Immunocytochemical localization, immunoblotting and zymographic analysis. *Thromb. Haemost.* 59: 529, 1988.
62. Park, S., Harker, L. A., Marzec, U. M., et al. Demonstration of single chain urokinase-type plasminogen activator on human platelet membrane. *Blood* 73:1421, 1989.
63. Miles, L. A., and Plow, E. F. Binding and activation of plasminogen on the platelet surface. *J. Biol. Chem.* 260:4303, 1985.
64. Silverstein, R. L., Leung, L. L., Harpel, P. C., et al. Complex formation of platelet thrombospondin with plasminogen. Modulation of activation by tissue activator. *J. Clin. Invest.* 74:1625, 1984.
65. Deguchi, K., Murashima, S., Shirakawa, S., et al. The potentiating effect of platelets on plasminogen activation by tissue plasminogen activator. *Thromb. Res.* 40:853, 1985.
66. Erickson, L. A., Ginsberg, M. H., and Loskutoff, D. J. Detection and partial characterization of an inhibitor of plasminogen activator in human platelets. *J. Clin. Invest.* 74:1465, 1984.
67. Plow, E. F., and Collen, D. The presence and release of alpha-2 antiplasmin from human platelets. *Blood* 58:1069, 1981.
68. Jang, I. K., Gold, H. K., Ziskind, A. A., et al. Differential sensitivity of erythrocyte-rich and platelet-rich arterial thrombi to lysis with recombinant tissue-type plasminogen activator. A possible explanation for resistance to coronary thrombolysis. *Circulation* 79:920, 1989.
69. ISIS-2 Collaborative Group. Randomized trial of intravenous streptokinase, oral aspirin, both, or neither among 17,187 cases of suspected acute myocardial infarction: ISIS-2. ISIS-2 (Second International Study of Infarct Survival) Collaborative Group. *Lancet* 2:349, 1988.
70. Fitzgerald, D. J., Catella, F., Roy, L., et al. Marked platelet activation in vivo after intravenous streptokinase in patients with acute myocardial infarction. *Circulation* 77:142, 1988.
71. Ohlstein, E. H., Storer, B., Fujita, T., et al. Tissue-type plasminogen activator and streptokinase-induced platelet hyperaggregability in the rabbit. *Thromb. Res.* 46:575, 1987.
72. Schafer, A. I., and Adelman, B. Plasmin inhibition of platelet function and of arachidonic acid metabolism. *J. Clin. Invest.* 75:456, 1985.
73. Loscalzo, J., and Vaughan, D. E. Tissue plasmino-

gen activator promotes platelet disaggregation in plasma. *J. Clin. Invest.* 79:1749, 1987.
74. Peerschke, E. I. The platelet fibrinogen receptor. *Semin. Hematol.* 22:241, 1985.
75. Rudd, M. A., George, D., Amarante, P., et al. Temporal effects of thrombolytic agents on platelet function in vivo and their modulation by prostaglandins. *Circ. Res.* 67:1175, 1990.
76. Kleiman, N. S., Ohman, E. M., Ellis, S. G., et al. Infarct vessel patency is enhanced by profound platelet inhibition with fibrinogen receptor blockade with 7E3 in patients receiving thrombolysis for acute myocardial infarction. (Abstract). *Circulation* 86(4):I-260, 1992.
77. Owen, J., Friedman, K. D., Grossman, B. A., et al. Thrombolytic therapy with tissue plasminogen activator or streptokinase induces transient thrombin activity. *Blood* 72:616, 1988.
78. Eisenberg, P. R., Sherman, L. A., and Jaffe, A. S. Paradoxic elevation of fibrinopeptide A after streptokinase: Evidence for continued thrombosis despite intense fibrinolysis. *J. Am. Coll. Cardiol.* 10:527, 1987.
79. Rapold, H. J., Kuemmerli, H., Weiss, M., et al. Monitoring of fibrin generation during thrombolytic therapy of acute myocardial infarction with recombinant tissue-type plasminogen activator. *Circulation* 79:980, 1989.
80. Rapold, H. J., deBono, D., Arnold, A. E., et al. Plasma fibrinopeptide A levels in patients with acute myocardial infarction treated with alteplase. Correlation with concomitant heparin coronary artery patency, and recurrent ischemia. The European Cooperative Study Group. *Circulation* 85:928, 1992.
81. Zahger, D., Maaravi, Y., Matzner, Y., et al. Partial resistance to anticoagulation after streptokinase treatment for acute myocardial infarction. *Am. J. Cardiol.* 66:28, 1990.
82. Shah, P. K. Thrombolytic therapy in acute myocardial infarction: Current limitations and future directions. *Learning Center Highlights,* 1992.
83. Takada, A., Takada, Y., and Sugawara, Y. The activation of Glu- and Lys-plasminogens by streptokinase: Effects of fibrin, fibrinogen and their degradation products. *Thromb. Res.* 37:465, 1985.
84. Cercek, B., Lew, A. S., Hod, H., et al. Pretreatment with heparin enhances thrombolysis by tissue type plasminogen activator. *Circulation* 74:683, 1986.
85. Rudd, M. A., George, D., Johnstone, M. T., et al. Effect of thrombin inhibition on the dynamics of thrombolysis and on platelet function during thrombolytic therapy. *Circ. Res.* 70:829, 1992.
86. Hirsh, J., O'Sullivan, E. F., and Martin, M. Evaluation of a standard dosage schedule with streptokinase. *Blood* 35:341, 1970.
87. Moran, D. M., Standring, R., Lavender, E. A., et al. Assessment of anti-streptokinase antibody levels in human sera using a microradioimmunoassay procedure. *Thromb. Haemost.* 52:281, 1984.
88. Elliot, J. M., Cross, D. B., Cederholm-Williams, S. A., et al. Neutralizing antibodies to streptokinase four years after intravenous thrombolytic therapy. *Am. J. Cardiol.* 71:640, 1993.
89. Lee, H.S., Davidson, R., Reid, T., et al. Raised levels of antistreptokinase antibody and neutralization titres from 4 days to 54 months after administration of streptokinase or anistreplase. *Europ. Heart J.* 14:84, 1993.
90. Fears, R., Ferres, H., Glasgow, E., et al. Monitoring of streptokinase resistance titre in acute myocardial infarction patients up to 30 months after giving streptokinase or anistreplase and related studies to measure specific antistreptokinase IgG. *Br. Heart J.* 68:167, 1992.
91. Lew, A. S., Neer, T., Rodriguez, L., et al. Clinical failure of streptokinase due to an unsuspected high titer of antistreptokinase antibody. *J. Am. Coll. Cardiol.* 4:183, 1984.
92. Fears, R., Hearn, J., Standring, R., et al. Lack of influence of pretreatment antistreptokinase antibody on efficacy in a multicenter patency comparison of intravenous streptokinase and anistreplase in acute myocardial infarction. *Am. Heart J.* 124 (2):305, 1992.
93. Gomez, M. A., Karagounis, L., and Andersen, J. L. Does an allergic-type reaction to streptokinase or anistreplase affect patency status following thrombolysis for acute myocardial infarction? (Abstract) *J. Am. Coll. Cardiol.* 21:348A, 1993.
94. Prowse, C. V., Hornsey, V., Ruckley, C. V., et al. A comparison of acylated streptokinase-plasminogen complex in healthy volunteers. *Thromb. Haemost.* 47:132, 1982.
95. Staniforth, D. H., Smith, R. A. G., and Hibbs, M. Streptokinase and anisoylated streptokinase-plasminogen complex: Their action on haemostasis in human volunteers. *Eur. J. Clin. Pharmacol.* 24: 751, 1983.
96. Marder, V. J., Rothbard, R. L., Fitzpatrick, P. G., et al. Rapid lysis of coronary artery thrombi with anisoylated plasminogen streptokinase activator complex: Treatment by bolus injection. *Ann. Intern. Med.* 104:304, 1986.
97. Timmis, A. D., Griffin, B., Crick, J. C. P., et al. Anisoylated plasminogen streptokinase activator in acute myocardial infarction: A placebo-controlled arteriographic coronary recanalization study. *J. Am. Coll. Cardiol.* 10:205, 1987.
98. ISIS-3 (Third International Study of Infarct Survival) Collaborative Group. ISIS-3: A randomized comparison of streptokinase vs tissue plasminogen activator vs anistreplase and of aspirin plus heparin vs aspirin alone among 41,299 cases of suspected acute myocardial infarction. *Lancet* 339(8796): 753, 1992.
99. Ganz, W., Ninomya, K., Hashida, J., et al. Intracoronary thrombolysis in acute myocardial infarction: Experimental background and clinical experience. *Am. Heart J.* 102:1145, 1981.

100. Garabedian, H. D., Gold, H. K., Leinbach, R. C., et al. Dose-dependent thrombolysis, pharmacokinetics and hemostatic effects of recombinant human tissue-type plasminogen activator for coronary thrombosis. *Am. J. Cardiol.* 58:673, 1986.
101. Collen, D. On the regulation and control of fibrinolysis. *Thromb. Haemost.* 73:77, 1980.
102. Woollard, K. V., Mews, G. C., Cope, G. D., et al. A comparison of intravenous and intracoronary streptokinase in acute myocardial infarction. *Aust. N.Z. J. Med.* 14:475, 1984.
103. Lew, A. S., Cercek, B., Hod, H., et al. A high residual plasma fibrinogen following intravenous streptokinase predicts delay or failure of reperfusion in acute myocardial infarction. *Am. J. Cardiol.* 58:680, 1986.
104. Six, A. J., Louwerenburg, H. W., Braams, R., et al. A double-blind randomized multicenter dose-ranging trial of intravenous streptokinase in acute myocardial infarction. *Am. J. Cardiol.* 65:119, 1990.
105. Lew, A. S., Laramee, P., Cercek, B., et al. The hypotensive effect of intravenous streptokinase in patients with acute myocardial infarction. *Circulation* 72:1321, 1985.
106. Davis, G. J., Chierchia, S., and Maseri, A. Prevention of myocardial infarction by very early treatment with intracoronary streptokinase. *N. Engl. J. Med.* 311:1488, 1984.
107. TIMI Study Group. The thrombolysis in myocardial infarction (TIMI) trial: Phase I findings. *N. Engl. J. Med.* 312:932, 1985.
108. Karagounis, L. A., Sorensen, S. G., Menlove, R. L., et al. Does Thrombolysis in Myocardial Infarction (TIMI) perfusion grade 2 represent a mostly patent artery or a mostly occluded artery? Enzymatic and electrocardiographic evidence from the TEAM-2 study. *J. Am. Coll. Cardiol.* 19:1, 1992.
109. Andersen, J. L., Karagounis, L. A., Becker, L. C., et al. TIMI perfusion grade 3 but not grade 2 results in improved outcome after thrombolysis for myocardial infarction. Ventriculographic, enzymatic and electrocardiographic evidence from the TEAM-3 study. *Circulation* 87:1829, 1993.
110. Lincoff, A. M., Ellis, S. G., Galeana, A., et al. Is a coronary artery with TIMI grade 2 flow "patent?" Outcome in the Thrombolysis and Angioplasty in Myocardial Infarction (TAMI) trial. (Abstract) *Circulation* 86(suppl I):I-268, 1992.
111. The GUSTO investigators. An international randomized trial comparing four thrombolytic strategies for acute myocardial infarction. *N. Engl. J. Med.* 329:673, 1993.
112. Tennant, S. N., Dixon, J., Venable, T. C., et al. Intracoronary thrombolysis in patients with acute myocardial infarction: Comparison of the efficacy of urokinase and with streptokinase. *Circulation* 69:756, 1984.
113. Van de Werf, F., Ludbrook, P. A.., Bergmann, S. R., et al. Coronary thrombolysis with tissue-type plasminogen activator in patients with evolving myocardial infarction. *N. Engl. J. Med.* 310:609, 1984.
114. Weinstein, J. The international registry to support approval of intracoronary streptokinase thrombolysis in the treatment of myocardial infarction. *Circulation* 68(Suppl I):61, 1983.
115. Blunda, M., Meister, S. G., Shechter, J. A., et al. Intravenous versus intracoronary streptokinase for acute transmural myocardial infarction. *Cathet. Cardiovasc. Diagn.* 10:319, 1984.
116. Chesebro, J. H., Knatterud, G., Roberts, R., et al. Thrombolysis in Myocardial Infarction (TIMI) trial, phase I: Comparison between intravenous tissue plasminogen activator and intravenous streptokinase. Clinical findings through hospital discharge. *Circulation* 76:142, 1987.
117. White, H. D., Norris, R. M., Brown, M. A., et al. Effect of intravenous streptokinase on left ventricular function and early survival after acute myocardial infarction. *N. Engl. J. Med.* 317:850, 1987.
118. Kennedy, J. W., Martin, G. V., Davis, K. B., et al. The Western Washington Trial of intravenous streptokinase in acute myocardial infarction randomized trial. *Circulation* 77:345, 1988.
119. PRIMI trial study group. Randomized double blind trial of recombinant prourokinase against streptokinase in acute myocardial infarction. *Lancet* 1:862, 1989.
120. Stack, R. S., O'Connor, C. M., Mark, D. B., et al. Coronary perfusion during acute myocardial infarction with a combined therapy of coronary angioplasty and high-dose intravenous streptokinase. *Circulation* 77:151, 1988.
121. Verstraete, M., Bory, M., Collen, D., et al. Randomized trial of intravenous recombinant tissue-type plasminogen activator versus intravenous streptokinase in acute myocardial infarction: Report from the European Cooperative Study Group for recombinant tissue-type plasminogen activator. *Lancet* 1:842, 1985.
122. Hogg, K. J., Gemmill, J. D., Burns, J., et al. Angiographic patency study of anistreplase versus streptokinase in acute myocardial infarction. *Lancet* 335:254, 1990.
123. Anderson, J. L., Sorensen, S. G., Moreno, F. L., et al. Multicenter patency trial of intravenous anistreplase compared with streptokinase in acute myocardial infarction. *Circulation* 83:126, 1991.
124. Ganz, W., and Shah, P. K. Temporal distribution of treatment to reperfusion times in patients with acute myocardial infarction: The effect of tissue plasminogen activator vs. streptokinase (Abstract). *J. Am. Coll. Cardiol.* 361A, 1992.
125. White, H. D., Rivers, J. T., Maslowski, A. H., et al. Effect of intravenous streptokinase as compared with that of tissue plasminogen activator on left ventricular function after first myocardial infarction. *N. Engl. J. Med.* 320:817, 1989.
126. Ganz, W., Geft, I., Shah, P. K., et al. Intravenous

streptokinase in evolving acute myocardial infarction. *Am. J. Cardiol.* 53:1209, 1984.

127. Bren, G. B., Wasserman, A. G., and Ross, A. M. The electrocardiogram in patients undergoing thrombolysis for myocardial infarction. *Circulation* 76(Suppl II):18, 1987.
128. Blanke, H., Scherff, F., Karsch, K. R., et al. Electrocardiographic changes after streptokinase-induced recanalization in patients with acute left anterior descending artery obstruction. *Circulation* 68:406, 1983.
129. Von Essen, R., Schmidt, W., Uebis, R., et al. Myocardial infarction and thrombolysis: Electrocardiographic short term and long term results using precordial mapping. *Br. Heart J.* 54:6, 1985.
130. Schwarz, F., Schuler, G., Katus, H., et al. Intracoronary thrombolysis in acute myocardial infarction: Correlations among serum enzymes, scintigraphic and hemodynamic findings. *Am. J. Cardiol.* 50:32, 1982.
131. Schwarz, F., Schuler, G., Katus, H., et al. Intracoronary thrombolysis in acute myocardial infarction: Duration of ischemia as a major determinant of late results after recanalization. *Am. J. Cardiol.* 50:933, 1982.
132. Tamaki, S., Murakami, T., Kadota, K., et al. Effects of coronary artery reperfusion on relation between creatine kinase-MB release and infarct size estimated by myocardial emission tomography with thallium-201 in man. *J. Am. Coll. Cardiol.* 2:1031, 1983.
133. Markis, J. E., Malagold, M., Parker, A., et al. Myocardial salvage after intracoronary thrombolysis with streptokinase in acute myocardial infarction: Assessment by intracoronary thallium-201. *N. Engl. J. Med.* 305:777, 1981.
134. Maddahi, J., Ganz, W., Ninomiya, K., et al. Myocardial salvage by intracoronary thrombolysis in evolving acute myocardial infarction: Evaluation using intracoronary injection of thallium-201. *Am. Heart J.* 102:664, 1981.
135. Weiss, A. T., Maddahi, J., Lew, A. S., et al. Reverse redistribution of thallium-201: A sign of nontransmural myocardial infarction with patency of the infarct-related coronary artery. *J. Am. Coll. Cardiol.* 7(1):61, 1986.
136. Schuler, G., Schwarz, F., Hofmann, M., et al. Thrombolysis in acute myocardial infarction using intracoronary streptokinase: Assessment by thallium-201 scintigraphy. *Circulation* 66:658, 1982.
137. Schofer, J., Mathey, D. G., Montz, R., et al. Use of dual intracoronary scintigraphy with thallium-201 and technetium-99m pyrophosphate to predict improvement in left ventricular wall motion immediately after intracoronary thrombolysis in acute myocardial infarction. *J. Am. Coll. Cardiol.* 2: 737, 1983.
138. De Coster, P. M., Melin, J. A., Detry, J. M. R., et al. Coronary artery reperfusion in acute myocardial infarction: Assessment by pre- and postintervention thallium-201 myocardial perfusion imaging. *Am. J. Cardiol.* 55:889, 1985.
139. Charuzi, Y., Beder, C., Marshall, L. A., et al. Improvement in regional and global left ventricular function after intracoronary thrombolysis: Assessment with two-dimensional endocardiography. *Am. J. Cardiol.* 53:662, 1984.
140. Serruys, P. W., Simoons, M. L., Suryapranata, H., et al. Preservation of global and regional left ventricular function after early thrombolysis in acute myocardial infarction. *J. Am. Coll. Cardiol.* 7:729, 1986.
141. Mahey, D. G., Sheehan, F. H., Schofer, J., et al. Time from onset of symptoms to thrombolytic therapy: A major determinant of myocardial salvage in patients with acute transmural myocardial infarction. *J. Am. Coll. Cardiol.* 6:518, 1985.
142. Koren, G., Weiss, A. T., Hasin, Y., et al. Prevention of myocardial damage in acute myocardial ischemia by early treatment with intravenous streptokinase. *N. Engl. J. Med.* 313:1384, 1985.
143. Rentrop, P., Blanke, H., Karsch, K. R., et al. Changes in left ventricular function after intracoronary streptokinase infusion in clinically evolving myocardial infarction. *Am. Heart J.* 102:1188, 1981.
144. Stack, R. S., Phillips, H. R., III, Grierson, D. S., et al. Functional improvement of jeopardized myocardium following intracoronary streptokinase infusion in acute myocardial infarction. *J. Clin. Invest.* 72:84, 1983.
145. Sobel, B. E., Geltman, E. M., Tiefenbrunn, A. J., et al. Improvement of regional myocardial metabolism after coronary thrombolysis induced with tissue-type plasminogen activator or streptokinase. *Circulation* 69:983, 1984.
146. Guth, B. D., Martin, J. F., Heusch, G., et al. Regional myocardial blood flow, function and metabolism using phosphorus-31 nuclear magnetic resonance spectoscopy during ischemia and reperfusion. *J. Am. Coll. Cardiol.* 10:673, 1987.
147. Ritchie, J. L., Davis, K. B., Williams, D. I., et al. Global and regional left ventricular function and tomographic radionuclide perfusion: The Western Washington Intracoronary Streptokinase in Myocardial Infarction Trial. *Circulation* 70:867, 1984.
148. Ferguson, D. W., White, C. W., Schwartz, J. L., et al. Influence of baseline ejection fraction and success of thrombolysis on mortality and ventricular function after acute myocardial infarction. *Am. J. Cardiol.* 54:705, 1984.
149. Sheehan, F. H., Mathey, D. G., Schofer, J., et al. Factors that determine recovery of left ventricular function after thrombolysis in patients with acute myocardial infarction. *Circulation* 71:1121, 1985.
150. Braunwald, E., and Kloner, R. A. The stunned myocardium: Prolonged, post-ischemic ventricular dysfunction. *Circulation* 66:1146, 1982.
151. Christian, T. F., Behrenbeck, T., Pellikka, P. A., et al. Mismatch of left ventricular function and infarct

size demonstrated by technetium-99m isonitrile imaging after reperfusion therapy for acute myocardial infarction: Identification of myocardial stunning and hyperkinesia. *J. Am. Coll. Cardiol.* 16:1632, 1990.

152. Ellis, S. G., Wynne, J., Braunwald, E., et al. Response of reperfusion-salvaged, stunned myocardium to inotropic stimulation. *Am. Heart J.* 107: 13, 1984.
153. Mercier, J. C., Lando, U., Kanmatsuse, K., et al. Divergent effects of inotropic stimulation on the ischemic and severely depressed reperfused myocardium. *Circulation* 66:397, 1982.
154. Arnold, J. M. O., Braunwald, E., Sandor, T., et al. Inotropic stimulation of reperfused myocardium with dopamine: Effects on infarct size and myocardial function. *J. Am. Coll. Cardiol.* 6:1026, 1985.
155. The Multicenter Postinfarction Research Group. Risk stratification and survival after myocardial infarction. *N. Engl. J. Med.* 309:331, 1983.
156. Kennedy, J. W., Ritchie, J. L., Davis, K. B., et al. Western Washington randomized trial of intracoronary streptokinase in acute myocardial infarction. *N. Engl. J. Med.* 309:1477, 1983.
157. Rentrop, K. P., Feit, F., Blanke, H., et al. Effects of intracoronary streptokinase and intracoronary nitroglycerin on coronary angiographic patterns and mortality in patients with acute myocardial infarction. *N. Engl. J. Med.* 311:1457, 1984.
158. ISAM study group. A prospective trial of intravenous streptokinase in acute myocardial infarction (ISAM): Mortality, morbidity and infarct size at 21 days. *N. Engl. J. Med.* 314:1465, 1986.
159. Simoons, M. L., van der Brand, M., de Zwaan, C., et al. Improved survival after early thrombolysis in acute myocardial infarction. *Lancet* 2:578, 1985.
160. Schroder, R., Neuhaus, K. L., Linderer, T., et al. Impact of late coronary artery reperfusion on left ventricular function one month after acute myocardial infarction (results from the ISAM study). *Am. J. Cardiol.* 64:878, 1989.
161. Rentrop, K. P., Feit, F., Sherman, W., et al. Late thrombolytic therapy preserves left ventricular function in patients with collateralized total coronary occlusion: Primary end point findings of the second Mount Sinai-New York University reperfusion trial. *J. Am. Coll. Cardiol.* 14:58, 1989.
162. Van de Werf, F., Arnold, A. E., for the European Cooperative Study Group for Recombinant Tissue Type Plasminogen Activator. Intravenous tissue plasminogen activator and size of infarct, left ventricular function and survival in acute myocardial infarction. *B.M.J.* 297:1374, 1988.
163. Van de Werf, F. Discrepancies between the effects of coronary reperfusion on survival and left ventricular function. *Lancet* 1:1367, 1989.
164. Simoons, M. L., Scrruys, P. W., van der Brand, M., et al. Early thrombolysis in acute myocardial infarction: Limitation of infarct size and improved survival. *J. Am. Coll. Cardiol.* 7:717, 1986.
165. Gruppo Italiano per lo Studio della Streptochinasi nell'Infarto Miocardico (GISSI). Effectiveness of intravenous streptokinase thrombolytic treatment in acute myocardial infarction. *Lancet* 1:397, 1986.
166. Gruppo Italiano per lo Studio della Streptochinasi nell-Infarto Miocardico (GISSI). Long-term effects of intravenous thrombolysis in acute myocardial infarction: Final report of the GISSI study. *Lancet* 2:871–4, 1987.
167. Cerqueira, M. D., Maynard, C., Ritchie, J. L., et al. Long-term survival in 618 patients from the Western Washington Streptokinase in Myocardial Infarction trials. *J. Am. Coll. Cardiol.* 20:1452, 1992.
168. Simoons, M. L., Vos, J., Tijssen, J. G., et al. Long-term benefit of early thrombolytic therapy in patients with acute myocardial infarction: 5 year follow-up of a trial conducted by the Interuniversity Cardiology Institute of the Netherlands. *J. Am. Coll. Cardiol.* 14:1609, 1989.
169. Hochman, J. S., and Choo, H. Limitation of myocardial infarct expansion by reperfusion independent of myocardial salvage. *Circulation* 75:299, 1987.
170. Eigler, N., Maurer, G., and Shah, P. K. Effect of early systemic thrombolytic therapy on left ventricular mural thrombus formation in acute anterior myocardial infarction. *Am. J. Cardiol.* 54:261, 1984.
171. Gang, E. S., Lew, A. S., Hong, M., et al. Decreased incidence of ventricular late potentials after successful thrombolytic therapy for acute myocardial infarction. *N. Engl. J. Med.* 321:712, 1989.
172. Bourke, J. P., Young, A. A., Richards, D. A. B., et al. Reduction in incidence of inducible ventricular tachycardia after myocardial infarction by treatment with streptokinase during infarct evolution. *J. Am. Coll. Cardiol.* 16:1703, 1990.
173. Braunwald, E., and Sobel, B. E. Coronary blood flow and myocardial ischemia. In E. Braunwald (ed.), *Heart Disease* (4th ed.). Philadelphia: W. B. Saunders, 1992. Pp. 1161–99.
174. Sheehan, F. H., Braunwald, E., Canner, P., et al. The effect of intravenous thrombolytic therapy on left ventricular function: A report on tissue-type plasminogen activator and streptokinase from the Thrombolysis in Myocardial Infarction (TIMI phase I) trial. *Circulation* 75:817, 1987.
175. Sabia, P. J., Powers, E. R., Ragosta, M., et al. An association between collateral blood flow and myocardial viability in patients with recent myocardial infarction. *N. Engl. J. Med.* 327:1825, 1992.
176. Fine, D. G., Weiss, A. T., Sapoznikov, D., et al. Importance of early initiation of intravenous streptokinase therapy for acute myocardial infarction. *Am. J. Cardiol.* 58:411, 1986.
177. Gruppo Italiano per lo Studio della Streptokinasi nell'Infarto Miocardico II. GISSI-2: A factorial randomized trial of alteplase versus streptokinase and heparin versus no heparin among 12,490 patients with acute myocardial infarction. *Lancet* 336 (8707):65, 1990.

178. Honan, M. B., Harrell, F. E., Reimer, K. A., et al. Cardiac rupture, mortality and the timing of thrombolytic therapy: A meta-analysis. *J. Am. Coll. Cardiol.* 16:359, 1990.
179. Sane, D. C., Califf, R. M., Topol, E. J., et al. Bleeding during thrombolytic therapy for acute myocardial infarction: Mechanisms and management. *Ann. Int. Med.* 111:1010, 1989.
180. The International Study Group. In-hospital mortality and clinical course of 20,891 patients with suspected acute myocardial infarction randomized between alteplase and streptokinase with or without heparin. *Lancet* 336(8707):71, 1990.
181. Califf, R. M., Topol, E. J., George, B. S., et al. Hemorrhagic complications associated with the use of intravenous tissue plasminogen activator in treatment of acute myocardial infarction. *Am. J. Med.* 85:353, 1988.
182. Bovill, E. G., Terrin, M. L., Stump, D. C., et al. Hemorrhagic events during therapy with recombinant tissue-type plasminogen activator for acute myocardial infarction. Results of the Thrombolysis in Myocardial Infarction (TIMI), Phase II Trial. *Ann. Int. Med.* 115:256, 1991.
183. Lupinetti, F. M., Stoney, W. S., Alford, W. C., Jr., et al. Cryoprecipitate-topical thrombin glue: Initial experience in patients undergoing cardiac operations. *J. Thorac. Cardiovasc. Surg.* 90:502, 1985.
184. Mentzer, R. L., Budzynski, A. Z., and Sherry, S. High-dose, brief-duration intravenous infusion of streptokinase in acute myocardial infarction: Description of effects in the circulation. *Am. J. Cardiol.* 57:1220, 1986.
185. Renkin, J., De Bruyne, B., Benit, E., et al. Cardiac tamponade early after thrombolysis for acute myocardial infarction: A rare but not reported hemorrhagic complication. *J. Am. Coll. Cardiol.* 17: 280, 1991.
186. Maggioni, A. P., Franzosi, M. G., Santoro, E., et al. GISSI-2 and the International Study. Risk of stroke in patients with acute myocardial infarction after thrombolytic and antithrombotic treatment. *N. Engl. J. Med.* 327:1, 1992.
187. Kremer, P., Flebig, R., Tilsner, V., et al. Lysis of left ventricular thrombi with urokinase. *Circulation* 72:112, 1985.
188. Zahger, D., Weiss, A. T., Anner, H., et al. Systemic embolization following thrombolytic therapy for acute myocardial infarction. *Chest* 97:754, 1990.
189. Freimark, D., Leor, R., Hod, H., et al. Impaired hepatic function tests after thrombolysis for acute myocardial infarction. *Am. J. Cardiol.* 67:535, 1991.
190. Queen, M., Biem, H. J., Moe, G. W., et al. Development of cholesterol embolization syndrome after intravenous streptokinase for acute myocardial infarction. *Am. J. Cardiol.* 65:1042, 1990.
191. Ohman, E. M., Califf, R. M., Topol, E. J., et al. Consequences of reocclusion after successful reperfusion therapy in acute myocardial infarction. *Circulation* 82:781, 1990.
192. Hsia, J., Kleiman, N., Aguirre, F., et al. Heparin-induced prolongation of partial thromboplastin time after thrombolysis: relation to coronary artery patency. *J. Am. Coll. Cardiol.* 20:31, 1992.
193. Meijer, A., Verheugt, F. W. A., Werter, C. J. P. J., et al. Aspirin versus coumadin in the prevention of reocclusion and recurrent ischemia after successful thrombolysis: A prospective, placebo controlled angiographic study. Results of the APRICOT study. *Circulation* 87:1524, 1993.
194. Ellis, S. G., Topol, E. J., George, B. S., et al. Recurrent ischemia without warning. Analysis of risk factors for in-hospital ischemic events following successful thrombolysis with intravenous tissue plasminogen activator. *Circulation* 80:1159, 1989.
195. Roberts, R., Rogers, W. J., Mueller, H. S., et al. Immediate versus deferred beta-blockade following thrombolytic therapy in patients with acute myocardial infarction. Results of the Thrombolysis in Myocardial Infarction (TIMI) II-B Study. *Circulation* 83:422, 1991.
196. Barbash, G. I., Hod, H., Roth, A., et al. Repeat infusion of recombinant tissue-type plasminogen activator in patients with acute myocardial infarction and early recurrent myocardial ischemia. *J. Am. Coll. Cardiol.* 16:779, 1990.
197. Neuhaus, K. L., Feuerer, W., Jeep-Tebbe, S., et al. Improved thrombolysis with a modified dose regimen of recombinant tissue-type plasminogen activator. *J. Am. Coll. Cardiol.* 14:1566, 1989.
198. Roux, S., Christeller, S., and Ludin, E. Effects of aspirin on coronary reocclusion and recurrent ischemia after thrombolysis: A meta-analysis. *J. Am. Coll. Cardiol.* 19:671, 1992.
199. Hsia, J., Hamilton, W. P., Kleiman, N., et al. A comparison between heparin and low-dose aspirin as adjunctive therapy with tissue plasminogen activator for acute myocardial infarction. Heparin-Aspirin Reperfusion Trial (HART) Investigators. *N. Engl. J. Med.* 323:1433, 1990.
200. Col, J., Decoster, O., Hanique, G., et al. Infusion of heparin conjunct to streptokinase accelerates reperfusion of acute myocardial infarction: results of a double-blind randomized trial (OSIRIS) (Abstract). *Circulation* 86(Suppl I):I259, 1992.
201. Granger, C. B., Califf, R. M., Hirsh, J., et al. APTT's after thrombolysis and standard intravenous heparin are often low and correlate with body weight, age and sex: Experience from the GUSTO trial (Abstract). *Circulation* 86(4):I-258, 1992.
202. Rudd, M. A., George, D., Johnstone, M. T., et al. Effect of thrombin inhibition on the dynamics of thrombolysis and on platelet function during thrombolytic therapy. *Circ. Res.* 70:829, 1992.
203. Cannon, C. P., McCabe, C. H., Henry, T. D., et al. Hirudin reduces reocclusion compared to heparin following thrombolysis in acute myocardial infarction: Results of the TIMI-5 trial (Abstract). *J. Am. Coll. Cardiol.* 21:136A, 1993.
204. Yusuf, S., Slieght, P., Held, P., et al. Routine medical management of acute myocardial infarction. *Circulation* 82(Suppl II):II-117, 1990.

205. Krumholtz, H. M., Paternak, R. C., Weinstein, M. C., et al. Cost effectiveness of thrombolytic therapy with streptokinase in elderly patients with suspected acute myocardial infarction. *N. Engl. J. Med.* 327:7, 1992.
206. Becker, R. C. Hemodynamic, mechanical, and metabolic determinants of thrombolytic efficacy: A theoretic framework for assessing the limitations of thrombolysis in patients with cardiogenic shock. *Am. Heart J.* 125:919, 1993.
207. Topol, E. J., Califf, R. M., Vandormael, M., et al. A randomized trial of late reperfusion therapy for acute myocardial infarction. *Circulation* 85:2090, 1992.
208. Gil, V., Antunese, A., Ventosa, A., et al. Late thrombolysis with alteplase improves left ventricular ejection fraction at 1 month after acute myocardial infarction—A double blind, placebo controlled study (Abstract). *J. Am. Coll. Cardiol.* 21:300A, 1993.
209. Morgan, C. D., Hochman, J. S., Burns, R. J., et al. The effect of late thrombolytic therapy on left ventricular function following acute myocardial infarction (Abstract). *J. Am. Coll. Cardiol.* 21:224A, 1993.
210. Bouten, M. J., Simoons, M. L., Hartman, J. A. M., et al. Prehospital thrombolysis with alteplase (rt-PA) in acute myocardial infarction. *European Heart J.* 13:925, 1992.
211. BEPS Collaborative Group. Prehospital thrombolysis in acute myocardial infarction: the Belgian Eminase Prehospital Study (BEPS). *European Heart J.* 12:965, 1991.
212. Weaver, W. D., Eisenberg, M. S., Martin, J. S., et al. Myocardial Infarction Triage and Intervention project-Phase I: Patient characteristics and feasibility of prehospital initiation of thrombolytic therapy. *J. Am. Coll. Cardiol.* 15:925, 1990.
213. The European Myocardial Infarction Project Group. Prehospital thrombolytic therapy in patients with suspected acute myocardial infarction. *N. Engl. J. Med.* 329:383, 1993.
214. Beller, G. A., Hood, W. B., Jr., and Smith, T. W. Effects of ischemia and coronary reperfusion on regional myocardial blood flow and the epicardial electrogram. *Cardiovasc. Res.* 11:489, 1977.
215. Krucoff, M. W., Green, C. E., Satler, L. F., et al. Noninvasive detection of coronary artery patency using continuous ST-segment monitoring. *Am. J. Cardiol.* 57:916, 1986.
216. Mikell, F. L., Petrovich, J., Snyder, M. C., et al. Reliability of Q-wave formation and QRS score in predicting regional and global left ventricular performance in acute myocardial infarction with successful reperfusion. *Am. J. Cardiol.* 57:923, 1986.
217. Shah, P. K., Cercek, B., Lew, A. S., et al. Angiographic validation of bedside markers of reperfusion. *J. Am. Coll. Cardiol.* 21:55, 1993.
218. Shechter, M., Rabinowitz, B., Beker, B., et al. Additional ST segment elevation during the first hour of thrombolytic therapy: An electrocardiographic sign predicting a favorable clinical outcome. *J. Am. Coll. Cardiol.* 20:1460, 1992.
219. Shah, P. K., Cercek, B., and Ganz, W. Marked transient worsening of ST segment elevation during thrombolytic therapy: a marker of impending reperfusion (Abstract). *Circulation* 86(Suppl I):I-268, 1992.
220. Wilber, D., Walton, J., O'Neill, W., et al. Effects of reperfusion on complete heart block complicating anterior myocardial infarction. *J. Am. Coll. Cardiol.* 4:1315, 1984.
221. Wei, J. Y., Markis, J. E., Malagold, M., et al. Cardiovascular reflexes stimulated by reperfusion of ischemic myocardium in acute myocardial infarction. *Circulation* 67:796, 1983.
222. Esente, P., Giambartolomei, A., Gensini, G. G., et al. Coronary reperfusion and Bezold-Jarisch reflex (bradycardia and hypotension). *Am. J. Cardiol.* 52:221, 1983.
223. Cercek, B., Lew, A. S., Laramee, P., et al. Time course and characteristics of ventricular arrhythmias following reperfusion in acute myocardial infarction. *Am. J. Cardiol.* 60:214, 1987.
224. Goldberg, S., Greenspon, A. J., Urban, P. I., et al. Reperfusion arrhythmia: A marker of restoration of antegrade flow during intracoronary thrombolysis for acute myocardial infarction. *Am. Heart J.* 105: 26, 1983.
225. Gorgels, A. P., Vos, M. A., Letsch, I. S., et al. Usefulness of the accelerated idioventricular rhythm as a marker for myocardial necrosis and reperfusion during thrombolytic therapy in acute myocardial infarction. *Am. J. Cardiol.* 61:231, 1988.
226. Corr, P. B., and Witkowski, F. X. Potential electrophysiologic mechanisms responsible for dysrhythmias associated with reperfusion of ischemic myocardium. *Circulation* 68(Suppl I):16, 1983.
227. Fujimoto, T., Peter, T., Hamamoto, H., et al. Electrophysiological observations on ventricular tachyarrhythmias following reperfusion. *Am. Heart J.* 105:201, 1983.
228. Garabedian, H. D., Gold, H. K., Yasuda, T., et al. Detection of coronary artery reperfusion with creatine kinase-MB determinations during thrombolytic therapy: Correlation with acute angiography. *J. Am. Coll. Cardiol.* 11:729, 1988.
229. Blanke, H., von Hardenberg, D., Cohen, M., et al. Patterns of creatine kinase release during acute myocardial infarction after nonsurgical reperfusion: Comparison with conventional treatment and correlation with infarct size. *J. Am. Coll. Cardiol.* 3:675, 1984.
230. Van der Laarse, A., Vermeer, F., Hermens, W. T., et al. Effects of early intracoronary streptokinase on infarct size estimated from cumulative enzyme release and on enzyme release rate: A randomized trial of 533 patients with acute myocardial infarction. *Am. Heart J.* 112:672, 1986.
231. Ellis, A. K., Little, T., Masud, A. Z., et al. Early

noninvasive detection of successful reperfusion in patients with acute myocardial infarction. *Circulation* 78:1352, 1988.

232. Laperche, T., Steg, P. G., Benessiano, J., et al. Patterns of myoglobin and MM creatine kinase isoforms release early after intravenous thrombolysis or direct percutaneous transluminal coronary angioplasty for acute myocardial infarction, and implications for the early noninvasive diagnosis of reperfusion. *Am. J. Cardiol.* 70:1129, 1992.
233. Devries, S. R., Sobel, B. E., and Abendschein, D. R. Early detection of myocardial reperfusion by assay of plasma MM-creatine kinase isoforms in dogs. *Circulation* 74:567, 1986.
234. Puleo, P. R., and Perryman, M. B. Noninvasive detection of reperfusion in acute myocardial infarction based on plasma activity of creatine kinase MB subforms. *J. Am. Coll. Cardiol.* 17(5):1047, 1991.
235. Herlitz, J., Hjalmarson, A., and Waldenstrom, J. Time lapse from estimated onset of acute myocardial infarction to peak serum enzyme activity. *Clin. Cardiol.* 7:433, 1984.
236. Roberts, R., and Ishikawa, Y. Enzymatic estimation of infarct size during reperfusion. *Circulation* 68(Suppl 1):83, 1983.
237. Habib, G. B., Heibig, J., Forman, S. A., et al. Influence of coronary collateral vessels on myocardial infarct size in humans. *Circulation* 83:739, 1991.
238. Hohnloser, S. H., Zabel, M., Kasper, W., et al. Assessment of coronary artery patency after thrombolytic therapy: Accurate prediction utilizing the combined analysis of three noninvasive markers. *J. Am. Coll. Cardiol.* 18:44, 1991.
239. Downie, A. C., Frost, P. G., Fielden, P., et al. Bedside measurement of creatine kinase to guide thrombolysis on the coronary care unit. *Lancet* 341:452, 1993.
240. Lewis, B. S., Ganz, W., Laramee, P., et al. Usefulness of a rapid initial increase in plasma creatine kinase activity as a marker of reperfusion during thrombolytic therapy acute myocardial infarction. *Am. J. Cardiol.* 62:20, 1988.

26. Tissue-type Plasminogen Activator in Acute Myocardial Infarction

Douglas E. Vaughan, Eugene R. Passamani, and Joseph Loscalzo

Tissue-type plasminogen activator (t-PA) is a serine protease found in trace concentrations in plasma. Endothelial cells appear to be the primary sites of synthesis and secretion of t-PA, and the liver is the principal clearance site of circulating t-PA. Although t-PA is a relatively inefficient plasminogen activator in solution, its activity is markedly enhanced by the presence of fibrin. This property prompted the efforts to develop t-PA as a pharmacologic agent and to apply it to the treatment of acute myocardial infarction.

Properties of t-PA

Intravascular clot formation (hemostasis) and dissolution (fibrinolysis) are finely balanced processes; pathophysiologic accentuation of either mechanism can result in vascular occlusion from thrombosis or hemorrhage, respectively. The molecular systems underlying these processes are quite similar in that each requires the activation of a key protease from an inert precursor, which in the case of thrombus formation is thrombin and in the case of thrombolysis is plasmin. Under physiologic conditions, the presence of specific circulating inhibitors of these two proteases limits their activities to the vicinity of the clot [1]. Endogenous or exogenous factors can lead to the production of excessive quantities of thrombin or plasmin, which in turn can trigger significant distortions of normal function of both the clotting and clot-dissolving systems.

t-PA is the most important activator of the fibrinolytic system in the circulation and is synthesized as a 72-kilodalton single-chain polypeptide composed of 527 amino acids. The primary structure of the protein is illustrated in Figure 26-1. This plasminogen activator has several distinct functional domains, and the unique structure and properties of the molecule have been extensively reviewed [2]. The aminoterminus of the protein is the location of domains that possess affinity for fibrin, including the second kringle domain (K_2) and the fibronectin-like finger domain (F). The carboxyterminal portion of the protein contains the serine protease active site, which is capable of converting plasminogen to plasmin by cleaving the Arg_{560}-Val_{561} bond. The property of t-PA that distinguishes it from other plasminogen activators is that its enzymatic activity is greatly enhanced by the presence of fibrin [3]. The enhancement of t-PA activity by fibrin appears to be the result of a conformational change in t-PA itself, in plasminogen, or in both molecules, simultaneously brought about by their binding to fibrin. These changes in protein conformation and affinity induce a nearly 1000-fold increase in the catalytic efficiency of t-PA.

The t-PA that has been used in clinical studies and more recently in clinical practice is produced by recombinant techniques [4]. The generic name for t-PA is alteplase, and this agent is produced by several manufacturers throughout the world, although most available information is based on studies performed with Activase, manufactured by Genentech, Inc. (San Francisco, CA). The molecular weight of the recombinant product is slightly less than the naturally occurring substance, and the specific activity of the drug is approximately 500,000 U/mg. The first human studies involved the administration of a preparation of t-PA that was predominantly double-chain in structure. For the last several years, production methods have changed and yield a predominantly single-chain form of t-PA, which is the form available for clinical use in the U.S. A

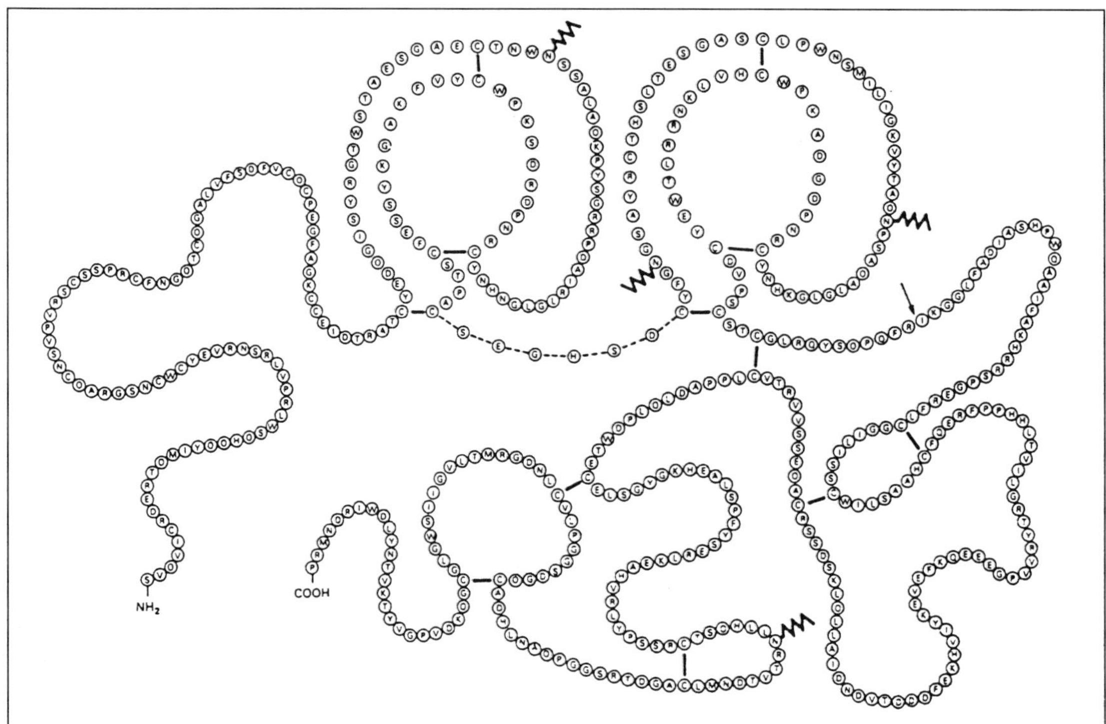

Fig. 26-1
Primary structure of the t-PA protein.

two-chain form of t-PA is available in Europe and has been applied in clinical investigation, as well; this form of t-PA has been given the generic name duteplase and is manufactured by Burroughs-Wellcome, Inc. (London, U.K.).

Under normal circumstances, the clearance of t-PA from plasma is quite rapid and its initial half-life is approximately 5 minutes in duration. The liver plays the key role in the clearance of t-PA from the circulation and, at present, two clearance mechanisms have been described. These include a protein-specific uptake system in hepatic parenchymal cells and a mannose-specific uptake system in hepatic endothelial and Kupffer cells [5]. Even though t-PA has a short life in plasma, there is evidence that fibrinolytic activity continues for hours after the administration of the drug [6], presumably because of retained plasminogen activator activity on the surface of a thrombus, gradual release into the circulation of t-PA initially bound to specific t-PA receptors on the surface of vascular endothelial cells [7], and the longer plasma half-life of plasmin itself.

Clinical Trials

Reperfusion Trials

In clinical trials, t-PA has been shown to be a useful thrombolytic agent in patients with acute myocardial infarction and in 1987 was approved by the Food and Drug Administration (FDA) for use. Its approval was based on studies demonstrating that administration of t-PA was capable of improving ventricular function and reducing the incidence of congestive heart failure in patients with acute myocardial infarction.

Most of the early studies in patients with acute myocardial infarction examined the efficacy of t-PA in opening obstructed coronary arteries and did not examine its effects on mortality or on the preservation of ventricular function. A number of relatively small clinical trials performed over the last several years were designed to demonstrate that t-PA can re-establish blood flow in occluded coronary arteries. This objective was viewed to be a fundamental requirement after the pathophysiologic relationship between coronary artery thrombosis and myocardial infarction was established in the 1980s by DeWood [8]. In reviewing the literature on coronary thrombolysis, it is necessary to distinguish "patency trials" from "recanalization trials" [9]. In patency trials, coronary angiography is performed either during or after the administration of thrombolytic therapy; no baseline angiographic data are available in these trials. By contrast, in recanalization trials, patients with angiographically documented occlusion of infarct-related vessels are selected for thrombolytic therapy, subsequently treated, and subjected to a second angiographic study after thrombolytic therapy is administered. Results of these trials have been summarized and reviewed on multiple occasions and consistently demonstrate that t-PA can induce reperfusion in occluded coronary arteries in approximately 69 percent of patients who are treated with the agent [9–11]. Clinical trials have also confirmed the efficacy of t-PA in promoting the patency of infarct-related arteries; in over 1500 patients, the 90-minute patency rate for t-PA approached 75 percent [12]. The cumulative data that are available at present with regard to patency suggest that t-PA is a slightly superior agent at achieving patency at 90 minutes than is streptokinase. In nearly 30 angiographic studies, the coronary patency at approximately 90 minutes following streptokinase treatment appears to be approximately 50 percent. The relative advantage of t-PA in re-establishing coronary artery patency appears to diminish with time, and other trials have shown no significant difference in patency between t-PA-treated and anisoylated plasminogen streptokinase activator complex (APSAC)-treated patients at 24 hours or at 7 days [12].

In the area of reperfusion, there are two widely referenced trials that are now considered major milestones in the development of t-PA as a thrombolytic agent. In the Thrombolysis in Myocardial Infarction (TIMI-I) Trial the efficacy of 80 mg of t-PA given intravenously was compared with that of 1.5 million units of streptokinase in a double-blind, randomized study of 290 patients with acute myocardial infarction [13]. This trial was conducted under the auspices of the National Heart, Lung, and Blood Institute. Patients were treated on average nearly 5 hours after the onset of pain, and all patients underwent pretreatment coronary angiograms; thus, this is a reperfusion or recanalization trial. Ninety minutes after the start of therapy, the patients treated with t-PA had nearly twice the frequency of reperfused infarct-related arteries than did those treated with streptokinase (62 percent versus 31 percent, respectively). In a similar trial conducted by the European Cooperative Study Group (ECSG), the efficacy of t-PA was compared with that of streptokinase in establishing coronary artery patency [14]. The trial randomized over 400 patients and reported a 90-minute patency rate for the t-PA group of approximately 70 percent, and a 90-minute patency rate of 56 percent for the streptokinase-treated group.

Left Ventricular Function Trials

Two major placebo-controlled trials of t-PA that were designed to examine left ventricular (LV) function as a primary endpoint have demonstrated substantial benefit related to the administration of the plasminogen activator. White and colleagues [15] randomized 136 patients who presented with ST segment elevation within 2 1/2 hours of the onset of chest pain. The mean time from onset of chest pain to initiation of intravenous therapy was 1.9 hours in the patients with a first myocardial infarction. The left ventricular ejection fraction (LVEF), determined by contrast left ventriculography 3 weeks from the time of infarction, was 62 percent in patients treated with t-PA versus 54 percent in the patients treated with placebo. In a similar placebo-controlled trial, investigators at Johns Hopkins University [16] randomized 138 patients with chest pain and ST elevation to t-PA or placebo. LVEF determined by radionuclide ventriculography at the time of hospital discharge, was 54 percent in the t-PA patients versus 48 percent in placebo patients. These two placebo-controlled trials demonstrated that t-PA is an effective agent in preserving LV function following acute myocardial infarction and were important factors in the November 1987 FDA decision to approve t-PA for use in patients with acute myocardial infarction.

More recently, there have been 11 direct comparative trials designed to assess the relative efficacy of various thrombolytic agents in preserving ventricular function. The results of these trials have been summarized by Topol [12] with the critical finding that no trial showed a significant difference in EF among thrombolytic agents or strategies.

Mortality Trials

The beneficial effect of thrombolytic therapy in reducing mortality following myocardial infarction was convincingly demonstrated in the landmark Gruppo Italino per lo Studio della Streptochinas: nell'Infarto Miocardico (GISSI-I) trial [17]. This trial showed an 18 percent reduction in mortality for patients who received intravenous streptokinase compared with those who received placebo among nearly 12,000 patients. These findings were confirmed by the ISIS-2 Trial [18] in which 17,000 patients showed a nearly 23 percent reduction in mortality after treatment with streptokinase. Two trials have been performed thus far that demonstrate the efficacy of t-PA in improving survival when compared with placebo treatment. In the Anglo-Scandinavian Study of Early Thrombolysis (ASSET) [19], patients were considered for inclusion in the study if the trial medication could be instituted within 5 hours of the onset of chest pain. This trial demonstrated a reduction in mortality of 26 percent at 1 month with t-PA treatment, with mortality rates of 7.2 percent and 9.8 percent in the t-PA and placebo groups, respectively.

The relative superiority of t-PA in establishing coronary artery patency prompted major discussion with regard to the values and benefits of currently available thrombolytic agents, in particular, streptokinase versus t-PA. This discussion has triggered interest worldwide and has led to the performance of three extremely large clinical trials that have been designed to compare the relative efficacy of these commonly used thrombolytic agents in terms of mortality. The GISSI-2 trial [20] and its international extension [21] examined over 20,000 patients with acute myocardial infarction within 6 hours of the onset of symptoms. Patients were enrolled and randomized to receive either streptokinase (1.5 million units over 60 minutes) or t-PA (100 mg over 3 hours). All patients were given aspirin (325 mg daily) for the first month after hospitalization and were also randomly assigned to receive either subcutaneous heparin (12,500 U bid) or no heparin. This trial was designed to compare mortality between the treatment regimens at 35 days. Overall, there was no statistically significant difference in mortality in the t-PA and the streptokinase treatment groups (9.6 percent versus 9.2 percent).

These findings were essentially confirmed by the Third International Study of Infarct Survival (ISIS-3) [22]. This trial involved a comparison of all three thrombolytic agents that are currently available: streptokinase, t-PA, and APSAC. In this study, over 41,000 patients were randomly assigned to streptokinase (1.5 million units over 1 hour), t-PA (duteplase, 0.6 million U/kg body weight over 4 hours), and APSAC (30 units over 3 minutes). In addition, patients were randomly assigned to receive either subcutaneous heparin (12,500 U bid for 1 week) starting 4 hours after randomization or no heparin. All patients also received aspirin at a dose of 162.5 mg daily. The ISIS-3 trial showed no difference in mortality rates among the three thrombolytic arms. Taken together, these two trials (GISSI-2 and ISIS-3) included more than 47,000 patients who were randomly assigned to receive either streptokinase or t-PA. The overall mortality rates for the two agents at 35 days, based on the pooled information from these two trials, is 10 percent [23].

In early 1993, a third trial was completed that compared an accelerated dose of t-PA to streptokinase for effects on mortality following myocardial infarction. This trial, the Global Utilization of Streptokinase and Tissue Plasminogen Activator to Treat Occluded Arteries (GUSTO-1) [24], involved the random assignment of over 41,000 patients within 6 hours of acute myocardial infarction to one of four treatment regimens: (1) streptokinase combined with intravenous (IV) heparin; (2) streptokinase combined with subcutaneous heparin; (3) accelerated dose t-PA combined with IV heparin; and (4) accelerated t-PA combined with streptokinase and IV heparin. These investigators reported a 1-month mortality rate of 6.3 percent for the accelerated t-PA plus IV heparin group. This represents a significant reduction in overall mortality when compared with that seen in the streptokinase plus subcutaneous heparin group (7.2 percent), the streptokinase plus IV heparin group (7.4 percent), and the accelerated t-PA plus streptokinase and IV heparin group (7.0 percent).

With regard to complications, t-PA has some distinct advantages and disadvantages when compared to other thrombolytic agents. In contrast with streptokinase, which provokes hypotension in 5 to

10 percent of patients [22], t-PA has considerably fewer hemodynamic effects. Bleeding remains a significant problem in patients treated with t-PA in spite of the relative selectivity of this agent for fibrin. At pharmacologic doses, t-PA is not exclusively fibrin-selective and does result in some activation of circulating plasminogen. For these reasons, successful coronary thrombolysis may be complicated by bleeding from sites of recent vascular puncture or trauma. All patients who receive t-PA or other thrombolytic agents must, therefore, be carefully monitored for bleeding from sites where the vascular tree has been invaded.

A more worrisome complication associated with the administration of t-PA is stroke. In the GISSI-2 trial [20, 21], there was a small but statistically significant excess of total strokes associated with t-PA compared to streptokinase (1.33 percent versus 0.94 percent, respectively; $p = .008$). In the ISIS-3 trial [22], patients assigned to streptokinase had fewer total strokes and intracranial bleeds than did those assigned to the t-PA arm. When the ISIS-3 and GISSI-2 data for streptokinase and t-PA are combined, the total stroke rate for t-PA is 1.4 percent versus 1.0 percent for streptokinase ($p < .001$) [22]. This trend toward a higher stroke rate was also seen in the GUSTO-1 trial in which the group of patients treated with accelerated dose t-PA plus IV heparin had a stroke rate of 1.55 percent compared with a rate of 1.22 percent in the group treated with streptokinase plus subcutaneous heparin [23, 24].

Adjunctive Therapy

A great deal of effort has been expended in recent years in identifying and refining the types of adjunctive therapies that are appropriate for administration to patients who receive thrombolytic treatment with t-PA. The use of aspirin and heparin as adjuncts to t-PA in the setting of acute myocardial infarction remains controversial. One of the most frequently tendered explanations for the equivalent effect of streptokinase and t-PA on mortality has been ascribed to the failure of the GISSI-2 and ISIS-3 trials to include high-dose IV heparin after treatment with t-PA [12]. There are some data to suggest that IV heparin increases the coronary artery patency rate in patients treated with t-PA. In a study of 83 patients treated with t-PA with or without IV heparin, initial angiograms showed coronary patency in a higher proportion of patients who received heparin than in those who did not (71 percent versus 43 percent, respectively; $p = .015$) [25]. Many of the patients enrolled in this study were not treated with aspirin. The other trial that is widely quoted as evidence supporting the requirement for IV heparin following treatment with t-PA is the Heparin-Aspirin Reperfusion Trial (HART) [26]. This trial compared t-PA plus early IV heparin to t-PA plus 80 mg aspirin. Coronary artery patency rates, determined approximately 18 hours after therapy, were higher in the heparin than in the aspirin group (82 percent versus 52 percent; $p < .001$). There are, however, some conflicting data on this issue. A trial of 241 patients performed by the National Heart Foundation compared 1-week patency rates in patients treated with t-PA and IV heparin to t-PA and aspirin (300 mg aspirin plus dipyridamole, 300 mg daily, for a week) [27]. This trial showed no difference in coronary artery patency rates between groups.

Similar results were reported in two additional trials that examined the contribution of heparin in maintaining coronary artery patency in patients treated with t-PA and full-dose aspirin. In these trials (TAMI-3 and ECSG-VI), the comparative coronary artery patency rates in patients treated with or without IV heparin and t-PA are relatively comparable [28, 29]. Thus, the data available at this time are not overwhelmingly convincing that patients treated with t-PA require IV heparin following therapy to maintain coronary artery patency.

In contrast, the benefit of aspirin in combination with thrombolytic therapy is now very well accepted [30, 31]. The role of aspirin in the treatment of patients with acute myocardial infarction was established best by the ISIS-2 trial [18] in which patients treated with aspirin showed a 23 percent reduction in total mortality compared with the placebo group. This outcome compared quite favorably with the reduction in mortality with streptokinase alone (25 percent), and the combination of aspirin and streptokinase resulted in a 42 percent reduction in overall mortality; the effects of aspirin and streptokinase are largely additive in terms of reducing mortality following myocardial infarction. Unfortunately, similar studies with regard to the role of aspirin in combination with t-PA have not been performed. However, based on the results of the ISIS-2 trial, the administration of aspirin to patients with acute myocardial infarction has been widely accepted into clinical practice and is generally recommended in the absence of clinical contraindications. This conclusion represents an extrapolation of existing data, however, and some concern remains that the administration of aspirin with t-PA may enhance the rate of hemorrhagic complications following therapy. In fact, in animal models of thrombolysis, the combined administration of t-PA and aspirin resulted in a marked reduction in platelet function and a prolongation of bleeding time much greater than that produced by either agent alone [32]. This prohemorrhagic effect has also been noted in some patients who received a combination of t-PA and aspirin and experienced bleeding complications after therapy [33].

Recent Developments in t-PA Therapy

In 1989, Neuhaus and colleagues reported the enhanced clinical efficacy of a "front-loaded," accelerated regimen of t-PA in the treatment of patients with acute myocardial infarction [34]. This regimen differs from the standard regimen of t-PA, and several important aspects are summarized in Figure 26-2. In terms of clinical efficacy, defined as angiographic patency at 90 minutes, the accelerated regimen offers nearly 20 percent improvement over the standard regimen. The improved efficacy of the regimen was confirmed in a larger trial (the rt-PA–APSAC Patency Study [TAPS]) that compared APSAC to t-PA with the accelerated regimen; the accelerated t-PA regimen provided 90-minute patency rates greater than 80 percent [35]. This value approximates the optimal, expected rate of thrombolysis, given that thrombi are identified in 80 to 85 percent of patients with acute myocardial infarction. The front-loaded, accelerated regimen of t-PA produced maximal levels of the drug in plasma of approximately 4 μg/ml after the bolus, and plasma levels greater than 3 μg/ml were maintained during the first 30 minutes of the infusion [36]. These values are approximately 30 to 50 percent higher than those achieved with the standard dosage regimens of t-PA. Plasma levels of this magnitude are likely to reduce any attenuating effects of plasminogen activator inhibitor-1 (PAI-1) on t-PA activity in plasma and may, therefore, contribute to the improved patency rates reported with accelerated infusions [37].

The derived pharmacokinetic variables for the front-loaded, accelerated regimens of t-PA are nearly identical with those published for the standard regimen, indicating that the hepatic t-PA clearance mechanisms have the capacity to deal with the elevated plasma levels that accompany accelerated drug administration. Despite the increased plasma levels of t-PA produced by the front-loaded regimen, the systemic effects of the enzyme, as mea-

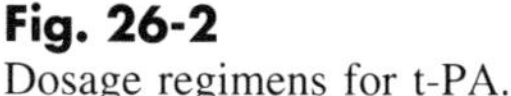

Fig. 26-2
Dosage regimens for t-PA.

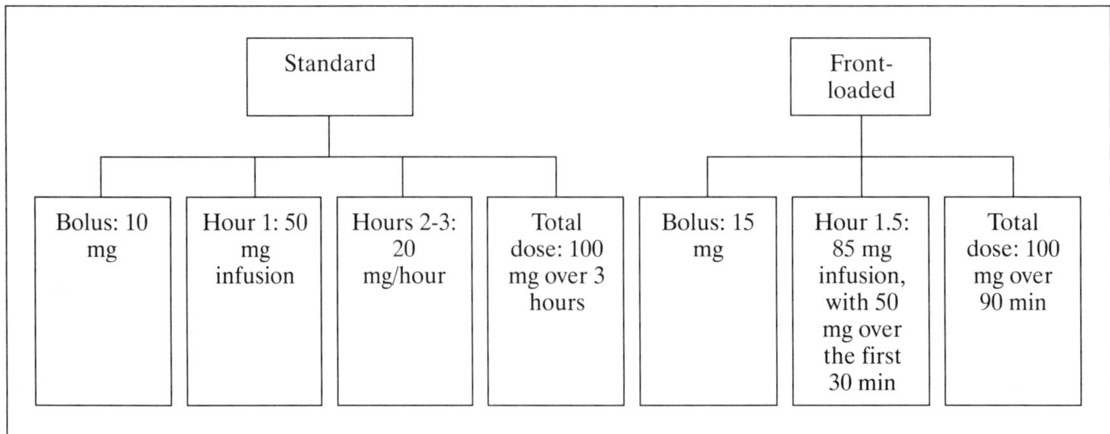

sured by decrements in circulating levels of fibrinogen, plasminogen, and alpha$_2$-antiplasmin, are similar to those obtained with the standard dosage regimen. This finding confirms that t-PA is a fibrin-specific agent, and is a relatively inefficient activator of circulating plasminogen.

New Directions

Efforts are continuing to develop new forms of t-PA that are safer and more efficacious than the currently available forms of the agent. These efforts include many different approaches, but fundamentally involve the development of new forms of the protein. At this point, only one of the second-generation forms of t-PA has been tested in clinical trials (Boehringer-Ingelheim [Ingelheim, Germany], analysis of trial results pending). Some of the more interesting forms of t-PA that are being developed include a t-PA deletion mutant that has a longer circulating half-life in plasma [38]. Another particularly interesting form of t-PA involves the development of a mutated protein form that lacks secondary binding sites for the specific inhibitor of t-PA in plasma (i.e., PAI-1) [39]. As noted earlier, there are some data supporting the hypothesis that PAI-1 can attenuate the fibrinolytic effects of t-PA [37]. Thus, the development of mutant forms of t-PA resistant to inhibition by this serpin may show improved efficacy over standard forms of t-PA, but this hypothesis remains to be tested.

References

1. Collen, D. On the regulation and control of fibrinolysis. *Thromb. Haemost.* 43:77, 1980.
2. Rijken, D. C., and Groeneveld, E. Isolation and functional characterization of the heavy and light chains of tissue-type plasminogen activator. *J. Biol. Chem.* 261:3098, 1986.
3. Hoylaerts, M., Rijken, D. C., Lijnen, H. R., et al. Kinetics of the activation of plasminogen by human tissue plasminogen activator: Role of fibrin. *J. Biol. Chem.* 257:2912, 1982.
4. Pennica, D., Holmes, W. E., Kohr, W. J., et al. Cloning and expression of human tissue-type plasminogen activator cDNA in *E. coli. Nature* 301:214, 1983.
5. Kuiper, J., Oher, M., Rijken, D. C., et al. Characterization of the interaction *in vivo* of tissue-type plasminogen activator with liver cells. *J. Biol. Chem.* 263:18220, 1988.
6. Eisenberg, P. R., Sherman, L. A., Tiefenbrunn, A. J., et al. Sustained fibrinolysis after administration of t-PA despite its short half-life in the circulation. *Thromb. Haemost.* 57:35, 1987.
7. Hajjar, K. A., Harpel, P. C., and Nachman, R. L. Binding of tissue plasminogen activator to cultured human endothelial cells. *J. Clin. Invest.* 80:1712, 1988.
8. DeWood, M. A., Spores, J., Notske, R., et al. Prevalence of total coronary occlusion during the early hours of transmural myocardial infarction. *N. Engl. J. Med.* 303:897, 1980.
9. Verstraete, M. Thrombolytic treatment in acute myocardial infarction. *Circulation* 82:II-96, 1990.
10. Loscalzo, J., and Braunwald, E. Tissue plasminogen activator. *N. Engl. J. Med.* 319:925, 1988.
11. Collen, D., Lijnen, H. R., Todd, P. A., et al. Tissue-type plasminogen activator. A review of its pharmacology and therapeutic use as a thrombolytic agent. *Drugs* 38:346, 1989.
12. Topol, E. J. Which thrombolytic agent should we choose? *Prog. Cardiovasc. Dis.* 24:165, 1991.
13. The TIMI Study Group. The thrombolysis in myocardial (TIMI) trial: Phase I findings. *N. Engl. J. Med.* 312:932, 1985.
14. Verstraete, M., Bernard, R., Borg, M., et al. Randomized trial of intravenous recombinant tissue-type plasminogen activator versus intravenous streptokinase in acute myocardial infarction: Report from the European Cooperative Study Group for Recombinant Tissue-type Plasminogen Activator. *Lancet* 1: 842, 1985.
15. White, H. D., Norris, R. M., Brown, M. A., et al. Effect of intravenous streptokinase on left ventricular function and early survival after acute myocardial infarction. *N. Engl. J. Med.* 317:850, 1987.
16. Guerci, A., Gerstenblith, G., Brinker, J. A., et al. A randomized trial of intravenous tissue plasminogen activator for acute myocardial infarction with subsequent randomization to elective coronary angioplasty. *N. Engl. J. Med.* 317:1613, 1987.
17. Gruppo Italiano per lo Studio della Streptochinasi nell'Infarto Miocardico (GISSI). Effectiveness of intravenous thrombolytic treatment in acute myocardial infarction. *Lancet* 1:397, 1986.
18. ISIS-2 Collaborative Group. Randomized trial of intravenous streptokinase, oral aspirin, both, or neither among 17,187 cases of suspected acute myocardial infarction: ISIS-2. *Lancet* 2:349, 1988.
19. Wilcox, R. G., von der Lippe, G., Olsson, C. G., et al. Trial of tissue plasminogen activator for mortality reduction in acute myocardial infarction. *Lancet* 2: 525, 1988.
20. Gruppo Italiano per lo Studio della Sopravvivenza nell'Infarto Miocardico (GISSI-II). GISSI-2: A factorial randomised trial of alteplase versus streptokinase and heparin versus no heparin among 12,490 patients with acute myocardial infarction. *Lancet* 336:65, 1990.
21. The International Study Group. In-hospital mortality

and clinical course of 20,891 patients with suspected acute myocardial infarction randomised between alteplase and streptokinase with or without heparin. *Lancet* 336:71, 1990.
22. ISIS-3 (Third International Study of Infarct Survival Collaborative Group). ISIS-3: A randomized comparison of streptokinase vs. tissue plasminogen activator vs. anistreplase and of aspirin and heparin vs. heparin alone among 41,299 cases of suspected acute myocardial infarction. *Lancet* 339: 753, 1992.
23. Ridker, P. M., Marder, V. J., and Hennekens, C. H. Large-scale trials of thrombolytic therapy for acute myocardial infarction: GISSI-2, ISIS-3, and GUSTO-1. *Ann. Int. Med.* 1993 (In press).
24. The GUSTO Investigators. An international randomized trial comparing four thrombolytic strategies for acute myocardial infarction. *N. Engl. J. Med.* 329: 673, 1993.
25. Bleich, S. D., Nichols, T. C., Schumacher, P. R., et al. Effect of heparin on coronary arterial patency after thrombolysis with tissue-plasminogen activator in acute myocardial infarction. *Am. J. Cardiol.* 66: 1412, 1990.
26. Hsia, J., Hamilton, W. P., Kleirman, N., et al. A comparison between heparin and low-dose aspirin as adjunctive therapy with tissue plasminogen activator for acute myocardial infarction. *N. Engl. J. Med.* 323:1433, 1990.
27. Thompson, P. L., Aylward, P. E., Federman, J., et al. A randomized trial of intravenous heparin with oral aspirin and dipyridamole 24 hours after recombinant tissue-type plasminogen activator for acute myocardial infarction. *Circulation* 83:1534 1991.
28. Topol, E. J., George, B. S., Keieaikes, D. J., et al. A randomized controlled trial of intravenous tissue plasminogen activator and early intravenous heparin in acute myocardial infarction. *Circulation* 79:281, 1989.
29. deBono, D. P., Simoons, M. L., Tijssen, J., et al. The effect of early intravenous heparin on coronary patency, infarct size, and bleeding complications after alteplase thrombolysis: Results of a randomized double-blind European Cooperative Study Group trial. *B. Heart J.* 67:122, 1992.
30. Ridker, P. M., Hebert, P. R., Fuster, V., et al. Are aspirin and heparin justified as adjuncts to thrombolytic therapy for acute myocardial infarction? *Lancet* 341:1574, 1993.
31. Roux, S., Christeller, S., and Ludin, E. Effects of aspirin on coronary reocclusion and recurrent ischemia after thrombolysis: a meta-analysis. *J. Am. Coll. Cardiol.* 19:671, 1992.
32. Vaughan, D. E., Declerck, P. J., De Mol, M., et al. Recombinant plasminogen activator inhibitor-1 (PAI-1) reverses the bleeding tendency associated with combined administration of tissue-type plasminogen activator and aspirin in rabbits. *J. Clin. Invest.* 84:586, 1989.
33. Gimple, L. W., Gold, H. K., Leinbach, L., et al. Correlation between template bleeding times and spontaneous bleeding during treatment of acute myocardial infarction with recombinant tissue-type plasminogen activator. *Circulation* 80:581, 1989.
34. Neuhaus, K.-L., Feuerer, W., Jeep-Tedde, S., et al. Improved thrombolysis with a modified dose regimen of recombinant tissue-type plasminogen activator. *J. Am. Coll. Cardiol.* 14:1566, 1989.
35. Neuhaus, K.-L., von Essen, R., Tebbe, U., et al. Improved thrombolysis in acute myocardial infarction with front-loaded administration of alteplase: results of the rt-PA–APSAC patency study (TAPS). *J. Am. Coll. Cardiol.* 19:8853, 1992.
36. Tanswell, P., Tebbe, U., Neuhaus, K.-L., et al. Pharmacokinetics and fibrin specificity of alteplase during accelerated infusions in acute myocardial infarction. *J. Am. Coll. Cardiol.* 19:1071, 1992.
37. Lucore, C. L., and Sobel, B. E. Interactions of tissue-type plasminogen activator with plasma inhibitors and their pharmacologic implications. *Circulation* 77:660, 1988.
38. Collen, D. Toward improved thrombolytic therapy. *Lancet* 342:34, 1993.
39. Keyt, B. A., Paoini, N. F., Refino, C. J., et al. A faster-acting, and more potent form of tissue plasminogen activator. *Proc. Natl. Acad. Sci. USA* 91: 3670, 1994.

27. The Open Artery Hypothesis

K. Michael Zabel and Robert M. Califf

The last three decades have seen dramatic changes in the approach to the patient with acute myocardial infarction (AMI). During the 1960s, the development of specialized intensive care units with continuous cardiac monitoring led to a marked reduction in mortality associated with primary ventricular arrhythmias, the most common cause of early death after AMI. The expanding use of antiarrhythmic agents such as lidocaine and beta-blockers in the 1970s further decreased mortality due to arrhythmia. At the same time, the development of sophisticated hemodynamic monitoring techniques improved the outlook for patients developing ventricular failure. In the early 1980s evidence presented by a number of investigators, including DeWood and colleagues [1], suggested that the majority of myocardial infarctions (MI) were caused by thrombotic coronary occlusion. This discovery opened the door to the development of therapeutic measures addressing the primary problem in AMI, that of impaired myocardial blood flow, rather than simply the management of complications secondary to this impaired flow. Various types of reperfusion therapy including emergency coronary bypass surgery (CABG) [2], early percutaneous transluminal coronary angioplasty (PICA) [3], and thrombolytic agents delivered intravenously [4] or directly into the occluded coronary artery [5] have been used to attain patency of the occluded coronary artery and each has been found effective in decreasing short-term mortality for patients with AMI.

Clinical Benefit of an Open Infarct-Related Artery

Understandably, the beneficial effects observed with these approaches have been attributed chiefly to their success in re-establishing blood flow to ischemic myocardium. This assumption has been supported by dozens of studies demonstrating that improved outcome is associated with patency of the infarct-related artery following AMI. These studies initially involved patients treated conservatively, that is, without specific intervention to facilitate reperfusion. In such patients, approximately 35 percent of infarct-related coronary arteries were patent at 12 to 24 hours [1] and up to 50 percent were patent by 2 to 8 weeks [6] following infarction. In patients treated without attempted revascularization at Parkland Memorial Hospital in Dallas in the late 1970s and early 1980s, 24 percent had perfusion of the infarct artery and 76 percent had minimal or no perfusion at the time of cardiac catheterization (mean, 27 days following AMI) [7]. Although the two groups were similar in terms of age, sex, atherosclerotic risk factors, medications, and ventricular function, there was a marked decrease in unstable angina (9 percent versus 27 percent), recurrent infarction (0 percent versus 12 percent), congestive heart failure (CHF) (0 percent versus 18 percent), and mortality (0 percent versus 17 percent) in patients with patent infarct arteries compared with those having occluded arteries (mean follow-up, 52 months).

Mechanical Reperfusion

Mechanical reperfusion with CABG or angioplasty results in quicker reperfusion and a higher rate of infarct-artery patency than conservative therapy. Patients with successful mechanical reperfusion have an improved outcome following AMI compared with those who have persistent occlusion of the artery. In a nonrandomized study of 382 patients assigned to conservative therapy or emergency CABG for treatment of AMI, patients receiving surgical reperfusion had a significant reduction in the incidence of sudden death and death from recurrent infarction as compared with the conventional treatment group [8]. The difference in morbid events was seen in spite of the similarity between the surgical and conservative groups with regard to age, gender, location of infarction, number of diseased vessels, and Killip class. Bernardi and Whitlow reported results of patients receiving cardiac catheterization at Cleveland Clinic within 6 weeks of an AMI [9]. In their retrospective study, 84 percent of patients with a patent infarct artery or antegrade coronary flow had received either angioplasty or CABG. When this group was compared with patients having occlusion of the infarct artery over a follow-up period averaging 3 years, patients with a patent artery had significantly less mortality (8 percent) than those with an occluded artery (18 percent). The incidence of CHF was also less in the patients with a patent artery (11 percent versus 30 percent) as was the incidence of ventricular aneurysm, cardiogenic shock, and severe mitral regurgitation. In a multivariate analysis of this population, both left ventricular function and infarct-artery patency were independent predictors of survival.

A recent report demonstrates the relationship of a patent infarct artery to improved early survival in patients treated with direct angioplasty for AMI [10]. In this study patients with PTCA resulting in a patent infarct-related artery had a dramatic decrease in hospital mortality as compared with patients having persistent or recurrent occlusion of the artery following PTCA (5 percent versus 39 percent). It is still not clear, however, whether the increased mortality following failed PTCA was due to a closed infarct artery or to unrecognized factors that are themselves associated with a higher risk of angioplasty failure (e.g., an enhanced thrombotic tendency). More study is needed to support the hypothesis that a patent infarct-related artery following successful mechanical reperfusion decreases mortality and serious morbidity in postinfarction patients.

Thrombolytic Therapy

In spite of the success of mechanical reperfusion techniques for achieving patency of the infarct artery and improving outcome in selected patients with AMI, intravenous thrombolytic agents are the most readily available and commonly used technique to enhance coronary recanalization. There is no longer any question that the use of IV thrombolysis significantly decreases both short- and long-term mortality in patients with AMI [11, 12]. As noted with mechanical reperfusion techniques, there is a large body of evidence tying the beneficial effects of IV thrombolytic agents to the restoration of flow in the infarct-related vessel. Figure 27-1 illustrates the advantage for patients discharged with an open infarct artery following thrombolytic therapy. In each of the randomized trials [13–16], there was improvement in 1-year mortality for the patients with a patent artery versus those with an occluded infarct-related artery. This difference was statistically significant in all but the Thrombolysis Myocardial Infarction-I (TIMI-I) study, which showed a clear trend, in the presence of a small sample size, toward benefit for patients with a patent infarct artery. Mathey and colleagues [16] demonstrated that a similar degree of benefit persists for as long as 4 years. They reported a 16 percent mortality rate at 48 months in patients with complete reperfusion following thrombolysis, compared with 37 percent mortality in those with partial or no reperfusion. In a separate report of 173 patients with AMI and single vessel coronary disease followed for an average of 4 years, 15 of 16 patients suffering cardiac death after discharge had an occluded infarct artery on predischarge angiography [17]. Furthermore, of 15 measured demographic, clinical, and angiographic variables in this group,

Fig. 27-1
Mortality at 12 months according to status of infarct artery at discharge. (Adapted from D. F. Fortin and R. M. Califf. Long-term survival from acute myocardial infarction: salutary effect of an open coronary vessel. *Am. J. Med.* 88:1N, 1990 and D. G. Mathey et al. Improved survival up to four years after early coronary thrombosis. *Am. J. Cardiol.* 61:524, 1988.)

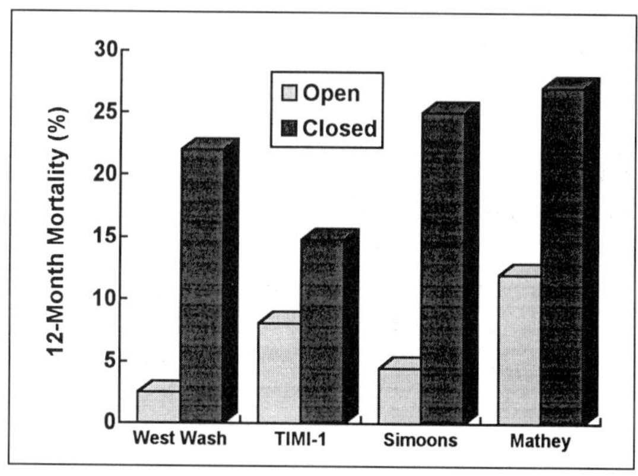

only infarct-artery patency and end-systolic volume index were independently related to survival.

Relation of Clinical Benefits to Duration of Coronary Occlusion

Although there is little disagreement that the benefits of thrombolytic agents stem from their ability to restore patency to occluded coronary arteries, there has been much debate over the specific mechanism that effects these benefits. The traditional view is that thrombolytic agents produce their beneficial effect on mortality by opening occluded coronary arteries within a time frame that allows salvage of at least a portion of jeopardized myocardium, thus resulting in improved ventricular function. Because ventricular function is closely tied to both short- and long-term mortality [18], myocardial salvage should result in a significant reduction in mortality. This model of thrombolytic benefit is strengthened by the strong inverse relationship between the clinical benefits observed following thrombolysis and the time to thrombolytic administration following coronary occlusion. For example, in the Second International Study of Infarct Survival (ISIS-2) study [12], the relative improvement in mortality for patients treated with thrombolysis 5 to 24 hours following symptom onset was 15 percent, but it was much greater (33 percent) for those treated within 4 hours of symptom onset. Patients receiving active treatment within 1 hour of symptom onset had an even more impressive 59 percent reduction in 35-day mortality. Combined data from the ISIS-2 and Gruppo Italiano per lo Studio della Streptochinasi nell'Infarto Miocardico (GISSI-I) studies regarding the improvement in mortality with IV streptokinase (SK) as a function of time-to-treatment is represented by the curve in Figure 27-2. Similar results were observed in the European Cooperative Study Group trial comparing tissue plasminogen activator (t-PA) to placebo [19]. In this trial the overall relative reduction in 3-month mortality for patients treated with t-PA within 5 hours was 35 percent while it was 59 percent for those treated within 3 hours of symptom onset.

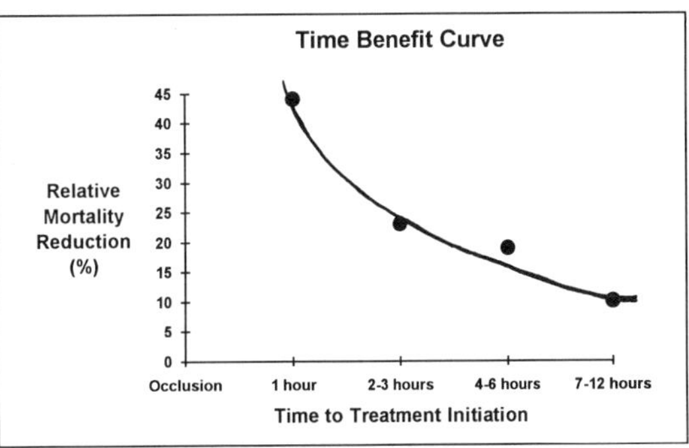

Fig. 27-2
Relative reduction in 30-day mortality in patients treated with thrombolysis compared with control patients, based on time from symptom onset to initiation of thrombolytic infusion. (Based on data from GISSI-I and ISIS-2 trials. Gruppo Italiano per lo Studio della Streptochinasi nell'Infarto Miocardico (GISSI). Effectiveness of intravenous thrombolytic treatment in acute myocardial infarction. *Lancet* 1:397, 1986 and Second International Study of Infarct Survival Collaborative Group. Randomized trial of intravenous streptokinase, oral aspirin, both, or neither among 17,187 cases of suspected acute myocardial infarction: ISIS-2. *Lancet* 2:349, 1988.)

Although intuitively appealing, the argument that the clinical benefits conferred by thrombolytic therapy are due only to myocardial salvage ignores the discrepancy between the impressive reduction in mortality and the relative lack of improved LV function in patients receiving thrombolysis. This discrepancy is typified by the experience of the Interuniversity Study Group in which 533 patients were randomized to placebo or SK [15]. Although the benefit in short-term mortality for the SK-treated patients was impressive (5 percent for SK versus 10 percent for placebo), the improvement in left ventricular ejection fraction (LVEF) was not (0.48 versus 0.44). Similarly, a study comparing IV anisoylated plasminogen streptokinase activator complex (APSAC) to heparin found a 56 percent relative reduction in short-term mortality (13 percent to 6 percent) in the APSAC group but virtually no difference in ventricular function (EF 0.53 versus 0.54) [20]. The Western Washington [5] and TIMI-I [13] trials also demonstrated marked improvement in mortality following thrombolytic therapy with minimal or no improvement in LV function. Since studies of AMI patients before the advent of thrombolysis suggest that a 10 percent absolute improvement in LVEF results in a 50 percent reduction in 1-year cardiac mortality [18], the improvements in EF noted in the above trials appear much too small to explain the substantial reduction in mortality exclusively on the basis of improved ventricular function.

Califf [21] has argued that ventricular function measurement is inherently unreliable in the postinfarction population, in part because of the large numbers of patients who die before data can be obtained or who undergo technically inadequate studies. In addition, because the group of patients with missing or inadequate contractility data mostly comprises the more seriously ill or dead patients who probably represent a group with worse LV function, such studies may provide an unreliable estimate of true ventricular function of any AMI population. Furthermore, if patients with poor LV function survive because of thrombolytic therapy, their low EF will tend to decrease the assessed EF in the thrombolytic-treated groups, adding another source of bias to the measurement.

Although mortality improvements do not correlate well with improved global ventricular function, mortality has been closely tied to the attainment of an open infarct-related artery following thrombolysis. This observation has led to the study of salvage-independent benefits of infarct-artery patency and has been strengthened by the observation that administration of thrombolytic agents late in the course of an MI results in improved patient outcome, even when therapy is given after significant myocardial salvage could be expected. In the ISIS-2 study of SK and aspirin, for example, patients receiving active therapy 5 to 12 hours following onset of AMI symptoms benefited from a decrease in 5-week cardiovascular mortality of 16 percent relative to placebo [12]. The Late Assessment of Thrombolytic Efficacy (LATE) study randomized 5700 patients presenting between 6 and 24 hours from symptom onset of AMI to either t-PA or placebo [22]. In patients presenting between 6 and 12 hours from symptom onset, the 35-day mortality was reduced by 26 percent (from 12.0 percent to 8.9 percent) among those receiving thrombolytic therapy; there was no significant benefit for those treated later than 12 hours from symptom onset. In a similar study, the Estudio Multicentrico Estreptoquinasa Republicas de America del Sur (EMERAS) group randomized 3900 patients presenting with AMI after 6 hours to either SK or placebo [23]. Although the results did not reach statistical significance, again there was a clear trend toward lower in-hospital mortality among patients receiving thrombolytic therapy 7 to 12 hours after symptom onset but no such trend for patients treated later than 12 hours. These well-designed studies demonstrate the benefit of initiating thrombolytic treatment in patients between 7 and 12 hours following the onset of symptoms in spite of the minimal myocardial salvage that can be expected from restoration of coronary flow during this relatively late period.

Table 27-1
Benefits of an open infarct-related artery, divided into "time-dependent" and "time-independent" components

TIME-DEPENDENT MECHANISMS
Myocardial salvage
Decreased infarct size
Improved ventricular function
TIME-INDEPENDENT MECHANISMS
Improved infarct healing
Decreased infarct expansion
Decreased aneurysm formation
Decreased mural thrombosis
Improved scar strength
Decreased rupture of LV
Improved electrical stability
Decreased arrhythmic death
Salvage of hibernating myocardium
Improved ventricular function
Improved collateral flow
Decreased incidence of recurrent infarction
Decreased severity of recurrent infarction

LV = left ventricle.

It is apparent that, although time-sensitive mechanisms of reperfusion (such as myocardial salvage) may explain a portion of the clinical benefits from thrombolysis, other less time-sensitive mechanisms also play a role. This observation has led some reviewers to suggest that the advantages of an open infarct artery following AMI can be divided into "time-dependent" and "time-independent" components [24]. An outline of this model is seen in Table 27-1. While we believe this classification is somewhat artificial, it nonetheless provides a useful model for the discussion of the data available to support each of these mechanisms.

Mechanisms of Clinical Benefit

Limitation of Infarct Size

Animal Models

The concept that early restoration of coronary flow can result in salvage of threatened ischemic myocardium is rooted in pathologic studies of infarction performed in animal models. Such models have demonstrated that reperfusion of a coronary artery following transient occlusion leads to a smaller infarct than that observed when the vessel is permanently obstructed [25]. The work performed by Reimer and Jennings in the mid-1970s clarified the pattern of myocyte death during an MI by providing evidence that infarction progresses in a wavefront pattern from the subendocardium to the subepicardium while the lateral extent of infarcted myocardium remains relatively constant over time [26]. The speed at which the wavefront progresses from the endocardial to epicardial surface depends on several factors, including myocardial oxygen requirement and the amount of collateral flow into the region of jeopardized tissue. In the dog model, about 50 percent of the myocardium at risk can be salvaged if reperfusion occurs 60 minutes after coronary artery ligation. This ratio decreases to about 35 percent at 3 hours and to less than 20 percent at 6 hours after ligation [26]. Similar results have been shown in dogs with experimentally induced thrombotic coronary artery occlusion and subsequent reperfusion with SK-induced thrombolysis [27]. In this model, reperfusion within 2 hours salvaged approximately 50 percent of jeopardized myocardium but reperfusion after 6 hours resulted in no significant salvage of tissue.

Results from these reperfusion models suggest a window of opportunity for the salvage of threatened myocardium in the patient presenting early in the course of AMI. Although the extent of this window cannot be extrapolated from animal models, we would expect that earlier recanalization of the infarct-associated coronary vessel would be associated with larger amounts of salvaged myocardium and ultimately with improved ventricular function. We would predict that reperfusion after some period of occlusion would not result in appreciable salvage of myocardium, recognizing that this time may differ according to a plethora of variables. Data from many trials of reperfusion therapy strongly support this theory.

Clinical Trials

The dependence of myocardial salvage on the duration of coronary occlusion has been measured in several clinical trials. The Western Washington Intravenous Streptokinase Trial [28] and the Intravenous Streptokinase in Acute Myocardial Infarction (ISAM) study [29] both demonstrated that patients who are treated within 3 hours of symptom onset have a larger LVEF than those treated later. Among patients treated with thrombolysis in the TIMI-II trial, the percentage with a normal or nearly normal predischarge EF (>0.55) was significantly greater for patients treated within 1 hour of symptoms than for those treated later [30]. Similarly, patients treated with t-PA in the National Heart Foundation of Australia trial had a gain in LV function if treated within 2 hours of symptom onset (mean EF of 0.72 versus 0.49 for patients receiving placebo) but had a much less impressive benefit if treated after 2 hours (0.57 versus 0.52) [31]. In a study of IV SK, patients treated within 90 minutes of symptom onset had a higher mean EF (0.56) than those treated after this time (0.47) [32].

In accordance with the open artery hypothesis of myocardial salvage, LV function is even more closely associated with early and sustained vessel patency than with the timing of thrombolytic treatment. In the Tissue Plasminogen Activator: Toronto (TPAT) trial the infarct size as measured by thallium scintigraphy was smaller, and the infarct-region ventricular function superior, in patients with a patent infarct artery 15 to 20 hours following treatment compared with patients having persistent occlusion of the artery [33]. Among TIMI-I patients with total occlusion of the infarct artery at baseline, only those who achieved reperfusion within 90 minutes after treatment with either SK or t-PA experienced an increase in EF before discharge [34]. These patients also had a marked improvement in regional wall motion that was not seen in the patients experiencing late reperfusion (>90 minutes following treatment) or no reperfusion. In an analysis of 542 patients studied by the Thrombolysis and Angioplasty in Myocardial Infarction (TAMI) group, Harrison and colleagues observed a modest but statistically significant improvement of LV function within 7 days of AMI in patients with a patent infarct artery at both 90 minutes and 7 days after initiation of thrombolytic therapy [35]. This was in contrast to a decrease in ventricular function over the same period in patients with delayed (> 90 minutes) or unsustained recanalization of the infarct vessel.

In an attempt to quantify the amount of myocardium amenable to salvage with reperfusion therapy, Christian and colleagues [36] used radioisotopic techniques to determine the ratio of salvaged to jeopardized myocardium in patients treated with either primary angioplasty or IV thrombolysis early in the course of AMI. Mean time to treatment was 3.7 hours in those receiving angioplasty (N = 22) and 2.8 hours in those receiving thrombolysis (N = 15). Among patients with a patent infarct artery following intervention, the mean proportion of salvaged myocardium was 50 to 60 percent of that initially at risk. No significant salvage was observed in patients with persistent occlusion of the infarct artery. This same group found that duration of coronary occlusion, degree of collateral flow during occlusion, and amount of myocardium at risk were each independently associated with final infarct size in a group of 89 patients with a first AMI [37]. This model closely replicates the basic findings of Reimer and Jennings in the animal model.

Relation of Patency to Survival

The above data provide a compelling argument in support of a beneficial effect of early reperfusion on LV function. Improved ventricular inotropy is probably the primary explanation for the time-sensitive component of improved mortality observed in patients receiving thrombolytic therapy (Fig. 27-2). One notable problem in this model of thrombolytic efficacy is the disparity between coronary patency and mortality among different thrombolytic agents. Although the patency rates of SK, APSAC, and t-PA are quite similar when measured at 3 hours or more following thrombolytic administration, most studies have shown patency rates before this time to be significantly higher with t-PA or APSAC ($\approx$70 percent at 90 minutes) compared with streptokinase ($\approx$50 percent at 90 minutes) [38]. In spite of the superiority of the newer agents in terms of early coronary patency, no difference in mortality was seen between groups treated with these agents in the randomized ISIS-3 or GISSI-2 trials, which together included over 62,000 patients [39, 40]. This observation has been used by some to discount the benefit of early coronary reperfusion and suggest that late (>3 hour) patency is responsible for the bulk of the mortality benefit attained with thrombolytic therapy.

The GUSTO Trial

It was in part to study the relative contribution of early coronary patency to post-MI mortality that the GUSTO (Global Utilization of Streptokinase and t-PA for Occluded Coronary Arteries) study was designed [41]. In this international study over 41,000 patients were enrolled at over 1000 hospitals within 6 hours of AMI symptoms and ST segment elevation. Patients were randomized into one of four thrombolytic strategies: SK, t-PA, or both thrombolytics (each of these groups also received IV heparin), or SK plus subcutaneous heparin. The primary endpoint for the trial was mortality at 30 days. In order to test the hypothesis that early coronary reperfusion results in improved clinical outcomes, the t-PA group received an accelerated dosing regimen consisting of a 15 mg bolus, followed by 0.75 mg/kg [maximum 50 mg] infusion over 30 minutes, followed by 0.50 mg/kg [maximum 35 mg] over 1 hour. This regimen had previously been shown to achieve a 90-minute patency rate of about 85 percent [42].

In order to document differences in infarct artery perfusion over time, an angiographic substudy was performed in parallel with the main mortality study [43]. This involved 2431 patients randomly assigned to one of the four reperfusion strategies and also randomized to coronary and LV angiography at 90 minutes, 180 minutes, 24 hours, or 5 to 7 days following initiation of thrombolysis. Coronary patency was defined as either TIMI flow grade 3 (normal flow) or grade 2 (vessel patency with delayed contrast entry into or out of the distal vessel). The patency rates over time (Fig. 27-3) showed no significant difference at 3 hours or more between t-PA and any other thrombolytic strategy. In contrast, there was a marked improvement in early patency (90 minutes) in the accelerated t-PA group (81 percent) compared with either SK alone (57 percent) or the combination of SK and nonaccelerated t-PA (73 percent). These differences were highly significant ($p < .001$ for t-PA versus SK, and $p < .04$ for t-PA versus combination) [43]. The relative advantage of accelerated t-PA over the other regimens was enhanced when the proportion of patients with complete reperfusion only (TIMI grade 3 flow) at 90 minutes was compared: 54 percent for t-PA versus 31 percent for SK ($p < .001$) and 38 percent for combination therapy ($p < .001$). Here, too, the benefit for accelerated t-PA was markedly diminished by 3 hours and was completely gone by 24 hours after initiation of therapy.

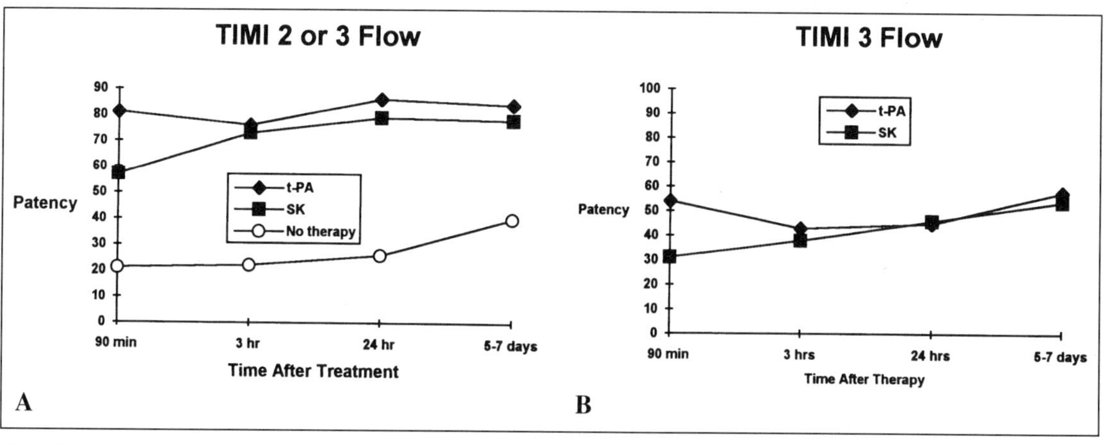

Fig. 27-3
(*A*) Percentage of patients with patency (TIMI grade 2 or 3) and (*B*) percentage of patients with normal (TIMI grade 3) flow of the infarct-related artery at various times after treatment with either intravenous t-PA or streptokinase or managed without thrombolytic therapy. (Data adapted from the GUSTO Angiographic Investigators. The effects of tissue plasminogen activator, streptokinase, or both on coronary-artery patency, ventricular function, and survival after acute myocardial infarction. *N. Engl. J. Med.* 329:1615, 1993 and C. B. Granger et al. Thrombolytic therapy for acute myocardial infarction: A review. *Drugs* 44:293, 1992.)

Table 27-2
Relation of global and regional ventricular function 5 to 7 days after AMI to infarct-related coronary flow 90 minutes after t-PA infusion

Ventricular function	TIMI flow grade 0 or 1	TIMI flow grade 2	TIMI flow grade 3
Ejection fraction	0.55	0.56	0.61
End-systolic volume index (ml/m^2)	33	30	26
Infarct-zone wall motion index	−2.6	−2.3	−1.8
No. abnormal chords	24	22	15
Preserved regional motion (%)	20	27	39

AMI = acute myocardial infarction; t-PA = tissue plasminogen activator; TIMI = Thrombolysis in Myocardial Infarction study.
Source: Adapted from the GUSTO Angiographic Investigators. The effects of tissue plasminogen activator, streptokinase, or both on coronary-artery patency, ventricular function, and survival after acute myocardial infarction. *N. Engl. J. Med.* 329:1615, 1993.

Patients having angiography at 90 minutes received repeat cardiac catheterization at 5 to 7 days postinfarction with measurement of LV function. There was a surprisingly strong correlation between the degree of infarct-artery patency at 90 minutes and measures of ventricular function at 5 to 7 days. As seen in Table 27-2, both global ventricular systolic function (measured by EF) and regional function (measured by the magnitude of depressed motion within the infarct zone and the number of chords with diminished motion) were superior in patients with complete reperfusion at 90 minutes (TIMI grade 3) as compared with those without perfusion (TIMI grades 0 or 1). For each index, the ventricular function of patients with partial reperfusion (TIMI grade 2) fell between those with no reperfusion and those with complete reperfusion. Furthermore, the relation of ventricular function and adequacy of reperfusion correlated well with the observed 30-day mortality in the angiographic substudy subjects (Fig. 27-4).

The GUSTO study was the first large clinical trial to document a difference between any of the three available thrombolytic agents [41]. It demon-

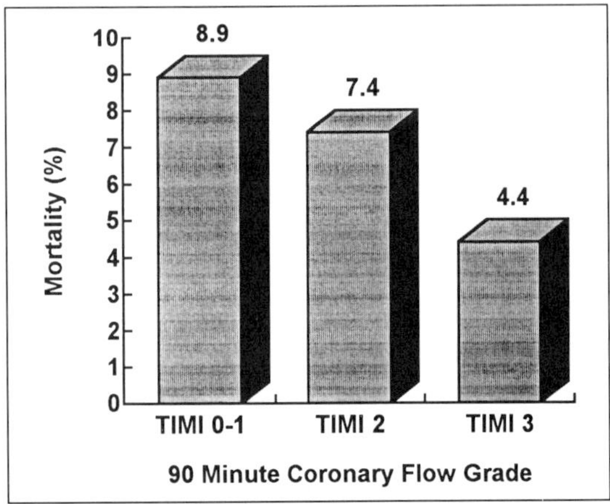

Fig. 27-4
Mortality rate at 30 days among patients with different degrees of patency as assessed by angiography 90 minutes after intravenous thrombolysis. (Data adapted from the GUSTO Angiographic Investigators. The effects of tissue plasminogen activator, streptokinase, or both on coronary-artery patency, ventricular function, and survival after acute myocardial infarction. *N. Engl. J. Med.* 329:1615, 1993.)

strated a 30-day mortality of 6.3 percent for patients treated with the accelerated t-PA regimen versus 7.3 percent ($p = .001$) for those receiving SK (there was no difference between the IV and subcutaneous heparin arms) and 7.0 percent for patients receiving the combination of SK and nonaccelerated t-PA. This improvement can be put into perspective by noting that therapy with SK (instead of placebo) in the GISSI-I trial resulted in the saving of 23 patient lives per 1000 treated. The GUSTO trial showed that an additional 10 lives in a group of 1000 may be saved if patients are treated with accelerated t-PA instead of SK.

The relative decrease in mortality of 14 percent with the use of accelerated t-PA as compared with SK mirrors the striking increase in complete early (90-minute) reperfusion with this regimen and the improvement in LV function in patients with complete early reperfusion. These data give strong support to the hypothesis that *early* coronary recanalization with myocardial reperfusion leads to rescue of myocardium that would otherwise become irreversibly damaged and that this myocardial salvage contributes to preservation of LV function which, in turn, results in decreased cardiac mortality. In fact, logistic regression analysis has shown that virtually all improvement in 30-day mortality within the t-PA treatment group can be accounted for by the improved 90-minute reperfusion rate [44].

Evidence of Nonsalvage Effects

Although early coronary patency seems necessary to demonstrate the largest decrease in mortality following AMI, there is strong evidence that the time-sensitive mechanism of myocardial salvage is not the only means by which an open infarct artery contributes to an improved clinical response. The LATE [22] and EMERAS [23] trials have demonstrated benefit to thrombolytic administration as late as 12 hours following coronary occlusion even though it is highly unlikely that significant myocardial salvage occurs after the coronary vessel has been closed for more than 4 to 6 hours. In addition, in spite of the significant improvement in ventricular function documented by the GUSTO angiographic trial in patients with complete early coronary reperfusion, the mortality benefit experienced from thrombolytic therapy exceeds that expected from myocardial salvage alone. Thus, there is evidence that some beneficial effects of reperfusion in AMI may be the consequence of other, perhaps less time-sensitive, mechanisms *in addition* to the salvage of ischemic myocardium. Several possible mechanisms for this additional benefit are listed in Table 27-1 and data supporting the most plausible of these mechanisms are discussed below.

Improved Ventricular Remodeling

Definition of Remodeling

An MI involves the death of a portion of the heart's muscular wall. This results in a change in the ventricular chamber configuration as the infarcted tissue is replaced by noncontractile connective tissue (i.e., a scar). If the patient survives, further changes in ventricular size, wall thickness, and histological composition occur over time in response to the dynamic forces acting on the heart and an attempt by the body to compensate for the lost myocardium. The process of infarct healing and subsequent structural changes to the heart are referred to as *ventricular remodeling.*

Although the process of ventricular remodeling is fluid and continuous, it can be conceived as a series of processes beginning at the time of infarction and proceeding for many years. Within days to weeks after AMI, the area of infarction thins as myocytes are replaced by connective tissue in the form of a scar. Along with this thinning may come *infarct expansion,* a dilation of the infarcted region. (This dilation is the result of hemodynamic forces acting on a thinned ventricular wall and *not* from new necrosis of previously viable myocytes, a process known as *infarct extension.*) Regional expansion of the ventricular wall has been observed as early as 3 days after infarction and may progress for weeks or even months [45]. The mechanical stress caused by dilation of the infarct segment can result in myocyte slippage and stretching in the adjacent noninfarcted myocardium, thus increasing the region of ventricular wall thinning and expansion [46]. Early infarct expansion and regional ventricular dilation after MI may be followed by a phase of global ventricular dilation occurring over several months to years. The extent of this global dilation is largely dependent on the degree of early infarct expansion. Using serial two-dimensional echocardiography, Erlebacher and colleagues demonstrated continuing global LV dilation up to 30 months following acute transmural infarction that resulted in early expansion of the infarct region [47]. In contrast, no global dilation was observed in patients without initial infarct expansion.

Remodeling also may involve hypertrophy of the noninfarcted myocardium as the heart attempts to compensate for the nonfunctional infarcted wall segments. In contrast to the hypertrophy associated with pressure overload, where sarcomeres are added in parallel, hypertrophy associated with remodeling after AMI is generally caused by volume overload where sarcomeres are added in series. The series hypertrophy results in chamber enlargement and can lead to impaired ventricular filling and impaired systolic function.

Consequences of Remodeling

Remodeling is not always detrimental. Moderate compensatory hypertrophy of the noninfarcted ventricle may help to preserve cardiac output in the patient with a sizable infarction. Furthermore, remodeling may be so subtle as to go undetected except by detailed pathologic analysis. Unfortunately, much of the ventricular remodeling that occurs following an AMI is both substantial and deleterious. Distortion of the normal ellipsoidal ventricular shape through ventricular remodeling can result in ventricular enlargement, aneurysm formation, mural thrombosis, diminished systolic and diastolic function, valvular incompetence, and cardiac rupture. Clinical consequences of these changes include decreased functional class, poor exercise capacity, and an increased risk of stroke, ventricular arrhythmia, recurrent infarction, and death. The ultimate extent and impact of remodeling in a given patient depends on several factors, including the size of the infarct (both the transmurality (thickness) and the circumferential extent of damage), the loading conditions on the ventricle, and the state of the infarct-associated coronary artery (occluded or patent) during the period of cardiac healing. In one study involving serial evaluation of volume changes in patients not receiving reperfusion therapy, early infarct expansion (day 2 to 10) occurred in approximately 20 percent of patients and resulted in an average 34 percent increase in LV volume. Over the ensuing 6 months, an additional 20 percent of patients developed a similar increase in ventricular volume, and those with early expansion continued to experience progressive global LV dilatation [48]. Patients suffering large anterior infarcts were more likely to have both early regional expansion and delayed global dilation of the ventricular wall. Furthermore, there was a greatly increased risk of death in patients having substantial ventricular dilation.

Effect of an Open Artery on Remodeling

Recanalization of an occluded coronary artery following AMI can decrease ventricular remodeling either by decreasing the size of the infarct (early reperfusion) or by modifying the subsequent healing process (both early and late reperfusion). The first mechanism requires that coronary recanalization occur while a significant volume of ischemic myocardium within the infarct zone is still viable: probably 3 to 6 hours. The second mechanism does not require recanalization in time to salvage jeopardized myocardium but it must occur in time to alter the healing process. The duration of this second "window of opportunity" for reperfusion is extensively debated, as there are few clinical trials that help to define it in humans. There are a number of animal models that have been studied in this regard, however.

Studies have been performed in rats using transient coronary occlusion to determine the effect of reperfusion timing on ultimate infarct size and the degree of infarct expansion. At least two groups have demonstrated that coronary reperfusion 30 minutes after ligation of the vessel results in a marked decrease in infarct size compared with permanent coronary ligation [49, 50]. After 90 to 120 minutes of coronary occlusion there was no discernible reduction in infarct size compared with permanent ligation; however, there was a marked decrease in the degree of infarct expansion over 6 weeks compared with rats that had infarcts of similar size but had *permanent* occlusion of the coronary artery. In addition, although there was no difference in transmurality between those with permanent occlusion and those with 90-minute reperfusion, the ensuing infarct scar was substantially thicker in rats receiving late reperfusion [49].

One criticism of the rat model for MI is its relative lack of collateral coronary flow. Although this distinction from humans is unlikely to affect the general conclusion that delayed coronary reperfusion can modify ventricular remodeling even it if occurs too late for significant myocardial salvage, it may offer a distorted view of the crucial time intervals involved in this process. Patients with extensive collateral flow to an infarct zone have less infarct expansion than those with minimal or no collateral flow. Therefore, it is reassuring that experiments using dogs (whose coronary collateral flow is similar to that of humans) also show an increase in infarct stiffness and a decrease in both early infarct expansion and global ventricular enlargement with reperfusion compared with animals without coronary reperfusion. These benefits have been documented in the dog model even when reperfusion occurs 6 hours after coronary occlusion [51].

The etiology for the observed benefit of reperfusion in the remodeling process has received much attention, but little consensus. Some suggest that reperfusion leads to intramyocardial hemorrhage, cellular swelling, and intracellular edema that serves to increase wall stiffness in the infarct region, thus reducing ventricular expansion for a given hemodynamic load [52]. Others suggest that even late reperfusion may salvage a thin (perhaps clinically undetectable) rim of epicardium that reinforces the infarct region [52]. Still others suggest that the blood-filled vessels themselves may serve to buttress necrotic myocardium [53]. Although there is little experimental data to support many of these theories, reperfusion of the infarct artery results in an almost immediate decrease in the circumferential size of the infarct zone. Brown and colleagues have presented evidence that this effect is due to calcium activation of the actin–myosin complex within damaged myocytes, leading to regional ventricular contracture [50]. Their pathologic studies have documented contraction-band necrosis in the infarct region of dogs with experimentally induced infarcts followed by reperfusion. The number of contraction bands decreases as reperfusion occurs after progressively longer periods of ischemia, suggesting that this potentially beneficial infarct contraction is a time-sensitive phenomenon.

There is a wealth of clinical data supporting the hypothesis that the remodeling process is altered in patients with an open infarct artery after AMI. Studies performed before the techniques of thrombolysis and angioplasty were available demonstrated the predictive value of an open infarct artery on early ventricular size and shape. In one study, all 14 patients with a persistently closed infarct artery developed ventricular dilation (an increase of at least 20 percent in ventricular volume) within 30 days of infarct, but only 2 of 26 patients with perfusion of the infarct artery at predischarge angiography developed dilation [54]. Further analysis of these patients revealed that perfusion status of the infarct artery was more predictive of ventricular dilation than even infarct size. Another study demonstrated that patients with a patent infarct vessel at a mean of 17 days following infarction subsequently had a significant decrease in LV end-diastolic and end-systolic volumes, decreased dyskinesis, and decreased sphericity as compared with those with persistent occlusion of the infarct artery [52].

Studies of patients entered into thrombolytic trials have shown a similar relation of coronary patency to reduced ventricular dilation. In a small trial of patients receiving SK at the University of Virginia [55], angiography was performed immediately after thrombolytic infusion and patients were followed with serial two-dimensional echocardiography for 10 days. Those with patent infarct arteries early after thrombolysis not only had a marked improvement in regional ventricular function, but avoided significant expansion of the infarct region during this brief period, in contrast to those with persistent coronary occlusion. A study performed by Siu and colleagues demonstrated a similar correlation between ventricular expansion and *late* patency of the infarct vessel in 30 patients treated with thrombolysis [56]. In this group, LV cavity size increased significantly over 12 weeks in patients with an occluded infarct-related artery at the time of coronary angiography 8 days after AMI. In contrast, patients with coronary patency at this time had no change in ventricular volume. In the GISSI-I study, thrombolytic therapy administered at a mean of 6 hours did not improve global EF but did result in lower end-systolic and end-diastolic volumes after the patients had a 6-month convalescence [57]. Even when infarct size was controlled for, patients receiving thrombolytic therapy (and therefore having a higher incidence of infarct-artery patency) had less ventricular expansion than those not receiving SK. GUSTO collaborators reported that LV volume is inversely associated with the extent of infarct-related coronary flow at both 90 minutes and 5 days (see Table 27-2) [43]. At 5 days, a moderate degree of patency (TIMI grade 2 flow) was associated with an 8 percent reduction in end-systolic volume and a 20 percent reduction was found in those with full reperfusion (TIMI grade 3) as compared with those who had either minimal or no patency (TIMI grades 0 or 1).

Hirayama and colleagues published preliminary data on patients with early reperfusion (≤ 6 hours from symptom onset), late reperfusion (> 6 hours from symptom onset), and no reperfusion after thrombolytic therapy [58]. They found that early reperfusion resulted in a smaller infarct size (as measured by T1-201 single photon emission computed tomography (SPECT), improved systolic function (measured by EF), and less ventricular expansion as compared with no reperfusion. Patients with late reperfusion, in contrast, had no benefit in terms of infarct size or systolic function but did have significantly less ventricular dilation compared with those who had no evidence of recanalization.

Effect of Open Artery on Formation of Aneurysm

The development of a ventricular wall aneurysm after infarction predisposes the patient to a variety of adverse consequences such as formation of mural thrombus with subsequent embolization, an increased risk of ventricular dysrhythmia, and depressed systolic function leading to CHF. Aneurysmal dilation involving an infarct scar is more likely with large infarctions and those that undergo significant early expansion. In this regard an open infarct artery may decrease the subsequent risk of aneurysm formation because of its effect on remodeling and decreased early expansion in addition to its effect on decreasing infarction size. Data supporting this hypothesis has been published by Forman et al. who studied 79 patients who had experienced anterior AMI [59]. Forman et al. reported formation of ventricular aneurysm in 25 of 52 patients (48 percent) with persistent occlusion of the left anterior descending (LAD) artery as compared with 4 of 27 (15 percent) who had recanalization of this vessel. In a similar study, Hirai found that 7 of 12 patients with failed reperfusion of the infarct artery after administration of thrombolytic therapy and without collateral flow to the infarct zone had developed aneurysmal dilation of the left ventricle when catheterization was repeated 35 days after infarction [60]. The remaining 5 patients with thrombolytic failure did not develop an aneurysm and all 5 had developed either spontaneous reperfusion or collateral flow to the infarct region by the late catheterization period. In contrast, only 1 of 25 patients with successful reperfusion developed an aneurysm within the same time frame.

In summary, ventricular remodeling following AMI frequently involves deleterious elements such as infarct expansion, global ventricular dilation, volume-overload hypertrophy, and aneurysm formation. Each of these elements has been associated with increased morbidity and mortality in the postinfarction period. Therefore, the observation that a patent infarct artery may modify the remodeling process provides one explanation for the observed beneficial effect of the open artery that is independent of its effect on myocardial salvage.

Improved Electrical Stability

Coronary artery patency favorably influences the electrical stability of the heart and may be another factor involved in reducing postinfarction mortality, independent of myocardial salvage. In the dog model, reperfusion of an occluded coronary artery within 4 hours resulted in a decrease of spontaneous ventricular arrhythmias in the early postinfarction period [61]. This effect was not observed if reperfusion was delayed until 6 hours after infarction, even though there was no discernible difference in ventricular function between dogs reperfused at 4 or 6 hours. Some have suggested this beneficial effect of coronary reperfusion on electrical stability is due to amelioration of the postinfarction imbalance in sympathetic and parasympathetic stimulation of the myocardium [62]. Animal models have shown sympathetic denervation of viable myocardium apical to a transmural MI [63]. This denervation results in catecholamine hypersensitivity, which may render that portion of the heart more susceptible to circulating catecholamines and increased arrhythmogenesis when the patient exercises or has emotional stress. Early recanalization of the infarct artery following AMI may reduce the loss of sympathetic fibers and thus prevent exaggerated catecholamine sensitivity. In support of this concept, Herre and colleagues found that dogs with completed infarcts had a sympathetic imbalance that increased the inducibility of ventricular tachycardia and fibrillation during sympathetic stimulation [63]. If the infarction was confined to the subendocardium by timely coronary reperfusion, it became more difficult to induce ventricular arrhythmia. In addition to the potential beneficial effect on sympathetic myocardial innervation, coronary reperfusion may enhance electrical stability by decreasing variations in refractoriness within the heart and by reducing aneurysmal dilation of the ventricular wall [64].

Effect on Late Potentials

Signal averaging is a method of generating a high resolution electrocardiographic tracing from standard surface electrodes. Using this technique, microvolt signals, known as late potentials, can be recorded from some patients following MI. Such signals are thought to be produced by conduction of the depolarization current through damaged myocardial tissue. These circuits are often capable of supporting a re-entrant ventricular arrhythmia. The presence of late potentials has been associated with an increased risk of ventricular tachyarrhythmia and sudden death in patients following AMI [65].

Several studies have shown an increased incidence of late potentials among patients with persistent occlusion of the infarct-related artery following MI. Vatterott et al. studied 124 consecutive patients presenting with AMI in Rochester, Minnesota and performed both coronary angiography and a signal-averaged electrocardiogram (ECG) on each during their initial hospital stay [66]. They found a twofold increase in the incidence of late potentials in patients with a closed infarct artery compared with those having a patent artery at the time of angiography (65 percent versus 34 percent; $p = .001$). In the subgroup of patients receiving thrombolytic therapy within 4 hours of symptom onset, the incidence of late potentials was 24 percent in patients with an open artery and 83 percent in those with persistent coronary occlusion. Stepwise logistic regression analysis found the status of the infarct artery was a powerful independent predictor of late potentials. It was, in fact, the only predictive variable among patients receiving thrombolytic therapy. Gang and colleagues found the incidence of late potentials was 5 percent among patients treated within 4 hours of symptom onset with t-PA and 23 percent among those not receiving thrombolytic therapy [67]. Furthermore, in the subgroup receiving t-PA, late potentials were seen only in patients with persistent occlusion of the infarct vessel within 24 hours of admission. None of the 38 patients with a patent infarct artery was found to have this marker for ventricular arrhythmia and sudden death. Moreno et al. studied 101 consecutive patients presenting with AMI and found that the risk of developing late potentials during the index hospital admission was decreased in patients receiving thrombolytic therapy compared with those treated conservatively (22 percent versus 43 percent; $p < .05$) [68]. In a detailed analysis they found that all the effect of thrombolysis on the prevention of late potentials was secondary to reperfusion or patency of the infarct-related coronary artery. Even long after completion of an infarction, the status of the infarct artery predicted the presence of late potentials on the signal-averaged ECG. Lange found late potentials in 40 percent of patients with occluded infarct vessels but in only 8 percent of those with patent vessels when angiography was performed as long as 24 months after AMI [69].

Effect on Inducible Tachyarrhythmias

Several investigations have focused on the incidence of inducible ventricular tachycardia using programmed electrical stimulation and its relationship to the status of the infarct vessel. A study of patients with transmural anterior MI complicated by LV aneurysm formation found that 8 of 16 patients not receiving thrombolytic therapy died suddenly or developed sustained ventricular tachycardia within a mean follow-up time of 11 months [70]. In spite of similar EF and other clinical characteristics, none of the 16 patients receiving thrombolytic agents had a clinical arrhythmic event during this period (p = .002). The disparity in clinical outcomes reflected the results of electrophysiologic study in a subgroup of these patients shortly after MI. In these patients, inducible ventricular tachycardia was observed in over 80 percent of patients not receiving thrombolytic agents as compared with only 8 percent of those given reperfusion therapy. Similar findings have been reported by Kerrschot and colleagues who noted inducible ventricular tachycardia following AMI in 48 percent of patients receiving thrombolytic therapy and 100 percent of patients managed without reperfusion therapy [71]. Reperfusion of the infarct zone by CABG may also be effective in improving the electrical stability of the heart. In patients in the nonrandomized Coronary Artery Surgery Study registry, those receiving revascularization with CABG had a dramatic reduction in the incidence of sudden death as compared with patients treated with medical therapy but no revascularization [72]. The largest reduction in sudden death was observed in the subgroup at highest risk for an arrhythmic event, those with LV dysfunction and a history of clinical CHF.

Data concerning the effect of coronary patency on antiarrhythmic therapy also came from the Cardiac Arrhythmia Suppression Trial (CAST) [73]. In patients treated with either encainide or flecainide after MI, the risk of arrhythmia-related death was significantly higher in patients not receiving thrombolytic reperfusion therapy than in those treated with thrombolytic agents. Similarly, Hii reported a study involving 64 consecutive patients with a remote MI who presented with sustained ventricular tachycardia or fibrillation [74]. Following angiography, serial programmed stimulation studies were performed on each patient in an attempt to identify an effective antiarrhythmic agent. Those patients with a patent infarct-related artery were significantly more likely to have effective antiarrhythmic therapy identified than those with a closed infarct artery (45 percent versus 9 percent), again suggesting a more stable electrical milieu in patients achieving reperfusion.

Rescue of Hibernating Myocardium

Some patients may have ongoing ischemia in the area of infarction even after a "completed" infarction. This may be due to intermittent flow in the infarct artery or collateral flow insufficient to relieve ischemia but adequate to prevent further myocardial death. In these cases, delayed reperfusion of the infarct artery would relieve ischemia and could lead to functional recovery of the ischemic region. Recent data concerning the presence of viable but nonfunctional myocardium (often called "hibernating" myocardium) in some patients following AMI lends support to this theory. Such myocardium is thought to be chronically ischemic, though not infarcted, and may regain its functional status if ischemia is relieved by late reperfusion of the infarct artery. Sabia and colleagues reported improved ventricular function with delayed (average 12 days after AMI) angioplasty of a totally occluded infarct artery when significant collateral flow to the infarct region was present during the period of occlusion [75]. Montalescot et al. noted improved peri-infarction wall motion following angioplasty of a patent but markedly stenotic infarct-related vessel 6 or more weeks after AMI [76]. Although these data are promising, further study is needed to determine the contribution of rescued hibernating myocardium to the clinical benefits attributable to coronary reperfusion.

Protection Against Future Ischemic Events

Even after a completed infarct, recanalization of the infarct artery may provide a conduit for blood flow to regions of the heart that may become jeopardized by ischemia in the future. By augmenting collateral flow in the noninfarct region, an open coronary artery may attenuate the effect of a future infarction, or even prevent it altogether. For example, a patient with a previous occlusion of the right coronary artery resulting in infarction of the inferior ventricular wall may have an improved prognosis after a subsequent occlusion of the LAD artery if the right coronary artery has recanalized and can provide collateral flow to a portion of the anterior wall. Obviously, such a benefit would be difficult to demonstrate in clinical trials because it could be seen only many years after the index infarction.

(Re)Definition of the Open Artery Hypothesis

Two groups of thought have driven previous definitions of the open artery hypothesis. One group, believing that myocardial salvage and improved ventricular function are the key to improved clinical outcome in patients with a patent infarct-related artery, has defined the hypothesis as the beneficial effect attributable to early restoration of coronary flow sufficient to induce significant myocardial salvage. Others, troubled by the lack of demonstrable improvement in ventricular function following reperfusion therapy but impressed with the correlation between an open infarct artery and improved survival, have stressed nonsalvage mechanisms to explain this correlation. The latter group defines the open artery hypothesis as a beneficial effect attributable to late coronary recanalization that is not contingent upon the salvage of myocardium nor necessarily reflected by improved LV function [24]. Reviewing the available data indicates that there are a number of potential mechanisms by which an open infarct artery may improve patient outcome. These mechanisms are not coexclusive, and several may function concurrently to improve the outlook for patients achieving reperfusion following AMI. Furthermore, classifying these mechanisms into time-sensitive and time-insensitive groups, as shown in Figure 27-1 for the purpose of discussion, is overly simplistic and fails to consider the overlap between groups in terms of the window of opportunity for achieving benefit.

The various possible mechanisms should be viewed as stretching along a time continuum extending from the onset of myocardial ischemia to the future (Fig. 27-5). At any time after coronary occlusion and the onset of ischemia, sustained re-

Fig. 27-5
Relative contribution of different mechanisms to overall improvement in clinical outcome in patients with a patent infarct-artery as a function of time to reperfusion.

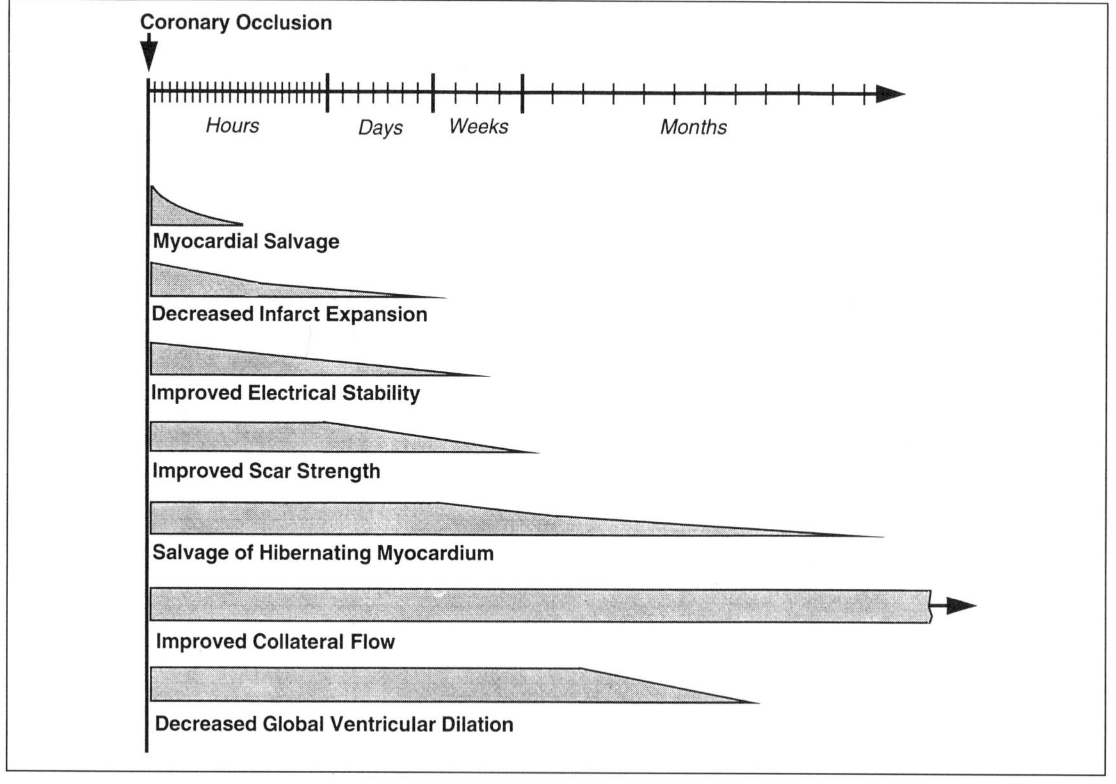

perfusion of the infarct artery provides benefit by a number of mechanisms. The duration of occlusion before reperfusion determines which of these mechanisms will operate in a particular patient. For example, a patient attaining recanalization of an infarct-related artery 24 hours after its occlusion is not likely to have a substantial degree of myocardial salvage and may or may not benefit from an improvement in electrical stability. This patient may well benefit, however, from improved infarct-scar strength, a decrease in global ventricular dilation, and improved collateral blood flow to noninfarcted myocardium. With the possible exception of myocardial salvage, available data do not allow for precise determination of the timing or shape of these benefit curves. Nevertheless, this model more accurately depicts the relation of each mechanism to the duration of coronary occlusion than does an attempt to group them according to time-dependent and time-independent mechanisms.

One should not interpret Fig. 27-5 as suggesting that the benefit of an open infarct artery is independent of the time to reperfusion. In fact, rapid reperfusion is critical to attain the maximum benefit with coronary patency. To illustrate this, Tiefenbrunn and Sobel used data from animal models and clinical trials to construct a curve representing the degree of benefit from reperfusion with increasing periods of occlusion (Fig. 27-6) [24]. Their model is supported by other clinical studies that suggest a profound loss of benefit with increasing time to reperfusion, especially early in the course of AMI. The rationale for this observation is that early recanalization of an occluded artery allows more of the mechanisms (see Fig. 27-5) to function in decreasing mortality. In addition, time-sensitive mechanisms (such as myocardial salvage) probably contribute more to the overall benefit of an open coronary artery than do less time-dependent ones. Thus, although there may be a benefit associated with late recanalization of an artery, this benefit will be less than if the artery had been reperfused earlier.

Fig. 27-6
Relative benefit observed in patients with coronary reperfusion after myocardial infarction as a function of time to reperfusion.

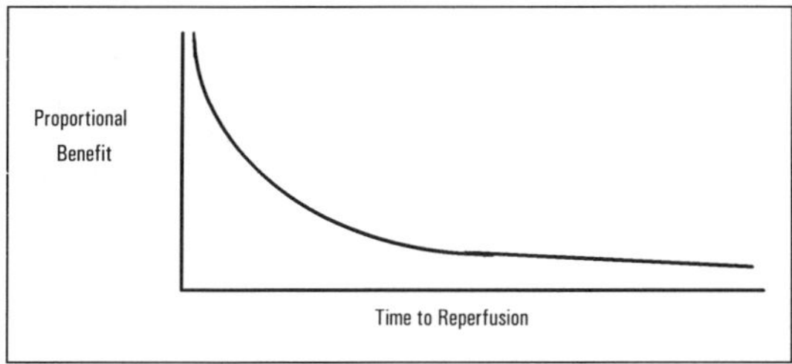

Clinical Implications of the Open Artery Hypothesis

The clinician caring for a patient with acute myocardial ischemia should remember that maintenance of perfusion to the myocardium is the fundamental tenet of clinical practice intended to improve outcome. This benefit must be weighed against the risk associated with opening an occluded artery. In the case of antithrombotic or fibrinolytic therapy, this risk is dominated by bleeding, particularly intracranial bleeding. For mechanical interventions, the primary concern is the risk of increased ischemic events such as MI and stroke. It is important to note that the risk of bleeding following thrombolysis appears to remain constant as a function of time after coronary occlusion, but the risk of ventricular rupture actually increases over time [77]. Because many of the benefits of coronary reperfusion decline significantly over time, the risk/benefit ratio for reperfusion therapy becomes less favorable with increased delay of treatment. At each phase of care for a patient with evolving infarction, including primary reperfusion, rescue interventions after failed thrombolysis, and later decisions about elective revascularization, the physician must carefully weigh the therapeutic options with a detailed assessment of likely benefits and risks for the patient.

Primary Reperfusion Therapy

Multiple approaches to achieving coronary perfusion following AMI have been advocated, including thrombolytic agents (delivered into the coronary artery or intravenously), bypass surgery, balloon angioplasty, and a number of other percutaneous, catheter-based techniques. Of these, only IV thrombolytic therapy lends itself to widespread use in a timely fashion. Currently, three thrombolytic agents are licensed for use within the United States for the treatment of AMI: SK, t-PA, and APSAC. All these agents activate the body's intrinsic fibrinolytic system, which leads to degradation of fibrin into fragments that can no longer form thrombi. There are, however, substantial differences in the three agents at the molecular level, resulting in variation in pharmacodynamics and thrombolytic efficiency. Several small studies have suggested that t-PA, when administered in the most efficacious manner, results in faster recanalization of occluded coronary vessels among patients suffering AMI as compared with SK or APSAC [42, 78, 79]. Nevertheless, the ISIS-3 and GISSI-2 trials failed to show an incremental benefit from t-PA in terms of short-term survival following AMI. This may be partially because neither study employed a front-loaded t-PA regimen (shown to result in the most rapid recanalization) and neither employed IV heparin in conjunction with thrombolytic therapy. The latter may be essential in maintaining patency with t-PA due to its relatively short half-life and limited systemic fibrinolytic effect.

The GUSTO study, in which t-PA was given in a front-loaded manner and IV heparin was used in all patients receiving t-PA, documented an improvement in clinical outcome (30-day mortality) in patients receiving t-PA compared with those receiving SK. The large angiographic substudy further confirmed an association between this improved clinical outcome and early coronary patency; both were increased with a regimen of accelerated t-PA. This study is the first to illustrate conclusively that different patency rates result in different outcomes and that patency rates vary with different thrombolytic strategies. Future studies may uncover other effective strategies combining efficient thrombolytic agents with more effective thrombin inhibitors and antiplatelet agents to achieve even higher early patency rates and improved outcomes.

The efficiency of any thrombolytic strategy can only affect a portion of the total coronary occlusion time in AMI because total occlusion time comprises many factors: patient delays in seeking treatment, delays in bringing the patient to the hospital, and delay in initiation of definitive therapy after the patient arrives at the hospital. Gersh and Anderson have shown that, on average, 3.7 hours elapse from the onset of AMI symptoms to reperfusion secondary to thrombolytic therapy in a hospital emergency room [80]. Of this time 22 percent is attributable to patient delay in seeking medical assistance, 21 percent to transportation of the patient to the hospital, 38 percent to delay after the patient arrives, and 19 percent to delay of reperfusion after thrombolytic administration. This analysis reveals the limitations of strategies that address only thrombolytic regimens; they impact only the final component (i.e., delay of reperfusion following thrombolytic administration) of total coronary occlusion time. Decreasing the patient's delay in seeking medical care and decreasing delays in the administration of thrombolytic therapy are also important.

Prehospital Thrombolysis

Prehospital initiation of thrombolytic therapy holds promise for significantly decreasing the overall time to definitive treatment for some patients with AMI. Two studies designed to test the feasibility and effectiveness of this strategy have been reported recently. The European Myocardial Infarction Project (EMIP) involved 5454 patients randomized to in-hospital or in-field treatment with APSAC [81]. Patients randomized to the in-field group received thrombolytic therapy about 1 hour earlier than those randomized to the in-hospital group. This resulted in a reduction of 13 percent in total 30-day mortality and 17 percent in cardiac mortality for the patients treated in-field. The Seattle Myocardial Infarction Triage and Intervention (MITI) study collected data on 360 patients who received in-field or in-hospital treatment with t-PA [82]. The difference in time to treatment between the MITI groups was about 30 minutes less than that for the EMIP groups and, perhaps because of the time difference, there was not a significant benefit documented for MITI patients treated in-field. The importance of early therapy was nonetheless confirmed by the observation that thrombolytic treatment initiated within 70 minutes of symptom onset resulted in decreased infarct size, improved EF, and decreased mortality as compared with therapy initiated later than 70 minutes.

The largest single component of treatment delay is the time from a patient's hospital presentation to the time of thrombolytic administration. Fortunately, this component is also one of the most amenable to improvements in delivery of care. Simple measures such as placing the decision to administer thrombolytic agents with the emergency department physician, creating a fast-track registration and triage system (including expeditious ECG) for patients with suspected AMI, initiating therapy in the emergency department rather than in the intensive care unit, and stocking thrombolytic agents within the emergency department as well as in the hospital pharmacy have the potential to greatly improve time-to-treatment measures. The median in-hospital time to thrombolytic administration for patients enrolled in the GUSTO trial was 66 minutes. Although this is an improvement over previous studies that showed average delays of 90 minutes or more, there can be further improvement by increasing the sense of urgency when a patient presents with suspected MI and by adopting the measures suggested above. The MITI trial has served as a benchmark in this regard, as patients in the in-hospital treatment group received thrombolytic therapy an average of only 20 minutes after they reached the hospital [82].

Rescue Reperfusion Therapy

Even with optimal use of thrombolytic and anticoagulant agents, 15 to 20 percent of patients fail to achieve reperfusion within 90 minutes of treatment. The best treatment strategy for this subgroup of patients remains controversial. The open artery hypothesis dictates that patients failing thrombolytic therapy should benefit from mechanical recanalization of the infarct artery even if it is delayed by 2 to 3 hours. This is especially true if the patient received thrombolytic therapy early in the infarct course and is still on the steep portion on the benefit curve (see Fig. 27-6). An argument for the use of emergency angioplasty in patients with failed thrombolysis can be made with increasing support from medical literature. Angioplasty can be performed safely in the peri-infarct period with reported success rates approaching 95 percent [83]. Low long-term mortality rates have been reported with a strategy of rescue angioplasty for failed thrombolysis [44], and studies indicate an improved clinical outcome for patients successfully reperfused with angioplasty following failed thrombolysis [84, 85].

TAMI-5 randomized 575 AMI patients receiving IV thrombolytic therapy to either emergency angiography with rescue angioplasty, if the infarct vessel were closed, or delayed angiography at 5 to 7 days [86]. Patients randomized to the aggressive strategy had a somewhat higher predischarge infarct-artery patency rate (94 percent versus 90 percent; $p = .65$) as well as a greater improvement of regional wall motion within the infarct zone. There was no difference in bleeding complications between the two groups. Although the TAMI-5 study was not specifically designed to test the efficacy of rescue angioplasty (which would require randomization of those with closed infarct arteries to either PTCA or control), it did find the strategy of emergent intervention following thrombolysis to be practicable and of relatively low risk.

The RESCUE trial was designed specifically to determine the efficacy of rescue angioplasty for patients with anterior AMI failing thrombolytic therapy [87]. In this trial, 150 patients with persistent occlusion of the LAD artery following thrombolytic administration were randomized to PTCA or no PTCA. Preliminary results indicate a lower incidence of death or CHF within 30 days among patients receiving rescue angioplasty (6.5 percent) versus control (16.4 percent; $p = .055$). Although there was no difference in the incidence of ventricular arrhythmia or resting LVEF between the groups, patients receiving rescue PTCA had a somewhat higher exercise EF (0.45 versus 0.40; $p = .04$).

If rescue angioplasty is to be a viable strategy, accurate, noninvasive techniques are needed to ascertain the status of the infarct artery following thrombolysis. Fortunately, several promising techniques are emerging in this area. The first involves continuous 12-lead ST segment monitoring. This approach has been employed for several years and is useful in the prediction of coronary patency following thrombolysis [88, 89]. Myocardial imaging using radiopharmaceutical agents, such as ^{99m}Tc-sestamibi, that do not redistribute may be used to define the area of myocardium at risk early in the course of infarction and subsequently to determine the extent of reperfusion [90]. Finally, the measurement of creatine kinase-MB (CK-MB) isoenzyme subforms may prove useful in determining vessel patency if this analysis can be performed reliably and quickly [91]. Until one or more of these techniques is completely developed, a reasonable marker for coronary reperfusion following thrombolytic administration is 50 percent resolution of the baseline ST segment elevation in a standard 12-lead ECG. In such patients, 85 to 95 percent can be shown to have reperfusion of the infarct-related artery [92].

Further investigation into rescue angioplasty is required before recommendations regarding this strategy can be made with assurance. At present, however, it seems reasonable to consider mechanical revascularization in patients with evidence of ongoing ischemia (e.g., persistent chest pain and ST segment elevation) 90 minutes or more after administration of thrombolytic therapy, especially in those with evidence of a large infarction, previous ventricular dysfunction, or acute CHF on presentation.

Delayed Reperfusion Therapy

Although no large clinical study has documented improved clinical outcomes in patients receiving reperfusion therapy more than 12 hours after onset of AMI symptoms, the open artery hypothesis suggests that patients achieving and maintaining an open infarct artery long after 12 hours may benefit by nonsalvage mechanisms. Two reports suggest delayed PTCA of persistently occluded coronary arteries may improve patient outcome following MI [93, 94]. Bernardi and Whitlow reported a retrospective study of 300 patients undergoing cardiac catheterization within 6 weeks following AMI [93]. They found occlusion of the infarct-related coronary artery in 145 patients, of whom 111 received mechanical intervention 6 to 42 days after infarction to open the infarct artery. Three-year survival was improved in the patients receiving late reperfusion (93 percent) as compared with patients having persistent infarct-artery occlusion (80 percent; $p < .01$). Multivariate analysis showed this benefit to be independent of LV function. A small randomized trial evaluating mechanical reperfusion late after AMI has been reported in preliminary form by Dzavik et al. [94]. In this study, patients within 5 and 42 days of their first transmural MI underwent coronary angiography. Those with an occluded infarct artery were randomized to attempted PTCA versus no PTCA and angiography was repeated after 4 months. The primary success rate of delayed PTCA in this setting was 77 percent. After 4 months, however, half the dilated arteries were occluded. Although only 18 patients had full 4-month follow-up data at the time of this report, patients with patency of the infarct artery at 4 months had a significant improvement in LVEF (mean, 0.51 at baseline; 0.60 at 4-month follow-up), whereas those with occlusion of the infarct vessel had no change in EF.

Although such studies are encouraging, more investigation in this area is needed before late mechanical revascularization without evidence of continued or inducible ischemia can be recommended.

Ancillary Interventions

Intelligent use of interventions that enhance or extend the benefits of an open coronary artery can significantly improve patient outcome following MI. Rapid use of beta-blocking agents, for example, limits the oxygen demand of ischemic myocardium, possibly shifting the time–benefit curve (Fig. 27-6) to the right and extending the window of opportunity of benefit from coronary reperfusion. Other interventions may enhance the beneficial effects of an open infarct vessel on infarct expansion, ventricular remodeling, or electrical stability. For example, the beneficial effect of angiotension-converting enzyme (ACE) inhibitors following AMI may be at least partly due to their ability to reduce ventricular wall stress during the healing phase, decreasing infarct expansion, and mitigating subsequent remodeling. Future developments may include agents that can modify the healing phase of AMI, perhaps by increasing the strength of the infarct scar or limiting electrical re-entry within the peri-infarction region.

Recent clinical trials have expanded our understanding of the benefits resulting from the patency of an infarct-associated artery after AMI. There is no longer any reasonable doubt that early reperfusion of the infarct-related artery is associated with improved ventricular function and a significant improvement in clinical outcome. Evidence is accumulating that delayed recanalization (by natural, pharmacological, or mechanical means) may also result in clinical benefit by modification of the ventricular remodeling process, improved electrical stability of the heart, improved collateral flow, or other mechanisms. While these studies are not definitive, they provide an incentive for further study into the clinical impact of delayed reperfusion and reaffirm the goal of interventional cardiology to develop more successful means of establishing and maintaining patency of coronary arteries after AMI.

References

1. DeWood, M. A., Spores, J., Notske, R., et al. Prevalence of total coronary occlusion during the early hours of transmural myocardial infarction. *N. Engl. J. Med.* 303:897, 1980.
2. DeWood, M. A., Notske, R. N., Berg R., et al. Medical and surgical management of early Q wave myocardial infarction. I. Effects of surgical reperfusion on survival, recurrent myocardial infarction, sudden death and functional class at 10 or more years of follow-up. *J. Am. Coll. Cardiol.* 13:65, 1989.
3. Hartzler, G. O., Rutherford, B. D., McConahay, D. R., et al. Percutaneous transluminal coronary angioplasty with and without thrombolytic therapy for treatment of acute myocardial infarction. *Am. Heart J.* 106:965, 1983.
4. Laffel, G. L., and Braunwald, E. Thrombolytic therapy: a new strategy for the treatment of acute myocardial infarction. *N. Engl. J. Med.* 311:710, 1984.
5. Kennedy, J. W., Ritchie, J. L., Davis, K. B., et al. Western Washington randomized trial of intracoronary streptokinase in acute myocardial infarction. *N. Engl. J. Med.* 309:1477, 1983.
6. Serruys, P. W., Simoons, M. L., Suryapranata, H., et al. Preservation of global and regional left ventricular function after early thrombolysis in acute myocardial infarction. *J. Am. Coll. Cardiol.* 7:729, 1986.
7. Cigarroa, R. G., Lange, R. A., and Hills, D. L. Prognosis after acute myocardial infarction in patients with and without residual anterograde coronary blood flow. *Am. J. Cardiol.* 64:155, 1989.
8. DeWood, M. A., Leonard, J., Grunwald, R. P., et al. Medical and surgical management of early Q wave myocardial infarction. II. Effects on mortality and global and regional left ventricular function at 10 or more years of follow-up. *J. Am. Coll. Cardiol.* 14:78, 1989.
9. Bernardi, M. M., and Whitlow, P. L. Infarct related artery patency: An independent predictor of three-year survival after acute myocardial infarction. (Abstract) *J. Am. Coll. Cardiol.* 17:214A, 1991.
10. Brodie, B. R., Stuckey, T. D., Hansen, C. J., et al. Importance of a patent infarct-related artery for hospital and late survival after direct coronary angioplasty for acute myocardial infarction. *Am. J. Cardiol.* 69:1113, 1992.
11. Gruppo Italiano per lo Studio della Streptochinasi nell'Infarto Miocardico (GISSI). Effectiveness of intravenous thrombolytic treatment in acute myocardial infarction. *Lancet* 1:397, 1986.
12. ISIS-2 (Second International Study of Infarct Survival) Collaborative Group. Randomized trial of intravenous streptokinase, oral aspirin, both, or or neither among 17,187 cases of suspected acute myocardial infarction: ISIS-2. *Lancet* 2:349, 1988.
13. Dalen, J. E., Gore, J. M., Braunwald, E., et al. Six- and twelve-month follow-up of the phase I thrombolysis in myocardial infarction (TIMI) trial. *Am. J. Cardiol.* 62:179, 1988.
14. Stadius, M. L., Davis, K., Maynard, C., et al. Risk stratification for 1 year survival based on characteristics identified in the early hours of acute myocardial infarction: The Western Washington intracoronary streptokinase trial. *Circulation* 74:703, 1986.
15. Simoons, M. L., Serruys, P. W., van den Brand, M., et al. for the Working Group on Thrombolytic Therapy in Acute Myocardial Infarction of the Netherlands Interuniversity Cardiology Institute. Early thrombolysis in acute myocardial infarction: Limitation of infarct size and improved survival. *J. Am. Coll. Cardiol.* 7:717, 1986.
16. Mathey, D. G., Schofer, J, Sheehan, F. H., et al. Improved survival up to four years after early coronary thrombolysis. *Am. J. Cardiol.* 61:524, 1988.
17. Galvani, M., Ottani, F., Ferrini, D., et al. Patency of the infarct-related artery and left ventricular function as the major determinants of survival after Q-wave acute myocardial infarction. *Am. J. Cardiol.* 71:1, 1993.
18. The Multicenter Postinfarction Research Group. Risk stratification and survival after myocardial infarction. *N. Engl. J. Med.* 309:331, 1983.
19. Van de Werf, F., and Arnold, A. E. R. Intravenous tissue plasminogen activator and size of infarct, left ventricular function, and survival in acute myocardial infarction. *B.M.J.* 297, 1374, 1988.
20. Meinertz, T., Kasper, W., Schumacher, M., et al. The German Multicenter Trial of anisoylated plasminogen streptokinase activator complex versus heparin for acute myocardial infarction. *Am. J. Cardiol.* 62:347, 1988.
21. Califf, R. M., Harrelson-Woodlief, L., and Topol, E. J. Left ventricular ejection fraction may not be useful as an end point of thrombolytic therapy comparative trials. *Circulation* 82:1847, 1990.
22. LATE Study Group. Late Assessment of Thrombolytic Efficacy (LATE) study with alteplase 6-24 hours after onset of acute myocardial infarction. *Lancet* 342:759, 1993.
23. EMERAS (Estudio Multicentrico Estreptoquinasa Republicas de America del Sur) Collaborative Group. Randomized trial of late thrombolysis in patients with suspected acute myocardial infarction. *Lancet* 342:767, 1993.
24. Tiefenbrunn, A. J., and Sobel, B. E. Timing of coronary recanalization: Paradigms, paradoxes, and pertinence. *Circulation* 85:2311, 1992.
25. Braunwald, E. The path to myocardial salvage by thrombolytic therapy. *Circulation* 76 (Suppl II):II-2, 1987.
26. Reimer, K. A., Lowe, J. E., Rasmussen, M. M., et al. The "wavefront phenomenon" of ischemic cell death. I. Myocardial infarct size versus duration of coronary occlusion in dogs. *Circulation* 56:786, 1977.
27. Bergmann, S. R., Lerch, R. A., Fox, K. A. A., et al. Temporal dependence of beneficial effects of coro-

nary thrombolysis characterized by positron tomography. *Am. J. Med.* 73:573, 1982.
28. Kennedy, J. W., Martin, G. V., Davis, K. B., et al. The Western Washington intravenous streptokinase in acute myocardial infarction randomized trial. *Circulation* 77:345, 1988.
29. ISAM Study Group. A prospective trial of intravenous streptokinase in acute myocardial infarction (ISAM). Mortality, morbidity and infarct size at 21 days. *N. Engl. J. Med.* 314:1465, 1986.
30. Timm, T. C., Ross, R., McKendal, G. R., et al. Left ventricular function and early cardiac events as a function of time to treatment with t-PA: A report from TIMI II. (Abstract) *Circulation* 84(Suppl II): II-230, 1991.
31. The National Heart Foundation of Australia Coronary Thrombolysis Group. Coronary thrombolysis and myocardial salvage by tissue plasminogen activator up to 4 hours after onset of myocardial infarction. *Lancet* 1:203, 1988.
32. Koren, G., Weiss, A. T., Hasin, Y., et al. Prevention of myocardial damage in acute myocardial ischemia by early treatment with intravenous streptokinase. *N. Engl. J. Med.* 313:1384, 1985.
33. Morgan, C. D., Roberts, R. S., Haq, A., et al. Coronary patency, infarct size and left ventricular function after thrombolytic therapy for acute myocardial infarction: Results from the tissue plasminogen activator: Toronto (TPAT) placebo-controlled trial. *J. Am. Coll. Cardiol.* 17:1451, 1991.
34. Sheehan, F. H., Braunwald, E., Canner, P., et al. The effect of intravenous thrombolytic therapy on left ventricular function: A report on tissue-type plasminogen activator and streptokinase from the thrombolysis in myocardial infarction (TIMI phase I) trial. *Circulation* 75:817, 1987.
35. Harrison, J. K., Califf, R. M., Woodlief, L. H., et al. Systolic left ventricular function after reperfusion therapy for acute myocardial infarction. *Circulation* 87:1531, 1993.
36. Christian, T. F., Gibbons, R. J., and Gersh, B. J. Effect of infarct location on myocardial salvage assessed by technetium-99m isonitrile. *J. Am. Coll. Cardiol.* 17:1303, 1991.
37. Christian, T. F., Schwartz, R. S., and Gibbons, R. J. Determinants of infarct size in reperfusion therapy for acute myocardial infarction. *Circulation* 86:81, 1992.
38. Granger, C. B., Califf, R. M., and Topol, E. J. Thrombolytic therapy for acute myocardial infarction: A review. *Drugs* 44:293, 1992.
39. ISIS-3 (Third International Study of Infarct Survival) Collaborative Group. ISIS-3: A randomized comparison of streptokinase vs tissue plasminogen activator vs anistreplase and of aspirin plus heparin vs aspirin alone among 41,229 cases of suspected acute myocardial infarction. *Lancet* 339:753, 1992.
40. The International Study Group. In-hospital mortality and clinical course of 20,891 patients with suspected acute myocardial infarction randomized between alteplase and streptokinase with or without heparin. *Lancet* 336:71, 1990.
41. The GUSTO Investigators. An international randomized trial comparing four thrombolytic strategies for acute myocardial infarction. *N. Engl. J. Med.* 329: 673, 1993.
42. Wall, T. C., Califf, R. M., George, B. S., et al. for the TAMI-7 Study Group. Accelerated plasminogen activator dose regimens for coronary thrombolysis. *J. Am. Coll. Cardiol.* 19:482, 1992.
43. The GUSTO Angiographic Investigators. The effects of tissue plasminogen activator, streptokinase, or both on coronary-artery patency, ventricular function, and survival after acute myocardial infarction. *N. Engl. J. Med.* 329:1615, 1993.
44. Mark, D. B., Hlatky, M. A., and O'Connor, C. M. Administration of thrombolytic therapy in the community hospital: Established principles and unresolved issues. *J. Am. Coll. Cardiol.* 12:32A, 1988.
45. Sharpe, N. Ventricular remodeling following myocardial infarction. *Am. J. Cardiol.* 70:20C, 1992.
46. Weisman, H. F., Bush, D. E., Mannisi, J. A., et al. Cellular mechanisms of myocardial infarct expansion. *Circulation* 78:186, 1988.
47. Erlebacher, J. A., Weiss, J. L., Eaton, L. W., et al. Late effects of acute infarct dilation on heart size. A two-dimensional echocardiographic study. *Am. J. Cardiol.* 49:1120, 1982.
48. Jeremy, R. W., Allman, K. C., Bautovitch, G., et al. Patterns of left ventricular dilatation during the six months after myocardial infarction. *J. Am. Coll. Cardiol.* 13:304, 1989.
49. Hockman, J. S., and Choo, H. Limitation of myocardial infarct expansion by reperfusion independent of myocardial salvage. *Circulation* 75:299, 1987.
50. Hale, S. L., and Kloner, R. A. Left ventricular topographic alterations in the completely healed rat infarct caused by early and late coronary artery reperfusion. *Am. Heart J.* 116:1508, 1988.
51. Brown, E. J., Swinford, R. D., Gadde, P., et al. Acute effects of delayed reperfusion on myocardial infarct shape and left ventricular volume: A potential mechanism of additional benefits from thrombolytic therapy. *J. Am. Coll. Cardiol.* 17:1641, 1991.
52. Califf, R. M., Topol, E. J., and Gersh, B. J. From myocardial salvage to patient salvage in acute myocardial infarction: The role of reperfusion therapy. *J. Am. Coll. Cardiol.* 14:1382, 1989.
53. Lamas, G. A., Pfeffer, M. A., and Braunwald, E. Patency of the infarct-related coronary artery and ventricular geometry. *Am. J. Cardiol.* 68:41D, 1991.
54. Jeremy, R. W., Hackworthy, R. A., Bautovich, G., et al. Infarct artery perfusion and changes in left ventricular volume in the month after acute myocardial infarction. *J. Am. Coll. Cardiol.* 9:989, 1987.
55. Touchstone, D. A., Beller, G. A., Nygaard, T. W., et al. Effects of successful intravenous reperfusion therapy on regional myocardial function and geometry in humans: A tomographic assessment using two-

dimensional echocardiography. *J. Am.Coll. Cardiol.* 13:1506, 1989.
56. Siu, S. C., Nidorf, S. M., Galambos, G. S., et al. The effect of late patency of the infarct-related coronary artery on left ventricular morphology and regional function after thrombolysis. *Am. Heart J.* 124:265, 1992.
57. Marino, P., Zanolla, L., Zardini, P., on behalf of the Gruppo Italiano per lo Studio della Streptochinasi nell'Infarto Miocardico (GISSI). Effect of streptokinase on left ventricular modeling and function after myocardial infarction: The GISSI (Gruppo Italiano per lo Studio della Streptochinasi nell'Infarto Miocardico) Trial. *J. Am. Coll. Cardiol.* 14:1149, 1989.
58. Hirayama, A., Mishima, M., Nanto, S., et al. Limitation of infarct expansion by late reperfusion independent of myocardial salvage in patients with acute myocardial infarction (Abstract). *Circulation* 84 (Suppl II):II-232, 1991.
59. Forman, M. B., Collins, H. W., Kopelman, H. A., et al. Determinants of left ventricular aneurysm formation after anterior myocardial infarction: A clinical and angiographic study. *J. Am. Coll. Cardiol.* 8:1256, 1986.
60. Hirai T., Fujita, M., Nakajima, H., et al. Importance of collateral circulation for prevention of left ventricular aneurysm formation in acute myocardial infarction. *Circulation* 79:791, 1989.
61. Arnold, J. M. O., Antman, E. M., Przyklenk, K., et al. Differential effects of reperfusion on incidence of ventricular arrhythmias and recovery of ventricular function at 4 days following coronary occlusion. *Am. Heart J.* 113:1055, 1987.
62. Fortin, D. F., and Califf, R. M. Long-term survival from acute myocardial infarction: Salutary effect of an open coronary vessel. *Am. J. Med.* 88:IN, 1990.
63. Herre, J. M., Wetstein, L., Lin, Y. L., et al. Effect of transmural versus nontransmural myocardial infarction on inducibility of ventricular arrhythmias during sympathetic stimulation in dogs. *J. Am. Coll. Cardiol.* 11:414, 1988.
64. Bates, E. R. Is survival in acute myocardial infarction related to thrombolytic efficacy or the open-artery hypothesis? A controversy to be investigated with GUSTO. *Chest* 4(Suppl):140S, 1992.
65. Denniss, A. R., Richards, D. A., Cody, D. V., et al. Prognostic significance of ventricular tachycardia and fibrillation induced at programmed stimulation and delayed potentials detected on the signal-averaged electrocardiograms of survivors of acute myocardial infarction. *Circulation* 74:731, 1986.
66. Vatterott, P. J., Hammill, S. C., Bailey, K. R., et al. Late potentials on signal-averaged electrocardiograms and patency of the infarct-related artery in survivors of acute myocardial infarction. *J. Am. Coll. Cardiol.* 17:330, 1991.
67. Gang, E. S., Lew, A. S., Hong, M., et al. Decreased incidence of ventricular late potentials after successful thrombolytic therapy for acute myocardial infarction. *N. Engl. J. Med.* 321:712, 1989.
68. Moreno, F. L. L., Karagounis, L., Marshall, H., et al. Thrombolysis-related early patency reduces ECG late potentials after acute myocardial infarction. *Am. Heart J.* 124:557, 1992.
69. Lange, R. A., Cigarroa, R. G., Wells, P. J., et al. Influence of anterograde flow in the infarct artery on the incidence of late potentials after acute myocardial infarction. *Am. J. Cardiol.* 65:554, 1990.
70. Sager, P. T., Perlmutter, R. A., Rosenfeld, L. E., et al. Electrophysiologic effects of thrombolytic therapy in patients with a transmural anterior myocardial infarction complicated by left ventricular aneurysm formation. *J. Am. Coll. Cardiol.* 12:19, 1988.
71. Kerrschot, I. E., Brugada, P., Ramentol, M., et al. Effects of early reperfusion in acute myocardial infarction on arrhythmias induced by programmed stimulation: A prospective randomized study. *J. Am. Coll. Cardiol.* 7:1234, 1986.
72. Holmes, D. R., Davis, K. B., Mock, M. B., et al. The effect of medical and surgical treatment on subsequent sudden cardiac death in patients with coronary artery disease: A report from the coronary artery surgery study. *Circulation* 73:1254, 1986.
73. The CAST Study Group. Preliminary report: Effect of encainide and flecainide on mortality in a randomized trial of arrhythmia suppression after myocardial infarction. *N. Engl. J. Med.* 321:406, 1989.
74. Hii, J. T. Y., Traboulsi, M., Mitchell, B., et al. Infarct artery patency predicts outcome of serial electropharmacological studies in patients with malignant ventricular tachyarrhythmias. *Circulation* 87:764, 1993.
75. Sabia, P. J., Powers, E. R., Ragosta, M., et al. An association between collateral blood flow and myocardial viability in patients with recent myocardial infarction. *N. Engl. J. Med.* 327:1825, 1992.
76. Montalescot, G., Faraggi, M., Drobinski, G., et al. Myocardial viability in patients with Q wave myocardial infarction and no residual ischemia. *Circulation* 86:47, 1992.
77. Honan, M. B., Harrell, F. E., Reimer, K. A., et al. Cardiac rupture, mortality and the timing of thrombolytic therapy: A meta-analysis. *J. Am. Coll. Cardiol.* 16:359, 1990.
78. Neuhaus, K. L., Feuerer, W., Jeep-Teebe, S., et al. Improved thrombolysis with a modified dose regimen of recombinant tissue-type plasminogen activator. *J. Am. Coll. Cardiol.* 14:1566, 1989.
79. McKendall, G. R., Attubato, M., Drew, T. M., et al. Improved infarct artery patency using a new modified regimen of t-PA: Results of the pre-hospital administration of t-PA (PATS) pilot trial (Abstract). *J. Am. Coll. Cardiol.* 15(Suppl A):3A, 1989.
80. Gersh, B. J., and Anderson, J. L. Thrombolysis and myocardial salvage. Results of clinical trials and the animal paradigm—paradoxic or predictable? *Circulation* 88:296, 1993.
81. The European Myocardial Infarction Group. Prehospital thrombolytic therapy in patients with suspected acute myocardial infarction. *N. Engl. J. Med.* 329:383, 1993.

82. Weaver, W. D., Cerqueria, M., Hallstrom, A. P., et al. for the Myocardial Infarction Triage and Intervention Project Group. Prehospital-initiated vs hospital-initiated thrombolytic therapy: The myocardial infarction triage and intervention trial. *J.A.M.A.* 270:1211, 1993.
83. Stack, R. S., Califf, R. M., Hinohara, T., et al. Survival and cardiac event rates in the first year after emergency coronary angioplasty for acute myocardial infarction. *J. Am. Coll. Cardiol.* 11:1141, 1988.
84. Whitlow, P. L. for the CRAFT Study Group. Catheterization/rescue angioplasty following thrombolysis (CRAFT): Results of rescue angioplasty (Abstract). *Circulation* 82(Suppl III):III-308, 1990.
85. Abbotsmith, C. W., Topol, E. J., George, B. S., et al. Fate of patients with acute myocardial infarction with patency of the infarct-related vessel achieved with successful thrombolysis versus rescue angioplasty. *J. Am. Coll. Cardiol.* 16:770, 1990.
86. Califf, R. M., Topol, E. J., Stack, R. S., et al. for the TAMI Study Group. Evaluation of combination thrombolytic therapy and timing of cardiac catheterization in acute myocardial infarction. *Circulation* 83:1543, 1991.
87. Ellis, S. G., da Silva, E. R., Heyndricks, G., et al. for the RESCUE Investigators. Final results of the randomized RESCUE study evaluating PTCA after failed thrombolysis for patients with anterior infarction. (Abstract). *Circulation* 88(Suppl I):I-106, 1993.
88. Krucoff, M. W., Green, C. E., Satler, L. F., et al. Noninvasive detection of coronary artery patency using continuous ST-segment monitoring. *Am. J. Cardiol.* 57:916, 1986.
89. Saran, R. K., Been, M., Furness, S. S., et al. Reduction in ST segment elevation after thrombolysis predicts either coronary reperfusion or preservation of left ventricular function. *Br. Heart J.* 64:113, 1990.
90. Santoro, G. M., Bisi, G., Sciagra, R., et al. Single-photon emission computed tomography with technetium-99m hexakis 2-methoxyisobutyl isonitril in acute myocardial infarction before and after thrombolytic treatment: Assessment of salvaged myocardium and prediction of late functional recovery. *J. Am. Coll. Cardiol.* 15:301, 1990.
91. Puleo, P. R., Guadagno, P. A., Roberts, R., et al. Early diagnosis of acute myocardial infarction based on assay of subforms of creatine kinase-MB. *Circulation* 82:759, 1990.
92. Califf, R. M., O'Neil, W., Stack, R. S., et al. Failure of simple clinical measurements to predict perfusion status after intravenous thrombolysis. *Ann. Int. Med.* 108:658, 1988.
93. Bernardi, M. M., and Whitlow, P. L. Reperfusion later than five days after acute myocardial infarction improves three-year survival (Abstract). *Circulation* 84:II-232, 1991.
94. Dzavik, V., Beanlands, D. S., Davies, R. F., et al. Beneficial effect of successful late PTCA on LV ejection fraction in patients with a recent infarct related coronary artery occlusion. *J. Am. Coll. Cardiol.* (Abstract). 19:229A, 1992.

28. Echocardiography in Acute Myocardial Infarction

Anne M. Hepner and William F. Armstrong

Acute myocardial infarction (AMI) is a leading cause of morbidity and mortality in the United States and other industrialized nations. Modern therapy includes emergent hospitalization with stabilization of hemodynamics and close observation for arrhythmias and other complications of myocardial infarction (MI). Moreover, today, emergent intervention in an effort to reverse the course of AMI and preserve myocardial function is often undertaken. Because of the immediate and dramatic sequelae of acute coronary occlusion, speed of diagnosis and rapid institution of therapy is of utmost importance. Diagnostic studies that allow rapid assessment of MI location and size and the likelihood of complications are of paramount importance in the initial management of these patients. In most institutions this assessment is performed by a combination of studies, including electrocardiography (ECG), enzyme determinations, and some form of cardiac imaging.

Because cardiac imaging provides a direct assessment of MI size and location, it is playing an increasing role in evaluating patients and in decision-making regarding emergent therapy. Of the multiple forms of cardiac imaging available, two-dimensional echocardiography is probably the one most often associated with cardiology but, paradoxically, in many institutions is the one least often used in patients with coronary artery disease. Although the ability of two-dimensional echocardiography to accurately diagnose congenital, pericardial, valvular, and primary myocardial disease is well known, its utility in patients with acute and chronic manifestations of coronary artery disease is less well appreciated by those not intimately involved in the technique.

In this chapter we first review the principles of registering a two-dimensional echocardiogram and then the practical data that can be gained from echocardiography in patients with known or suspected MI. Finally, we review some investigational techniques that may have future applicability in patients with coronary disease. It should be noted that all the echocardiographic illustrations in this chapter are taken from the frozen image of a video screen. In reality, interpretation of the echocardiographic examination is done in real time from the videotaped image of the beating heart. The real-time image is of higher visual quality than the single frozen frame images presented here and generally contains substantially more diagnostic information.

Two-Dimensional Echocardiographic Examination

Echocardiographic examination involves the combined utilization of three interdependent modalities. The primary imaging technique is two-dimensional echocardiography, which serves as the routine screening tool for defining chamber size, anatomic abnormalities, and detection and quantification of wall motion abnormalities. M-mode echocardiography, the older imaging technique, provides only a limited "ice pick" view of the heart and now plays little or no role in the evaluation of patients with coronary artery disease. Doppler ultrasound techniques allow determination of the direction and velocity of blood flow, from which information concerning intracardiac physiology can be deduced. The newer technique of color Doppler flow imaging allows visualization for intracardiac shunts and can be used to detect ventricular septal defects (VSD) and regurgitant valvular lesions developing as a consequence of MI.

The Transthoracic Echocardiographic Examination

The transthoracic echocardiographic examination can be performed using equipment of only moderate cost and with relatively limited requirements with respect to personnel and laboratory space. Modern echocardiographic equipment is portable, and the examination can be performed in the emergency room, coronary care unit, catheterization laboratory, echocardiography laboratory, or physician's office. Information concerning coincident valvular, pericardial, myocardial, or congenital heart disease is immediately obtained with a high degree of accuracy. Because the examination affords an excellent view of all areas of the heart, two-dimensional echocardiography combined with Doppler interrogation can be used for detection of all mechanical complications of MI.

The examination is generally performed by a single sonographer-technician. A transducer directs an array of ultrasound beams into the chest. These rays are then reflected from intracardiac structures and converted into a real-time, two-dimensional image of the beating heart. This examination is performed in multiple tomographic views. Most diagnoses rely on a series of parasternal long- and short-axis views and apical two- and four-chamber views. The orientation of the more common echocardiographic views with respect to external cardiac anatomy is presented in Figures 28-1 and 28-2. An example of a normal two-dimensional echocardiogram is presented in Figures 28-3 and 28-4.

Transthoracic echocardiography has several advantages compared with other imaging modalities that are often used in patients with AMI. Among these advantages are its relatively low cost, the versatility of the examination with respect to being able to assist in the diagnosis of virtually any form of heart disease, the portability of the equipment, the short time required to accomplish an examination, and the totally noninvasive and risk-free nature of the examination, which allows it to be repeated at short intervals if necessary. Disadvantages include the user-interactive nature of the examination, which requires skilled sonographers to perform the examination and highly trained personnel for interpretation. The success with which the complete examination is adequately accomplished in adult patients is less than it is in pediatric populations; however, in the majority of experienced laboratories, diagnostic information is available for more than 95 percent of patients.

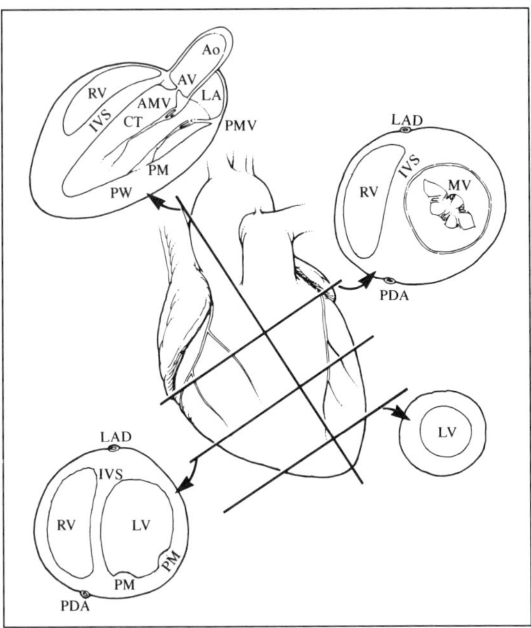

Fig. 28-1
Parasternal echocardiographic imaging planes. The topography of the heart is illustrated along with the plane of imaging for the parasternal long-axis view (*upper left*) and parasternal short-axis view at the mitral level (*upper right*), papillary muscle level (*middle right*), and apical level (*lower right*). Ao = aorta; LA, RA = left and right atria; LV, RV = left and right ventricles; MV = mitral valve; AV = aortic valve; IVS = intraventricular septum; PW = posterior wall; AMV, PMV = anterior and posterior mitral valves; CT = chordae tendineae; LAD = left anterior descending artery; PDA = posterior descending artery.

The Transesophageal Echocardiographic Examination

The transesophageal echocardiographic examination typically is performed with a 5 mHz imaging transducer attached to a modified gastroscope. The transesophageal transducer is then linked to the standard echocardiographic machine. The examination is performed by a physician echocardiographer in combination with a sonographer-technician who is responsible for operating the echocardiography machine. After the patient has had a 6-hour fast, in-

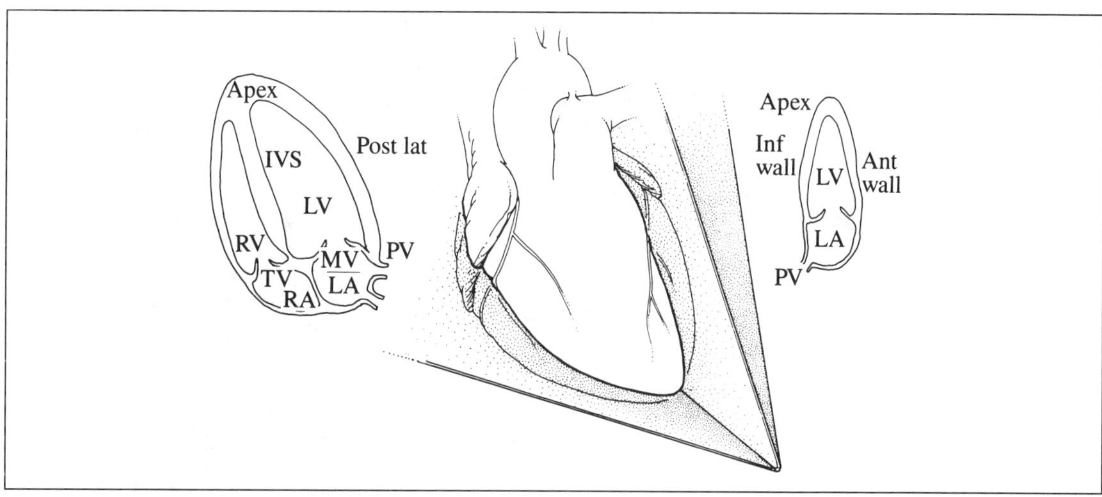

Fig. 28-2
Apical imaging planes. The two traditional apical views are the four-chamber and two-chamber views and are schematized to the left and right of the heart, respectively. See Figure 28-1 for abbreviations.

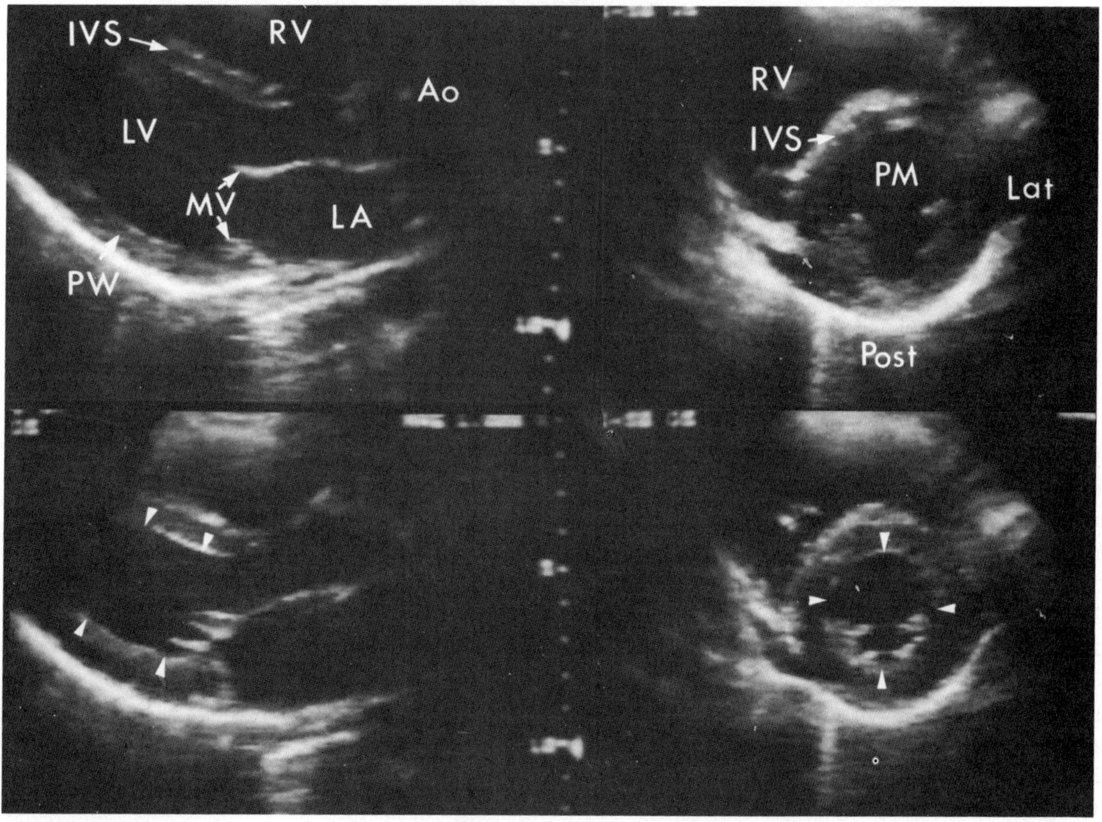

Fig. 28-3
Normal parasternal long- and short-axis views of the left ventricle. Note the normal thickness of all regions of visualized myocardium and the inward motion and thickening of the myocardium that have occurred with systole. See Figure 28-1 for abbreviations.

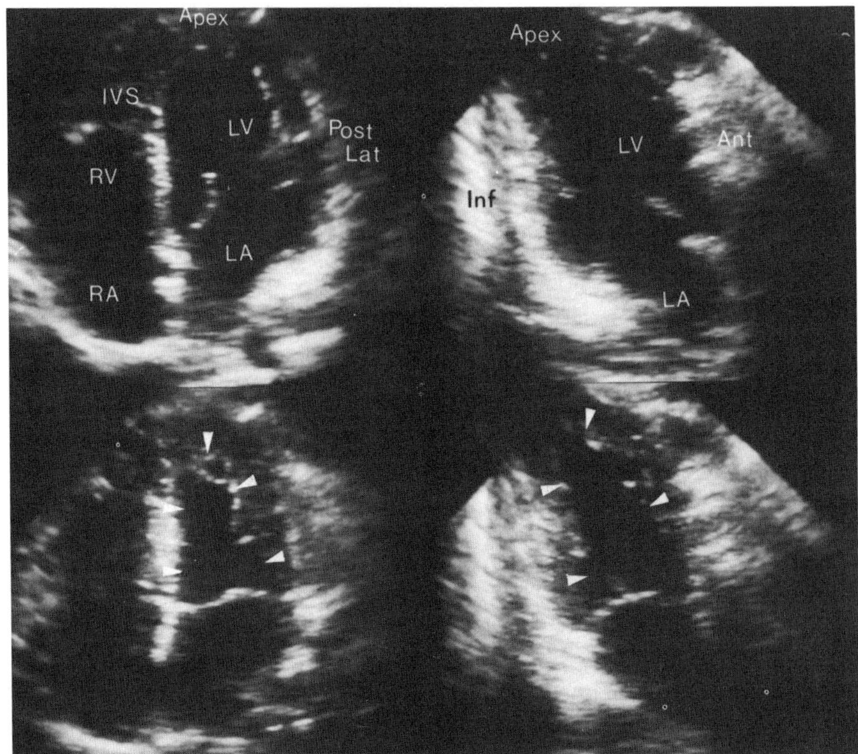

Fig. 28-4
Normal four- and two-chamber apical views. Note the normal "bullet" shape of the left ventricle and the more triangular geometry of the right ventricle during both diastole and systole. All regions of myocardium appropriately thicken and move inward with ventricular systole. See Figure 28-1 for abbreviations.

formed consent is obtained and the patient's throat is anesthetized with a topical aerosol anesthetic. Intravenous sedation is administered and the patient is rotated to a left lateral decubitus position. A plastic bite guard is placed in the patient's mouth and the transesophageal probe is passed into the patient's esophagus. The array of ultrasound beams is directed toward the heart via the esophageal probe. These rays are then reflected from intracardiac structures and converted into a real-time, two-dimensional image of the beating heart. Multiple views of intracardiac structures are obtained by advancing and withdrawing the probe or by flexing and retroflexing the scope (Figs. 28-5 through 28-7). Because the probe is close to cardiac structures and a high-frequency transducer is used, artifact is kept to a minimum and clear images of all cardiac structures can be obtained. Exceptional views of the mitral and submitral apparatus, left atrial appendage, interatrial septum, and ascending and descending aorta are routinely obtained. The use of a biplane or multiplane probe affords additional views, including the proximal superior vena cava, inferior vena cava, ascending aortic root, and pulmonary artery.

Transesophageal echocardiography is especially useful in patients with AMI and new hemodynamic compromise or new murmurs when the diagnosis is still in question after a transthoracic echocardiogram. Patients with aortic dissection and associated MI, as well as ventilated or obese patients with difficult transthoracic windows, represent subsets in which transesophageal echocardiography can provide unique and critical clinical information.

Transesophageal echocardiography has several advantages over other conventional imaging modalities, including cardiac catheterization and magnetic resonance imaging (MRI). It is portable, does not require the use of nephrotoxic contrast dye, can be performed within a short period of time on an

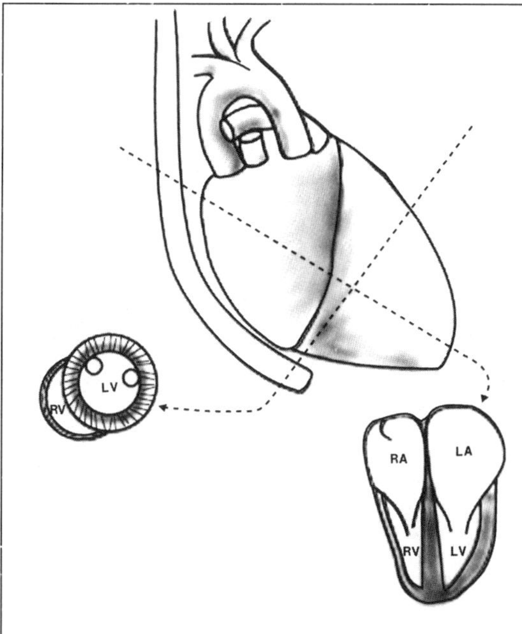

Fig. 28-5
Schematic diagram representing the transesophageal probe in position within the esophagus. Short- and long-axis views are obtained by altering the position of the probe in the esophagus. LA = left atrium; RA = right atrium; LV = left ventricle; RV = right ventricle.

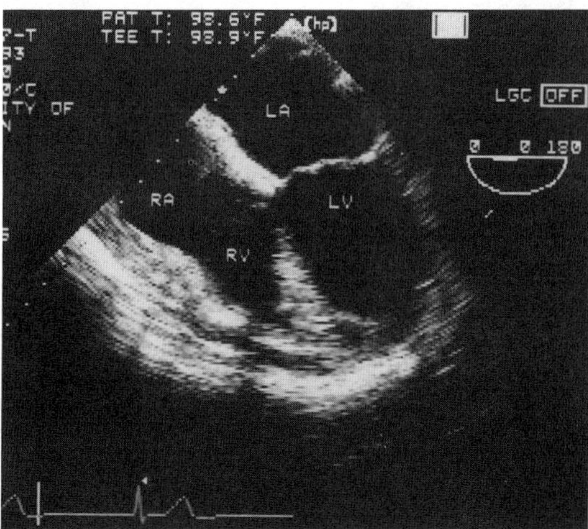

Fig. 28-6
Standard four-chamber view illustrating all four chambers and mitral and tricuspid valves. MV = mitral valve; TV = tricuspid valve; LA = left atrium; RA = right atrium; LV = left ventricle; RV = right ventricle.

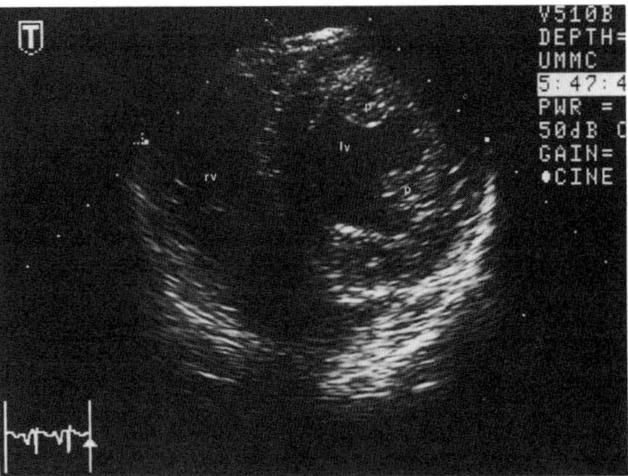

Fig. 28-7
Standard transgastric view of the left ventricle at papillary muscle level. LV = left ventricle; RV = right ventricle; P = papillary muscle.

emergent basis, and does not require multiple staff members to complete the study. Disadvantages include the need for intravenous sedation and the inability to perform the test in patients with significant esophageal pathology.

Sensitivity of Echocardiography in Detecting Coronary Artery Disease

The premise underlying the utilization of echocardiography for coronary disease is that myocardial ischemia or MI results in abnormal left ventricular (LV) wall motion that can then be detected by echocardiography. That the wall motion becomes abnormal almost immediately after onset of myocardial ischemia was first described by Tennant and Wiggers in 1935 [1]. Two-dimensional echocardiography can detect wall motion abnormalities associated with transient myocardial ischemia or AMI and those that result from established remote MI. Abnormal wall motion with ischemia or MI has subsequently been documented by a number of other techniques including ventriculography, radionuclide angiography, and electrocardiography [2–4].

The advent of percutaneous balloon angioplasty afforded the opportunity to evaluate the timing of onset of wall motion abnormalities after interruption of coronary flow in patients. These studies have confirmed earlier animal work that showed almost immediate onset of wall motion abnormalities after coronary occlusion. After coronary occlusion by balloon at the time of angioplasty, wall motion becomes almost immediately abnormal, preceding the onset of ECG changes or angina [4–6]. In this setting, wall motion abnormalities may also occur in the absence of typical symptoms or ECG changes.

As imaged with two-dimensional echocardiography, normal LV wall motion includes two interrelated phenomena: myocardial thickening and concurrent motion of the endocardial border toward the center of the left ventricle, both of which contribute to shrinking of the ventricular cavity and ejection of blood during systole. Myocardial thickening and endocardial motion can be detected with echocardiography. With mild degrees of ischemia, myocardial thickening is diminished and, coincident with the inward endocardial motion, the affected segment first diminishes (hypokinesis) and then moves paradoxically (dyskinesis) with more advanced stages of ischemia [7–11]. This two-stage abnormality of wall motion is a simplification; in reality, there is marked heterogeneity over the time course of systole, such that the wall may initially move paradoxically but later during systole have more appropriate motion [12].

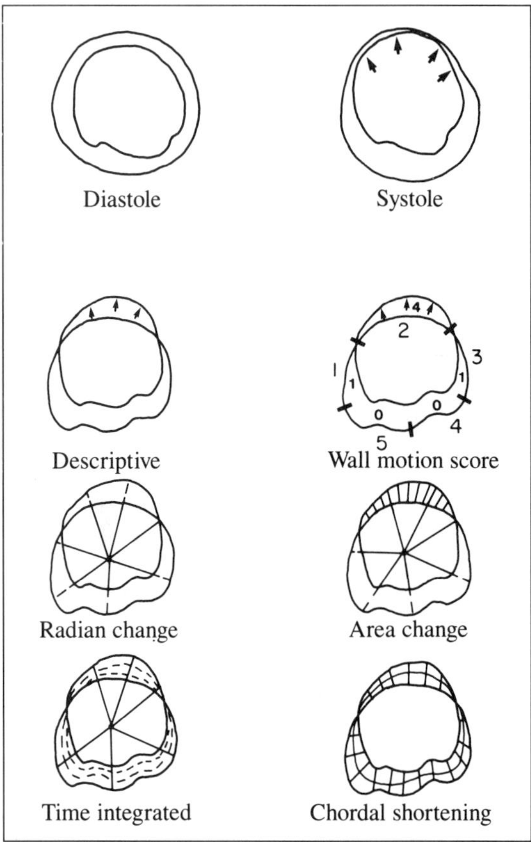

Fig. 28-8
Multiple algorithms by which wall motion can be graded. An example of anterior dyskinesis is presented that can be described in a purely descriptive manner as dyskinetic or quantified by any of the five demonstrated algorithms. See text for full details. (From W. F. Armstrong. Echocardiography in coronary artery disease. *Prog. Cardiovasc. Dis.* 30:267, 1988. With permission.)

Methods of Wall Motion Analysis

Early studies relied on visual assessment of wall motion abnormalities and classified them by subjective criteria as normal, hypokinetic, akinetic, or dyskinetic. The exact methodology for analyzing and quantifying wall motion is not uniformly accepted among echocardiographers; reports using different schemes for analysis of wall motion are often generated.

Figure 28-8 shows several such methods. Superimposed on any of these schemes is the understanding that LV regions are perfused by different coronary arteries. The general relation of the perfusion beds of the three major epicardial coronary arteries to the echocardiographic walls is presented in Figure 28-9. The simplest method is visual assessment of normal versus akinetic, dyskinetic, or hypokinetic motion, which can then be semiquantified by dividing the left ventricle into predefined regions and assigning a numerical hierarchy to increasing degrees of wall motion abnormality in each of the regions. These numbers can be summed to form a wall motion score or indexed to the number of segments to form a wall motion score index [13]. Figures 28-10 and 28-11 are examples of the wall motion score index generated for two patients with small inferior and large anteroapical infarctions, respectively. This semiquantitative method for quantifying wall motion abnormalities thus takes into account both the severity of the abnormality and its extent in the left ventricle. This technique of determining a wall motion score has found its most practical use in clinical assessment of patients with AMI.

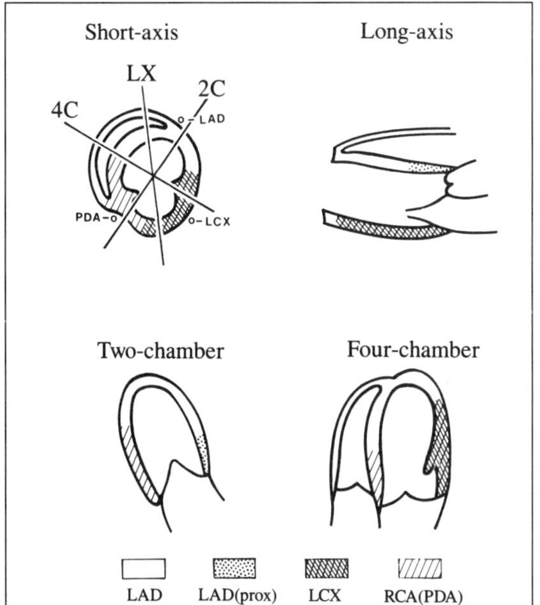

Fig. 28-9
General distribution of the coronary arteries versus the echocardiographic wall segments. (From H. Feigenbaum. *Echocardiography* [4th ed.]. Philadelphia: Lea & Febiger, 1986. With permission.)

More detailed and quantitative schemes have also been developed. They rely on outlining the endocardial border at end diastole and end systole and then creating a series of radians from the center of the mass of the left ventricle. The left ventricle is then subdivided into any number of regions (typically 16 to 100) that can be quantitatively evaluated by shortening individual radians or shrinking individual subtended areas [14]. Methodologic problems arise in defining the center of the mass of the ventricle during diastole and systole. In addition, the left ventricle rotates around both its long and short axes during contraction, which may cause nonequivalent regions to be compared during diastole and systole. Several methods have been proposed to correct for this phenomenon, none of which has been uniformly accepted by echocardiographers [15].

Newer methods for analyzing wall motion include analysis of the entire contraction sequence as suggested by Weyman, Gillam, and their colleagues [12, 16, 17] and the centerline chordal shortening method originally developed for angiography but subsequently applied to two-dimensional echocardiography [18, 19]. The detailed studies by Weyman and others explain many of the problems previously encountered with analysis of wall motion. These workers demonstrated that there is a temporal heterogeneity to LV wall motion in the presence of myocardial ischemia. When the entire contraction sequence of the left ventricle is analyzed at 17-msec intervals from end diastole to end systole, it becomes apparent that dyskinesis occurs at different points during systole depending on the duration of myocardial ischemia. This results in a phenomenon in which endocardial position may be frankly dyskinetic during early systole but move to appropriate end-systolic points later in the contraction sequence. Dyskinesis has the effect of masking areas of wall motion abnormality present during early systole but not present at end systole.

The most recent method for quantitation of LV wall motion involves creation of an endocardial map. The left ventricle is "filleted" open and the area of abnormal wall motion is mapped by transferring its longitudinal and circumferential extent in multiple views onto the planar map of the ventricle. The surface area of the ventricular endocardium and the surface area of the wall motion abnormality can be quantified. This technique has provided valuable information regarding ventricular geometry and infarct remodeling [20–22].

Detection of Abnormal Wall Motion in Clinical Syndromes

Experimentally induced myocardial ischemia results in abnormal LV wall motion. Identical abnormalities occur with spontaneous ischemia in patients with coronary disease. Wall motion abnormalities associated with transient myocardial ischemia and MI are identical in appearance, the only difference being that those associated with MI persist, whereas those associated with transient ischemia (e.g., angina pectoris) disappear.

Several centers have evaluated the use of two-dimensional echocardiography at the time of variant angina, either spontaneous or induced with ergonovine [23–26]. The most extensive experience in this field is that of Distante and his colleagues from Pisa [25]. They noted that each of 37 spontaneous and 18 ergonovine-induced attacks of angina was associated with abnormalities of LV wall motion,

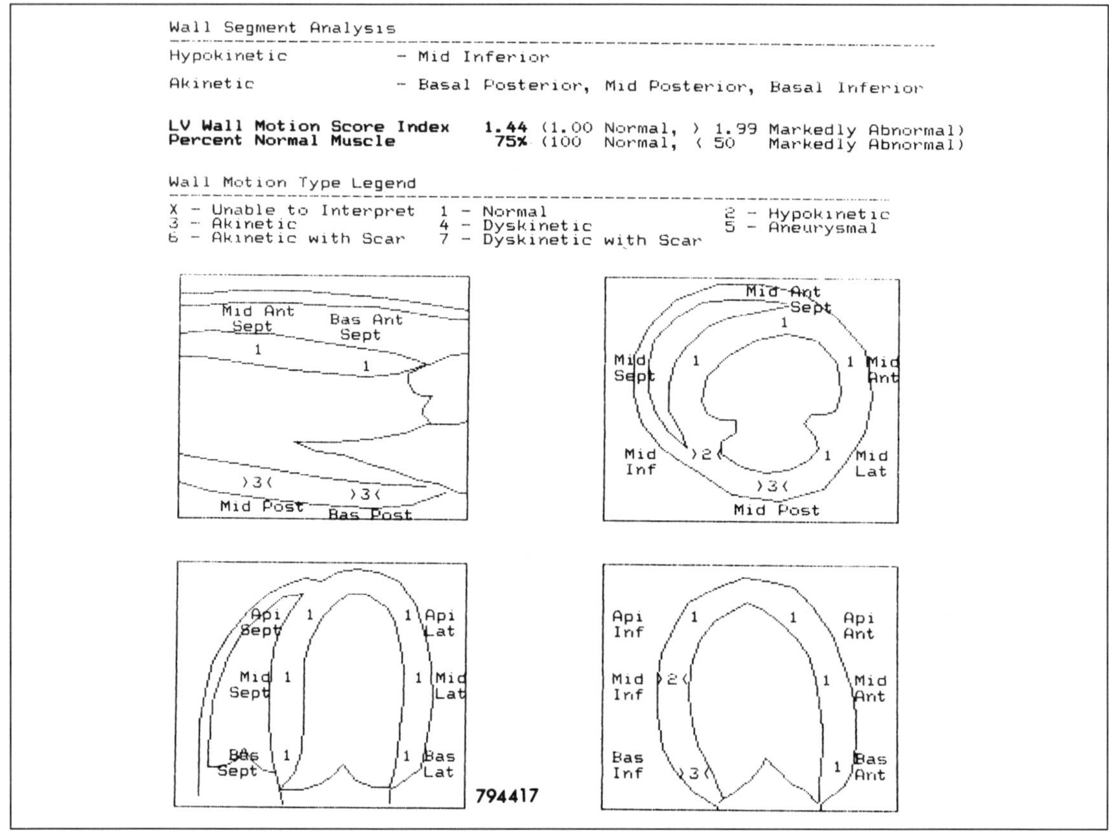

Fig. 28-10
Wall motion score generated by the patient presented in Figure 28-13. Note in the schematic portion that the inferoposterior and inferior walls are either hypokinetic (score 2) or akinetic (score 3) and that the remaining wall motion is normal. This pattern is consistent with a limited-extent electrocardiographic inferior infarction.

which generally preceded the onset of chest pain. Wall motion abnormalities were occasionally seen in the absence of chest pain or diagnostic ECG changes. Their data suggest that detection of wall motion abnormalities may be an early indicator of myocardial ischemia and that ECG monitoring during ergonovine challenge may allow detection of coronary spasm at a point before more advanced stages of ischemia are established, as is required when traditional endpoints are used.

Abnormal wall motion is often seen in patients presenting with unstable angina. Unlike variant angina, which has a clear onset and resolution of both the clinical syndrome and the wall motion abnormalities, unstable angina tends to be associated with more profound and long-lasting ischemia. Nixon and colleagues demonstrated that many patients with unstable angina have persistent wall motion abnormalities [27]. Some of the more long-lasting abnormalities may represent subclinical MI rather than active transient ischemia. Unlike the profound ischemia of unstable or preinfarction angina, milder attacks of angina may be associated with shorter-lived periods of abnormal wall motion, which are more difficult to detect because of their transient nature. Figure 28-12 was recorded in a patient with a spontaneous episode of angina during the echocardiographic examination and demonstrates a reversible wall motion abnormality of the anterior ventricular septum.

Comparison with Other Techniques

Two-dimensional echocardiography has been compared with other imaging techniques for detecting abnormal wall motion. The first large comparative

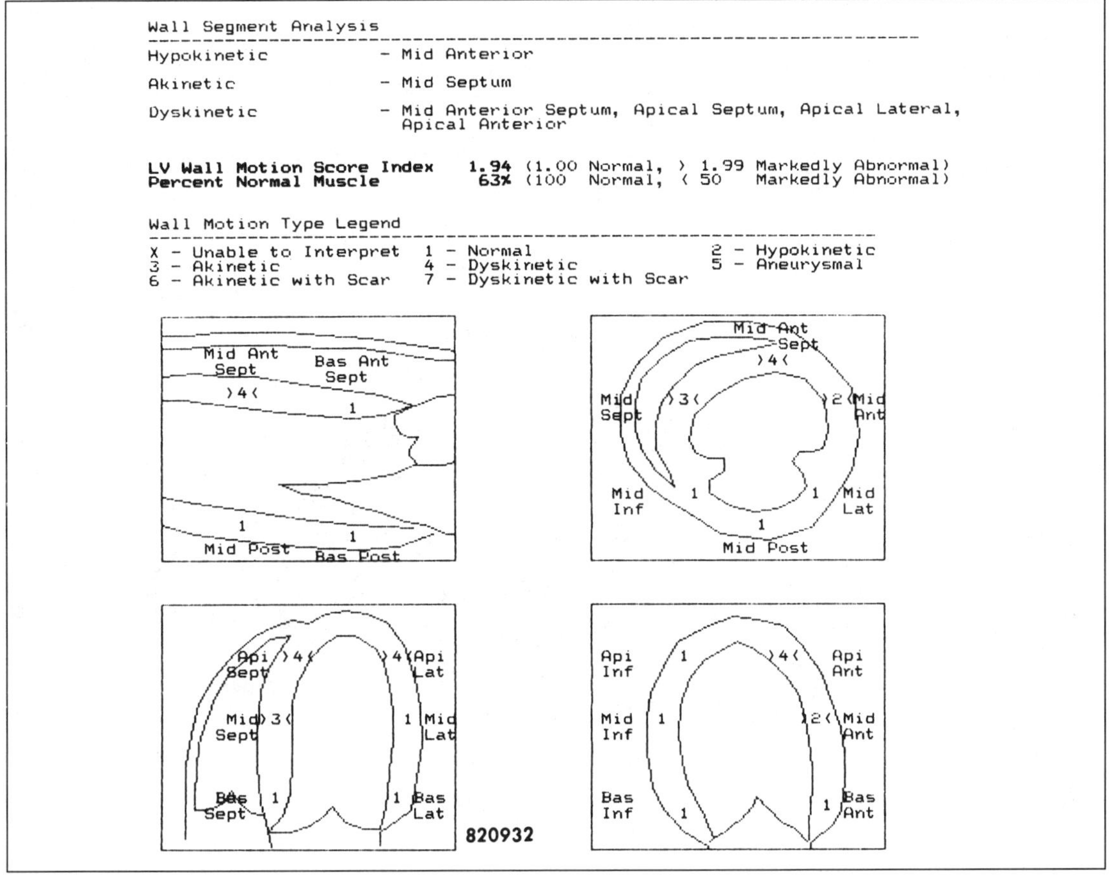

Fig. 28-11
Wall motion score generated in the patient presented in Figures 28-14 and 28-15. A large anteroapical infarction is present with a wall motion score index of 1.94.

study of echocardiography and biplane angiography was performed by Kisslo et al. in 105 patients [28]. Using early-generation scanning equipment, Kisslo and colleagues were able to obtain images adequate for analysis in 430 of 525 cardiac regions (82 percent) in their study patients. Comparing the two techniques, they noted concordance of observations with respect to the presence or absence of wall motion abnormalities in 375 of the 430 analyzable regions. Similar studies have been repeated by other investigators who have also included radionuclide techniques for comparison [3, 29–33]. Nixon and colleagues compared the presence of LV wall motion abnormalities and the distribution of thallium perfusion deficits in 32 consecutive patients admitted with AMI [33]. They found close correlations between two-dimensional echocardiographic wall motion scores and estimates of MI by both thallium scintigraphy and technetium pyrophosphate scanning.

Use in Diagnosis of Acute Myocardial Infarction

Given the sensitivity of echocardiographic scanning to detect ischemia-induced wall motion abnormalities, one obvious utilization of echocardiography is to assist in the initial diagnosis of AMI in the patient presenting with chest pain. One of the earliest demonstrations of this use was by Heger et al. These investigators performed two-dimensional echocardiograms within 48 hours of admission in 44 patients with chest pain and AMI [34]. Using early-generation equipment, wall motion abnormal-

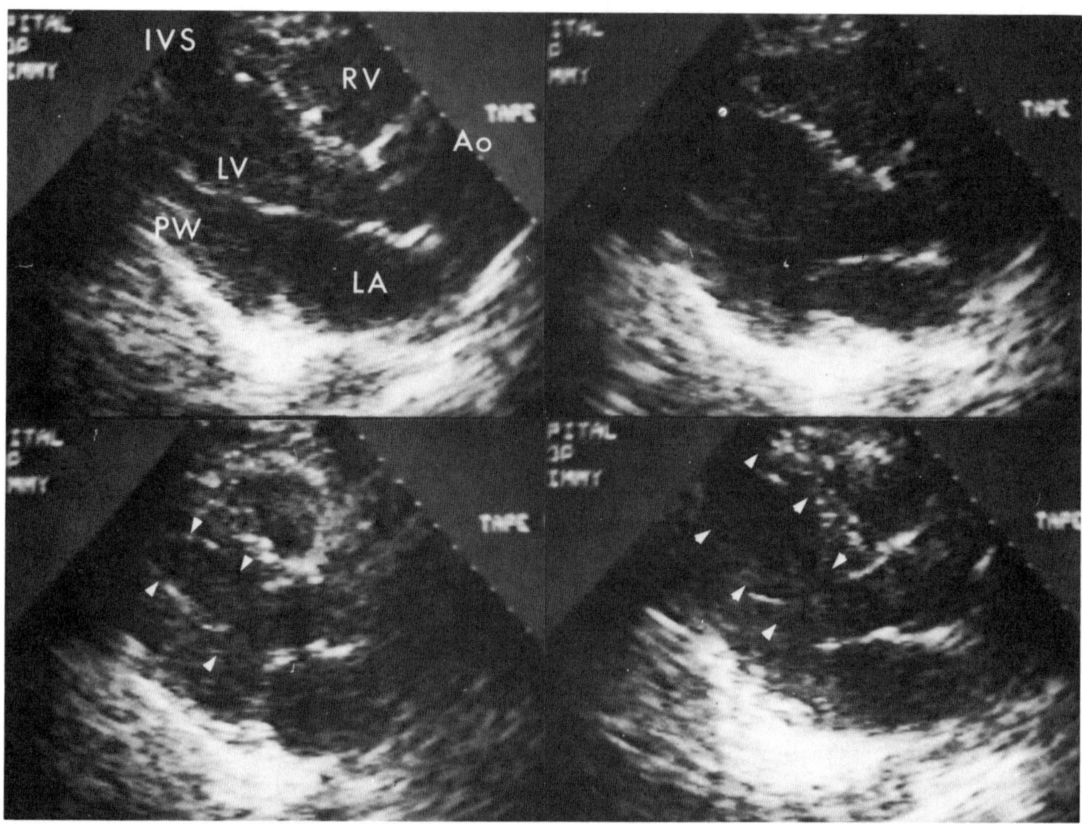

Fig. 28-12
Two-dimensional echocardiogram recorded in a patient with spontaneous angina. The parasternal long-axis views during diastole (*upper panels*) and systole (*lower panels*) in a pain-free state (*left panels*) and during a spontaneous episode of angina (*right panels*) are shown. During angina the distal anterior septum is dyskinetic, whereas wall motion remains normal in the inferoposterior wall.

ities were identified in 37 patients in whom complete echocardiographic studies could be recorded. There was generally good agreement between the ECG location of the MI and the echocardiographic wall motion abnormality. The patients with inferior MIs had wall motion abnormalities bordering on the posterior interventricular groove in the basal and mid portions of the left ventricle. The patients with either inferoposterior or inferolateral MIs on the echocardiogram had wall motion abnormalities in the continuous posterolateral regions of the left ventricle. Patients with anteroseptal MIs had apical, anterior wall, and septal involvement at the level of the mid ventricle. Those with anterolateral involvement had anterior septal, apical, and lateral wall involvement. Three patients with both anterior and inferior ECG changes had diffuse wall motion abnormalities, including (in each case) the apex, inferior wall, septum, lateral, and anterior walls at the mid ventricle, and the more proximal lateral and inferior walls.

In a similar study, Stamm and his colleagues evaluated 51 patients with recent MIs and single-vessel coronary disease subsequently proven with angiography [35]. Using a more detailed 11-segment ventricular model, they demonstrated a similar distribution of wall motion abnormalities. Their patients with single-vessel disease had localized wall motion abnormalities, whereas 17 of 20 patients with multivessel disease at subsequent cardiac catheterization had multiple regions of wall motion abnormality. The regions of remote wall motion abnormalities often normalized over the course of MI. The authors termed this phenomenon "remote asynergy" and demonstrated a link between this phenomenon and adverse clinical outcome. In a subsequent study from this same group, the presence of remote asynergy statistically correlated with subsequent angina, reinfarction, congestive failure, arrhythmia, and death [36].

Horowitz and colleagues from Philadelphia evaluated the ability of two-dimensional echocardiography to assist in the initial diagnosis of AMI in patients presenting with chest pain [37]. Their study was performed in 80 consecutive patients, 65 of whom (81 percent) had adequate two-dimensional echocardiograms recorded within 8 hours of admission. Abnormal regional wall motion was found in 36 of these patients, 31 of whom developed clinical MI as assessed by routine enzymatic and ECG criteria. Five patients with wall motion abnormalities failed to develop clinical MI; three of them subsequently underwent angiography, and coronary disease was demonstrated in each. These patients in all likelihood had unstable angina with wall motion abnormalities. LV wall motion was normal in 29 patients presenting with chest pain, and in 27 no

Fig. 28-13
Parasternal long-axis views recorded in a patient with an acute inferoposterior myocardial infarction. *Upper panel.* Note the full thickness of the inferoposterior wall during diastole (*black and white arrows*). *Lower panel.* With systole the anterior septum thickens and moves downward (*white arrows*), but the inferoposterior wall moves posteriorly and thins (*white arrows*). The wall motion score for this patient is presented in Figure 28-10.

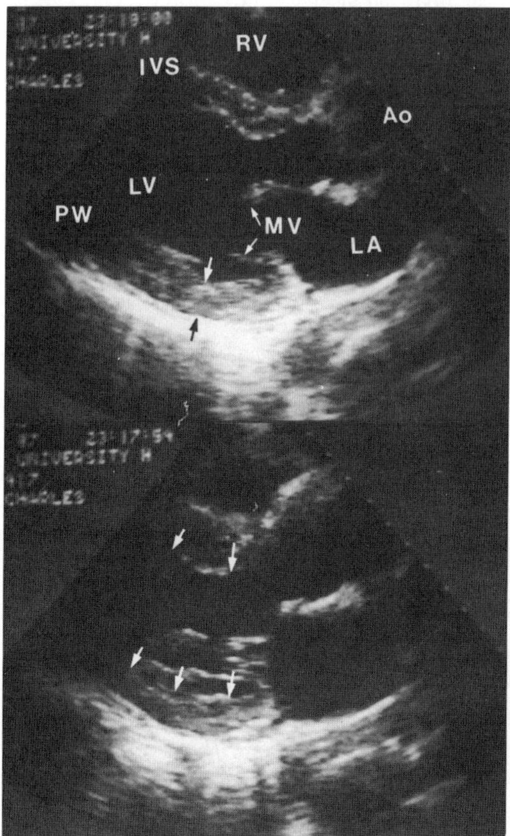

Fig. 28-14
Parasternal long-axis view during diastole (*upper panel*) and systole (*lower panel*) recorded in a patient presenting with a large anterior myocardial infarction. Note the preserved thickness of the ventricular septum and that the distal 90 percent of the anterior septum is dyskinetic during systole (*upward-pointing white arrows*), whereas the proximal portion of the ventricular septum moves normally.

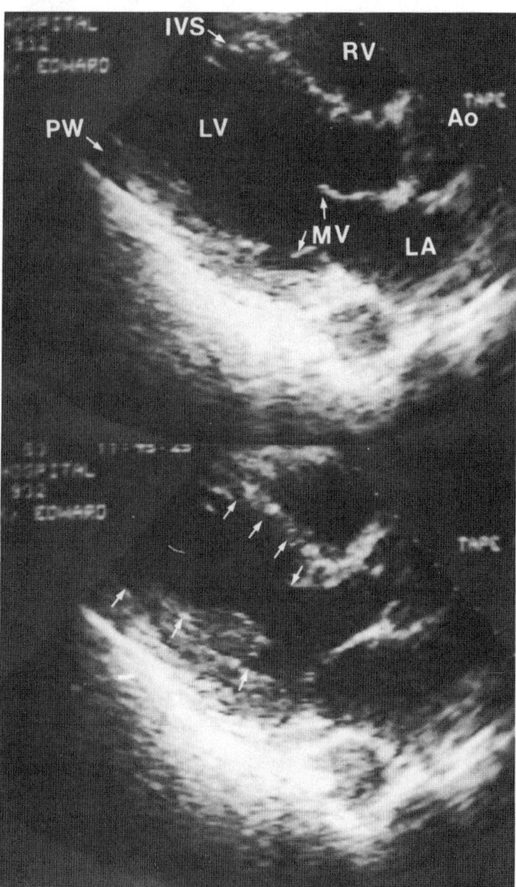

clinical MI developed. Two patients developed limited (by enzyme criteria) non-Q-wave MIs.

Cardiac complications occurred in ten patients in the cohort of 65 patients, all of whom had abnormal regional wall motion on echocardiography performed early after admission. Figures 28-13 through 28-17 were recorded in patients with either AMI or remote MI and demonstrate the range of abnormalities seen in MI.

Echocardiography has been shown to provide diagnostic and prognostic information in patients presenting to the emergency room with chest pain syndromes [38]. Sabia et al. followed 171 consecutive patients presenting to the emergency room with chest pain syndromes [39]. The average follow-up for these patients was two years. Two-dimensional echocardiography was performed in all patients in addition to routine ECG, history, and physical examination. One-third of patients suffered a major cardiac event during follow-up. Less than 10 percent of patients with normal LV systolic function suffered an event versus 50 percent in the group with abnormal LV systolic function (Fig. 28-18). ECG was an insensitive predictor of MI in this group, with only 9 of 29 patients demonstrating ST elevation in the presence of documented MI. Late events (after 48 hours) were also more frequent in patients with abnormal wall motion as seen by two-dimensional echocardiography (Fig. 28-19).

Patients presenting with typical chest pain and classic ECG changes of Q-wave MI rarely present a diagnostic dilemma. The patients with smaller non-Q-wave MI remain problematic by all diagnostic imaging techniques. This subset of patients has

Fig. 28-15
Apical four- and two-chamber views in the patient presented in Figure 28-14, demonstrating dyskinesis of the anterior wall, anterior septum, and apex (*arrows*). The wall motion score for this patient can be found in Figure 28-11.

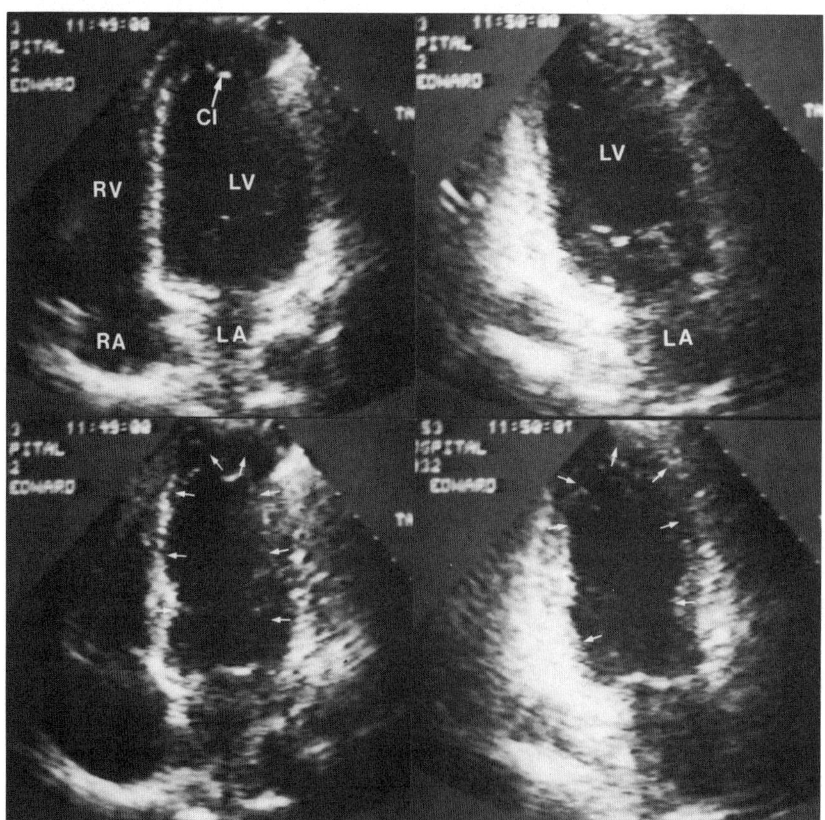

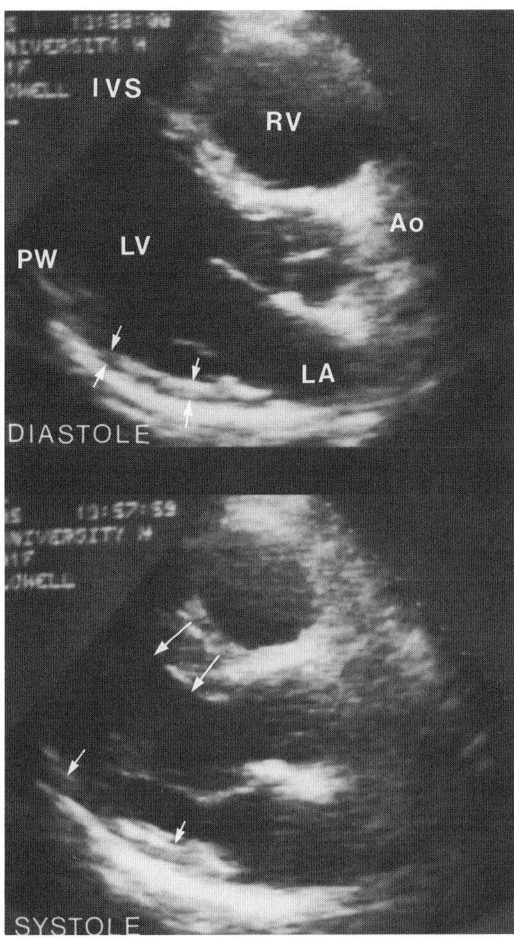

Fig. 28-16
Parasternal long-axis view recorded in a patient with a remote inferior myocardial infarction. During diastole (*upper panel*) note the normal-thickness ventricular septum with a thin, scarred inferoposterior wall (*arrows*). With systole the anterior septum thickens and moves normally, whereas the inferoposterior wall remains pathologically thinned and is dyskinetic.

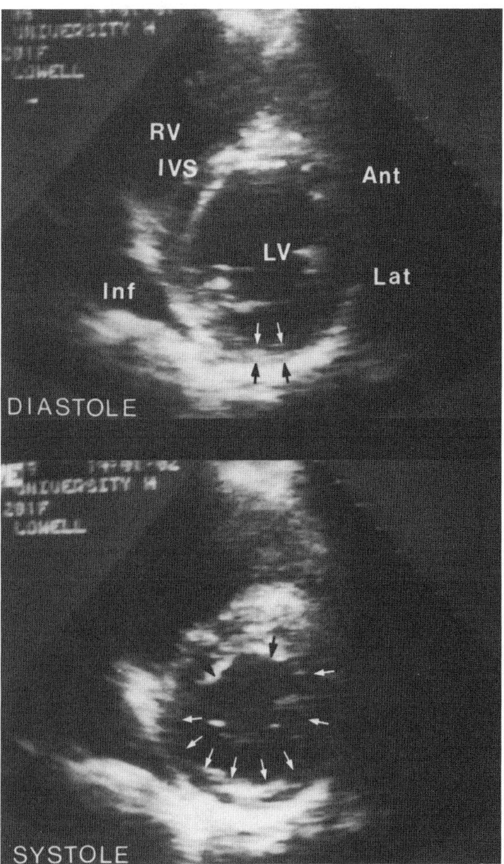

Fig. 28-17
Parasternal short-axis views in a patient with a remote inferior myocardial infarction (same as in Figure 28-16). Note the full thickness of the septum and the anterior and lateral walls and the pathologically thinned and scarred inferoposterior wall (*white and black arrows*). With systole (*lower panel*) the inferoposterior and inferior walls are dyskinetic.

been specifically evaluated with echocardiography by several investigators [39–41]. There is a threshold mass of myocardium and a degree of transmural infarction that must be exceeded before abnormal wall motion is detected by echocardiography; thus, the frequency of wall motion abnormalities in non-Q-wave MI is expected to be less than that seen in Q-wave MI.

Loh et al. evaluated this problem in 30 patients studied within 12.5 hours after the onset of chest pain [41]. Wall motion abnormalities were seen in 10 of 12 patients (83 percent) who were subsequently shown to have myocardial necrosis. Wall motion abnormalities were absent in all 18 patients who failed to develop clinical MI. A similar study was undertaken in 50 patients by Arvan and Varat [40]. Sensitivity for identifying patients who subsequently developed enzymatic evidence of a non-Q-wave MI was 67 percent for echocardiographic imaging versus 52 percent for ECG; respective specificities were 91 percent and 95 percent. Combining the results of the two studies increased the

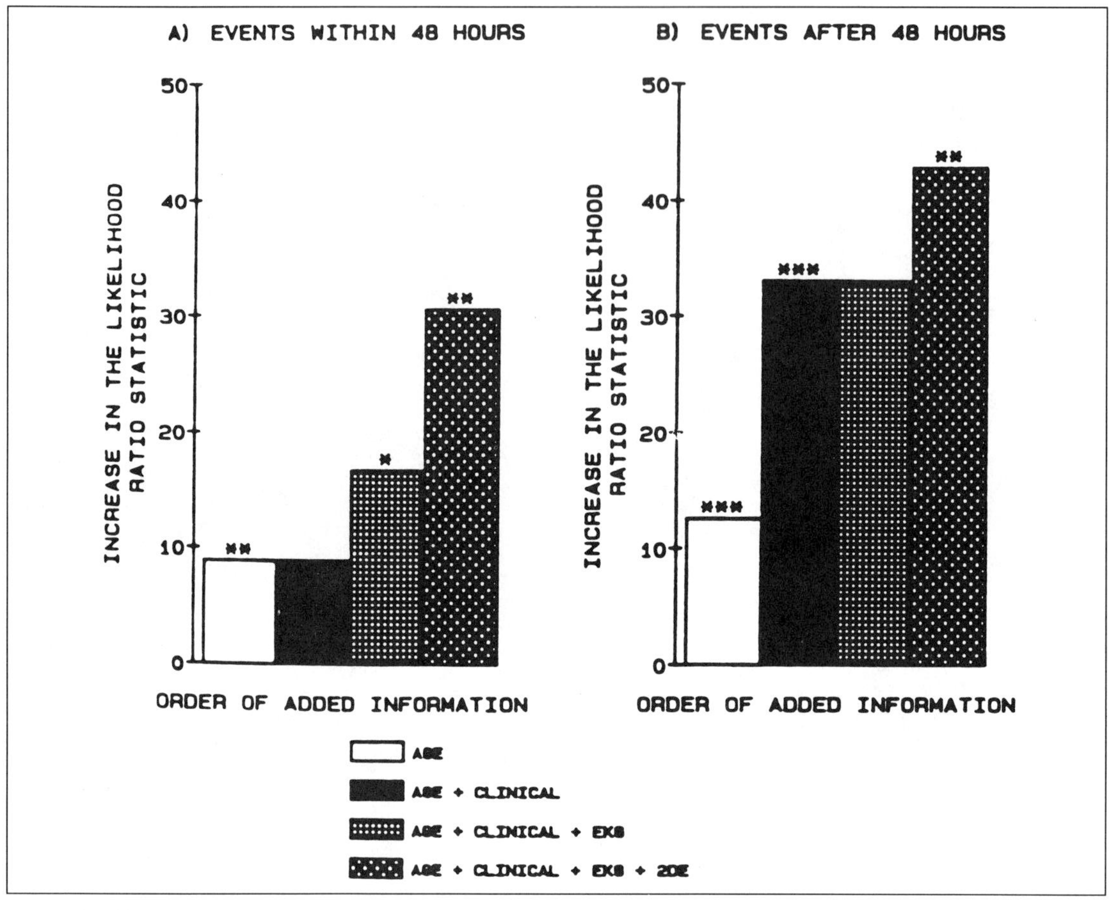

Fig. 28-18
Bar graphs showing comparison of additional prognostic value of tests (depicted as increase in likelihood ratio statistic) performed in succession for determining early (*A*) and late (*B*) events. Age alone is compared with age and clinical variables; with age, clinical, and electrocardiographic (EKG) variables; and with age, clinical, EKG, and two-dimensional echocardiographic (2DE) variables. Significant increases in the likelihood ratio statistic correspond to the following p values: * = $p < .05$, ** = $p < .01$, and *** = $p < .001$. (Reproduced from Sabia et al. The importance of two-dimensional echocardiographic assessment of left ventricular systolic function in patients presenting to the emergency room with cardiac-related symptoms. *Circulation* 84:1615, 1991. With permission.)

sensitivity for detecting non-Q-wave MI to 76 percent.

Thus, it appears that wall motion abnormalities are often present in non-Q-wave MI, but as noted with other imaging techniques or ECG the diagnosis of MI is less precise for non-Q-wave MI than it is for Q-wave MI. Although wall motion abnormalities, once established, tend to persist in Q-wave MI [38], there may be spontaneous improvement in patients with non-Q-wave infarctions [39].

The problem of perioperative MI has been addressed by Force and his colleagues [42, 43]. As expected, Q-wave MIs after coronary artery bypass surgery (CABG) are associated with a high likelihood of wall motion abnormalities. These authors

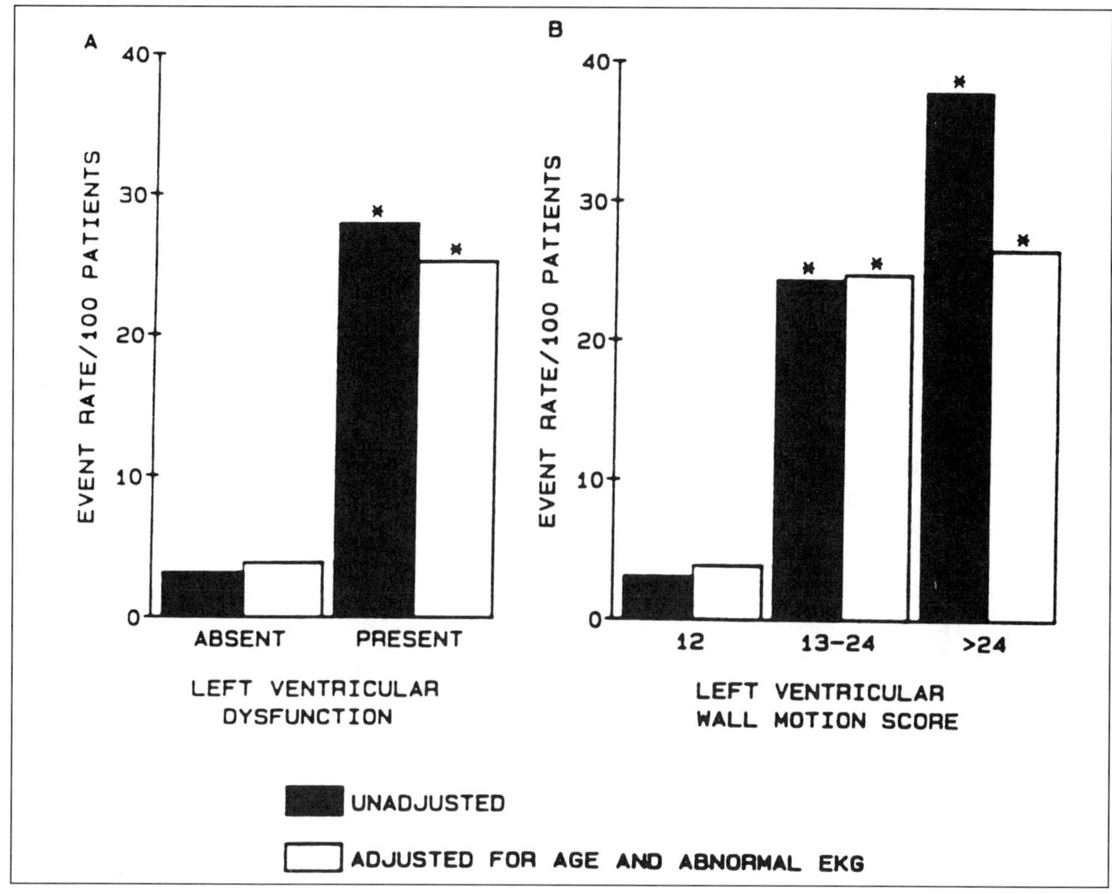

Fig. 28-19
Bar graphs showing event rates within 48 hours of presentation to the emergency room for those with and without left ventricular systolic dysfunction (*A*), and for those with different degrees of left ventricular systolic dysfunction (*B*). Unadjusted rates and rates adjusted for age and the presence of an abnormal electrocardiogram (EKG) are depicted. $* = p < .01$ compared with no left ventricular systolic dysfunction and with a left ventricular wall motion score of 12. (Reproduced from Sabia et al. The importance of two-dimensional echocardiographic assessment of left ventricular systolic function in patients presenting to the emergency room with cardiac-related symptoms. *Circulation* 84:1615, 1991. With permission.)

noted a similar severity of wall motion abnormality in patients with perioperative non-Q-wave MIs.

There has been substantial interest in the problem of reciprocal ST segment depression seen in the anterior leads in patients with inferior AMI. Two possible explanations for the reciprocal precordial ST segment depression are that it represents a pure reciprocal phenomenon from inferior ST segment elevation or that it represents concurrent anterior myocardial ischemia. Analysis of LV wall motion with echocardiography suggests that the ST segment depression seen in the anterior precordium most often reflects larger inferior MIs, generally with posterolateral extension, and is not due to coincident anterior wall ischemia [44, 45].

Persistent ST segment elevation after anterior AMI has also been evaluated with two-dimensional echocardiography. In a limited series of patients this observation appears to correlate with marked dyskinesis of the anterior and apical wall segments rather than indicate frank formation of aneurysm [46].

Detection of Infarct Size

The ability of echocardiography to detect wall motion abnormalities due to MI has been evaluated in numerous studies. When experimentally controlled and evaluated with high-resolution techniques such as sonomicrometry, abnormalities of LV wall motion occur with reductions in resting coronary flow of 20 percent or more [7]. Further reduction in flow results in more marked abnormalities, including systolic thinning of the myocardium and endocardial dyskinesis [7–9]. There are thresholds with respect to the degree of flow reduction required before wall motion abnormalities develop. Furthermore, thresholds exist with respect to the absolute amount of myocardium as well as the transmural degree of involvement required to produce abnormalities detectable with echocardiography. It should be noted that the subtle abnormalities present with reductions of only 20 percent or less may not be detectable with two-dimensional echocardiography, but acute flow reductions of 50 percent or more consistently result in wall motion abnormalities of sufficient magnitude to be visually detected with two-dimensional scanning [8–12, 47].

Weiss and colleagues directly compared the extent of LV akinesis or dyskinesis in 11 patients whose hearts were subsequently examined pathologically at autopsy [2]. They found a correlation of r = .9 for pathologic percent circumference of an infarcted left ventricle versus the percent circumference of a left ventricle that was akinetic or dyskinetic on echocardiography (Fig. 28-20). As seen in experimental animal studies, echocardiography tended to overestimate the anatomic size of MI.

Both myocardial thickening and endocardial motion have been evaluated with two-dimensional echocardiography and compared with experimental MI size [9–11, 48–54]. Virtually all studies concur that the extent of abnormal wall motion overestimates the anatomic size of MI [9–11, 50, 53]. It has been well demonstrated that normally perfused viable myocardium at the border of ischemic or infarcted myocardium may have abnormal systolic function [52–55]. Thus, although there is generally a good correlation between histologic infarction size and the extent of wall motion abnormalities, the echocardiographic technique detects functionally abnormal border areas, which results in overestimation of the anatomic infarction size. The most

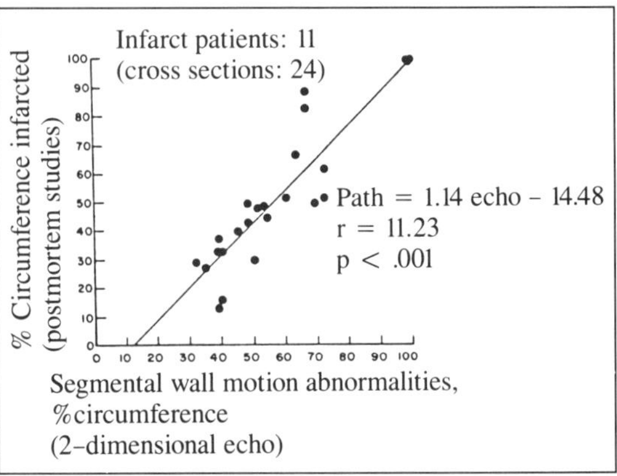

Fig. 28-20
Comparison of the extent of the left ventricular circumference demonstrating akinesis or dyskinesis on an antemortem echocardiogram and the percent of transmurally infarcted left ventricular circumference by postmortem examination in 11 patients subsequently examined at autopsy. (From J. L. Weiss et al. Two-dimensional echocardiographic recognition of myocardial injury in man: Comparison with postmortem studies. *Circulation* 63:401, 1981. With permission of the American Heart Association, Inc.)

likely explanation for this is that the adjacent, nonischemic areas are "tethered" to the ischemic region and passively reflect the abnormal motion of the infarction area [52]. The method used to analyze wall motion can also introduce errors that add to this overestimation because of their dependence on a fixed or floating reference point to which the endocardial motion is then referenced. As the infarct or ischemic area expands and moves during systole, the center of the mass shifts; nonequivalent areas may then be compared, resulting in overestimation of the ischemic zone [56].

Just as the degree of flow reduction required to produce abnormal wall motion is important, so is the absolute size of the MI. Pandian and colleagues evaluated this phenomenon in an animal model and demonstrated that small subendocardial MIs, involving 1 to 6 percent of LV mass, were not likely to be associated with wall motion abnormalities of sufficient magnitude to be detected by routine echocardiography [51]. The clinical correlate of this situation is that in humans smaller MIs may not be detected by two-dimensional echocardiography.

The role of the extent of transmural involvement has been specifically explored by several investigators. Lieberman and colleagues demonstrated that regions of myocardium with 1 to 20 percent of transmural involvement had reduced thickening as compared with noninfarcted remote segments. Furthermore, they demonstrated a threshold effect, in that segments with over 20 percent myocardial involvement showed frank systolic thinning and the degree of thinning did not increase with degrees of transmural involvement above 21 percent of wall thickness [10]. Thus, from an experimental standpoint, it appears that MI is reflected accurately by the presence of echocardiographic wall motion abnormalities.

Use of Echocardiography in AMI Interventions

Modern therapy for AMI includes not only observation and maintenance of hemodynamics during the natural history of the ischemic event but often involves urgent efforts at reperfusion. Reperfusion is currently done by thrombolysis with tissue plasminogen activator, streptokinase, or emergent balloon dilation of a coronary artery. Two-dimensional echocardiography can be used to document the return of function following such intervention.

The study by Topol and colleagues was one of the first using echocardiography to document return of function following reperfusion [57]. These authors demonstrated that LV wall motion was more likely to improve in segments distal to coronary arteries that not only had been subject to thrombolysis but also to acute dilation with balloon angioplasty.

Early data from other investigators also demonstrated myocardial salvage following emergent balloon angioplasty [58]. Serial two-dimensional echocardiograms were performed in 19 patients who underwent emergent reperfusion and in eight patients who received only conventional noninterventional therapy. Examples of echocardiograms from such patients are presented in Figures 28-21 through 28-23. Figures 28-21 and 28-22 are two-dimensional echocardiograms recorded in patients at the time of presentation and again several days after reperfusion via coronary angioplasty. Both studies demonstrate return of LV function following reperfusion. Figure 28-23 is a computer-generated outline of the diastolic-systolic endocardial contours before and after angioplasty of the case presented in Figure 28-22. The global ejection fraction (EF) has been calculated and is shown to increase after return of ventricular function. Overall results of this study, presented in Figure 28-24, demonstrate that in patients who did not receive any form of reperfusion therapy the wall motion abnormalities, as quantified by a wall motion score index, remained stable over a minimum 6-day period, whereas there was a statistically significant improvement in wall motion in the patients undergoing reperfusion. In this study, a wall motion score index that confirmed return of regional function was generated; however, a return of global function has also been demonstrated by other investigators by calculation of the EF from echocardiograms [59, 60].

In addition to its role in demonstrating return of function following reperfusion, two-dimensional echocardiography may play a role in identifying patients who are appropriate candidates for aggressive therapy [61]. As previously discussed, echocardiography can make the initial diagnosis of infarction and estimate its size. As such, an earlier diagnosis is feasible, and those patients with large infarcts who are most likely to benefit from aggressive management can be immediately identified.

Aortic Dissection and Acute Myocardial Infarction

On occasion patients present with chest pain and other clinical parameters suggesting an acute cardiovascular process. Dissecting aortic aneurysm is one such clinical problem and one which may coexist with MI. Coronary artery involvement due to antegrade dissection or obstruction by a flap occurs in about 10 to 20 percent of cases. Several studies have used transesophageal echocardiography to evaluate the proximal coronary vessels. Pearce et al. [62] identified the proximal left main coronary artery 86 percent of the time and the right coronary artery 82 percent of the time when an experienced operator specifically attempted to image these arteries. The presence of coronary involvement and the relationship of the dissection to the origin of the coronary artery are important when surgical repair is being contemplated in the case of an ascending aortic root dissection. Coronary artery involvement in a proximal aortic root dissection is an indication

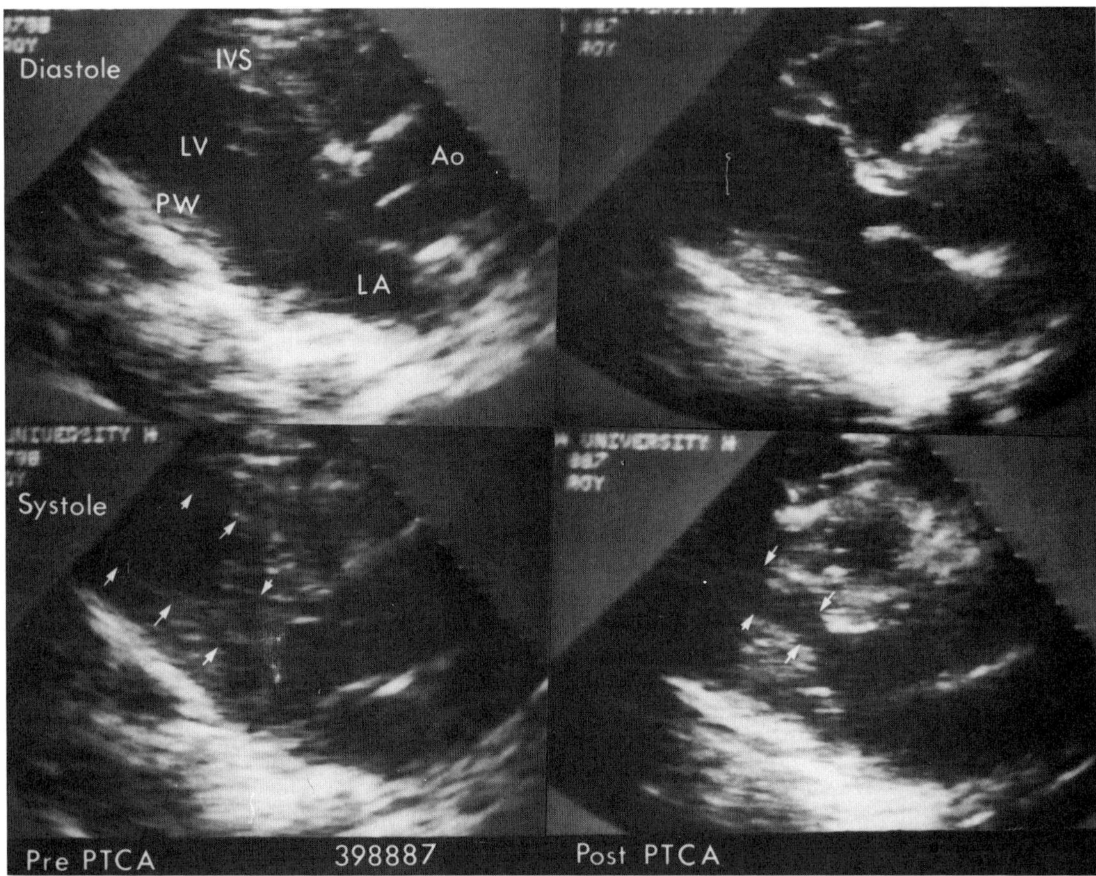

Fig. 28-21
Parasternal long-axis views during diastole and systole recorded in a patient with impending anterior myocardial infarction. The panels on the left were recorded at the time of presentation and those on the right 5 days after successful angioplasty of the left anterior descending coronary artery. Note that at the time of presentation the distal septum is dyskinetic (*upward-pointing arrows*), and the inferoposterior wall is relatively hypokinetic. Five days after successful angioplasty the inferoposterior wall moves normally and there has been restitution of normal wall motion in the entire ventricular septum. (From W. F. Armstrong. Echocardiography in patients with coronary artery disease. In R. Schlant, et al. *New Concepts in Cardiac Imaging 1988.* Chicago: Year Book Medical Publishers, 1988. With permission.)

for surgery. The patient in Figure 28-25 presented with severe substernal chest pain and ST segment elevation in the inferior leads. He received intravenous lytic therapy with resolution of pain, then developed postinfarction angina associated with anterior ST segment elevation two days later. Cardiac catherization was interrupted because a previously unsuspected dissection flap was found. Transesophageal echocardiography identified a large ascending aortic root with severe aortic insufficiency and a redundant dissection flap emanating from the proximal right coronary artery origin. The flap nearly occluded the left main coronary artery in diastole when it was pulled anteriorly by the severe aortic insufficiency. Transesophageal echocardiography has become an important modality for evaluating patients with suspected aortic dissection. Because the procedure is performed portably, without the risk of contrast dye, a rapid diagnosis including the presence or absence of dissection, aortic insufficiency, and involvement of the proximal coronary vessels can be made.

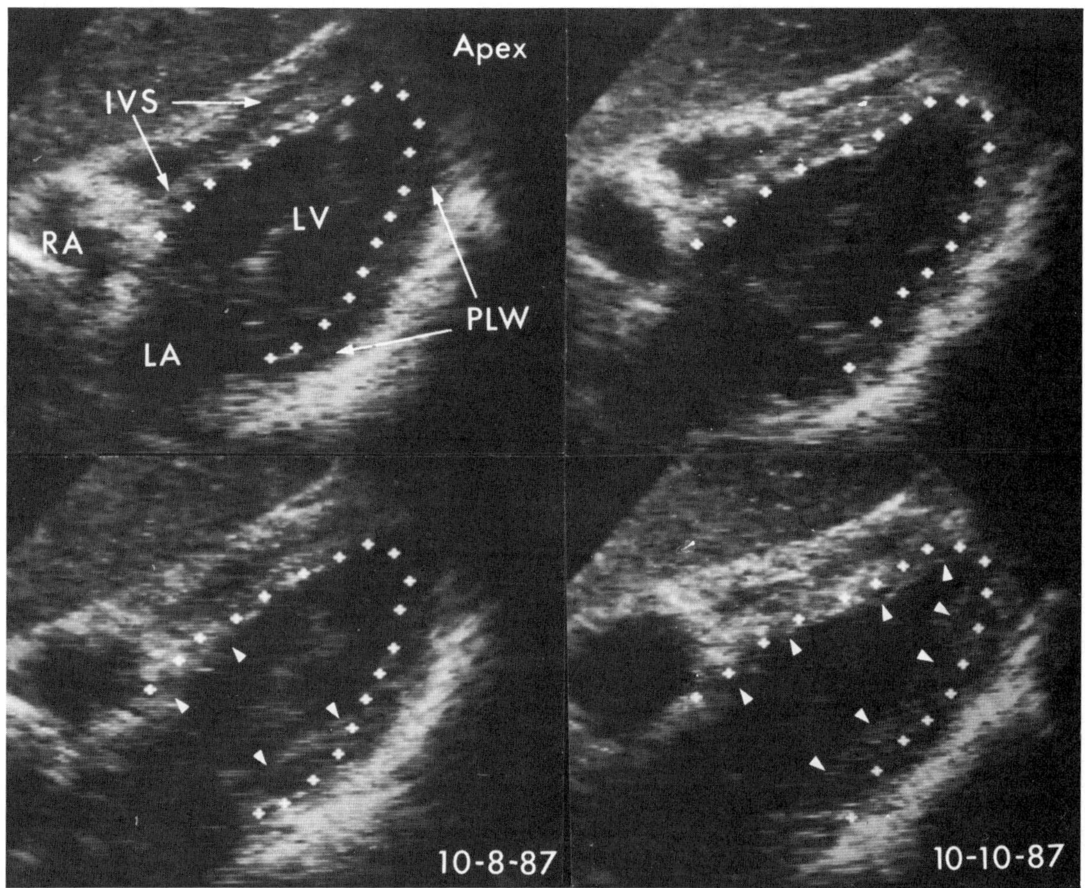

Fig. 28-22
Subcostal two-dimensional echocardiograms in a patient with impending myocardial infarction. The upper panels are end-diastolic images. The lower panels are recorded at end systole. The asterisks outline the endocardial position at end diastole. At presentation (*left panels*) only the basal septum and proximal posterolateral wall (PLW) move inward with systole (*arrows*). Two days after angioplasty (*right panels*) there has been return of normal systolic function of the distal septum, apex, and posterolateral wall (*arrows*). See Figure 28-1 for abbreviations. (From W. F. Armstrong. Echocardiography in coronary artery disease. *Prog. Cardiovasc. Dis.* 30:267, 1988. With permission.)

Use of Echocardiography in Assessing Prognosis After AMI

Although simple detection of wall motion abnormalities in a patient with chest pain implies coronary artery disease, their mere presence does not assist in the assessment of prognosis. For the latter analysis, the distribution of wall motion abnormalities must be quantified. It should be stressed that with echocardiography (or any other imaging technique that relies on ventricular function) what is assessed is the functional extent of the wall motion abnormality, not necessarily the anatomic extent of infarction, which often tends to be somewhat smaller. As noted previously in the discussion of methods for wall motion analysis, multiple schemes for quantitating wall motion abnormalities have been proposed. The scheme utilized most often by studies evaluating prognosis after AMI is calculation of a wall motion score or score index, in which the motion of multiple predefined ventricular wall areas is graded by a hierarchical score [16]. These

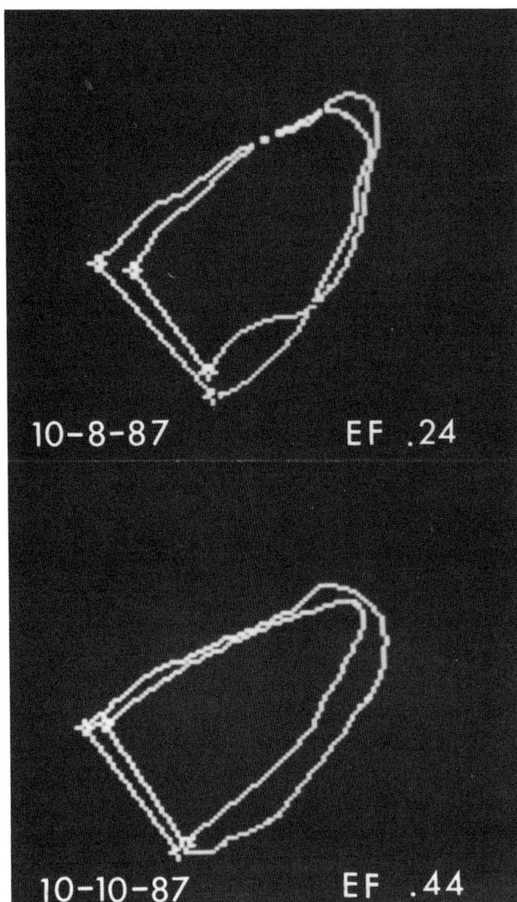

Fig. 28-23
Computer-generated endocardial outlines for the patient in Figure 28-22. The ejection fraction (EF) increased from 0.24 to 0.44 between the two studies. The apex is no longer dyskinetic, and there is normal motion of the lateral wall.

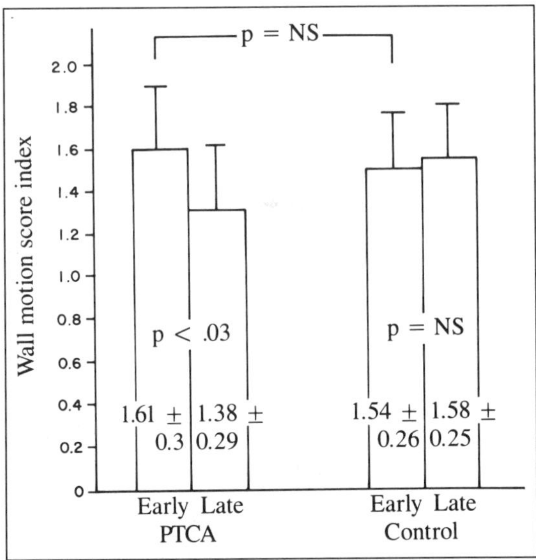

Fig. 28-24
Changes in wall motion score index in patients undergoing emergent percutaneous transluminal coronary angioplasty (PTCA) and a control group of patients without intervention. There were 19 patients in the PTCA group and 8 in the control group. (From W. F. Armstrong. Echocardiography and coronary artery disease. *Int. J. Card. Imaging* 2:241, 1987. With permission.)

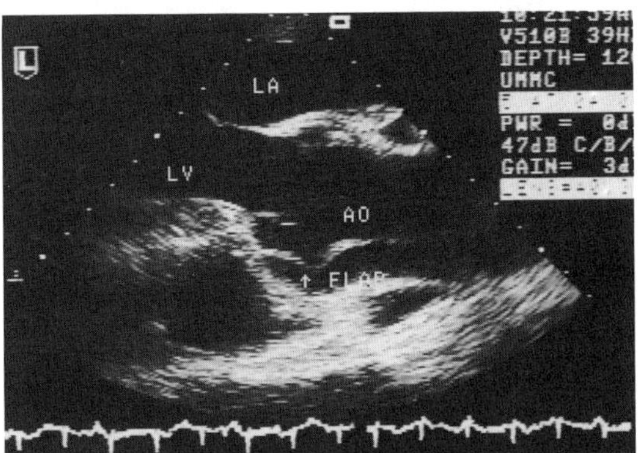

Fig. 28-25
Ascending aortic dissection in inferior myocardial infarction. Dissection flap is seen emanating from the right sinus of Valsalva. LA = left atrium; LV = left ventricle; Ao = ascending aorta; Flap = dissection flap.

scores are then summed and indexed to the number of segments evaluated. The more diffuse and extensive the wall motion abnormalities, the higher the wall motion score or score index. Examples of this type of wall motion score are shown in Figures 28-10 and 28-11, which were derived from the patients presented in Figures 28-13 through 28-15.

The first attempt at correlating the extent of LV wall motion abnormalities with clinical outcome was reported by Heger et al. in 1980 [13]. This study comprised 44 consecutive patients with AMI evaluated with early-generation two-dimensional scanning equipment. The left ventricle was divided into nine predefined segments and the wall motion characterized as normal (score 0) to dyskinetic (score 3). These individual scores were then summed for all nine segments to a wall motion score. Analysis of the two-dimensional echocardiograms revealed that regional wall motion abnormalities were present in all 44 patients. An uncomplicated clinical course was seen in 13 patients who had a mean wall motion score of 3.2 ± 2.4. This wall motion score was statistically less ($p < .001$) than that seen in 12 patients with isolated pulmonary congestion (9.7 ± 3.1) or 10 patients with hypotension and pulmonary congestion (10.6 ± 4.8).

A similar study was performed in 75 patients by Gibson et al. [36]. Their patients underwent echocardiographic imaging an average of 7.9 hours after admission for AMI, and the results of the echocardiograms were analyzed in a fashion similar to that noted above. The authors used a more complicated 11-segment scheme and indexed the wall motion scores to the number of segments. This initial wall motion score index was then correlated with the admission and maximum Killip classifications for each patient during hospitalization. In the Gibson study, 41 patients were classified on admission as Killip class I, and their initial wall motion score index was 1.08 ± 0.38. Twenty-two patients with a mean wall motion score of 0.93 ± 0.37 remained in Killip class I during their hospitalization. Eighteen patients who initially were in Killip class I progressed to Killip class II, and one patient progressed from Killip class I to Killip class IV. The wall motion score indexes in these patients were 1.23 ± 0.29 and 1.91 ± 0.00, respectively. The data from this study are presented in Figure 28-26. The higher wall motion score indexes were seen in patients with large infarctions and in those with remote areas of wall motion abnormality in addition to the index infarction. Remote wall motion abnormalities were seen in 32 patients. Their presence had a statistical association with a number of complications, including death, cardiogenic shock, reinfarction, progression of Killip classification, and postinfarction angina. The ability of two-dimensional echocardiography to assess prognosis after MI has been demonstrated in numerous other laboratories [63–68]. Table 28-1 summarizes results of these studies.

Doppler Assessment of Systolic Function

Echocardiography provides direct visualization of wall motion abnormalities and their implications for detecting and quantifying MI as well as assess-

Fig. 28-26
Correlation of the echocardiographically derived wall motion index (mean + standard deviation) with admission and maximum Killip classes (I–IV). The number of patients (pts) in each subgroup appears in parentheses. See text for further details. (From R. S. Gibson et al. Value of early two-dimensional echocardiography in patients with acute myocardial infarction. *Am. J. Cardiol.* 49:110, 1982. With permission.)

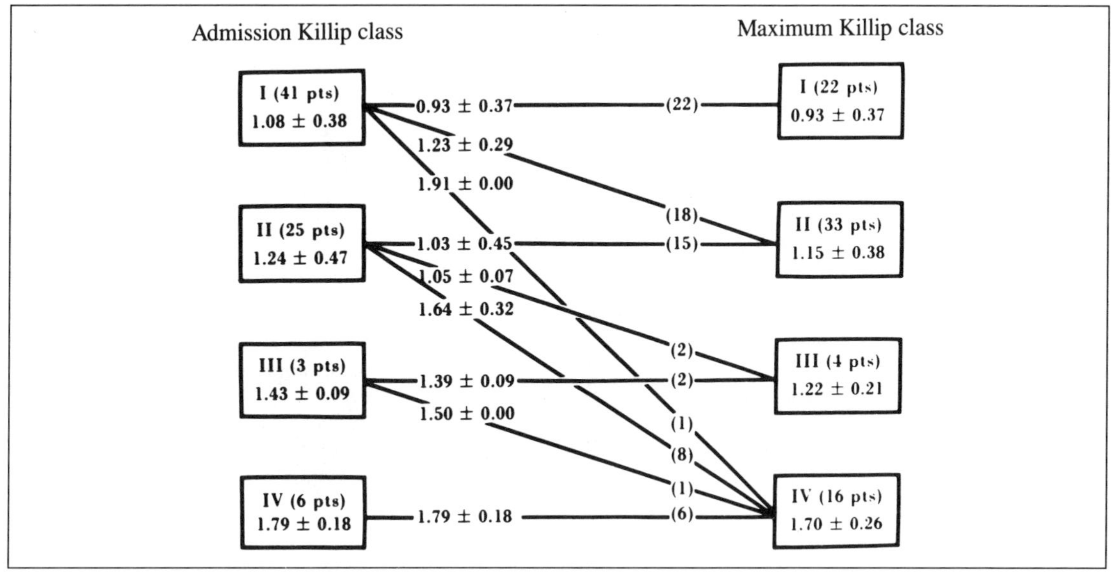

Table 28-1
Echocardiographic assessment of prognosis following myocardial infarction

Study	No. of patients	Timing[a]	Endpoint[b]	Analysis[c]	N[d]	Adverse outcome (%)	Analysis	N	Adverse outcome (%)
Heger [13]	39	E	C, D HP	WMS≥8	19	18 (95)	WMS<8	18	6 (33)
Horowitz [67]	43	E	HP, C, D, MA	WMS≥8	16	11 (69)	WMS<8	27	2 (7)
Abrams [68]	23	E	C, D, A, MI	WMS≥2	12	7 (58)	WMS<2	11	0 (0)
				EF<0.40	9	7 (78)	EF>0.40	14	0 (0)
VanReet [32]	93	E	D	WMS<0.5	25	10 (40)	WMS>0.5	68	1 (2)
				EF<0.35	27	10 (37)	EF≥0.95	60	1 (2)
Nishimura [64]	61	E	C, D, MA	WMS≥2	27	24 (89)	WMS<2	34	6 (18)
Bhatnagar [66]	47	P	A, MI	WMS≥8	16	14 (89)	WMS<8	31	3 (10)
Nishimura [65]	46	P	D, MI, C, A	WMS≥2	24	15 (63)	WMS<2	22	2 (9)

[a]Time frame for obtaining echocardiographic study. E = early: echocardiogram performed at time of presentation and short follow-up period (generally in hospital); P = predischarge echocardiogram and longer outpatient follow-up.
[b]D = death; MI = recurrent myocardial infarction; A = angina; C = congestive heart failure; HP = hypoperfusion/shock; MA = malignant arryhythmias or heart block.
[c]Type of echocardiographic analysis and threshold for favorable or adverse outcome. EF = ejection fraction; WMS = wall motion score (scoring systems are different for each study; therefore absolute numbers are *not* interchangeable among studies for WMS).
[d]Number of patients in each subset.

ment of infarct size expressed as a function of the amount of muscle with abnormal motion. Information concerning overall systolic function of the left ventricle can be obtained from Doppler ultrasound recordings of the aortic outflow. Stroke volume and cardiac output can be calculated as the product of LV outflow tract (or aortic) cross-sectional area and the systolic velocity integral [69, 70]. In a given patient when outflow tract or aortic dimensions are constant, global systolic performance is directly proportional to the Doppler-derived aortic flow velocity integral. In addition to the overall velocity integral, other parameters (e.g., peak acceleration and velocity) reflect systolic performance of the ventricle. The behavior of these parameters is shown in Figure 28-27. The behavior of the aortic flow velocity signals, under different conditions of contractility and loading conditions, has been experimentally evaluated [70]. Similar observations have been made in the clinical arena in patients with ventricular dysfunction undergoing therapy for congestive failure [71, 72]. Thus far, this application of Doppler ultrasound has seen only limited clinical utilization in the United States. Because of substantial deviation from cardiac output measured by thermodilution or other standard techniques when group data are compared, the role of Doppler ultrasound for precise prediction of output is limited. Doppler evaluation of aortic flow velocity may play a valuable role in detecting serial changes in a given patient, however.

Complications After Myocardial Infarction

Two-dimensional echocardiographic imaging combined with Doppler techniques allows rapid, noninvasive diagnosis of virtually any complication of MI. Table 28-2 presents common complications of MI that can be detected with cardiac ultrasound. The following discussion outlines many of these applications.

Pericardial Effusion

Perhaps the most common complication of MI is the development of transient pericarditis with effusion. When evaluated with serial echocardiograms, this complication occurs after 26 to 37 percent of MIs, usually 1 to 3 days after the acute event [73, 74]. The etiology of this type of pericarditis is an associated epicardial infarction and inflammation, and as such is a complication of transmural MI. Acute pericarditis following MI has been associated with a worse prognosis and more extensive infarction [74]. The incidence of pericardial effusion

Fig. 28-27
Aortic flow velocity under baseline circumstances (*left*), with increased cardiac output (*middle*), or with diminished output (*right*). Note that peak velocity, acceleration, and area under the curve increase with an increase in stroke volume and diminish with reduced left ventricular systolic function. (From W. F. Armstrong. Echocardiography in coronary artery disease. *Prog. Cardiovasc. Dis.* 30:267, 1988. With permission.)

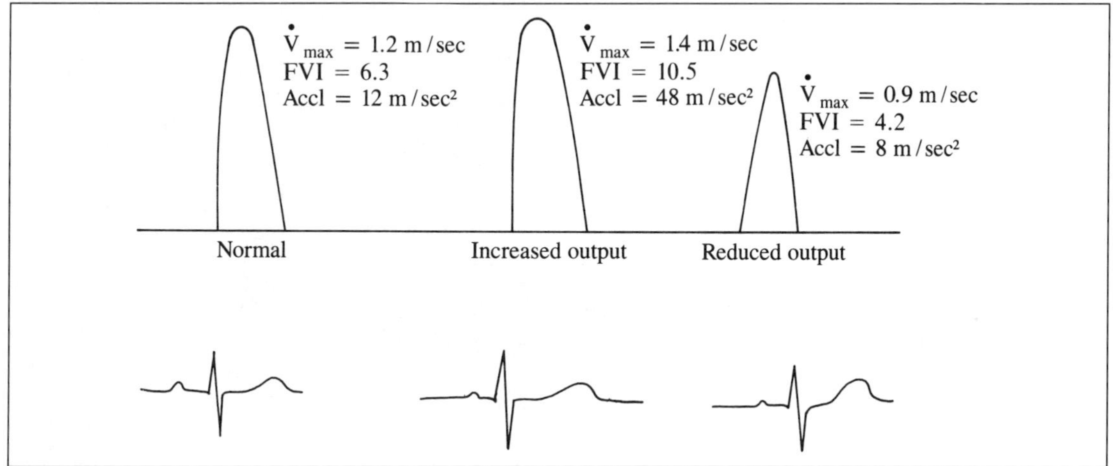

Table 28-2
Complications of myocardial infarction detectable with echocardiography and Doppler

Pericardial effusion (acute or delayed)
Aneurysm formation
Mural thrombus
Pseudoaneurysm
Infarct expansion
Papillary muscle rupture
Functional mitral regurgitation
Tricuspid regurgitation
Right ventricular infarction
Reinfarction

is similar in patients treated and not treated with thrombolytic therapy.

Aneurysm Formation

The definition and detection of aneurysms by two-dimensional echocardiography is based on the same criteria as those for contrast ventriculography. LV aneurysm refers to the formation of an area of myocardial scar with distinctly abnormal geometry during both diastole and systole compared with normal LV configuration [75–77]. This complication is more common after anterior and apical MIs, occurring in 20 to 40 percent of cases [76, 78]. Figure 28-28 illustrates a large anteroapical aneurysm in a patient after an anterior MI.

The detection of LV aneurysm by two-dimensional echocardiography was first demonstrated by Weyman and colleagues in 1976 [75]. In this small retrospective study there was excellent agreement between single plane angiography and two-dimensional echocardiography for localizing LV aneurysms. Similar reports have been generated in other laboratories [76–79]. The largest study comparing catheterization and echocardiography for detection of LV aneurysm was reported by Visser et al. These investigators studied 422 consecutive patients with documented MI [76]. Using recent-generation equipment, these authors obtained adequate two-dimensional echocardiograms in 91 percent of their patients. LV aneurysm was shown by echocardiography in 111 patients and by cineangiography in 118 patients. Concordance of the two studies was seen in 103 patients thought to have aneurysm and in 260 thought not to have aneurysm. Compared with cineangiography, echocardiography was 93 percent sensitive and 94 percent specific for detection of LV aneurysm.

It should be noted that many of the discrepancies between the two imaging techniques probably arise from the different loading conditions under which the examinations are performed rather than being true discrepancies of data. The adverse loading conditions present at the time of cardiac catheterization generally tend to magnify the extent of wall motion abnormalities as compared with abnormalities seen by noninvasive imaging studies.

Visser and colleagues also evaluated the time course of aneurysm formation after MI in 158 patients in whom serial studies were available [79]. Aneurysms formed in 35 of 158 patients (22 per-

Fig. 28-28
Apical four-chamber view in a patient with anteroapical aneurysm. Note the full thickness of the myocardium at the base with a distinct break from normal geometry (*arrows*) present during diastole and systole. (From W. F. Armstrong. Echocardiography in coronary artery disease. *Prog. Cardiovasc. Dis.* 30:267, 1988. With permission.)

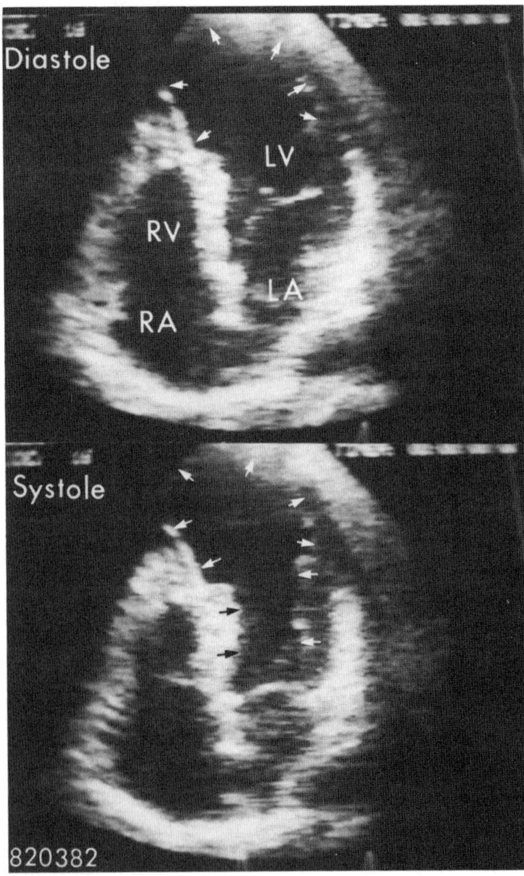

cent); particularly important is that all formed within the first 3 months after MI. The patient most likely to form an aneurysm was one who had marked acute anterior dyskinesis after MI. Aneurysms formed in 27 of 84 patients (32.1 percent) with anterior wall motion abnormalities and in 6 of 68 patients (8.8 percent) with posterior wall motion abnormalities. Marked anterior dyskinesis was present in 25 of the 27 patients who formed aneurysms but was evident in only 5 of the 57 who had anterior infarctions and did not form aneurysms. Of particular note in this study, 15 patients formed aneurysms within the first 5 days after MI. Early aneurysm formation probably represents infarct expansion (see below) rather than formation of a true fibrous aneurysm. Other investigators had previously suggested that expansion carried a poor prognosis for spontaneous myocardial rupture [80]. In the Visser et al. study, 3-month mortality was 66 percent and 1-year mortality 80 percent for patients with early formation of aneurysm [79].

The size of an LV aneurysm can be quantified by defining the boundary between normal and abnormal wall motion and then measuring the normal and abnormal areas either linearly, as a function of the circumference of the ventricle, or by area, as a function of the total endocardial area. With either procedure, an index of the residual myocardium can be generated. Patients with greater amounts of residual normal myocardium tend to have a better prognosis [77, 78]. The ability of echocardiography to predict surgical survival and improvement after aneurysmectomy has also been investigated [81, 82]. Ryan et al. reported 37 patients studied with two-dimensional echocardiography before aneurysmectomy and demonstrated that an echocardiographic index of functioning myocardium at the base of the heart accurately separated the patients likely to survive surgery and improve by at least one clinical classification from those who subsequently died at surgery or did not improve [82]. In comparison, global EF from ventriculography did not distinguish those with favorable outcomes from those with poor clinical outcomes. Virtually identical data were reported by Visser et al. in a cohort of 56 patients [81]. These workers calculated an index of aneurysm size versus normal functioning muscle by quantifying the linear extent of normal muscle along the anterior, posterior, lateral, and septal walls of the ventricle. From this index they calculated a percent of functioning muscle. Their data suggested that patients with less than 40 percent functioning muscle were at high risk after aneurysm resection.

For patients who are not undergoing surgical resection, echocardiographic aneurysm size also correlates with clinical status. This parameter has been retrospectively evaluated by Matsumoto et al. in 68 patients studied with serial echocardiograms after their first MI [78]. These investigators noted a significantly higher incidence of heart failure and mortality in patients with large aneurysms (functioning muscle < 40 percent) than in those with small aneurysms.

Infarct Expansion

Formation of a true ventricular aneurysm with a fibrous wall generally occurs over a period of weeks to several months after MI. A second, superficially similar, phenomenon is that of infarct expansion [80, 83–86]. This term refers to the acute thinning and stretching of infarcted myocardium, which from a cardiac imaging standpoint produces an abnormality suggestive of ventricular aneurysm acutely rather than more slowly after MI. Clinically, this phenomenon is suggested when a patient has recurrent chest pain and increasing ST segment elevation without enzymatic evidence of reinfarction [86]. Pathologically, it is associated with an acutely thinned area of necrotic myocardium devoid of a dense fibrous wall, as seen in chronically forming aneurysms. It has been associated with a higher likelihood of rupture in the zone of expansion [85]. Infarct expansion can be recognized by two-dimensional echocardiography when wall dilation occurs within the first several days after MI [83, 84]. An example of acute aneurysm formation 1 day after anterior MI is shown in Figure 28-29. This patient subsequently experienced fatal cardiac rupture near the apex.

Infarct expansion can be quantified in the short axis of the left ventricle by using internal landmarks such as the papillary muscles and then quantifying the circumferential distance between them or the arc subtended by their centers. With this technique, it appears that acute expansion and dilation of the infarct segment is a common cause of global cardiac enlargement during the first 3 days after MI [84]. Recent data suggest that development of myocardial expansion, independent of ECG or enzyme estimates of MI size, predicts a greater short-term

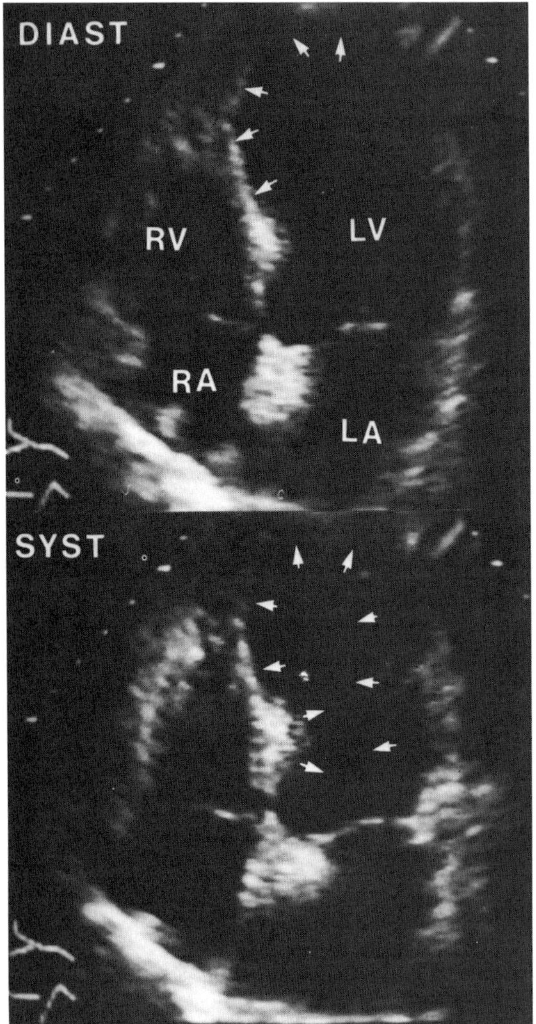

Fig. 28-29
Apical four-chamber view in a patient with acute infarct expansion. During diastole the left ventricle is clearly dilated, and there is abnormal geometry of the left ventricle (*arrowheads*) produced by acute dilation and thinning of the distal septum and apex. During systole the abnormal geometry is more marked.

mortality, specifically with the likelihood of frank myocardial rupture being substantially greater [80, 83–85].

Pseudoaneurysm

A pseudoaneurysm is the short-term result of a walled-off or contained myocardial rupture. In contrast to true aneurysm, which has a fibrous wall of high tensile strength and which is unlikely to rupture, a pseudoaneurysm is a walled-off myocardial rupture that has a low-strength wall and a reasonably high likelihood of recurring rupture leading to cardiac tamponade and death. Both true and pseudoaneurysms cause an abnormal bulge of the ventricular contour when imaged by echocardiography or other imaging techniques. Pathologically, a pseudoaneurysm is connected to the left ventricular cavity by a narrow orifice. Because of the high-resolution and tomographic imaging nature of echocardiography, this diagnostic feature of a pseudoaneurysm can be accurately identified [87, 88]. It has been suggested that aneurysms that appear external to the cardiac silhouette and that connect with the LV cavity by a narrow orifice (less than one-third the maximum dimension of the body of the aneurysm) represent a false aneurysm rather than a true aneurysm. Pseudoaneurysms are frequently filled with fresh thrombus. Figure 28-30 was recorded

Fig. 28-30
Parasternal long-axis and apical two-chamber views in a patient with an inferior myocardial infarction 3 months prior to admission. Rupture of the inferior wall leading to pseudoaneurysm formation is evident. Note the communication between the cavity of the left ventricle and the extra cardiac space (*long white arrow*) and the border of the pseudoaneurysm (*small white arrows*), which is partially filled with thrombus.

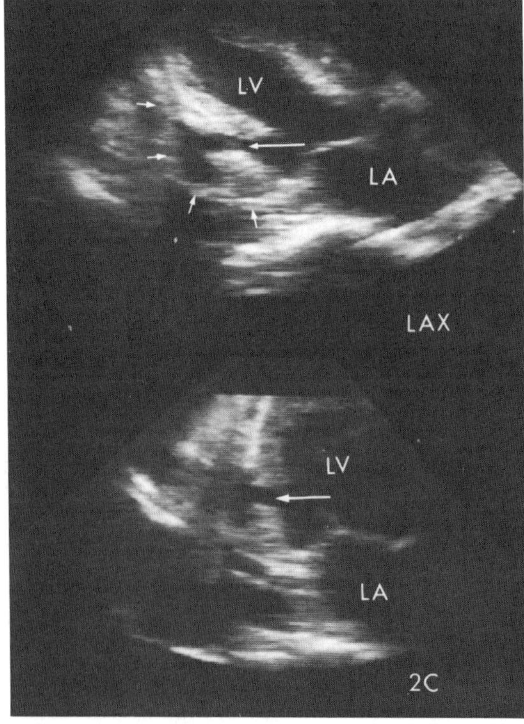

in a patient with a posterior wall pseudoaneurysm detected two months after a clinical inferior infarction.

Mural Thrombus

Two-dimensional echocardiography is an excellent tool for evaluating intracardiac masses, not only intracardiac tumors but also mural thrombi after AMI. Its sensitivity, specificity, and overall accuracy compare favorably with those of postmortem examination [89, 90], direct examination in the operating room [90, 91], contrast ventriculography [90], or indium 113 labeled platelet studies [89, 90]. Because echocardiography allows simultaneous assessment of LV wall motion and the remainder of the cardiac anatomy, it is probably the preferred examination when screening for mural thrombi. Its sensitivity is reported as 97 percent in experimentally induced thrombus [90] and 95 percent in patients [89, 91]. Specificity has ranged from 86 percent [94] to 92 percent [91]. Experimentally, early abnormalities of blood flow suggesting stasis occur within minutes to hours of coronary occlusion [92]. Mural thrombi are most likely to form within the first 72 hours after MI [93, 94] and may form during administration of therapeutic anticoagulation [95–97]. They are found after approximately 40 percent of anterior MIs but are rarely seen after inferior MI [93, 94, 98, 99]. Figure 28-31 illustrates the range of thrombus formation seen with MI. There may be substantial day-to-day variation in size and shape of the thrombus.

Fig. 28-31
Two-dimensional echocardiograms from four patients with mural thrombi complicating infarction or aneurysm. *A.* There is a small, round, filling defect in the apex of the left ventricle that is neither pedunculated nor mobile. *B.* There is a larger mass filling approximately one-third of the ventricular cavity. *C.* Pedunculated apical thrombus with free edges. Note that this thrombus is not adherent along its entire length and that it protudes into the ventricular cavity. *D.* Pedunculated and mobile thrombus. This thrombus has a free edge that during the real-time examination was mobile. (From W. F. Armstrong. Echocardiography in coronary artery disease. *Prog. Cardiovasc. Dis.* 30:267, 1988. With permission.)

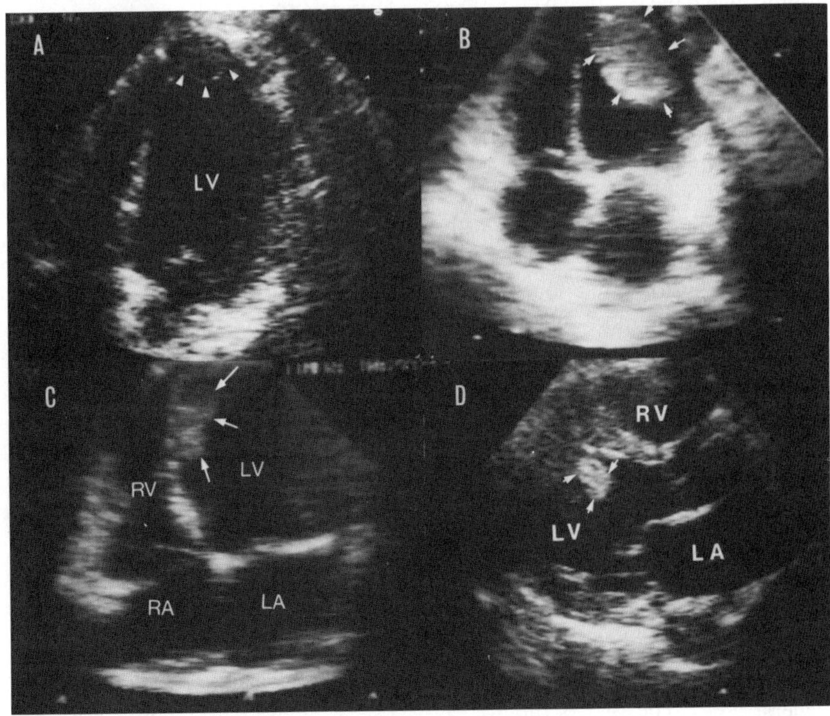

The likelihood of clinical embolization is greater in those patients with echocardiographically demonstrated mural thrombi than in those without documented thrombus formation [89, 98, 100, 101]. Additional characteristics of the thrombus can be defined by echocardiography, including its size, whether it is sessile or protruding, and whether it has mobility within the cavity. Subsequent embolization is more likely if the underlying ventricular thrombus is either pedunculated (protruding into the cavity) or mobile [101–103]. Therapeutic anticoagulation, although having only a minimal effect on thrombus formation, may protect from embolic events [100, 104].

Right Ventricular Infarction

Right ventricular (RV) infarction is a relatively common complication seen almost exclusively in the presence of inferior MI. It generally occurs in the presence of proximal right coronary artery lesions, often in patients with transient heart block and large inferior MIs [105]. It should be suspected clinically when hypotension disproportionate to the suspected infarct size is seen in a patient with an inferior MI. From an echocardiographic standpoint, RV infarction is diagnosed when the right ventricle is dilated and wall motion abnormalities are present in both the inferior wall and the RV free wall [106–109]. Figure 28-32 shows an RV infarction diagnosed with two-dimensional echocardiography. RV infarction consists of a spectrum of abnormalities ranging from subclinical RV dysfunction to marked RV dilation with necrosis of the entire RV wall [105, 109]. RV infarctions with only subtle degrees of systolic dysfunction may not be detected with echocardiography. In addition to the obvious primary problems with RV systolic function, RV infarction may be associated with more subtle abnormalities. Among them is transient right-to-left intracardiac shunting through a patent foramen ovale, which manifests only after RV and right atrial pressures rise. This results in systemic hypoxia and can be documented using contrast echocardiography [110, 111] in conjunction with either transthoracic or transesophageal echocardiography.

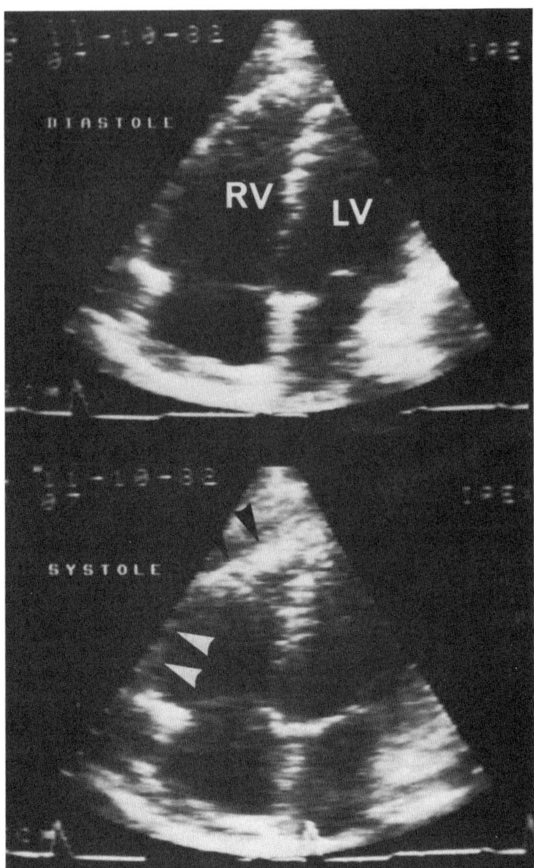

Fig. 28-32
Apical four-chamber view of a patient with a right ventricular infarction. During systole the more apical portions of the right ventricle appropriately move inward (*black arrowheads*), whereas the more basal portion of the wall is frankly dyskinetic (*white arrows*). (From W. F. Armstrong. Echocardiography in coronary artery disease. *Prog. Cardiovasc. Dis.* 30:267, 1988. With permission.)

Ventricular Septal Defect

Rupture of infarcted myocardium can occur in one of three general areas. The first is rupture of the free wall, which usually results in immediate cardiac tamponade and death, but in a minority of patients results in formation of a pseudoaneurysm. In the usual case, in which rupture leads to tamponade and death, two-dimensional echocardiography may be used to visualize the point of rupture [112]. Rupture of the free wall may also occur over hours or days. In such patients there is often an episode of chest pain or hypotension that prompts the cardiologist to order echocardiography. Findings by echocardiography may include tampondae, pericardial hematoma, and, rarely, the site of rupture.

The second form of myocardial rupture is that of the ventricular septum, leading to an acquired

VSD; the third is rupture of a papillary muscle (most commonly of the mitral valve), resulting in severe valvular regurgitation. Ventricular septal rupture or papillary muscle rupture should be suspected in a patient with AMI who develops a new, loud, holosystolic murmur. Often the two entities can be accurately distinguished by echocardiography when one is directly imaged [113–117]. Figure 28-33 shows a large VSD that occurred after an inferior MI. Because the septum may be dissected over much of its length, color Doppler is often very useful.

Most VSDs are associated with aneurysm formation, and early rupture usually occurs at the margin of the aneurysm. As such, the area of rupture is usually immediately adjacent to a major wall motion abnormality [113–116]. With use of modern

Fig. 28-33
Apical views in a patient with an inferior myocardial infarction and an acute ventricular septal defect. In the view at the left there is an area of distinct thinning and aneurysm formation in the proximal ventricular septum (*arrows*). With a slightly different angulation a large ventricular septal defect is seen (*arrows*).

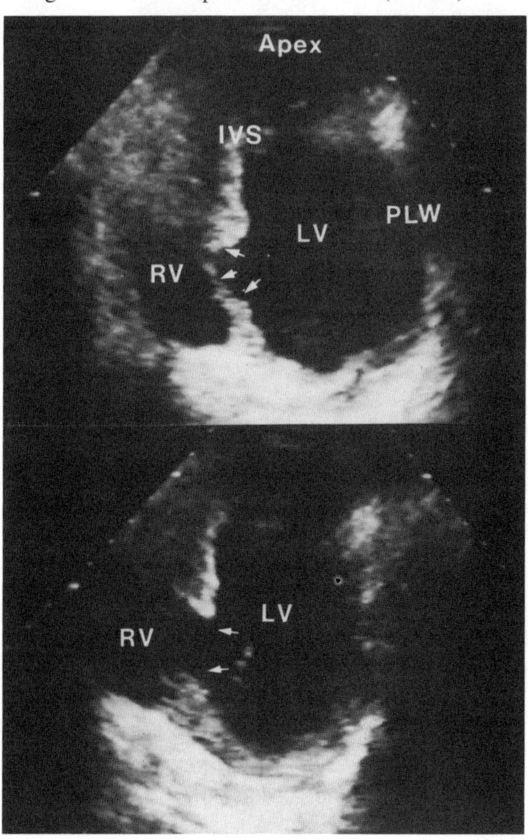

scanning equipment and multiple views, most of the larger (i.e., > 1 cm) VSDs should be directly imaged. These defects occur in locations different from congenital VSDs, and the scanning planes for their detection are different from those used for the congenital defects. Careful attention is required to scan all areas of the ventricular septum, especially along regions of wall motion abnormality.

If the VSD is anatomically small, it may evade detection by routine two-dimensional echocardiography. Investigation with color Doppler flow imaging is an effective method for localizing postinfarction VSD [118–121]. An example is presented in Plate 1. In addition to establishing the diagnosis of VSD, echocardiography may play a role in determining prognosis. Patients with well preserved ventricular function and normal hyperdynamic wall motion outside the infarct zone have a better prognosis than those with diffuse wall motion abnormalities and depressed systolic function [113].

When transthoracic echocardiography with color flow Doppler fails to demonstrate a VSD, transesophageal echocardiography often allows a definitive diagnosis to be made. The unimpeded visualization and higher resolution images can often identify abnormal left-to-right flow, if not show the defect itself. Koenig et al. [122] described a patient with suspected VSD who had a transthoracic echocardiogram that revealed only an akinetic septum. Transesophageal echocardiography clearly demonstrated a defect in the lower third of the septum [121]. An example of a patient who presented with hypotension in the setting of an AMI and was found to have a VSD by transesophageal echocardiography is presented in Figure 28-34 and Plate 2. Smyllie et al. [119] compared cardiac catheterization with color flow Doppler and with continuous wave and pulsed Doppler. Cross-sectional echocardiography correctly predicted the infarct territory in all cases but visualized the rupture in only 35 to 45 percent. Spectral Doppler detected the rupture in 95 percent but could not localize it. Color mapping identified the defect and localized it in 100 percent (N = 20) and defined the presence of single or multiple jets in all patients. Improvements in two-dimensional echocardiography imaging and color Doppler have made this a highly sensitive and specific technique in the diagnosis of postinfarction VSD (sensitivity 100 percent, specificity 100 percent), thus obviating the need for high-risk cardiac catheterization in the majority of patients.

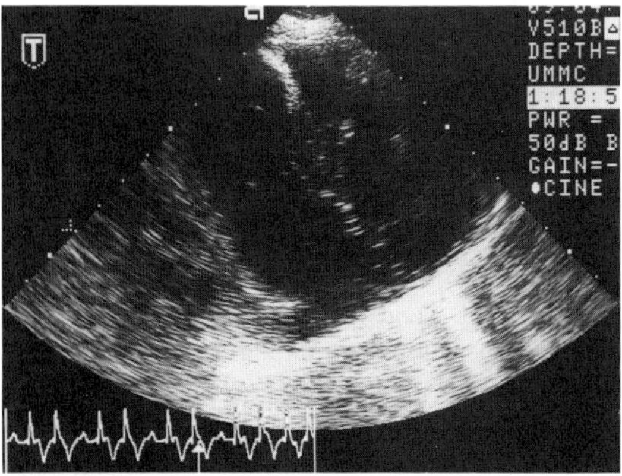

Fig. 28-34
Transesophageal echocardiogram recorded from a transgastric approach in a short-axis view in a patient with inferior infarction and cardiogenic shock. Note, at 12 o'clock, the distinct loss of tissue consistent with a fairly large ventricular septal defect.

Table 28-3
Clinical syndromes associated with chest discomfort and a murmur

Associated with myocardial infarction
Ventricular septal rupture[a]
Papillary muscle rupture (mitral)[a]
Papillary muscle dysfunction without rupture[a]
Acute tricuspid regurgitation[a]
Free wall rupture[a]
Nonischemic syndromes
Valvular aortic stenosis[a]
Bacterial endocarditis[b]
Hypertrophic myopathy[a]
Acute myocarditis with mitral regurgitation[b]
Chordal rupture (spontaneous or traumatic)[a]
Pulmonary embolus with tricuspid regurgitation[b]
Mitral valve prolapse[a]

[a]Entities for which echocardiography/Doppler provides definitive data.
[b]Entities for which echocardiography/Doppler provides supportive data.

Complications Involving the Mitral Apparatus

Necrosis of the papillary muscle can lead to rupture of the muscle. Frank rupture of a papillary muscle is generally associated with immediate onset of severe mitral regurgitation and pulmonary edema. The papillary muscles are complicated structures with multiple heads, and rupture can produce variable degrees of papillary muscle disruption. Rupture leads to a spectrum of mitral regurgitation depending on the exact location of the rupture. Mitral valve papillary muscle rupture should be clinically suspected in patients with acute pulmonary edema, hypotension, recurrent chest pain, and a new murmur after MI (Table 28-3). From an echocardiographic standpoint, a spectrum of abnormalities can be visualized including actual rupture of the papillary muscle body (Fig. 28-35) and detection of a flail mitral valve leaflet (Fig. 28-36) [116, 123–126]. When either of these entities is noted in the presence of AMI and a loud systolic murmur, a diagnosis of rupture of the papillary muscle can be established. When technical considerations preclude adequate imaging or when the rupture involves only one small head of a papillary muscle, two-dimensional imaging may not be diagnostic. In these cases Doppler interrogation along the plane of the mitral valve can document the presence of mitral regurgitation as the cause of a newly noted murmur.

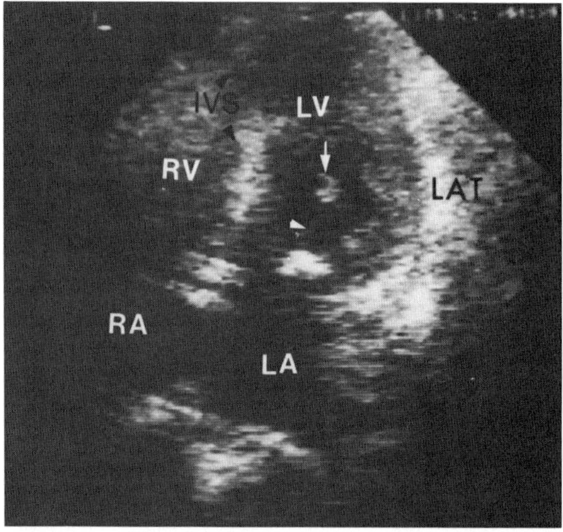

Fig. 28-35
Apical four-chamber view in a patient with flail mitral valve due to acute myocardial infarction. The papillary muscle has ruptured, and the tip of the muscle can be seen as a free-floating structure attached only by its chordae (*arrowhead*) in the cavity of the left ventricle.

A chronically infarcted papillary muscle may not demonstrate frank rupture but only reduction in its length, leading to papillary muscle dysfunction. Echocardiographically, this appears as abnormal

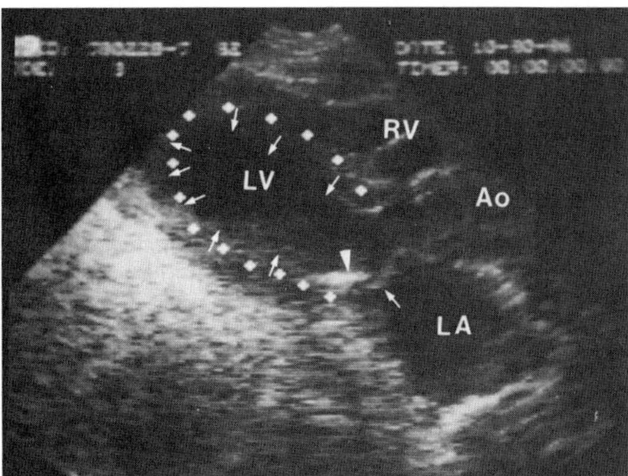

Fig. 28-36
Parasternal long-axis view during systole in a patient with an inferoapical myocardial infarction and papillary muscle rupture. The cross marks note the diastolic position of the ventricular endocardium. Note that during systole the anterior septum has moved appropriately, as has the proximal inferoposterior wall. There is dyskinesis of the inferoapical area (*outward-pointing arrows*). The anterior mitral valve leaflet is flail, and its tip (*small white arrow*) can be seen in the left atrium behind the mitral annulus (*white arrowhead*).

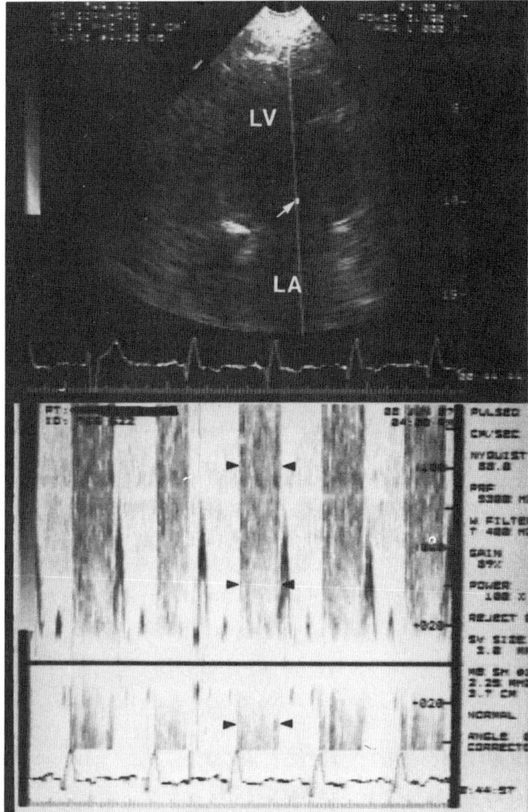

Fig. 28-37
Apical four-chamber view recorded in a patient with a remote myocardial infarction and a holosystolic murmur. Note the abnormal mitral valve closure with bowing of the leaflets toward the ventricular cavity during systole. With the Doppler sample volume immediately behind the mitral valve, an abnormal high velocity regurgitant jet is noted, diagnostic of mitral regurgitation.

closure of the mitral valve such that it tends to bow into the cavity of the left ventricle and become functionally incompetent [127, 128]. This form of papillary muscle dysfunction can be accurately identified with two-dimensional echocardiography; furthermore, the degree of mitral regurgitation can be assessed using Doppler interrogation. Figure 28-37 shows a patient with a known inferior MI and a loud holosystolic murmur. No abnormalities of the ventricular septum were visualized. The mitral valve had abnormal coaptation, and Doppler interrogation revealed abnormal systolic flow in the left atrium consistent with mitral regurgitation.

Transesophageal echocardiography has rapidly become the imaging modality of choice in the assessment of mitral valvular disease. In the setting of an AMI with hypotension or a new murmur, transesophageal echocardiography can provide rapid and detailed assessment of the mitral and submitral apparatus. The presence of ruptured chords and/or rupture of a portion or all of a papillary muscle can be clearly delineated and the degree of mitral regurgitation can be evaluated. Not only can the diagnosis be made accurately and quickly, but the valve apparatus can be evaluated preoperatively for possible repair versus replacement. The patient in Figure 28-38 presented with an acute lateral wall infarction with onset of a new murmur. The transthoracic echocardiogram was limited by the patient's body habitus, ventilatory support, and supine position on the catheterization table. Transesophageal echocardiogram revealed partial rupture of the posterolateral papillary muscle with severe mitral regurgitation in an eccentric anteriorly directed jet with reversal of flow with the pulmonary veins. Several reports have outlined the ability of transesophageal echocardiography to accurately assess papillary muscle rupture and the resultant mitral regurgitation it produces [123, 124].

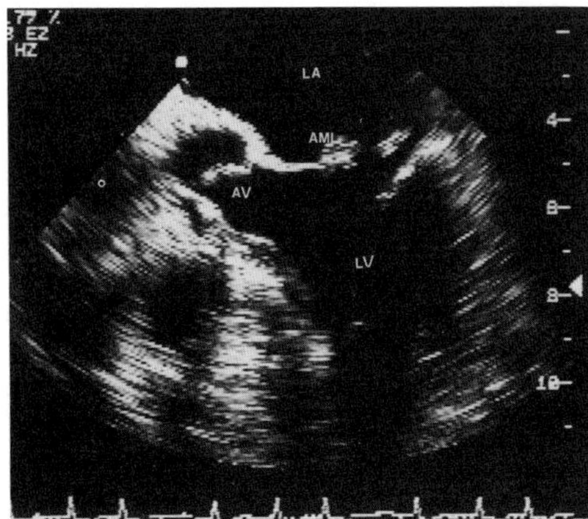

Fig. 28-38
Transesophageal echocardiogram illustrating anterior mitral leaflet flail with a thickened distal leaflet tip suspicious for partial papillary muscle rupture. LA = left atrium; LV = left ventricle; AV = aortic valve; AML = anterior mitral leaflet.

Remodeling After Acute Myocardial Infarction

Accurate, reproducible measurements of endocardial surface area and the area of segmental dysfunction have contributed greatly to our understanding of the remodeling process after AMI. Guyer et al. demonstrated the use of this endocardial mapping technique in accurately quantifying the global extent of abnormal systolic function in a canine model in the postinfarction setting [22]. Regions of dyssynergy were measured in two perpendicular planes and then plotted in the appropriate location on the endocardial map. The extent of left ventricle with abnormal wall motion correlated closely with the fraction of endocardial area overlying the infarction ($r = .92$; $p \leq .001$) and the fraction of myocardial volume infarcted ($r = .86$; $p \leq .001$) when evaluated in the canine model. With the use of this validated technique for measuring endocardial surface area and percentage of abnormal wall motion, Picard et al. followed 57 patients with a first MI for 1 year [20]. They noted variable increases in endocardial surface area over the first 3 months related to the size and location of the infarction. Marked increases in endocardial surface area occurred in infarctions complicated by expansion. Between 3 months and 1 year, however, the mean endocardial surface area decreased in all groups. Although the endocardial surface area differed at 3 months among patients with Q-wave anterior and inferior infarctions, the absolute change in endocardial surface area from 3 months to 1 year was not influenced by infarct size, location, or the presence or absence of expansion. In addition, despite lack of intervention, regional dysfunction for most patients demonstrated improvement over time regardless of the location (anterior or inferior) or type of MI (Q-wave, non-Q-wave). The authors concluded that, if followed for at least 1 year, LV structure (by endocardial surface area), and LV regional function (by extent of abnormal wall motion) demonstrate variable but continued improvement even in the absence of intervention. Nidorf et al. in a similar study of patients with infarction requiring early intervention noted ventricular remodeling was influenced by extent of abnormal wall motion and adequacy of perfusion to the infarct bed [21] (Fig. 28-39).

Exercise Echocardiography After Myocardial Infarction

The resting echocardiogram provides valuable prognostic information in patients after MI. Prognosis is determined on the basis of established wall motion abnormalities. Exercise echocardiography refers to the technique of echocardiographic imaging in conjunction with stress testing to detect inducible wall motion abnormalities that imply exercise-induced ischemia and additional jeopardized myocardium. This technique has been shown by a number of investigators to be an accurate means of detecting patients with coronary artery disease [129, 130]. More recently, it has been performed in conjunction with low-level exercise in patients recovering from MI [131–133].

Jaarsma et al. reported results in 49 patients [131] in which new exercise-induced wall motion abnormalities during the convalescent period were associated with a higher likelihood of recurrent angina or infarction. Ryan and colleagues reported virtually identical results [133]. In their study, 16 of 17 patients with new or worsening abnormalities after exercise experienced a complication versus 4 of 23 patients with stable wall motion abnormalities. Figure 28-40 shows a patient with a non-Q-

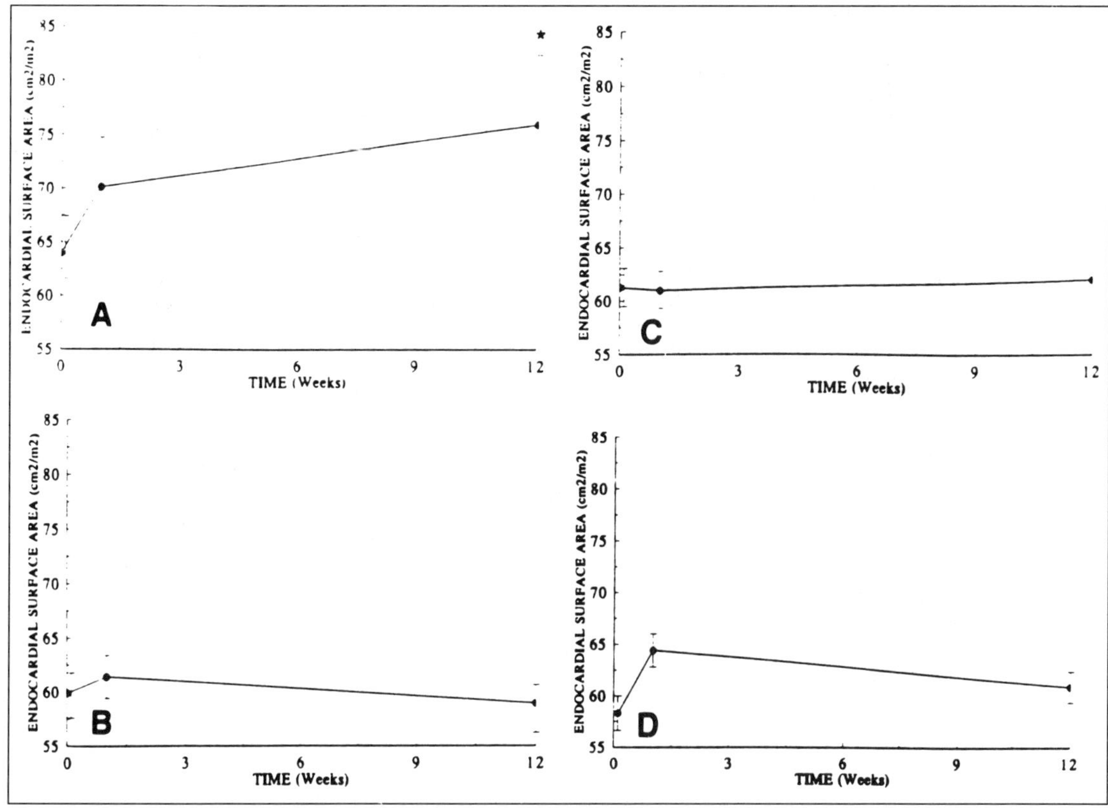

Fig. 28-39
Endocardial surface area of a patient at entry, at 1 week, and at 3 months. *A.* Group Ia: persistent occlusion and no collateral flow; *B.* Group Ib: persistent occlusion and collateral flow; *C.* Group II: early coronary reperfusion; *D.* Group III: late coronary reperfusion. * = t test; entry versus late follow-up, p < .005. (Reproduced from Nidorf et al. Benefit of late coronary reperfusion on ventricular morphology and function after myocardial infarction. *J. Am. Coll. Cardiol.* 21:683, 1993. With permission.)

wave infarction evaluated during the convalescent period. Wall motion is preserved in the septum at rest but becomes markedly abnormal after low-intensity exercise.

Future Developments in Echocardiography

The current capabilities of two-dimensional echocardiography and Doppler ultrasound techniques in patients with chest pain syndromes who develop AMI have been discussed above. Other applications now under investigation include attempts at tissue characterization, myocardial perfusion contrast echocardiography, and direct coronary visualization.

Tissue Characterization

Tissue characterization relies on computerized analysis of the gray levels of myocardium in an effort to detect ischemic or necrotic myocardium [134–137]. Multiple algorithms have been used successfully to this end, although they all appear closely linked to wall motion. To provide truly valuable information tissue characterization parameters must be developed that allow demonstration of functionally abnormal but potentially viable ischemic myocardium, which would then assist in decisions for emergent reperfusion.

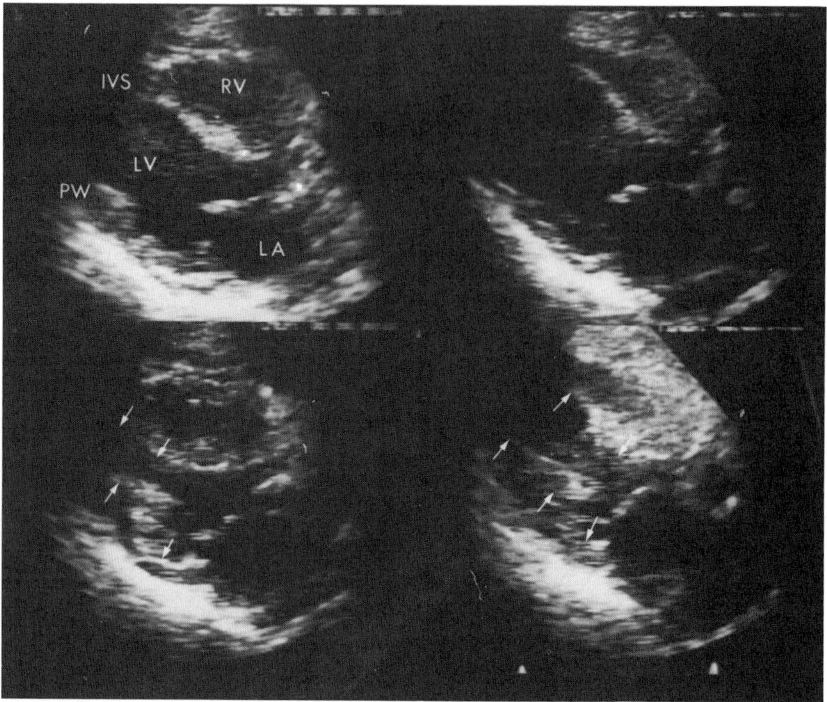

Fig. 28-40
Rest and postexercise echocardiograms recorded in the parasternal long-axis view. The study was performed 14 days after an uncomplicated myocardial infarction. At rest the proximal inferoposterior wall is akinetic. With exercise, the patient developed no chest pain, and the test was stopped for fatigue and dyspnea. After exercise, the entire inferoposterior wall and distal ventricular septum become dyskinetic, implying multivessel coronary disease, which was confirmed at subsequent catheterization.

Direct Coronary Visualization

The proximal right and left coronary arteries can be imaged by transthoracic ultrasound, and this imaging plays a role in the pediatric population for diagnosing aberrant coronary arteries and coronary arterial aneurysm [138]. In the adult population, the feasibility of detecting atherosclerotic plaque in the proximal coronary arteries has been demonstrated in several laboratories [139, 140, 155]; however, its clinical impact is yet to be defined. More recently, the feasibility of visualizing the proximal coronary arteries with transesophageal echo has also been demonstrated. The technique may eventually play a role in screening patients for high-risk lesions such as left main or proximal left anterior descending coronary artery obstructions.

Imaging Diastolic Properties of the Left Ventricle

Although the abnormalities of systolic function are often thought of as the major abnormality produced by myocardial ischemia, abnormalities of diastolic relaxation occur almost universally with ischemia and may play a role in clinical deterioration [141, 142]. These abnormalities are reflected in the pattern of LV inflow through the mitral valve. With normal LV compliance, mitral inflow is biphasic with inflow velocities more rapid early in diastole. There is an immediate reversal in this ratio with the onset of myocardial ischemia. This picture is seen experimentally in the animal laboratory [141] and at the time of balloon angioplasty in patients [142]. Although these changes are generally thought to reflect altered diastolic compliance of the left ventricle, they do not correlate highly with any of the more well accepted hemodynamic parameters of a diastolic function [141], and their magnitude is highly dependent on ventricular loading conditions.

Assessment of Myocardial Perfusion

Contrast echocardiography was initially developed for assessing chamber boundaries and intracardiac shunts. Development of new myocardial contrast agents now allows assessment of myocardial perfusion with two-dimensional echocardiography [143–154]. This technique, initially developed in the animal laboratory, has been demonstrated to be an accurate means of determining MI size [145] and, more recently, an accurate means of identifying reperfusion hyperemia. Figure 28-41 is a composite showing the range of observations that have been noted with myocardial contrast echocardiography. The ultimate goal of this technique is to develop contrast agents and methodology to determine absolute myocardial perfusion levels. Although approximated in animal laboratories, precisely determining perfusion levels is not yet feasible with this technique.

Myocardial contrast echocardiography has been used in patients on an investigational basis and was demonstrated to be safe [147–154]. Newer agents currently under development should increase the margin of safety for this technique. Current data suggest that the distribution of coronary arteries can be determined with myocardial perfusion contrast echocardiography [147], that severe coronary artery narrowings can be documented, and that return of flow after reperfusion can be demonstrated [148].

Fig. 28-41
Myocardial contrast echocardiograms recorded at baseline (*B*), during coronary occlusion (*C*), and immediately after release of the occlusion, demonstrating reactive hyperemia (*D*). *A*. Recorded at baseline prior to contrast injection or any coronary manipulation. *C*. There is an area (*arrows*) that has not increased in image intensity and that corresponds to a nonperfused region of myocardium. This same area shows preferential uptake of the contrast during the phase of reactive hyperemia.

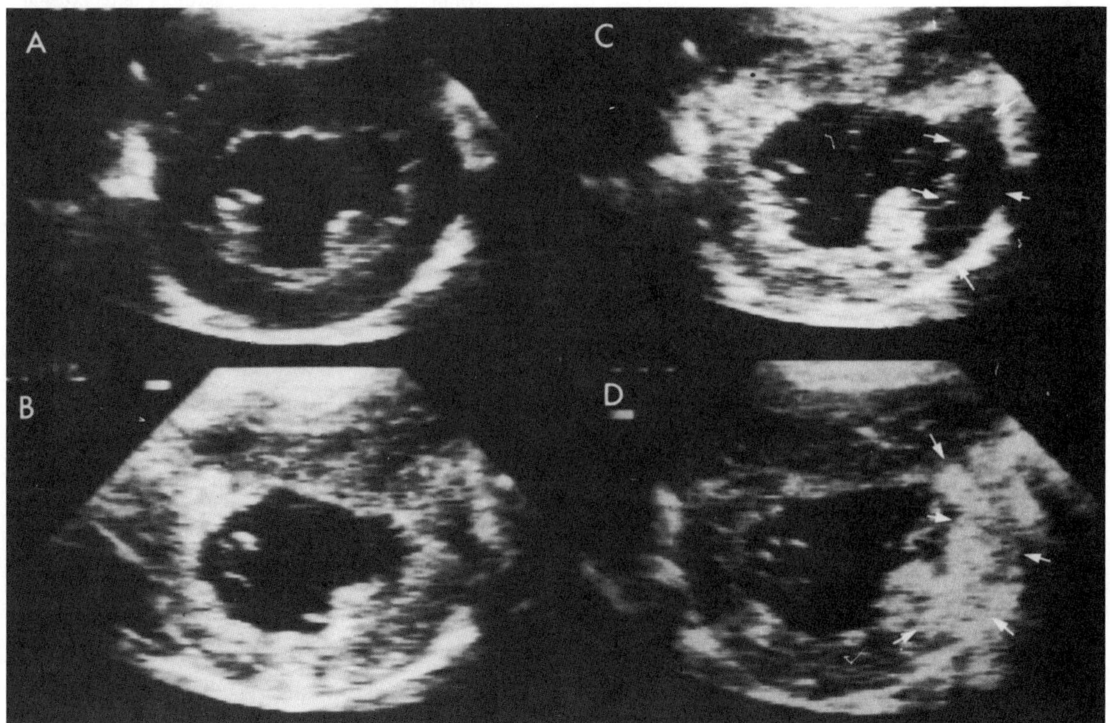

Recent laboratory and clinical studies have demonstrated that this technique can identify collateral perfusion distal to total coronary obstructions and that demonstration of preserved collateral flow is an accurate marker for myocardial viability and eventual recovery of function. Myocardial contrast echocardiography shows tremendous promise for allowing simultaneous assessment of perfusion and ventricular function.

Modern ultrasound techniques are highly versatile, relatively inexpensive, and noninvasive, and they allow visualization of all areas of the human heart. When dealing with patients with coronary artery disease, wall motion abnormalities are the hallmark of myocardial ischemia and can be accurately identified and quantified. Echocardiography may provide the initial diagnosis of acute ischemic syndromes, quantitation of MI size, and assessment of short- and long-term prognosis. In addition, two-dimensional echocardiography combined with Doppler techniques can diagnose most complications arising after MI. Future developments may allow assessment of the diastolic properties of the heart and of myocardial perfusion itself.

References

1. Tennant, R., and Wiggers, C. J. The effect of coronary occlusion on myocardial contraction. *A.J.P.* 112:351, 1935.
2. Weiss, J. L., Bulkley, B. H., Hutchins, C. M., et al. Two-dimensional echocardiographic recognition of myocardial injury in man: Comparison with postmortem studies. *Circulation* 63:401, 1981.
3. Hecht, H. S., Taylor, R., Wong, M., et al. Comparative evaluation of segmental asynergy in remote myocardial infarction by radionuclide angiography, two-dimensional echocardiography, and contrast ventriculography. *Am. Heart J.* 101:740, 1981.
4. Wohlgelernter, D., Cleman, M., Highman, H. A., et al. Regional myocardial dysfunction during coronary angioplasty: Evaluation by two-dimensional echocardiography and 12-lead electrocardiography. *J. Am. Coll. Cardiol.* 7:1245, 1986.
5. Labovitz, A. J., Lewen, M. K., Kern, M., et al. Evaluation of left ventricular systolic and diastolic dysfunction during transient myocardial ischemia produced by angioplasty. *J. Am. Coll. Cardiol.* 10:748, 1987.
6. Hauser, A. M., Gangadharan, V., Ramos, R. G., et al. Sequence of mechanical, electrocardiographic and clinical effects of repeated coronary artery occlusion in human beings: Echocardiographic observations during coronary angioplasty. *J. Am. Coll. Cardiol.* 5:193, 1985.
7. Vatner, S. F. Correlation between acute reductions in myocardial blood flow and function in conscious dogs. *Circ. Res.* 47:201, 1980.
8. Wyatt, H. L., Forrester, J. S., and Tyberg, J. V. Effect of graded reductions in regional coronary perfusion on regional and total cardiac function. *Am. J. Cardiol.* 36:185, 1975.
9. Buda, A. J., Zotz, R. J., Pace, D. P., et al. Comparison of two-dimensional echocardiographic wall motion and wall thickening abnormalities in relation to the myocardium at risk. *Am. Heart J.* 111: 587, 1986.
10. Lieberman, A. N., Weiss, J. L., and Jugdutt, B. I. Two-dimensional echocardiography and infarct size relationship of regional wall motion and thickening to the extent of myocardial infarction in the dog. *Circulation* 63:739, 1981.
11. Nieminen, M., Parisi, A. F., and O'Boyle, J. E. Serial evaluation of myocardial thickening and thinning in acute experimental infarction: Identification and quantification using two-dimensional echocardiography. *Circulation* 66:174, 1982.
12. Weyman, A. E., Franklin, T. D., and Hogan, R. D. Importance of temporal heterogeneity in assessing the contraction abnormalities associated with acute myocardial ischemia. *Circulation* 70:102, 1984.
13. Heger, J. J., Weyman, A. E., Wann, L. S., et al. Cross-sectional echocardiographic analysis of the extent of left ventricular asynergy in acute myocardial infarction. *Circulation* 61:1113, 1980.
14. Parisi, A. F., Moynihan, P. F., Folland, E. D., et al. Quantitative detection of regional left ventricular contraction abnormalities by two-dimensional echocardiography. *Circulation* 63:761, 1981.
15. Mann, D. L., Gillam, D., and Weyman, A. E. Cross-sectional echocardiographic assessment of regional left ventricular performance and myocardial perfusion. *Prog. Cardiovasc. Dis.* 29:1, 1986.
16. Gillam, L. D., Hogan, R. D., Foale, R. A., et al. A comparison of quantitative echocardiographic methods for delineating infarct induced abnormal wall motion. *Circulation* 70:113, 1984.
17. Gillam, L. D., Franklin, T. D., Foale, R. A., et al. The natural history of regional wall motion in the acutely infarcted canine ventricle. *J. Am. Coll. Cardiol.* 7:1325, 1986.
18. Sheehan, F. H., et al. Advantages and applications of the centerline method for characterizing regional ventricular function. *Circulation* 74:293, 1986.
19. McGillem, M. J., Mancini, J., DeBoe, S. F., et al. Modification of the centerline method for assessment of echocardiographic wall thickening and motion: A comparison with areas of risk. *J. Am. Coll. Cardiol.* 11:861, 1988.
20. Picard, M. H., Wilkins, G. T., Ray, P. A., et al. Natural history of left ventricular size and function

after acute myocardial infarction. *Circulation* 82:484, 1990.

21. Nidorf, S. M., Siu, S. C., Galambos, G., et al. Benefit of late coronary reperfusion on ventricular morphology and function after myocardial infarction. *J. Am. Coll. Cardiol.* 21:683, 1993.
22. Guyer, D. E., Foale, F. A., Gillam, L. D., et al. An echocardiographic technique for quantifying and displaying the extent of regional left ventricular dyssynergy. *J. Am. Coll. Cardiol.* 8:830, 1990.
23. Gerson, M. C., Noble, R. J., Wann, L. S., et al. Noninvasive documentation of Prinzmetal's angina. *Am. J. Cardiol.* 43:329, 1979.
24. Widlansky, S., McHenry, P. L., Corya, B. C., et al. Coronary angiographic, echocardiographic and electrocardiographic studies on a patient with variant angina due to coronary artery spasm. *Am. Heart J.* 90:631, 1975.
25. Distante, A., Rovai, D., Picano, E., et al. Transient changes in left ventricular mechanics during attacks of Prinzmetal angina: A two-dimensional echocardiographic study. *Am. Heart J.* 108:440, 1984.
26. Distante, A., Picano, E., Moscarelli, E., et al. Echocardiographic versus hemodynamic monitoring during attacks of variant angina pectoris. *Am. J. Cardiol.* 55:1319, 1985.
27. Nixon, J. V., Brown, C. N., and Smitherman, T. C. Identification of transient and persistent segmental wall motion abnormalities in patients with unstable angina by two-dimensional echocardiography. *Circulation* 65:1497, 1982.
28. Kisslo, J. A., Robertson, D., Gilbert, B. W., et al. A comparison of real-time, two-dimensional echocardiography and cineangiography in detecting left ventricular asynergy. *Circulation* 55:134, 1977.
29. Linduall, K., Hamsten, A., Landou, C., et al. Comparative study of echo- and angiocardiographically determined regional left ventricular wall motion in recent myocardial infarction. *Eur. Heart J.* 5: 533, 1984.
30. Erbel, R., Schweizer, P., Meyer, J., et al. Sensitivity of cross-sectional echocardiography in detection of impaired global and regional left ventricular function: Prospective study. *Int. J. Cardiol.* 7:375, 1985.
31. Freeman, A. P., Giles, R. W., Walsh, W. F., et al. Regional left ventricular wall motion assessment: Comparison of two-dimensional echocardiography and radionuclide angiography with contrast angiography in healed myocardial infarction. *Am. J. Cardiol.* 56:8, 1985.
32. VanReet, R. E., Quinones, M. A., Poliner, L. R., et al. Comparison of two-dimensional echocardiography with gated radionuclide ventriculography in the evaluation of global and regional left ventricular function in acute myocardial infarction. *J. Am. Coll. Cardiol.* 3:243, 1984.
33. Nixon, J. V., Narahara, K. A., and Smitherman, T. C. Estimation of myocardial involvement in patients with acute myocardial infarction by two-dimensional echocardiography. *Circulation* 62: 1248, 1980.
34. Heger, J., Weyman, A. E., Wann, L. S., et al. Cross-sectional echocardiography in acute myocardial infarction: Detection and localization of regional left ventricular asynergy. *Circulation* 60:531, 1979.
35. Stamm, R. B., Gibson, R. S., Bishop, H. L., et al. Echocardiographic detection of infarct localized asynergy and remote asynergy during acute myocardial infarction: Correlation with the extent of angiographic coronary disease. *Circulation* 67:233, 1983.
36. Gibson, R. S., Bishop, H. L., Stamm, R. B., et al. Value of early two-dimensional echocardiography in patients with acute myocardial infarction. *Am. J. Cardiol.* 49:1110, 1982.
37. Horowitz, B. S., Morganroth, J., Parrotto, C., et al. Immediate diagnosis of acute myocardial infarction by two-dimensional echocardiography. *Circulation* 65:323, 1982.
38. Jaarsma, W., Visser, C. A., Van Eengie, M. J., et al. Left ventricular wall motion with and without Q-wave disappearance after acute myocardial infarction. *Am. J. Cardiol.* 59:516, 1987.
39. Sabia, P., Abbott, R. D., Afrookteh, A., et al. The importance of two-dimensional echocardiographic assessment of left ventricular systolic function in patients presenting to the emergency room with cardiac-related symptoms. *Circulation* 84:1615, 1991.
40. Arvan, S., and Varat, M. A. Two-dimensional echocardiography versus surface electrocardiography for the diagnosis of acute non-Q wave myocardial infarction. *Am. Heart J.* 110:44, 1985.
41. Loh, I. K., Charuzi, Y., Beeder, C., et al. Early diagnosis of nontransmural myocardial infarction by two-dimensional echocardiography. *Am. Heart J.* 104:963, 1982.
42. Force, T., Kemper, A. J., Bloomfield, P., et al. Non-Q wave perioperative myocardial infarction: Assessment of the incidence and severity of regional dysfunction with quantitative two-dimensional echocardiography. *Circulation* 72:781, 1985.
43. Force, T., Bloomfield, P., O'Boyle, J. E., et al. Quantitative two-dimensional echocardiographic analysis of regional wall motion in patients with perioperative myocardial infarction. *Circulation* 70:233, 1984.
44. Camara, E. J., Chandra, N., Ouyang, P., et al. Reciprocal ST change in acute myocardial infarction: Assessment by electrocardiography and echocardiography. *J. Am. Coll. Cardiol.* 2:251, 1983.
45. Pierard, L. A., Sprynger, M., Cilis, F., et al. Significance of precordial ST-segment depression in inferior acute myocardial infarction as determined by echocardiography. *Am. J. Cardiol.* 57:82, 1986.
46. Arvan, S., and Varat, M. A. Persistent ST-segment elevation and left ventricular wall abnormalities: A two-dimensional echocardiographic study. *Am. J. Cardiol.* 53:1542, 1984.

47. Kerber, R. E., Marcus, M. L., Ehrhardt, J., et al. Correlation between echocardiographically demonstrated segmental dyskinesis and regional myocardial perfusion. *Circulation* 52:1097, 1975.
48. O'Boyle, J. E., Parisi, A. F., Nieminen, M., et al. Quantitative detection of regional left ventricular contraction abnormalities by 2-dimensional echocardiography. *Am. J. Cardiol.* 51:1732, 1985.
49. Pandian, N. G., Koyanagi, S., Skorton, D. J., et al. Relations between 2-dimensional echocardiographic wall thickening abnormalities, myocardial infarct size and coronary risk area in normal and hypertrophied myocardium in dogs. *Am. J. Cardiol.* 52:1318, 1983.
50. Wyatt, H. L., Meerbaum, S., Heng, M. K., et al. Experimental evaluation of the extent of myocardial dyssynergy and infarct size by two-dimensional echocardiography. *Circulation* 63:607, 1981.
51. Pandian, N. G., Skorton, D. J., Collins, S. M., et al. Myocardial infarct size threshold for two-dimensional echocardiographic detection: Sensitivity of systolic wall thickening and endocardial motion abnormalities in small versus large infarcts. *Am. J. Cardiol.* 55:551, 1985.
52. Wyatt, H. L., Forrester, J. S., da Luz, P. L., et al. Functional abnormalities in nonoccluded regions of myocardium after experimental coronary occlusion. *Am. J. Cardiol.* 37:366, 1976.
53. Homans, D. C., Asinger, R., Elsperger, K. J., et al. Regional function and perfusion at the lateral border of ischemic myocardium. *Circulation* 71:1038, 1985.
54. Guth, B. D., White, F. C., Gallagher, K. P., et al. Decreased systolic wall thickening in myocardium adjacent to ischemic zones in conscious swine during brief coronary artery occlusion. *Am. Heart J.* 107:458, 1984.
55. Lima, J. A. C., Becker, L. C., Melin, J. A., et al. Impaired thickening of nonischemic myocardium during acute regional ischemia in the dog. *Circulation* 71:1048, 1985.
56. Force, T., Kemper, A., Perkins, L., et al. Overestimation of infarct size by quantitative two-dimensional echocardiography: The role of tethering and of analytic procedures. *Circulation* 73:1360, 1986.
57. Topol, E. J., Weiss, J. L., Brinker, J. A., et al. Regional wall motion improvement after coronary thrombolysis with recombinant tissue plasminogen activator: Importance of coronary angioplasty. *J. Am. Coll. Cardiol.* 6:426, 1985.
58. Presti, C. F., Gentile, R., Armstrong, W. F., et al. Demonstration of myocardial salvage by percutaneous transluminal coronary angioplasty using two-dimensional echocardiography (Abstract). *Clin. Res.* 35:315A, 1987.
59. Otto, C. M., Stratton, J. R., Maynard, C., et al. Echocardiographic evaluation of segmental wall motion early and late after thrombolytic therapy in acute myocardial infarction: The western Washington tissue plasminogen activator emergency room trial. *Am. J. Cardiol.* 65:132, 1990.
60. Charuzi, Y., Beeder, C., Marshall, L. A., et al. Improvement in regional and global left ventricular function after intracoronary thrombolysis: Assessment with two-dimensional echocardiography. *Am. J. Cardiol.* 53:622, 1984.
61. Oh, J. K., Miller, F. A., Shub, C., et al. Evaluation of acute chest pain syndromes by two dimensional echocardiography: Its potential application in the selection of patients for acute reperfusion therapy. *Mayo Clin. Proc.* 62:59, 1987.
62. Pearce, F. B., Sheikh, K. H., deBruijn, N. P., et al. Imaging of the coronary arteries by transesophageal echocardiography. *J. Am. Soc. Echo.* 2:76, 1982.
63. Kan, G., Visser, C. A., Lie, K. I., et al. Early two-dimensional echocardiographic measurement of left ventricular ejection fraction of acute myocardial infarction. *Eur. Heart J.* 5:210, 1984.
64. Nishimura, R. A., Tajik, A. J., Shub, C., et al. Role of two-dimensional echocardiography in the prediction of in-hospital complications after acute myocardial infarction. *J. Am. Coll. Cardiol.* 4: 1080, 1984.
65. Nishimura, R. A., Reeder, G. S., Miller, F. A., et al. Prognostic value of predischarge two-dimensional echocardiogram after acute myocardial infarction. *Am. J. Cardiol.* 53:429, 1984.
66. Bhatnagar, S. K., Moussa, M. A. A., and Al-Yusuf, A. R. The role of prehospital discharge two-dimensional echocardiography in determining the prognosis of survivors of first myocardial infarction. *Am. Heart J.* 109:472, 1985.
67. Horowitz, R. S., and Morganroth, J. Immediate detection of early high-risk patients with acute myocardial infarction using two-dimensional echocardiographic evaluation of left ventricular regional wall motion abnormalities. *Am. Heart J.* 103:814, 1982.
68. Abrams, D. S., Starling, M. R., Crawford, M. H., et al. Value of noninvasive techniques for predicting early complications in patients with clinical class II acute myocardial infarction. *J. Am. Coll. Cardiol.* 2:818, 1983.
69. Huntsman, L. L., Stewart, D. K., Barnes, S. R., et al. Noninvasive Doppler determination of cardiac output in man. *Circulation* 67:593, 1983.
70. Wallmeyer, K., Wann, L. S., Sagar, K. B., et al. The influence of preload and heart rate on Doppler echocardiographic indexes of left ventricular performance: Comparison with invasive indexes in an experimental preparation. *Circulation* 74:181, 1986.
71. Buchtal, A., Hanson, G. C., and Pleisach, A. R. Transcutaneous aortovelography—potentially useful technique in management of critically ill patients. *Br. Heart J.* 38:451, 1976.
72. Mehta, N., and Bennett, D. E. Impaired left ventricular function in acute myocardial infarction assessed by Doppler measurement of ascending aortic blood velocity and maximum acceleration. *Am. J. Cardiol.* 57:1052, 1986.
73. Kaplan, K., Davison, R., Parker, M., et al. Frequency of pericardial effusion as determined by M-

mode echocardiography in acute myocardial infarction. *Am. J. Cardiol.* 55:335, 1985.
74. Pierard, L. A., Albert, A., Henrard, L., et al. Incidence and significance of pericardial effusion in acute myocardial infarction as determined by two-dimensional echocardiography. *J. Am. Coll. Cardiol.* 8:517, 1986.
75. Weyman, A. E., Peskoe, S. M., Williams, E. S., et al. Detection of left ventricular aneurysms by cross-sectional echocardiography. *Circulation* 54:936, 1976.
76. Visser, C. A., Kan, C., David, G. K., et al. Echocardiographic-cineangiographic correlation in detecting left ventricular aneurysm: A prospective study of 422 patients. *Am. J. Cardiol.* 50:337, 1982.
77. Jugdutt, B. I. Identification of patients prone to infarct expansion by the degree of regional shape distortion on an early two-dimensional echocardiogram after myocardial infarction. *Clin. Cardiol.* 13:28, 1990.
78. Matsumoto, M., Watanabe, F., Goto, A., et al. Left ventricular aneurysm and the prediction of left ventricular enlargement studied by two-dimensional echocardiography: Quantitative assessment of aneurysm size in relation to clinical course. *Circulation* 72:280, 1985.
79. Visser, C. A., Kan, G., Meltzer, R. S., et al. Incidence, timing and prognostic value of left ventricular aneurysm formation after myocardial infarction: A prospective, serial echocardiographic study of 158 patients. *Am. J. Cardiol.* 57:729, 1986.
80. Eaton, L. W., Weiss, J. L., Bulkley, B., et al. Regional cardiac dilatation after acute myocardial infarction. *N. Engl. J. Med.* 300:57, 1979.
81. Visser, C. A., Kan, G., Meltzer, R. S., et al. Assessment of left ventricular aneurysm resectability by two-dimensional echocardiography. *Am. J. Cardiol.* 56:857, 1985.
82. Ryan, T., Petrovic, Q., Armstrong, W. F., et al. Quantitative two-dimensional echocardiographic assessment of patients undergoing left ventricular aneurysmectomy. *Am. Heart J.* 111:714, 1986.
83. Erlebacher, J. A., Weiss, J. L., Eaton, L. W., et al. Late effects of acute infarct dilation on heart size: A two-dimensional echocardiographic study. *Am. J. Cardiol.* 49:1120, 1982.
84. Erlebacher, J. A., Weiss, J. L., Weisfeldt, M. L., et al. Early dilation of the infarcted segment in acute transmural myocardial infarction: Role of infarct expansion in acute left ventricular enlargement. *J. Am. Coll. Cardiol.* 4:201, 1984.
85. Schuster, E. H., and Bulkley, B. H. Expansion of transmural myocardial infarction: A pathophysiologic factor in cardiac rupture. *Circulation* 60:1532, 1979.
86. Hutchins, G. M., and Bulkley, B. H. Infarct expansion versus extension: Two different complications of acute myocardial infarction. *Am. J. Cardiol.* 41:1127, 1978.
87. Gatewood, R. P., and Nanda, N. C. Differentiation of left ventricular pseudoaneurysm from true aneurysm with two-dimensional echocardiography. *Am. J. Cardiol.* 46:869, 1980.
88. Catherwood, E., Mintz, G. S., Kotler, M. N., et al. Two-dimensional echocardiographic recognition of left ventricular pseudoaneurysm. *Circulation* 62: 294, 1980.
89. Stratton, J. R., Lighty, G. W., Pearlman, A. S., et al. Detection of left ventricular thrombus by two-dimensional echocardiography: Sensitivity, specificity, and causes of uncertainty. *Circulation* 1:156, 1966.
90. Seabold, J. E., Schroder, E., Conrad, G. R., et al. Indium-111 platelet scintigraphy and two-dimensional echocardiography for detection of left ventricular thrombus: Influence of clot size and age. *J. Am. Coll. Cardiol.* 9:1057, 1987.
91. Keren, A., Goldberg, S., Gottlieb, S., et al. Natural history of left ventricular thrombi: Their appearance and resolution in the posthospitalization period of acute myocardial infarction. *J. Am. Coll. Cardiol.* 15:790, 1990.
92. Mikell, F. L., Asinger, R. W., Elsperger, K. J., et al. Tissue acoustic properties of fresh left ventricular thrombi and visualization by two-dimensional echocardiography: Experimental observations. *Am. J. Cardiol.* 49:1157, 1982.
93. Spirito, P., Bellotti, P., Chiarella, F., et al. Prognostic significance and natural history of left ventricular thrombi in patients with acute anterior myocardial infarction: A two-dimensional echocardiographic study. *Circulation* 72:774, 1985.
94. Visser, C. A., Kan, D. G., Meltzer, R. S., et al. Long-term follow-up of left ventricular thrombus after acute myocardial infarction. *Chest* 86:532, 1984.
95. Gueret, P., Dubourg, O., Ferrier, A., et al. Effects of full-dose heparin anticoagulation on the development of left ventricular thrombosis in acute transmural myocardial infarction. *J. Am. Coll. Cardiol.* 8:419, 1986.
96. Arvan, S., and Boscha, K. Prophylactic anticoagulation for left ventricular thrombi after acute myocardial infarction: A prospective randomized trial. *Am. Heart J.* 113:688, 1987.
97. Sharma, B., Carvalho, A., Wyeth, R., et al. Left ventricular thrombi diagnosed by echocardiography in patients with acute myocardial infarction treated with intracoronary streptokinase followed by intravenous heparin. *Am. J. Cardiol.* 56:422, 1985.
98. Weinreich, D. J., Burke, J. F., and Pauletto, F. J. Left ventricular mural thrombi complicating acute myocardial infarction. *Ann. Intern. Med.* 100:789, 1984.
99. Asinger, R. W., Mikell, F. L., Elsperger, J., et al. Incidence of left-ventricular thrombosis after acute transmural myocardial infarction. *N. Engl. J. Med.* 305:797, 1981.
100. Keating, E. C., Gross, S. A., Schlamowitz, R. A., et al. Mural thrombi in myocardial infarctions. *Am. J. Med.* 74:989, 1983.
101. Stratton, J. R., and Resnick, A. D. Increased em-

bolic risk in patients with left ventricular thrombi. *Circulation* 75:1004, 1987.
102. Visser, C. A., Kan, G., Meltzer, R. S., et al. Embolic potential of left ventricular thrombus after myocardial infarction: A two-dimensional echocardiographic study of 119 patients. *J. Am. Coll. Cardiol.* 5:1276, 1985.
103. Meltzer, R. S., Visser, C. A., and Fuster, V. Intracardiac thrombi and systemic embolization. *Ann. Intern. Med.* 104:689, 1986.
104. Tramarin, R., Pozzoli, M., Opasich, F. C., et al. Two-dimensional echocardiographic assessment of anticoagulant therapy in left ventricular thrombosis early after acute myocardial infarction. *Eur. Heart J.* 7:482, 1986.
105. Isner, J. M., and Roberts, W. C. Right ventricular infarction complicating left ventricular infarction secondary to coronary heart disease. *Am. J. Cardiol.* 42:885, 1978.
106. Panidis, I. P., Kotler, M. N., Mintz, G. S., et al. Right ventricular function in coronary artery disease as assessed by two-dimensional echocardiography. *Am. Heart J.* 107:1187, 1984.
107. Lopez-Sendon, J., Garcia-Fernandez, A., Coma-Canella, I., et al. Segmental right ventricular function after acute myocardial infarction: Two-dimensional echocardiographic study in 63 patients. *Am. J. Cardiol.* 51:390, 1983.
108. Jugdutt, B. I., Haraphongse, M., Basualdo, C. A., et al. Evaluation of biventricular involvement in hypotensive patients with transmural inferior infarction by two-dimensional echocardiography. *Am. Heart J.* 108:1417, 1984.
109. Dell'Italia, L. J., Starling, M. R., Crawford, M. H., et al. Right ventricular infarction: Identification by hemodynamic measurements before and after volume loading and correlation with noninvasive technique. *J. Am. Coll. Cardiol.* 4:931, 1984.
110. Rietveld, A. P., Merrman, L., Essed, C. E., et al. Right to left shunt, with severe hypoxemia, at the atrial level in a patient with hemodynamically important right ventricular infarction. *J. Am. Coll. Cardiol.* 4:776, 1983.
111. Bansal, R. C., Marsa, R. J., Holland, D., et al. Severe hypoxemia due to shunting through a patent foramen ovale: A correctable complication of right ventricular infarction. *J. Am. Coll. Cardiol.* 5:188, 1985.
112. Desoutter, P., Halphen, C., and Haiat, R. Two-dimensional echocardiographic visualization of free ventricular wall rupture in acute anterior myocardial infarction. *Am. Heart J.* 108:1360, 1984.
113. Bishop, H. L., Gibson, R. S., Stamm, R. B., et al. Role of two-dimensional echocardiography in the evaluation of patients with ventricular septal rupture postmyocardial infarction. *Am. Heart J.* 102:965, 1981.
114. Bansal, R. C., Eng, A. K., and Shakudo, M. Role of two-dimensional echocardiography, pulsed, continuous wave and color flow Doppler techniques in the assessment of ventricular septal rupture after myocardial infarction. *Am. J. Cardiol.* 65:852, 1990.
115. Rogers, E. W., Glassman, R. D., Feigenbaum, H., et al. Aneurysms of the posterior interventricular septum with postinfarction ventricular septal defect. *Chest* 78:741, 1980.
116. Mintz, G. S., Victor, M. F., Kotler, M. N., et al. Two-dimensional echocardiographic identification of surgically correctable complications of acute myocardial infarction. *Circulation* 64:91, 1981.
117. Drobac, M., Gilbert, B., Howard, R., et al. Ventricular septal defect after myocardial infarction: Diagnosis by two-dimensional contrast echocardiography. *Circulation* 67:335, 1983.
118. Pollak, H., Spiel, R., Enenkel, W., et al. Early diagnosis of subacute free wall rupture complicating acute myocardial infarction. *Eur. Heart J.* 14:640, 1993.
119. Smyllie, J., Dawkins, K., Conway, N., et al. Diagnosis of ventricular septal rupture after myocardial infarction: Value of colour flow mapping. *Br. Heart J.* 62:260, 1989.
120. Smyllie, J. H., Sutherland, G. R., Geuskens, R., et al. Doppler color flow mapping in the diagnosis of ventricular septal rupture and acute mitral regurgitation after myocardial infarction. *J. Am. Coll. Cardiol.* 15:1449, 1990.
121. Miyatake, K., Okamoto, M., Kinoshita, N., et al. Doppler echocardiographic features of ventricular septal rupture in myocardial infarction. *J. Am. Coll. Cardiol.* 5:182, 1985.
122. Koenig, K., Kasper, W., Hofman, T., et al. Transesophageal echocardiography for diagnosis of rupture of the ventricular septum or LV papillary muscle during acute MI. *Am. J. Cardiol.* 59:362, 1987.
123. Barzilai, B., Davis, V. G., Stone, P. H., et al. Prognostic significance of mitral regurgitation in acute myocardial infarction. *Am. J. Cardiol.* 65:1169, 1990.
124. Jackman, J. D., Tcheng, J. E., Califf, R. M., et al. Current concepts in the management of ischemic mitral regurgitation. *Cardio* 76, 1991.
125. Erbel, R., Schweizer, P., Besdos, P., et al. Two-dimensional echocardiographic diagnosis of papillary muscle rupture. *Chest* 79:595, 1981.
126. Come, P. C., Riley, M. F., and Weintraub, R. Echocardiographic detection of complete and partial papillary muscle rupture during acute myocardial infarction. *Am. J. Cardiol.* 56:787, 1985.
127. Godley, R. W., Wann, L. S., Rogers, E. W., et al. Incomplete mitral leaflet closure in patients with papillary muscle dysfunction. *Circulation* 63:565, 1981.
128. Ogawa, S., Hubbard, F. E., Mardelli, T. J., et al. Cross-sectional echocardiographic spectrum of papillary muscle dysfunction. *Am. Heart J.* 97:312, 1979.
129. Limacher, M. C., Quinones, M. A., Poliner, L. R., et al. Detection of coronary artery disease with

exercise two-dimensional echocardiography. *Circulation* 67:1211, 1983.

130. Armstrong, W. F., O'Donnell, J., Ryan, T., et al. Effect of prior myocardial infarction and extent and location of coronary disease on accuracy of exercise echocardiography. *J. Am. Coll. Cardiol.* 10:531, 1987.
131. Jaarsma, W., Visser, C. A., Funke Kupper, A. J., et al. Usefulness of two-dimensional exercise echocardiography shortly after myocardial infarction. *Am. J. Cardiol.* 57:86, 1986.
132. Applegate, R. J., Dell'Italia, L. J., and Crawford, M. H. Usefulness of two-dimensional echocardiography during low-level exercise testing early after uncomplicated acute myocardial infarction. *Am. J. Cardiol.* 60:10, 1987.
133. Ryan, T., Armstrong, W. F., O'Donnell, J., et al. Risk stratification following myocardial infarction using exercise echocardiography. *Am. Heart J.* 114: 1305, 1987.
134. Milunski, M. R., Mohr, G. A., Perez, J. E., et al. Ultrasonic tissue characterization with integrated backscatter. *Circulation* 80:491, 1989.
135. Glueck, R. M., Mottley, J. G., Miller, J. G., et al. Effects of coronary artery occlusion and reperfusion on cardiac cycle-dependent variation of myocardial ultrasonic backscatter. *Circ. Res.* 56:683, 1985.
136. Skorton, D. J., Melton, H., Pandian, N. G., et al. Detection of acute myocardial infarction in closed-chest dogs by analysis of regional two-dimensional echocardiographic gray-level distributions. *Circ. Res.* 52:36, 1983.
137. Haendchen, R. V., Ong, K., Fishbein, M. C., et al. Early differentiation of infarcted and noninfarcted reperfused myocardium in dogs by quantitative analysis of regional myocardial echo amplitudes. *Circ. Res.* 57:718, 1985.
138. Caldwell, R. L., Hurwitz, R. A., Girod, D. A., et al. Two-dimensional echocardiographic differentiation of anomalous left coronary artery from congestive cardiomyopathy. *Am. Heart J.* 106:710, 1983.
139. Ryan, T., Armstrong, W. F., and Feigenbaum, H. Prospective evaluation of the left main coronary artery using digital two-dimensional echocardiography. *J. Am. Coll. Cardiol.* 7:807, 1986.
140. Chen, C. C., Morganroth, J., Ogawa, S., et al. Detecting left main coronary artery disease by apical, cross-sectional echocardiography. *Circulation* 62: 288, 1980.
141. Friedman, B. J., Drinkovic, N., Miles, H., et al. Assessment of left ventricular diastolic function: Comparison of Doppler echocardiography and gated blood pool scintigraphy. *J. Am. Coll. Cardiol.* 8:1348, 1986.
142. Fujii, J., Yaxaki, Y., Sawada, H., et al. Noninvasive assessment of left and right ventricular filling in myocardial infarction with a two-dimensional Doppler echocardiographic method. *J. Am. Coll. Cardiol.* 5:1155, 1985.
143. Armstrong, W. F. Assessment of myocardial perfusion with contrast enhanced echocardiography. *Echocardiography* 3:355, 1986.
144. Armstrong, W. F., Mueller, T. M., Kinney, E. L., et al. Assessment of myocardial perfusion abnormalities with contrast-enhanced two-dimensional echocardiography. *Circulation* 66:166, 1982.
145. Armstrong, W. F., West, S. R., Dillon, J. C., et al. Assessment of location and size of myocardial infarction with contrast-enhanced echocardiography. II. Application of digital imaging techniques. *J. Am. Coll. Cardiol.* 4:141, 1984.
146. Kemper, A. J., Force, T., Kloner, R., et al. Contrast echocardiographic estimation of regional myocardial blood flow after acute coronary occlusion. *Circulation* 72:1115, 1985.
147. Moore, C. A., Smucker, M. L., and Kaul, S. Myocardial contrast echocardiography in humans. I. Safety—a comparison with routine coronary arteriography. *J. Am. Coll. Cardiol.* 8:1066, 1986.
148. Lang, R. M., Feinstein, S. B., Feldman, T., et al. Contrast echocardiography for evaluation of myocardial perfusion: Effects of coronary angioplasty. *J. Am. Coll. Cardiol.* 8:232, 1986.
149. Feinstein, S. B., Lang, R. M., Dick, C., et al. Contrast echocardiographic perfusion studies in humans. *Am. J. Card. Imaging* 1:29, 1986.
150. Lim, Y., Nanto, S., Masuyama, T., et al. Coronary collaterals assessed with myocardial contrast echocardiography in healed myocardial infarction. *Am. J. Cardiol.* 66:556, 1990.
151. Lim, Y., Nanto, S., Masuyama, T., et al. Visualization of subendocardial myocardial ischemia with myocardial contrast echocardiography in humans. *Circulation* 79:233, 1989.
152. Villanueva, F. S., Glasheen, W. P., Sklenar, J., et al. Assessment of risk area during coronary occlusion and infarct size after reperfusion with myocardial contrast echocardiography using left and right atrial injections of contrast. *Circulation* 88:596, 1993.
153. Sabia, P. J., Powers, E. R., Jayaweera, A. R., et al. Functional significance of collateral blood flow in patients with recent acute myocardial infarction. *Circulation* 85:2080, 1992.
154. Sabia, P. J., Powers, E. R., Ragosta, M., et al. An association between collateral blood flow and myocardial viability in patients with recent myocardial infarction. *N. Engl. J. Med.* 327:1825, 1992.
155. Weyman, A. E., Feigenbaum, H., Dillon, J. C., et al. Noninvasive visualization of the left main coronary artery by cross-sectional echocardiography. *Circulation* 54:169, 1976.

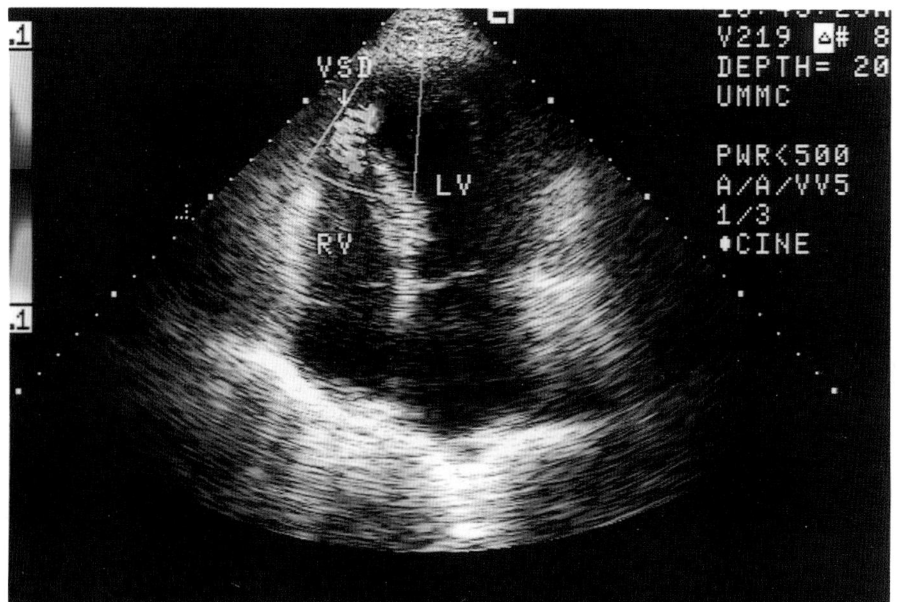

Plate 1
Apical four-chamber view recorded in a patient with anteroapical myocardial infarction and systolic murmur. With routine scanning, no ventricular septal defect was visualized. After activation of color flow imaging, a definite jet can be seen near the apex of the left ventricle consistent with pathological left-to-right flow through a ventricular septal rupture associated with the myocardial infarction. VSD = ventricular septal defect; RV = right ventricle; LV = left ventricle.

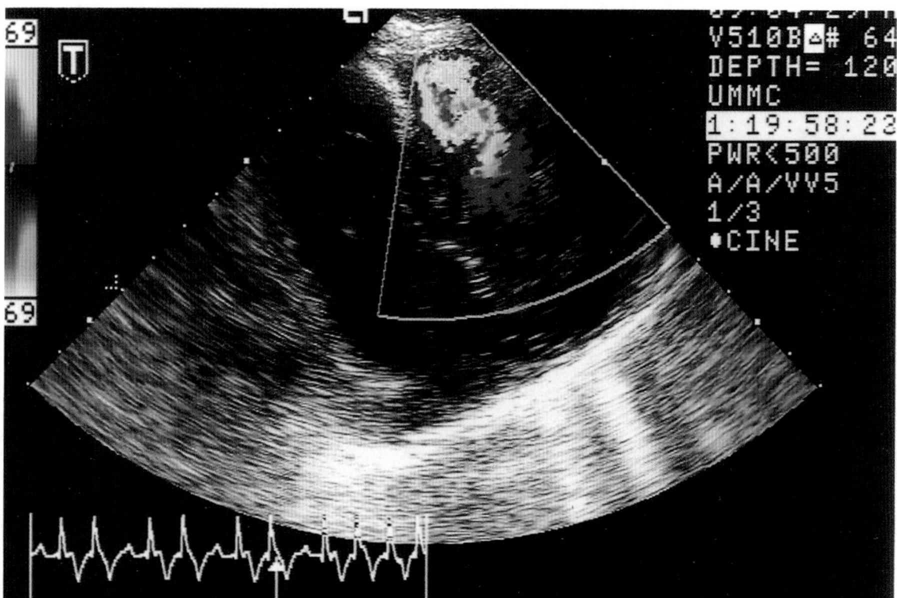

Plate 2
Same patient as presented in Figure 28-34 with color Doppler flow imaging superimposed. Note the large color flow jet directed from the left ventricle into the right ventricle in the area of the tissue drop-out.

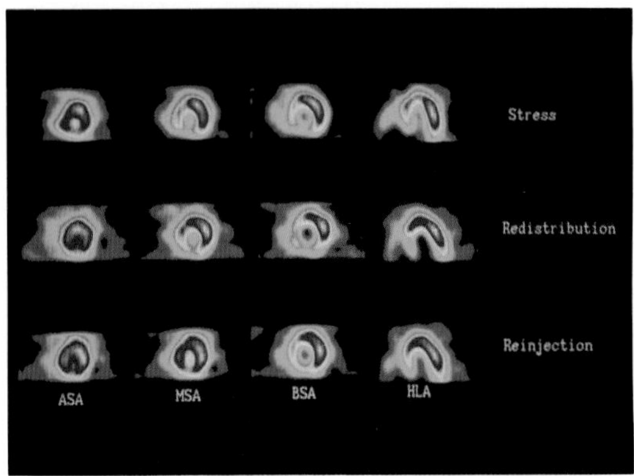

Plate 3
Stress-redistribution-reinjection Tl 201 images. Stress images (*upper panel*) show areas of hypoperfusion involving the anteroseptal and inferoposterior portions of the left ventricle. There is minimal redistribution (*middle panel*) in these areas after 3 hours. However, following reinjection (*lower panel*) there is evidence of significant reversibility in all areas. ASA = apical, MSA = midventricular, and BSA = basal short-axis sections.

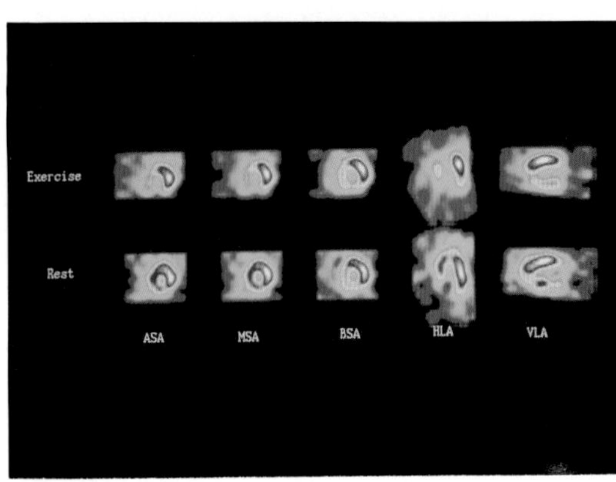

Plate 4
Stress-redistribution Tl 201 images from a patient with a recent non-Q-wave myocardial infarction. Stress images (*upper panel*) show areas of severe hypoperfusion with a multivessel distribution involving the anterior, septal and inferoposterior portions of the left ventricle. There is significant redistribution (*lower panel*) in all areas after 3 hours. Coronary arteriography confirmed severe disease in the left anterior descending, left circumflex and right coronary arteries. ASA = apical, MSA = midventricular, and BSA = basal short-axis sections; HLA = horizontal and VLA = vertical long-axis sections.

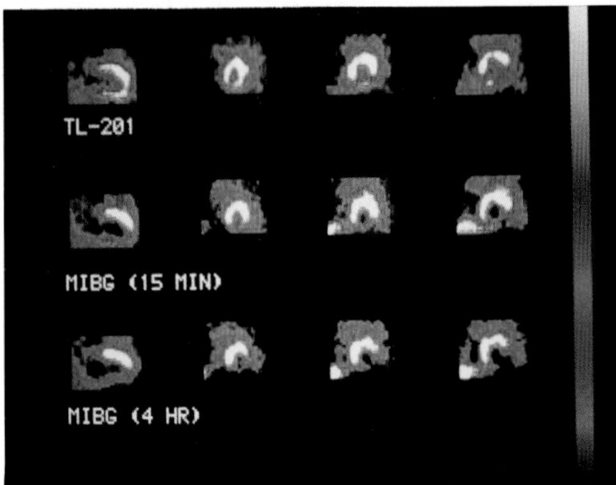

Plate 5
Representative sets of T1 201 and metaiodobenzylguanidine (MIBG) tomograms from a patient who sustained a recent inferior wall myocardial infarction. The first column shows vertical long-axis sections, and the second, third and fourth columns show apical, midventricular, and basal ventricular short-axis sections, respectively. Images in the top row are T1 201 tomograms and the middle and lower images are the 15-minute and 4-hour tomograms, respectively. Note the obvious disparity between the size of the myocardial perfusion defect and the larger area of sympathetic denervation reflected by the 4-hour MIBG images. (Adapted from A. I. McGhie et al. Regional cardiac adrenergic function using I-123 meta-iodobenzylguanidine tomographic imaging after acute myocardial infarction. *Am. J. Cardiol.* 67:236, 1991. With permission.)

29. Nuclear Imaging Techniques in Patients with Acute Myocardial Infarction

A. Iain McGhie, James R. Corbett, and James T. Willerson

Nuclear imaging techniques play an integral role in managing patients with acute coronary syndromes. Radionuclide ventriculography (RVG) is widely used as an accurate technique to assess left and right ventricular function in patients after myocardial infarction (MI). Increased use of thrombolysis has led to a need to develop techniques that allow for the detection of viable myocardium in the area subtended by the infarct-related artery. Several nuclear techniques, with either perfusion agents or metabolic tracers, appear to have a role in this regard. For example, the new technetium 99m (Tc 99m) radiopharmaceutical, 2-methoxyisobutyl isonitril (sestamibi), with its unique myocardial kinetics has been used to evaluate the efficacy of thrombolytic agents and coronary angioplasty in salvaging myocardium in acute myocardial infarction (AMI). Infarct-avid imaging techniques can also be used to identify and localize areas of myocardial necrosis. In addition, when combined with perfusion imaging, infarct-avid imaging may be of value in risk stratification for patients with AMI and unstable angina [1–4].

Assessment of Ventricular Function by Use of Radionuclide Ventriculography

One of the most important prognostic variables following AMI is the extent of left ventricular (LV) dysfunction. Once the discharge left ventricular ejection fraction (LVEF) falls below 0.40, there is a progressive increase in cardiac mortality over the subsequent year. Patients with an LVEF below 0.30 have a fivefold increase in mortality in the first year (Fig. 29-1) [5]. RVG is an accurate and reproducible method for assessing global and segmental left and right ventricular function [6–12]. The patient's red blood cells are labeled with Tc 99m to allow visualization of the cardiovascular blood pool and subsequent measurement of right and left ventricular EFs and volumes using an interactive computer (Fig. 29-2). Technical details relative to methodology for performing RVG are given elsewhere [6–12].

RVG has been used to estimate the functional impact of MI on left and right ventricular performance in patients during the first few hours following their infarction [13]. Within the first 8 hours from onset of symptoms, RVG can provide an objective estimate of the severity of LV dysfunction in patients with MI. This technique is superior to clinical assessments, including physical examination, chest radiograph, and estimation of severity of LV dysfunction by Killip classification (Table 29-1, Fig. 29-3) [13].

Several studies have analyzed serial changes in LV function after MI in patients treated with thrombolytic therapy [14–18]. These studies demonstrated the shortcomings of global indexes of ventricular function, showing that changes in regional ventricular function are often not reflected by changes in the LVEF. Characteristically, early in the evolution of MI, severe asynergy is present in the segment supplied by the occluded artery with compensatory hyperkinesis in segments distant from the infarct zone. If reperfusion occurs and results in salvage of myocardium, function improves with time in the infarct region, accompanied by normalization of the hyperkinetic segments. The net effect is that global ventricular function is preserved or improved at time of follow-up. Con-

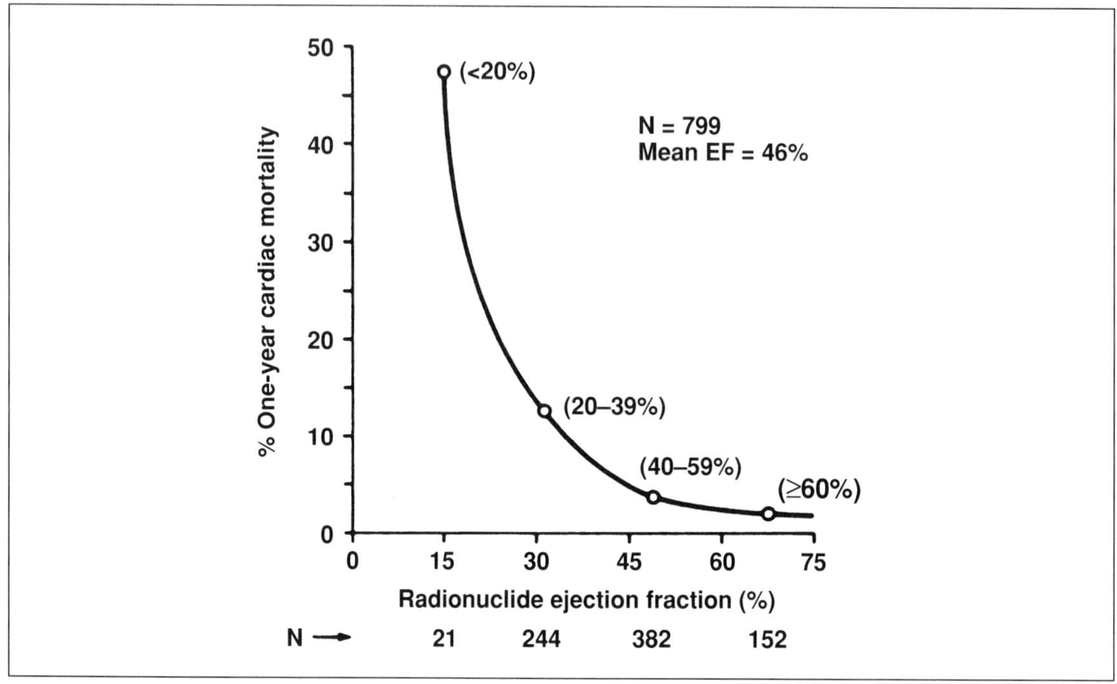

Fig. 29-1
Prognostic importance of the predischarge left ventricular ejection fraction (EF) as measured by radionuclide ventriculography in patients with recent myocardial infarction. Note the exponential increase in mortality when the left ventricular ejection fraction falls below 0.40. (From the Multicenter Postinfarction Research Group. Risk stratification and survival after myocardial infarction. *N. Engl. J. Med.* 309:331, 1983. Reprinted by permission.)

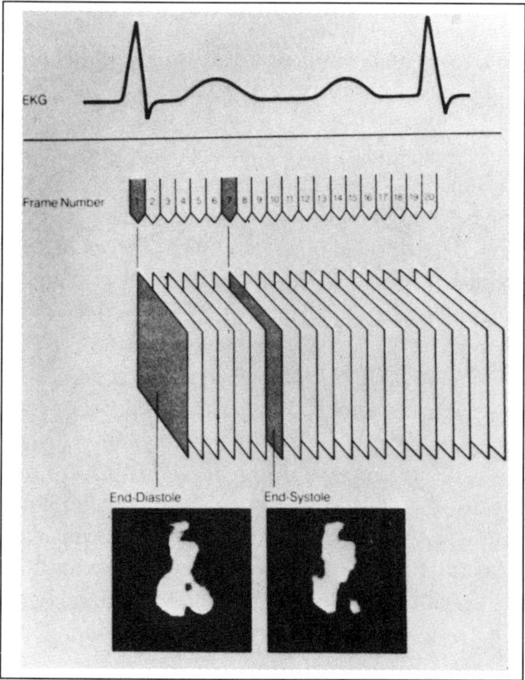

Fig. 29-2
Radionuclide ventriculogram obtained by summing radionuclide counts from various portions of the cardiac cycle from the subsequent display of the radionuclide ventriculogram and end-diastolic (*bottom left*) and end-systolic (*bottom right*) frames. This type of imaging is often referred to as MUGA imaging.

Table 29-1
Radionuclide left ventricular volumes and ejection fraction according to Killip classification

	LVEF			
Killip class	All patients	Patients with volume data	LVEDVI (ml/m²)	LVESVI (ml/m²)
I	0.50 ± 0.14 (N = 41)	0.52 ± 0.14 (N = 27)	75 ± 29 (N = 27)	39 ± 24 (N = 27)
II	0.42 ± 0.17 (N = 52)	0.43 ± 0.17 (N = 43)	82 ± 33 (N = 43)	49 ± 28 (N = 43)
III	0.27 ± 0.07 (N = 7)	0.27 ± 0.07 (N = 6)	110 ± 52 (N = 6)	80 ± 41 (N = 6)

LVEDVI and LVESVI = left ventricular end-diastolic and left ventricular end-systolic volume index, respectively; LVEF = left ventricular ejection fraction; N = number of patients.
Source: C. F. Sanford et al. Value of radionuclide ventriculography in the immediate characterization of patients with acute myocardial infarction. *Am. J. Cardiol.* 49:637, 1982. With permission.

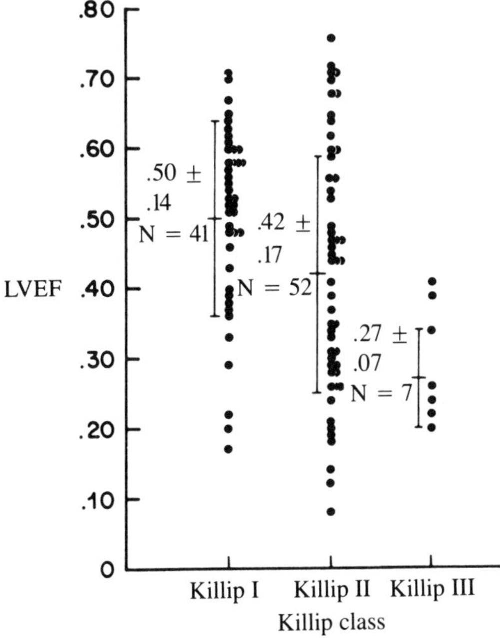

Fig. 29-3
Left ventricular ejection fraction (LVEF) determined by MUGA imaging compared to the clinical Killip classification. Mean values ± standard deviation are presented for each classification. A higher Killip classification is associated with a significantly lower mean ejection fraction ($p < .001$). Please note, however, that some patients with Killip I classification have severe impairment of their LVEFs and a few patients with Killip III classification have relatively well preserved LVEFs. (From C. F. Sanford et al. Value of radionuclide ventriculography in the immediate characterization of patients with acute myocardial infarction. *Am. J. Cardiol.* 49:637, 1982. With permission.)

versely, without reperfusion and myocardial salvage, function is unchanged in the segments subtended by the infarct-related artery, and normalization of the hyperkinetic segments does not occur, which results in deterioration in global ventricular function (Fig. 29-4).

Alterations in the topography of the left ventricle as a result of infarct expansion have an adverse effect on morbidity and mortality [19]. This is not an uncommon complication of AMI, particularly when the anterior and septal LV walls are involved [20]. Meizlish et al. successfully used planar RVG to detect functional aneurysm formation in patients soon after anterior MI [21]. In this study, patients with evidence of early functional aneurysm formation had a threefold increase in mortality in the first year compared with those without early aneurysm formation. Other studies have successfully utilized RVG to evaluate the effects of remodeling on ventricular volume after MI. In a study investigating the time course of remodeling in patients following infarction, Warren et al. demonstrated that in 55 percent of patients (20 of 36) there was a more than 20 percent increase in end-diastolic volume, with the greatest increase in volume occurring in the 10 months following hospital discharge [22]. It was also noted that the increase in end-diastolic volume was more common and more severe following occlusion of the left anterior descending (LAD) coronary artery. Using RVG, Jeremy et al. evaluated the effect of patency of the infarct-related artery on ventricular volumes [23]. In patients without perfusion of the infarct-related artery, there was an increase in ventricular volume in the month follow-

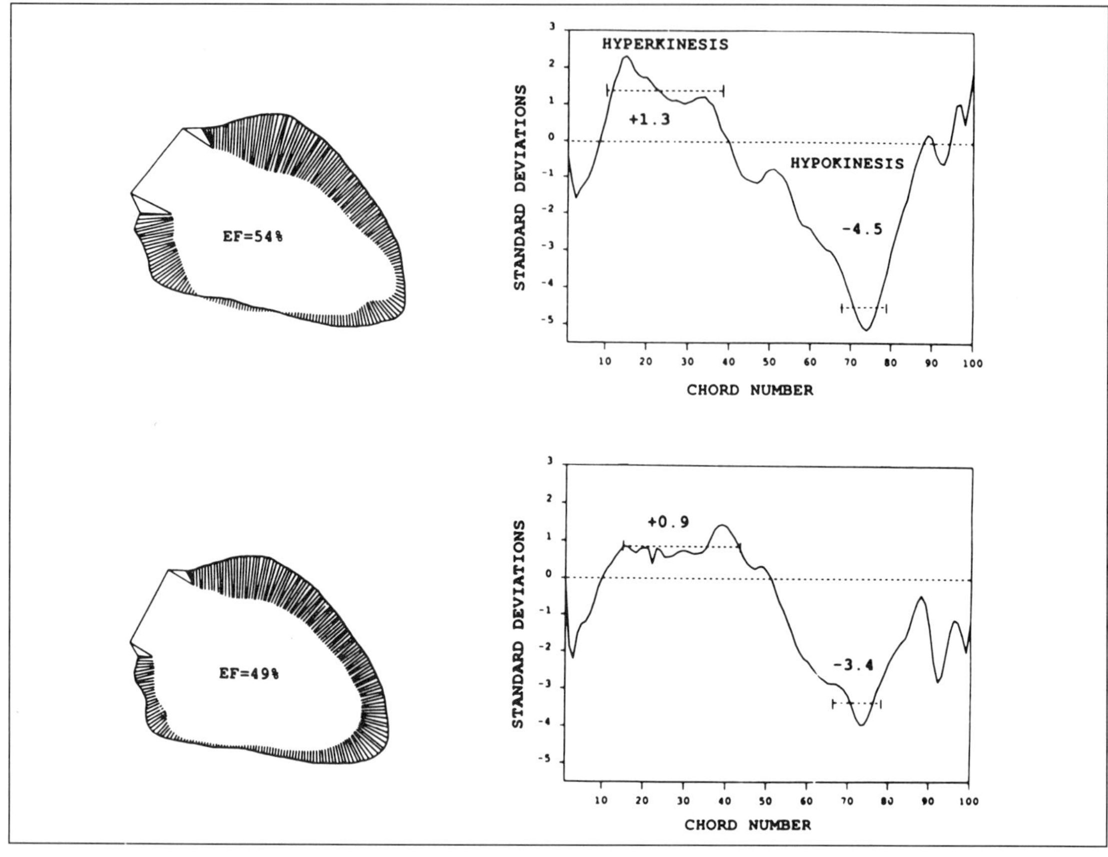

Fig. 29-4
Assessment of regional ventricular function, using the centerline method, in a patient with acute myocardial infarction treated with thrombolytic therapy. Global left ventricular function improves because of the development of anterior hyperkinesis (*top panel*) despite a severe regional wall motion inferiorly in the region of the infarct. However, with time there is a return to baseline in the previously hyperkinetic region, leading to a slight reduction in the global ejection fraction despite functional recovery in the infarct region (see text for further details). (From F. Sheehan. Cardiac angiography. In M. L. Marcus, H. R. Schelbert, D. J. Skorton and G. L. Wolf, eds., *Cardiac Imaging—Principles and Practice,* Philadelphia: W. B. Saunders, 1991. Pp. 109–148. Reprinted by permission.)

ing infarction. In contrast, in patients in whom perfusion to the infarct-related artery was restored, there was a 20 percent or more reduction in ventricular volume.

RVG is uniquely suited to the evaluation of right ventricular function [24–27]. The gated equilibrium and first-pass techniques have both been used. However, because of methodologic considerations, the gated first-pass technique is a good compromise [28]. Technetium 99m is injected as a bolus with scintigraphic data acquired in a gated mode during the time the bolus travels from the superior vena cava to the pulmonary artery. Infarction of the right ventricle can occur in association with inferior wall MI and may result in the clinical syndrome of "right ventricular infarction," a form of cardiogenic shock originally described by Cohn et al. [29]. Identification of this condition is important because if it is identified and treated correctly, prognosis is relatively good as compared with cardiogenic shock resulting from infarction of the left ventricle [30, 31].

Determining Myocardial Viability After Myocardial Infarction

The increasing use of thrombolytic therapy and, to a lesser extent, coronary angioplasty in managing patients with AMI has led to an expanded role for nuclear techniques. These techniques are of value in identifying viable myocardium in areas subtended by the infarct-related artery, and they allow assessment of the efficacy of such therapies in salvaging myocardium. The radiopharmaceuticals used for this purpose can be broadly categorized into two groups, namely, markers of myocardial perfusion or of myocardial metabolism.

Markers of Myocardial Perfusion

Thallium 201

Thallium 201 (Tl 201) is a potassium-analog radioisotope taken up by myocardium by both active and passive mechanisms involving NaK-ATPase [32, 33]. Uptake of Tl 201 by the myocyte does not appear to be affected by either ischemia or hypoxia unless these processes result in cell death [34–37]. Similarly, in experimental models of postischemic dysfunction (myocardial stunning) and chronic ischemia with dysfunction (hibernating myocardium), no effect on myocardial kinetics of Tl 201 has been shown [38, 39]. There is a linear relationship between Tl 201 uptake and regional coronary blood flow, with a tendency toward underestimation and overestimation at the upper and lower limits of the physiologic range, respectively [40–43]. After myocardial uptake of Tl 201, a dynamic exchange of thallium occurs between the myocardium and blood. The rate at which thallium washes out of the myocardium primarily depends on the Tl 201 concentration gradient between the myocardium and the blood [44, 45]. Tl 201 has an approximate half-life in the myocardium of 4 to 8 hours.

Following a resting injection, thallium is distributed according to resting flow as long as the myocyte sarcolemmal membrane is intact. Less Tl 201 is distributed to areas of myocardium with lower coronary flows, producing a perfusion defect. This differential uptake of Tl 201 results in heterogeneous Tl 201 myocardial concentration gradients, and therefore, differences in washout rates between areas of myocardium with normal and abnormal resting flows; i.e., there is faster washout of Tl 201 from normally perfused myocardium because of a greater myocardial-to-blood concentration gradient. With the passage of time, myocardial content of Tl 201 in the normally and abnormally perfused myocardium tends to equalize. This "redistribution" of thallium explains why resting perfusion defects can reverse when imaging is repeated after approximately 4 hours. Areas showing incomplete redistribution of Tl 201 can result from an area of mixed viable and infarcted myocardium, e.g., subendocardial infarct with normal epicardial myocardium, subtended by a stenosed coronary artery, or alternatively, because an inadequate time has elapsed for sufficient redistribution to occur for complete reversal of the defect.

Although Tl 201 kinetics are not inherently altered by coronary occlusion followed by reperfusion, several important observations have been made in this situation. Although there is a close correlation between Tl 201 uptake and functional recovery following reperfusion [46, 47], myocardial viability and salvage are overestimated because of the hyperemic flow that occurs following reperfusion [48–50]. Initially, infarcted myocardium takes up Tl 201. However, the myocardium is unable to retain it, resulting in accelerated clearance from these regions. This has important implications for clinical imaging protocols. Sufficient time between injection of Tl 201 and imaging should be allowed for Tl 201 to wash out of infarcted myocardium and to wash in to areas of myocardium with low flow. Some have suggested that Tl 201 imaging should be delayed for at least 24 to 48 hours to avoid overestimation of myocardial salvage [51], but others argue that a postdischarge stress Tl 201 study can be used for evaluating myocardial salvage and viability in the region of the infarct-related coronary artery and detecting myocardial ischemia [47].

Several studies have used rest-redistribution Tl 201 imaging for identifying viable myocardium in patients with coronary artery disease [52–54]. In a recent study, patients undergoing coronary artery bypass surgery (CABG) with LV dysfunction were evaluated using rest-redistribution Tl 201 to predict viability in LV segments that were asynergic [54]. In severely dyssynergic segments, 62 percent of segments with normal viability, as determined by Tl 201 imaging, and 54 percent with mildly reduced viability improved following surgery, but only 23 percent with severely reduced viability improved after surgery. When segments that were adequately vascularized were considered separately, i.e., those demonstrating Tl 201 uptake following surgery, the positive and negative predictive values for this technique were 73 percent and 77 percent, respectively. These findings appear to be lower than those quoted for stress-redistribution-reinjection imaging. Similar findings have been reported for patients with severe chronic stable angina pectoris or unstable angina who underwent rest-redistribution Tl 201 imaging before revascularization [52, 53].

Recently, there has been interest in the use of 24-hour Tl 201 redistribution imaging or imaging following reinjection of another dose of Tl 201 after 4-hour redistribution imaging. This latter method is generally referred to as "reinjection" imaging and it has been shown to enhance the predictive value of Tl 201 in recognizing myocardial viability in patients with coronary artery disease and LV dysfunction [55–58]. Previously, conventional stress Tl 201 imaging was performed following an injection of Tl 201 at peak stress, and redistribution imaging was performed 3 to 4 hours later. A perfusion defect noted after stress that had resolved by the time of redistribution imaging was considered to represent ischemic but viable myocardium; a defect still present at the time of redistribution imaging was interpreted as representing nonviable scar tissue. However, several studies, using improvement in regional ventricular function following revascularization or positron emission tomography (PET) with fluorodeoxyglucose F 18 (FDG) (see below), have shown that 40 to 60 percent of irreversible perfusion defects contain viable myocardium [59–61]. Studies from Bonow and associates have shown that reinjection of Tl 201 following stress-redistribution imaging can greatly enhance the value of Tl 201 defects imaging in determining viability in areas of hypoperfused myocardium in patients with coronary artery disease and LV dysfunction. Reinjection imaging performed after 4-hour redistribution imaging enhanced the detection of viable myocardium in 1/4 to 1/3 of defects that were classified as being irreversible at time of 4-hour redistribution imaging. The positive and negative predictive value of stress-redistribution-reinjection Tl 201 imaging was found to be greater than 80 percent and comparable with findings using FDG imaging (Plate 3).

Rubidium 82

Like Tl 201, this positron-emitting radioisotope is a potassium analog, but with a very much shorter half-life than Tl 201—only 90 seconds. In an experimental model of coronary occlusion and reperfusion, Goldstein observed that myocardial viability could be determined by analyzing the Rb 82 washout curves [62]. Areas of necrotic nonviable myocardium have accelerated washout because the sarcolemmal membranes are not intact and are unable to retain Rb 82. Preliminary clinical studies in patients have produced encouraging results [63].

Technetium Tc 99m Sestamibi

Tc 99m sestamibi is a lipophilic cation which is initially distributed in the myocardium according to blood flow. Myocardial uptake occurs primarily by diffusion, mainly from negative electrical gradients across sarcolemmal and inner mitochondrial membranes, and to a lesser extent by concentration gradients [64, 65]. Approximately 90 percent of Tc 99m sestamibi activity can be found in the mitochondria as the original free cationic complex [66]. Therefore, although delivery of sestamibi depends on myocardial perfusion, retention depends on membrane integrity, i.e., on myocardial viability [67–71]. Initial studies suggested that Tc 99m sestamibi, unlike Tl 201, did not undergo significant redistribution and was slowly cleared from the myocardium [65]. Studies both in animals and in humans have demonstrated that infarct size can be accurately determined using sestamibi imaging [72, 73].

The myocardial kinetics of sestamibi are particularly suited for assessing the amount of myocardial salvage after thrombolytic therapy or acute revascularization in patients with AMI; they have also been used to assess the efficacy of thrombolytic regimes and acute revascularization procedures [73–77]. The paradigm is as follows: sestamibi is given immediately before administration of thrombolytic therapy or before the revascularization procedure. The lack of redistribution allows imaging to be performed within 6 hours after the intervention.

The size of the perfusion defect at this time is an estimate of the amount of jeopardized myocardium before intervention. Days later, imaging is repeated after administration of a second dose of sestamibi; this gives an estimate of final infarct size. The amount of salvaged myocardium is estimated by subtracting the final infarct size estimate from the estimate of jeopardized myocardium.

A close relation was found between the size of the early sestamibi perfusion defect and the EF at 6 weeks and also between the size of the defect at early sestamibi imaging and the EF and end-systolic volume at 1 year [78, 79]. However, Gibbons and associates confirmed that mismatch between infarct size and LV function can occur in patients with AMI soon after reperfusion therapy [78]. In a study of 32 patients with AMI treated either by thrombolysis or primary angioplasty, there was no change in LVEF between hospital discharge and 6 weeks later for the group as a whole. However, 5 of 32 patients had a significant increase (8 EF units) and 6 of 32 a significant decrease (8 EF units) in ventricular function during this time. Patients with an increase in EF had a discharge EF lower than that estimated for the infarct size, probably as a result of myocardial stunning. Conversely, patients with a decrease in EF had a higher than anticipated discharge EF that probably resulted from hyperkinesis of noninfarcted areas of myocardium at the time of hospital discharge.

Pellikka et al. performed serial single photon emission computer tomography (SPECT) imaging with sestamibi at three time points in patients after AMI (Fig. 29-5) [74]. No significant decrease in the perfusion defect size was seen in 6 of 25 patients with occluded infarct-related arteries. In comparison, patients with patent arteries showed a decrease in defect size; 9 of 19 at 18 to 48 hours and another six patients by time of hospital discharge. Using planar sestamibi imaging techniques, Wackers et al. also showed larger decreases in the size of the perfusion defect in patients with patent as compared with occluded infarct-related arteries, 45 percent less and 8 percent less, respectively [80]. In addition to quantifying the area of risk and the final infarct size, Gibbons and associates showed how collateral flow, an important determinant of infarct size, can also be estimated noninvasively using SPECT im-

Fig. 29-5
Mean change in perfusion defect size as a percentage of the left ventricle (%LV) at the time of the 18- to 48-hour and 6- to 14-day studies is plotted for the 19 patients with patent arteries and the six patients with occluded arteries. NS = not significant. (From P. A. Pellikka et al. Serial changes in myocardial perfusion using tomographic technetium-99m-hexakis-2-methoxy-methopropyl-isonitrile imaging following reperfusion therapy of myocardial infarction. *J. Nucl. Med.* 31:1269, 1990. With permission.)

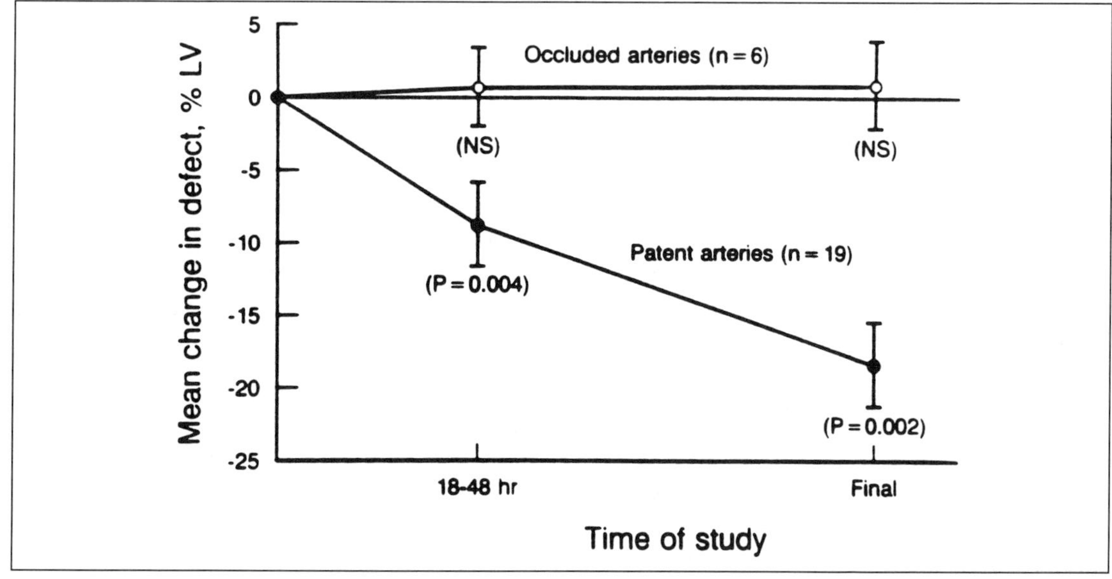

aging with sestamibi [75]. By quantitating the severity of the acute perfusion defect, they demonstrated an inverse correlation between the severity of the perfusion defect and the angiographic collateral grade. In this study, the radionuclide estimate of myocardium at risk ($r = .61$; $p < .0001$), angiographic collateral grade ($p = .0003$), and radionuclide estimates of collateral flow ($r = .70$, $p < .0001$) were all significantly associated with final infarct size.

Tc 99m sestamibi can also simultaneously evaluate ventricular function [81]. Both right and left ventricular EFs can be calculated by injecting Tc 99m sestamibi and acquiring the data using a first-pass technique; the myocardial perfusion images are acquired later. Ventricular function can also be assessed by acquiring the planar or tomographic perfusion images gated to the electrocardiogram (ECG). This technique allows assessment of both global ventricular function and the regional variables of endocardial wall motion and wall thickening [82–84].

Therefore, Tc 99m sestamibi continues to be used in studies evaluating the efficacy of interventions used to salvage myocardium in AMI [76, 77]. However, it is doubtful whether Tc 99m sestamibi will find application in routine care of patients with AMI because of logistic and financial constraints. Nevertheless, present data show conclusively that Tc 99m sestamibi has an important role in determining the effects of coronary occlusion and reperfusion in settings in which a mismatch between perfusion and function can occur, i.e., with myocardial stunning. In contrast, the utility of Tc 99m sestamibi in determining myocardial viability in the setting of chronic ischemia, in which there is often a matched reduction in both myocardial perfusion and function, i.e., hibernating myocardium, is less clear [85, 86]. However, there is increasing experimental and clinical evidence to support the hypothesis that resting uptake of sestamibi may be of value in determining myocardial viability in this situation, particularly if quantitative SPECT techniques are utilized [87, 88].

Water-Perfusable Tissue Index

Water-perfusable tissue index (PTI) has been proposed as an alternate means for evaluating myocardial viability with use of PET [89]. The paradigm for this methodology is that viable myocardium exchanges water rapidly but necrotic myocardium does not. The PTI is calculated from the transmission data and emission data from blood volume (carbon monoxide O 15 labeled red cells) and myocardial blood flow (water O 15) studies. For any particular region of interest, the PTI is expressed as the ratio of the water O 15 perfusable fraction to total anatomical tissue fraction. Using this technique, Yamamoto et al. showed that a PTI of 0.70 or more was predictive of functional recovery following AMI treated with thrombolysis [89]. Similarly, patients with previous MI segments with perfusion-metabolism mismatch by ammonia N 13-FDG imaging had higher PTI than segments considered to be nonviable because of matched defects. These workers also confirmed that absolute myocardial blood flow is not predictive of functional recovery in this situation.

Tracers of Myocardial Metabolism

Fluorodeoxyglucose F 18

Under fasting conditions, fatty acids are the main energy source for normal myocardium. In the presence of ischemia, the myocardium increases its utilization of glucose as a source of high-energy phosphates. This enhanced utilization of glucose as an energy source by ischemic myocardium can be estimated with PET with use of fluorodeoxyglucose F 18 (FDG). This radiolabeled intermediary undergoes phosphorylation by the hexokinase reaction, but it is not metabolized further in the glycolytic pathway. The phosphorylated FDG is essentially trapped in the cytosol and accumulates in proportion to exogenous metabolism of glucose [90, 91]. Mismatch of metabolism and perfusion, i.e., myocardium with metabolic activity in areas with severely reduced perfusion, was first demonstrated by Marshall et al. in patients with previous MI [92]. Two subsequent studies demonstrated that this technique is of value in predicting the functional outcome of revascularization in patients undergoing CABG; the positive and negative predictive accuracies were 78 to 81 percent and 78 to 92 percent, respectively [61, 93]. A more recent study confirmed the high negative predictive accuracy of this technique, but found that functional recovery following revascularization in myocardium with metabolism-perfusion mismatch was variable [94].

The value of FDG in determining myocardial viability in patients who have sustained a recent MI is uncertain [95–97]. The studies by Marshall and other investigators demonstrate that myocardium with severely reduced perfusion and a matched absence of metabolic activity is strongly predictive of lack of functional recovery either with time or after revascularization. However, the predictive value of finding myocardial perfusion-metabolism mismatch, i.e., metabolically active myocardium with severely reduced perfusion, is much lower. In the study by Schwaiger et al., functional recovery occurred in only 50 percent of segments with severely reduced perfusion and enhanced FDG uptake [95]. The reasons for the differences in these findings is unclear and requires further study. Reasons may relate to the methodology of the study or possibly to differences in substrate utilization by reperfused and nonreperfused myocardium, which may also change with time [98, 99].

Carbon C 11 Acetate

Carbon 11 acetate (C 11), a radiolabeled intermediary of oxidative phosphorylation, has also been used to study myocardial metabolism [100–105]. Myocardium avidly extracts acetate and is activated to acetylcoenzyme A in the cytosol and oxidized in mitochondria via the tricarboxylic acid cycle, which is the final common pathway of oxidative metabolism. Regional time–activity curves show biexponential clearance independent of blood flow. The rapid, early phase reflects oxidative phosphorylation; a slower, late clearance represents incorporation into the amino acid and lipid pool. Rate constants obtained from the rapid clearance of C 11 acetate are closely related to the rate of myocardial oxygen consumption over a wide range of physiologic values. In the presence of myocardial ischemia, uptake is reduced in proportion to flow, and clearance is reduced in proportion to oxidative metabolism [100–105]. As noted with other radiolabeled markers of metabolism, interpretation of data is complex and requires making certain assumptions [106].

Oxidative metabolism is depressed after infarction, both in infarcted and adjacent segments. This has been observed even after restoration of myocardial blood flow [103, 107, 108]. Buxton et al. in their study of reperfused canine myocardium found that oxidative metabolism and regional ventricular function demonstrated a parallel recovery with time [107]. Similarly, Groper et al. found that oxidative metabolism was a predictor of functional recovery in patients after AMI and also in patients with chronic coronary artery disease, and that this technique was a more reliable predictor than was FDG [94, 97]. Schelbert's group evaluated regional blood flow, oxidative metabolism, and glucose metabolism in patients with recent MI [109]. Blood flow (normal, 0.83 ± 0.20 ml/g/min) was significantly lower in areas of areas of matched and mismatched perfusion-glucose uptake, 0.32 ± 0.12 and 0.57 ± 0.20 ml/g/min, respectively. Oxidative metabolism was less severely reduced than blood flow in areas with perfusion-glucose uptake mismatch, but was reduced in proportion to blood flow in matched regions. The authors hypothesized that the preserved oxidative metabolism observed in areas with enhanced glucose uptake may signify a regional increase in oxygen extraction. In patients with AMI following reperfusion, Henes et al. observed that although myocardial blood flow returned to normal within hours (18 ± 6 hours), oxidative metabolism improved more gradually (9 ± 7 days) and often remained depressed [108].

Possible explanations for the discrepancy between flow and oxidative metabolism are probably multifactorial. They include presence of heterogeneous myocardium (normal, irreversibly damaged, and reversibly damaged), residual coronary artery stenosis, and microvascular reperfusion injury. In another study with somewhat conflicting findings by Vanoverschelde et al., regional oxidative metabolism and its relation to myocardial perfusion (ammonia N 13) and metabolism (FDG) were studied in patients 2 weeks and 3 months after AMI [110]. These workers found that regional oxidative metabolism was reduced in proportion to residual myocardial blood flow and that oxidative metabolism was not predictive of functional recovery. In addition, they noted that regional oxidative metabolism was not significantly different among similarly hypoperfused segments with and without flow (ammonia N 13) metabolism (FDG) mismatch. The differences observed between this group's findings and previous studies may relate to the longer time interval between MI and imaging in Vanoverschelde's study. The differences in the findings may also be related to the temporal sequence of alterations in myocardial metabolism following MI and reperfusion, which highlights the need for further investigation.

Radiolabeled Fatty Acids

As discussed previously, fatty acids are the preferred substrate of the myocardium under fasting conditions and account for approximately 90 percent of oxygen consumed under aerobic conditions. Therefore, radiolabeled fatty acids may be of value in studying myocardial metabolism. Currently, the most widely used radiolabeled fatty acids are iodophenylpentadecanoic acid I 123 and palmitate C 11 with conventional nuclear imaging techniques and PET, respectively [111–120].

Uptake of these agents primarily depends on blood flow. However, inferences about beta oxidation can be made by studying the subsequent washout of the radiolabeled fatty acids from the myocardium. Clearance from the myocardium is biexponential, with an early fast and a slower second component. The early phase is a reflection of beta oxidation of the fatty acids; the slower clearance results from incorporation of the fatty acids into the endogenous lipid pool. Myocardial ischemia reduces the early myocardial clearance of fatty acids because of decreased beta oxidation and increases in the proportion of fatty acid incorporated into the lipid pool [115, 116]. These changes can be detected noninvasively by using radiolabeled fatty acids. Sobel's group has published extensively regarding the effects of MI on palmitate C 11 kinetics and its value in delineating the amount of salvaged and jeopardized myocardium following reperfusion both in experimental models and in humans [117–121]. However, interpreting myocardial kinetics of radiolabeled fatty acids is complex due to several compounding variables, including blood flow, competition with alternate substrates, back diffusion of unmetabolized tracer into the vascular space, availability of other intermediate compounds, and the activity of key enzymes [121, 122]. These problems along with limited availability and lack of evidence demonstrating superiority over other readily available radiotracers have prevented widespread use of these radiopharmaceuticals.

Infarct-Avid Myocardial Scintigraphy

Detection of AMI ordinarily relies on a classic clinical history, a typical evolution of cardiac enzymes, and diagnostic changes in the ECG. However, some patients delay their hospital admissions or are unable to provide an accurate history, making recognition of MI more difficult. In some of these same circumstances, the temporal limitations related to infarct detection by cardiac enzyme measurements make them unreliable for establishing whether an infarct has occurred. Some patients have preexisting ECG alterations that preclude using it to detect AMI; this includes patients with left bundle branch block and those with previous infarctions. Moreover, patients with non-Q-wave MIs do not demonstrate diagnostic ECG changes; the best hope is ST wave changes typical of non-Q-wave infarction; however, similar ECG alterations occur in patients with subendocardial ischemia, rapid heart rates, ventricular hypertrophy, electrolyte abnormalities, subarachnoid hemorrhage, and intracardiac conduction abnormalities. Therefore, it is important to have alternative means for detecting MI when it occurs. Moreover, because infarct size is an important determinant of future prognosis, it is also important to have methods that allow accurate estimates of infarct size to be made independent of its location.

Technetium Tc 99m Stannous Pyrophosphate Imaging

Technetium Tc 99m stannous pyrophosphate (^{99m}Tc-PPi) has been shown to be a sensitive method for detecting AMIs [123–136]. ^{99m}Tc-PPi is incorporated into regions of myocardial necrosis with some residual myocardial blood flow (10 to 40 percent of control values) and increased calcium concentration in the hours to days following MI (Figs. 29-6 and 29-7). With permanent coronary artery occlusion, ^{99m}Tc-PPi deposition increases in the irreversibly injured myocardial cells between 10 to 12 hours and 24 to 72 hours after MI. Approximately one-half of ^{99m}Tc-PPi myocardial scintigrams become negative within 5 days of the event. The sequence of events correlates with calcium deposition and increases in coronary blood flow to

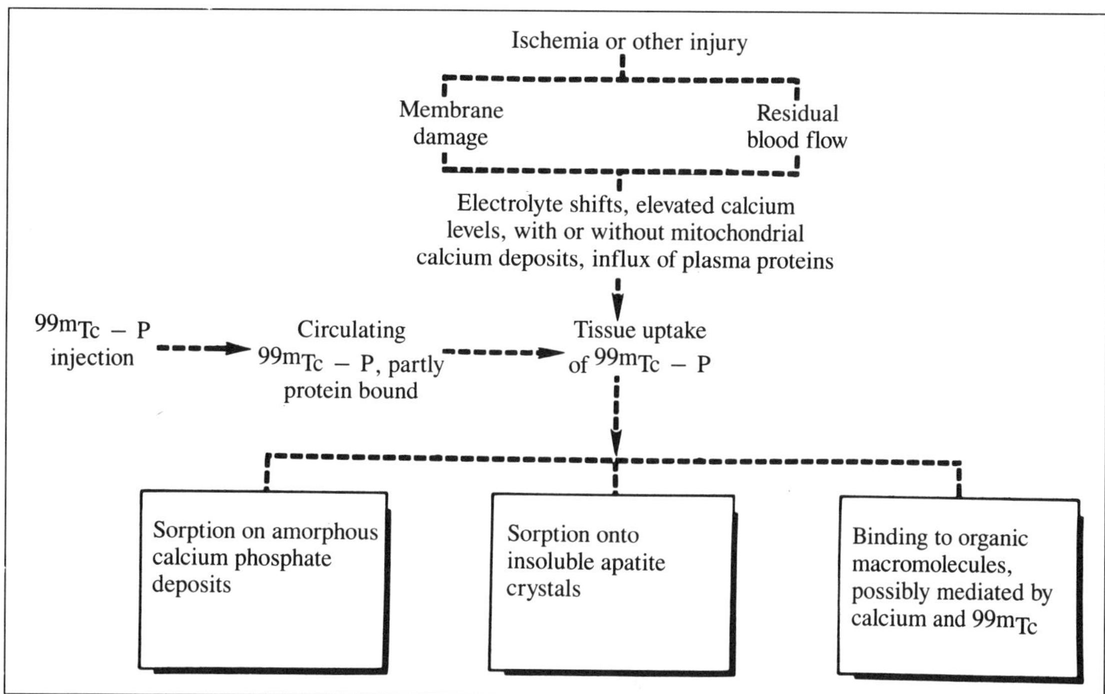

Fig. 29-6
Scheme for explaining abnormal technetium 99m stannous pyrophosphate (^{99m}Tc-P) myocardial scintigrams following the onset of acute myocardial infarction (or other injury). With severe ischemia or other cellular injury, there are alterations in membrane permeability followed by the entry of excess calcium into irreversibly damaged myocardial cells where it is deposited in mitochondria. Subsequently, the intravenous injection of ^{99m}Tc-P is bound to albumin and taken up in the injured myocardial cells where it complexes with calcium phosphate in soluble and insoluble form. (Reproduced from *The Journal of Clinical Investigation,* 1977, 60:724, by copyright permission of The American Society for Clinical Investigation.)

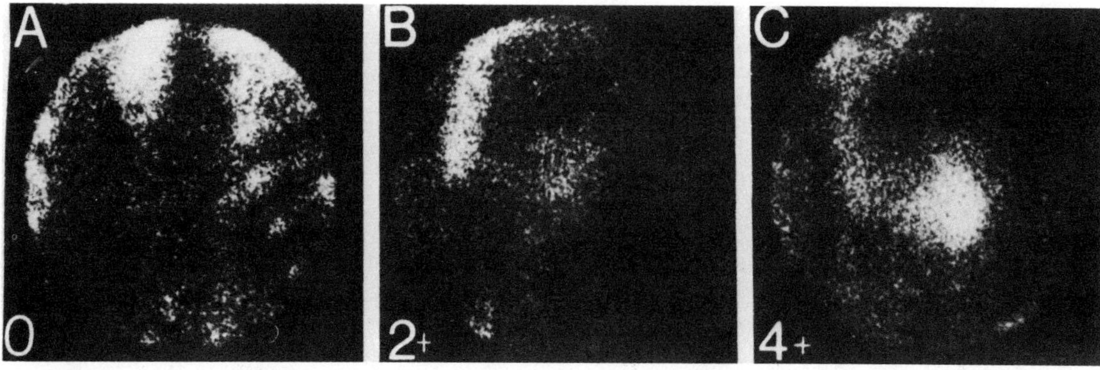

Fig. 29-7
Varying intensity of technetium 99m stannous pyrophosphate from faintly positive (2+) to intensely positive (4+). Typically, acute myocardial infarcts associated with adequate flow to the area of necrosis show the intensely positive pattern, but infarcts with very severely reduced residual myocardial flow show the faintly positive patterns. Often the faintly positive pattern of abnormal technetium 99m stannous pyrophosphate uptake is found during the first 10 to 24 hours after a Q-wave infarct followed by a more intense uptake of the radiopharmaceutical at 2 to 4 days after the event. With non-Q-wave infarcts, perhaps 33 to 40 percent have the faintly positive pattern.

the damaged area followed by the resorption of calcium during the reparative phase after the infarction (see Fig. 29-6). Temporary coronary artery occlusion and reperfusion, such as occur with thrombolytic therapy, may cause the ^{99m}Tc-PPi myocardial scintigrams to become abnormal within 1 to 2 hours of the event, but they may return to a normal pattern within 2 to 3 days [137]. Rapid deposition of ^{99m}Tc-PPi is associated with increased coronary blood flow to the damaged myocardial region, as occurs with thrombolytic therapy; thus any delay in the development of an abnormal ^{99m}Tc-PPi myocardial scintigram relates to the relative inadequacy of coronary blood flow to the damaged region within the first few hours to days after the event. With thrombolytic therapy or spontaneous thrombolysis, improved coronary blood flow to the damaged myocardial region allows early detection of the region of MI by ^{99m}Tc-PPi (Fig. 29-8).

Planar (two-dimensional) ^{99m}Tc-PPi myocardial scintigraphy generally detects infarction 3 gm or larger in size, but it may fail to detect smaller infarctions, especially those that are subendocardial or inferior in location. However, SPECT imaging allows the detection of infarctions as small as 1 gm in size, including most subendocardial and inferior infarctions after permanent or temporary coronary artery occlusion followed by reperfusion. An overlay of the ^{99m}Tc-PPi myocardial scintigram to the blood pool background using SPECT imaging allows more precise identification of MIs and eliminates blood pool activity as a cause of an apparently

Fig. 29-8
A. A markedly abnormal technetium 99m stannous pyrophosphate myocardial scintigram may occur with immediate reperfusion of an acute anterolateral infarct in the anterior (*top left*), slight left anterior oblique (*top right*), steep left anterior oblique (*bottom left*), and left lateral (*bottom right*) imaging projection images.
B. Effect of blood flow on accumulation of technetium 99m stannous pyrophosphate in acutely infarcted canine myocardium after an intravenous injection. Open bars represent pyrophosphate uptake in animals with permanent left anterior descending coronary artery occlusions for 3 hours; filled bars represent pyrophosphate uptake in animals that had reperfusion after 3 hours of temporary coronary artery occlusion. There was a marked increase in pyrophosphate uptake by the injured tissue when reflow was provided, such that mean technetium 99m stannous pyrophosphate uptake in the damaged tissue was 40 times that in normal myocardium in the reflow model. (*B.* from R. W. Parkey et al. Effect of coronary blood flow and site of injection of Tc99m-PPi detection of early canine myocardial infarcts. *J. Nucl. Med.* 22:134, 1981. With permission.)

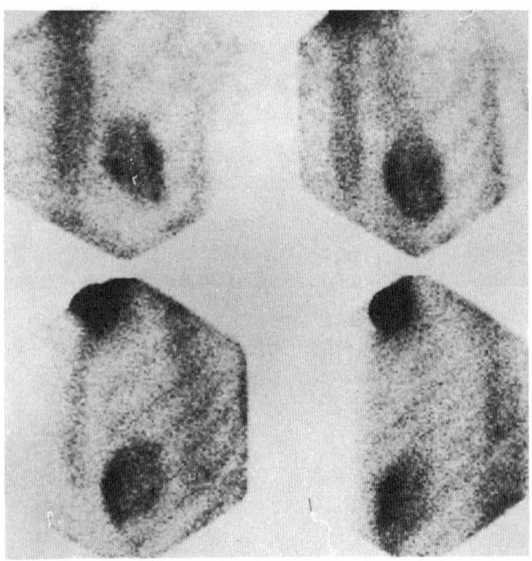
A

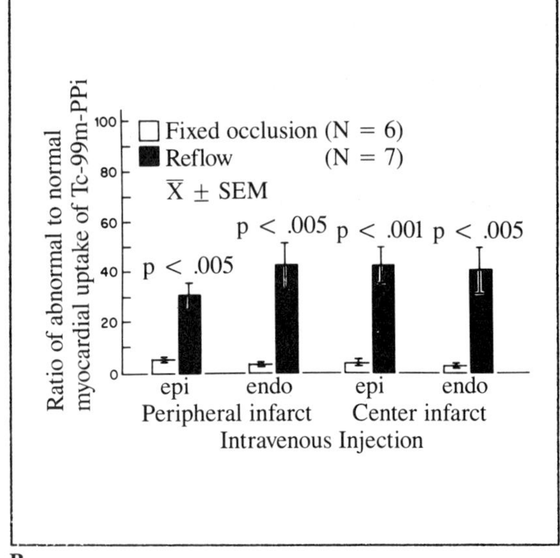

B

abnormal ^{99m}Tc-PPi study. However, acute myocardial necrosis of any etiology that results in confluent necrosis of more than 1 gm of myocardial tissue may be detected by ^{99m}Tc-PPi myocardial scintigraphy with SPECT. Thus, trauma, infection, cardioversion-induced myocardial injury, and invasive tumor may all cause abnormal ^{99m}Tc-PPi myocardial scintigrams.

^{99m}Tc-PPi with SPECT has also been used to estimate the extent of MIs. This technique provides an accurate estimate of the size of MIs with permanent coronary artery occlusion (Fig. 29-9) [129–131] and with temporary coronary artery occlusion followed by reperfusion (Fig. 29-10) [132]. With reperfused infarctions, it is important to inject the ^{99m}Tc-PPi approximately 90 minutes after reperfusion to avoid overestimating infarct size (see Fig. 29-10) [132]. It is possible to measure infarct size using ^{99m}Tc-PPi and express the measurement as a percentage of total LV mass or as the "infarction fraction" [130]. With this approach, one may estimate the extent of normally perfused LV myocardium by using a perfusion marker such as Tl 201, and estimate the size of the MI by using ^{99m}Tc-PPi SPECT measurements. An overlay of the Tl 201 and ^{99m}Tc-PPi myocardial scintigrams allows one to estimate infarct size as a percentage of the LV mass (Fig. 29-11) [130]. This approach allows one to normalize infarct size for the size of the heart.

Radiolabeled Antimyosin Scintigraphy

Radiolabeled antimyosin antibody can be used as an alternative to ^{99m}Tc-PPi imaging to detect MI [138–141]. Irreversible cellular damage with loss of integrity of the sarcolemmal membrane allows penetration of the antimyosin antibodies into the interior of the injured myocytes. Following MI, myosin is slowly degraded, allowing antibody directed to the heavy chain of myosin to complex with it. The attached label allows detection of that region of myocardium, by use of conventional imaging techniques, as infarct-avid uptake. Imaging with radiolabeled antimyosin antibody has sensitivity similar to ^{99m}Tc-PPi for detecting infarcted myocardium [142] and persistently abnormal antimyosin antibody images. The significance and duration

Fig. 29-9
Scatter plots of scintigraphic (SPECT) versus postmortem-determined infarct weight in dogs with the corresponding data fit by linear regression for all infarcts (*A*), infarcts caused by left anterior descending coronary artery occlusions (*B*), and infarcts caused by circumflex coronary artery occlusions (*C*). (From S. E. Lewis et al. Measurement of infarct size in acute canine myocardial infarction by single photon emission computed tomography with technetium-99m pyrophosphate. *Am. J. Cardiol.* 54:195, 1984. With permission.)

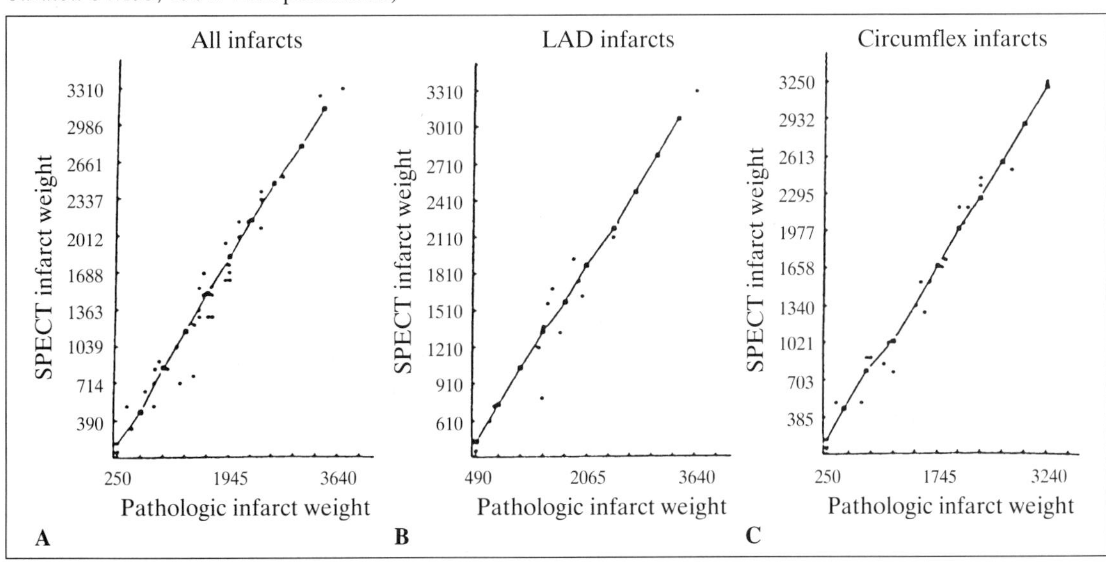

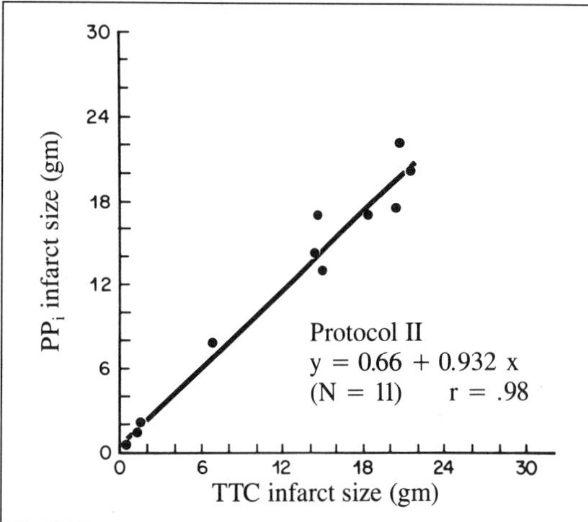

Fig. 29-10
Comparison of infarct size as estimated by the triphenyltetrazolium chloride (TTC) method and by technetium 99m stannous pyrophosphate myocardial scintigraphy with SPECT (PPi infarct size) in anesthetized dogs with a temporary occlusion (3 hours) of the left anterior descending coronary artery followed by 2 hours of reflow. The pyrophosphate was injected in 11 dogs 90 minutes after reflow. Using SPECT imaging, an excellent estimate of infarct size was obtained. (From D. E. Jansen et al. Quantification of myocardial injury produced by temporary coronary artery occlusion and reflow with technetium-99m-pyrophosphate. *Circulation* 75:613, 1987. By permission of the American Heart Association, Inc.)

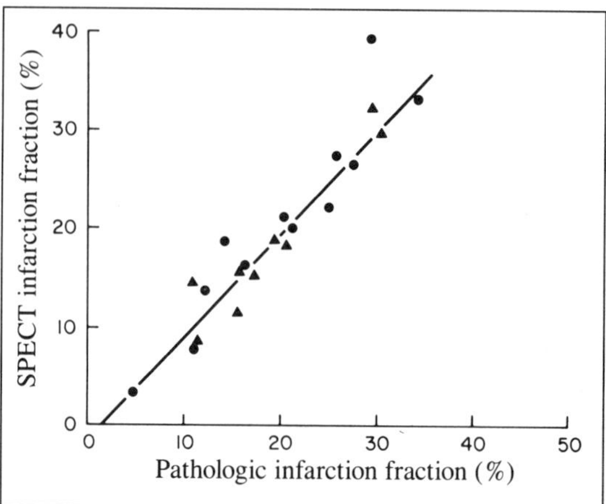

Fig. 29-11
Correlation between postmortem-determined infarction fraction and SPECT determinations of infarction fraction in 21 dogs with circumflex (12 dogs) or left anterior descending (9 dogs) coronary artery occlusions. Myocardial imaging for detection of infarction fraction was done with a combination of thallium 201 and technetium 99m stannous pyrophosphate with overlay images. (Reprinted with permission from the American College of Cardiology. *J. Am. Coll. Cardiol.* 6:149, 1985.)

of persistently abnormal antimyosin antibody scans have yet to be determined, but this observation suggests the need for serial imaging in some patients. Antimyosin antibody uptake also occurs with any condition that causes irreversible cellular injury in the heart, including myocarditis, which can mimic the clinical features of AMI [143, 144].

Assessment of Prognosis After Myocardial Infarction

Thallium 201 Myocardial Scintigraphy

Perfusion imaging with Tl 201 myocardial scintigraphy and submaximal exercise testing provides several advantages over exercise ECG alone. These include a higher predictive accuracy, the ability to identify specific coronary distributions, detection of multivessel disease, and the detection of ischemia in the infarct zone. Gibson et al. demonstrated that patients could be stratified into low- and high-risk groups on the basis of the results of submaximal exercise Tl 201 imaging (Fig. 29-12) [145]. Reversible defects, defects involving multiple vascular territories, and increased lung uptake were independent predictors of increased risk for patients for future coronary events, including MI, death, and need for a future surgical intervention (CABG or percutaneous transluminal coronary angioplasty) because of recurrent acute coronary heart disease syndromes (Plate 4). Subsequent studies have confirmed the predictive value of submaximal stress testing, although not all demonstrated the findings from Tl 201 imaging to be of independent predictive value [146–148]. In patients with unstable angina managed with medical therapy, the presence of reversible Tl 201 perfusion defects is also an important independent predictor of an adverse outcome [149, 150].

Johnson et al. used dual isotope Tl 201 and indium In 111 (In 111) antimyosin SPECT imaging performed 72 to 96 hours after the onset of chest pain to identify patients at risk of further ischemic

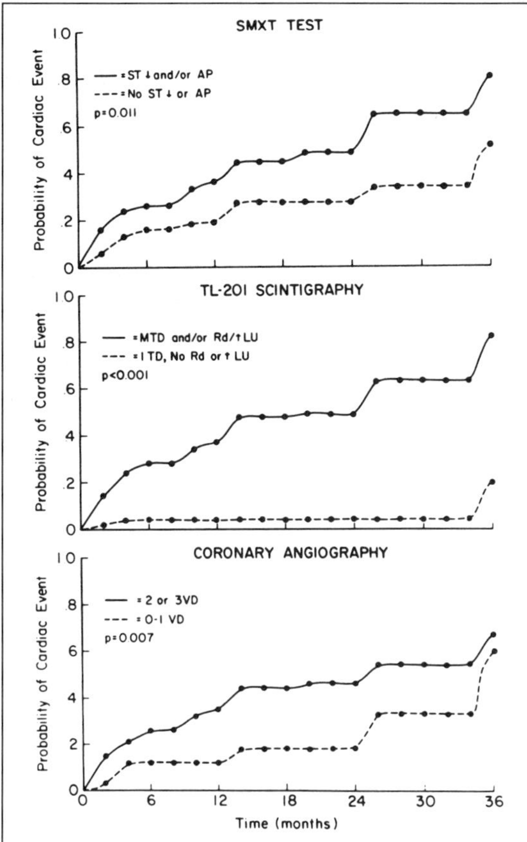

Fig. 29-12
Line graphs showing the cumulative probability of a cardiac event in the 36 months following myocardial infarction. Patients are categorized into high- and low-risk groups according to results of their submaximal exercise test (SMXT), Tl 201 scintigraphy, and coronary arteriography. AP = angina pectoris; ST = ST segment; MTD = multiple transient defects, Rd = redistribution; LU = lung uptake of T1 201; VD = vessel disease. (From R. S. Gibson et al. Prediction of cardiac events after uncomplicated myocardial infarction: A prospective study comparing predischarge exercise thallium-201 scintigraphy and coronary angioplasty. *Circulation* 68:321, 1983. With permission.)

events soon after MI [151]. Patients with matching Tl 201 defects and In 111 antimyosin uptake (N = 14) had a benign course with no ischemic in-hospital events. In contrast, 16 of 23 patients (70 percent) with mismatched Tl 201 defects and antimyosin uptake developed evidence of further ischemic events.

Recently, dipyridamole has been used as an alternative means to produce stress after recent MI [152–154]. Dipyridamole produces maximal stress with minimal increases in myocardial oxygen demand; this effect can be rapidly reversed by use of aminophylline. Since dipyridamole produces greater increases in coronary flow rate than does submaximal exercise, it should be more sensitive for detecting myocardial ischemia. Similar data have been reported with use of adenosine [155]. Dipyridamole Tl 201 imaging has also been used soon (1 to 4 days) after MI to predict both in-hospital and out-of-hospital events [156]. Fifty patients were studied, providing clinical, ECG, and Tl 201 data for multivariate analysis. Redistribution of Tl 201 in the infarct zone was found to be associated with both in-hospital and out-of-hospital events.

Therefore, stress Tl 201 myocardial imaging is an effective means of stratifying survivors of MI for risk. The presence of redistribution defects, defects indicative of a multivessel distribution, or increased lung uptake of Tl 201 is a harbinger of poor prognosis after MI. Candell-Riera et al. evaluated various predischarge noninvasive strategies for risk stratification of patients after AMI [157]. They found that the combination of submaximal exercise Tl 201 imaging and rest RVG was the most effective noninvasive strategy and that use of cardiac catheterization did not provide additional prognostic information. However, many of these studies of Tl 201 imaging after AMI were performed before thrombolysis was used. There have been questions regarding the prognostic importance of Tl 201 imaging in patients who have received thrombolytic therapy during a recent MI [158–160].

Rest and Exercise Radionuclide Ventriculography

In addition to evaluating resting LV function, RVG allows assessment of the LV response to exercise after MI. The normal response to exercise is characterized by an increase in EF by more than 5 EF units, a decrease in end-systolic volume, an increase in the systolic pressure/volume index, and more vigorous segmental contraction. Using RVG combined with submaximal exercise testing, we and others demonstrated that patients with depressed resting LV function and those with abnormal LV responses to exercise at low levels have increased morbidity and mortality [161–166]. These patients are at increased risk for future coronary heart disease events, including MI, sudden death, refractory heart failure, or new myocardial ischemia requiring some form of surgical intervention in the 6 to 24 months after hospital discharge (Fig. 29-13; Tables 29-2 and 29-3). Patients with moderate to severe reduction in LVEF (< 0.35 to 0.40), either at rest or during submaximal exercise, have a significantly higher risk of subsequent cardiac death. However, in patients with preserved global LVEF (> 0.35 to 0.40), the response to exercise and the functional indexes measured during submaximal exercise gave better characterization than the resting LVEF. Cardiac events in patients with an abnormal response in this group had more nonfatal ischemic events, including MI, than cardiac death.

Future Directions

There is great interest in developing techniques that allow detection of intra-arterial thrombus. Some workers have used radiolabeled monoclonal antifibrin antibodies to image thrombus formation in peripheral arteries [167]. Recently, a radiolabeled antibody to glycoprotein (GP)-140 has been used to image activated platelets in vivo at sites of endothelial injury [168, 169]. GP-140 is a glycoprotein found predominately in the membrane of the alpha-granule of platelets, which only becomes externalized after platelets are activated [170]. This radiolabeled monoclonal antibody has an advantage over conventional platelet labeling techniques because

Fig. 29-13
Left ventricular ejection fraction (LVEF), end-systolic volume index (*middle panel*), and pressure volume (P/V) index (*right panel*) at rest (R) and during peak submaximal exercise (SE) in patients with and without cardiac events during the 8 months after myocardial infarction. Note that patients who did not have future cardiac events usually had normal left ventricular global functional responses to submaximal exercise, whereas patients destined to have future cardiac events usually had abnormal left ventricular functional responses to low-level exercise. (From J. R. Corbett et al. Prognostic value of submaximal exercise radionuclide ventriculography following acute transmural and nontransmural myocardial infarction. *Am. J. Cardiol.* 52:82A, 1983. With permission.)

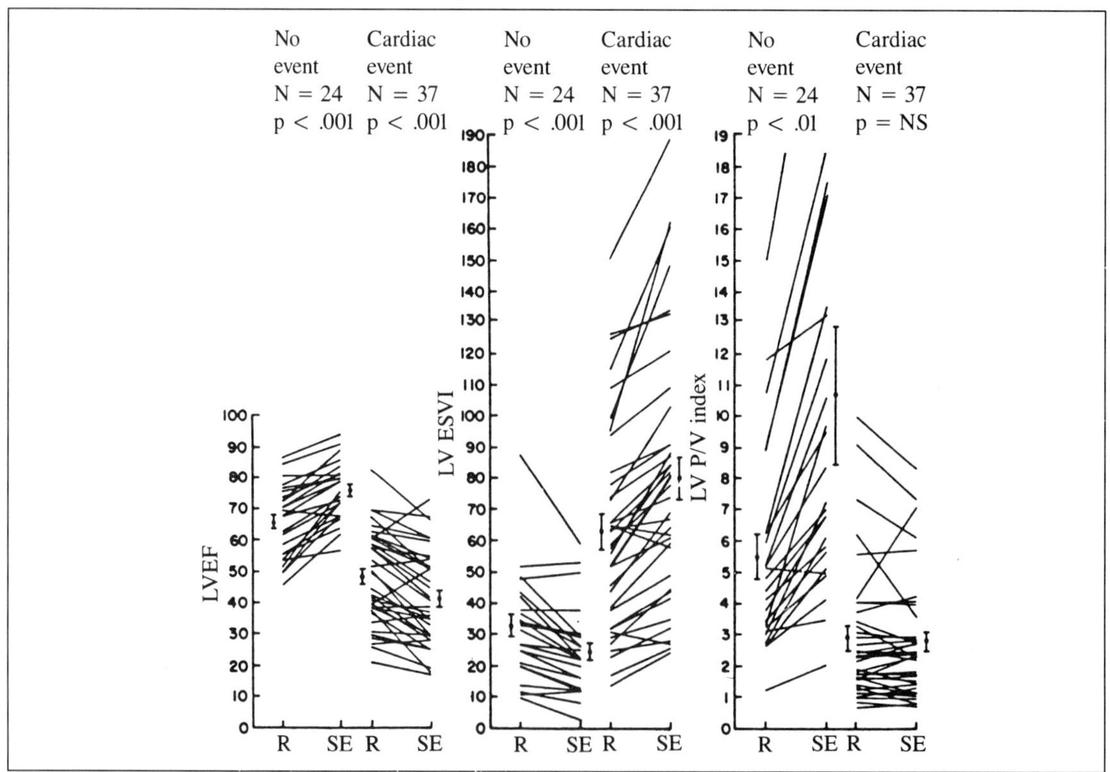

Table 29-2
Results of multivariate, discriminant-function analysis according to degree of left ventricular dysfunction

	LVEF <0.40 (N = 29)		LVEF ≥0.40 (N = 88)	
No event versus any event	1. Peak LVEF	0.90	1. ΔLVEF	0.89
	2. ΔESVI	0.97	2. Peak LVEF	0.93
	3. Killip class	1.00		

ESVI = left ventricular end-systolic volume index; LVEF = left ventricular ejection fraction.
Source: J. R. Corbett et al. Prognostic value of submaximal exercise radionuclide ventriculography following acute transmural and nontransmural myocardial infarction. *Am. J. Cardiol.* 52:82A, 1983. With permission.

Table 29-3
Results of multivariate, discriminant-function analysis of all clinical, exercise, and scintigraphic variables at 6-month follow-up

	All patients (N = 117)		Anterior TM (N = 33)		Inferior TM (N = 39)		Limited NT (N = 18)		Extensive NT (N = 24)	
No event versus any event	1. ΔLVEF	0.89	1. Peak LVEF	0.84	1. ΔLVEF	0.87	1. ΔESVI	84%	1. ΔESVI	96%
	2. Peak LVEF	0.91	2. Age	90%	2. WMS	90%	2. SE pain	89%	2. ΔWMS	96%
			3. ΔLVEF	0.94			3. ST changes	89%	3. SE pain	100%
							4. ST ↓ 0.1 mV	94%		
							5. ΔBP	94%		
							6. ΔWMS	100%		

BP = systolic blood pressure; ESVI = left ventricular end-systolic volume index; LVEF = left ventricular ejection fraction; NT = nontransmural; SE = submaximal exercise; ST = ST segment; TM = transmural; WMS = wall motion score; Δ = change with exercise; ↓ = depression; N = number of patients.
Source: J. R. Corbett et al. Prognostic value of submaximal exercise radionuclide ventriculography following acute transmural and nontransmural myocardial infarction. *Am. J. Cardiol.* 52:82A, 1983. With permission.

only activated platelets are imaged, which optimizes the target-to-background ratio. Whether the limited spatial and contrast resolution of current imaging devices will be sufficient to image thrombus formation in human coronary arteries is uncertain. Nevertheless, the ability to detect activated platelets in a coronary artery, possibly indicating the presence of an unstable atherosclerotic plaque, is an intriguing possibility with potentially important implications. For example, detection of activated platelets in patients with coronary artery disease may be a potent predictor of adverse prognoses, possibly indicating that more aggressive management is required. Use of a radiolabeled thrombolytic agent, such as tissue plasminogen activator, may allow both detection by noninvasive techniques and treatment of thrombus formation [171].

Areas of sympathetic denervation occur after AMI, often more extensive than the area associated with infarction [172]. This results in areas of noninfarcted but denervated myocardium. These areas are supersensitive to catecholamines and may provide the substrate for arrhythmogenesis [173]. Radiolabeled analogs of norepinephrine, such as metaiodobenzylguanidine I 123 and hydroxyephedrine C 11, allow the study of cardiac pathophysiology of the sympathetic nervous system in patients with recent MI (Plate 5) [174–176]. These imaging techniques may allow the identification of high-risk individuals with a propensity for arrhythmic death. Further prospective studies are needed to evaluate the potential use of norepinephrine analogs to identify patients at risk of life-threatening ventricular arrhythmias.

Nuclear imaging techniques continue to play an important role in the care of patients with AMI. Infarct-avid imaging agents, such as ^{99m}Tc-PPi or In 111 antimyosin, are used for detecting an MI or for estimating its size. When used in combination with a myocardial perfusion agent, the technique may be of value in identifying areas of jeopardized myocardium. RVG is a readily available technique that provides accurate evaluation of both right and left ventricular function at rest and during exercise.

By allowing calculation of indexes of global ventricular function, i.e., EF and ventricular volumes and assessments of regional ventricular function, RVG provides an accurate and comprehensive noninvasive characterization of ventricular function in patients during the acute and convalescent phases of MI. The accuracy of this technique can be enhanced further with tomographic acquisition [12]. The exponential increase in the use of interventions to salvage myocardium in AMI has led to the use of radionuclide tracers of perfusion, metabolism, or both to identify viable myocardium within the distribution of the reperfused coronary artery. In particular, Tc 99m sestamibi has proved to be valuable in determining the amount of myocardial salvage achieved by reperfusion therapies and has also been used to evaluate the efficacy of these interventions. Predischarge stress testing, by exercise or pharmacologic means, combined with RVG or myocardial perfusion agents continues to play an important role in the identification of patients who are at increased risk of future cardiac events after AMI. With the increasing number of radiopharmaceuticals becoming available and the improvements in imaging hardware and software, nuclear cardiology will continue to play an important role in routine clinical evaluation and in predicting prognosis for patients with AMI.

References

1. Johnson, L. L., Seldin, D. W., Keller, A. M., et al. Dual isotope thallium and indium antimyosin SPECT imaging to identify acute infarct patients at further ischemic risk. *Circulation* 80:37, 1990.
2. Bonte, F. J., Parkey, R. W., Graham, K. D., et al. A new method for radionuclide imaging of myocardial infarcts. *Radiology* 110:473, 1974.
3. Willerson, J. T., Parkey, R. W., Bonte, F. J., et al. Technetium stannous pyrophosphate myocardial scintigrams in patients with chest pain of varying etiology. *Circulation* 51:1046, 1975.
4. Willerson, J. T., Parkey, R. W., Bonte, F. J., et al. Acute subendocardial myocardial infarction in patients: Its detection by technetium 99m stannous pyrophosphate myocardial scintigrams. *Circulation* 51:436, 1975.
5. Multicenter Postinfarction Research Group. Risk stratification and survival after myocardial infarction. *N. Engl. J. Med.* 309:331, 1983.
6. Okada, R. D., Kirshenbaum, H. D., Kushner, F. G., et al. Observer variance in the qualitative evaluation of left ventricular wall motion and the quantitation of left ventricular ejection fraction using rest and exercise multigated blood pool imaging. *Circulation* 61:128, 1980.
7. Okada, R. D., Pohost, G. M., Nichols, A. B., et al. Left ventricular regional wall motion assessment by multigated and end-diastolic, end-systolic gated radionuclide left ventriculography. *Am. J. Cardiol.* 45:1211, 1980.
8. Parker, J. A., Secker-Walker, R., Hill, R., et al. A new technique for the calculation of left ventricular ejection fraction. *J. Nucl. Med.* 13:585, 1972.
9. Borer, J. S., Kent, K. M., Bacharach, S. L., et al. Sensitivity, specificity and predictive accuracy of radionuclide cineangiography during exercise in patients with coronary artery disease. *Circulation* 60:572, 1979.
10. Dehmer, G. J., Firth, B. G., Lewis, S. E., et al. Direct measurement of cardiac output by gated equilibrium blood pool scintigraphy: Validation of scintigraphic volume measurements by a nongeometric technique. *Am. J. Cardiol.* 47:1061, 1981.
11. Konstam, M. A., Wynne, J., Holman, B. L., et al. Use of equilibrium (gated) radionuclide ventriculography to quantitate left ventricular output in patients with and without left-sided valvular regurgitation. *Circulation* 64:578, 1981.
12. Corbett, J. R., Jansen, D. E., Lewis, S. E., et al. Tomographic gated blood pool radionuclide ventriculography: Analysis of wall motion and left ventricular volumes in patients with coronary artery disease. *J. Am. Coll. Cardiol.* 6:349, 1985.
13. Sanford, C. F., Corbett, J., Curry, G. L., et al. Value of radionuclide ventriculography in the immediate characterization of patients with acute myocardial infarction. *Am. J. Cardiol.* 49:637, 1982.
14. Sheehan, F. H., Mathey, D. G., Schofer, J., et al. Effect of interventions in salvaging left ventricular function in acute myocardial infarction: A study of intracoronary streptokinase. *Am. J. Cardiol.* 52: 431, 1983.
15. Stack, R. S., Philips, H. R., Grierson, D. S., et al. Functional improvement of jeopardized myocardium following intracoronary streptokinase infusion in acute myocardial infarction. *J. Clin. Invest.* 72:84, 1983.
16. Cribier, A., Berland, J., Champoud, O., et al. Intracoronary thrombolysis in evolving myocardial infarction: Sequential angiographic analysis of left ventricular performance. *Br. Heart J.* 50:401, 1983.
17. Serruys, P. W., Simoons, M. L., Suryapranata, H., et al. Preservation of global and regional left ventricular function after early thrombolysis in acute myocardial infarction. *J. Am. Coll. Cardiol.* 7:729, 1986.
18. Wackers, F. J., Terrin, M. L., Kayden, D. S., et al. Quantitative radionuclide assessment of regional ventricular function after thrombolytic therapy for

acute myocardial infarction: Results of Phase I Thrombolysis in Myocardial Infarction (TIMI) Trial. *J. Am. Coll. Cardiol.* 13:998, 1989.

19. Hutchins, G. M., and Bulkley, B. H. Infarct expansion versus extension: Two different complications of acute myocardial infarction. *Am. J. Cardiol.* 41:1127, 1978.
20. Weisman, H. F., and Healy, B. Myocardial infarct expansion, infarct extension, and reinfarction: Pathophysiologic concepts. *Prog. Cardiovasc. Dis.* 30:73, 1987.
21. Meizlish, J. L., Berger, H. J., Plankey, M., et al. Functional aneurysm formation after acute anterior myocardial infarction. *N. Engl. J. Med.* 311:1001, 1984.
22. Warren, S. E., Royal, H. D., Markis, J. E., et al. Time course of left ventricular dilation after myocardial infarction: Influence of infarct-related artery and success of coronary thrombolysis. *J. Am. Coll. Cardiol.* 11:12, 1988.
23. Jeremy, R. W., Hackworthy, R. A., Bautovich, G., et al. Infarct artery perfusion and change in left ventricular volume in the month after acute myocardial infarction. *J. Am. Coll. Cardiol.* 9:989, 1987.
24. Maddahi, J., Berman, D. S., Masouka, D. T., et al. A new technique for assessing right ventricular ejection fraction using rapid multiple-gated equilibrium cardiac blood pool scintigraphy. Description, validation and findings in chronic coronary artery disease. *Circulation* 60:581, 1979.
25. Rigo, P., Murray, M., Taylor, D., et al. Right ventricular dysfunction in patients with acute inferior infarction. *Circulation* 32:268, 1975.
26. Slutsky, R., Hooper, W., and Gerber, K. Assessment of right ventricular function at rest and during exercise in patients with coronary heart disease: A new approach using equilibrium radionuclide ventriculography. *Am. J. Cardiol.* 45:63, 1980.
27. Starling, M. R., Dell'Italia, L. J., Chaudhuri, T. K., et al. First transit and equilibrium radionuclide angiocardiography in patients with inferior transmural myocardial infarction: Criteria for diagnosis of associated hemodynamically significant right ventricular infarction. *J. Am. Coll. Cardiol.* 4:923, 1984.
28. Winzelberg, C. G., Boucher, C. A., Pohost, G. M., et al. Right ventricular function in aortic and mitral disease: Relation of gated first-pass radionuclide angiography to clinical and hemodynamic findings. *Chest* 79:520, 1981.
29. Cohn, J. N., Guilia, N. H., Broder, M. I., et al. Right ventricular infarction. *Am. J. Cardiol.* 33: 209, 1978.
30. Dell'Italia, L. J., Starling, M. R., Blunhardt, R., et al. Comparative effects of volume loading, dobutamine and nitroprusside in patients with predominate right ventricular infarction. *Circulation* 72: 1327, 1985.
31. Shah, P., Maddahi, J., Berman, D., et al. Scintigraphically detected predominant right ventricular dysfunction in acute myocardial infarction: Clinical and hemodynamic correlates and implications for therapy and prognosis. *J. Am. Coll. Cardiol.* 6: 1264, 1985.
32. Weich, H. F., Strauss, H. W., and Pitt, B. Extraction of thallium-201 by the myocardium. *Circulation* 56:188, 1977.
33. McCall, D., Zimmer, L. J., and Katy, A. M. Kinetics of thallium exchange in cultured rat cells. *Circ. Res.* 56:370, 1985.
34. Goldhaber, S. Z., Newell, J. B., Alpert, N. M., et al. Effects of ischemic-like insult on myocardial thallium-201 accumulation. *Circulation* 67:778, 1983.
35. Leppo, J. A., MacNeil, P. B., Moring, A. F., et al. Separate effects of ischemia, hypoxia and contractility on thallium-201 kinetics in rabbit myocardium. *J. Nucl. Med.* 27:66, 1986.
36. Pohost, G. M., Alpert, N. S., Ingwall, J. S., et al. Thallium redistribution: Mechanisms and clinical utility. *Semin. Nucl. Med.* 20:70, 1980.
37. Leppo, J. A. Myocardial uptake of thallium and rubidium during alterations in perfusion and oxygenation in isolated rabbit hearts. *J. Nucl. Med.* 28:878, 1987.
38. Sinusas, A. J., Watson, D. D., Cannon, J. M., Jr., et al. Effect of ischemia and postischemic dysfunction on myocardial uptake of technetium-99m-labeled methoxyisobutyl isonitrile and thallium-201. *J. Am. Coll. Cardiol.* 14:1785, 1989.
39. Moore, C. A., Cannon, J., Watson, D. D., et al. Thallium 201 kinetics in stunned myocardium characterized by severe postischemic dysfunction. *Circulation* 81:1622, 1990.
40. Strauss, H. W., Harrison, K., Langan, V. K., et al. Thallium-201 for myocardial imaging: Relation of thallium-201 to regional myocardial perfusion. *Circulation* 51:641, 1975.
41. Chu, A., Murdock, R. H., and Cobb, F. R. Relationship between regional distribution of thallium-201 and myocardial blood flow in normal, acutely ischemic and infarcted myocardium. *Am. J. Cardiol.* 50:1141, 1982.
42. Nielsen, A. P., Morris, K. G., Murdock, R. H., et al. Linear relationship between the distribution of thallium-201 and blood flow in ischemic and nonischemic myocardium during exercise. *Circulation* 61:797, 1980.
43. Pohost, G. M., Okada, R. D., O'Keefe, D. D., et al. Thallium redistribution in dogs with severe coronary artery stenosis of fixed caliper. *Circ. Res.* 48: 439, 1981.
44. Gewirtz, H., O'Keefe, D. D., Pohost, G. M., et al. The effect of ischemia on thallium-201 clearance from the myocardium. *Circulation* 58:216, 1978.
45. Kaul, S., Chester, D. A., Pohost, G. M., et al. Influence of peak exercise heart rate on normal thallium-201 myocardial clearance. *J. Nucl. Med.* 2726, 1986.
46. Markis, J. E., Malagold, M., Parker, J. A., et al. Myocardial salvage after intracoronary thrombol-

ysis with streptokinase in acute myocardial infarction. *N. Engl. J. Med.* 305:777, 1981.
47. Beller, G. A. Role of myocardial perfusion imaging in evaluating thrombolytic therapy for acute myocardial infarction. *J. Am. Coll. Cardiol.* 9:661, 1987.
48. Melin, J. A., Becker, L. C., and Bulkley, B. H. Differences in thallium-201 uptake in reperfused and nonreperfused myocardial infarction. *Circ. Res.* 53:414, 1983.
49. Okada, R. D., and Pohost, G. M. The use of preintervention and postintervention thallium imaging for assessing the early and late effects of experimental coronary arterial reperfusion in dogs. *Circulation* 69:1153, 1984.
50. Granato, J. E., Watson, D. D., Flanagan, T. L., et al. Myocardial thallium-201 kinetics during coronary occlusion and reperfusion: Influence of method of reflow and timing of thallium-201 administration. *Circulation* 73:150, 1986.
51. Schwartz, F., Schuler, G., Katus, H., et al. Intracoronary thrombolysis in acute myocardial infarction: Correlation among serum enzyme, scintigraphic and hemodynamic findings. *Am. J. Cardiol.* 50:30, 1982.
52. Berger, B. C., Watson, D. D., Burwell, L. R., et al. Redistribution of thallium at rest in patients with stable and unstable angina and the effect of coronary artery bypass surgery. *Circulation* 60:1114, 1979.
53. Mori, T., Minamiji, K., Kurogane, H., et al. Rest-injected thallium-201 imaging for assessing viability of severe asynergic regions. *J. Nucl. Med.* 32:1718, 1991.
54. Ragosta, M., Beller, G. A., Watson, D. D., et al. Quantitative planar rest-redistribution 201Tl imaging in detection of myocardial viability and prediction of improvement in left ventricular function after coronary bypass surgery in patients with severely depressed left ventricular function. *Circulation* 87:1630, 1993.
55. Dilsizian, V., Rocco, T. P., Freedman, N. M., et al. Enhanced detection of ischemic but viable myocardium by the reinjection of thallium after stress-redistribution imaging. *N. Engl. J. Med.* 323:141, 1990.
56. Dilsizian, V., Smeltzer, W. R., Freedman, N. M., et al. Thallium reinjection after stress-reinjection imaging: Does 24-hour delayed imaging after reinjection enhance detection of viable myocardium? *Circulation* 83:1247, 1991.
57. Bonow, R. O., Dilsizian, V., Cuocolo, A., et al. Identification of viable myocardium in patients with chronic coronary artery disease and left ventricular dysfunction: Comparison of thallium scintigraphy with reinjection and PET imaging with ^{18}F-Fluro-deoxyglucose. *Circulation* 83:26, 1991.
58. Perrone-Filardi, P., Bacharach, S. L., Dilsizian, V., et al. Regional left ventricular wall thickening: Relation to regional uptake of ^{18}Fluorodeoxyglucose and 201Tl in patients with chronic coronary artery disease. *Circulation* 86:1125, 1992.
59. Brunken, R., Tillisch, J., Schwaiger, M., et al. Regional perfusion, glucose metabolism, and wall motion in patients with chronic electrocardiographic Q wave infarctions: Evidence for persistence of viable tissue in infarct regions by positron emission tomography. *Circulation* 73:951, 1986.
60. Brunken, R., Schwaiger, M., Grover-McKay, M., et al. Positron emission tomography detects tissue metabolic activity in myocardial segments with persistent thallium perfusion defects. *J. Am. Coll. Cardiol.* 10:557, 1987.
61. Tillisch, J., Brunken, R., Marshall, R., et al. Reversibility of cardiac wall-motion abnormalities predicted by positron emission tomography. *N. Engl. J. Med.* 314:884, 1986.
62. Goldstein, R. A. Kinetics of rubidium-82 after coronary occlusion and reperfusion. *J. Clin. Invest.* 75:1131, 1985.
63. Gould, L., Yoshida, K., Hess, M., et al. Myocardial metabolism of fluorodeoxyglucose compared to cell membrane integrity for the potassium analogue rubidium-82 for assessing infarct size in man by PET. *J. Nucl. Med.* 32:1, 1991.
64. Beanlands, R. S., Dawood, F., Wen, W. H., et al. Are the kinetics of Technetium-99m methoxyisobutyl isonitrile affected by cell metabolism and viability? *Circulation* 82:1802, 1990.
65. Beller, G. A., and Sinusas, A. J. Experimental studies of the physiologic properties of technetium-99m isonitriles. *Am. J. Cardiol.* 66:5E, 1990.
66. Carvalho, P. A., Chui, M. L., Kronauge, J. F., et al. Subcellular distribution and analysis of technetium-99m-MIBI in isolated perfused rat hearts. *J. Nucl. Med.* 33:1516, 1992.
67. Freeman, I., Grunwald, A. M., Hoory, S., et al. Effect of coronary occlusion and myocardial viability on myocardial activity of Tc-99m-sestamibi. *J. Nucl. Med.* 32:292, 1991.
68. Beanlands, R. S., Dawood, F., Wen-Hu, W., et al. Are the kinetics of technetium-99m methoxyisobutyl isonitrile affected by cell metabolism and viability? *Circulation* 82:1802, 1990.
69. Wackers, F. J., Gibbons, R. J., Verani, M. S., et al. Serial quantitative planar technetium-99m hexakis 2-methoxy-isobutyl isonitrile imaging in acute myocardial infarction: Efficacy for noninvasive assessment of thrombolytic therapy. *J. Am. Coll. Cardiol.* 14:861, 1989.
70. Rocco, T. P., Dilsizian, V., Strauss, H. W., et al. Technetium-99m isonitrile myocardial uptake at rest II: Relationship to clinical markers of potential viability. *J. Am. Coll. Cardiol.* 14:1678, 1989.
71. Kahn, J. K., McGhie, I., Faber, T. L., et al. Assessment of myocardial viability with technetium-99m 2-methoxy isobutyl isonitrile and gated tomography in patients with coronary artery disease. *J. Am. Coll. Cardiol.* 13:31A, 1989.
72. Verani, M. S., Jeroudi, M. O., Mahmarian, J. J., et al. Quantification of myocardial salvage during coronary occlusion and myocardial salvage using cardiac imaging with technetium-99m hexakis 2-

methoxy-isobutyl isonitrile. *J. Am. Coll. Cardiol.* 12:1573, 1988.

73. Gibbons, R. J., Verani, M. S., Behrenbeck, T., et al. Feasibility of tomographic technetium-99m-hexakis-2methoxy-methopropyl-isonitrile imaging for the assessment of myocardial area at risk and the effect of acute treatment in myocardial infarction. *Circulation* 80:1277, 1989.
74. Pellikka, P. A., Behrenbeck, T., Verani, M. S., et al. Serial changes in myocardial perfusion using tomographic technetium-99m-hexakis-2-methoxy-methopropyl-isonitrile imaging following reperfusion therapy of myocardial infarction. *J. Nucl. Med.* 31:1269, 1990.
75. Christian, T. F., Schwartz, R. S., and Gibbons, R. J. Determinants of infarct size in reperfusion therapy for acute myocardial infarction. *Circulation* 86:81, 1992.
76. Gibbons, R. J., Holmes, D. R., Reeder, G. S., et al. Immediate angioplasty compared with the administration of a thrombolytic agent followed by conservative treatment for myocardial infarction. *N. Engl. J. Med.* 328:726, 1993.
77. Behrenbeck, T., Pellikka, P. A., Huber, K. C., et al. Primary PTCA in myocardial infarction: Assessment of myocardial salvage with Tc-99m sestamibi. *J. Am. Coll. Cardiol.* 17:365, 1991.
78. Christian, T. F., Behrenbeck, T., Pellikka, P. A., et al. Mismatch of left ventricular function and infarct size demonstrated by technetium-99m isonitrile imaging after reperfusion therapy for acute myocardial infarction: Identification of myocardial stunning and hyperkinesia. *J. Am. Coll. Cardiol.* 16:1632, 1990.
79. Christian, T. F., Behrenbeck, T., Gersh, B. J., et al. Relation of left ventricular volume and function one year after acute myocardial infarction to infarct size determined by technetium-99m sestamibi. *Am. J. Cardiol.* 68:21, 1991.
80. Wackers. F. J., Gibbons, R. J., Verani, M. S., et al. Serial quantitative planar technetium-99m-isonitrile imaging in acute myocardial infarction: Efficacy for noninvasive assessment of thrombolytic therapy. *J. Am. Coll. Cardiol.* 14:861, 1989.
81. Leppo, J. A., DePuey, E. G., and Johnson, L. L. A review of cardiac imaging with sestamibi and teboroxime. *J. Nucl. Med.* 32:2012, 1991.
82. Najm, Y. C., Timmis, A. D., Maisey, M. N., et al. The evaluation of ventricular function using gated myocardial imaging with Tc-99m MIBI. *Eur. Heart J.* 10:142, 1989.
83. Clausen, M., Henze, E., Schmidt, A., et al. The contraction fraction in myocardial studies with technetium-99m isonitrile correlations with radionuclide ventriculography and infarct size measured by SPECT. *Eur. J. Nucl. Med.* 15:61, 1989.
84. Faber, T. L., Akers, M. S., Peshock, R. M., et al. Three-dimensional and perfusion quantification in gated single-photon emission computed tomograms. *J. Nucl. Med.* 32:2311, 1991.
85. Cuocolo, A., Pace, L., Ricciardelli, B., et al. Identification of myocardium in patient with chronic artery disease: Comparison of thallium-201 scintigraphy with reinjection and technetium-99m methoxyisobutyl isonitrile. *J. Nucl. Med.* 33:505, 1992.
86. Bonow, R. O., and Dilsizian, V. Thallium-201 and Technetium-99m-sestamibi for assessing viable myocardium. *J. Nucl. Med.* 33:815, 1992.
87. Coleman, P., Metherall, J., Pandian, N., et al. Predicting enhanced regional ventricular function post-revascularization: Comparison of thallium-201 and sestamibi in patients with left ventricular dysfunction (Abstract). *Circulation* 86:I-108, 1992.
88. Arrighi, J., Dodati, J., Bacharach, S., et al. The detection of viable myocardium by Tc-99m sestamibi is enhanced when the severity of irreversible defects are assessed (Abstract). *Circulation* 86:I-108, 1992.
89. Yamamoto, Y., de Silva, R., Rhodes, C. G., et al. A new strategy for assessment of viable myocardium and regional myocardial blood flow using ^{15}O-water and dynamic positron emission tomography. *Circulation* 86:167, 1992.
90. Krivokapich, J., Huang, S. C., Selin, C. E., et al. Fluorodeoxyglucose rate constants, lumped constant, and glucose metabolic rate in rabbit heart. *Am. J. Physiol.* 252:H777, 1987.
91. Ratib, O., Phelps, M. E., Huang, S. C., et al. Positron emission tomography with deoxyglucose for estimating local myocardial glucose metabolism. *J. Nucl. Med.* 23:577, 1982.
92. Marshall, R. C., Tillisch, J. H., Phelps, M. E., et al. Identification and differentiation of resting myocardial ischemia in man with positron computed tomography, 18F-labeled flurodeoxyglucose and N-13-ammonia. *Circulation* 67:766, 1983.
93. Tamaki, N., Yonekura, Y., Yamashita, K., et al. Positron emission tomography using fluorine-18 deoxyglucose in evaluation of coronary artery bypass grafting. *Am. J. Cardiol.* 64:860, 1989.
94. Groper, R. J., Geltman, E. M., Sampathkumaran, K., et al. Functional recovery after coronary revascularization for chronic coronary artery disease is dependent on maintenance of oxidative metabolism. *J. Am. Coll. Cardiol.* 20:569, 1992.
95. Schwaiger, M., Brunken, R., Grover-McKay, M., et al. Regional myocardial metabolism in patients with acute myocardial infarction assessed by positron emission tomography. *J. Am. Coll. Cardiol.* 8:800, 1986.
96. Pierard, L. A., De Landsheere, C. M., Berthe, C., et al. Identification of viable myocardium by echocardiography during dobutamine infusion in patients with myocardial infarction after thrombolytic therapy: Comparison with positron emission tomography. *J. Am. Coll. Cardiol.* 15:1021, 1990.
97. Gropler, R. J., Siegel, B. A., Sampathkumaran, K., et al. Dependence of recovery of contractile function on maintenance of oxidative metabolism after myocardial infarction. *J. Am. Coll. Cardiol.* 19:989, 1992.

98. Buxton, D. B., Vaghaiwalla, M. F., Krivokapich, J., et al. Quantitative measurement of sustained metabolic abnormalities in reperfused canine myocardium (Abstract). *J. Nucl. Med.* 31:795, 1990.
99. Myears, D. W., Sobel, B. E., and Bergmann, S. R. Substrate use in ischemic and reperfused canine myocardium: Quantitative considerations. *Am. J. Physiol.* 253:H107, 1987.
100. Brown, M., Myears, D., and Bergmann, S. Validity of estimates of myocardial oxidative metabolism with carbon-11-acetate and positron emission tomography despite altered patterns of substrate utilization. *J. Nucl. Med.* 30:187, 1989.
101. Brown, M., Marshall, D., Sobel, B., et al. Delineation of myocardial oxygen utilization with carbon-11-labeled acetate. *Circulation* 76:687, 1987.
102. Brown, M., Myears, D., and Bergmann, S. Noninvasive assessment of canine myocardial oxidative metabolism with carbon-11-acetate and positron emission tomography. *J. Am. Coll. Cardiol.* 12: 1054, 1988.
103. Walsh, M., Geltman, E., Brown, M., et al. Noninvasive estimation of regional myocardial oxygen consumption by positron emission tomography with carbon-11-acetate in patients with myocardial infarction. *J. Nucl. Med.* 30:1798, 1989.
104. Buxton, D. B., Nienaber, C. A., Luxen, A., et al. Noninvasive quantitation of regional myocardial oxygen consumption in vivo with [1-^{11}C] acetate and dynamic positron emission tomography. *Circulation* 79:134, 1989.
105. Armbrecht, J. J., Buxton, D. B., and Schelbert, H. R. Validation of [1-^{11}C] acetate kinetics as a tracer for noninvasive assessment of oxidative metabolism with positron emission tomography in normal, ischemic, postischemic, and hyperemic canine myocardium. *Circulation* 81:1594, 1990.
106. Lear, J. L. Relationship between myocardial clearance rates of carbon-11-acetate-derived radiolabel and oxidative metabolism: Physiologic basis and clinical significance (Editorial). *J. Nucl. Med.* 32: 1957, 1991.
107. Buxton, D. B., Mody, F. V., Krivokapich, J., et al. Quantitative assessment of prolonged metabolic abnormalities in reperfused myocardium. *Circulation* 85:1842, 1992.
108. Henes, C. G., Bergmann, S. R., Perez, J. E., et al. The time course of restoration of nutritive perfusion, myocardial oxygen consumption, and regional function after coronary thrombolysis. *Cor. Artery Dis.* 1:687, 1990.
109. Czernin, J., Porenta, G., Brunken, R., et al. Regional blood flow, oxidative metabolism, and glucose utilization in patients with recent myocardial infarction. *Circulation* 88:884, 1993.
110. Vanoverschelde, J. L. J., Melin, J. A., Bol, A., et al. Regional oxidative metabolism in patients after recovery from reperfused anterior myocardial infarction: Relation to regional blood flow and glucose uptake. *Circulation* 85:9, 1992.
111. Jansen, D. E., Gabliani, G., Wolfe, C., et al. Determination of viable myocardial mass with iodinated phenylpentadecanoic acid and single photon emission computed tomography. *Circulation* 70:449, 1984.
112. Hansen, C. L., Corbett, J. R., Pippin, J., et al. Iodine-123 phenylpentadecanoic acid and single photon emission tomography in identifying left ventricular regional abnormalities in patients with coronary heart disease: Comparison with thallium scintigraphy. *J. Am. Coll. Cardiol.* 12:78, 1988.
113. Kennedy, P., Corbett, J. R., Kulkarni, P. V., et al. 123I-phenylpentadecanoic acid myocardial scintigraphy: Usefulness in identification of myocardial ischemia. *Circulation* 74:1007, 1986.
114. Schon, H., Schelbert, H. R., Najafi, A., et al. C-11-labeled palmitic acid for noninvasive evaluation of regional myocardial fatty acid metabolism with positron computed tomography. II. Kinetics of C-11-palmitic acid in acutely ischemic myocardium. *Am. Heart J.* 1103:548, 1982.
115. Schelbert, H. R., Henze, E., Schon, H., et al. C-11-labeled palmitic acid for noninvasive evaluation of regional myocardial fatty acid metabolism with positron computed tomography. III. In vivo demonstration of the effects of substrate availability on myocardial metabolism. *Am. Heart J.* 105:492, 1983.
116. Bergmann, S. R., Fox, K. A. A., Ter-Pogossian, M. M., et al. Clot-selective coronary thrombolysis with tissue-type plasminogen activator. *Science* 220:1181, 1983.
117. Van de Werf, F., Bergmann, S. R., Fox, K. A. A., et al. Coronary thrombolysis with intravenously administered human tissue-type plasminogen activator produced by recombinant DNA technology. *Circulation* 69:605, 1984.
118. Sobel, B. E., Geltman, E. M., Tiefenbrunn, A. J., et al. Improvement of regional myocardial metabolism after coronary thrombolysis induced with tissue-type plasminogen activator or streptokinase. *Circulation* 69:983, 1984.
119. Bergmann, S. R., Lerch, R. A., Fox, K. A. A., et al. Temporal dependence of beneficial effects of coronary thrombolysis characterized by positron emission tomography. *Am. J. Med.* 73:573, 1982.
120. Knabb, R. M., Bergmann, S. R., Fox, K. A. A., et al. The temporal pattern of recovery of myocardial perfusion and metabolism delineated by positron emission tomography following coronary thrombolysis. *J. Nucl. Med.* 28:1563, 1987.
121. Fox, K. A., Abendschein, D. R., Ambos, H. D., et al. Efflux of metabolized and nonmetabolized fatty acid from canine myocardium. Implications for quantifying myocardium metabolism tomographically. *Circ. Res.* 57:232, 1985.
122. Rosamond, T. L., Abendschein, D. R., Sobel, B., et al. Metabolic fate of radiolabeled palmitate in ischemic canine myocardium: Implications for pos-

itron emission tomography. *J. Nucl. Med.* 28:1322, 1987.
123. Buja, L. M., Parkey, R. W., Stokely, E. M., et al. Pathophysiology of technetium-99m stannous pyrophosphate and thallium-201 scintigraphy of acute anterior myocardial infarcts in dogs. *J. Clin. Invest.* 57:1508, 1976.
124. Buja, L. M., Tofe, A. J., Kulkarni, P. V., et al. Sites and mechanisms of localization of technetium-99m phosphorus radiopharmaceuticals in acute myocardial infarcts and other tissues. *J. Clin. Invest.* 60: 724, 1977.
125. Buja, L. M., Poliner, L. R., Parkey, R. W., et al. Clinicopathologic study of persistently positive technetium-99m stannous pyrophosphate myocardial scintigrams and mycocytolytic degeneration after acute myocardial infarction. *Circulation* 56:1016, 1977.
126. Poliner, L. R., Buja, L. M., Parkey, R. W., et al. Clinicopathologic findings in 52 patients studied by technetium-99m stannous pyrophosphate myocardial scintigrams. *Circulation* 59:257, 1979.
127. Willerson, J. T., Parkey, R. W., Bonte, F. J., et al. Pathophysiologic considerations and clinicopathological correlates of technetium-99m stannous pyrophosphate myocardial scintigraphy. *Semin. Nucl. Med.* 10:54, 1980.
128. Chien, K. R., Reeves, J. P., Buja, L. M., et al. Phospholipid alterations in ischemic myocardium: Temporal and topographical correlations with Tc-99m-PPi accumulation and in vitro sarcolemmal Ca^{2+} permeability defect. *Circ. Res.* 48:711, 1981.
129. Parkey, R. W., Kulkarni, P., Lewis, S., et al. Effect of coronary blood flow and site of injection on ^{99m}Tc-PPi detection of early canine myocardial infarcts. *J. Nucl. Med.* 22(2):133, 1981.
130. Lewis, S. E., Devous, M. D., Sr., Corbett, J. R., et al. Measurement of infarct size in acute canine myocardial infarction by single photon emission computed tomography with technetium-99m pyrophosphate. *Am. J. Cardiol.* 54:193, 1984.
131. Croft, C., Rude, R. E., Lewis, S. E., et al. Comparison of left ventricular function and infarct size in patients with and without persistently positive technetium-99m pyrophosphate myocardial scintigrams after myocardial infarction: Analysis of 357 patients. *Am. J. Cardiol.* 53:421, 1984.
132. Corbett, J. R., Lewis, M., Willerson, J. T., et al. Technetium-99m pyrophosphate imaging in patients with acute myocardial infarction: Comparison of planar images with single-photon tomography with and without blood pool overlay. *Circulation* 69:1120, 1984.
133. Corbett, J. R., Lewis, S. E., Wolfe, C. L., et al. Measurement of myocardial infarct size in patients by technetium pyrophosphate single photon tomography. *Am. J. Cardiol.* 54:1231, 1984.
134. Wolfe, C. L., Lewis, S. E., Corbett, J. R., et al. Measurement of infarction using single photon emission computed tomography. *J. Am. Coll. Cardiol.* 6:145, 1985.
135. Wheelan, K., Wolfe, C., Corbett, J., et al. Early positive technetium-99m stannous pyrophosphate images as a marker of reperfusion in patients receiving thrombolytic therapy for acute myocardial infarction. *Am. J. Cardiol.* 56:252, 1985.
136. Jansen, D. E., Corbett, J. R., Lewis, S. E., et al. Quantification of myocardial infarction: A comparison of single photon emission computed tomography with pyrophosphate to serial plasma MB-CK measurements. *Circulation* 72:327, 1985.
137. Jansen, D. E., Corbett, J. R., Buja, L. M., et al. Quantification of myocardial injury produced by temporary coronary artery occlusion and reflow with technetium-99m-pyrophosphate. *Circulation* 75:611, 1987.
138. Khaw, B. A., and Haber, E. Imaging necrotic myocardium: detection with ^{99m}Tc-pyrophosphate and radiolabeled antimyosin. *Cardiol. Clin.* 7:577, 1989.
139. Khaw, B. A., Yasuda, T., Gold, H. K., et al. Acute myocardial infarct imaging with Indium-111-labeled monoclonal antimyosin Fab. *J. Nucl. Med.* 28:1671, 1987.
140. Khaw, B. A., Strauss, H. W., Moore, R., et al. Myocardial damage delineated by indium-111 antimyosin Fab and technetium-99m pyrophosphate. *J. Nucl. Med.* 28:76, 1987.
141. Takeda, K., LaFrance, N. D., Weissman, H. F., et al. Comparison of indium-111 antimyosin antibody and technetium-99m pyrophosphate localization in reperfused and nonreperfused myocardial infarction. *J. Am. Coll. Cardiol.* 17:519, 1991.
142. Beller, G. A., Khaw, B. A., Haber, E., et al. Localization of radiolabeled cardiac myosin-specific antibody in myocardial infarcts: Comparison with technetium-99m stannous pyrophosphate. *Circulation* 55:74, 1977.
143. Dec, G. W., Palacios, I., Yasuda, T., et al. Antimyosin antibody cardiac imaging: Its role in the diagnosis of myocarditis. *J. Am. Coll. Cardiol.* 16:97, 1990.
144. Narula, J., Khaw, B. A., Dec, G. W., et al. Brief report: Recognition of acute myocarditis masquerading as acute myocardial infarction. *N. Engl. J. Med.* 328:100, 1993.
145. Gibson, R. S., Watson, D. D., Craddock, G. B., et al. Prediction of cardiac events after uncomplicated myocardial infarction: A prospective study comparing predischarge exercise thallium-201 scintigraphy and coronary angiography. *Circulation* 68:321, 1983.
146. Wilson, W. W., Gibson, R. S., Nygaard, T. W., et al. Acute myocardial infarction associated with single vessel disease: An analysis of clinical outcome and the prognostic importance of vessel patency and residual ischemic myocardium. *J. Am. Coll. Cardiol.* 11:223, 1988.
147. Hung, J., Goris, M. L., Nash, E., et al. Comparative

value of maximal treadmill testing, exercise thallium myocardial perfusion scintigraphy and exercise radionuclide ventriculography for distinguishing high- and low-risk patients soon after acute myocardial infarction. *Am. J. Cardiol.* 53:1221, 1984.

148. Abraham, R. D., Freedman, S. B., Dunn, R. F., et al. Prediction of multivessel coronary artery disease and prognosis early after acute infarction by exercise electrocardiography and thallium-201 myocardial perfusion scanning. *Am. J. Cardiol.* 58:423, 1986.
149. Marmur, J. D., Freeman, M. R., Langer, A., et al. Prognosis in medically stabilized unstable angina: Early Holter ST-segment monitoring compared with predischarge thallium tomography. *Ann. Intern. Med.* 114:336, 1991.
150. Brown, K. A. Prognostic value of thallium-201 myocardial perfusion imaging in patients with unstable angina who respond to medical treatment. *J. Am. Coll. Cardiol.* 17:1053, 1991.
151. Johnson, L. L., Seldin, D. W., Keller, A. M., et al. Dual isotope thallium and indium antimyosin SPECT imaging to identify acute infarct patients at further ischemic risk. *Circulation* 80:37, 1990.
152. Leppo, J. A., O'Brien, J., Rothendler, J. A., et al. Dipyridamole-thallium-201 scintigraphy in the prediction of future cardiac events after acute myocardial infarction. *N. Engl. J. Med.* 310:1014, 1984.
153. Younis, L. T., Byers, S., Shaw, L., et al. Prognostic value of intravenous dipyridamole thallium scintigraphy after an acute ischemic event. *Am. J. Cardiol.* 64:161, 1989.
154. Gimble, L. W., Hutter, A. M., Guiney, T. E., et al. Prognostic utility of predischarge dipyridamole-thallium imaging compared to predischarge submaximal exercise electrocardiography and maximal exercise thallium imaging after uncomplicated acute myocardial infarction. *Am. J. Cardiol.* 64: 1243, 1989.
155. Mahmarian, J. J., Pratt, C. M., Nishimura, S., et al. Quantitative adenosine 201-Tl single-photon emission computed tomography for the early assessment of patients surviving acute myocardial infarction. *Circulation* 87:1197, 1993.
156. Brown, K. A., O'Meara, J., Chambers, C. E., et al. Ability of dipyridamole-thallium-201 imaging 1 to 4 days after acute myocardial infarction to predict in-hospital and late recurrent myocardial ischemic events. *Am. J. Cardiol.* 65:160, 1990.
157. Candell, R. J., Permanyer, M. G., Castell, J., et al. Uncomplicated first myocardial infarction: Strategy for comprehensive prognostic studies. *J. Am. Coll. Cardiol.* 18:1220, 1991.
158. Tilkemeier, P. L., Guiney, T. E., LaRaia, P. J., et al. Prognostic value of predischarge low-level exercise thallium testing after thrombolytic treatment of acute myocardial infarction. *Am. J. Cardiol.* 66:1203, 1990.
159. Sutton, J. M., and Topol, E. J. Significance of a negative exercise thallium test in the presence of a critical residual stenosis after thrombolysis for acute myocardial infarction. *Circulation* 83:1278, 1991.
160. Haber, H. L., Beller, G. A., Watson, D. D., et al. Exercise thallium-201 scintigraphy after thrombolytic therapy with or without angioplasty for acute myocardial infarction. *Am. J. Cardiol.* 71:1257, 1993.
161. Corbett, J. R., Nicod, P. H., Huxley, R. L., et al. Left ventricular functional alterations at rest and during submaximal exercise in patients with recent myocardial infarction. *Am. J. Med.* 74:577, 1983.
162. Corbett, J. R., Dehmer, G. J., Lewis, S. E., et al. The prognostic value of submaximal exercise testing with radionuclide ventriculography before hospital discharge in patients with recent myocardial infarction. *Circulation* 64:535, 1981.
163. Borer, J. S., Rosing, D. R., Miller, R. H., et al. Natural history of left ventricular function during the year after acute myocardial infarction: Comparison with clinical, electrocardiographic and biochemical determinations. *Am. J. Cardiol.* 46:1, 1980.
164. Dewhurst, N. G., and Muir, A. L. Comparative prognostic value of radionuclide ventriculography at rest and during exercise in 100 patients after first myocardial infarction. *Br. Heart J.* 49:111, 1983.
165. Corbett, J. R., Nicod, P., Lewis, S. E., et al. Prognostic value of submaximal exercise radionuclide ventriculography after myocardial infarction. *Am. J. Cardiol.* 52:82A, 1983.
166. Morris, K. G., Palmeri, S. T., Califf, R. M., et al. Value of radionuclide angiography for predicting specific cardiac events after acute myocardial infarction. *Am. J. Cardiol.* 55:318, 1985.
167. Cerqueria, M. D., Stratton, J., Vracko, R., et al. Noninvasive arterial thrombus imaging in ^{99m}Tc monoclonal antifibrin antibody. *Circulation* 85:298, 1992.
168. Miller, D. D., Boulet, A. J., Tio, F. O., et al. In vivo technetium-99m S12 antibody imaging of platelet-granules in rabbit endothelial neointimal proliferation after angioplasty. *Circulation* 83:224, 1991.
169. Miller, D. D., Rivera, F. J., Garcia, O. J., et al. Imaging of vascular injury with ^{99m}Tc-labeled monoclonal antiplatelet antibody S12: Preliminary experience in human percutaneous transluminal angioplasty. *Circulation* 85:1354, 1992.
170. Sternberg, P. E., McEver, R. P., Shuman, M. A., et al. A platelet alpha-granule membrane protein (GMP-140) is expressed on the plasma membrane after activation. *J. Cell. Biol.* 101:880, 1985.
171. Ord, J. M., Hasapes, J., Daughtery, A., et al. Imaging of thrombi with tissue-type plasminogen activator rendered enzymatically inactive and conjugated to a residualizing label. *Circulation* 85:288, 1992.
172. Barber, M. J., Mueller, T. H., Henry, D. P., et al. Transmural myocardial infarction in dog produces

sympathectomy in non-infarcted myocardium. *Circulation* 67:796, 1983.

173. Inoue, H., and Zipes, D. P. Results of sympathetic denervation in the canine heart: Supersensitivity that may be arrhythmogenic. *Circulation* 75:877, 1987.
174. Stanton, M., Tuli, M. M., Radtke, N., et al. Regional sympathetic denervation after myocardial infarction: Humans detected non-invasively using I-123 metaiodobenzylguanidine. *J. Am. Coll. Cardiol.* 14:1519, 1989.
175. McGhie, A. I., Corbett, J. R., Akers, M. S., et al. Regional cardiac adrenergic function using I-123 meta-iodobenzylguanidine tomographic imaging after acute myocardial infarction. *Am. J. Cardiol.* 67:236, 1991.
176. Rosenspire, K., Haka, M., Van Dort, M. E., et al. Synthesis and preliminary evaluation of ^{11}C-meta-hydroxyephedrine: A false transmitter agent for heart neuronal imaging. *J. Nucl. Med.* 31:1328, 1990.

VII. Therapeutic Interventions During and After Acute Myocardial Infarction

30. Beta Blockers During and After Acute Myocardial Infarction

Robert P. Byington and Curt D. Furberg

Coronary heart disease continues to occupy a position of prominence as a cause of death and morbidity in the United States and other Western nations. Although a reduction in coronary heart disease mortality was observed and well documented during the 1970s and 1980s [1], the acute and chronic sequelae of coronary atherosclerosis are still responsible for 1,500,000 people having a myocardial infarction (MI) each year in the United States [2]. Among these events are 500,000 deaths, 250,000 of which occur before the patients reach the hospital. Furthermore, survivors of a documented MI are known to have an increased risk of premature death relative to the general population.

In 1992 there were 747,000 patients in the United States admitted to a hospital with the primary diagnosis of acute myocardial infarction (AMI) [3], and 666,000 were discharged alive [4]. Thus 81,000 patients died during hospitalization, which corresponds to an overall in-hospital mortality rate of 10.8 percent. More than 90 percent of the patients with an AMI who survive the hospital phase and who eventually die, die of cardiac causes [5]. Identifying preventive interventions that can reduce this toll represents a major public health challenge.

Morbid Mechanisms Behind Coronary Deaths of Postmyocardial Infarction Patients and Interventions Aimed at These Mechanisms

It is apparent that to effectively improve survival, either during AMI itself or in the long term following an MI, an intervention must favorably influence one or more of the morbid mechanisms behind the coronary deaths. In principle, there are six morbid mechanisms behind these deaths.

1. Progressive coronary atherosclerosis
2. Coronary thrombosis
3. Electrical complications (e.g., ventricular fibrillation)
4. Mechanical complications (e.g., congestive heart failure)
5. Recurrent ischemia (resulting from an imbalance between oxygen supply and demand)
6. Plaque instability

These mechanisms are related and often overlapping. Progression of the underlying coronary atherosclerosis operates only in the long term, whereas the other mechanisms operate both acutely and over the long term.

Interventions with the potential for counteracting these morbid mechanisms have been and continue to be evaluated in a large number of randomized clinical trials. Extensive review articles are available that provide detailed information concerning the interventions and the findings of the trials [6–11]. These interventions may be summarized as follows:

1. The most fundamental cause of myocardial infarction is coronary atherosclerosis. Lipid-lowering regimens of diet, or medication, or both have been tested with the hope of retarding the rate of progression via a reduction in serum cholesterol levels. The benefits of treatment are a function of the magnitude of the reduction in serum cholesterol and the duration of treatment. The Lipid Research Clinics (LRC) trial of cholestyramine [12] and the Finnish trial of gemfibrozil [13] were two of the earliest trials to demonstrate the primary preventive effects of

lipid-lowering. Evidence has been mounting for the secondary preventive effects of these agents [14]. Particularly exciting are the new HMG Co-A reductase inhibitors, also known as "statins." For example, the Pravastatin, Lipids, and Atherosclerosis in the Carotids (PLAC-2) trial of pravastatin in 151 coronary patients followed for 3 years found an approximate 60 percent reduction in coronary events attributable to the agent [15]. Possible explanations for this greater than expected reduction in events include improved plaque stability and endothelial function.

2. Three types of intervention have been explored aimed at preventing extension of an existing thrombus or achieving thrombolysis. These interventions are conventional anticoagulants (e.g., heparin), platelet-active drugs (e.g., aspirin, sulfinpyrazone, dipyridamole), and thrombolytic agents (e.g., tissue plasminogen activator [t-PA] and streptokinase [SK]). As acute interventions, all three classes have well documented effects on survival [7, 10, 11, 16–19], although there is no clear evidence that thrombolytic therapy benefits the patient during the first day after MI. Furthermore, it appears that their mechanisms are different and that the effects of a platelet-active agent (e.g., aspirin) and a thrombolytic agent (e.g., SK) are almost additive [18]. Although aspirin appears to have a small beneficial long-term effect on survival in MI patients, there is no strong evidence for the long-term beneficial effects of the other agents.
3. With the observation that more than one-half of all deaths among coronary patients are sudden, presumably due to ventricular arrhythmias, various classes of antiarrhythmic agents have been tested. Intravenous (IV) and oral agents have been tested with the expectation of reducing the risk of ventricular fibrillation. Unfortunately, many antiarrhythmic drugs can paradoxically also be arrhythmogenic (such as the class I drugs), and their use can lead to serious adverse effects. Overall, a reduction in short- or long-term mortality has not been demonstrated for most antiarrhythmics [20], possibly because (1) a reduction in ventricular arrhythmias does not translate into a reduction in mortality (an explanation that is contrary to other experimental evidence), (2) a true beneficial effect is hidden by the deficiencies in the methodology of the conducted studies, or (3) the arrhythmogenic effect outweighs the antiarrhythmic effect. However, there are a few antiarrhythmic treatments that have recently been receiving positive attention. For example, the class III agent amiodarone is currently being tested and a recently published meta-analysis of 1557 patients in nine completed clinical trials indicated a 29 percent reduction in mortality [20]. Also, meta-analyses of a few small trials of magnesium suggest that this agent reduces arrhythmias and possibly mortality [21, 22].
4. Until recently, limited attention was paid to patients with the most complicated MIs, primarily because it was difficult enough to find appropriate treatment for patients with uncomplicated infarctions. These patient groups include those with congestive heart failure (CHF), hypotension, and shock. Of potential interest are the direct-acting vasodilators (e.g., nitrates/nitroglycerin) [11, 23] and the angiotensin-converting enzyme (ACE) inhibitors (e.g., enalapril, captopril, and ramipril). Two recent trials demonstrated the efficacy of ACE inhibitors for postinfarction patients with heart failure. The first, the Survival and Ventricular Enlargement (SAVE) trial of captopril in 2231 postinfarction patients with poor ventricular function, showed a 19 percent reduction in all-cause mortality attributable to the agent [24]. Similarly, the Acute Infarction Ramipril Efficacy (AIRE) trial of ramipril in 2006 postinfarction patients with clinical evidence of failure showed a 27 percent reduction [25]. The roles of alpha blockers, diuretics, and inotropic agents (e.g., digitalis) in secondary prevention following an MI are still unclear. It is known, however, that long-term therapy with high-dose thiazide diuretics may lead to K^+ and Mg^+ depletion, which in turn can lead to serious arrhythmias.
5. Because an improvement in the balance between oxygen supply and demand can reduce the risk of recurrent ischemic events as well as of certain arrhythmias and mechanical failure, interventions that may improve this balance have been sought. Three types of such intervention have been evaluated in patients with AMI: physical exercise, calcium channel blockers, and beta blockers. Favorable evidence exists for the beneficial effects of moderate physical exercise [26], but the major problem with this intervention is the cooperation of the patient. Calcium channel

blockers (e.g., nifedipine, verapamil, diltiazem, and lidoflazine) have the ability to reduce vasospasm, but there is no proved benefit on short- or long-term mortality. In fact, pooled analyses suggest there is a slight increased risk of death and reinfarction with these agents [11, 27], particularly those calcium channel blockers that increase heart rate (the dihydropyridines) [20, 28]. On the other hand, a great deal of evidence has accrued demonstrating that beta blockers are the most effective prophylactic agents for the short- and long-term treatment of MI patients. If given within the first 24 hours of an AMI, first as an IV bolus then orally, beta blockers clearly and consistently have been shown to reduce in-hospital mortality [9, 11, 20, 29, 30]. In the long term, these agents have also been shown to be the most effective treatment for patients who have survived the acute phase of the MI.

Thus, the presumed major mechanisms for increased coronary mortality during the postinfarction period include cardiac arrhythmias, left ventricular (LV) dysfunction, persistent myocardial ischemia, and plaque instability. Increased levels of circulating catecholamines or enhanced sympathetic drive can increase both the severity of myocardial ischemia and the frequency of ventricular arrhythmias. After the clinical introduction of the beta blocker propranolol for angina pectoris and arrhythmias in 1963, it was conceived that beta blocker administration might favorably influence the acute and long-term course of MI patients by attenuating the undesirable consequences of increased sympathetic nervous system activity. However, because these drugs could also depress LV function, another major factor contributing to mortality after an MI, beta blockers were initially avoided in patients with AMI or were used in small doses for fear of causing, or aggravating existing, CHF.

Treatment During the Early 1970s: Recognized Need for a Prophylactic Agent

Through the middle of the twentieth century and up to and during the early 1970s, the primary treatment for an MI patient (who survived long enough to make it to the hospital) was bed rest. Drugs such as nitroglycerin were given symptomatically to alleviate pain, and early antiarrhythmics were given to reduce ventricular arrhythmias. New diagnostic and monitoring procedures became available and were more widely used. Innovative monitoring strategies such as the coronary care unit were also becoming more widely available. However, even as late as the early 1970s there still was no proved medical therapy available with a documented effect on the improved survival of MI patients.

In 1976 an international panel of experts in the field of coronary heart disease was brought together by the National Heart, Lung, and Blood Institute (NHLBI) to consider primary and secondary prevention strategies aimed at dealing with coronary heart disease mortality [31]. Particular emphasis was placed on the prevention of sudden cardiac death. A number of therapeutic regimens were considered, all of which were directed toward either the treatment and prevention of arrhythmias or the use of agents that might limit the extent of myocardial ischemia.

The panel recommended examining the possible effectiveness of the long-term administration of a beta blocker in survivors of AMI. The panelists recognized, as noted above, that an agent that could block the sympathetic nervous activity thought to be involved in precipitating sudden death and that also had nonneurologic antiarrhythmic properties would be of value to MI patients. In fact, beta blockers were already being prescribed for angina and arrhythmias. Moreover, a number of small clinical trials conducted primarily in Europe had already suggested that beta blockers may have a beneficial effect on the mortality rate (particularly the rate of sudden death) in patients who had experienced an AMI. However, clear proof of efficacy was lacking because of the small sample size and some methodologic deficiencies of these first-generation trials.

Based on the recommendation of the panel, the NHLBI initiated the Beta-Blocker Heart Attack Trial (BHAT) in 1977 [31]. This trial was to be a large-scale (about 4000 patients), double-blind, placebo-controlled, multicentered, long-term (up to 4 years) clinical trial of the efficacy of a particular beta blocker, propranolol (the only approved beta blocker in the United States at that time), given to survivors of AMI.

At approximately the same time, a number of other second-generation, large-scale, long-term studies of other beta blockers in post-MI patients were beginning or were just under way. For example, Merck Sharp & Dohme was beginning a large trial of timolol in Norway [32]; Julian and coworkers were examining the effects of sotalol [33]; and Taylor and coworkers were studying oxprenolol [34]. (These and other trials are described below.) Also, investigators were examining the short-term effects of beta-blocker therapy and the effects of different modes of administration. The results of all these investigations indicated that beta blockers are effective prophylactic agents in post-MI patients in both the short and the long term.

Pharmacology of Beta Blockers

The pharmacodynamic properties and cardiac effects of most of the commonly used and studied beta blockers are listed in Table 30-1 [35]. The differences in the agents may be useful for explaining the observed differences in the short- and long-term effects of the agents. It is clear now that, although there is a general class effect for beta blockers, this effect may be improved or diminished by the properties of a particular beta blocker, as is described below in the section outlining the results of the clinical trials of the drugs.

Beta blockers, also referred to as beta-adrenergic receptor blockers, are competitive inhibitors of the adrenergic receptors in the body. Two properties shared by all the agents are the ability to lower resting blood pressure and the existence of an antiarrhythmic effect. Three other important properties that a beta blocker may or may not have are cardioselectivity, intrinsic sympathomimetic activity (ISA), and membrane-stabilizing activity.

Cardioselectivity refers to the ability of some beta blockers to preferentially block the adrenergic receptors of the heart (the beta-1 receptors). Other beta blockers block the adrenergic receptors of both the heart (beta-1 receptors) and the bronchi and blood vessels (beta-2 receptors). These substances are often referred to as "unselective" agents.

Although it may appear that a cardioselective beta blocker would be preferable (to avoid the known effects of beta-2 blockers that can depress LV function and can cause or aggravate pulmonary problems), it may be that the generalized effect of the beta-2 blockers may benefit the MI patient. For example, it has been speculated that the hypokalemic effect of stress-induced adrenaline release and diuretic use could reduce serum potassium to dangerously low levels, which in turn could elicit

Table 30-1
Pharmacodynamic properties and cardiac effects of beta-blocking drugs

β-blocker	Cardioselectivity[a]	ISA[b]	Membrane-stabilizing activity	Resting heart rate	Myocardial contractility	Resting AV conduction	Antiarrhythmic effect	Potency ratio[c]
Acebutolol	Yes	+	+	↓	↓	↓	+	0.3
Alprenolol	No	++	+	↓↔	↓↔	↓↔	+	0.3
Atenolol	Yes	0	0	↓	↓	↓	+	1.0
Metoprolol	Yes	0	±	↓	↓	↓	+	1.0
Oxprenolol	No	++	+	↓↔	↓↔	↓↔	+	0.7
Pindolol	No	+++	+	↓↔	↓↔	↓↔	+	6.0
Practolol	Yes	++	0	↓↔	↓↔	↓↔	+	0.3
Propranolol	No	0	++	↓	↓	↓	+	1.0
Sotalol	No	0	0	↓	↓	↓	+	0.3
Timolol	No	±	0	↓	↓	↓	+	6.0

\+ = β-blocker has a positive effect; ± = β-blocker has mixed effects; ↓ = β-blocker decreases the activity; ↔ = β-blocker has no effect on the activity.
[a]Cardioselectivity is generally noted only at therapeutic doses.
[b]ISA = intrinsic sympathomimetic activity.
[c]β-blockade potency ratio (propranolol = 1.0).
Source: W. H. Frishman and R. Silverman. Physiologic and metabolic effects. In W. H. Frishman (ed.). *Clinical Pharmacology of the β-Adrenoceptor Blocking Drugs* (2nd ed.). Norwalk, CN: Appleton-Century-Crofts, 1984. With permission.

potentially life-threatening ventricular arrhythmias [36]. Theoretically, through beta-2-receptor blockade, a nonselective blocker could prevent the hypokalemic effects by slowing the cellular uptake of potassium.

Intrinsic sympathomimetic activity of beta blockers refers to the ability of some of the agents to partially stimulate adrenergic receptors. These agents are still referred to as receptor antagonists because while bound to the receptors (and partially stimulating them) they prevent the binding of more powerful stimulators, e.g., epinephrine and norepinephrine.

The theoretical advantages of beta blockers with ISA may be noted in Table 30-1. Note in Table 30-1 that all beta blockers can lower (or at least leave unchanged) the resting heart rate, myocardial contractility (i.e., cardiac output), and resting atrioventricular conduction. However, the agents with at least a moderate ISA effect may or may not lower these parameters. Thus, it may be hypothesized that patients taking these agents would have a lower incidence of cardiac mechanical problems compared with patients on beta blockers without ISA.

Membrane-stabilizing activity of a beta blocker refers to the ability of the agent to retard the rate of the rise of the intracardiac action potential while leaving the resting potential and the spike duration unchanged. This anesthetic, electrophysiologic effect is not mediated by beta receptors. Although a number of the agents can produce this effect, no beta blocker at therapeutic doses exhibits this activity. It is therefore questionable whether membrane-stablizing activity is of any clinical or therapeutic use.

Review of Clinical Trials of Postmyocardial Infarction Patients

Methods

The major outcome data of beta-blocker trials in AMI and over the long term following hospital discharge are presented below. We chose to consider those trials reported prior to November 1993 in which both intervention and follow-up were carried out during or beyond the time of hospital discharge. Mortality trials were included in this review if they met the following criteria: (1) random assignment of subjects to either a beta blocker or a control group, and (2) a total sample size of at least 100. These criteria were chosen for two important reasons. First, we wanted to restrict the review to trials that incorporated in their design some protection against treatment group allocation bias. Randomization provides this protection. Second, we wanted to focus on trials that possibly could have had sufficient statistical power, as judged by a relatively large sample size, to discern a clinically important effect or trend.

In this review, total mortality has been used whenever possible as the primary response variable, regardless of whether it was the choice in the published report. This point minimizes the potential bias inherent in endpoint determination, as total mortality relies only on a simple count, with no element of judgment.

To reduce the bias that may come about from the differential withdrawal of patients, we have followed the "intention-to-treat principle" for the analyses. That is, all patients who were randomized in a trial were included in the mortality estimates (to the extent the data were available).

Because many of the trials presented only the number of deaths for each treatment group, classic survival curves could not be computed. Therefore, we chose to compare the proportion of deaths in each treatment group by a χ^2 test so that there might be some consistency in the analyses. We recognize that this method provides only an approximation to the comparison of survival curves, but it is our experience that the results are usually similar.

Other endpoints presented in this review are serum enzyme levels (as a surrogate for infarct size) and nonfatal reinfarction. Because the trials that examined the effect of a beta blocker on serum enzymes were not always large, we did not restrict the trials we present to only those with more than 100 patients.

When differences for endpoints other than total mortality are said in this review to be statistically significant, in most instances this is the conclusion of the published report and usually denotes a conventional p value of less than .05.

In this review we also present data examining the short-term versus the long-term effects of beta-blocker administration, as well as data examining the differences between the intravenous and oral administration of the agents.

Results

Short-Term Oral Trials

Eight published trials meeting the review criteria [37–44] evaluated the effect of short-term, oral administration of beta blockers (Table 30-2). In three of the trials, treatment continued beyond the hospital stay or for more than 28 days. The early trials represent the first-generation beta-blocker trials. The beta-blocking doses were generally low compared with those shown to be effective in subsequent trials. In seven of the eight trials the patients were enrolled within 24 hours of the onset of symptoms. The other trial enrolled patients within 72 hours. Propranolol was tested in five trials; alprenolol, practolol, atenolol, and oxprenolol were tested in one trial each. One trial evaluated two beta blockers. All the trials were fairly small, the largest enrolling 454 patients.

In none of the trials was beta-blocker therapy shown to be effective (Table 30-3). Overall, there were 101 deaths among 1147 patients (8.8 percent) allocated to the beta-blocker groups compared with 100 deaths among 1017 control patients (9.8 percent). The overall relative efficacy is thus a 10 percent difference in mortality among the beta-blocker patients (not statistically significant).

Five other published and unpublished trials did not meet review criteria. However, their overall mortality trends were similar to those of the reviewed trials.

Table 30-2
Eight short-term mortality trials of oral beta blockers

Investigator	Year of report	β-blocker	Dose (mg)	Initiation of treatment	Days of treatment
Balcon [37]	1966	Propranolol	20 qid	Admission	28
Clausen [38]	1966	Propranolol	10 qid	Pain <24 hr	14
Multicentre [39]	1966	Propranolol	20 qid	Pain <24 hr	28
Norris [40]	1968	Propranolol	20 qid	Pain <72 hr	21
Briant [41]	1970	Alprenolol	100 qid	Admission	3 (mean)
Barber [42]	1976	Practolol	300 bid	Admission	90
Wilcox [43]	1980	Propranolol/ atenolol	40 tid 50 bid	Pain < 24 hr	42
Wilcox [44]	1980	Oxprenolol	40 tid	Pain <24 hr	42

Table 30-3
Eight short-term mortality trials of oral beta blockers: Mortality experience

		Control group		β-blocker group				
Investigator	β-blocker	Deaths/no. of pts.	%	Deaths/no. of pts.	%	Absolute efficacy (/100)	Relative efficacy (%)	p
Balcon	Propranolol	15/58	25.9	14/56	25.0	0.9	−3	NS
Clausen	Propranolol	19/64	29.7	18/66	27.3	2.4	−8	NS
Multicentre	Propranolol	12/95	12.6	15/100	15.0	−2.4	+19	NS
Norris	Propranolol	24/228	10.5	21/226	9.3	1.2	−12	NS
Briant	Alprenolol	4/57	7.0	5/62	8.1	−1.1	+15	NS
Barber	Practolol	15/228	6.6	14/221	6.3	0.3	−4	NS
Wilcox	Propranolol/ atenolol	7/129	5.4	8/259	3.1	2.3	−43	NS
Wilcox	Oxprenolol	4/158	2.5	6/157	3.8	−1.3	+51	NS
Total		100/1017	9.8	101/1147	8.8	1.0	−10	

pts. = patients; p = p value.

Short-Term Intravenous/Oral Trials: Mortality and Serum Enzyme Changes

In 14 trials that met our review criteria for mortality analysis [29, 45–57], an initial IV loading dose was given during the acute phase of the MI and was followed by oral medication for the remainder of the trial (Table 30-4). The trials, reported between 1979 and 1986, comprise the second-generation beta-blocker trials. In contrast to the previous trials that initiated treatment with an oral dose generally within 24 hours of symptoms, the patients in the new trials were enrolled as early as possible, usually within 6 to 8 hours. Although treatment varied from 27 hours to 1 year for these trials, the data presented below reflect 7-day mortality. Seven beta blockers were tested. The differences in drug dosages reflect varying beta-blocking potency.

The results of our review are presented in Table 30-5. Two trials reported a statistically significant benefit of beta-blocker use. In the larger trial (International Study of Infarct Survival [ISIS]), 317 of the 8037 patients allocated to receive atenolol died (3.9 percent) compared with 367 of the 7990 control patients (4.6 percent), a 14 percent relative reduction in mortality. A pooled analysis shows that in the 14 reviewed trials 497 of 13,442 beta-blocker patients died (3.7 percent) compared with 569 of 13,358 control patients (4.3 percent). Thirteen trials that did not meet our review criteria would have added a total of approximately 700 patients to the database. Their overall mortality trends were similar to those of the reviewed trials.

Further analyses of the ISIS data and of pooled trial results indicate that the benefit of intravenous/oral beta-blocker use in AMI patients is seen primarily within the first 24 hours when the mortality rate is the highest.

Low 7-day mortality rates may be noted among the control patients with an AMI in these trials (see Table 30-5). This finding may be explained by the trial eligibility criteria that were employed. As many as one-half the patients admitted to a hospital with an AMI had absolute or relative contraindications to beta-blocker therapy. For example, the excluded patients had a higher prevalence of CHF.

Unfortunately, the data do not allow a comparison of the effects on mortality among the various beta blockers. It may be said, however, that atenolol had a well documented benefit, and that there is no evidence that metoprolol, a beta blocker without ISA, is more effective than other beta blockers without this activity.

A previous review of beta blockers presented data on the effects of IV beta blockade on serum enzyme levels (as a surrogate for infarct size) in

Table 30-4
Fourteen short-term mortality trials of IV/oral beta blockers

Investigator	Year of report	β-blocker	Dose (mg) IV	Dose (mg) PO (daily)	Initiation of treatment (hr)	Duration of treatment
Andersen [45]	1979	Alprenolol	5	400	6 (median)	1 year
Hjalmarson [46]	1983	Metoprolol	15	200	11.3 (mean)	3 months
Yusuf [47]	1983	Atenolol	5	100	<12	10 days
UKCSG [48]	1984	Timolol	2 + 14[a]	10	<6	In hosp.
ICSG [49]	1984	Timolol	2 +14[a]	10	<6	In hosp.
Federman [50]	1984	Timolol	5.5	20	<6	28 days
Heber [51]	1984	Labetalol	[b]	[b]	<6	5 days
Norris [52]	1984	Propranolol	0.1/kg	320	<6	27 hours
MILIS [53]	1984	Propranolol	0.1/kg	[c]	8 (mean)	9 days
Owensby [54]	1984	Pindolol	3	15	<12	3 days
MIAMI [55]	1985	Metoprolol	15	200	<24	16 days
Salathia [56]	1985	Metoprolol	15	200	<6	1 year
TIARA [57]	1986	Timolol	5.5	20	<6	1 month
ISIS [29]	1986	Atenolol	5–10	100	<12	7 days

[a]Infused over 24 hours.
[b]Dose-dependent on blood pressure.
[c]Dose-dependent on blood pressure and heart rate.

28 short-term trials [9]. Eleven of the trials met our review criteria [47, 49, 53, 55, 58–64] and are presented in Table 30-6. Eight of the eleven trials began beta-blocker treatment within 12 hours of the onset of pain. Most of the trials were small, with fewer than 50 patients allocated to the beta-blocker group.

Overall, beta blockers appear to have a moderate effect on enzyme levels, especially those trials that began beta-blocker therapy within 12 hours. For the three trials that began therapy after 12 hours, there was no reduction in the level of the serum enzymes. Also, the wide variety of such agents that produce the observed effect suggests that it is a function of beta blockade in general and not a function of cardioselectivity or ISA.

For the 17 trials that did not meet our strict review criteria, the overall trends in enzyme reduc-

Table 30-5
Fourteen short-term mortality trials of IV/oral beta blockers: Mortality experience

		Control group		β-blocker group				
Investigator	β-blocker	Deaths/no. of pts.	%	Deaths/no. of pts.	%	Absolute efficacy (/100)	Relative efficacy (%)	p
Andersen	Alprenolol	24/242	9.9	28/238	11.8	−1.9	+19	NS
Hjalmarson	Metoprolol	23/697	3.3	18/698	2.6	0.7	−22	NS
Yusuf	Atenolol	16/233	6.9	6/244	2.5	4.4	−64	<.05
UKCSG	Timolol	5/52	9.6	4/56	7.1	2.5	−26	NS
ICSG	Timolol	4/71	5.6	3/73	4.1	1.5	−27	NS
Federman	Timolol	0/51	0.0	1/50	2.0	—	—	—
Heber	Labetalol	0/83	0.0	3/83	3.6	—	—	—
Norris	Propranolol	10/371	2.7	12/364	3.3	−0.6	+22	NS
MILIS	Propranolol	4/135	3.0	4/134	3.0	0.0	0	NS
Owensby	Pindolol	1/50	2.0	1/50	2.0	0.0	0	NS
MIAMI	Metoprolol	93/2901	3.2	79/2877	2.7	0.5	−14	NS
Salathia	Metoprolol	17/384	4.4	18/416	4.3	0.1	−2	NS
TIARA	Timolol	5/98	5.1	3/102	2.9	2.2	−42	NS
ISIS	Atenolol	367/7990	4.6	317/8037	3.9	0.7	−14	<.05
Total		569/13,358	4.3	497/13,422	3.7	0.6	−13	

pts. = patients; p = p value.

Table 30-6
Effects of IV beta blockade on serum enzyme levels in short-term trials

Investigator	β-blocker	Entered pts. within 12 hr of pain	No. on β-blocker	Enzyme	Observed reduction (%)	p
Waagstein [58]	Practolol or H87/07 or metoprolol	Yes	39	Max GOT	−5 (increase)	NS
Evemy [59]	Practolol	No	46	AST	0	NS
Peter [60]	Propranolol	Yes	47	CK	10	NS
Norris [61]	Propranolol	Yes	20	CK	52	NS
Norris [62]	Propranolol	Yes	33	CK	25	<.05
Mueller [63]	Propranolol	Yes	44	CK, CK-MB	"No change"	NS
Azancot [64]	Acebutolol	No	14	CK-MB	0	NS
Yusuf [47]	Atenolol	Yes	244	CK-MB	30	<.001
ICSG [49]	Timolol	Yes	73	CK	30	<.05
MILIS [53]	Propranolol	No	134	CK-MB	−2 (increase)	NS
MIAMI [55]	Metoprolol	Yes	2877	ASAT	11	<.05

pts. = patients; p = p value.

tion were almost identical to those of the reviewed trials.

Long-Term Oral Trials: Mortality and Reinfarction

Twenty published and unpublished randomized controlled trials have evaluated the long-term effect of beta blockers on all-cause mortality [32–34, 42, 43, 45, 56, 65–77]. For this review, long-term has arbitrarily been defined as at least 1 year of treatment and follow-up. Again, our review was restricted to trials that had a total sample size of more than 100 patients. Thus, four trials were excluded because they were less than a year in duration, and two were excluded because they had fewer than 100 patients. One trial that was included in the list was actually slightly less than a year in average duration (mean, 318 days) because the trial was terminated early [77].

The 20 trials we selected were reported between the years 1974 and 1990 and are described in Table 30-7. Treatment was usually initiated prior to hospital discharge. Only four trials had a mean duration of treatment of more than 2 years. Ten beta blockers were tested, although the largest databases exist for propranolol, metoprolol, oxprenolol, practolol, and timolol.

The mortality results are presented in Table 30-8. Five trials showed a statistically significant reduction in all-cause mortality: the Norwegian Timolol Trial, the BHAT (propranolol) trial, the trial by Schwartz and coworkers (oxprenolol), the trial by Salathia and coworkers (metoprolol), and the trial by Boissel and coworkers (acebutolol). In the Lopressor Intervention Trial (LIT) of metoprolol statistical significance emerges only if deaths during the first week of therapy are excluded.

Overall, there were 1042 deaths among 10,480 control patients. This figure corresponds to an average mortality of 9.9 percent. The mortality was 21 percent lower among the beta-blocker-treated patients. Among the 11,021 beta-blocker patients there were 858 deaths, corresponding to an average mortality rate of 7.8 percent. The average relative mortality reduction in the trials of beta blockers without ISA was 40 percent higher than that of the trials with ISA (25 percent reduction versus 18

Table 30-7
Twenty long-term (1 year or longer) mortality trials of oral beta blockers

Investigator	Year of report	β-blocker	Daily dose (mg)	Initiation of treatment post-MI	Duration of treatment
Wilhelmsson [65]	1974	Alprenolol	400	6 weeks	2 years
Ahlmark [66]	1974	Alprenolol	400	2 weeks	2 years
Barber [42]	1976	Practolol	600	3 hr (median)	2 years
Multicentre [67]	1977	Practolol	400	13 days (mean)	15 mo (mean)
Andersen [45]	1979	Alprenolol	400	6 hr (median)	1 year
Wilcox [43]	1980	Propranolol/ atenolol	120 100	<24 hr	1 year
Rehnqvist [68]	1980	Metoprolol	200	Discharge	1 year
Norwegian [32]	1981	Timolol	20	7–28 days	17 mo (mean)
Taylor [34]	1982	Oxprenolol	80	13 mo (mean)	4 years (mean)
Hansteen [69]	1982	Propranolol	160	5 days (mean)	1 year
BHAT [70]	1982	Propranolol	180/240	10 days (mean)	25 mo (mean)
Julian [33]	1982	Sotalol	320	5 days	1 year
Australian-Swedish [71]	1983	Pindolol	15	2–21 days	2 years
Manger Cats [72]	1983	Metoprolol	200	4 weeks (mean)	1 year
EIS [73]	1984	Oxprenolol	320	24 days (median)	1 year
Olsson [74]	1985	Metoprolol	200	Before discharge	3 years
Salathia [56]	1985	Metoprolol	200	<6 hr	1 year
Schwartz [75]	1985	Oxprenolol	160	Not available	~4 years
LIT [76]	1987	Metoprolol	200	10 days (mean)	1 year
Boissel [77]	1990	Acebutolol	400	10.5 days (mean)	up to 1 year

Table 30-8
Twenty long-term (1 year or longer) mortality trials of oral beta blockers: Mortality experience

		Control group		β-blocker group				
Investigator	β-blocker	Deaths/no. of pts.	%	Deaths/no. of pts.	%	Absolute efficacy (/100)	Relative efficacy (%)	p
Wilhelmsson	Alprenolol	14/116	12.1	7/114	6.1	6.0	−49	NS
Ahlmark	Alprenolol	11/93	11.8	5/69	7.2	4.6	−39	NS
Barber	Practolol	38/213	17.8	33/207	15.9	1.9	−11	NS
Multicentre	Practolol	127/1520	8.4	102/1533	6.7	1.7	−20	NS
Andersen	Alprenolol	40/218	18.3	32/209	15.3	3.0	−17	NS
Wilcox	Propranolol/atenolol	12/122	9.8	28/251	11.2	−1.4	+13	NS
Rehnqvist	Metoprolol	6/52	11.5	4/59	6.8	4.7	−41	NS
Norwegian	Timolol	152/939	16.2	98/945	10.4	5.8	−36	<.001
Taylor	Oxprenolol	48/471	10.2	60/632	9.5	0.7	−7	NS
Hansteen	Propranolol	37/282	13.1	25/278	9.0	4.1	−31	NS
BHAT	Propranolol	188/1921	9.8	138/1916	7.2	2.6	−26	<.01
Julian	Sotalol	52/583	8.9	64/873	7.3	1.6	−18	NS
Australian-Swedish	Pindolol	47/266	17.7	45/263	17.1	0.6	−3	NS
Manger Cats	Metoprolol	16/293	5.5	9/291	3.1	2.4	−43	NS
EIS	Oxprenolol	45/883	5.1	57/858	6.6	−1.5	+30	NS
Olsson	Metoprolol	31/147	21.1	25/154	16.2	4.9	−23	NS
Salathia	Metoprolol	43/364	11.8	27/391	6.9	4.9	−42	<.05
Schwartz	Oxprenolol	39/488	8.0	17/485	3.5	4.5	−56	<.01
LIT	Metoprolol	62/1200	5.2	65/1195	5.4	−0.2	+5	NS
Boissel	Acebutolol	34/309	11.0	17/298	5.7	5.3	−48	<.02
Total		1042/10,480	9.9	858/11,021	7.8	2.1	−21	

pts. = patients; p = p value.

Table 30-9
Nonfatal reinfarction experience in 15 long-term (1 year or longer) trials of oral beta blockers

		Control group		β-blocker group				
Investigator	β-blocker	Events/no. of pts.	%	Events/no. of pts.	%	Absolute efficacy (/100)	Relative efficacy (%)	p
Wilhelmsson [52]	Alprenolol	18/116	15.5	16/114	14.0	1.5	−10	NS
Ahlmark [53]	Alprenolol	14/93	15.1	3/69	4.3	10.8	−71	<.05
Barber [29]	Practolol	21/226	9.3	9/222	4.1	5.2	−56	<.05
Multicentre [54]	Practolol	97/1520	6.4	75/1533	4.9	1.5	−23	NS
Rehnqvist [55]	Metoprolol	5/52	9.6	3/59	5.1	4.5	−47	NS
Norwegian [19]	Timolol	131/939	14.0	90/945	9.5	4.5	−32	<.01
Taylor [21]	Oxprenolol	58/471	12.3	67/632	10.6	1.7	−14	NS
Hansteen [56]	Propranolol	21/282	7.4	16/278	5.8	1.6	−23	NS
BHAT [64]	Propranolol	121/1921	6.3	103/1916	5.4	0.9	−15	NS
Julian [20]	Sotalol	22/583	3.8	24/873	2.7	1.1	−27	NS
Australian-Swedish [58]	Pindolol	28/266	10.5	25/263	9.5	1.0	−10	NS
Manger Cats [59]	Metoprolol	20/293	6.8	16/291	5.5	1.3	−19	NS
EIS [60]	Oxprenolol	38/883	4.3	36/858	4.2	0.1	−3	NS
Olsson [61]	Metoprolol	31/147	21.1	18/154	11.7	9.4	−45	<.05
Boissel [77]	Acebutolol	4/309	1.3	6/298	2.0	−0.7	+56	NS
Total		629/8101	7.8	507/8505	6.0	1.8	−23	

pts. = patients; p = p value.

percent reduction). The average mortality reduction of the unselective beta blockers was almost identical to that of the selective beta blockers (22 percent reduction versus 21 percent reduction).

The long-term effect of oral beta blockers on the rate of nonfatal reinfarction was also examined. Fifteen of the long-term mortality trials that met our review criteria also presented reinfarction data [32–34, 42, 65–69, 71–74, 77, 78]. The results are presented in Table 30-9. (Descriptions of the trials are found in Table 30-7.)

Most trials found a favorable trend with long-term oral beta-blocker use. Four trials showed a statistically significant reduction in events among the beta-blocker patients. In pooled analysis, there was an overall 24 percent reduction in the incidence of nonfatal reinfarction.

The accumulation of data from all the short- and long-term trials indicates clearly that beta blockers, whether given acutely or over the long term, reduce all-cause mortality and nonfatal reinfarction. Specifically, although there is no specific evidence that short-term oral therapy alone is effective, there is strong evidence that a combination of intravenous (especially soon after the onset of symptoms) and oral beta blockers effectively prevents premature mortality. There is also evidence that in the short term beta blockers can reduce serum enzymes, a finding suggestive that beta blockers can reduce infarct size. Finally, there is overwhelming scientific evidence that in the long term beta blockers reduce both the incidence of nonfatal reinfarction and the occurrence of all-cause mortality.

The trials also raised several questions, many of which relate directly to clinical care. Data from the trials will be used in an attempt to address the questions.

Beta Blockers During and After Acute Myocardial Infarction: Evidence from Trials

What Are the Mechanisms of Beta-Blocker Action?

The reduction in all-cause mortality was due to a reduction in atherosclerotic cardiovascular deaths. The benefit is explained particularly by prevention of sudden cardiac deaths. For example, the mortality experience of BHAT is presented in Table 30-10 [70]. These data are typical of the long-term trials and demonstrate that not only do post-MI patients die more frequently of cardiovascular problems than of noncardiovascular problems but that propranolol is significantly effective in reducing the absolute and relative risks of atherosclerotic death in general and sudden atherosclerotic death in particular.

These data suggest that beta blockers exert their favorable effect by reducing the frequency and severity of arrhythmias. Such a statement is further

Table 30-10
Cause-specific mortality by treatment group: BHAT[a]

Cause of death	Placebo group (N = 1921) No. of deaths	Placebo group (N = 1921) Rate (%)	Propranolol group (N = 1916) No. of deaths	Propranolol group (N = 1916) Rate (%)	Absolute efficacy (/100)	Relative efficacy (%)	p
Total mortality	188	9.8	138	7.2	2.6	−26	<.01
Noncardiovascular	17	0.9	11	0.6	0.3	−35	NS
Cardiovascular	171	8.9	127	6.6	2.3	−26	<.01
Nonatherosclerotic	7	0.4	8	0.4	0.0	0	NS
Atherosclerotic	164	8.5	119	6.2	2.3	−27	<.01
Nonsudden	75	3.9	55	2.9	1.0	−26	NS
Sudden[b]	89	4.6	64	3.3	1.3	−28	<.05

p = p value.
[a]Average length of follow-up was 25 months.
[b]Atherosclerotic death within 1 hour of symptoms.
Source: Beta-Blocker Heart Attack Trial Research Group. A randomized trial of propranolol in patients with acute myocardial infarction. I. Mortality results. *J.A.M.A.* 247:1707, 1982. Copyright 1982. American Medical Association.

supported in Table 30-11 by an examination of the instantaneous death rates in BHAT [79], the Norwegian Timolol Trial [32], and a propranolol study reported by Hansteen et al. in 1982 [69]. In all three trials, there was again a large reduction in both the absolute and relative risks due to beta blocker use.

Furthermore, the prevalence of ventricular arrhythmias at baseline and 6 weeks after randomization was examined per treatment group in a sample of BHAT patients [80] (Table 30-12). Although the prevalence of arrhythmia at 6 weeks was higher in both treatment groups among patients with arrhythmias at baseline, there was still an overall 40 percent reduction of arrhythmia among the propranolol patients (19.9 percent prevalence among the propranolol patients versus 33.0 percent prevalence among the placebo patients).

Stratifying the BHAT patients by the presence or absence of complex ventricular premature beats (VPBs) at baseline reveals that there is a greater relative reduction in mortality among patients with VPBs [81]. As may be noted in Figure 30-1, there is a 31 percent propranolol-attributable reduction in total mortality among patients with complex VPBs and a 28 percent reduction in sudden death. For patients without the arrhythmia, the respective figures are lower: 25 and 16 percent.

Finally, experimental studies have shown that beta blockers raise the threshold for ventricular fibrillation in ischemic myocardium. A reduction in the incidence of ventricular fibrillation (cardiac arrest) during beta blockade has also been noted in some trials (Table 30-13), although the effect in two of the trials is small.

There is much evidence that beta blockers exert their effect by an antiarrhythmic mechanism, but it should be noted that there is also evidence that other mechanisms may be operating as well. For example, the observed reductions in nonsudden death (see Table 30-10) and nonfatal reinfarctions (see Table 30-9) suggest an anti-ischemic effect. This mechanism may be separate from the antianginal effect of the beta blockers, as other compounds with antianginal properties do not influence survival (e.g., calcium channel blockers).

Table 30-11
Instantaneous death rates in three long-term beta-blocker trials

			Instantaneous death rate (%)			
Trial	Year of report	β-blocker	Control group	β-blocker group	Absolute efficacy (/100)	Relative efficacy (%)
Norwegian [32]	1981	Timolol	4.7	1.9	2.8	−60
Hansteen [69]	1982	Propranolol	6.0	3.2	2.8	−47
BHAT [79]	1987	Propranolol	3.5	2.2	1.3	−37
Total			4.1	2.2	1.9	−46

Table 30-12
Prevalence of ventricular arrhythmia at 6 weeks postrandomization by presence of ventricular arrhythmia at baseline and by treatment group: BHAT

	Placebo group		Propranolol group		
VA at baseline	VA at 6 wk/no. of pts.	%	VA at 6 wk/no. of pts.	%	% difference in VA
Yes	44/59	74.6	25/52	48.1	−36
No	92/353	26.1	60/376	16.0	−39
Total	136/412	33.0	85/428	19.9	−40

VA = ventricular arrhythmia (defined as at least 10 VPBs/hr on a 24-hour ambulatory electrocardiogram; pts. = patients.
Source: J. Morganroth et al. Beta-Blocker Heart Attack Trial—impact of propranolol therapy on ventricular arrhythmias. *Prev. Med.* 14:346, 1985. With permission.

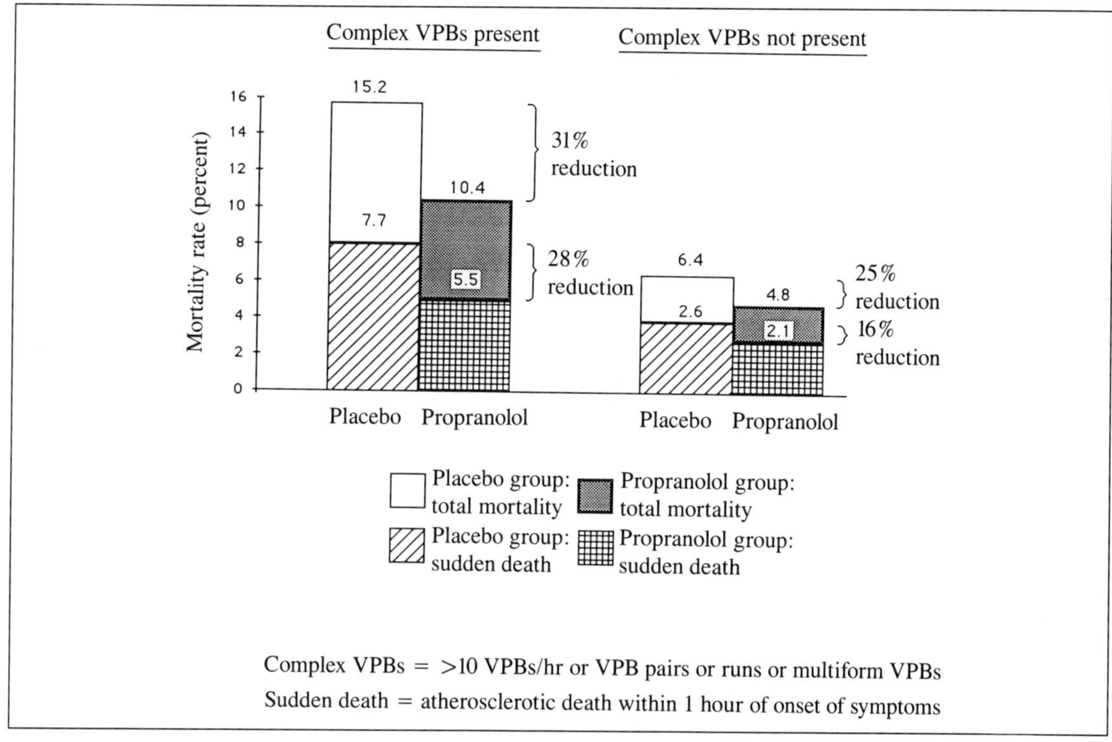

Fig. 30-1
Total mortality and sudden death rates (percent) by the presence of complex ventricular premature beats (VPBs) at baseline, by treatment group in the Beta-Blocker Heart Attack Trial. The average length of follow-up was 25 months. (From L. M. Friedman et al. Effect of propranolol in patients with myocardial infarction and ventricular arrhythmia. *J. Am. Coll. Cardiol.* 7:1, 1986. With permission.)

Table 30-13
Incidence of ventricular fibrillation in acute beta-blocker trials

		Control group		β-blocker group			
Investigator (length of follow-up)	β-blocker	Events/no. of pts.	%	Events/no. of pts.	%	Absolute efficacy (/100)	Relative efficacy (%)
ISIS [29] (7 days)	Atenolol	198/7990	2.5	189/8037	2.4	0.1	−5
MIAMI [55] (15 days)	Metoprolol	52/2901	1.8	48/2877	1.7	0.1	−7
Norris [52] (48 hr)	Propranolol	14/371	3.8	2/364	0.5	3.3	−85

pts. = patients.

Other mechanisms for the beta blockers have also been hypothesized, although there is no experimental evidence for them [9]. They include an infarct reduction mechanism, increased vascularity mechanisms, scar reduction mechanisms, and antiplatelet mechanisms.

Who Should Get a Beta Blocker?

For an MI patient who does not have any contraindication to a beta blocker (discussed below), the question naturally arises: Which of these patients would benefit the most from beta-blocker therapy and which would benefit the least? The overall clinical trial experience indicates that beta blockers have a greater effect in some patients than in others and that the effect is, to a large extent, a function of how complicated the MI is.

For example, post hoc analyses of the BHAT data suggest that the patients with uncomplicated MIs (and an already low annual mortality) benefit to a small degree from propranolol therapy [82]. The BHAT all-cause mortality rates are stratified by treatment group and by the presence or absence of transient electrical or mechanical cardiac complications at baseline in Table 30-14. In the large subgroup of patients with no complications, the observed relative benefit of propranolol was only 6 percent (relative risk 0.94). The most pronounced relative difference in mortality between the two study groups was observed in the subgroup with electrical problems only. Here, the mortality in the propranolol group was roughly one-half that in the placebo group (relative risk 0.48). In the two risk groups with mechanical complications, the relative difference in mortality was 38 and 25 percent, respectively. These relative differences remained basically unchanged after adjustment for possible confounding variables. The highest absolute risk reduction was found in the subgroup with either electrical or mechanical problems: four to six lives were prolonged for every 100 patients treated over an average period of 25 months.

A more detailed analysis of the individual electrical and mechanical complications in these patients is shown in Table 30-15. Patients who had suffered an episode of ventricular tachycardia during hospitalization made up the single largest subgroup. Among these patients, mortality was 44 percent lower in the propranolol group than in the control group. The greatest absolute efficacy and the lowest relative risk, which suggest that patients received special benefit from propranolol therapy, were observed in the small subgroup of patients who had experienced ventricular fibrillation (23 lives prolonged for every 200 such patients treated, a 63 percent reduction in mortality). The smallest absolute efficacy and the highest relative risk, which suggest little benefit from propranolol therapy, were observed in the small subgroup of patients who had experienced pulmonary edema (only one life prolonged for every 200 such patients treated, or a 2 percent reduction in mortality).

The cumulative life table curves for the BHAT data stratified by treatment group and by the presence/absence of any electrical/mechanical problem are shown in Figure 30-2. The difference in the treatment group curves for the high-risk patients is

Table 30-14
All-cause mortality by risk and treatment groups: BHAT[a]

	Placebo group		Propranolol group				
Risk group	No. of pts.	Mortality rate (%)	No. of pts.	Mortality rate (%)	Absolute efficacy (/100)	Relative efficacy (%)	Adjusted relative efficacy[b] (%)
No electrical or mechanical complications	1079	6.6	1047	6.2	0.4	−6	−4
Electrical complications only	423	10.9	443	5.2	5.7	−52	−57
Mechanical complications only	202	16.8	201	10.4	6.4	−38	−43
Both electrical and mechanical complications	217	17.1	225	12.9	4.2	−25	−30

pts. = patients.
[a]Average length of follow-up was 25 months.
[b]Adjusted for 13 variables predictive of mortality.
Source: C. D. Furberg et al. Effect of propranolol in post-infarction patients with mechanical or electrical complications. *Circulation* 69:761, 1984. By permission of the American Heart Association, Inc.

Table 30-15
All-cause mortality by reported complication during hospitalization before enrollment and by treatment group: BHAT*

Complication	Placebo group		Propranolol group		Absolute efficacy (/100)	Relative efficacy (%)
	No. of pts.	Mortality rate (%)	No. of pts.	Mortality rate (%)		
Electrical						
Ventricular fibrillation	99	18.2	104	6.7	11.5	−63
Ventricular tachycardia	446	12.1	441	6.8	5.3	−44
Complete AV block	44	15.9	54	9.3	6.6	−42
Incomplete AV block	153	12.4	158	8.9	3.5	−28
Atrial fibrillation	109	14.7	131	11.5	3.2	−22
Mechanical						
Pulmonary edema	51	19.6	52	19.2	0.4	−2
Cardiogenic shock	21	14.3	29	10.3	4.0	−28
Persistent hypotension	133	12.0	142	9.2	2.8	−23
Basilar rales	57	22.8	58	13.8	9.0	−39
Signs/symptoms of CHF	287	17.4	274	13.5	3.9	−22

pts. = patients.
*Average length of follow-up was 25 months.
Source: C. D. Furberg et al. Effect of propranolol in post-infarction patients with mechanical or electrical complications. *Circulation* 69:761, 1984. By permission of the American Heart Association, Inc.

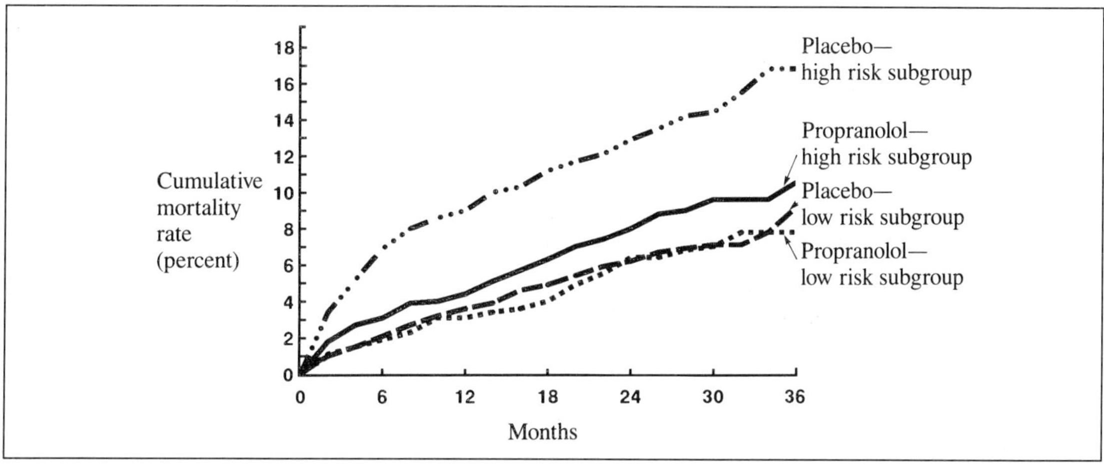

Fig. 30-2
Cumulative life table mortality curves by risk group and by treatment group in the Beta-Blocker Heart Attack Trial. High risk = presence of any of the following at baseline: complete or incomplete AV block, ventricular fibrillation or tachycardia, atrial fibrillation, pulmonary edema, cardiogenic shock, persistent hypotension, congestive heart failure, or basilar rates. (From C. D. Furberg et al. Effect of propranolol in post-infarction patients with mechanical or electrical complications. *Circulation* 69:761, 1984. By permission of the American Heart Association, Inc.)

dramatic, whereas there is little difference in the treatment group curves for the low-risk patients.

Similar observations have been noted in other trials, although a common problem in all the trials is inadequate subgroup design and the lack of statistical power to detect real benefit in any subgroup of patients. The Beta-Blocker Pooling Project (BBPP) published its results in 1988 [83]. The overall goals for the BBPP were to overcome the problems inherent in the analysis of one trial and to combine the results of the nine largest long-term secondary-prevention trials of beta blockers to determine whether there were subgroups of MI patients who benefited the most from beta-blocker therapy.

When the results of nine large trials were combined, the investigators of the BBPP found that patients with a high risk of mortality were those most likely to benefit both absolutely and relatively from beta-blocker therapy. All the trials specifically included patients with nonsevere electrical or mechanical complications at the time of their infarction. Furthermore, the investigators found that lower-risk MI patients also benefited from beta-blocker therapy, although the absolute and relative benefits were small.

The clinical trial experience of beta-blocker use in the elderly is limited, but there seems to be good rationale to extrapolate overall results to this population, if only because the proportion of complicated MI increases with age. For example, in the BHAT a trend toward an even greater benefit was observed in patients 60 years of age or older when compared to MI patients younger than 60 [84]. Table 30-16 presents BHAT mortality statistics for MI patients 30 to 59 years of age (N = 2589) and 60 to 69 years of age (N = 1248). For patients less than 60 years of age, approximately 90 percent of all deaths were atherosclerotic in nature, and the observed benefit from propranolol was largely due to a decrease in sudden deaths. For patients 60 years or older, approximately 83 percent of all deaths were atherosclerotic in nature, and the overall reduction in mortality in the propranolol group was due primarily to a large reduction of atherosclerotic sudden and nonsudden deaths.

The BBPP produced similar results [83], with some refinement. For patients younger than 50 years of age, the pooled data provided no evidence of beta-blocker benefit (relative risk 0.97, only a 3 percent reduction in mortality). For patients 60 years of age or older, there was evidence of a moderate benefit (relative risk 0.83, a 17 percent reduction in mortality). For patients 50 to 59 years of age, however, there was evidence of relatively large

Table 30-16
Cause-specific mortality by age and treatment groups: BHAT[a]

Cause of death	Mortality rate (%): Placebo group	Mortality rate (%): Propranolol group	Absolute efficacy (/100)	Relative efficacy (%)
Age 30–59 years				
Total mortality	7.4	6.0	1.4	−19
Cardiovascular	6.8	5.7	1.1	−16
Atherosclerotic	6.5	5.5	1.0	−15
Nonsudden	2.7	2.5	0.2	−7
Sudden[b]	3.8	3.1	0.7	−18
Age 60–69 years				
Total mortality	14.7	9.8	4.9	−33
Cardiovascular	13.1	8.6	4.5	−34
Atherosclerotic	12.6	7.6	5.0	−40
Nonsudden	6.3	3.7	2.6	−41
Sudden[b]	6.3	3.9	2.4	−38

Propranolol group 30–59 years = 1301 patients; propranolol group 60–69 years = 615 patients; placebo group 30–59 years = 1288 patients; placebo group 60–69 years = 633 patients.
[a]Average length of follow-up was 25 months.
[b]Atherosclerotic death within 1 hour of symptoms.
Source: From C. M. Hawkins et al. Effect of propranolol in reducing mortality in older myocardial infarction patients. *Circulation* 67(Suppl I):94, 1983. By permission of the American Heart Association, Inc.

benefit (relative risk 0.63, a 37 percent reduction in mortality).

Finally, when deciding which patients to treat prophylactically, one should keep in mind that there are other indications for long-term beta-blocker use, e.g., angina pectoris, hypertension, and the presence of ventricular arrhythmias.

Who Should Not Get a Beta Blocker?

From the early trials of beta blockers, it is known that approximately one-half of all patients admitted early with an AMI and about 20 percent of those surviving 1 to 3 weeks have relative or absolute contraindications to beta-blocker treatment. Contraindications include hypotension, bradycardia, severe CHF, atrioventricular conduction disorders, and obstructive lung disease.

Although most of the large clinical trials actively avoided recruiting MI patients who had any of these problems to a severe extent, the results from the trials are still instructive. For example, most of the nine trials comprising the BBPP excluded patients with such problems as severe CHF and severe hypotension. With the remaining patient population, the question arises: Is there a subgroup of beta-blocker patients who experience greater mortality than the control patients? The BBPP investigators found that of the 36 patient subgroups examined for beta-blocker benefit only one small subgroup had a relative risk greater than 1, indicating a possible contraindication to the agents [83]. However, even this difference was not statistically significant. The investigators concluded that they could not find, among the patients enrolled in the trials, any subgroup in which beta-blocker therapy was conclusively a problem.

It should also be noted that not all patients with a "contraindication" should be excluded a priori from beta-blocker treatment. It is a question of degree. For example, the mortality data from BHAT show that patients with a history of mild or moderate CHF also benefit from beta-blocker therapy [85]. Table 30-17 shows that the placebo patients had consistently higher mortality rates. In fact, the results mirror what was seen in Table 30-14: the patients with CHF actually experienced greater benefit from beta blockade than did patients without CHF.

We can also examine the incidence of CHF during the course of a trial. Table 30-18 indicates that in BHAT overall there was no difference in the incidence of CHF between the propranolol and placebo groups. Both groups had a 25-month incidence of 6.7 percent. Stratified by history of CHF, the propranolol patients with a history of CHF had a 17 percent higher rate of recurrent CHF (14.8 percent versus 12.6 percent), but the difference is not statistically significant. In fact, a life table analysis of these data indicates that the recurrent failure was

Table 30-17
Cause-specific mortality by history of CHF and by treatment group: BHAT*

	Placebo group		Propranolol group			
Cause of death	Deaths/no. of pts.	%	Deaths/no. of pts.	%	Absolute efficacy (/100)	Relative efficacy (%)
Total mortality						
Hx of CHF	67/365	18.4	46/345	13.3	5.1	−27
No Hx of CHF	121/1556	7.8	92/1571	5.9	1.9	−25
Atherosclerosis						
Hx of CHF	65/365	17.8	40/345	11.6	6.2	−35
No Hx of CHF	99/1556	6.4	79/1571	5.0	1.4	−21
Sudden death (<1 hr of symptoms)						
Hx of CHF	38/365	10.4	19/345	5.5	4.9	−47
No Hx of CHF	51/1556	3.3	45/1571	2.9	0.4	−13

Hx = history; CHF = congestive heart failure; pts. = patients.
*Average length of follow-up was 25 months.
Source: K. Chadda et al. Effect of propranolol after myocardial infarction in patients with congestive heart failure. *Circulation* 73:503, 1986. By permission of the American Heart Association, Inc.

Table 30-18
Incidence of CHF during the follow-up period, by treatment group: BHAT

	Placebo group		Propranolol group				
History of CHF	Events/no. of pts.	%	Events/no. of pts.	%	Absolute efficacy (/100)	Relative efficacy (%)	p
Yes	46/365	12.6	51/345	14.8	−2.2	+17	NS
No	82/1556	5.3	78/1571	5.0	0.3	−6	NS
Total	128/1921	6.7	129/1916	6.7	0.0	0	NS

pts. = patients; p = p value.
Source: K. Chadda et al. Effect of propranolol after myocardial infarction in patients with congestive heart failure. *Circulation* 73:503, 1986. By permission of the American Heart Association, Inc.

more frequent early and that after 5 months the rates began to equalize.

What Are the Adverse Effects of Beta-Blocker Therapy?

Related to the issue of which patients should not receive a beta blocker is the issue of the possible risks among the patients who do receive a beta blocker. When deciding to treat patients with beta blockers after an MI, one must weigh the risks of therapy against the potential benefits. In studies of patients with no absolute or relative contraindications to beta-blocker treatment, severe adverse reactions leading to discontinuation of therapy were fairly infrequent. The proportion of patients taken off active treatment for medical reasons ranged from 5 to 20 percent. However, the composition of the patient populations, the drug dosages and duration of treatment, and the methods of ascertaining and reporting adverse effects are factors that need to be considered when comparing these percentages. A notable finding in these reports, however, is the observation that so-called side effects are also common among placebo patients. Often signs and symptoms are attributed to a patient's treatment rather than to the condition being treated.

Adverse beta-blocker effects have been categorized into two types: those pharmacologically related to beta blockade and those not related [86]. Reactions of the first type are more common, simply because of the importance of the sympathetic nervous system in controlling metabolic functions. Related to the pharmacology of the beta blockers, there is still little evidence whether cardioselective beta blockers or those with partial ISA are associated with a lower incidence of adverse reactions than are the nonselective beta blockers or those without ISA.

Review of the large beta-blocker clinical trials reveals that cardiovascular problems accounted for the largest number of severe reactions in the beta-blocker groups. These problems included symptomatic CHF, hypotension with and without dizziness, bradycardia, and atrioventricular block. CHF, as noted above, was less common than expected, perhaps because most of the trials excluded from participation those patients with moderate to severe heart failure.

The trials also showed a higher frequency among beta-blocker patients of minor side effects that did not lead to discontinuation of the treatment, such as cold extremities, nausea, constipation, asthma, fatigue, mental depression, impotence, and dry eyes. In BHAT [87] long-term propranolol use was associated with a slight gain in weight (< 3 lbs).

If one accepts that high-risk patients are the prime candidates for preventive therapy, one must be prepared to pay a price: a higher incidence of adverse effects. Figure 30-3 presents BHAT data stratifying the incidence of CHF leading to discontinuation of treatment by treatment group and risk group. The incidence of CHF in the uncomplicated group and the group with electrical complications was only about 4 to 6 percent over 25 months, regardless of whether the patients received beta blockers. Among the patients with a history of mechanical complications and assigned to the placebo group, the risk of CHF was about twice these rates (9 to 11 percent). If these patients were taking propranolol, the rates increased (15 to 16 percent). However, this figure is outweighed by the 30 to 40

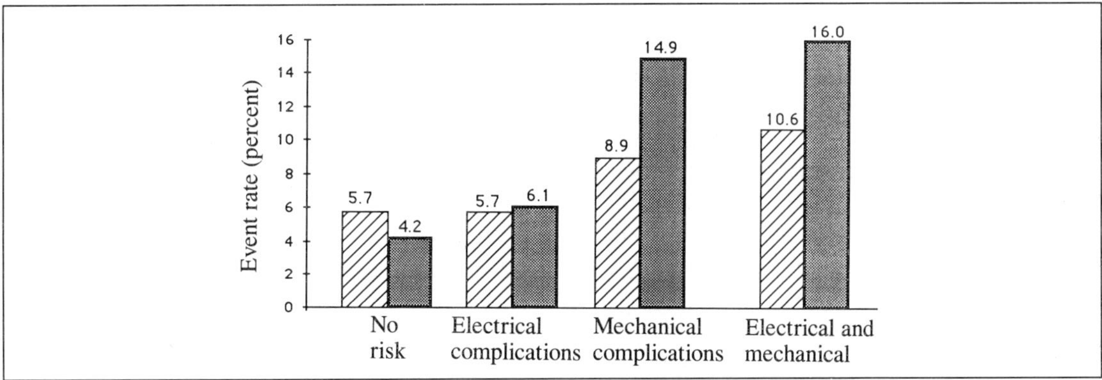

Fig. 30-3
Incidence of congestive heart failure (leading to temporary or permanent discontinuation of treatment), according to the presence of complications at baseline, by treatment group, in the Beta-Blocker Heart Attack Trial. The average length of follow-up was 25 months. Hatched bars = placebo group; dotted bars = propranolol group. (From C. D. Furberg et al. Effect of propranolol in post-infarction patients with mechanical or electrical complications. *Circulation* 69:761, 1984. By permission of the American Heart Association, Inc.)

percent reduction in mortality among these patients attributed to beta-blocker therapy (see Table 30-14).

Beta Blockers and Blood Lipids in Postinfarction Patients

Beta blockers without ISA, such as propranolol, are known to decrease high-density lipoprotein (HDL) cholesterol and increase triglyceride levels, both of which are associated with the development of atherosclerosis and clinical coronary disease. For this reason, it has been hypothesized that some of the benefit of the long-term use of beta blockers is offset by the lipid effect [88, 89].

Most of the literature on this topic focuses on noninfarction populations, such as patients with hypertension or angina. Postinfarction patients, however, are different because the risk factors for postinfarction events (e.g., electrical instability) are not the same as the traditional risk factors for first coronary events (e.g., a decreased HDL level). Therefore, it may be asked whether there is any evidence to indicate that altered lipid levels attenuate any of the documented effects of beta blockers in postmyocardial infarction patients. The BHAT data were examined to address this question [90]. After 6 months of follow-up, the mean serum HDL level was 6 percent lower among the propranolol patients compared with the placebo patients (41.8 mg/dl versus 44.4 mg/dl, $p < .01$). Multivariate survival models showed that for every 1 mg decrease in HDL there was a 0.7 percent increase in mortality, giving a total theoretical increase of about 2 percent for the propranolol patients (2 percent = 0.7 percent × 2.6 mg/dl). These same models also showed that the overall estimated reduction in mortality attributable to propranolol remained about 20 percent, even after adjustment for the lipid changes. Therefore, the estimated benefit of using beta blockers was 10 times the estimated hazard. It was also noted that propranolol had no discernible effect on the most atherogenic lipid fraction, low-density lipoprotein (LDL) cholesterol.

Regardless of the lipid-altering effects of some of the beta blockers, animal studies have shown that at least one, propranolol, actually retards the development of atherosclerosis [91, 92]. The mechanisms that have been proposed to explain this observed effect include inhibition of endothelial permeability to lipoproteins, altered hemodynamic factors, and a reduction of plaque calcium content [93].

Choosing a Beta Blocker and Its Dosage

The questions of which beta blocker to use and what dosage to prescribe are difficult because no large clinical trial has formally compared the preventive and adverse effects of two beta blockers given to post-MI patients. Comparing trials can be problematic because several nonpharmacologic factors can explain observed numerical differences in treatment effects across trials. For example, inclusion of a high proportion of low-risk, uncomplicated infarctions would tend to dilute the benefit in the high-risk groups. True equipotency is also difficult to determine. It is clearly possible that for some beta blockers and some trials (particularly the early ones), a less than optimal dose was tested. Statistically, chance is an important factor to consider when comparing relative and absolute risks and benefits.

However, there may be ancillary pharmacologic properties that could be important. It appears that beta blockers with ISA are slightly less effective than those without ISA. For example, in Table 30-8, the ten trials that studied a beta blocker with ISA (e.g., alprenolol and oxprenolol) have a pooled relative benefit of 18 percent reduction in mortality. Of the ten trials that studied a beta blocker without ISA (e.g., propranolol, timolol, and metoprolol), the pooled relative benefit is a 25 percent reduction in deaths. There is no scientific evidence that the cardioselective blockers (e.g., atenolol and metoprolol) are more effective than the nonselective blockers (e.g., propranolol and timolol). In fact, the strongest data on the favorable long-term mortality effects come from trials of propranolol and timolol. As noted above, there is some speculation that beta-2 blockade may enhance the antiarrhythmic action of beta-1 blockade.

Reviews of clinical trial evidence can offer more unbiased insights into drug mechanisms and how the drugs compare than individual trial reports. Based on the review presented here, the beta blockers recommended for the prophylactic treatment of MI are timolol, propranolol, atenolol, and metoprolol. The side effect profile may be most favorable for atenolol [94]. The recommended daily doses are those evaluated in the trials: timolol 20 mg/day, propranolol 180 to 240 mg/day, atenolol 100 mg/day, and metoprolol 200 mg/day.

When to Begin and End Beta-Blocker Therapy

Review of the acute short-term trials (see Tables 30-4 and 30-5) clearly indicates that if beta-blocker therapy is contemplated it should be initiated with an IV bolus within 6 to 8 hours of the onset of pain. However, the relatively low 7-day mortality among patients without complications to beta blockers (approximately 4 percent, as shown in Table 30-5) and the small relative benefit (approximately 13 percent, as shown in Table 30-5) raise the issue of cost versus benefit. In light of the larger benefit associated with thrombolytic therapy and aspirin [18], the role of beta blockers in the early phase of an MI is debatable. However, because there is no clear benefit of thrombolytic therapy during the first day postinfarction and because a beta blocker such as atenolol has its primary effect during the first day, it would seem to make scientific sense to combine beta-blocker and thrombolytic therapies.

This hypothesis, whether immediate or deferred beta-blocker therapy adds an additional benefit to IV thrombolytic therapy, was addressed in the Thrombolysis in Myocardial Infarction (TIMI II-B) study [30]. All patients in this substudy received IV recombinant tissue-type plasminogen activator (rt-PA). Patients were randomly assigned to receive immediate IV metoprolol (plus oral metoprolol after the third IV dose) or to receive oral metoprolol beginning on day 6. In the short term there was a reduction in rates of reinfarction and chest pain in the group receiving immediate IV beta-blocker therapy but no difference in all-cause mortality. Over a 1-year follow-up period the two groups had comparable rates of mortality, reinfarction, and chest pain. It was concluded that among MI patients on thrombolytic therapy, immediate IV beta-blocker therapy did not have an advantage over deferred therapy in reducing mortality.

For the long term, the choices are relatively limited at this time because only beta-blocker therapy, aspirin, and ACE inhibitors (in selected patients) have documented effects on survival and risk of reinfarction. In most of the long-term trials, beta-blocker therapy was started 1 to 3 weeks after the infarction, while the patient was still hospitalized (see Table 30-7). It was a clear advantage in these trials to initiate treatment by the time the patient had begun to recover, was in a stable condition, and could be observed.

It seems prudent to recommend that oral beta-blocker therapy be initiated 6 to 9 days after AMI in patients who are hemodynamically stable, have no major contraindications to beta blockers, and are at increased risk of mortality. These patients are prime candidates for beta-blocker therapy.

With respect to the duration of treatment, the long-term trials provide substantial data for the assessment of treatment benefit up to 2 years. Beyond this time, the data are limited, and a recommendation for continued treatment would have to be based on the extrapolation of the 2-year data. Because the cumulative mortality curves for the propranolol and placebo groups continue to diverge even at 36 months for patients with a complicated MI in BHAT (see Fig. 30-2) and because most postinfarction patients have angina pectoris and ventricular arrhythmias, it seems prudent, in the absence of any troublesome adverse reaction, to continue treatment indefinitely.

Clinical Impact and Public Health Impact of Beta Blockers

To the clinician and the patient, the absolute benefit of a preventive measure appears to be more important than the relative treatment effect. Table 30-19 demonstrates this principle. In a low-risk population, a reduction of the annual mortality from 2.0 percent to 1.5 percent means that 200 such patients would have to be treated for 1 year to prolong one life. The relative benefit is 25 percent (i.e., the relative risk is 0.75). A similar relative benefit in a high-risk population with a 20 percent annual mortality rate would reduce this mortality rate to 15 percent, which corresponds to five lives prolonged for every 100 such patients treated. Thus, a 25 percent relative morality reduction in a high-risk group is preferable to a 25 percent reduction in a low-risk group. In fact, among high-risk patients a lower relative reduction can actually translate to a greater absolute efficacy. An apparent paradox is that among high-risk patients a smaller (10 percent) relative reduction (from 20 to 18 percent) still gives a better absolute reduction (two lives prolonged for every 100 treated) than a 25 percent relative reduction in a low-risk group (from 2.0 to 1.5 percent mortality, or one life prolonged for every 200 treated.)

This principle is illustrated in Table 30-14, where the greatest absolute benefit of propranolol therapy was among those patients with transient mechanical problems. Therefore, clinically, beta blockers exert their greatest benefit on patients at high risk of death.

The public health implications are clear. As noted at the beginning of the chapter, there are approximately 80,000 in-hospital heart attack deaths in the United States each year and 666,000 patients who survive hospitalization. Based on the data available from the assembled beta-blocker trials, it is conservatively estimated that among the hospital survivors 17,000 deaths could be postponed during the first year postinfarction and that more than 50,000 deaths could be averted over the first 5 years postinfarction. Furthermore, a cost-effectiveness analysis indicated that there is clear evidence of benefit from beta-blocker treatment of medium- to high-risk MI hospital survivors and suggestive evidence of benefit for the treatment of some low-risk patients [95].

Beta blockers were the first agents to have a demonstrated effect on mortality following an MI and they continue to play an important role in the treatment of postinfarction patients. The next goals are to reduce this toll even more through improved secondary prevention and, more importantly, to engage in research aimed at the primary prevention of coronary disease.

Table 30-19
Efficacy measures and their clinical usefulness (hypothetical data)

Population	Annual mortality rate (%) Placebo	Annual mortality rate (%) Intervention	Relative efficacy (%)	Absolute efficacy (efficacy by no. of pts. treated)
Low risk	2.0	1.5	−25	0.5/100 = 1/200
High risk	20.0	15.0	−25	5/100
High risk	20.0	18.0	−10	2/100

pts. = patients.

References

1. Stamler, J. The marked decline in coronary heart disease mortality rates in the United States, 1968–1981: Summary of findings and possible explanations. *Cardiology* 72:11, 1985.
2. American Heart Association. *Heart and Stroke Facts: 1995 Statistical Supplement.* Dallas: AHA, 1995.
3. National Center for Health Statistics. Detailed diagnoses and procedures, National Hospital Discharge Survey, 1992. *Vital Health Stat.* [13] No. 118, August 1994.
4. National Center for Health Statistics. National Hospital Discharge Survey: Annual Summary, 1992. *Vital Health Stat.* [13] No. 119, October 1994.
5. Canner, P. L., Berge, K. G., Wenger, N. K., et al. Fifteen year mortality in Coronary Drug Project patients—long-term benefit from niacin. *J. Am. Coll. Cardiol.* 8:1245, 1986.
6. May, G. S., Eberlein, K. A., Furberg, C. D., et al. Secondary prevention after myocardial infarction: A review of long-term trials. *Prog. Cardiovasc. Dis.* 24:331, 1982.
7. May, G. S., Furberg, C. D., Eberlein, K. A., and Geraci, B. Secondary prevention after myocardial infarction: A review of short-term acute phase trials. *Prog. Cardiovasc. Dis.* 25:335, 1983.
8. Furberg, C. D. Effect of antiarrhythmic drugs on mortality after myocardial infarction. *Am. J. Cardiol.* 52:32C, 1983.
9. Yusuf, S., Peto, R., Lewis, J., et al. Beta-blockade during and after myocardial infarction—an overview of the randomized trials. *Prog. Cardiovasc. Dis.* 27:335, 1985.
10. Yusuf, S., Collins, R., Peto, R., et al. Intravenous and intracoronary fibrinolytic therapy in acute myocardial infarction—overview of results on mortality, reinfarction and side-effects from 33 randomized controlled trials. *Eur. Heart J.* 6:556, 1985.
11. Yusuf, S. Interventions that potentially limit myocardial infarct size: Overview of clinical trials. *Am. J. Cardiol.* 60:11A, 1987.
12. Lipid Research Clinics Coronary Primary Prevention Trial Results. I. Reduction in incidence of coronary heart disease. *J.A.M.A.* 251:351, 1984.
13. Frick, M. H., Elo, O., Haapa, K., et al. Helsinki Heart Study—primary prevention trial with gemfibrozil in middle-aged men with dyslipidemia. *N. Engl. J. Med.* 317:1237, 1987.
14. Brown, B. G., Zhao, X.-Q., Sacco, D. E., et al. Lipid lowering and plaque regression—new insights into prevention of plaque disruption and clinical events in coronary disease. *Circulation* 87:1781, 1993.
15. Furberg, C. D., Byington, R. P., Crouse, J. R., et al. Pravastatin, lipids, and major coronary events. *Am. J. Cardiol.* 73:1133, 1994.
16. Gruppo Italiano per lo Studio Della Streptochinasi Nell'Infarto Miocardico (GISSI): Effectiveness of intravenous thrombolytic treatment in acute myocardial infarction. *Lancet* 1:397, 1986.
17. Antiplatelet trialists' collaboration: Secondary prevention of vascular disease by prolonged antiplatelet treatment. *Br. Med. J.* 296:320, 1988.
18. ISIS Collaborative Group: Results of a large randomized trial of intravenous streptokinase and oral aspirin in acute myocardial infarction (Abstract). *J. Am. Coll. Cardiol.* 11:232A, 1988.
19. GUSTO Angiographic Investigators. The effects of tissue plasminogen activator, streptokinase, or both on coronary-artery patency, ventricular function, and survival after acute myocardial infarction. *N. Engl. J. Med.* 329:1615, 1993.
20. Teo, K. K., Yusuf, S., and Furberg, C. D. Effects of prophylactic antiarrhythmic drug therapy in acute myocardial infarction. *J.A.M.A.* 270:1589, 1993.
21. Teo, K. K., Yusuf, S., Collins, R., et al. Effects of intravenous magnesium in suspected acute myocardial infarction—overview of randomized trials. *B.M.J.* 303:1499, 1991.
22. Horner, S. M. Efficacy of intravenous magnesium in acute myocardial infarction in reducing arrhythmias and mortality—meta-analysis of magnesium in acute myocardial infarction. *Circulation* 86:774, 1992.
23. Held, P. H., Teo, K. K., and Yusuf, S. Effects of beta-blockers, calcium channel blockers, and nitrates in acute myocardial infarction and unstable angina pectoris. In E. J. Topol (ed.). *Textbook of Interventional Cardiology.* Philadelphia: W. B. Saunders, 1991. Pp. 49–65.
24. Pfeffer, M. A., Braunwald, E., Moye, L. A., et al. Effect of captopril on mortality and morbidity in patients with left ventricular dysfunction after myocardial infarction—results of the Survival and Ventricular Enlargement Trial. *N. Engl. J. Med.* 327:669, 1992.
25. Acute Infarction Ramipril Efficacy (AIRE) Study Investigators. Effect of ramipril on mortality and morbidity of survivors of acute myocardial infarction with clinical evidence of heart failure. *Lancet* 342:821, 1993.
26. O'Connor, G. T., Buring, J. E., Yusuf, S., et al. An overview of randomized trials of rehabilitation with exercise after myocardial infarction. *Circulation* 80:234, 1989.
27. Held, P. H., Yusuf, S., and Furberg, C. D. Calcium channel blockers in acute myocardial infarction and unstable angina—an overview. *B.M.J.* 299:1187, 1989.
28. Messerli, F. H., and Weiner, D. A. Are all calcium antagonists equally effective for reducing reinfarction rate? *Am. J. Cardiol.* 72:818, 1993.
29. ISIS-1 (First International Study of Infarct Survival) Collaborative Group: Randomised trial of intravenous atenolol among 16,027 cases of suspected acute myocardial infarction: ISIS-1. *Lancet* 2:57, 1986.
30. Roberts, R., Rogers, W. J., Mueller, H. S., et al. Immediate versus deferred β-blockade following thrombolytic therapy in patients with acute myocar-

dial infarction—results of the Thrombolysis in Myocardial Infarction (TIMI) II-B Study. *Circulation* 83:422, 1991.

31. Byington, R. P. for the Beta-Blocker Heart Attack Trial Research Group: Beta-Blocker Heart Attack Trial: Design, methods, and baseline results. *Controlled Clin. Trials* 5:382, 1984.
32. Norwegian Multicenter Study Group: Timolol-induced reduction in mortality and reinfarction in patients surviving acute myocardial infarction. *N. Engl. J. Med.* 304:801, 1981.
33. Julian, D. G., Prescott, R. J., Jackson, F. S., et al. Controlled trial of sotalol for one year after myocardial infarction. *Lancet* 1:1142, 1982.
34. Taylor, S. H., Silke, B., Ebutt, A., et al. A long-term prevention study with oxprenolol in coronary heart disease. *N. Engl. J. Med.* 307:1293, 1982.
35. Frishman, W. H., and Silverman, P. Physiologic and metabolic effects. In W. H. Frishman (ed.), *Clinical Pharmacology of the β-Adrenoceptor Blocking Drugs* (2nd ed.). Norwalk, CN: Appleton-Century-Crofts, 1984.
36. Furberg, C. D., Byington, R. P., Prineas, R. J., et al. Potassium, beta-2 receptor blockade and mortality: The BHAT experience (Abstract). *Circulation* 70 (Suppl II):7, 1984.
37. Balcon, R., Jewitt, D. E., Davies, J. P. H., et al. A controlled trial of propranolol in acute myocardial infarction. *Lancet* 2:917, 1966.
38. Clausen, J., Felsby, M., Jorgensen, F. S., et al. Absence of prophylactic effect of propranolol in myocardial infarction. *Lancet* 2:920, 1966.
39. Multicenter Trial: Propranolol in acute myocardial infarction. *Lancet* 2:1435, 1966.
40. Norris, R. M., Caughey, D. E., and Scott, P. J. Trial of propranolol in acute myocardial infarction. *B.M.J.* 2:398, 1968.
41. Briant, R. B., and Norris, R. M. Alprenolol in acute myocardial infarction: Double-blind trial. *N. Z. Med. J.* 71:135, 1970.
42. Barber, J. M., Boyle, D. M., Chaturvedi, N. C., et al. Practolol in acute myocardial infarction. *Acta Med. Scand.* [Suppl] 587:213, 1976.
43. Wilcox, R. G., Roland, J. M., Banks, D. C., et al. Randomised trial comparing propranolol with atenolol in immediate treatment of suspected myocardial infarction. *B.M.J.* 280:885, 1980.
44. Wilcox, R. G., Rowley, J. M., Hampton, J. R., et al. Randomised placebo-controlled trial comparing oxprenolol with disopyramide phosphate in immediate treatment of suspected myocardial infarction. *Lancet* 2:765, 1980.
45. Andersen, M. P., Bechsgaard, P., et al. Effect of alprenolol on mortality among patients with definite or suspected acute myocardial infarction, preliminary results. *Lancet* 2:865, 1979.
46. Hjalmarson, A., Herlitz, J., Holmberg, S., et al. The Goteborg Metoprolol Trial: Effects on mortality and morbidity in acute myocardial infarction. *Circulation* 67(Suppl I):26, 1983.
47. Yusuf, S., Sleight, P., Rossi, P., et al. Reduction in infarct size, arrhythmias and chest pain by early intravenous beta-blockade in suspected acute myocardial infarction. *Circulation* 67(Suppl I):32, 1983.
48. UK Collaborative Study Group. Mortality results from timolol trials in various British hospitals. Personal communication from W. D. Cooper, MSD Coordinator, and E. J. Flint to the authors of reference 9, 1984.
49. The International Collaborative Study Group. Reduction of infarct size with the early use of timolol in acute myocardial infarction. *N. Engl. J. Med.* 310: 9, 1984.
50. Federman, J., Pitt, A., Harris, P., et al. Mortality results from Australian Timolol Trial, Personal communication to authors of reference 9, 1984.
51. Heber, M. E., Rosenthal, E., Thomas, N. B., et al. Effect of labetalol on indices of myocardial necrosis in patients with suspected acute infarction. Unpublished manuscript, results presented in reference 9, 1984.
52. Norris, R. M., Barnaby, P. F., Brown, M. A., et al. Prevention of ventricular fibrillation during acute myocardial infarction by intravenous propranolol. *Lancet* 2:883, 1984.
53. Roberts, R., Croft, C., Gold, H. K., et al. Effect of propranolol on myocardial infarct size in a randomized blinded multicenter trial. *N. Engl. J. Med.* 311:218, 1984.
54. Owensby, D. A., and O'Rourke, M. F. Failure of pindolol to alter determinants of myocardial oxygen requirements, enzyme release or clinical course in acute myocardial infarction (Abstract). *Circulation* 70(Suppl II):156, 1984.
55. The MIAMI Trial Research Group. Metoprolol in Acute Myocardial Infarction (MIAMI): A randomised placebo-controlled international trial. *Eur. Heart J.* 6:199, 1985.
56. Salathia, K. S., Barber, J. M., McIlmoyle, E. L., et al. Very early intervention with metoprolol in suspected acute myocardial infarction. *Eur. Heart J.* 6:190, 1985.
57. Roque, F., for the TIARA Group Investigators. Limitation of infarct size and reduction of late ventricular arrhythmias with early administered timolol in acute myocardial infarction: A one-month follow-up study (Abstract). *J. Am. Coll. Cardiol.* 7:67A, 1986.
58. Waagstein, F., and Hjalmarson, A. C. Double-blind study of the effect of cardioselective beta-blockade on chest pain in acute myocardial infarction. *Acta Med. Scand.* [Suppl] 587:201, 1975.
59. Evemy, K. L., and Pentecost, B. L. Intravenous and oral practolol in the acute stages of myocardial infarction. *Eur. J. Cardiol.* 7:391, 1978.
60. Peter, T., Norris, R. M., Clarke, E. D., et al. Reduction of enzyme levels by propranolol after acute myocardial infarction. *Circulation* 57:1091, 1978.
61. Norris, R. M., Clarke, E. D., Sammel, N. J., et al. Protective effect of propranolol in threatened myocardial infarction. *Lancet* 2:907, 1978.

62. Norris, R. M., Sammel, N. L., Clarke, E. D., et al. Treatment of acute myocardial infarction with propranolol: Further studies on enzyme appearance and subsequent left ventricular function in treated and control patients with developing infarcts. *Br. Heart J.* 43:617, 1980.
63. Mueller, H. S., and Ayres, S. M. Propranolol decreases sympathetic nervous activity reflected by plasma catecholamines during evolution of myocardial infarction in man. *J. Clin. Invest.* 65:338, 1980.
64. Azancot, I., Lorente, P., Georgiopoulis, G., et al. Effects of acebutolol on myocardial infarct extension: A randomized electrocardiographic, enzymatic, and angiographic study. *Circulation* 66:986, 1982.
65. Wilhelmsson, C., Vedin, J. A., Wilhelmsen, L., et al. Reduction of sudden deaths after myocardial infarction by treatment with alprenolol. *Lancet* 2: 1157, 1974.
66. Ahlmark, G., Saetre, H., and Korsgren, M. Reduction of sudden deaths after myocardial infarction. *Lancet* 2:1563, 1974.
67. Multicentre International Study: Supplementary report: Reduction in mortality after myocardial infarction with long-term beta-adrenoreceptor blockade. *B.M.J.* 2:419, 1977.
68. Rehnqvist, N., Ahnve, S., Erhardt, L., et al. Effect of metoprolol after acute myocardial infarction (Abstract). *Proc. Eur. Cong. Cardiol.* 16:16, 1980.
69. Hansteen, V., Moinichen, E., Lorentsen, E., et al. One year's treatment with propranolol after myocardial infarction: Preliminary report of Norwegian Multicentre Trial. *B.M.J.* 284:155, 1982.
70. Beta-Blocker Heart Attack Trial Research Group. A randomized trial of propranolol in patients with acute myocardial infarction. I. Mortality results. *J.A.M.A.* 247:1707, 1982.
71. Australian and Swedish Pindolol Study Group. The effect of pindolol on the two years mortality after complicated myocardial infarction. *Eur. Heart J.* 4:367, 1983.
72. Manger Cats, V., van Capelle, F. J. L., Lie, K. I., et al. Effect of treatment with 2 × 100 mg metoprolol on mortality in a single-center study with low placebo—mortality rate after infarction (Abstract). *Circulation* 68(Suppl III):181, 1983. Also personal communication to authors of reference 9.
73. European Infarction Study Group. A secondary prevention study with slow-release oxprenolol after myocardial infarction: Morbidity and mortality. *Eur. Heart J.* 5:189, 1984.
74. Olsson, G., Rehnqvist, N., et al. Long-term treatment with metoprolol after myocardial infarction: Report on 3 year mortality and morbidity. *J. Am. Coll. Cardiol.* 5:1428, 1985.
75. Schwartz, P. J., Motolese, M., Pollavini, G., et al. Surgical and pharmacological antiadrenergic interventions in the prevention of sudden death after a first myocardial infarction (Abstract). *Circulation* 72(Suppl III): 358, 1985.
76. The Lopressor Intervention Research Group. The Lopressor Intervention Trial: Multicentre study of metoprolol in survivors of acute myocardial infarction. *Eur. Heart J.* 8:1056, 1987.
77. Boissel, J. P., Leizorovicz, A., Picolet, H., et al. Secondary prevention after high-risk acute myocardial infarction with low-dose acebutolol. *Am. J. Cardiol.* 66:251, 1990.
78. Beta-Blocker Heart Attack Trial Research Group. A randomized trial of propranolol in patients with acute myocardial infarction. II. Morbidity results. *J.A.M.A.* 250:2814, 1983.
79. Peters, R. W., Byington, R., Arensberg, D., et al. Mortality in the Beta-Blocker Heart Attack Trial: The circumstances surrounding death. *J. Chronic Dis.* 40:75, 1987.
80. Morganroth, J., Lichstein, E., Byington, R., et al. Beta-Blocker Heart Attack Trial: Impact of propranolol therapy on ventricular arrhythmias. *Prev. Med.* 14:346, 1985.
81. Friedman, L. M., Byington, R. P., Capone, R. J., et al. Effect of propranolol in patients with myocardial infarction and ventricular arrhythmia. *J. Am. Coll. Cardiol.* 7:1, 1986.
82. Furberg, C. D., Hawkins, C. M., Lichstein, E., et al. Effect of propranolol in post-infarction patients with mechanical or electrical complications. *Circulation* 69:761, 1984.
83. Beta-Blocker Pooling Project Research Group. The Beta-Blocker Pooling Project (BBPP): Subgroup findings from randomized trials in post-infarction patients. *Eur. Heart J.* 9:8, 1988.
84. Hawkins, C. M., Richardson, D. W., Vokonas, P. S., et al. Effect of propranolol in reducing mortality in older myocardial infarction patients. *Circulation* 67(Suppl I):94, 1983.
85. Chadda, K., Goldstein, S., Byington, R., and Curb, J. D. Effect of propranolol after myocardial infarction in patients with congestive heart failure. *Circulation* 73:503, 1986.
86. Frishman, W. H. Beta-adrenergic receptor blockers: Adverse effects and drug interactions. *Hypertension* (Suppl II):21, 1988.
87. Rossner, S., Taylor, C. L., Byington, R. P., et al. Long-term propranolol treatment and changes in body weight after myocardial infarction. *B.M.J.* 300: 902, 1990.
88. Northcote, R. J. β-blockers, lipids, and coronary atherosclerosis—fact or fiction? *B.M.J.* 296, 731, 1988.
89. van Brummelen, P. The relevance of intrinsic sympathomimetic activity for β-blocker-induced changes in plasma lipids. *J. Cardiovasc. Pharmacol.* 5:S51, 1983.
90. Byington, R. P., Worthy, J., Craven, T., et al: Propranolol-induced lipid changes and their prognostic significance after a myocardial infarction—the Beta-Blocker Heart Attack Trial Experience. *Am. J. Cardiol.* 65:1287, 1990.
91. Kaplan, J. R., Manuck, S. B., Adams, M. R., et al. Inhibition of coronary atherosclerosis by propranolol

in behaviorally predisposed monkeys fed an atherogenic diet. *Circulation* 76:1364, 1987.

92. Pick, R., and Glick, G. Effects of propranolol, minoxidil, and clofibrate on cholesterol-induced atherosclerosis in Stumptail Macaques. *Atherosclerosis* 27:71, 1977.
93. Cruickshank, J. M. β-Blockers, plasma lipids, and coronary heart disease. *Circulation* 82(Suppl II):II-60, 1990.
94. Kostis, J. B., and Rosen, R. C. Central nervous system effects of β-adrenergic-blocking drugs: The role of ancillary properties. *Circulation* 75:204, 1987.
95. Goldman, L., Benjamin Sia, S. T., Cook, E. F., et al. Costs and effectiveness of routine therapy with long-term beta-adrenergic antagonists after acute myocardial infarction. *N. Engl. J. Med.* 319:152, 1988.

31. Anticoagulant and Platelet Inhibitory Agents for Myocardial Infarction

Antonio Fernández-Ortiz, Ik-Kyung Jang, and Valentin Fuster

Atherosclerotic plaque rupture with subsequent thrombosis is the predominant cause of acute myocardial infarction (AMI) [1, 2]. The exposure of plaque components to flowing blood in the coronary arteries leads within minutes to the development of a thrombus that anchors firmly to the arterial wall, extends into the lumen, and may occlude the artery, or dissolve or embolize distally, depending on local and systemic factors and antithrombotic therapy [3, 4]. Platelets are predominant at the site of the stenosis, whereas fibrin is the main component of the thrombus distal to the stenosis and in the initial layers of thrombus that overlie the deep injury; this is consistent with the higher concentration of thrombin observed in thrombus adjacent to deeply injured arteries [4].

The role of antithrombotic agents in relation to AMI includes (1) primary prevention of myocardial infarction (MI) and cardiovascular morbidity and mortality, (2) treatment of the acute and early phases of MI with or without coronary thrombolysis, and (3) secondary prevention of myocardial ischemia and MI. Recommendations for the use of current antithrombotic agents and consideration of potential applications for new anticoagulants and antiplatelet agents in MI are important aspects of this role.

Primary Prevention of Myocardial Infarction and Cardiovascular Mortality

The role of aspirin in the primary prevention of AMI has been studied in two large randomized trials: the United States Physicians' Health Study [5, 6] and the British Doctors' Trial [7]. The Physicians' Health Study was a large, double-blind, placebo-controlled trial conducted among 22,071 U.S. male physicians, aged 40 to 84 years. At an average of 5 years follow-up, a 44 percent reduction in risk of a first MI was observed in the aspirin-treated group (325 mg every other day). There was, however, a trend indicating an increase in the frequency of hemorrhagic strokes in the aspirin group (13 cases in the aspirin group versus 6 in the placebo group). The British Doctors' Trial, which tested 500 mg of aspirin daily among 5139 male physicians aged 50 to 78 years at baseline, did not find significant differences between the treatment groups in the incidence of MI at a follow-up of 6 years. However, a significant increase in disabling strokes was observed among those assigned to aspirin. A number of differences in the designs of these two primary prevention trials may have influenced their results, the most important difference being the much larger sample size of the Physicians' Health Study and the aspirin dosage used. In addition, the clinical relevance of risk reductions reported as percentages when the absolute prevalence of events is low requires careful interpretation [8, 9]. Although the rate of nonfatal MI was reduced by 44 percent in the Physicians' trial, the absolute risk reduction was less than two events per thousand per year.

The role of low-dose oral anticoagulants in the primary prevention of ischemic heart disease in patients with coronary risk factors is addressed in the ongoing Thrombosis Prevention Trial (TPT) [10]. In this study, anticoagulation was induced with a starting dose of 2.5 mg of warfarin (or placebo) daily and increased by 0.5 or 1 mg/day at monthly intervals until the appropriate stable dose was individually achieved (International Normalized Ratio [INR] of about 1.5). The aspirin component of the trial was a 75-mg controlled-release preparation administered daily. Recruitment was completed in early 1994 with the entry of 5,493 men; follow-up will continue until 1997. The annual risk of serious bleeding requiring transfusion or surgery may be about 1:500 for those in active treatment, whether it consists of aspirin and warfarin or either alone [10]. A benefit can probably be achieved without an unacceptable increase in the risk of serious bleeding.

Current Recommendations

Because the effects of aspirin on cardiovascular death and stroke remain inconclusive, any decision to prescribe aspirin to prevent a first MI should be based on individual clinical judgment, taking into account the patient's cardiovascular risk profile as well as side effects of the drug. The prescription of aspirin at a dose of 160 to 325 mg a day should be considered in patients with significant risk factors that cannot be modified or reduced, if no specific contraindications to long-term aspirin treatment are present. No data are available regarding the use of warfarin at the present time.

Treatment of the Acute and Early Phases of Myocardial Infarction

Antithrombotic agents may play their role during and early after AMI by (1) preventing deep venous thrombosis and pulmonary embolism, (2) preventing arterial embolism, (3) reducing early recurrence or extension of MI and death in patients not receiving thrombolytic therapy, and (4) reducing early reocclusion or death after successful reperfusion with thrombolytic therapy.

Prevention of Deep Venous Thrombosis and Pulmonary Embolism

The incidence of deep venous thrombosis in the lower extremities of patients with AMI ranges from 17 to 38 percent [11–20] (Table 31-1), which is similar to the incidence in patients considered at moderate risk for venous thrombosis after surgery [21, 22]. This observation, coupled with the increased risk of recurrent MI within 3 months of an initial infarction in patients undergoing noncardiac surgery [23], suggests the presence of a hypercoagulable state soon after AMI, similar to that present after major surgery [24]. Deep venous thrombi form soon after MI (half or more within 3 days) [12, 13, 16]. The incidence is greater after a large or recurrent infarction with congestive heart failure (CHF) or cardiogenic shock [13, 17, 25]; after prolonged immobilization [25]; and among certain subsets of patients, particularly those older than 70 years [17, 26] (see Table 31-1). Clinically obvious pulmonary emboli occurred in 5 percent of nonanticoagulated patients (0.6 percent fatal) in the Veterans Administration Cooperative Study (VACS) of anticoagulants for AMI [27]. Similarly, clinical evidence of pulmonary emboli was present in 4 percent of nonanticoagulated patients in a trial of intravenous (IV) streptokinase (SK) for AMI [28]. These studies were conducted, however, before the current practice of early mobilization after MI.

Table 31-1
Incidence of deep venous thrombosis in patients admitted for acute myocardial infarction

Condition	Deep venous thrombosis (%)
Chest pain, no myocardial infarction	7–10
Myocardial infarction	17–38
Within 5–7 days	13–29
Mobilization within 1 to 3 days	
No heart failure	9
With heart failure	22
Bed rest for 5 days	
No heart failure	63
With heart failure	80
Age	
<50	13
>70	70

Although anticoagulant therapy is highly effective, two-thirds of patients who die from pulmonary embolism succumb abruptly or within 2 hours after embolism [29]; prevention is the key to reduce mortality and morbidity from pulmonary embolism. The best noninvasive test for determining the incidence of early, asymptomatic, deep venous thrombosis is ultrasonography. In a prospective study of 220 patients [30], real-time B-mode ultrasonography, with the single criterion of vein compressibility with the ultrasound transducer probe, resulted in 100 percent sensitivity and 99 percent specificity in detecting proximal venous thrombosis (above the knee). In another study [31], color Doppler ultrasound was shown to accurately diagnose thrombosis within the femoropopliteal veins with a sensitivity and a specificity of 100 percent each, and within the calf veins with a sensitivity and specificity of 95 percent and 100 percent, respectively.

Clinical trials have shown that a reduction in the rate of venous thrombosis by anticoagulation also results in a decreased incidence of pulmonary embolism. Acute IV heparinization followed by oral anticoagulation reduced the incidence of venous thrombi to 6 percent or less [12, 14, 16]. It also decreased the incidence of pulmonary embolism from 5 percent to less than 2 percent in clinical studies [32, 33] and from between 6 and 32 percent to between 0 and 5 percent at autopsy [32–34]. Low-dose subcutaneous heparin started within 12 to 18 hours of the onset of symptoms of AMI and continued for 10 days has also successfully reduced the incidence of venous thrombosis from a mean of 23 percent to 4 percent [18–20], and the incidence of fatal pulmonary embolism from 0.7 to 0.1 percent [21]. Although the use of low-molecular-weight heparin has been successful in preventing venous thrombosis in surgical patients [35–37], its role in patients undergoing AMI has yet to be determined.

Current Recommendations

Early mobilization of patients, within 1 to 3 days after MI, is important in the prevention of deep venous thrombosis and pulmonary embolism. For patients at high risk of venous thrombosis (age greater than 70, necessity for long immobilization, previous deep venous thrombosis or pulmonary emboli, obesity, or evidence of chronic venous insufficiency) immediate subcutaneous heparin (5000 IU every 12 hours) should be administered unless full-dose anticoagulant therapy has been initiated in association with thrombolytic therapy or to prevent arterial embolism.

Prevention of Arterial Embolism

Without antithrombotic therapy, the overall incidence of mural thrombosis after AMI is about 20 percent; with anterior MI the incidence increases to 40 percent and to as high as 60 percent with large anterior MIs [38]. Because the incidence of systemic embolism is about 10 percent with mural thrombosis, the embolism rates are approximately 2 percent, 4 percent, and 6 percent, respectively, in each of the above-mentioned groups [38]. Autopsy studies of fatal MIs, which represent the largest infarctions, have found the incidence of mural thrombi in the range of 40 to 70 percent when anticoagulant therapy was not given [39–41], but this incidence is substantially reduced to 22 to 24 percent by anticoagulant treatment [27, 34]. Although more than one-third of patients with AMI develop left ventricular (LV) thrombi, this complication occurs in less than 5 percent of those with inferior infarction (Table 31-2).

A propensity for thrombus formation probably begins at the onset of myocardial necrosis, when endocardial inflammation creates a thrombogenic surface [42]. The incidence of embolism is highest during the period of active thrombus formation in the first 1 to 3 months after AMI, but the risk of embolism remains substantial even beyond the acute phase in patients with persistent myocardial dysfunction, CHF, or atrial fibrillation. In terms of survival, the significance of echocardiographic detection of mural thrombus in patients with AMI is still controversial. Most studies suggest that the prognosis for survival of patients developing LV mural thrombi in the course of AMI is less favorable than for those who do not have this finding [41, 43]. However, other authors have suggested that the prognosis for survival is better in patients with evidence of thrombus formation, because of a pro-

Table 31-2
Prevalence of mural thrombus formation and systemic embolism in patients with acute myocardial infarction and chronic left ventricular dysfunction

Condition	Mural thrombi (%)	Embolism (% per year)
Acute myocardial infarction		
All	10–20	1–3
Anterior	30–40	2–6
Large apical	60–70	10–20
Inferior	<5	<1
Chronic ventricular aneurysm	50	1
Dilated cardiomyopathy		
Diffuse	30	3–4
Segmental	15	3

tective effect of mural thrombi in preventing myocardial rupture [44].

Two-dimensional echocardiography, with a sensitivity of 77 to 92 percent and a specificity of 85 to 94 percent [45–49], is the most accurate method of detecting LV mural thrombus. Invasive techniques, such as LV cineangiography, have only 31 percent sensitivity and 75 percent specificity [38, 50, 51], and carry with them the risk of catheter-induced embolism. Protrusion and mobility of intracavitary thrombi and the combination of regions of stasis and motion within the cardiac chambers in the echocardiographic study have been correlated with increased risk of thromboembolism [52–54].

Over the past 20 years, three large trials involving patients with anterior and inferior AMIs concluded that initial treatment with heparin followed by administration of an oral anticoagulant reduced the occurrence of cerebral embolism from 3 percent to 1 percent when compared with no anticoagulation (Table 31-3) [27, 33, 55]. Within the past decade, six randomized studies involving patients with AMI have addressed the relation of echocardiographically detected LV thrombi and anticoagulant treatment [56–61]. In aggregate, the use of high-dose IV or subcutaneous heparin reduced by more than 50 percent the incidence of thrombus formation in AMI; individually, however, each trial had insufficient sample size to detect significant differences. Anticoagulant therapy has been effective if given on admission to the hospital; delay until a mural thrombus is demonstrated echocardiographically may miss the time in which therapy can be most valuable [38]. It is uncertain whether thrombolytic therapy will reduce the likelihood that a patient will develop ventricular thrombi. Data from available studies are conflicting, either because the patients tested had reduced infarct size or the studies used concomitant anticoagulant medication. In 96 patients with AMI from the Thrombolysis in Myocardial Infarction (TIMI) study [62], echocardiograms performed 48 to 72 hours after patients were hospitalized showed that the rate of thrombus formation was approximately 30 percent lower in patients who were given lytic therapy than in those who were not, but this difference was not statistically different. The Gruppo Italiano per lo Studio della Sopravvivenza nell'Infarto Miocardico-II (GISSI-2) study suggested benefit from the lytic agents themselves [63].

Table 31-3
Prevention of systemic embolism by short-term anticoagulation

Trial	No. of patients	Systemic embolism (%)		
		Anticoagulant	Control	Reduction
BMRC [55]	1427	1.3	3.4	62*
BMH [33]	1136	1.7	2.3	26
VACS [27]	999	0.8	5.4	85*

BMRC = British Medical Research Council; BMH = Bronx Municipal Hospital; VACS = Veterans Administration Cooperative Study.
*$p < .01$.

Current Recommendations

Patients with large anterior MI should be treated with anticoagulant therapy aimed at preventing mural thrombosis and arterial embolization. Immediate subcutaneous or IV heparin, in a dose sufficient to prolong the activated partial thromboplastin time (APTT) ratio to 1.5 to 2 times control, should be administered in these patients and continued until discharge. In patients with ventricular mural thrombi identified by echocardiography or those with large akinetic regions, heparin therapy may be followed by warfarin. Therapy with warfarin is associated with resolution of LV thrombi in the majority of cases, and the oral anticoagulation is usually stopped after 3 months unless the risk of thromboembolism remains elevated as a result of CHF, impaired LV function, or persistent evidence of LV thrombus.

Reduction of Early Recurrence or Extension of MI and Death in Patients Not Receiving Thrombolytic Therapy

Before the advent of thrombolytic therapy, the incidence of early recurrence of MI was 14 to 30 percent, an incidence comparable to that found at necropsy (17 percent) [64–72]. More than half of early recurrences occurred within 10 days and the remainder within 14 to 18 days after the initial MI [68]. Reinfarction is generally accepted as a re-elevation or reappearance of creatine kinase-MB in the serum after an initial peak [65, 67]. Neither chest pain nor electrocardiogram (ECG) changes provide accurate markers for recognizing reinfarction, as both occur in only about half of patients with extension. The clinical impact of early recurrence of MI is important because it results in significant reduction in LV function [64] and survival [64, 65, 67–71]. The incidence of reinfarction is much higher in patients with non-Q-wave MI (approximately 40 percent) than in those with Q-wave infarction (approximately 10 percent) [68], and also higher in patients with small infarctions than in those with large ones [64]. Clinical risk factors associated with reinfarction in patients with non-Q-wave infarction are female sex, obesity, and recurrent chest pain with associated ST-T changes [64, 68, 70]. Instability in patients with non-Q-wave infarctions may be partially related to the high incidence of subtotal occlusion or transient episodes of reperfusion-reocclusion in the infarct-related artery, leaving an area of myocardium in jeopardy for ischemia [73, 74]. Early reocclusion may also be related to the association of high-grade complex lesions with ruptured plaque and thrombus, both of which are thrombogenic surfaces [1, 2, 75, 76], and the apparent hypercoagulable state that may follow AMI [23, 77, 78]. Vasoconstriction may play an additional role in reocclusion, which may explain the reduction in early reinfarction (from 9.0 percent to 5.2 percent) in patients with non-Q-wave MI treated with diltiazem [79].

The role of platelet inhibitor therapy in patients with AMI was addressed by the Second International Study of Infarct Survival (ISIS-2) [32]. In this study, more than 17,000 patients with suspected MI were randomized within 24 hours of the onset of symptoms to receive IV SK (1.5 million U), oral aspirin (160 mg daily), both, or neither. In this large trial, aspirin alone reduced vascular mortality by 23 percent compared with placebo, as assessed at 5 weeks ($p < .00001$); 160 mg of aspirin reduced mortality as much as full-dose SK given alone; and the two active agents were additive, reducing the death rate from 13.2 percent for double placebo to 8 percent. The beneficial effect of aspirin was probably related to a reduction of early reinfarction rate once spontaneous or SK-induced vessel recanalization had occurred. Indeed, aspirin reduced the rates of nonfatal reinfarction and stroke by 49 percent and 46 percent, respectively. The benefit had been maintained at median follow-up of 15 months [32].

The antithrombotic effects of heparin have been utilized for decades in the treatment of AMI, but formerly as much for its demonstrated benefits in reducing complications (deep venous thrombosis, pulmonary embolism, and LV mural thrombosis) as for its potential adjunctive role in treating the proximate cause of MI, thrombotic coronary occlusion. During the 1960s and 1970s, there were several randomized studies of short-term anticoagulation after AMI. Only three were of sufficient size to detect a significant effect of therapy: the British Medical Research Council (BMRC) study [55], the Bronx Municipal Hospital (BMH) study [33], and the Veterans Administration Cooperative Study (VACS) [27]. Mortality and reinfarction rates among anticoagulant-treated patients were not significantly different from controls except for mortality in women in the BMH study (Table 31-4). Therefore, it ap-

Table 31-4
Short-term anticoagulation in acute myocardial infarction

		Mortality (%)		Reinfarction (%)	
Study	No. of patients	Control	Treated	Control	Treated
BMRC [55]	1427	18	16	13.0	9.7
BMH [33]	1136				
Men	745	16	15	10.3	11.0
Women	391	31	15*	18.6	13.4
VACS [27]	999	11	10	6.0	4.0

BMRC = British Medical Research Council; BMH = Bronx Municipal Hospital; VACS = Veterans Administration Cooperative Study.
*$p < .01$.

peared that high-dose anticoagulation did not significantly reduce in-hospital mortality or reinfarction, an observation which led to the general belief that short-term in-hospital anticoagulation after MI was not worthwhile.

Three studies during the 1970s stimulated new enthusiasm for the short-term use of anticoagulants [80–82]. These retrospective epidemiologic studies reported that hospitalized patients treated with anticoagulants had two- to threefold lower mortality rates than those who were not treated. A significant criticism of these studies, however, is related to patient selection bias. In another similar retrospective study, differences between treatment groups disappeared when groups were adjusted for the severity of MI [83]. Although admitting that prospective randomization is a more valid study procedure, the authors of both these retrospective studies concluded that their data were strong enough to justify a re-evaluation of short-term anticoagulation in patients with MI. Chalmers et al. [84] reanalyzed the randomized, controlled trials of anticoagulants for AMI and found that, when case fatality ratios were pooled, anticoagulants reduced mortality by a significant 21 percent. They urged that all patients without specific contraindications be given anticoagulants during hospitalization for MI.

In comparisons of risk reductions between aspirin and anticoagulants in AMI without thrombolytic therapy, the beneficial effects on mortality appear similar: there was a 23 percent reduction in overall mortality in ISIS-2 [32] compared with a 16 to 22 percent reduction in studies using heparin, oral anticoagulants, or both [86, 87]. Attributing risk reductions to administration of aspirin, however, is more certain because it is based on a single-line randomized trial, whereas attributing risk reductions to administration of anticoagulants is based on an overview of numerous smaller trials, most of which were conducted more than 30 years ago when clinical trial methodology was far less rigorous. The scientific limitations of pooling data and the fact that percentages rather than exact numbers were pooled have prompted such methodology to be described as "pooling, drowning, and floating" [85]. Nevertheless, the pooled approach may be helpful for detecting beneficial trends, which, if not convincing, may at least serve as guidelines for future, better designed, prospective trials.

Current Recommendations

Regardless of whether thrombolytic therapy is planned, all patients with AMI and no contraindications should immediately receive aspirin at a dose of 160 to 325 mg a day. There are no convincing data to indicate that short-term anticoagulation after MI prevents early recurrence better than aspirin alone. Because anticoagulation appears to produce some net benefit, trials aimed at evaluating the effects of short-term antithrombotic regimens (e.g., anticoagulants plus platelet inhibitors) should be considered.

Reduction of Early Reocclusion or Death after Successful Reperfusion with Thrombolytic Therapy

In the past decade, several controlled trials in patients with AMI demonstrated that IV thrombolytic agents recanalize occluded arteries, reduce the size of the infarct, preserve LV function, and reduce mortality [32, 88–94]. Earlier reopening of the artery is associated with better outcome; however, late reopening of the artery may also contribute to clinical benefit through mechanisms other than acute rescue of stunned myocardium, such as late recovery of borderline areas of myocardial hibernation [95]. In addition, the potential benefits of thrombolytic therapy may be reduced if reocclusion of a patent infarct-related artery occurs. Some clinical evidence suggests that the long-term mortality rate may be related to patency of the infarct-related artery at the time of discharge [88, 95–97], independent of standard measures of LV function. Therefore, the most rational treatment of patients with AMI would consist of rapid and persistent recanalization of the occluded coronary artery [98].

In the Thrombolysis and Angioplasty in Myocardial Infarction (TAMI) trials, reported by Ohman et al. [98], the highest frequency of acute reclosure occurred within 12 hours after reperfusion, and 50 percent of all identified reocclusions were within the first 24 hours. After the first day, the rate declined substantially to about 1 percent per day for the remainder of the first week. The overall incidence of reocclusion was 12 percent. It is important to note that only half these events were clinically recognizable. Persistent patency was associated with a 4.5 percent mortality rate, whereas reocclusion led to an 11 percent mortality rate. Reocclusion was also associated with worsened infarct-zone regional function at follow-up.

Antithrombotic agents may limit MI after thrombolytic therapy by promoting the lysis of an occlusive thrombus or by preventing reocclusion. The combination of aspirin and SK in the ISIS-2 study [32] decreased the death rate by 42 percent. The salutary effects of aspirin were probably caused by prevention of coronary reocclusion after vessel patency was achieved through spontaneous or pharmacologic lysis, because the highest rate of reinfarction was in the active SK nonaspirin group. A recent meta-analysis study [99]of 932 patients with angiographic data on reocclusion also showed a dramatically lower reocclusion rate in groups treated with aspirin than in groups treated without aspirin (11 percent versus 29 percent, $p < .001$).

Regarding the combination of heparin and thrombolytic therapy, there are no mortality trials of adequate sample size that assess heparin as the sole adjunctive therapy to thrombolysis; in fact, once the effectiveness of aspirin was successfully demonstrated, no heparin trial could be designed without a comparison with aspirin. The Studio sulla Calciparina nell'Angina e nella Trombosi Ventricolare nell'Infarto (SCATI) trial [61], although not designed as a mortality trial and the population analyzed was relatively small (433 patients received IV SK), showed additional benefit in short-term survival when subcutaneous heparin was added to SK. Mortality during hospitalization was 8.8 percent in control patients (no heparin) and 4.5 percent in the heparin group. No patient received aspirin in this trial. The Heparin-Aspirin Reperfusion Trial (HART) [100] randomized 205 patients to receive either IV heparin (5000 U bolus, then 1000 U/hour to maintain APTT 1.5 to 2 times control), or oral aspirin (80 mg) together with tissue plasminogen activator (t-PA) (100 mg infusion) initiated within 6 hours of the onset of symptoms of AMI. The investigators evaluated the patency rate by angiography in the first 24 hours. At the time of the angiogram, the patency rate was 82 percent in the patients assigned to heparin, but only 52 percent in the aspirin group ($p < .0001$). However, there has been some criticism of the study for having selected such a small dose of aspirin (80 mg) as the alternative to heparin. The possibility that a higher aspirin dose would have substantially altered the outcome in the HART study remains speculative.

The issue of additional benefit of heparin to full-dose aspirin combined with thrombolytic therapy has been largely debated. The sixth trial of the European Cooperative Study Group (ECSG-6) [101], which randomized 652 patients with AMI treated with alteplase and aspirin (250 mg intravenously or 300 mg orally) to either concomitant IV heparin or placebo, demonstrated that allocation to heparin is associated with a real, though possibly small, higher patency rate at 48 to 120 hours (83 percent versus 75 percent, $p = .02$). However, the mortality rate was similar to those receiving only t-PA plus aspirin. In the GISSI-2/International [102] and ISIS-3 [103] trials, subcutaneous heparin, added to thrombolytic therapy plus full-dose aspirin, was associated with 0.5 percent benefit in early mortality, but this benefit was lost after discontinuation of heparin, with no significant mortality advantage at 1 month. Such use of subcutaneous heparin has been questioned on the basis of delayed administration (4 to 12 hours after thrombolytic therapy), erratic absorption, and the relatively suboptimal anticoagulant state achieved [104].

Further information about the risk and benefits of heparin and its route of administration when combined with aspirin and thrombolytic therapy has been provided by the recently finished Global Utilization of Streptokinase and t-PA for Occluded Arteries (GUSTO) trial [105]. This study enrolled 41,021 patients with AMIs from 1081 centers in 15 countries. Patients were randomized into four treatment groups: (1) accelerated t-PA plus IV heparin, (2) SK plus subcutaneous heparin, (3) SK plus IV heparin, or (4) both thrombolytics (t-PA in nonaccelerated fashion and lower-dose SK) with IV heparin. All patients received 160 mg aspirin daily. The results have shown no clinical benefit of immediate IV heparin versus subcutaneous heparin for SK when added to aspirin; the trial did not test such a comparison for t-PA. Furthermore, no available angiographic patency data support the additional use of IV heparin once full-dose aspirin has been given with SK [106] or anisoylated plasminogen streptokinase activator complex (APSAC) [107]. Large-scale randomized trials of mortality, testing IV heparin versus no heparin in the setting of adequate aspirin, are still necessary to address this important issue.

Interestingly, Theroux et al. [108] recently reported reactivation of unstable angina and occurrence of MI after the discontinuation of heparin in a large clinical trial comparing aspirin and heparin for 6 days during the acute phase of unstable angina. This phenomenon appears to result from an imbalance between ongoing prothrombotic forces and decreasing antithrombotic activity after the withdrawal of heparin. Clinicians should be aware of the potential for reactivation after treatment with IV heparin in many other situations: for example, AMI, heparin cessation before bypass surgery, or cessation of heparin after an allergic reaction.

Current Recommendations

All patients with AMI seen within 12 hours of the onset of symptoms and without specific contraindications should receive oral aspirin (160 to 325 mg daily) along with an IV thrombolytic agent without delay. The adjunctive use of IV heparin should be considered when t-PA is used; however when SK or APSAC is used, data regarding efficacy are contradictory. Clinicians should be aware of the possibility of a true rebound phenomenon when heparin is discontinued after thrombolytic therapy.

Secondary Prevention of Late Recurrence of Myocardial Infarction and Mortality

With respect to secondary prevention of cardiovascular disease, ten large, randomized, placebo-controlled trials of the use of platelet inhibitory drugs after MI have been conducted [109–118] (Table 31-5). In seven of them, aspirin was used alone at a dose of 300 to 1500 mg daily or in combination with dipyridamole. Sulfinpyrazone was used in two of the studies, and ticlopidine in one. Although no significant differences among the various platelet inhibitory regimens were found, available data do not support the additional cost and increased frequency of administration of dipyridamole or sulfinpyrazone [119]. The pooled analysis of these trials concluded that platelet inhibitors significantly reduced vascular mortality by 13 percent, nonfatal reinfarction by 31 percent, nonfatal stroke by 42 percent, and all important vascular events by 25 percent [119, 120].

During the 1950s and 1960s many trials were performed to test the hypothesis that long-term anticoagulation prevents reinfarction and death in patients after MI. Because the incidence of these events decreases after the patient is discharged from the hospital, long-term trials require a large number of patients to detect benefit. Unfortunately, most of the early trials had inadequate numbers of patients. In 1970, an International Anticoagulant Review Group [121] attempted to overcome the problem of inadequate study size by pooling data from nine controlled, long-term anticoagulant trials involving 2205 men and 282 women. This collective review group concluded that mortality was reduced by 20 percent in men given long-term anticoagulants; however, given the problem of trial heterogeneity and inadequate design, this result must be interpreted with caution.

In 1980, the Sixty-Plus Reinfarction Study from The Netherlands revived study of the value of long-term anticoagulation after MI [122]. Ambulatory patients over the age of 60 years were studied. All patients had been receiving anticoagulants after documented MI that had occurred a minimum of 6 months earlier. Eligible patients were randomized to continue anticoagulants or to substitute placebo. The median interval from the time of the initial infarction was 6 years. There was a dramatic 55 percent reduction in the incidence of fatal and nonfatal recurrence of MI in the anticoagulant group, as well as a trend toward lower mortality (Table 31-6). The greater benefit of anticoagulants in this trial was probably related to better control of anticoagulant dosage therapy and to the fact that, in this relatively stable group of patients studied 6 years postinfarction, recurrent thrombotic events were important determinants of survival. In another review of 19 previous trials of oral anticoagulants in the prevention of death and recurrence of MI, Loeliger [123] found that, in trials with a level of anticoagulation mainly within the INR range of 2.5 to 5.0, the average risk of death was lowered by 40 percent and the average risk of nonfatal reinfarction was reduced by approximately two-thirds. In contrast, studies with inadequate or poor documentation of the level of anticoagulation found no difference in mortality but identified a trend favoring anticoagulant therapy in the prevention of reinfarction.

Table 31-5
Platelet inhibitory drugs after myocardial infarction

Study	Follow-up (mo.)	Drug	Dosage (mg/day)	No. of patients	Results of therapy
MRC-I [112]	12	ASA	300	1239	Trend toward less total death
CDP [113]	22	ASA	927	1529	Trend toward less total and vascular mortality
GARS [114]	24	ASA	1500	946	Trend toward lower myocardial infarction and cardiac death
MRC-II [115]	12	ASA	900	1682	Trend toward less total and coronary mortality
AMIS [116]	38	ASA	1000	4524	No benefit
PARIS-I [117]	41	ASA	972	2026	Trend toward less total and coronary mortality
ART [118]	16	SULF	800	1558	Reduction in sudden death only
ARIS [111]	19	SULF	800	727	Decreased reinfarction
PARIS-II [110]	23	ASA plus DIP	972 225	3128	Decreased reinfarction, trend toward lower total and coronary death
STAI [119]	6	TICL	500	652	Trend toward less cardiovascular mortality

MRC = Medical Research Council; CDP = Coronary Drug Project; GARS = German-Austrian Reinfarction Study; AMIS = Aspirin Myocardial Infarction Study; PARIS = Persantine-Aspirin Reinfarction Study; ART = Anturane Reinfarction Trial; ARIS = Anturane Reinfarction Italian Study; STAI = Studio sulla Ticlopidina nell'Agina Inestable; ASA = aspirin; DIP = dipyridamole; SULF = sulfinpyrazone; TICL = ticlopidine.

Table 31-6
Sixty-plus reinfarction study

Parameter	Placebo	Anticoagulant	p value
No. of patients	439	439	
Mean age (yr)	67	67	
Time since infarction (yr)	5	6	
Total recurrence infarction	64	29	.0005
Fatal recurrence infarction	28	11	
Total deaths	69	51	.071
Sudden deaths	20	22	
Total cerebrovascular events	21	13	.16
Intracerebral hemorrhage	1	9	
Nonhemorrhagic events	13	2	
Not identified	6	1	

In 1990, the Warfarin Reinfarction Study (WARIS) [124] appeared in response to the debate on long-term oral anticoagulation following the Sixty-Plus Study. WARIS was a prospective, double-blind, placebo-controlled study of 1214 survivors of AMI treated with warfarin (to an INR 2.8 to 4.8 times control) or placebo for an average of 37 months. Reductions in mortality of 24 percent, reinfarction of 34 percent, and stroke of 55 percent were observed among the warfarin-treated patients. Considering the results of these trials, aspirin and oral anticoagulants should be directly compared to establish if there is really a difference in efficacy. The benefit of warfarin plus aspirin has not been documented in a prospective study of patients after MI. The Coumadin Aspirin Reinfarction Study (CARS) was initiated to evaluate the effectiveness of warfarin plus aspirin versus aspirin alone for the prevention of reinfarction, death, and stroke.

Current Recommendations

Aspirin appears to have a protective effect for the prevention of coronary and cerebrovascular events in patients after MI. Aspirin, at a dose of 325 mg daily, is devoid of significant side effects and is, therefore, recommended. Furthermore, the long-term benefit of aspirin in patients in the chronic

Table 31-7
Antithrombotic therapy for myocardial infarction

Myocardial infarction	Risk	ASA	AC	ASA + AC
Primary prevention	Low	±	Unknown	–
Acute phase:				
No lysis	High	+	±	±
Lysis (SK/APSAC)	High	+	±	±
Lysis (t-PA)	High	+	+ (IVH)	±
Prevention DVT	Low	–	+ (SH)	–
Prevention LVT	Medium	–	+ (SH)	–
Secondary prevention	Medium	+	+	±*

ASA = aspirin; AC = anticoagulant; APSAC = anisoylated plasminogen streptokinase activator complex; SK = streptokinase; DVT = deep venous thrombosis; LVT = left ventricular thrombosis; IVH = intravenous heparin; SH = subcutaneous heparin; t-PA = tissue plasminogen activator; + = indicated, considered useful/effective; ± = acceptable, uncertain efficacy; – = not indicated.
*Evolving trials.

phase of unstable angina [125, 126] supports this recommendation. Chronic anticoagulant therapy may also reduce the rate of reinfarction and death in patients after an MI. Summarized recommendations for antithrombotic therapy for MI are outlined in Table 31-7.

Future Applications of New Anticoagulants and Antiplatelet Agents in Myocardial Infarction

The pivotal role of thrombin in the pathogenesis of platelet-rich thrombosis after deep arterial injury or thrombolytic therapy is supported by several independent studies. Specific thrombin inhibition can completely prevent formation [127] and accelerate lysis [128] of platelet-rich thrombi after deep arterial injury, suggesting that thrombosis after deep arterial injury is thrombin-dependent. Heparin [129] and the specific antithrombins [130] are thought to act mainly by blocking thrombin generation through interruption of the positive feedback that thrombin exerts on its own generation. Heparin must form a transient ternary complex with antithrombin-III and thrombin to inhibit thrombosis. The assembly of this complex within the thrombus is hindered by the relatively large size of antithrombin-III (molecular weight 58,000). This may be a key factor in the limited antithrombin efficacy of the heparinoids [131]. In contrast, direct antithrombins such as hirudin, DuP-714, hirulog, D-phenylalanyl-L-prolyl-L-arginylchloromethylketone (PPACK), argatroban, and hirugen have low molecular weight, do not depend on antithrombin-III, and effectively inhibit clot-bound thrombin [132].

Hirudin, a 65-residue polypeptide derived from the salivary gland of the medicinal leech *Hirudo medicinalis,* has the highest affinity for thrombin, is well tolerated in humans, and is nonimmunogenic [132, 133]. Hirudin binds thrombin with 1:1 stoichiometry; therefore, the plasma concentration of hirudin required to totally prevent thrombus formation is proportional to the amount of thrombin generated [131]. In a porcine preparation of platelet-rich occlusive thrombus after deep carotid artery injury, hirudin (at APTT 2 to 3 times baseline) significantly accelerated lysis by rt-PA compared with heparin (at APTT greater than 5 times baseline) and increased the incidence of reperfusion [128]. Preliminary clinical data from the TIMI-5 study [134] showed hirudin to have advantages over heparin as adjunctive therapy to t-PA and aspirin for the treatment of AMI. Hirudin was effective in preventing reocclusion by reducing the reocclusion rate from 7 percent to 1 percent in the heparin group, without an increase in spontaneous hemorrhage.

Multiple antiplatelet agents have been investigated for the prevention of arterial thrombosis and the enhancement of arterial thrombolysis with thrombolytic agents. Although there are preliminary results from clinical pilot studies, the role of such agents in patients with AMI is not yet established. Thromboxane synthase inhibitors have a theoretic advantage of preserving prostacyclin production from the endothelium [135, 136], whereas thromboxane A_2-prostaglandin endoperoxide receptor antagonists can block these products at the receptor level [137]. Agents that have both thromboxane synthase inhibition and endoperoxide receptor blocking actions have been developed [138] and tested in patients with AMI [139]. Serotonin antagonists have been studied alone and in conjunction with thromboxane A_2-prostaglandin endoperoxide receptor blockers [140]. Prostacyclin and prostaglandin E_1 may also reduce platelet aggregation by increasing platelet 5′-cyclic adenosine monophosphate (cAMP) levels [141]. The last step of the pathway can be blocked by a monoclonal antibody against glycoprotein IIb/IIIa receptor, or synthetic or natural peptides that have the arginine-glycine-aspartic acid sequence or the fibrinogen gamma-chain carboxyl-terminal sequence [142]. Results of the TAMI-8 pilot study have shown the combination of the monoclonal antibody m7E3 Fab with t-PA, heparin, and aspirin to be a promising and safe strategy for patients with AMI [143]. The combination of t-PA, thrombin inhibitor, and glycoprotein IIb/IIIa receptor blocker has also been shown to be effective in lysing resistant platelet-rich thrombus [144].

References

1. Falk, E. Plaque rupture with severe pre-existing stenosis precipitating coronary thrombosis: Characteristics of coronary atherosclerotic plaques underlying fatal occlusive thrombi. *Br. Heart J.* 50: 127, 1983.
2. Davies, M. J., and Thomas, A. C. Plaque fissuring—the cause of acute myocardial infarction, sudden ischemic death and crescendo angina. *Br. Heart J.* 53:363, 1985.
3. Fuster, V., Badimon, L., Badimon, J. J., et al. The pathogenesis of coronary artery disease and the acute coronary syndromes. *N. Engl. J. Med.* 326: 252; 318, 1992.
4. Chesebro, J. H., Badimon, J. J., Badimon, L., et al. Anticoagulant and antiplatelet therapy in acute coronary syndromes and atrial fibrillation. *Cardiol. Rev.* 3:167, 1993.
5. The Steering Committee of the Physicians' Health Study Research Group. Preliminary report: Findings from the aspirin component of the ongoing Physicians' Health Study. *N. Engl. J. Med.* 318: 262, 1988.
6. The Steering Committee of the Physicians' Health Study Research Group. Final report on the aspirin component of the ongoing Physicians' Health Study. *N. Engl. J. Med.* 321:129, 1989.
7. Peto, R., Gray, R., Collins, R., et al. A randomized trial of the effect of prophylactic daily aspirin in British male doctors. *B.M.J.* 296:313, 1988.
8. Feinstein, A. R. Statistical significance versus clinical importance. *Qual. Life Cardiovasc. Care.* Autumn:99, 1988.
9. Weissler, A. M., Miller, B. I., and Boudoulas, H. The need of clarification of percent risk reduction data in clinical cardiovascular trial reports. *J. Am. Coll. Cardiol.* 13:764, 1989.
10. Meade, T. W., and Miller, G. J. Combined use of aspirin and warfarin in primary prevention of ischemic heart disease in men at high risk. *Am. J. Cardiol.* 75:23B, 1995.
11. Murray, T. S., Lorimer, A. R., Cox, F. C., et al. Leg-vein thrombosis following myocardial infarction. *Lancet* 2:792, 1970.
12. Nicolaides, A. N., Kakkar, V. V., Renney, J. T. G., et al. Myocardial infarction and deep vein thrombosis. *B.M.J.* 1:432, 1971.
13. Maurer, B. J., Wray, R., Shillingford, J. P. Frequency of venous thrombosis after myocardial infarction. *Lancet* 2:1385, 1971.
14. Handley, A. J., Emerson, P. A., Fleming, P. R. Heparin in the prevention of deep vein thrombosis after myocardial infarction. *B.M.J.* 2:436, 1972.
15. Handley, A. J. Low-dose heparin after myocardial infarction. *Lancet* 2:623, 1972.
16. Wray, R., Maurer, B., and Shillingford, J. Prophylactic anticoagulant therapy in the prevention of calf vein thrombosis after myocardial infarction. *N. Engl. J. Med.* 288:815, 1973.
17. Simmons, A. V., Sheppard, M. A., and Cox, A. F. Deep venous thrombosis after myocardial infarction predisposing factors. *Br. Heart J.* 35:623, 1973.
18. Gallus, A. S., Hirsh, J., Tuttle, R. J., et al. Small subcutaneous doses of heparin in prevention of venous thrombosis. *N. Engl. J. Med.* 288:545, 1973.
19. Warlow, C., Beattie, A. G., Terry, G., et al. A double-blind trial of low doses of subcutaneous heparin in the prevention of deep vein thrombosis after myocardial infarction. *Lancet* 2:934, 1973.
20. Emerson, P. A., and Marks, P. Preventing thromboembolism after myocardial infarction: Effect of low-dose heparin or smoking. *B.M.J.* 1:18, 1977.
21. International Multicenter Trial. Prevention of fatal postoperative pulmonary embolism by low doses of heparin. *Lancet* 2:45, 1975.
22. Consensus Conference. Prevention of venous thrombosis and pulmonary embolism. *J.A.M.A.* 256: 744, 1986.
23. Tarhan, S., Moffitt, E. A., Taylor, W. F., et al. Myocardial infarction after general anesthesia. *J. Am. Coll. Cardiol.* 220:1451, 1972.
24. Ygge, J. Changes in blood coagulation and fibrinolysis during the postoperative period. *Am. J. Surg.* 119:225, 1970.

25. Miller, R. R., Lies, J. E., Caretta, R. F., et al. Prevention of lower extremity venous thrombosis by early mobilization: Confirmation in patients with acute myocardial infarction by ^{125}I fibrinogen uptake and venography. *Ann. Intern. Med.* 84:700, 1976.
26. Emerson, P. A., Teather, D., and Handley, A. J. The application of decision theory to the prevention of deep vein thrombosis following myocardial infarction. *Q. J. Med.* 43:389, 1974.
27. Veterans Administration Cooperative Investigators. Anticoagulant in acute myocardial infarction: Results of a cooperative clinical trial. *J.A.M.A.* 225:724, 1973.
28. Aber, C. P., Bass, N. M., Berry, C. L., et al. Streptokinase in acute myocardial infarction: A controlled multicenter study in the United Kingdom. *B.M.J.* 2:1100, 1976.
29. Donaldson, G. A., Williams, C., Scanell, J., et al. A reappraisal of the application of the Trendelenburg operation to massive fatal embolism. *N. Engl. J. Med.* 268:171, 1963.
30. Lensing, A. W., Prandoni, P., Brandjes, D., et al. Detection of deep vein thrombosis by real-time B-mode ultrasonography. *N. Engl. J. Med.* 320:342, 1989.
31. Baxter, G. M., Duffy, P., and Partridge, E. Color flow imaging of calf vein thrombosis. *Clin. Radiol.* 46:198, 1992.
32. ISIS-2 (Second International Study of Infarct Survival). Collaborative Group. Randomized trial of intravenous streptokinase, oral aspirin, both or neither among 17,187 cases of suspected acute myocardial infarction: ISIS-2. *Lancet* 2:349, 1988.
33. Drapkin, A., and Merskey, C. Anticoagulation therapy after acute myocardial infarction: Relation of therapeutic benefit to patient's age, sex, and severity of infarction. *J.A.M.A.* 222:541, 1972.
34. Hilden, T., Iversen, K., Raaschou, F., et al. Anticoagulants in acute myocardial infarction. *Lancet* 2:327, 1961.
35. Kakkar, V. V., and Murray, W. J. G. Efficacy and safety of low-molecular-weight heparin (CY216) in preventing postoperative venous thromboembolism: A co-operative study. *Br. J. Surg.* 72:786, 1985.
36. Koller, M., Schoch, U., Buchmann, P., et al. Low molecular weight heparin as thromboprophylaxis in elective visceral surgery. *Thromb. Haemost.* 56: 243, 1986.
37. The European Fraxiparin Study Group. Comparison of low molecular weight heparin and unfractionated heparin for the prevention of deep vein thrombosis in patients undergoing abdominal surgery. *Br. J. Surg.* 75:1058, 1988.
38. Meltzer, R. S., Visser, C. A., and Fuster, V. Intracardiac thrombi and systemic embolization. *Ann. Intern. Med.* 104:689, 1986.
39. Mikell, F. L., Asinger, R. W., Elsperger, K. J., et al. Regional stasis of blood in the dysfunctional left ventricle: Echocardiographic detection and differentiation from early thrombosis. *Circulation* 66: 755, 1982.
40. Asinger, R. W., Mikell, F. L., Elsperger, J., et al. Incidence of left ventricular thrombosis after acute transmural myocardial infarction: Serial evaluation by two-dimensional echocardiography. *N. Engl. J. Med.* 305:297, 1981.
41. Funke-Kupper, A. J., Verheugt, F. W. A., Peels, C. H., et al. Left ventricular thrombus incidence and behavior studied by serial two-dimensional echocardiography in acute anterior myocardial infarction: Left ventricular motion, systemic embolism and oral anticoagulation. *J. Am. Coll. Cardiol.* 13:1514, 1989.
42. Johnson, R. C., Crissman, R. S., and Didio, L. J. A. Endocardial alterations in myocardial infarction. *Lab. Invest.* 40:183, 1979.
43. Spirito, P., Bellotti, P., Chiarella, F., et al. Prognostic significance and natural history of left ventricular thrombi in patients with acute anterior myocardial infarction: A two-dimensional echocardiographic study. *Circulation* 72:774, 1985.
44. Nihoyannopoulus, P., Smith, G. C., Maseri, A., et al. The natural history of left ventricular thrombus in myocardial infarction: A rationale in support of masterly inactivity. *J. Am. Coll. Cardiol.* 14:903, 1989.
45. DeMaria, A. N., Bommer, W., Neumann, A., et al. Left ventricular thrombi identified by cross-sectional echocardiography. *Ann. Intern. Med.* 100: 29, 1979.
46. Reeder, G. S., Tajik, A. J., and Seward, J. B. Left ventricular mural thrombus. Two-dimensional echocardiographic diagnosis. *Mayo Clin. Proc.* 56:82, 1981.
47. Asinger, R. W., Mikell, F. L., Sharma, B., et al. Observations on detecting left ventricular thrombus with two-dimensional echocardiography: Emphasis on avoidance of false positive diagnoses. *Am. J. Cardiol.* 47:145, 1981.
48. Ezekowitz, M. D., Wilson, D. A., Smith, E. O., et al. Comparison of ^{111}indium scintigraphy and two-dimensional echocardiography in the diagnosis of left ventricular thrombi. *N. Engl. J. Med.* 306: 1509, 1982.
49. Visser, C. A., Kan, G., David, G. K., et al. Two-dimensional echocardiography in the diagnosis of left ventricular thrombus: A prospective study of 67 patients with anatomic validation. *Chest* 83: 228, 1983.
50. Swan, J. H. C., Magnusson, P. T., Buchbinder, N. A., et al. Aneurysm of the cardiac ventricle: Its management by medical and surgical intervention. *West. J. Med.* 129:26, 1978.
51. Reeder, G. S., Lengyel, M., Tajik, A. J., et al. Mural thrombus in left ventricular aneurysm: Incidence, role of angiography, and relation between anticoagulation and embolization. *Mayo Clin. Proc.* 56: 77, 1981.
52. Visser, C. A., Kan, G., Meltzer, R. S., et al. Embolic

potential of left ventricular thrombus after myocardial infarction: A two-dimensional echocardiographic study of 119 patients. *J. Am. Coll. Cardiol.* 5:1276, 1985.

53. Stratton, J. R., Nemanich, J. W., Johannessen, K. A., et al. Fate of left ventricular thrombi in patients with remote myocardial infarction or idiopathic cardiomyopathy. *Circulation* 78:1388, 1988.
54. Judgutt, B. I., Sivaram, C. A., Wortman, C., et al. Prospective two-dimensional echocardiographic evaluation of left ventricular thrombus and embolism after acute myocardial infarction. *J. Am. Coll. Cardiol.* 13:554, 1989.
55. Report of the Working Party on Anticoagulant Therapy in Coronary Thrombosis to the Medical Research Council: Assessment of short-term anticoagulant administration after cardiac infarction. *B.M.J.* 1:335, 1969.
56. Nordrehaug, J. E., Johenessen, K.-A., vor der Lippe, G., et al. Usefulness of high-dose anticoagulants in preventing left ventricular thrombus in acute myocardial infarction. *Am. J. Cardiol.* 55:1491, 1985.
57. Davis, M. J. E., and Ireland, M. A. Effects of early anticoagulation on the frequency of left ventricular thrombi after anterior myocardial infarction. *Am. J. Cardiol.* 57:1244, 1986.
58. Gueret, P., Dubourg, O., Ferrier, E., et al. Effects of full-dose heparin anticoagulation on the development of left ventricular thrombosis in acute transmural myocardial infarction. *J. Am. Coll. Cardiol.* 8:419, 1986.
59. Arvan, S., and Boscha, K. Prophylactic anticoagulation for left ventricular thrombi after acute myocardial infarction: A prospective randomized trial. *Am. Heart J.* 113:688, 1987.
60. Turpie, A. G. G., Robinson, J. G., and Doyle, D. J. Comparison of high-dose with low-dose subcutaneous heparin in the prevention of left ventricular mural thrombosis in patients with acute transmural anterior myocardial infarction. *N. Engl. J. Med.* 320:352, 1989.
61. SCATI (Studio sulla Calciparina nell'Angina e nella Trombosi Ventricolare nell'Infarto) Group. Randomized controlled trial of subcutaneous calcium-heparin in acute myocardial infarction. *Lancet* 2:182, 1989.
62. Held, A. C., Gore, J. M., Paraskos, J., et al. Impact of thrombolytic therapy on left ventricular mural thrombi in acute myocardial infarction. *Am. J. Cardiol.* 62:310, 1988.
63. Vecchio, C., Chiarella, F., Lupi, G., et al. Left ventricular thrombus in anterior acute myocardial infarction after thrombolysis: A GISSI-2 connected study. *Circulation* 84:512, 1991.
64. Marmos, A., Sobel, B., and Roberts, R. Factors presaging early recurrence myocardial infarction ("extension"). *Am. J. Cardiol.* 48:603, 1981.
65. Rothkopf, M., Boerner, J., Stone, M. J., et al. Detection of myocardial infarct extension by CKB radioimmunoassay. *Circulation* 59:268, 1979.
66. Fraker, T. D., Jr., Wagner, G. S., and Rosati, R. Extension of myocardial infarction: Incidence and prognosis. *Circulation* 60:1126, 1979.
67. Nasser, F. N., Chesebro, J. H., Homburger, H. A., et al. Myocardial infarct extension diagnosis by CK-MB radioimmunoassay and clinical significance. *Clin. Res.* 29:226, 1981.
68. Marmos, A., Geltman, E. M., Schechuman, K., et al. Recurrent myocardial infarction: Clinical predictors and prognostic implications. *Circulation* 66: 415, 1982.
69. Baker, J. T., Bramlet, D. A., Lester, R. M., et al. Myocardial infarct extension: Incidence and relationship to survival. *Circulation* 65:918, 1982.
70. Strauss, H. D. Myocardial infarction extension: Clinical significance. *Primary Cardiol.* 8:14, 1982.
71. Buda, A. J., MacDonald, I. L., Dubbin, J. D., et al. Myocardial infarct extension: Prevalence, clinical significance, and problems in diagnosis. *Am. Heart J.* 105:744, 1983.
72. Hutchins, G. M., and Bulkley, B. H. Infarct expansion versus extension: Two different complications of acute myocardial infarction. *Am. J. Cardiol.* 41: 1127, 1978.
73. DeWood, M., Stifter, W. F., Simpson, C. S., et al. Coronary arteriographic findings soon after non-Q wave myocardial infarction. *N. Engl. J. Med.* 315:417, 1986.
74. Gibson, R. S. Clinical, functional, and angiographic distinctions between Q wave and non-Q wave myocardial infarction: Evidence of spontaneous reperfusion and implications for intervention trials. *Circulation* 75(Suppl V):128, 1987.
75. Ambrose, J. A., Monsen, C., Borrico, S., et al. Angiographic demonstration of a common link between unstable angina pectoris and non-Q wave myocardial infarction. *Am. J. Cardiol.* 61:224, 1988.
76. Fuster, V., Badimon, L., Cohen, M., et al. Insights into the pathogenesis of acute ischemic syndromes. *Circulation* 77:1213, 1988.
77. Fuster, V., and Chesebro, J. H. Pharmacologic effects of platelet inhibitor drugs. *Mayo Clin. Proc.* 56:185, 1981.
78. Chesebro, J. H., Fuster, V., Pumphrey, C. W., et al. Improvement of shortened platelet survival half-life from the early to the late phase of myocardial infarction. *Circulation* 64(Suppl IV):197, 1981.
79. Gibson, R. S., Boden, W. E., Theroux, P., et al. Diltiazem and reinfarction in patients with non-Q wave myocardial infarction: Results of a double blind, randomized, multicenter trial. *N. Engl. J. Med.* 315:423, 1986.
80. Modan, B., Shani, S., Schor, S., et al. Reduction of hospital mortality from acute myocardial infarction by anticoagulant therapy. *N. Engl. J. Med.* 292:1359, 1975.
81. Tonascia, J., Gordis, L., and Schmerler, H. Retrospective evidence favoring use of anticoagulants for myocardial infarction. *N. Engl. J. Med.* 292: 1362, 1975.

82. Szklo, M., Tonascia, J. A., Goldberg, R., et al. Additional data favoring use of anticoagulant therapy in acute myocardial infarction: A population-based study. *J.A.M.A.* 242:1261, 1979.
83. Ravid, M., Kleiman, N., Shapira, J., et al. Anticoagulant therapy in acute myocardial infarction: Demonstration of a selection bias in a retrospective study. *Thromb. Res.* 18:753, 1980.
84. Chalmers, T. C., Matta, R., Smith H., Jr., et al. Evidence favoring the use of anticoagulants in the hospital phase of acute myocardial infarction. *N. Engl. J. Med.* 297:1091, 1977.
85. Goldman, L., and Feinstein, A. R. Anticoagulants and myocardial infarction: the problems of pooling, drowning and floating. *Ann. Intern. Med.* 90:92, 1979.
86. Yusuf, S., Wittes, J., and Friedman, L. Overview of results of randomized clinical trials in heart disease: I. Treatments following myocardial infarction. *J.A.M.A.* 60:2088, 1988.
87. MacMahon, S., Collins, R., Knight, C., et al. Reduction in major morbidity and mortality by heparin in acute myocardial infarction. *Circulation* 78:II-98, 1988.
88. Kennedy, J. W., Ritchie, J. L., Davis, K. B., et al. Western Washington randomized trial of intracoronary streptokinase in acute myocardial infarction. *N. Engl. J. Med.* 309:1477, 1983.
89. Kennedy, J. W., Ritchie, J. L., Davis, K. B., et al. Western Washington randomized trial of intracoronary streptokinase in acute myocardial infarction. A 12-month follow up report. *N. Engl. J. Med.* 312: 1073, 1985.
90. Simoons, M. L., Serruys, P. W., van den Brand, M., et al. Early thrombolysis in acute myocardial infarction: Limitations of infarct size and improved survival. *J. Am. Coll. Cardiol.* 7:717, 1986.
91. Schroder, R., Neahaus, K.-L., Leizorovick, A., et al. A prospective placebo-controlled double-blind multicenter trial of intravenous streptokinase in acute myocardial infarction (ISAM): Long-term mortality and morbidity. *J. Am. Coll. Cardiol.* 9: 197, 1987.
92. Gruppo Italiano per lo Studio della Streptochinasi nell'Infarto Miocardico (GISSI). Effectiveness of intravenous thrombolytic treatment in acute myocardial infarction. *Lancet* 1:397, 1986.
93. Wilcox, R. G., von der Lippe, G., Olsson C. G., et al. Trial of tissue plasminogen activator for mortality reduction in acute myocardial infarction: Anglo-Scandinavian Study of Early Thrombolysis (ASSET). *Lancet* 2:525, 1988.
94. AIMS Trial Study Group. Effect of intravenous APSAC on mortality after acute myocardial infarction: Preliminary report of a placebo-controlled clinical trial. *Lancet* 1:545, 1988.
95. Braunwald, E. Myocardial reperfusion, limitation of infarct size, reduction of left ventricular dysfunction, and improved survival: Should the paradigm be expanded? *Circulation* 79:441, 1989.
96. Van de Werf, F. Discrepancies between the effects of coronary reperfusion on survival and left ventricular function. *Lancet* 1:1367, 1989.
97. Califf, R. M., Topol, E. J., Gersh, B. J., et al. From myocardial salvage to patient salvage in acute myocardial infarction: The role of reperfusion therapy. *J. Am. Coll. Cardiol.* 14:1382, 1989.
98. Ohman, E. M., Califf, R. M., Topol, E. J., et al. Consequences of reocclusion after successful reperfusion therapy in acute myocardial infarction. *Circulation* 82:781, 1990.
99. Roux, S., Christeller, S., and Lüdin, E. Effects of aspirin on coronary reocclusion and recurrent ischemia after thrombolysis: A meta-analysis. *J. Am. Coll. Cardiol.* 19:671, 1992.
100. Hsia, J., Hamilton, W. P., Kleiman, N., et al. A comparison between heparin and low-dose aspirin as adjunctive therapy with tissue plasminogen activator for acute myocardial infarction. (HART). *N. Engl. J. Med.* 323:1433, 1990.
101. De Bono, D. P., Simoons, M. L., Tijssen, J., et al. Effect of early intravenous heparin on coronary patency, infarct size and bleeding complications after alteplase thrombolysis: Results of a randomized double blind European Cooperative Study Group trial. *Br. Heart J.* 67:122, 1992.
102. Gruppo Italiano per lo Studio della Sopravvivenza nell'Infarto Miocardico-II: GISSI-2: A factorial randomized trial of alteplase versus streptokinase and heparin versus no heparin among 12,490 patients with acute myocardial infarction. *Lancet* 336:65, 1990.
103. ISIS-3 (Third International Study of Infarct Survival) Collaborative Group. ISIS-3: A randomized comparison of streptokinase vs tissue plasminogen activator vs anistreplase and of aspirin plus heparin vs aspirin alone among 41,299 cases of suspected acute myocardial infarction. *Lancet* 339:753, 1992.
104. Kroon, C., ten Hove, W. R., de Boer, A., et al. Highly variable anticoagulant response after subcutaneous administration of high dose (12,500 IU) heparin in patients with myocardial infarction and healthy volunteers. *Circulation* 86:1370, 1992.
105. The GUSTO (Global Utilization of Streptokinase and t-PA for Occluded Arteries) Investigators. A comparison of four thrombolytic regimens consisting of tissue plasminogen activator, streptokinase, or both with subcutaneous intravenous heparin for acute myocardial infarction. *N. Engl. J. Med.* 329:673, 1993.
106. Col, J., Decoster, O., Hanique, G., et al. Infusion of heparin conjunct to streptokinase accelerates reperfusion of acute myocardial infarction: Results of a double blind randomized study (OSIRIS) (Abstract). *Circulation* 86:I-259, 1992.
107. O'Connor, C., for the DUCCS Study Group. Duke University Clinical Cardiology Studies (DUCCS-1). Presented at the American Heart Association, Anaheim, California, 1992.

108. Theroux, P., Waters, D., Lam, J., et al. Reactivation of unstable angina after the discontinuation of heparin. *N. Engl. J. Med.* 327:141, 1992.
109. Klimt, C. R., Knatterud, G. L., Stamler, J., et al. Part II: Secondary prevention with persantine and aspirin. *J. Am. Coll. Cardiol.* 7:251, 1986.
110. Report from the Anturane Reinfarction Italian Study: Sulfinpyrazone in post-myocardial infarction. *Lancet* 1:237, 1982.
111. Elwood, P. C., Cochrane, A. L., Burr, M. L., et al. A randomized controlled trial of acetyl salicylic acid in the second prevention of mortality from myocardial infarction. *B.M.J.* 1:436, 1974.
112. Coronary Drug Project Group. Aspirin in coronary heart disease. *J. Chronic Dis.* 29:625, 1976.
113. Breddin, K., Loew, D., Lechner, K., et al. Secondary prevention of myocardial infarction: Comparison of acetylsalicylic acid, phenprocoumon and placebo: A multicenter two year prospective study. *Thromb. Haemost.* 40:225, 1979.
114. Elwood, P. C., and Sweetnam, P. M. Aspirin and secondary mortality after myocardial infarction. *Lancet* 2:1313, 1979.
115. Aspirin Myocardial Infarction Study Research Group. A randomized, controlled trial of aspirin in persons recovered from myocardial infarction. *J.A.M.A.* 243:661, 1980.
116. Persantine-Aspirin Reinfarction Study Research Group. Persantine and aspirin in coronary heart disease. *Circulation* 62:449, 1980.
117. Anturane Reinfarction Trial Research Group. Sulfinpyrazone in the prevention of sudden death after myocardial infarction. *N. Engl. J. Med.* 302:250, 1980.
118. Balsano, F., Rizzon, P., Violi, F., et al. Antiplatelet treatment with ticlopidine in unstable angina. *Circulation* 82:17, 1990.
119. Antiplatelets Trialists' Collaboration. Secondary prevention of vascular disease by prolonged antiplatelet treatment. *B.M.J.* 296:320, 1988.
120. Canner, P. L. Aspirin in coronary heart disease: Comparison of six clinical trials. *Isr. J. Med. Sci.* 19:413, 1983.
121. International Anticoagulant Review Group. Collaborative analysis of long-term anticoagulant administration after acute myocardial infarction. *Lancet* 1:203, 1970.
122. Report of the Sixty Plus Reinfarction Study Research Group. A double-blind trial to assess long term oral anticoagulant therapy in elderly patients after myocardial infarction. *Lancet* 2:989, 1980.
123. Loeliger, E. A. Oral anticoagulation in patients surviving myocardial infarction: A new approach to old data. *Eur. J. Clin. Pharmacol.* 26:137, 1984.
124. Smith, P., Arnesen, H., and Holme, I. The effect of warfarin on mortality and reinfarction after myocardial infarction. *N. Engl. J. Med.* 323:147, 1990.
125. Lewis, H. D., Jr., Davis, J. W., Archibald, D. G., et al. Protective effects of aspirin against acute myocardial infarction and death in men with unstable angina: Results of Veterans Administration Cooperative Study. *N. Engl. J. Med.* 309:396, 1983.
126. Cairns, J. A., Gent, M., Singer, J., et al. Aspirin, sulfinpyrazone or both in unstable angina. *N. Engl. J. Med.* 313:1369, 1985.
127. Heras, M., Chesebro, J. H., Penny, W. J., et al. Effects of thrombin inhibition on the development of acute platelet-thrombus deposition during angioplasty in pigs: Heparin versus recombinant hirudin, a specific thrombin inhibitor. *Circulation* 79: 657, 1989.
128. Zoldhelyi, P., Chesebro, J. H., Mruk, J. S., et al. Failure of aspirin compared with heparin or hirudin to enhance lysis by rt-PA of platelet-rich thrombus after deep arterial injury in the pig (Abstract). *J. Am. Coll. Cardiol.* 19A:91, 1992.
129. Hirsh, J. Heparin. *N. Engl. J. Med.* 324:1565, 1991.
130. Fenton, J. W. II, Villanueva, G. B., Ofosu, F. A., et al. Thrombin inhibition by hirudin: How hirudin inhibits thrombin. *Haemostasis* 21(1):27, 1991.
131. Weitz, J. L., Hudoba, M., Massel, D., et al. Clot-bound thrombin is protected from inhibition by heparin-antithrombin III but is susceptible to inactivation by antithrombin III-independent inhibitors. *J. Clin. Invest.* 86:385, 1990.
132. Markwardt, F., Nowak, G., Stürzebecher, J., et al. Pharmacokinetics and anticoagulant effect of hirudin in man. *Thromb. Haemost.* 52:160, 1984.
133. Verstraete, M., Hoet, B., Tornai, I., et al. Hirudin, a specific thrombin inhibitor: Pharmacokinetics and haemostatic effects in man. *Circulation* 80(II): 421, 1989.
134. Cannon, C. P., McCabe, C. H., Henry, T. D., et al. Hirudin reduces reocclusion compared to heparin following thrombolysis in acute myocardial infarction: Results of the TIMI-5 Trial (Abstract). *J. Am. Coll. Cardiol.* 21:136A, 1993.
135. Bush, L. R., Campbell, W. B., Buja, L. M., et al. Effects of the selective thromboxane inhibitor dazoxibin on variations in cyclic blood flow in stenosed canine coronary arteries. *Circulation* 69: 1161, 1984.
136. Hook, B. G., Schumacher, W. A., Lee, D. L., et al. Experimental coronary artery thrombosis in the absence of thromboxane A_2 synthesis: Evidence for alternate pathway for coronary thrombosis. *J. Cardiovasc. Pharmacol.* 7:174, 1985.
137. Shebuski, R. J., Smith, J. M., Storer, B. L., et al. Influence of selective endoperoxide/thromboxane A_2 receptor antagonism with sulotroban on lysis time and reocclusion rate after tissue plasminogen activator-induced coronary thrombolysis in the dog. *J. Pharmacol. Exp. Ther.* 246:790, 1988.
138. Vandeplassche, G., Hermans, C., Van de Walter, A., et al. Differential effects of thromboxane A_2 synthase inhibition, singly or combined with thromboxane A_2-prostaglandin endoperoxide receptor antagonism, on occlusive thrombosis elicited by endothelial cell injury or by deep vascular damage in canine coronary arteries. *Circ. Res.* 69:313, 1991.

139. Tranchesi, B., Caramelli, B., Gebara, O., et al. Efficacy and safety of ridogrel versus aspirin in coronary thrombolysis with alteplase for myocardial infarction (Abstract). *J. Am. Coll. Cardiol.* 19:92A, 1992.
140. Golino, P., Asthon, J. H., McNatt, J., et al. Simultaneous administration of thromboxane A_2- and serotonin S_2-receptor antagonists markedly enhances thrombolysis and prevents or delays reocclusion after tissue-type plasminogen activator in a canine model of coronary thrombosis. *Circulation* 79: 911, 1989.
141. Topol, E. J., Ellis, S. G., Califf, R. M., et al. Combined tissue-type plasminogen and prostacyclin therapy for acute myocardial infarction. *J. Am. Coll. Cardiol.* 14:877, 1989.
142. Coller, B. S. Inhibitors of the platelet glycoprotein IIb/IIIa receptor as conjunctive therapy for coronary artery thrombolysis. *Cor. Art. Dis.* 3:1016, 1992.
143. Kleiman, N. S., Ohman, M., Califf, R. M., et al. Profound inhibition of platelet aggregation with monoclonal antibody 7E3 Fab after thrombolytic therapy. Results of the Thrombolysis and Angioplasty in Myocardial Infarction (TAMI) 8 Pilot Study. *J. Am. Coll. Cardiol.* 22:381, 1993.
144. Jang, I. K., Gold, H. K., Leinbach, R. C., et al. Lysis of resistant thrombus by t-PA combined with platelet IIb/IIIa receptor blocking synthetic pentapeptide (G4210) and selective thrombin inhibitor, Argatroban. (Abstract). *Circulation* 84:II-599, 1991.

32. Management of Persistent Heart Failure After Acute Myocardial Infarction

Milton Packer

Patients who develop congestive heart failure (CHF) during acute myocardial infarction (AMI) have three possible clinical outcomes. They may die as a result of progressive CHF or a malignant ventricular tachyarrhythmia. Alternatively, the hemodynamic and clinical manifestations of CHF may resolve because of the administration of effective therapy or due to spontaneous resolution of the systolic or diastolic abnormalities seen in the acutely ischemic left ventricle. Finally, the CHF state may persist, even though the patient has received (and may be continuing to receive) appropriate therapy with intravenous diuretics, vasodilators, and positive inotropic agents.

Management of the patient with persistent CHF after AMI is more difficult than treatment of the patient with chronic CHF. The course of patients with persistent postinfarction CHF is characterized by a striking degree of instability. Their clinical status may deteriorate rapidly and with little warning; hence, drugs that require days to weeks to exert their beneficial effects may fail to act with sufficient rapidity to be clinically useful in this setting. The postinfarction patient may also be particularly susceptible to the side effects of pharmacologic interventions; as a result, orally active agents must be used cautiously, as their actions (if unfavorable) cannot be rapidly terminated. Finally, compared with the patient with chronic CHF, postinfarction patients are more likely to be receiving drugs that may adversely affect left ventricular (LV) function. All of these factors make management of the postinfarction patient with persistent CHF a special therapeutic challenge.

Pathophysiology of Postinfarction Heart Failure

In postinfarction patients the hemodynamic abnormalities that underlie the syndrome of CHF may result from loss of viable myocardium, mechanical stresses that increase loading conditions in the heart, impaired ventricular relaxation, or a combination of these mechanisms. It is important to elucidate the contribution of each of these factors to the development of CHF in each patient because each mechanism responds differently to therapeutic interventions. Fortunately, the pathophysiology of postinfarction CHF can be characterized in most patients with the use of noninvasive cardiac imaging techniques.

Two-dimensional echocardiography or radionuclide ventriculography (RVG) (or both) should be performed in every patient with persistent CHF after an AMI. These techniques can detect and quantify the loss of functioning myocardium [1, 2]; patients whose CHF is the result of systolic dysfunction generally have a left ventricular ejection fraction (LVEF) less than 0.35 [3]. Noninvasive techniques can also be used to confirm the presence and estimate the severity of mechanical lesions that may contribute importantly to the development of CHF, such as the occurrence of mitral regurgitation in patients with papillary muscle rupture or the presence of an intracardiac left-to-right shunt in patients with ventricular septal rupture [4, 5]. Every effort should be made to detect such structural defects, as they are amenable to surgical correction and respond poorly to medical therapy [6–8].

Structural defects must be considered in any patient with postinfarction CHF who develops a new systolic murmur or whose LVEF is more than 0.35. Although the CHF state in patients with preserved systolic function may be related to abnormalities of diastolic function (which may also be qualified by noninvasive techniques), such diastolic abnormalities improve rapidly during the first week of the infarction and require no specific therapy [9–11]. In contrast, mechanical defects produce a precarious hemodynamic state that is likely to deteriorate (rather than resolve) with time [6–8]. Because the presence of a structural defect cannot be ruled out by bedside examination, echocardiography provides essential information in every patient with persistent CHF and preserved systolic function. If any doubt exists about the diagnosis, right heart catheterization should be performed immediately to look for the presence of regurgitant waves on the pulmonary wedge pressure tracing or to detect a large increase in oxygen saturation in blood collected from the right ventricle and pulmonary artery compared with that obtained from the right atrium.

Factors Contributing to the Development of Postinfarction Heart Failure

Factors that may exacerbate the development of CHF are more likely to be present in the patient who develops the syndrome immediately after an AMI than in the patient who develops CHF gradually over long periods of time.

Cardiac Arrhythmias

Most arrhythmias that can worsen the hemodynamic and clinical status of patients with CHF are supraventricular in origin and include sinus tachycardia, paroxysmal supraventricular or junctional tachycardia, atrial flutter, and atrial fibrillation. These tachyarrhythmias reduce the time available for ventricular filling, an event that is particularly deleterious in patients with impaired ventricular relaxation. Tachycardias may also increase myocardial oxygen consumption and decrease the time available for myocardial perfusion; these factors may act in concert to exacerbate myocardial ischemia. The most common causes of sinus and supraventricular tachycardias are anxiety, persistent pain, fever, pericarditis, atrial infarction, and pulmonary embolism. Most importantly, the occurrence of supraventricular tachyarrhythmias may be the only clue to the presence of LV failure. Hence attempts to treat supraventricular arrhythmias in the postinfarction patient must address the underlying cause and must assume (unless proved otherwise) that LV function is markedly impaired.

Myocardial Ischemia

The poor systolic function that is seen in some patients following an AMI may not only be the result of myocardial necrosis but may occur as a consequence of reversible myocardial ischemia. Such ischemia may manifest as episodes of typical angina, or it may occur without symptoms [12, 13]. An aggressive approach to the treatment of recurrent angina in patients with LV dysfunction is warranted [14], but the therapeutic implications of silent ischemia in this patient subset remain unclear. Although some investigators would differ [15], silent ischemia appears to be a rare event in patients with severe LV dysfunction following an AMI. Fewer than 5 percent of such patients have evidence of asymptomatic ST segment changes during ambulatory monitoring (M. Pfeffer, personal communication). Nevertheless, recurrent ischemic events are likely to be an important cause of disease progression in patients with postinfarction CHF. This may explain why coronary artery bypass surgery (CABG) favorably modifies the long-term outcome of patients with multiple-vessel disease and LV dysfunction [14].

Pharmacologic Agents

Several agents that are commonly used in patients with an AMI may exacerbate the symptoms of heart failure.

Anti-inflammatory drugs that are commonly given for the treatment of pericarditis may contribute to the development of CHF. Corticosteroids as well as nonsteroidal anti-inflammatory drugs may cause sodium retention; the latter may also antagonize the compensatory actions of endogenous vasodilators and reduce the efficacy of diuretic drugs [16, 17]. Both steroids and nonsteroidal agents may increase the severity of infarct expansion, an event that may contribute importantly to the development of CHF [18, 19]. Low-dose aspirin therapy does not produce such deleterious hemodynamic effects, however, and may be particularly useful in preventing the recurrence of myocardial ischemic events [20].

Antiarrhythmic drugs are commonly given for the treatment of asymptomatic ventricular arrhythmias in patients with LV dysfunction, even though nearly all antiarrhythmic drugs exert important cardiodepressant effects. The negative inotropic actions of agents such as disopyramide and flecainide are well established [21–23], but cardiac performance may also deteriorate following the administration of encainide, mexiletene, tocainide, procainamide, and lidocaine [23–27]. All antiarrhythmic drugs may exacerbate ventricular arrhythmias [28], especially in patients with LV dysfunction. The established risks of antiarrhythmic drug therapy outweigh the unproved benefits of these agents in preventing sudden death in most patients with postinfarction CHF.

Calcium channel blocking drugs may be used in postinfarction patients for the treatment of myocardial ischemia or supraventricular arrhythmias. All calcium channel blockers (including the dihydropyridines), however, exert important negative inotropic effects and may exacerbate the symptoms of CHF in patients with advanced LV dysfunction [29]. This observation may explain why the administration of these agents to patients with postinfarction CHF appears to affect their long-term outcome unfavorably [30].

Beta-adrenergic blocking drugs may be used during the postinfarction period for the treatment of myocardial ischemia and the prevention of future ischemic events. Beta blockers, however, may exacerbate the CHF state in patients with impaired LV dysfunction after an AMI [31]. If the beta blockers are withdrawn as a consequence of this adverse reaction, attempts should be made to reinstitute therapy with these drugs once the CHF state is under better control because the long-term prognosis of such patients may be altered favorably by interventions that interfere with the activity of the sympathetic nervous system [31, 32].

Treatment of Postinfarction Heart Failure

The major goals of the treatment of patients with persistent CHF following an AMI are to improve functional capacity and reduce long-term morbidity and mortality. The treatment of the postinfarction patient with heart failure can be divided into three phases: the first 48 hours, 3 to 21 days, and more than 3 weeks after the acute infarction.

First 48 Hours

Patients with CHF after an AMI are usually treated acutely with short-acting intravenous (IV) drugs in an effort to achieve rapid hemodynamic stability. Should the syndrome of CHF persist despite IV therapy or recur when IV drugs are withdrawn, the patient will require long-term treatment with oral agents. The concurrent use of IV drugs, however, considerably complicates the initiation of oral therapy, as the actions of and reactions to oral agents may be enhanced or obscured by concurrently administered IV drugs. Hence, before the initiation of oral therapy, it is advisable to discontinue the use of IV agents whenever possible. Fortunately, this can be done in most patients with postinfarction CHF.

Withdrawal of Intravenous Vasodilators

Nitroglycerin and nitroprusside are used to lower cardiac filling pressures in patients with acute CHF following MI, but the need for these drugs commonly wanes within 72 hours of the acute event. Cardiac filling pressures may decline because of diuretic therapy or because the diastolic abnormalities seen during the acute phase subside [6, 7]. Hence, cardiac filling pressures are frequently low 48 hours after an AMI regardless of whether the patient has been treated with nitroprusside [33]. In addition, patients may develop tolerance to IV vasodilators, especially nitroglycerin, when they are administered continuously; under such circumstances, these drugs can be tapered without incident [34, 35]. The rapid withdrawal of IV vasodilators should always be avoided, however, as the abrupt discontinuation of both nitroprusside and nitrates can produce rebound hemodynamic and clinical events [36, 37]. The increases in cardiac filling pressures that are occasionally seen when these drugs are withdrawn in the postinfarction patient can usually be controlled with IV diuretic therapy.

Withdrawal of Intravenous Positive Inotropic Agents

Dobutamine and amrinone can be used to enhance the inotropic state and improve the hemodynamic condition of patients with CHF after an MI [38, 39]. Many patients lose their dependency on these drugs, however, as the function of the acutely ischemic myocardium recovers [40]. Tolerance may also develop to the actions of continuous IV dobutamine, probably because of a progressive decrease in the density of myocardial beta receptors [41]. Consequently, the gradual withdrawal of IV positive inotropic agents usually produces few adverse hemodynamic and clinical effects. This is fortunate because no oral substitute for dobutamine or amrinone is presently available. Orally active beta agonists and phosphodiesterase inhibitors have yet to be proved clinically useful during long-term treatment [42–44].

Withdrawal of Intravenous Vasoconstrictors

The most difficult challenge in the management of the postinfarction patient with CHF is the withdrawal of drugs used to support systemic blood pressures, e.g., dopamine and norepinephrine. Orally active substitutes for these agents are not available, and the results of studies with experimental drugs (levodopa and ibopamine) that generate circulating levels of dopamine and its analogs have been disappointing [45, 46]. Occasionally, dopamine therapy can be successfully withdrawn only when the function of the ischemic myocardium can be improved with the use of surgical or nonsurgical revascularization techniques [47].

Days 3 to 21 After Infarction

Once therapy with an IV agent is withdrawn, treatment should be immediately initiated with long-term oral agents. The drugs of choice that should be considered in every patient with postinfarction CHF heart failure are (1) digitalis, (2) diuretics, (3) converting-enzyme inhibitors, and (4) isosorbide dinitrate.

Digitalis

Digitalis produces little hemodynamic effect within the first hours of an experimental or clinical MI, especially when ventricular function is not impaired [38, 48–50]. As time passes from the onset of the acute event, however, the ability of digitalis to produce favorable hemodynamic effects becomes more apparent [48, 50, 51]. What may account for this observation? Digitalis is most effective in patients with the most marked ventricular dilatation [52, 53], but patients within hours of an AMI have insufficient time for ventricular enlargement to occur. As the left ventricle dilates during the first week after the acute event, however, digitalis may begin to produce important hemodynamic benefits [48].

Are these hemodynamic effects translated into clinical improvement? Several controlled trials have now shown that digitalis is an effective agent for the treatment of patients with chronic CHF in normal sinus rhythm [44, 52, 54]. Digoxin improves exercise tolerance and reduces the need for diuretics, hospitalization, and emergency care for worsening CHF heart failure [54]; when digoxin is withdrawn, the clinical status of the patient deteriorates [44, 55]. These benefits have been observed primarily in patients with systolic dysfunction (as evidenced by a low ejection fraction (EF), LV dilatation, and a third heart sound) [52, 53]. In contrast, digoxin appears to be ineffective in patients with preserved systolic function, regardless of the severity of symptoms [56, 57]. This observation underscores the importance of characterizing the pathophysiology of CHF before deciding what drugs the patient should receive.

Despite concerns about its toxicity, digoxin appears to be well tolerated by most patients with chronic CHF. Although there have been concerns about the potential of digoxin to produce arrhythmias in subjects with acute ischemia, this risk appears to subside during the first week after the AMI [48]. In fact, digoxin may be less arrhythmogenic than other positive inotropic agents, particularly those that act by increasing intracellular cyclic adenosine monophosphate (AMP) [44].

Diuretics

Diuretics produce symptomatic benefits in patients with CHF following an AMI. Their major advantage is their rapidity of effect. Diuretics can relieve dyspnea and edema within hours or days, whereas the responses to many other therapeutic agents may take weeks or months. Diuretics alone appear to be insufficient to control the symptoms of CHF in most patients, however. A high proportion of patients whose symptoms are stabilized by diuretics alone deteriorate clinically during long-term follow-up, unless they also receive concurrent therapy with digitalis or converting-enzyme inhibitors [54]. Increments in the dose of diuretics may produce little hemodynamic benefit, perhaps because such high doses activate endogenous neurohormonal vasoconstrictor systems that may limit the benefits of these drugs [58]. Furthermore, the electrolyte depletion that may result from aggressive diuretic therapy may exacerbate the ventricular arrhythmias seen in patients with an AMI [59]. Hence, in most patients it seems preferable to add a second drug than to use high doses of diuretics.

Converting-Enzyme Inhibitors

The renin-angiotensin system is activated following an AMI and contributes importantly to the increase in ventricular wall stress that is seen in these patients [60]. Such augmented wall stress may initiate a process of ventricular enlargement that can lead to a progressive deterioration of LV function [61]. This sequence of events, however, can be interrupted by therapy with a converting-enzyme inhibitor [61, 62]. Patients with CHF following an AMI experience important hemodynamic benefits when treated with converting-enzyme inhibitors; early therapy appears to attenuate the development of ventricular enlargement and, thereby, acts to preserve ventricular function [63–65]. Similar benefits may not be achieved, however, if ventricular volumes are reduced by agents that stimulate endogenous neurohormonal systems [65].

Controlled clinical trials have demonstrated that converting-enzyme inhibitors can reduce the mortality of patients with a recent MI when initiated as early as 3 days and as late as 10 to 16 days following the acute event. In the Acute Infarction Ramipril Efficacy (AIRE) trial, ramipril reduced mortality by 27 percent in patients with established CHF (with or without LV dysfunction) when treatment was maintained for 6 to 15 months [66]. In the Survival and Ventricular Enlargement (SAVE) trial, captopril reduced mortality by 19 percent in patients with a LVEF less than 0.40 (with or without symptoms of CHF) when treatment was maintained for 24 to 60 months [67]. The results of these two studies indicate that when administered 3 to 21 days following the AMI, converting-enzyme inhibitors can favorably influence the natural history of patients who have hemodynamic or clinical evidence of LV dysfunction.

Should converting-enzyme inhibitors be administered before 3 to 21 days and should they be administered to all postinfarction patients—even those without evidence of LV dysfunction or CHF? These two questions have been addressed in two large-scale studies, the Fourth International Study of Infarct Survival (ISIS-4) and Gruppo Italiano per lo Studio della Sopravvivenza nell'Infarto Miocardico-3 (GISSI-3), which enrolled patients regardless of ventricular function or clinical symptoms, initiated therapy within 24 hours of the ischemic event, and continued therapy for 4 to 6 weeks. In these studies, captopril and lisinopril reduced mortality by 5 to 10 percent, which, although small in magnitude, was statistically significant. Subgroup analysis suggested that the small effect was related to the dilution of a large therapeutic effect in patients with LV dysfunction by the enrollment of patients without evidence of CHF. Hence, in patients with hemodynamic and clinical evidence of ventricular dysfunction, therapy with a converting-enzyme inhibitor should be initiated as soon as possible—even within the first 24 hours of the infarction. In contrast, in patients with normal ventricular function and without CHF, the benefits of treatment with a converting enzyme remain uncertain. Such early treatment may be harmful if the therapy with converting-enzyme inhibitor is initiated by using large doses or employing an IV route of administration [68].

Nitrates

In patients with postinfarction heart failure, nitroglycerin and isosorbide dinitrate produce hemodynamic effects similar to those seen with the converting-enzyme inhibitors, but it is unknown if long-term nitrate therapy can favorably modify the ventricular remodeling process. When the results of controlled trials with nitrates are pooled, treatment with nitrates appears to reduce mortality in patients with an AMI [69], but this effect was not confirmed in ISIS-4 and GISSI-3.

Even after the acute phase of the infarction has passed, the role of nitrates in the management of patients with persistent CHF remains uncertain. In the placebo-controlled trials carried out to date, long-term treatment with oral isosorbide dinitrate has produced some favorable effects, but nitrates failed to produce an increase in exercise capacity that was consistently better than placebo, and nitrate therapy was not reliably accompanied by the relief of symptoms [37, 70, 71]. Even when combined with hydralazine, isosorbide dinitrate failed to improve the clinical status or exercise tolerance of patients with chronic heart failure after 2 and 6 months of therapy [72].

After 3 Weeks

One of the major goals of long-term therapy in the patient with postinfarction CHF is to prolong life. Agents that may affect survival (favorably or unfavorably) include digitalis, direct-acting vasodilators, converting-enzyme inhibitors, beta blockers, and calcium channel blockers.

Digitalis

We know little about the effect of digitalis on the survival of patients with CHF following an AMI, as controlled trials with this agent have not been carried out. Retrospective analyses have identified digitalis therapy as a risk factor for enhanced mortality [73], but it is possible that this adverse association was related to the severity of CHF heart failure in treated patients and not to therapy with the drug. A large-scale trial to evaluate the impact of digitalis on survival is now being conducted by the National Heart, Lung, and Blood Institute.

Direct-Acting Vasodilators

The Veterans Administration Vasodilator Heart Failure Trial (V-HeFT) reported that a combination of hydralazine and isosorbide dinitrate can reduce mortality in patients with mild to moderate symptoms [74]. The combination of the two vasodilators was poorly tolerated, however. During the period of follow-up, one or both drugs were discontinued in 38 percent of patients because of side effects, and only 55 percent of patients were taking full doses of both drugs at the end of 6 months. These side effects appeared to be more frequent with hydralazine than with isosorbide dinitrate; hydralazine may also exacerbate ischemia in patients with CHF and active angina [75]. Consequently, many physicians have prescribed isosorbide dinitrate alone in an effort to gain the prognostic benefits reported in V-HeFT. Isosorbide dinitrate alone may not prolong life in patients with CHF, however. The reduction in mortality seen in V-HeFT was related to an increase in the LVEF [76], but such an increase is more likely to be seen with hydralazine than with isosorbide dinitrate [77]. In addition, the regression of cellular hypertrophy seen when the two vasodilators are combined can be achieved with hydralazine alone but not with isosorbide dinitrate alone [78]. Therefore, although one retrospective study noted an association between nitrate therapy and prolonged survival of patients after an AMI [79], the role of nitrate monotherapy in preventing future cardiovascular events in these patients remains uncertain.

Converting-Enzyme Inhibitors

Even if converting-enzyme inhibitors are not initiated early after an AMI they can be beneficial during the chronic phase—after ventricular dilatation has occurred. Converting-enzyme inhibitors reduce the symptoms of CHF, enhance exercise tolerance, and reduce mortality [54, 80–86]; these benefits are seen in patients with mild, moderate, or severe symptoms. Even in patients with LV systolic dysfunction but no symptoms of CHF, converting-enzyme inhibitors can reduce the risk of the development of CHF as well as the risk of a recurrent MI [67, 87]. Converting-enzyme inhibitors, however, cannot control the symptoms of CHF in the absence of diuretic therapy [88], but fortunately, these drugs can antagonize many of the adverse neurohormonal and metabolic effects of diuretics [82, 83]. On the other hand, diuretics appear to potentiate the side effects of the converting-enzyme inhibitors [89]. These observations suggest that although these two classes of drugs should almost always be combined, caution should be exercised (particularly in the postinfarction patient) to titrate the dose of diuretics so as to minimize the occurrence of symptomatic hypotension and functional renal insufficiency.

Beta-Adrenergic Blockers

Beta blockers have particular appeal in the postinfarction patient because they interfere with the potentially deleterious effects of adrenergic stimulation on the failing heart. A variety of beta blockers (primarily those without intrinsic sympathomimetic activity) have been shown to prolong life in patients following an AMI; this reduction in mortality appears to be most marked in patients with a history of CHF before or during their AMI [31, 32]. Despite these benefits, however, few physicians are using beta blockers in patients with LV dysfunction following an AMI because of fears that these drugs may aggravate the symptoms of CHF. Although this complication could conceivably be avoided by incorporating beta-agonist activity into the pharmacologic profile of the drug, the presence of such activity could potentially abolish the ability of a beta blocker to prolong survival [90].

Calcium Channel Blockers

Calcium channel blockers at first appear to be advantageous in patients with postinfarction CHF, as their anti-ischemic effects might prevent the development of ischemic necrosis, and their ability to retard entry of calcium into the cell might exert favorable long-term effects on the progression of CHF [91, 92]. Calcium channel blockers, however, exert important negative inotropic effects in patients with LV dysfunction [29]. Furthermore, their ability to stimulate neurohormonal systems may contribute to disease progression. These factors may explain why the administration of a calcium channel blocker to patients with postinfarction CHF was associated with an increase (rather than a decrease) in recurrent cardiac events and mortality [30]. These observations indicate that calcium channel blockers should be avoided in patients with postinfarction CHF.

The patient who develops CHF after an AMI presents a special challenge to the practicing physician. Every effort should be made to alleviate reversible causes of CHF in these patients and to minimize the contribution of potentially deleterious factors. A variety of pharmacologic interventions are available that can improve the hemodynamic status and the functional capacity of these patients; in addition, drugs have been developed that can reduce long-term morbidity and mortality in this disease. Above all, we must attempt to reduce the recurrence of future ischemic events in these high-risk patients with aspirin and by the judicious use of CABG in patients with multivessel disease [14, 20]. The benefits of surgery appear to be particularly striking in postinfarction patients with LV dysfunction [14].

References

1. Sanford, G. F., Corbett, J., Nicod, P., et al. Value of radionuclide ventriculography in the immediate characterization of patients with an acute myocardial infarction. *Am. J. Cardiol.* 49:637, 1982.
2. Nishimura, R. A., Tajik, A. J., Shub, C., et al. Role of two-dimensional echocardiography in the prediction of in-hospital complications after acute myocardial infarction. *J. Am. Coll. Cardiol.* 4:1080, 1984.
3. Mangschau, A., Rollag, A., Jonsbu, J., et al. Congestive heart failure and ejection fraction in acute myocardial infarction. *Acta Med. Scand.* 220:101, 1986.
4. Come, P. C., Riley, M. F., Weintraub, R., et al. Echocardiographic detection of complete and partial papillary muscle rupture during acute myocardial infarction. *Am. J. Cardiol.* 56:787, 1985.
5. Barzilai, B., Bessler, C., Jr., Perez, J. E., et al. Significance of Doppler-detected regurgitation in acute myocardial infarction. *Am. J. Cardiol.* 61:220, 1988.
6. Miller D. C., and Stinson, E. B. Surgical management of acute mechanical defects secondary to myocardial infarction. *Am. J. Surg.* 141:677, 1981.
7. Scanlon, P. J., Montoya, A., Johnson, S. A., et al. Urgent surgery for ventricular septal rupture complicating acute myocardial infarction. *Circulation* 72 (Suppl II):185, 1985.
8. Pinwica, A., Menasche, P., Beaufils, P., and Julliard, J. M. Long-term results of emergency surgery for postinfarction ventricular septal defect. *Ann. Thorac. Surg.* 44:274, 1987.
9. Murray, D. P., Corbei, H. M., Dunselman, P. H., et al. Natural evolution of left ventricular haemodynamics following uncomplicated acute myocardial infarction. *Int. J. Cardiol.* 11:175, 1986.
10. Pirzada, F. A., Ekong, E. A., Vokonas, P. S., et al. Experimental myocardial infarction. XIII. Sequential changes in left ventricular pressure-length relations in the acute phase. *Circulation* 53:970, 1976.
11. Fletcher, P. J., Pfeffer, J. M., Pfeffer, M. A., et al. Left ventricular diastolic pressure-volume relations in rats with healed myocardial infarction: Effects on systolic function. *Circ. Res.* 49:618, 1981.
12. Tavazzi, L., Giannuzzi, P., Giordano, A., et al. Is post-infarction angina related to poor residual left ventricular function? *Eur. Heart J.* 7(Suppl C):25, 1986.

13. Chierchia, S., Lazzari, M., Freedman, B., et al. Impairment of myocardial perfusion and function during painless myocardial ischemia. *J. Am. Coll. Cardiol.* 1:924, 1983.
14. Luchi, R. J., Scott, S. M., and Deupree, R. H. Comparison of medical and surgical treatment for unstable angina pectoris: Results of a Veterans Administration Cooperative Study. *N. Engl. J. Med.* 316:977, 1987.
15. Cohn, P. F. Silent myocardial ischemia. *Ann. Intern. Med.* 109:312, 1988.
16. Dzau, V. J., Packer, M., Lilly, L. S., et al. Prostaglandins in severe heart failure: Relation to activation of the renin-angiotensin system and hyponatremia. *N. Engl. J. Med.* 310:347, 1984.
17. Oliw, E., Kover, G., Larsson, C., et al. Reduction by indomethacin of furosemide effects in the rabbit. *Eur. J. Pharmacol.* 38:95, 1976.
18. Mannisi, J. A., Weisman, H. F., Bush, D. E., et al. Steroid administration after myocardial infarction promotes early infarct expansion: A study in the rat model. *J. Clin. Invest.* 79:1431, 1987.
19. Hammerman, H., Schoen, F. J., Braunwald, E., et al. Drug-induced expansion of infarct: Morphologic and functional correlations. *Circulation* 69:611, 1984.
20. Lewis, H. D., Davis, J. W., Archibald, D. G., et al. Protective effects of aspirin against acute myocardial infarction and death in men with unstable angina. *N. Engl. J. Med.* 309:396, 1983.
21. Jackson, N., Verma, S. P., Frais, M. A., et al. Hemodynamic dose-response effects of flecainide in acute myocardial infarction with and without left ventricular decompensation. *Clin. Pharmacol. Ther.* 37:619, 1985.
22. Cohen, A. A., Daru, V., Covelli, G., et al. Hemodynamic effects of intravenous flecainide in acute noncomplicated myocardial infarction. *Am. Heart J.* 110:1193, 1985.
23. Silke, B., Frais, M. A., Verna, S. P., et al. Comparative hemodynamic effects of intravenous lignocaine, disopyramide and flecainide in uncomplicated acute myocardial infarction. *Br. J. Clin. Pharmacol.* 22:707, 1986.
24. MacMahon, B., Bakshi, M., Branagan, P., et al. Pharmacokinetics and haemodynamic effects of tocainide in patients with acute myocardial infarction complicated by left ventricular failure. *Br. J. Clin. Pharmacol.* 19:429, 1985.
25. Lotto, A., Finzi, A., Massari, F. M., et al. Hemodynamic effects of antiarrhythmic drugs in acute myocardial infarction. *G. Ital. Cardiol.* 14:762, 1984.
26. Gottlieb, S. S., Kukin, M. L., Yushak, M., et al. Cardiodepressant effects of encainide in patients with severe left ventricular dysfunction. *Ann. Int. Med.* 110:505, 1989.
27. Gottlieb, S. S., Kukin, M. L., Wilson, P. B., et al. Loading doses of oral procainamide exert cardiodepressant effects and activate neurohormones in patients with left ventricular dysfunction (Abstract). *J. Am. Coll. Cardiol.* 11:91A, 1988.
28. Velebit, V., Podrid, P., Lown, B., et al. Aggravation and provocation of ventricular arrhythmias by antiarrhythmic drugs. *Circulation* 65:886, 1982.
29. Packer, M., Kessler, P. D., and Lee, W. H. Calcium channel blockade in the management of severe chronic congestive heart failure: A bridge too far. *Circulation* 75(Suppl V):56, 1987.
30. Multicenter Diltiazem Post-Infarction Research Group. The effect of diltiazem on mortality and reinfarction after myocardial infarction. *N. Engl. J. Med.* 319:385, 1988.
31. Chadda, K., Goldstein, S., Byington, R., and Curb, J. D. Effect of propranolol after acute myocardial infarction in patients with congestive heart failure. *Circulation* 73:503, 1986.
32. Olsson, G., and Rehnqvist, N. Effect of metoprolol in postinfarction patients with increased heart size. *Eur. Heart J.* 7:468, 1986.
33. Cohn, J. N., Franciosa, J. A., Francis, G. S., et al. Effect of short-term infusion of sodium nitroprusside on mortality rate in acute myocardial infarction complicated by left ventricular failure. *N. Engl. J. Med.* 306:1129, 1982.
34. Roth, A., Weber, L., Friedenberger, L., et al. Hemodynamic effects of intravenous isosorbide dinitrate and nitroglycerin in acute myocardial infarction and elevated pulmonary artery wedge pressure. *Chest* 91:190, 1987.
35. Packer, M., Lee, W. H., Kessler, P. D., et al. Prevention and reversal of nitrate tolerance in patients with congestive heart failure. *N. Engl. J. Med.* 317:799, 1987.
36. Packer, M., Meller, J., Medina, N., et al. Rebound hemodynamic events after the abrupt withdrawal of nitroprusside in patients with severe chronic heart failure. *N. Engl. J. Med.* 301:1193, 1979.
37. Franciosa, J. A., Nordstrom, L. A., and Cohn, J. N. Nitrate therapy for congestive heart failure. *J.A.M.A.* 240:443, 1978.
38. Goldstein, R. A., Passamani, E. R., and Roberts, R. A comparison of digoxin and dobutamine in patients with acute infarction and cardiac failure. *N. Engl. J. Med.* 303:846, 1980.
39. Taylor, S. H., Verna, S. P., Hussain, M., et al. Intravenous amrinone in left ventricular failure complicated by acute myocardial infarction. *Am. J. Cardiol.* 56:29B, 1985.
40. Braunwald, E., and Kloner, R. A. The stunned myocardium: Prolonged, postischemic ventricular dysfunction. *Circulation* 66:1150, 1982.
41. Unverferth, D. V., Blanford, M., Kates, R. E., et al. Tolerance to dobutamine after a 72 hour continuous infusion. *Am. J. Med.* 69:262, 1980.
42. Roubin, G. S., Choong, C. Y., Devenish-Meares, S., et al. Beta-adrenergic stimulation of the failing left ventricle: A double-blind, randomized trial of sustained oral therapy with prenalterol. *Circulation* 69:955, 1984.
43. Weber, K. T., Andrews, V., Janicki, J. S., et al. Pirbuterol, an oral beta-adrenergic receptor agonist,

in the treatment of chronic cardiac failure. *Circulation* 66:1262, 1982.
44. DiBianco, R., Shabetai, R., Kostuk, W., et al. Oral milrinone and digoxin in heart failure: Results of a placebo-controlled, prospective trial of each agent and the combination (Abstract). *Circulation* 76(Suppl IV):256, 1987.
45. Kasper, W., Meinertz, T., Busch, W., et al. Does long term oval levodopa therapy improve cardiac function in congestive heart failure? (Abstract). *Circulation* 72(Suppl III):302, 1985.
46. Rajfer, S. I., Rossen, J. D., Douglas, F. L., et al. Effects of long-term therapy with oral ibopamine on resting hemodynamics and exercise capacity in patients with heart failure: Relationship to the generation of N-methyldopamine and to plasma norepinephrine levels. *Circulation* 73:740, 1986.
47. Heuser, R. R., Maddoux, G. L., Goss, J. E., et al. Coronary angioplasty for acute mitral regurgitation due to myocardial infarction: A nonsurgical treatment preserving mitral valve integrity. *Ann. Intern. Med.* 107:852, 1987.
48. Kumar, R., Hood Jr., W. B., Joison, J., et al. Experimental myocardial infarction. VI. Efficacy and toxicity of digitalis in acute and healing phase in intact conscious dogs. *J. Clin. Invest.* 49:358, 1970.
49. Balcon, R., Hoy, J., and Sowton, E. Haemodynamic effects of rapid digitalization following acute myocardial infarction. *Br. Heart J.* 30:373, 1968.
50. Marchionni, N., Pini, R., Vannucci, A., et al. Hemodynamic effects of digoxin in acute myocardial infarction in man: A randomized controlled trial. *Am. Heart J.* 109:636, 1985.
51. Kurogane, K., Fujitani, K., and Fukuzaki, H. Hemodynamic effects of digoxin on congestive heart failure in old myocardial infarction, dilated cardiomyopathy, acute myocardial infarction and mitral stenosis. *Jpn. Heart J.* 26:155, 1985.
52. Guyatt, G. H., Sullivan, M. J. J., Fallen, E. L., et al. A controlled trial of digoxin in congestive heart failure. *Am. J. Cardiol.* 61:371, 1988.
53. Lee, D. C., Johnson, R. A., Bingham, J. B., et al. Heart failure in outpatients: A randomized trial of digoxin versus placebo. *N. Engl. J. Med.* 306:699, 1982.
54. Captopril-Digoxin Multicenter Research Group. Comparative effects of captopril and digoxin in patients with mild to moderate heart failure. *J.A.M.A.* 259: 539, 1988.
55. Arnold, S. B., Byrd, R. C., Meister, W., et al. Long-term digitalis therapy improves left ventricular function in heart failure. *N. Engl. J. Med.* 303:1443, 1980.
56. Fleg, J. L., Gottlieb, S. H., and Lakatta, E. G. Is digoxin really important in treatment of compensated heart failure? A placebo-controlled crossover trial in patients with sinus rhythm. *Am. J. Med.* 73:244, 1982.
57. Gheorghiade, M., and Beller, G. A. Effects of discontinuating maintenance digoxin therapy in patients with ischemic heart disease and congestive heart failure in sinus rhythm. *Am. J. Cardiol.* 51:1243, 1983.
58. Larsen, F. F. Haemodynamic effects of high or low doses of furosemide in acute myocardial infarction. *Eur. Heart J.* 9:125, 1988.
59. Nodrehaug, J. E., and von der Lippe, G. Hypokalemia and ventricular fibrillation in acute myocardial infarction. *Br. Heart J.* 50:525, 1983.
60. Dargie, H. J., McAlpine, H. M., and Morton, J. J. Neuroendocrine activation in acute myocardial infarction. *J Cardiovasc. Pharmacol.* 9(Suppl 2):S21, 1987.
61. Pfeffer, J. M., Pfeffer, M. A., and Braunwald, E. Influence of chronic captopril therapy on the infarcted left ventricle of the rat. *Circ. Res.* 57:84, 1985.
62. Pfeffer, M. A., Pfeffer, J. M., Steinberg, C., and Finn, P. Survival after an experimental infarction: Beneficial effect of long-term therapy with captopril. *Circulation* 72:406, 1985.
63. McAlpine, H. M., Morton, J. J., Leckie, B., et al. Haemodynamic effects of captopril in acute left ventricular failure complicating myocardial infarction. *J. Cardiovasc. Pharmacol.* 9(Suppl 2):S25, 1987.
64. Pfeffer, M. A., Lamas, G. A., Vaughn, D. E., et al. Effect of captopril on progressive ventricular dilatation after anterior myocardial infarction. *N. Engl. J. Med.* 319:80, 1988.
65. Sharpe, N., Murphy, J., Smith, H., and Hannan, S. Treatment of patients with symptomless left ventricular dysfunction after myocardial infarction. *Lancet* 1:255, 1988.
66. The Acute Infarction Ramipril Efficacy (AIRE) Study Investigators. Effect of ramipril on mortality and morbidity of survivors of acute myocardial infarction with clinical evidence of heart failure. *Lancet* 342: 821, 1992.
67. Pfeffer, M. A., Braunwald, E., Loye, L. A., et al. Effect of captopril on mortality and morbidity in patients with left ventricular dysfunction after myocardial infarction. Results of the Survival and Ventricular Enlargement Trial. *N. Engl. J. Med.* 327: 669, 1992.
68. Swedberg, K., Held, P., Kjekshus, J., et al. Effects of the early administration of enalapril on mortality in patients with acute myocardial infarction. *N. Engl. J. Med.* 327:678, 1992.
69. Yusuf, S., Collins, R., MacMahon, S., et al. Effect of intravenous nitrates on mortality in acute myocardial infarction: An overview of the randomized trials. *Lancet* 1:1088, 1988.
70. Leier, C. V., Huss, P., Magorien, R. D., et al. Improved exercise capacity and differing arterial and venous tolerance during chronic isosorbide dinitrate therapy for congestive heart failure. *Circulation* 67:817, 1983.
71. Franciosa, J. A., Goldsmith, S. R., and Cohn, J. N. Contrasting immediate and long-term effects of isosorbide dinitrate on exercise capacity in congestive heart failure. *Am. J. Med.* 69:559, 1980.

72. Cohn, J. N., Archibald, D. G., and Johnson, G. Effects of vasodilator therapy on peak exercise oxygen consumption in heart failure: V-HeFT (Abstract). *Circulation* 75(Suppl II):443, 1987.
73. Bigger Jr., J. T., Fleiss, J. L., Rolnitzky, L. M., et al. Effect of digitalis treatment on survival after acute myocardial infarction. *Am. J. Cardiol.* 55:623, 1985.
74. Cohn, J. N., Archibald, D. G., Ziesche, S., et al. Effect of vasodilator therapy on mortality in chronic congestive heart failure: Results of a Veterans Administration Cooperative Study. *N. Engl. J. Med.* 314:1547, 1986.
75. Packer, M., Meller, J., Medina, N., et al. Provocation of myocardial ischemic events during initiation of vasodilator therapy for severe chronic heart failure: Clinical and hemodynamic evaluation of 52 consecutive patients with ischemic cardiomyopathy. *Am. J. Cardiol.* 48:939, 1981.
76. Archibald, D. G., and Cohn, J. N. A treatment-associated increase in ejection fraction predicts long-term survival in congestive heart failure: The V-HeFT study (Abstract). *Circulation* 75(Suppl II):309, 1987.
77. Unverferth, D. V., Mehegan, J. P., Magorien, R. D., et al. Regression of myocardial cellular hypertrophy with vasodilatory therapy in chronic congestive heart failure associated with idiopathic cardiomyopathy. *Am. J. Cardiol.* 51:1392, 1983.
78. Magorien, R. D., Unverferth, D. V., and Leier, C. V. Hydralazine therapy in chronic congestive heart failure: Sustained central and regional hemodynamic responses. *Am. J. Med.* 77:267, 1984.
79. Rapaport, E. Influence on long-acting nitrate therapy on the risk of reinfarction, sudden death, and total mortality in survivors of acute myocardial infarction. *Am. Heart J.* 110:276, 1985.
80. Captopril Multicenter Research Group. A placebo-controlled trial of captopril in refractory chronic congestive heart failure. *J. Am. Coll. Cardiol.* 2:755, 1983.
81. Sharpe, D. N., Murphy, J., Coxon, R., and Hannan, S. F. Enalapril in patients with chronic heart failure: A placebo-controlled, randomized, double-blind study. *Circulation* 70:271, 1984.
82. Cleland, J. G. F., Dargie, H. J., Hodsman, G. P., et al. Captopril in heart failure: A double-blind controlled trial. *Br. Heart J.* 52:530, 1984.
83. Cleland, J. G. F., Dargie, H. J., Ball, S. G., et al. Effects of enalapril in heart failure: A double blind study of effects on exercise performance, renal function, hormones, and metabolic state. *Br. Heart J.* 54:305, 1985.
84. CONSENSUS Trial Study Group. Effect of enalapril on mortality in severe congestive heart failure: Results of the Cooperative North Scandinavian Enalapril Survival Study (CONSENSUS). *N. Engl. J. Med.* 316:1429, 1987.
85. Newman, T. J., Maskin, C. S., Dennick, L. G., et al. Effects of captopril on survival in patients with heart failure. *Am. J. Med.* 84(3A):140, 1988.
86. The SOLVD Investigators. Effect of enalapril on survival in patients with reduced left ventricular ejection fractions and congestive heart failure. *N. Engl. J. Med.* 325:293, 1991.
87. The SOLVD Investigators. Effect of enalapril on mortality and the development of heart failure in asymptomatic patients with reduced left ventricular ejection fractions. *N. Engl. J. Med.* 327:685, 1992.
88. Richardson, A., Bayliss, J., Scriven, A., et al. Double-blind comparison of captopril alone against furosemide plus amiloride in mild heart failure. *Lancet* 2:709, 1987.
89. Packer, M., Lee, W. H., Medina, M., et al. Functional renal insufficiency during long-term therapy with captopril or enalapril for severe chronic heart failure. *Ann. Intern. Med.* 106:346, 1987.
90. Yusuf, S., Peto, R., Lewis, J., et al. Beta blockade during and after myocardial infarction: An overview of the randomized trials. *Prog. Cardiovasc. Dis.* 27:335, 1985.
91. Sonnenblick, E. H., Fein, F., Capasso, J. M., et al. Microvascular spasm as a cause of cardiomyopathies and the calcium-blocking agent, verapamil, as potential primary therapy. *Am. J. Cardiol.* 55:179B, 1985.
92. Garrett, J. S., Wikman-Coffelt, J., Sievers, R., et al. Verapamil prevents the development of alcoholic dysfunction in hamster myocardium. *J. Am. Coll. Cardiol.* 9:1326, 1987.

33. Psychosocial and Behavioral Factors During Recovery from Myocardial Infarction

Ira S. Ockene, Lynn P. Clemow, and Judith K. Ockene

Improvements in medical therapy have led to increased survival among myocardial infarction (MI) patients, but many patients who survive experience social and psychological problems that can be as severe as or even worse than the physical disease itself [1–4]. Immediately after infarction, fear, anger, depression, and guilt are commonplace. Most patients experience rapid psychological recovery, but as many as one-third continue to suffer negative psychological effects that impair their quality of life [5]. For some patients the emotional distress is so pronounced that psychological intervention in the coronary care unit (CCU) is necessary [6]. After the initial distress associated with the infarction subsides, most patients function well psychosocially [7, 8]. A significant minority, however, continue to experience marked psychosocial difficulties as much as 2 years later [9–11].

Several reports indicate that patients who experience psychological problems (especially anxiety and depression) during early convalescence continue to demonstrate considerable long-term impairment [11–14]. Moreover, features of "invalidism" such as cessation of sexual activity and failure to return to work for nonphysical reasons generally develop during early convalescence. These psychosocial problems do not appear to be strongly related to the severity of acute MI [15]. Therefore psychological intervention should be initiated early, with specific attention paid to anxiety and depression.

Medical and psychosocial factors interact in a complex manner to influence the recovery process. Symptoms such as angina, dyspnea, and easy fatiguability attendant to an MI can produce deterioration in vocational (e.g., unemployment) or psychological (e.g., anxiety, depression) domains. Such manifestations of coronary heart disease (CHD) as arrhythmias or tachycardia, particularly when linked by the patient to the possibility of sudden death, can produce hypervigilance to body sensations, hypochondriasis, or a sense of "walking on egg shells." Medications that are commonly used to treat CHD can also impair psychosocial functioning. For example, antihypertensive and beta-blocking medications have the potential to cause depression or impair sexual performance [16].

Conversely, evidence suggests that psychosocial factors can adversely affect cardiac functioning after an MI. Immediately after an MI, the psychological state of the patient can influence physiologic events. During the hours and days following the infarction there is an increase in plasma levels of catecholamines, free fatty acids, and cortisol [17], which can contribute to potentially lethal complications (e.g., ventricular arrhythmias, cardiogenic shock, left ventricular failure). During this critical period, patients who are less anxious and more effectively cope with the stress of the event have lower elevations of catecholamines and free fatty acids [18]. Later during convalescence, prolonged depression and anxiety can lead to long-term invalidism because of unnecessary restriction of social and physical activity. Such inactivity may contribute to a decline in cardiac functioning due to the physiologic effects of deconditioning [19]. Social isolation, which is often a feature of depression, also appears to be related to increased rates of mortality and sudden death in patients who survive an MI [20]. Another factor that has been reported to affect physical condition after an MI is type A behavior. In a study of men with established coronary disease, those with type A behavior were at a significantly higher risk of subsequent coronary events than men who were type B, although these findings remain controversial (see "Type A" Personality) [21].

The occurrence of an MI is a serious life crisis that often dramatically alters the lives of patients and their families. Because many patients have been active and in fairly good health, the diagnosis of an MI suddenly arouses concerns about death and long-term disability. In the midst of such a crisis, emotional reactions such as anxiety, helplessness, despondency, and denial are to be expected [22]. As the patient's medical condition stabilizes and the fear of death recedes, other concerns emerge. Prominent among them are the financial drain of hospitalization, the ability to return to work, resumption of physical and sexual activity, and the necessity of making life style changes to reduce the risk of reinfarction [15, 23–26].

Clearly, recovery from MI requires complex social, vocational, and psychological adjustment for patients and their families. Although most MI patients adjust well to their illness after a period of disruption and distress [15, 22, 27, 28], some, perhaps as many as 25 percent, experience long-standing emotional distress, family turmoil, and occupational problems [1, 2, 15, 24, 28, 29]. Failure to recognize and intervene when such problems persist may lead to the development of serious disability and invalidism.

In addition to the direct behavioral effects of an infarct, the recovered patient must deal with the heightened need to address risk factor modification. Clear evidence exists that secondary prevention of CHD is of value, even if the patient has had an infarct or has already undergone coronary artery bypass surgery [30–34]. The patient is therefore under considerable pressure, both self-generated and from without, to quit smoking, change diet, exercise, and modify a stressful life style. This pressure has its own behavioral consequences, but the alteration of risk factors is in fact desirable, so the health care provider must have the skills needed to help the patient make appropriate changes without causing undue anxiety and stress.

The present chapter, which focuses on psychosocial problems that arise in the course of recovery after an MI, is organized into three sections: problems during the acute phase (hospitalization), problems after return to home and during the early convalescent period, and problems during the late convalescent/rehabilitation period. Because of the diversity of factors that have been related to recovery, we limit our discussion to problems that occur relatively frequently or that are particularly deleterious.

Psychological and Behavioral Adjustment During Hospitalization

Emotional Status

The symptoms of MI, especially chest pain and shortness of breath, usually arouse intense anxiety. The patient fears disability and death. Upon arrival at the hospital, the often previously well patient is suddenly immersed in the disorienting activity of the hospital. Coming to the CCU via the emergency room, the patient is rapidly interviewed, examined, and monitored while an intravenous line is placed, oxygen is administered, and blood samples are drawn, often from an artery as well as a vein. People and machinery swirl about the patient, and the disorientation is accentuated by the drugs used to treat anxiety and pain—sedatives such as diazepam (Valium) and potent narcotics such as morphine.

After initial evaluation in the emergency room, the patient is transferred to the CCU. In the past, therapy of MI was largely expectant, with the patient who was doing well being placed in bed and observed, but in the recent past interventional therapies to minimize infarct size (e.g., thrombolytic therapy and coronary angioplasty) have increasingly filled the patient's early hours in the hospital with procedures and discomfort. In the CCU itself the patient finds an unfamiliar environment filled with an array of distracting sounds, alarms, and lights.

For most patients, the procedures involved in the initial evaluation and admission to the CCU temporarily intensify emotional distress [35]. However, after becoming familiar with their surroundings, most patients are reassured by their treatment in the unit [2, 12].

Prior to arrival in the CCU, there is little opportunity to address the patient's emotional distress. In the emergency room the first priority is to manage the medical situation and stabilize the patient's medical condition. Treatment of fear and anxiety is usually limited to explaining the problem, administering medication to control ischemia and pain, and reassuring the patient [15]. Additional simple interventions that do not interfere with emergency room activities are possible.

If possible, the patient should not be left unattended. When left alone, the patient may imagine the worst, creating in his or her mind a situation far gloomier than reality. Anxiolytic medication should be provided to those patients who are unduly distressed, rather than waiting until they arrive in the CCU.

Anxiety

Once the patient arrives in the CCU, emotional distress can be more thoroughly assessed. The characteristics of anxiety (Fig. 33-1) that are frequently observed in MI patients include fear of death and disability, a sense of dread and foreboding, tremulousness, restlessness, and insomnia. Increased sympathetic nervous system activity is also observed, which can produce increased levels of catecholamines, resulting in tachycardia, tachypnea, diaphoresis, hypertension, or ventricular ectopy. Increases in cardiac output, peripheral resistance, and myocardial oxygen consumption may also result [36].

It is important to familiarize the patient with the CCU. This measure involves explaining equipment that is used, restrictions that are imposed (e.g., bed rest), and the unit's routine (e.g., regular monitoring of vital signs during the night). The patient is likely to be easily distracted and may have a short attention span. Therefore short, simple explanations are preferred. Even simple explanations may have to be repeated several times before they are comprehended. Environmental adjustments to minimize noise and disruption of sleep-wake cycles may also be helpful. For some patients, playing soothing music significantly reduces anxiety in a CCU [37].

Listening to the patient and providing appropriate reassurance are also important. Patients often harbor unrealistic fears that can be debilitating. Sometimes these fears are expressed directly, but more commonly they are expressed indirectly in comments about the need for others to care for the children or discussion of a will. The patient may not be immediately receptive to support and reassurance and may require encouragement to express his or her concerns.

It may be useful to consider the patient's family as a factor influencing the patient's anxiety in the CCU. In a preliminary study, the anxiety levels of CCU patients and those of their visiting family

Fig. 33-1
Typical time course of emotional reaction to a myocardial infarction. CCU = coronary care unit. (From N. H. Cassem and T. P. Hackett. Psychiatric consultation in a coronary care unit. *Ann. Intern. Med.* 75:9, 1971. With permission.)

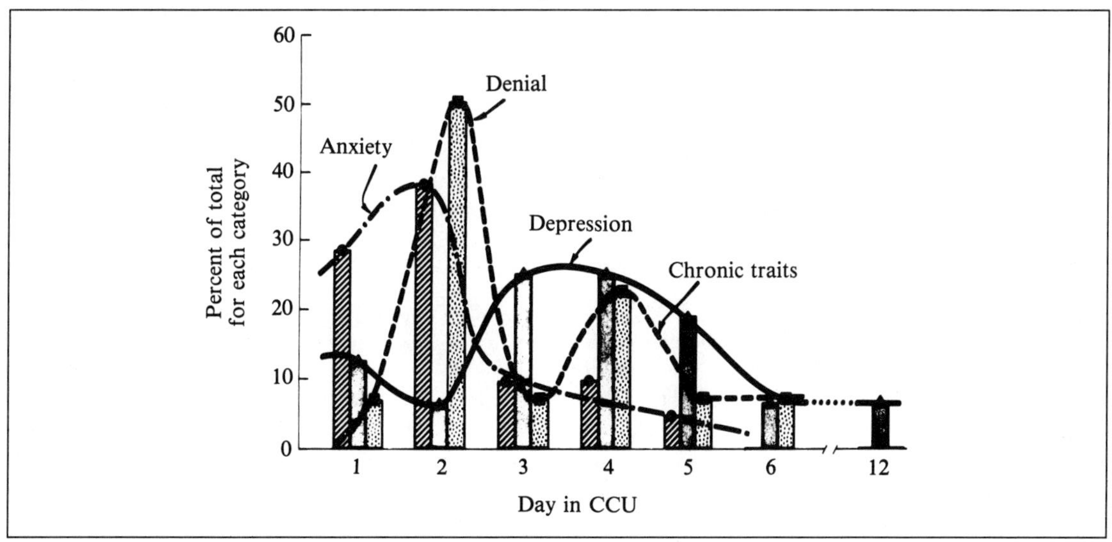

members were significantly correlated [38]. The results of a very small intervention study found that anxiety was lower in patients whose families had been prepared by the nursing staff prior to the visit than in control patients whose families had no such preparation [39]. In a larger study, a psychoeducational nursing intervention to counsel male MI patients and their wives together significantly reduced anxiety in the patients and their partners [40].

Pharmacologic treatment of anxiety should also be considered, especially for patients who exhibit heightened autonomic responses to stressful stimuli [15, 35]. Benzodiazepines are the drugs of choice for the treatment of anxiety. Diazepam 5 to 10 mg orally every 8 hours is recommended for MI patients [35]. When benzodiazepines are used, they should be ordered on a fixed-dose schedule rather than on an as-needed schedule because many patients who need medication fail to request it.

Overall, most patients cope with the emotional ordeal of the MI well. Elevated anxiety typically continues for the first day or two and then diminishes as the patient's medical condition stabilizes [6, 12, 18, 41]. As chest pain and shortness of breath decrease, fear of death abates and concern about the future begins to emerge. With the realization that he or she is physically limited and that life style changes are necessary, the patient may experience sadness and a sense of loss [6, 12, 41].

Depression

Depression is a common reaction to severe illness and is probably seen in about 50 percent of MI patients [42], but the depression observed at this early point in recovery is usually transient (see Fig. 33-1). Sometimes, however, the patient becomes despondent, pessimistic about the future, hopeless, or withdrawn. Often it is difficult to recognize that the patient is depressed because he or she does not complain about the symptoms or even denies the depression. If the patient is pessimistic about recovery or is withdrawn and inactive, rehabilitation may be compromised. The incidence of major depression may be as high as 19 percent within 10 days after an MI has occurred. The more severe depressive symptoms are seen most commonly in individuals with a history of mood disorders, in patients with large infarcts, and in those with significant functional impairment [43].

Patients' perceptions of their health status strongly influence depression. If they believe they will be severely restricted in their activities, they are more likely to become depressed. This situation is especially likely to occur if fatigue and weakness are interpreted as evidence of cardiac decline. For most patients, depression can be alleviated by education, early ambulation, involvement in rehabilitation activities, and reassurance from the medical staff [15]. Aside from preventing deconditioning and other complications of prolonged bed rest, early ambulation provides a clear message that patients are expected to regain their health and to become active again. With early ambulation, the patients' emotional status and self-image generally improve [4, 44, 45]. Early involvement in rehabilitative activities emphasizes that the patient is expected to recover and return to a normal or near-normal life style. Education should be initiated early, with the goal of helping the patient understand the infarction and its management. Information about the anatomy and function of the heart should be provided so that patients can understand why the infarct occurred and how healing takes place. Coronary risk factors must be discussed, with an emphasis on modifiable risk factors. The activities involved in rehabilitation should also be explained (exercise, smoking cessation, diet and weight control, medication).

Patients also should be given the opportunity to discuss their fears and concerns. During this early stage of recovery, worry about ability to support a family, resumption of sexual activity, loss of autonomy, and restriction of leisure activities are common. Patients often have misconceptions about the MI that contribute to depression [46]. Chief among them is the belief that the heart is fragile after infarction and that it will ''give out'' if subjected to stress [15]. Patients who harbor this belief are reluctant to exert themselves and consequently severely restrict their activities.

Denial and Other Coping Strategies

Denial of illness has been reported to be a common response to an acute MI (see Fig. 33-1) [2, 3, 6, 27, 28]. According to Cassem and Hackett [6], denial is mobilized as a reaction to heightened anxiety and fear of death and plays an important role in keeping the patient's emotional distress in check.

An implication of this argument is that patients who use denial experience less anxiety and depression than those who do not. Moreover, Hackett and Cassem [47] argued that deniers have better survival records in the CCU than nondeniers, although the studies done to date have insufficient statistical power to establish this point with certainty. Consistent with this position, research indicates that patients who use denial during hospitalization tend to be less anxious and have less morbidity and mortality in the CCU [41, 48, 49]. More recent investigators criticized the excessively broad and nonspecific definitions of denial in these classic studies [50–52]. Studies with more precise and behaviorally based definitions found less-protective influence of denial and focused more on the various coping strategies employed by post-MI patients. A recent study [53] identified many and varied coping strategies reported by patients in the first 3 to 5 days after an acute MI occurred. The strategies most frequently reported included optimistic thinking, confronting the challenges involved, and self-reliance. Relatively few used evasive or denial-based avoidance strategies, when strictly defined. The current research emphasizes the importance of a flexible approach to these patients, with an understanding that the needs and coping strategies will differ across individuals, and will evolve over time.

Tesar and Hackett [35] distinguished between two types of denial. Denial of illness occurs when patients contend that they have not sustained an MI or that their illness is not serious. This type of denial is maladaptive and sets the stage for noncompliance and inappropriate behavior. With the second type of denial, the patient accepts that he or she has sustained an MI but denies fear of its consequences. Patients who use denial in this manner cope by minimizing their fear.

Whatever the early effects of denial, it seems clear that excessive use of denial is maladaptive for long-term recovery [52]. Some of the maladaptive behaviors that have been linked to denial of illness are insistence on return to normal activities, inappropriate behavior (e.g., smoking, sexually provoking the nurses), and hostility [6]. When such problems arise, a concerted effort must be made to elicit the patient's cooperation [35]. Sometimes reassurance and clarification of misconceptions are sufficient to solve the problem. Repeated efforts to convince the patient of the gravity of the situation are rarely effective, however, and can exacerbate the problem. When such efforts fail, tactful confrontation may be necessary to change the inappropriate behavior. Caution must be exercised, however, so that staff do not express anger and frustration when confronting a problematic patient. Working with the staff to help them develop a constructive approach to this type of patient is productive.

Infrequent Psychosis-Like Features

Some seriously ill patients become agitated or delirious while in the CCU (see Fig. 33-1) [15, 36]. For some patients, delirium or agitation is a manifestation of extreme anxiety. Other determinants of these problems include metabolic disturbances, insufficient cerebral blood flow secondary to dropping cardiac output, hypoxia, adverse medication effects (including lidocaine toxicity, and the "paradoxical" agitation sometimes seen with sedatives and opiates), sleep deprivation, or environmental factors such as noise or monotony [3, 15, 35].

Appropriate intervention for these conditions depends on identification of the underlying cause. Depending on the etiology, treatment usually involves one or more of the following: discontinuing toxic drugs, correcting metabolic abnormalities, using neuroleptic medication, or ameliorating environmental factors.

Initial Risk Factor Management

Studies have demonstrated that interventions for risk factor change (e.g., smoking cessation) that are initiated while the patient is in the hospital produce higher continued cessation or maintenance rates than when counseling is delayed until after discharge (either because of hospital policy or because of the impact of the recent event) [54, 55]. As change has already often been initiated, the interventions used must include those oriented toward helping the patient to develop the skills needed to resist returning to old behaviors, that is, "relapse prevention" skills [56, 57]. Perhaps most importantly for the health care provider, it is essential that he or she deliver a strong message advising change. Without it the patient is likely to think that a risk factor change such as smoking cessation is not especially important, as the physician did not give the issue any weight. The physician and other health care providers can also spend a few minutes assisting the patient to decide on an appropriate approach to making or maintaining the change and to develop a plan. The more input and assistance provided by the physician and the health care team, the greater is the likelihood of change [58]. Perhaps the most important factor in change of behavior is the patient's commitment to change, and the health care team can provide support to facilitate this commitment. The topic of risk factor modification is more extensively discussed in the next section.

Psychological Adjustment During Early Convalescence

Emotional Status

Depression is one of the most significant problems confronted by MI patients during the weeks following discharge from the hospital [2, 15, 28, 46, 59]. Cessation of sexual activity, unwarranted restriction of activity, social withdrawal, insomnia, and failure to return to work are some of the problems that are related to depression [46]. The physical inactivity that often accompanies depression also may contribute to deterioration in medical status because of physical deconditioning [4, 45]. Early rehabilitation efforts instill optimism about a quick recovery, but this optimism may quickly dissipate when patients begin to confront the realities of their disability and struggle to implement life style changes. Patients test their physical capacities and reassess their health status [60]. During these early weeks following discharge, complaints about anxiety and nervousness, weakness, tearfulness, diminished appetite, fear of sexual arousal, social withdrawal, disturbed sleep, pessimism about the future, and a sense of uselessness are common [2, 15, 29, 46].

The patient may experience weakness and fatigue with increased activity [4, 45]. When patients return home, they are usually deconditioned because of extended bed rest. As a result, they may fatigue with ordinary activities, such as walking around the yard. Unaware that weakness is due to muscle atrophy and other effects of immobilization, MI patients attribute these symptoms to a damaged heart.

Unless patients are forewarned to expect this weakness and fatigue, they are likely to worry that their disease is more severe than they believed. When even minimal activity produces noticeable fatigue and weakness, it is difficult for the uninformed patient to imagine a return to normal activities. Coupled with the often severe restrictions on smoking, diet, and alcohol, patients may perceive a future marked by limitations.

Denial

As already discussed, denial can be a useful protective mechanism whereby the individual minimizes the importance of the cardiac event and can thereby more easily get on with life. Once the patient is beyond the acute event, however, he or she must deal with the need to go through an appropriate rehabilitation process and alter risk factors to diminish the likelihood of a recurrence. At this point denial beyond a level needed to minimize anxiety becomes counterproductive, with the individual resisting making necessary changes (continuing to smoke, permitting excessive physical stress) because "it isn't that serious," and avoiding problem-solving behavior [61, 62].

Levine et al. [52] developed a new scale for assessing denial that built on the Hackett-Cassem denial scale [63]. Using this instrument they demonstrated that increased denial led to more rapid recovery early on, but that these patients had more difficulty during the following year, being less compliant with rehabilitation regimens and requiring more days of hospitalization. Levine et al. concluded:

> Denial of illness is adaptive as a coping response in emergency situations when the cardiovascular system is dysfunctional or excessively stressed and no immediate action is necessary or possible. Under these conditions denial of illness blocks added stressor input. However, when the patient's medical condition has become stabilized, denial of illness is maladaptive because continued blocking or distortion of cognitive and affective processes prevents realistic appraisal and motivation for necessary action.

Social Support and Family Distress

Social support has in recent years taken on increasing significance as a major determinant of psychological outcome of disease [64–67]. A complex interaction occurs between patient, family, and professional staff. The family's ability to provide support to the patient is to a large extent dependent on family members' own psychological strength, the distress they are experiencing, and their assessment of the gravity of the patient's illness. The skill of the professional staff in providing support and information to the family members may significantly affect the latter's ability to provide the patient with much-needed support [68]. Family members also benefit from the opportunity to discuss their fears and concerns about caring for the MI patient.

Studies of social support in MI are relatively limited. Speedling [66] found that spouses were often more distressed than patients during the acute hospitalization and suggested that the medical structure may have a negative effect on families, restricting access to the patient by limiting visiting hours and surrounding the patient with layers of formidable technology and busy caregivers. Lack of control and unavailability of adequate information, fear of the hospital environment, and concern over changing family roles and altered finances also play important roles as family stressors [69, 70].

Sociocultural factors are also important. Ell and Haywood [71] looked at socioeconomic status and other variables among blacks, Hispanics, and Anglos as they related to coping mechanisms following an MI. In general, family support was associated with improved function, but among the Hispanic patients a supportive family and close attachments were most positively correlated with self-esteem and positive well-being but negatively associated with personal functioning, suggesting that perhaps the cared-for individual was being *overly* cared for. Although social networking was in general salutory, other cultural differences were seen. The authors emphasized the need to take cultural considerations into account when planning rehabilitative programs and pointed out the need for further research in this area.

It seems clear that family members should be incorporated into the therapeutic environment of the patient and given the information necessary so that they can play an informed, nonconflicting role. This point is true while the patient is in the hospital [67] and is even more evident once the patient returns home. Spouses and other family members can offer important support and understanding at a crucial time and be effective advocates for life style change to alter risk factor levels [71]. Often, however, the convalescent period is marked by conflict between the patient and spouse, with differing opinions on the timing of the patient's resumption of activity being the most common area of friction [72]. Again, providing adequate and clear information and guidance to both patient and family during the days prior to discharge is valuable and important. The entire team—physician, nurses, rehabilitation personnel—should be involved, with appropriate coordination so that different caregivers deliver the same message. Nothing causes more confusion and family friction than a conservative rehabilitation team saying "no driving for a month" whereas the patient's physician, unaware, says "you can drive in a week." Patients and families often have a sense of having been cast adrift during the first few weeks after discharge as they make the adjustment from intense contact and supervision in the hospital to the far more infrequent caregiver contact once the patient is home. The specific importance of the nurse in assisting the spouse and the specific opportunity provided by the peridischarge period were emphasized by Bramwell [70], who noted that the receptiveness of patient and spouse during this critical time should be effectively utilized.

In an interesting 3-year follow-up study of 2330 post-MI patients, Ruberman et al. [20] found that two major psychosocial factors affected subsequent mortality: stress level related to such traumatic events as marital separation, forced retirement, or financial difficulty; and social isolation, with a lack of contact with family, friends, or social organizations. Individuals with high levels of either stress or social isolation suffered an approximately twofold increase in mortality, especially that due to sudden death, and the two factors demonstrated an additive effect. Marital status alone also is associated with post-MI survival, with married patients having significantly better survival rates than nonmarried individuals [73].

The beneficial effect of social support may manifest through such "physical" forms as providing transportation, cooking heart-healthy meals, doing household work, providing financial support; through "moral support" mechanisms such as encouraging and supporting risk-factor alteration, stress reduction, and healthier work patterns; through the direct psychological effects of companionship; or through a combination of these mechanisms. More research is needed in this area.

As the spouse provides much of the social support for the patient, it is worth noting the particular stresses and issues with which this person may struggle. Most of the available studies examined wives of male MI patients and found that they face numerous problems: the threat of losing a partner, separation from family and friends, child or household care problems, financial strain, changes in role, and an uncertain future [74]. They also reported feeling a low level of control over events in the hospital, followed by a high sense of responsibility for patient care after discharge. Wives also feel there is little opportunity to ventilate their emotions [75]. The effects of this stress may be seen in the frequent reports of sleep and appetite problems, headaches, problems concentrating, and irritability. Though these initial symptoms generally subside, as many as 40 percent of the spouses continue to report physical and emotional distress a year after the husband's MI occurred [74]. Distress may be particularly acute in a subgroup of women (45 percent in one study [76]) who had not supported the husband's seeking help right away when he experienced the early signs of the MI. These women appeared more overwhelmed by the seriousness of the illness and presented with higher levels of denial, more confusion, and less ability to make plans [76].

Interventions directed at the family must be done with care and sensitivity lest they cause more harm than good. It is considered important to train family members of patients with CHD in resuscitative techniques [77]. However, in an interesting study Dracup et al. [78] demonstrated that patients whose family members had been taught cardiopulmonary resuscitation (CPR) were more anxious at 3 months' follow-up than were those whose family members had not been given such training, and the family members themselves derived no psychological benefit from the training. Thus breaking through a denial mechanism or increasing dependency/responsibility feelings of patients and family members may be counterproductive and must be done carefully.

On a more promising note, Taylor et al. [79] carried out an interesting intervention study directed at reducing spouse anxiety. During the patient's week 3 exercise test, spouses were randomized either to wait in the waiting room or to attend the exercise test and then go on the treadmill themselves for 3 minutes at their husband's maximum workload. The wives who experienced their husband's workload capabilities increased their ratings of their husband's ability to handle exercise and stress. This type of intervention should narrow the gap between husband's and wife's perceptions of what the post-MI patient can and cannot do.

Risk Factor Modification

Although the best prevention is primary prevention, the increasing success of our treatment of acute MI is resulting in a large pool of individuals who have had an infarct and in whom prevention of another clinical event is a primary goal. Within 5 years of an infarction, 13 percent of men and almost 40 percent of women suffer a second infarction [80]. The evidence in favor of the important role of risk factor modification in both primary and secondary prevention of CHD is overwhelming [81, 82]. Although the evidence in favor of secondary prevention is not as strong, numerous studies suggested that post-MI patients benefit from risk factor intervention. Cessation of cigarette smoking results in a 50 percent reduction of mortality in post-MI patients compared to those who continue to smoke [83–85]. Progression of coronary artery disease (CAD) as measured by quantitative angiography is significantly reduced by cholesterol reduction in patients with clinical CAD [32–34]. Although trials demonstrating a clear benefit of antihypertensive therapy in post-MI patients do not yet exist, such therapy appears logical in view of the known potency of hypertension as a risk factor for CHD and the increased risk of post-MI patients for congestive heart failure and stroke.

Smoking Cessation

Cigarette smoking is one of the most important modifiable risk factors for CAD in the United States today [86]. Certainly it is in the best interest of the post-MI patient to stop smoking, and fortunately as many as 50 percent do stop immediately after an infarction. However, many eventually resume smoking [87]. An important role of a cardiac rehabilitation program is to help those who have already quit to stay quit and to assist those who have not yet stopped in their efforts at cessation. A variety of smoking cessation techniques, ranging from individual and group sessions to aversive therapy, are available, with all having some short-term success [88–92]. The most effective methods are the multicomponent or "broad-spectrum" approaches that incorporate interventions to deal with the psychological, physiologic, and social aspects of smoking. Although there are many approaches available, most smokers do not go to formal smoking cessation programs, with fewer than 10 percent of smokers who quit having "attended" a special program. Thus the health care team and the setting to which the patient is exposed become important channels for intervention. Patients who are committed to change generally adhere to prescribed regimens and are more often successful. The health care provider may find a number of excellent self-help booklets available from the American Heart Association, the American Lung Association, and the American Cancer Society, all of which are of use to the patient and discuss available alternative options, such as formal smoking cessation programs. Other risk factors, such as nutrition, exercise, and stress, are also behaviorally related, and similar techniques should be of value for all [93].

"Type A" Personality

No discussion of psychological factors and MI would be complete without mention of the "type A" controversy. Since the 1950s Rosenman and Friedman and others [21, 94, 95] put forward the thesis that individuals who are "type A"—defined as hard-driving, competitive, time oriented, and aggressive—are at increased risk for the development of CAD. An independent panel in 1981 recognized type A behavior as a risk factor for CHD [96]. Nonetheless, other studies failed to replicate these findings, including the Multiple Risk Factor Intervention Trial, the Aspirin Myocardial Infarction Study, and the Beta Blocker Heart Attack Trial [20, 97, 98]. The proponents of the type A hypothesis have claimed methodologic error in these negative studies. In recent years, investigators have turned away from studying global type A behavior, and moved toward identifying the components of the behavior pattern most strongly associated with CAD. Most widely studied are measures of hostility and the findings are less equivocal than are those for the overall type A behavior studies. Expressive hostility and antagonistic interpersonal style appear to be the components of the type A pattern that are most strongly related to CAD. Other aspects of hostility, including cynicism and mistrust of others, have also been related to CAD morbidity and mortality [99]. It is interesting to note that several studies of psychological interventions to treat the type A behavior pattern reported success in reducing the characteristic type A behaviors and in reducing recurrent coronary events [100]. In an especially interesting study, Friedman et al. [101] reported on the results of a controlled study of a program (the Recurrent Coronary Prevention Program) designed to modify the type A characteristics of individuals after MI. They found that type A behavior could be modified, and that individuals exhibiting such behavior modification had significantly fewer recurrences of nonfatal infarction than did the control subjects given only cardiac counseling. At 4.5 years of follow-up, a significant difference in cardiac deaths was also noted [102]. In a later report Friedman et al. [103] noted that the individuals who had been in the type A counseling group maintained their lowered intensity of type A behavior and their lowered cardiac recurrence rates for the 1-year follow-up period after the end of the counseling program. When studied in further detail, the intervention program resulted in reductions in the core type A traits, such as hostility, impatience, and time urgency. It also decreased depression and anger, while increasing social support and general well-being [104]. A recent report [105] of 83 women with premature acute MI in the Recurrent Coronary Prevention Project suggested that there may be gender differences in the relationship between type A characteristics and coronary disease. Time urgency and emotional arousability were inversely related to mortality over an 8- to 10-year period, controlling for electrocardiographic (ECG) arrhythmias. The data suggested that a pattern of emotional suppression in the face of adversity (e.g., divorce, employment without a college degree) was a particularly lethal combination in these women. Alteration of hostility and other type A characteristics through intervention had no impact on survival in these women. This exploratory study with a relatively small number of women raised two key points: (1) the importance of studying CHD risk in women rather than generalizing from studies of men, and (2) the importance of studying behavioral or dispositional variables such as type A characteristics in their social contexts (i.e., social isolation, work environment) [106].

To date, the results of the Recurrent Coronary Prevention Program have not been reproduced, although there have been no attempts to do so. The study is of considerable importance, and an effort to confirm its findings is needed.

Ragland and Brand [107] returned to the original Western Collaborative Group Study [95] and looked at the survival patterns of 257 men from the original group. The average follow-up was 12.7 years among the 160 type A patients and 11.5 years among the 71 type B patients. Unexpectedly, the subsequent mortality in patients surviving more than 24 hours following the MI was significantly lower in the type A patients. An editorial accompanying that article [108] summarized the available literature, and concluded, "It is important to acknowledge that *something* is going on in terms of the relation between personality and heart disease. However, the nature of that influence is far more complex than is conveyed by the simple assertion that type A behavior is a risk factor for coronary heart disease."

Psychological and Behavioral Adjustment During Late Convalescence and Rehabilitation

Maintenance of Risk Factor Modification

Relapse or return to old behaviors is common among individuals who have made changes, even among those who had had an MI. Thus continued support and interventions aimed at maintenance of risk factor change continue to be important even after a year of maintained change. Several patterns of relapse occur. Typical patterns include the presence of extended withdrawal effects leading to a conscious decision to return to smoking; a slip under unusual circumstances (e.g., a family crisis) followed by a quick relapse; and a gradual return to regular smoking following rationalized use ("one won't hurt"). Smokers are often consistent in their relapse patterns; thus these patterns can be identified, and counseling can be directed toward their prevention.

Steps can be taken to ensure a greater likelihood of maintained cessation. First, the former smoker can identify previous "high-risk" situations that triggered smoking and prepare for them. Next, the former smoker can practice ways of dealing with these situations without cigarettes. Helping patients to develop healthy behaviors (e.g., exercise) in place of unhealthy behaviors such as smoking facilitates maintenance of risk factor change.

Sexual Adjustment

Sexual dysfunction following MI is common, occurring to some degree in as many as 50 percent of patients [2, 109]. Of the 30 percent of patients reporting sexual dysfunction in one study, half reported erectile dysfunction and half reported reduced libido [110]. Interestingly, the patients reporting sexual dysfunction in the 3 months following an uncomplicated MI had a higher rate of recurrent MI than did those with preserved sexual functioning. This may be a function of greater infarct size. Reasons for sexual dysfunction include fear of inducing another infarction during intercourse, fear that sexual activity may be excessively stressful, and a general spousal oversolicitousness that may contribute to the patient's lowered self-esteem [111]. Although physical causes for sexual dysfunction are also possible (decreased cardiac output, progressive atherosclerosis, drug effects such as beta blocker–induced impotence), they are considerably less common than psychogenic causes [112]. Also mentioned as a possible etiology for post-MI sexual dysfunction is the desire by one or both partners to use the infarction for discontinuing what was already an unsatisfactory relationship [113].

Providing adequate information and giving patients and their spouses permission to resume sexual activity is important. Excellent discussions of sex and the cardiac patient can be found in books written for the lay public by Alpert [113] and Cambre [114]. Patients and their partners need to understand that:

1. The risk of death during sexual activity is low. In a study of 5559 cases of sudden death, only 0.6 percent were related to sexual activity, and

most of these deaths involved extramarital partners averaging 20 years younger than the victim and occurred in unfamiliar surroundings [115].
2. Sexual activity is normally ''moderate'' in intensity, comparable to climbing stairs, as an exercise [116]. Peak heart rates rarely exceed 120 beats per minute and maintain this level for only 10 to 15 seconds. Therefore sexual activity can be resumed at about the same time stairclimbing can be resumed, generally 2 to 4 weeks after the infarction.
3. Although it is common for cardiac patients to be advised to assume the bottom position during sexual activity, there is little evidence that body position affects heart rate or blood pressure [117]. Therefore there is no reason to advise the patient and spouse to add the stress of unfamiliar positions.
4. Many of the normal physiologic consequences of sexual activity produce sensations that the patient is apt to interpret as related to heart disease. Heavy breathing, a rapid heart rate, a sense of congestion in the chest, and sweating are normal accompaniments of lovemaking, but the sensitized patient is liable to be frightened by them [59].

Other reasonable recommendations include avoiding sexual activity immediately after food or alcohol consumption, as both increase heart rate; avoiding temperature extremes; and avoiding sex when fatigued or upset [112].

Anxiety Disorders

Recent studies identified an increased incidence of anxiety disorders in post-MI patients. Anxiety disorders occur in approximately 15 percent of individuals with CAD, roughly two to three times the general population rate [118]. The persistent anxiety disorders (i.e., those that extend beyond the initial MI recovery period) described in the literature seem to occur in two specific forms: panic disorder and post-traumatic stress disorder. Panic disorder can cause symptoms that mimic angina even in the absence of coronary disease, and as many as 50 percent of patients with CAD and atypical angina may fulfill the criteria for panic disorder [119]. The experience of having an MI can have the effect of sensitizing the patient to any somatic anxiety symptoms that resemble the onset of the MI (e.g., chest pain, shortness of breath, light-headedness). Vigilance for these symptoms and the accompanying anxiety can set up an unfortunate cycle of heightened somatic concern and escalating anxiety symptoms. Two preliminary reports [120, 121] recently documented the symptoms of post-traumatic stress disorder in a number of post-MI patients, 6 to 12 months after the cardiac event occurred [120]. The symptoms included intrusive reexperiencing of the traumatic event, avoidance of stimuli associated with the event, a numbing of responsiveness to the outside world, and increased autonomic arousal. Significant symptoms of these traumatic reactions occurred in 18 percent of 50 MI and coronary artery bypass surgery patients who went through a cardiac rehabilitation program [121]. Though the findings are preliminary, these symptoms and the related problems of depression, generalized anxiety, and anger that can accompany them have a major impact on the patient's long-term quality of life.

Intervention Programs

Psychosocial intervention programs are an accepted part of present-day cardiac rehabilitation services, yet there are few well-controlled studies to support their use. Several studies suggested reduced morbidity and mortality from psychological intervention [122, 123]. In Rahe et al.'s study [123], patients in the intervention group attended six biweekly sessions beginning 1 month after hospital discharge. Spouses attended only one session. Patients who received group therapy were described as having significantly lower morbidity and mortality, although there was no difference in risk factor alteration. Educational information given to the intervention group was forgotten at follow-up. Of interest, and common to many studies of this type, was the small sample size: 22 patients in each group. In addition, the authors chose to define significance at the .15 level (the mortality difference was $p = .12$). Mumford et al. [124] reviewed 34 controlled studies of intervention in surgical and MI patients and concluded that the provision of information and emotional support during a medical crisis resulted in a shorter hospital stay than did routine medical care alone. In recent years, with increasing emphasis being placed on the cost-effectiveness of interventions, there has been an increasing tendency to shift from time- and personnel-intensive psychotherapy toward more broadly diffusible behavioral and educational interventions. Education alone can be effective in allaying patients' anxieties and fear: Mazzuca [125] concluded that patient education alone can be as therapeutic as more expensive psychological interventions.

Oldenburg et al. [126] carried out a controlled study in post-MI patients that compared two in-hospital interventions, education and counseling, with routine medical and nursing care. The educational intervention consisted of relaxation procedures and the provision of information about heart disease and its treatment. The counseling intervention included the educational interventions as well as six to ten counseling sessions. All of these interventions took place while the patient was in the hospital; no further intervention was provided once the patient was discharged. At 3, 6, and 12 months of follow-up, both intervention groups did significantly better than the control group on tests of psychological and life style functioning, and they were also less symptomatic and less dependent on medical treatment. The authors suggested that these results compare favorably with those seen in outpatient cardiac rehabilitation programs.

In a particularly interesting study, Stern et al. [127] randomized 106 post-MI patients to one of three groups: exercise therapy, group counseling, or control. Subjects who failed to reach a workload of 7 METs (multiples of resting oxygen consumption) on exercise testing were rated as anxious, depressed, or both. Each intervention lasted 12 weeks, with follow-up for 1 year. Exercise increased mean work capacity, decreased fatigue, lessened anxiety and depression, and promoted independence and sociability. Counseling substantially reduced depression, decreased interpersonal friction, and led to greater independence and sociability. The control group showed no significant changes. No mortality differences were seen. With time, however, these differences narrowed, and by the end of the follow-up period there was little difference between the three groups. The authors noted that an optimum rehabilitation program would probably include both exercise and counseling interventions.

In a recent study, Frasure-Smith [128] tested an interesting and cost-effective follow-up program for post-MI patients. Patients were assessed by a 20-item structured interview for psychological distress while they were in the hospital immediately following the MI. Once discharged, patients were contacted by telephone on a monthly basis and their distress was reassessed. When a high level of distress was reported on this index, the patient received a visit from a nurse to further assess the individual's needs and develop an appropriate brief intervention. The screening phone calls and interventions were available for a year after the MI occurred. At 5-year follow-up, the program significantly reduced both cardiac mortality and acute MI recurrence, but only for those patients who reported high levels of distress in the initial hospital assessment. This study suggests that cost-effective psychosocial interventions for post-MI patients can be developed and that the patients most in need of such services can be identified before they are discharged from the hospital.

The best cardiac rehabilitation programs do not separate behavioral interventions but integrate them into an interdisciplinary program that combines physical activity, risk factor intervention, education, nutrition, networking, and emotional support [129].

Return to Work

Within the first 6 months after an acute MI, approximately 75 percent of previously employed individuals return to work [2, 130]. A number of factors, including medical complications during hospitalization, higher age, lower education, higher perceived pre-MI job stress, and rural residence were found to correlate with a lesser likelihood of returning to work [131]. In a later study Mæland and Havik [132] evaluated the relation between likelihood of return to work 6 months after an MI and a series of psychological and other factors in 249 patients under 67 years old, with a number of interesting findings.

Patients characterized by marked hopelessness were less likely to return to work than those less pessimistic. Interestingly, there was a significant negative correlation between years of education and levels of hopelessness; both were independently related to return to work. Denial showed a bipolar response; patients in the lowest and the highest quartiles were less likely to return to work than were patients with moderate denial scores. The return-to-work rate was strongly related to levels of anxiety and depression as reported by the patients during hospitalization and at 6 weeks' follow-up, and it was independent of age, educational level, or severity of infarction.

The patients' basic knowledge about heart disease was unrelated to return to work, but levels of cardiac life style knowledge (risk factors, behavioral factors) were strongly related to return to work. However, the significance of this relationship disappeared when educational levels were taken into account; education and cardiac life style knowledge were closely related.

Expectation of future work capacity was strongly and linearly related to return to work; patients who anticipated few problems had a nearly threefold higher return-to-work rate than those who expected the greatest reduction in work capacity. This relationship was also independent of the patient's age or the severity of the infarction. Although expectation of future work capacity was correlated with educational level and level of perceived job stress, the association between expectation of future work capacity and return to work remained highly significant even after controlling for these potential confounders. This central role of patient expectation in predicting return to work was noted by others for both MI and coronary artery bypass surgery [35, 131, 133]. The lack of relation of expectation of return to work to severity of MI and to work-related factors makes it unlikely that the patients' expectations simply reflect the underlying reality of their situation; negative expectations may act as self-fulfilling prophecies by leading to passivity and feelings of helplessness.

In summary, discriminant function analysis reduced the number of variables independently predictive of failure to return to work to three: negative expectations, the experience of negative moods, and insufficient knowledge of the effect of life style on heart disease. Each represents a different set of the patient's psychological make-up: attitude, emotion, and knowledge. The best clinical predictor of return to work is the simple maneuver of asking the patient his or her own opinion of the likelihood of such an event occurring; such a finding is also seen in other areas of patient behavior, such as smoking cessation, where a potent predictor of success is a similar "do you believe you will be smoking one year from now" type of question [134]. In these areas, the patient knows himself or herself best.

Mæland and Havik [132] concluded that the patient's perceived illness plays a central role in the coping and readaptation process that occurs after the acute event. They suggested that early rehabilitative intervention may successfully alter the patient's initial expectations and facilitate recovery.

The importance of returning to work to the individual's well-being is emphasized by recent research [135]. Rost and Smith [135] demonstrated reductions in emotional distress in post-MI patients who returned to work, while distress increased over 12 months in those who did not return to work. This effect remained powerful even when controlling for initial psychological and physical status, social support, and sociodemographic variables. Emotional distress was reduced even in those who returned to jobs with which they had expressed dissatisfaction at the time of the MI.

References

1. Croog, S. H. Recovery and rehabilitation of heart patients: Psychosocial aspects. In D. S. Krantz, A. Baum, and J. E. Singer (eds.), *Handbook of Psychology and Health* (Vol. 3). Hillsdale, NJ: Erlbaum, 1983. Pp. 295–334.
2. Doehrman, S. R. Psycho-social aspects of recovery from coronary heart disease: A review. *Soc. Sci. Med.* 2:199, 1977.
3. Razin, A. M. Psychosocial intervention in coronary artery disease: A review. *Psychosom. Med.* 44:363, 1982.
4. Wenger, N. K., and Hellerstein, H. K. (eds.), *Rehabilitation of the Coronary Patient* (2nd ed.). New York: Wiley, 1984.
5. Mayou, R., Williamson, B., and Foster, A. Outcome two months after myocardial infarction. *J. Psychosom. Res.* 22:439, 1978.
6. Cassem, N. H., and Hackett, T. P. Psychiatric consultation in a coronary care unit. *Ann. Intern. Med.* 75:9, 1971.
7. Ott, C., Sivarajan, E. S., Newton, K. M., et al. A controlled randomized study of early cardiac rehabilitation: The sickness impact profile as an assessment tool. *Heart Lung* 12:162, 1983.
8. Stern, M., Pascale, L., and Ackerman, A. Life adjustment post-myocardial infarction: Determining predictive variables. *Arch. Intern. Med.* 137:1680, 1977.
9. Byrne, D. G. Psychological responses to illness and

outcome after survived myocardial infarction: A long term follow-up. *J. Psychosom. Res.* 26:105, 1982.

10. Mayou, R., Foster, A., and Williamson, B. Medical care after myocardial infarction. *J. Psychosom. Res.* 23:23, 1979.
11. Wiklund, I., Sanne, H., Vedin, A., and Wilhelmsson, C. Psychosocial outcome one year after a first myocardial infarction. *J. Psychosom. Res.* 28:309, 1984.
12. Cay, E. L., Vetter, N., Philip, A. E., and Dugard, P. Psychological status during recovery from acute heart attack. *J. Psychosom. Res.* 16:425, 1972.
13. Mayou, R. Prediction of emotional and social outcome after a heart attack. *J. Psychosom. Res.* 28: 17, 1984.
14. Stern, M. J., Pascale, L., and McLoone, J. B. Psychosocial adaptation following an acute myocardial infarction. *J. Chronic Dis.* 29:513, 1976.
15. Stern, M. J. Psychosocial rehabilitation following myocardial infarction and coronary artery bypass surgery. In N. K. Wenger and H. K. Hellerstein (eds.), *Rehabilitation of the Coronary Patient* (2nd ed.). New York: Wiley, 1984. Pp. 453–471.
16. Zelnik, T. Depressive effects of drugs. In N. Cameron (ed.), *Presentations of Depression.* New York: Wiley, 1987. Pp. 355–400.
17. Vetter, N. J., Strange, R. C., Adams, W., and Oliver, M. F. Initial metabolic and hormonal response to acute myocardial infarction. *Lancet* 1:284, 1974.
18. Klein, R. F., Garrity, T. F., and Gelein, J. Emotional adjustment and catecholamine excretion during early recovery from myocardial infarction. *J. Psychosom. Res.* 18:425, 1974.
19. Wenger, N. K. Early ambulation after myocardial infarction: Rationale, program components, and results. In N. K. Wenger and H. K. Hellerstein (eds.), *Rehabilitation of the Coronary Patient* (2nd ed.). New York: Wiley, 1984. Pp. 97–113.
20. Ruberman, W., Weinblatt, E., Goldberg, J. D., and Chaudhary, B. S. Psychosocial influences on mortality after myocardial infarction. *N. Engl. J. Med.* 311:552, 1984.
21. Jenkins, C. D., Zyzanski, S. J., and Rosenman, R. H. Risk of new myocardial infarction in middle aged men with manifest coronary heart disease. *Circulation* 53:342, 1976.
22. Moos, R. H. Coping with acute health crisis. In T. Millon, C. Green, and R. Meagher (eds.), *Handbook of Clinical Health Psychology.* New York: Plenum Press, 1982. Pp. 129–151.
23. Argondizzo, N. T. Education of the patient and family. In N. K. Wenger and H. K. Hellerstein (eds.), *Rehabilitation of the Coronary Patient* (2nd ed.). New York: Wiley, 1984. Pp. 161–178.
24. Bilodeau, C. B., and Hackett, T. P. Issues raised in a group setting by patients recovering from myocardial infarction. *Am. J. Psychiatry* 128:73, 1971.
25. Skelton, M., and Dominian, J. Psychological stress in wives of patients with myocardial infarction. *B.M.J.* 2:101, 1983.
26. Stern, M. J., and Pascale, L. Psychosocial adaptation post-myocardial infarction: The spouse's dilemma. *J. Psychosom. Res.* 23:83, 1979.
27. Krantz, D. S., and Deckel, W. Coping with coronary heart disease and stroke. In T. G. Burish and L. A. Bradley (eds.), *Coping with Chronic Disease.* New York: Academic Press, 1983. Pp. 85–112.
28. Razin, A. M. Coronary artery disease: Reducing risk and aiding recovery. In A. M. Razin (ed.), *Helping Cardiac Patients.* San Francisco: Jossey-Bass, 1985. Pp. 157–193.
29. Gulledge, A. D. The psychological aftermath of a myocardial infarction. In W. D. Gentry and R. B. Williams (eds.), *Psychological Aspects of Myocardial Infarction and Coronary Care.* St. Louis: Mosby, 1975. Pp. 107–123.
30. Weinblatt, E., Shapiro, S., Frank, C. W., and Sagar, R. V. Prognosis of men after myocardial infarction: Mortality and first recurrence in relation to selected parameters. *Am. J. Public Health* 58:1329, 1968.
31. Blankenhorn, D. H., Nessim, S. A., Johnson, R. L., et al. Beneficial effects of combined colestipol-niacin therapy on coronary atherosclerosis and coronary venous bypass grafts. *J.A.M.A.* 257:3233, 1987.
32. Cushin-Hemphill, C., Mack, W. J., Pogoda, J. M., et al. Beneficial effects of colestipol-niacin on coronary atherosclerosis: A 4-year follow-up. *J.A.M.A.* 264:3013, 1990.
33. Ornish, D., Brown, S. E., Scherwitz, L. W., et al. Lifestyle changes and heart disease. *Lancet* 336: 741, 1990.
34. Brown, G., Albers, J. J., Fisher, L. D., et al. Regression of coronary artery disease as a result of intensive lipid-lowering therapy in men with high levels of apolipoprotein-B. *N. Engl. J. Med.* 323:1289, 1990.
35. Tesar, G. E., and Hackett, T. Psychiatric management of the hospitalized cardiac patient. In D. S. Krantz and J. A. Blumenthal (eds.), *Behavioral Assessment and Management of Cardiovascular Disorders.* Sarasota, FL: Professional Resource Exchange, 1987. Pp. 67–80.
36. Tolson, W. W., Mason, J. W., Sachar, E. J., et al. Urinary catecholamine responses associated with hospital admission in normal human subjects. *J. Psychosom. Res.* 8:365, 1965.
37. White, J. Music therapy: An intervention to reduce anxiety in the myocardial infarction patient. *Clin. Nurse Specialist* 6:58, 1992.
38. Frederickson, K. Anxiety transmission in the patient with myocardial infarction. *Heart Lung* 18: 617, 1989.
39. Doerr, B., and James, J. Effects of family preparation on the state anxiety level of the CCU patient. *Nurs. Res.* 28:315, 1979.
40. Thompson, D. R. A randomized controlled trial of in-hospital nursing support for first-time myocardial infarction patients. *Br. J. Clin. Psychol.* 31:215, 1992.
41. Hackett, T. P., Cassem, N. H., and Wishnie, H. A.

The coronary-care unit: An appraisal of its psychologic hazards. *N. Engl. J. Med.* 279:1365, 1968.

42. Croog, S. H., and Levine, S. *The Heart Patient Recovers.* New York: Human Sciences Press, 1977. Pp. 102–106.
43. Forrester, A. W., Lipsey, J. R., Teitelbaum, M. L., et al. Depression following myocardial infarction. *Int. J. Psychiatry Med.* 22:33, 1992.
44. Sivarajan, E. S., Bruce, R. A., Almes, M. J., et al. In-hospital exercise after myocardial infarction does not improve treadmill performance. *N. Engl. J. Med.* 305:357, 1981.
45. Wenger, N. K. Rehabilitation of the patient with acute myocardial infarction during hospitalization: Early ambulation and patient education. In M. L. Pollock and D. H. Schmidt (eds.), *Heart Disease and Rehabilitation* (2nd ed.). New York: Wiley, 1986. Pp. 405–421.
46. Hackett, T. P. Depression following myocardial infarction. *Psychosomatics* 26(Suppl):23, 1985.
47. Hackett, T. P., and Cassem, N. H. Psychological adaptation to convalescence in myocardial infarction patients. In J. P. Naughton, H. K. Hellerstein, and I. C. Mohler (eds.), *Exercise Testing and Experience Training in Coronary Heart Disease.* New York: Academic Press, 1973.
48. Froese, A., Hackett, T. P., Cassem, N. H., and Silverberg, E. L. Trajectories of anxiety and depression in denying and nondenying acute myocardial infarction patients during hospitalization. *J. Psychosom. Res.* 18:413, 1974.
49. Gentry, W. D., Foster, S., and Haney, T. Denial as a determinant of anxiety and perceived health status in the coronary care unit. *Psychosom. Med.* 34:39, 1972.
50. Terry, D. J. Stress, coping and coping resources as correlates of adaptation in myocardial infarction patients. *Br. J. Clin. Psychol.* 31:215, 1992.
51. Lowery, B. J. Psychological stress, denial and myocardial infarction outcomes. *Image: J. Nurs. Scholarship* 23:51, 1991.
52. Levine, J., Warrenburg, S., Kerns, R., et al. The role of denial in recovery from coronary heart disease. *Psychosom. Med.* 49:109, 1987.
53. Scherck, K. A. Coping with acute myocardial infarction. *Heart Lung* 21:327, 1992.
54. Pozen, M. W., Steckmiller, J. A., Harris, W., et al. A nurse rehabilitator's impact on patients with myocardial infarction. *Med. Care* 15:830, 1977.
55. Johnson, B. L., Cantwell, J. D., and Fletcher, G. F. Eight steps to inpatient cardiac rehabilitation: The team effort—methodology and preliminary results. *Heart Lung* 5:97, 1976.
56. Marlatt, G., and Gordon, J. Determinants of relapse: Implications for the maintenance of behavior change. In W. Davidson (ed.), *Behavioral Medicine: Changing Health Lifestyles.* New York: Brunner/Mazel, 1979.
57. Shiffman, S. Relapse following smoking cessation: A situational analysis. *J. Consult. Clin. Psychol.* 500:71, 1982.
58. Ockene, J. K. Physician-delivered interventions for smoking cessation: Strategies for increasing effectiveness. *Prev. Med.* 16:723, 1987.
59. Hackett, T. P., and Cassem, N. H. Psychologic aspects of rehabilitation after myocardial infarction and coronary artery bypass surgery. In N. K. Wenger and H. K. Hellerstein (eds.), *Rehabilitation of the Coronary Patient* (2nd ed.). New York: Wiley, 1984. Pp. 437–471.
60. Garrity, T. F. Behavior adjustment after myocardial infarction: A selective review of recent descriptive, correlational, and intervention research. In S. M. Weiss, J. A. Herd, and B. H. Fox (eds.), *Perspectives on Behavioral Medicine.* New York: Academic Press, 1981. Pp. 67–87.
61. Lazarus, R. S. The costs and benefits of denial. In S. Breznitz (ed.), *The Denial of Stress.* New York: International Universities Press, 1983.
62. Janis, I. L. Preventing pathogenic denial by means of stress inoculation. In S. Breznitz (ed.), *The Denial of Stress.* New York: International Universities Press, 1983.
63. Hackett, T. P., and Cassem, N. H. Development of a quantitative rating scale to assess denial. *J. Psychosom. Res.* 18:93, 1974.
64. Bruhn, J. G. Effects of chronic illness on the family. *J. Fam. Pract.* 4:1057, 1977.
65. Davidson, D. M. The family and cardiac rehabilitation. *J. Fam. Pract.* 8:253, 1979.
66. Speedling, E. F. *Heart Attack: The Family Response at Home and in the Hospital.* New York: Tavistock, 1982.
67. Waltz, M. Type A, social context, and adaptation to serious illness: A longitudinal investigation of the role of the family in recovery from myocardial infarction. In T. H. Schmidt, T. M. Dembroski, and G. Blumchen (eds.), *Biological and Psychological Factors in Cardiovascular Disease.* Berlin: Springer, 1986.
68. Unger, D. G., and Powell, D. R. Supporting families under stress: The role of social networks. *Fam. Relat.* 29:566, 1980.
69. Bedsworth, J. A., and Molen, M. T. Psychological stress in spouses of patients with myocardial infarction. *Heart Lung* 11:450, 1982.
70. Bramwell, L. Wives' experiences in the support role after husbands' first myocardial infarction. *Heart Lung* 15:578, 1986.
71. Ell, K. O., and Haywood, L. J. Social support and recovery from myocardial infarction: A panel study. *J. Soc. Service Res.* 4:1, 1984.
72. Wishnie, H. A., Hackett, T. P., and Cassem, N. H. Psychological hazards of convalescence following myocardial infarction. In R. H. Moos (ed.), *Coping with Physical Illness.* New York: Plenum Press, 1977.
73. Chandra, V., Szklo, M., Goldberg, R., and Tonascia, J. The impact of marital status on survival after an acute myocardial infarction: A population-based study. *Am. J. Epidemiol.* 117:320, 1983.
74. Nyamathi, A. The coping response of female spouses

of patients with myocardial infarction. *Heart Lung* 16:86, 1987.
75. Sirles, A., and Selleck, C. Cardiac disease and the family: Impact, assessment, and implications. *J. Cardiovasc. Nurs.* 3:23, 1989.
76. Nyamathi, A. Coping and adjustment of spouses of critically ill patients with heart disease. *Heart Lung* 21:160, 1992.
77. Goldberg, R. J. Physicians and CPR training in high-risk family members. *Am. J. Public Health* 77:671, 1987.
78. Dracup, K., Guzy, P. M., Taylor, S. E., and Barry, J. Cardiopulmonary resuscitation (CPR) training: Consequences for family members of high-risk cardiac patients. *Arch. Intern. Med.* 146:1757, 1986.
79. Taylor, C. B., Bandura, A., Ewart, C. K., et al. Exercise testing to enhance wives' confidence in their husbands cardiac capability soon after clinically uncomplicated acute myocardial infarction. *Am. J. Cardiol.* 55:635, 1985.
80. Kannel, W. B., Thom, T. J., and Hurst, J. W. Incidence, prevalence, and mortality of cardiovascular diseases. In J. W. Willis (ed.), *The Heart* (6th ed.). New York: McGraw-Hill, 1986. P. 560.
81. Goldman, L., and Cook, E. F. The decline in ischemic heart disease mortality rates. *Ann. Intern. Med.* 101:825, 1984.
82. Expert Panel on Detection, Evaluation, and Treatment of High Blood Cholesterol in Adults. Summary of the second part of the National Cholesterol Education Program (NCEP) Expert Panel on Detection, Evaluation, and Treatment of High Blood Cholesterol in Adults (Adults Treatment Panel II). *J.A.M.A.* 269:3015, 1993.
83. Mulcahy, R., Hickey, N., Graham, I., et al. Factors influencing long-term prognosis in male patients surviving a first coronary heart attack. *Br. Heart J.* 37:158, 1975.
84. Wilhelmsson, C., Vedin, J. A., Elmfeldt, D., et al. Smoking and myocardial infarction. *Lancet* 1:415, 1975.
85. Sparrow, D., Dawber, T., and Colson, T. Influence of cigarette smoking on prognosis after first myocardial infarction. *J. Chronic Dis.* 31:425, 1978.
86. *The Health Consequences of Smoking: Cardiovascular Disease. A Report of the Surgeon General.* Washington, D.C.: U.S. Department of Health, Education and Welfare, Public Health Service, 1983.
87. Burt, A., Thornley, P., Illingworth, D., et al. Stopping smoking after myocardial infarction. *Lancet* 1:304, 1974.
88. Pechacek, T. F., and McAlister, A. Strategies for the modification of smoking behavior: Treatment and prevention. In J. Ferguson and B. Taylor (eds.), *A Comprehensive Handbook of Behavior Medicine.* New York: Spectrum, 1979.
89. Lichtenstein, E., and Danaher, B. G. Modification of smoking behavior: A critical analysis of theory, research and practice. In M. Hersen, R. M. Eisler, and P. M. Miller (eds.), *Advances in Behavior Modification.* New York: Academic Press, 1976. Pp. 79–132.
90. Bernstein, D. A., and Glasgow, R. E. The modification of smoking behavior. In O. F. Pomerleau and J. P. Brady (eds.), *Behavioral Medicine: Theory and Practice.* Baltimore: Williams & Wilkins, 1979.
91. Syme, S., and Alcahay, R. Control of cigarette smoking from a social perspective. *Annu. Rev. Public Health* 3:101, 1982.
92. Ockene, J. K., and Ockene, I. S. Nine ways to help your patient stop smoking. *Your Patient and Cancer* 2:47, 1982.
93. Suinn, R. M. Behavior therapy for cardiac patients. *Behav. Res. Ther.* 5:569, 1974.
94. Friedman, M., and Rosenman, R. H. *Type A Behavior and Your Heart.* New York: Alfred A. Knopf, 1974.
95. Rosenman, R. H., Brand, R. J., Jenkins, C. D., et al. Coronary heart disease in the Western Collaborative Group Study: Final follow-up experience of 8.5 years. *J.A.M.A.* 233:872, 1975.
96. Review Panel on Coronary-Prone Behavior and Coronary Heart Disease. Coronary-prone behavior and coronary heart disease: A critical review. *Circulation* 63:1199, 1981.
97. Shekelle, R. B., Hulley, S. B., Neaton, J. D., et al. The MRFIT behavior pattern study. II. Type A behavior and incidence of coronary heart disease. *Am. J. Epidemiol.* 122:559, 1985.
98. Shekelle, R. B., Gale, M., and Norusis, M. Type A score (Jenkins Activity Survey) and risk of recurrent coronary heart disease in the Aspirin Myocardial Infarction Study. *Am. J. Cardiol.* 56:221, 1985.
99. Goldstein, M. G., and Niaura, R. Psychological factors affecting physical conditions: Cardiovascular disease literature review. *Psychosomatics* 33: 143, 1992.
100. Nunes, E. V., Frank, K. A., and Kornfeld, D. S. Psychologic treatment for the type A behavior pattern and for coronary heart disease: A meta analysis of the literature. *Psychosom. Med.* 48:159, 1987.
101. Friedman, M., Thoresen, C. E., Gill, J. J., et al. Alteration of type A behavior and its effect upon cardiac recurrences in post myocardial infarction subjects: Summary results of the Recurrent Coronary Prevention Project. *Am. Heart J.* 112:653, 1986.
102. Powell, L. H., and Thoresen, C. E. Effects of type A behavioral counseling and severity of prior acute myocardial infarction on survival. *Am. J. Cardiol.* 62:1159, 1988.
103. Friedman, M., Powell, L. H., and Thoresen, C. E. Effect of discontinuance of type A behavioral counseling on type A behavior and cardiac recurrence rate of post myocardial infarction patients. *Am. Heart J.* 114:483, 1987.
104. Mendes de Leon, C. F., Powell, L. H., and Kaplan, B. H. Changes in coronary-prone behaviors in the Recurrent Coronary Prevention Project. *Psychosom. Med.* 53:407, 1991.

105. Powell, L. H., Shaker, L. A., Jones, B. A., et al. Psychosocial predictors of mortality in 83 women with premature acute myocardial infarction. *Psychosom. Med.* 55:426, 1993.
106. Chesney, M. A. Social isolation, depression and heart disease: Research on women broadens the agenda. *Psychosom. Med.* 55:434, 1993.
107. Ragland, D. R., and Brand, R. J. Type A behavior and mortality from coronary heart disease. *N. Engl. J. Med.* 318:65, 1988.
108. Dimsdale, J. E. A perspective on type A behavior and coronary disease. *N. Engl. J. Med.* 318:110, 1988.
109. Hellerstein, H. K., and Friedman, E. H. Sexual activity and the post-coronary patient. *Arch. Intern. Med.* 125:987, 1970.
110. Weizman, R., Eldar, M., Hod, H., et al. Effects of uncomplicated acute myocardial infarction on biochemical parameters of stress and sexual function. *Psychosomatics* 32:275, 1991.
111. Sanders, J. D., and Sprenkle, D. H. Sexual therapy for the post coronary patient. *J. Sex Marital Ther.* 6:174, 1980.
112. Bloch, A., Maeder, J., and Haissly, J. Sexual problems after myocardial infarction. *Am. Heart J.* 90: 536, 1975.
113. Alpert, J. S. *The Heart Attack Handbook* (2nd ed.). Boston: Little, Brown, 1985.
114. Cambre, S. *The Sensuous Heart.* Atlanta: Pritchett & Hull, 1978.
115. Ueno, M. The so-called coition death. *Jpn. J. Legal Med.* 17:535, 1963.
116. Hellerstein, H. K., and Friedman, E. H. Sexual activity and the post-coronary patient. *Med. Aspects Hum. Sexuality* 3:70, 1969.
117. Kavanaugh, T., and Shephard, R. J. Sexual activity after myocardial infarction. *Can. Med. J.* 116: 1250, 1977.
118. Wells, K. B., Golding, J. M., and Burnam, M. A. Chronic medical conditions in a sample of the general population with anxiety, affective and substance use disorders. *Am. J. Psychiatry* 146:1440, 1989.
119. Beitman, B. D., Mukerji, V., Alpert, M., et al. Panic disorder in cardiology patients. *Psychiatric Med.* 8:67, 1990.
120. Kutz, I., Garb, R., and David, D. Post traumatic stress disorder following myocardial infarction. *Gen. Hosp. Psychiatry* 10:169, 1988.
121. Doerfler, L. A., Pbert, L., and DeCosimo, D. Symptoms of post-traumatic stress disorder following myocardial infarction and coronary artery bypass surgery. Unpublished manuscript, 1990.
122. Ibrahim, M. A., Feldman, J. G., Sultz, H. A., et al. Management after myocardial infarction: A controlled trial of the effect of group psychotherapy. *Int. J. Psychiatry Med.* 5:253, 1974.
123. Rahe, R. H., Ward, H. W., and Hayes, V. Brief group therapy in myocardial infarction rehabilitation: Three to four-year follow-up of a controlled trial. *Psychosom. Med.* 41:229, 1979.
124. Mumford, E., Schlesinger, H. J., and Glass, G. The effect of psychological intervention on recovery from surgery and heart attacks: An analysis of the literature. *Am. J. Public Health* 72:141, 1982.
125. Mazzuca, S. A. Does patient education in chronic disease have therapeutic value? *J. Chronic Dis.* 35:521, 1982.
126. Oldenburg, B., Perkins, R. J., and Andrews, G. Controlled trial of psychological intervention in myocardial infarction. *J. Consult. Clin. Psychol.* 53:852, 1985.
127. Stern, M. J., Gorman, P. A., and Kaslow, L. The group counseling v exercise therapy study. *Arch. Intern. Med.* 143:1719, 1983.
128. Frasure-Smith, N. In-hospital symptoms of psychological stress as predictors of long-term outcome after acute myocardial infarction in men. *Am. J. Cardiol.* 67:121, 1991.
129. Davidson, D. M., and Maloney, C. A. Recovery after cardiac events. *Phys. Ther.* 65:1820, 1985.
130. Mæland, J. G., and Havik, O. E. Return to work after a myocardial infarction: The influence of background factors, work characteristics and illness severity. *Scand. J. Soc. Med.* 14:183, 1986.
131. Mayou, R. The course and determinants of reactions to myocardial infarction. *Br. J. Psychiatry* 134: 588, 1979.
132. Mæland, J. G., and Havik, O. E. Psychological predictors for return to work after a myocardial infarction. *J. Psychosom. Res.* 31:471, 1987.
133. Stanton, B. A., Jenkins, C. D., Denlinger, P., et al. Predictors of employment status after cardiac surgery. *J.A.M.A.* 249:907, 1983.
134. Ockene, J. K., Benfari, R. C., Hurwitz, I., et al. Relationship of psychosocial factors to smoking behavior change in an intervention program. *Prev. Med.* 11:13, 1982.
135. Rost, K., and Smith, R. Return to work after an initial myocardial infarction and subsequent emotional distress. *Arch. Intern. Med.* 152:381, 1992.

VIII.
Post–Myocardial Infarction Considerations

34. Exercise and Pharmacologic Testing After Acute Myocardial Infarction

Pierre Théroux and Martin Juneau

Exercise testing is now widely used for the investigation of the post-myocardial infarction patient. A task force of the American College of Cardiology and of the American Heart Association recently concluded that this test was indicated to evaluate prognosis and functional capacity soon after the occurrence of an uncomplicated myocardial infarction [1]. Fifteen years ago exercise testing was considered contraindicated in that clinical setting [2].

Pioneer works originating from the Scandinavian countries documented the applicability and the safety of the exercise test performed during the early rehabilitation period [3–6]. Subsequent studies confirmed the absence of complications and further described a prognostic implication of the various findings of the test, setting the stage for risk stratification after myocardial infarction and programs of active management of patients [7–22]. More recent studies refined the analyses of the various information provided by exercise testing, integrating them with results of other available investigational procedures [23–37]. Concomitant with these developments, therapeutic strategies have been tested to improve prognosis, and emphasis has been put on the positive aspects of early rehabilitation. In recent years, the management of myocardial infarction has become aggressive, with widespread use of acute interventional procedures. The impact of these procedures on prognosis and risk stratification is now being studied.

Exercise testing during the early postinfarction period should now be considered not only as a method for risk stratification but also and more importantly as an aid to direct the care of patients.

Factors Influencing Prognosis After Myocardial Infarction

Table 34-1 summarizes the cardiovascular variables associated with a poor prognosis after myocardial infarction has occurred and how they can be evaluated.

Myocardial dysfunction, the direct consequence of cell loss, is the main determinant of prognosis [27, 38–40]. The presence of electrical instability worsens the prognosis in this situation [41, 42] and also provides independent information [43]. Left ventricular function is conveniently quantified by the ejection fraction but end-systolic volume could provide a better appraisal. Electrical instability is measured by the mean hourly count of ventricular premature complexes (VPCs) on a 24-hour Holter recording and by the presence of ventricular tachycardia.

An important determinant of prognosis is residual ischemia. One early manifestation, spontaneous ischemia during hospitalization for an acute myocardial infarction, is observed in 18 percent of patients and is associated with a high rate of subsequent cardiac events [44, 45]. The ischemia may be located in the infarct zone or at a distance. In one-third of the patients, it is located at a distance from the infarct zone and marks multivessel disease. Most often, however, early ischemia is manifested in the infarct zone. It is then more frequently associated with anterior and non-Q-wave myocardial infarction; multivessel disease is not a prerequisite for this situation, but the artery responsible for the infarct is often patent, suggesting early reperfusion and salvage of a part of myocardium that remains at risk [46, 47]. Indeed, non-Q-wave myocar-

Table 34-1
Physiopathologic determinants of prognosis after myocardial infarction and tests used for their clinical investigation

Left ventricular dysfunction
Indexes of infarct size
Physical examination
Radionuclide ventriculography
Contrast ventriculography
Echocardiographic studies
Residual ischemia
Early spontaneous ischemia
Treadmill exercise test
Thallium scintigraphy during exercise
Dipyridamole test
Exercise radionuclide ventriculography
Coronary angiography
Ventricular arrhythmias
Holter monitoring
Electrophysiologic testing

dial infarction may be considered an unstable state because it is associated with a high risk of recurrent infarction during follow-up [48].

Information Derived from Exercise Testing

Exercise testing yields information on these various determinants of prognosis (Table 34-2). Thus, chest pain and ST segment depression are usually associated with residual ischemia and more extensive coronary disease [15, 19]. ST segment elevation may occur in regions of akinetic and dyskinetic wall motion and is often associated with a high QRS score and a large infarct [49]. Poor left ventricular function also influences the responses of heart rate and blood pressure and reduces exercise tolerance.

Table 34-2
Prognostic information derived from exercise testing

Left ventricular dysfunction
Tolerance to exercise
Blood pressure response
Heart rate response
ST segment elevation
Residual ischemia
ST segment depression
Anginal pain
Ventricular arrhythmias
Exercise-induced ventricular premature complexes

Exercise-induced ventricular premature beats are associated with more severe regional wall motion abnormalities in the infarcted area [50].

None of these findings, including the ST segment changes, is highly specific since each can be influenced by a variety of factors. Thus, in the context of the patient, the physician should consider not a single, but all parameters.

Heart Rate

The heart rate and blood pressure responses during exercise are complex; they are influenced by the level of physical fitness before the infarction occurred, the deconditioning effect of a period of rest, and the intensity of the early rehabilitation program. The physiologic responses may also be influenced by an altered autonomic tone or responsiveness often found during the early postinfarction period and also by the various medications used. One important determinant, however, is cardiac reserve; the compromised heart maintains its output by an increase in heart rate.

Various definitions of an inappropriate increase in heart rate have been used. Among studies showing a prognostic value of heart rate, some used a heart rate acceleration to 125 or 130 beats per minute or more at predefined workloads [6, 16]; others used the relative increase in heart rate from the preexercise value [17]. In a predischarge, symptom-limited test, the mean heart rate achieved was greater in nonsurvivors than in survivors [32]. Most of the studies, however, did not describe a prognostic value associated with the acceleration of heart rate [7, 10, 14, 15, 23, 25, 34]. Obviously, the heart rate response to exercise is not the best indicator of compromised left ventricular function. Use of this parameter for this purpose would require strictly standardized protocols, which is not now the case. Medications would have to be avoided, particularly beta blockers [11, 30]. The interval from the occurrence of the myocardial infarction to the time of the test would also have to be defined, as peak heart rate response increases significantly 3 and 7 weeks after the infarction and remains stable thereafter [51].

Blood Pressure

Exertional hypotension is a physiologic indicator of severe myocardial ischemia in patients with chronic ischemic disease. The specificity of this finding early after the occurrence of a myocardial infarction has been questioned because the incidence decreases over the following 4 to 11 weeks [52]. The attenuated heart rate and blood pressure response in patients with well-preserved left ventricular function could be caused by stimulation of left ventricular baroreceptors.

Many studies nevertheless described a worse prognosis when the blood pressure rise was inadequate [12, 17, 21]. In some of these studies, the abnormal response was an independent predictor of prognosis when the response was analyzed jointly with other parameters [30, 32–37]; the prognostic significance was not influenced by the concomitant administration of beta blockers [32, 34–37]. Again there is a lack of standardization in the study of this parameter because different criteria are used to define the inadequate rise, from an increase of less than 5 mm Hg [7], less than 10 mm Hg [34–36], or less than 30 mm Hg [32]. Other studies defined the inadequate rise as a peak blood pressure below 110 mm Hg [30].

Functional Capacity

Reduced exercise capacity is defined as the failure to reach a predetermined target workload or heart rate, or in a symptom-limited test, a certain level or duration of exercise. The reasons for this failure are usually cardiac and can consist of any symptom that renders the patient uncomfortable (e.g., chest pain, dyspnea, or fatigue) or any abnormal sign urging the physician to stop the test (e.g., marked ST segment depression, a fall in blood pressure, or significant arrhythmias). Reduced exercise capacity is nonspecific and can be caused by any of the determinants of prognosis. On the other hand, it is sensitive to all the determinants and, not surprisingly, it is a predictor of prognosis in most studies [11, 14, 22–24, 29, 30, 32–36]. When its value is assessed, the timing of the test is important because functional capacity increases markedly during the weeks following an acute myocardial infarction [53], even in the absence of changes in left ventricular ejection fraction [54].

Angina Pectoris

The frequency of angina pectoris during the exercise test varies with the protocol used and the timing of the exercise test after myocardial infarction [12, 17]. In one study, it occurred in 15 (21 percent) of 70 patients submitted to a symptom-limited protocol before hospital discharge; only 9 of these patients had angina in a test repeated 6 weeks later, whereas 12 others without angina during the early test developed new angina [12]. Angina is more reproducible in tests performed 3, 7, and 11 weeks after myocardial infarction has occurred [51].

A prognostic value of the presence of angina pectoris was described in early studies [6, 12, 13, 16–19]. More recent studies did not confirm these observations [32–37]. Its occurrence during the exercise test is, however, predictive of angina during follow-up [19], particularly when angina is also present before the infarction developed [55]. Angina occurs during follow-up in 96 percent of patients with both preinfarction angina and angina during the exercise test; it occurs in only 26 percent of patients without preinfarction angina and exercise test angina. Consistently, angina during the exercise test is predictive of the need for additional treatment, and often revascularization [11, 19, 29, 30]. In one study, coronary artery bypass surgery was performed in 20 percent of patients with angina during the exercise test compared to 9 percent of the patients without angina during the test ($p < .001$) [30]. Angina during the test also correlates with more frequent multivessel disease [19, 56].

ST Segment Depression

ST segment depression is observed during exercise in 30 to 40 percent of patients. It is associated with extensive coronary artery disease [15, 19, 56–59] and is the single most useful prognostic parameter (Table 34-3). ST segment depression can predict mortality [8, 21, 31], recurrent myocardial infarction [28, 36], and bypass surgery [30, 35–37]. The prognosis is worse when it occurs at a lower level of exercise [11]. The magnitude of ST segment depression is also important [7], and repeated tests may yield more prognostic data than a single test [10]. A symptom-limited exercise test results in more frequent and more reproducible detection of ST segment depression [10, 12, 17, 50].

ST segment depression may not be specific for ischemia. The use of radionuclide techniques during the treadmill test can help distinguish ischemic and nonischemic ST segment depression, as will be discussed.

Table 34-3
Prognostic value of parameters of exercise tests in various series (1972–1986)

First author	No. of patients	% with CABG	Heart rate	Blood pressure	Tolerance	Angina	ST segment shift	VPCs	Events: Death	Events: MI	Events: Angina
Granath [6]	205	0	*	–	–	*	–	*	×		
Markiewitz [7]	46	8.7	NS	NS	NS	–	*	*	×		
Théroux [8]	210	5.7	–	–	–	NS	*	*	×		
Smith [9]	62	?	–	–	–	–	*	NS	×	×	
Sami [10]	200	9.5	NS	NS	NS	NS	*	*	×	×	
Davidson [11]	195	9.7	–	–	*	*	*	NS	×	×	×
Starling [12]	89	0	–	*	–	*	*	–	×	×	×
Koppes [13]	90	?	–	–	–	*	*	–	×	×	×
Madsen [14]	205	0	NS	NS	*	–	NS	NS	×		
Schwartz [15]	48	?	NS	NS	NS	*	NS	NS	×		
Lindvall [16]	76	0	*	–	–	*	*	*	×	×	×
Velasco [17]	200	0	*	*	–	*	*	NS	×		
Fuller [19]	40	7.5	–	–	–	*	*	NS	×	×	×
Srinivasan [20]	154	0	–	–	–	–	*	–	×		
Saunamäki [21]	317	0	*	*	–	–	NS	*	×		
Weld [22]	236	0	–	–	*	–	NS	*	×		
Corbett [23]	60	?	NS	NS	*	*	*	NS	×	×	×
De Feyter [24]	179	13.4	–	–	*	NS	NS	NS	×	×	
Gibson [25]	165	15.2	NS	–	NS	*	*	NS	×	×	×
Rapaport [26]	75	?	–	–	–	–	NS	–	×	×	
Norris [27]	325	23.7	–	–	NS	NS	NS	–	×		
Dwyer [28]	658	12.8	–	–	NS	NS	NS	–	×	×	
Hung [29]	117	7.7	–	–	*	*	*	–	×	×	×
Krone [30]	667	12	*	*	*	*	NS	*	×	×	
Jespersen [31]	126	1	–	–	–	NS	*	–	×	×	
Fioretti [32]	300	15	*	*	*	NS	NS	NS	×		
Madsen [33]	466	0	–	NS	*	NS	*	NS	×	×	
Waters [34]	225	16	NS	*	*	NS	*	*	×		
Handler [35]	222	9	–	*	*	NS	NS	NS	×		
Starling [36]	72	15	–	*	NS	NS	*	NS	×	×	×
Fioretti [37]	351	21.7	NS	*	*	NS	NS	NS	×		

NS = nonsignificant; * = denotes statistical significance; × = event considered; – = not analyzed; ? = not reported; CABG = coronary artery bypass grafting; VPCs = ventricular premature complexes; MI = myocardial infarction.

ST Segment Elevation

ST segment elevation during the exercise test occurs mainly in electrocardiogram leads overlying the infarct area; its magnitude tends to decrease as time after infarction elapses [3]. It is associated with pathologic Q waves, lower ejection fractions, and a higher number of akinetic or dyskinetic segments [15, 60]. It is not an indicator of residual ischemia [60]. The prognostic value of ST segment elevation is thus more related to left ventricular dysfunction than to residual ischemia [15, 34, 60, 61]. Consequently, it is a weak predictor with no independent value when more accurate parameters of left ventricular function are also considered.

Ventricular Arrhythmias

Many studies have documented that exercise-induced ventricular arrhythmias predict mortality during follow-up [6, 7, 22, 30, 34] and more specifically, sudden death [8]. The independent prognostic value of exercise-induced ventricular arrhythmias was confirmed in multivariate analyses that included clinical characteristics and other findings of the exercise test [22, 30, 34]. The frequency of ventricular premature beats increases in tests performed between 3 and 11 weeks after infarction [62] and is stable thereafter [51]. The same is found in serial Holter monitoring recordings. The presence of a ventricular premature beat is determined more by the severity of regional wall motion contraction abnormalities in the infarct zone than by either the number of diseased vessels or global left ventricular dysfunction [50].

Prognostic Value of Exercise Testing

The Confusion

Some of the results published on the prognostic value of exercise testing after myocardial infarction has occurred are shown in Table 34-3. At first glance, these results appear confusing. For example, heart rate was predictive of future events in 6 studies and not predictive in 8; 10 studies reported a predictive value for blood pressure response and 6 reported no value; exercise tolerance had prognostic value in 12 studies and no value in 7; angina was predictive in half of the studies; the respective figures for ST segment shifts are 17 and 12 studies and for ventricular arrhythmias 9 and 14.

The results of exercise testing are thus clearly influenced by a variety of confounding factors and should be interpreted with caution. On the other hand, exercise testing provides information on the various pathophysiologic factors influencing prognosis, and the integration of these data can be useful for the overall assessment of patients. The results are also influenced by the characteristics of the populations studied, the protocol used, the parameters most clearly scrutinized, the end points used, and the concomitant medication administered. Other factors such as the influence of test results on subsequent patient management, the nature of the cardiac events considered during follow-up, and the duration of the follow-up also influence the conclusions.

Toward Cohesion

Despite the apparent confusion, many important and conclusive observations can be drawn from the available literature. First, 6 of the 9 studies that showed a prognostic value for the presence of ventricular premature beats had mortality alone as the end point, whereas 8 of the 14 negative studies had multiple end points including myocardial infarction and angina. The last two end points clearly cannot be related to arrhythmias and using them could be misleading. The positive studies included a multivariate analysis that documented an independent prognostic value of VPCs. The presence of VPCs increased the mortality risk twofold to threefold. As indicated in Table 34-3, the prognostic value observed with the presence of VPCs was not influenced by the year the study was performed, probably because no well-defined therapeutic strategies exist for management of ventricular beats after myocardial infarction. The results of the Cardiac Arrhythmia Suppression Trial (CAST) conducted to determine whether control of ventricular arrhythmias could reduce mortality dramatically demonstrate this point [62].

Conversely, time-dependent results are found when the prognostic value of ST segment depression is examined. Eighteen of the 26 studies documented a prognostic value: 75 percent of the 13 published before 1982 and 43 percent of the studies published after 1982. This apparently declining value of ST segment depression can easily be explained by the more liberal use of anti-ischemic treatment and be correlated with the increasing use of bypass surgery and coronary angioplasty. In the studies conducted before 1982, coronary artery surgery was performed in 0 to 9.7 percent of patients (mean, 3 percent). The studies performed after 1982 reported an incidence of bypass surgery as high as 24 percent (mean, 12.6 percent).

In the SAVE trial which tested the effectiveness of captopril in post-myocardial infarction patients with an ejection fraction lower than 40 percent, 31 percent of patients had a revascularization procedure as early as 3 to 16 days after the myocardial infarction occurred [63]. After 43 months, 43 percent of the patients had undergone coronary angioplasty or coronary artery bypass surgery in the US centers participating in the study.

Medical treatment has also improved enormously during these years, with strict control of risk factors, comprehensive rehabilitation programs, and liberal use of beta blockers, converting enzyme inhibitors, and acetylsalicylic acid. The impact of these medical interventions on prognosis could be greater than that of surgical treatment and coronary angioplasty.

It is also of interest to note that over this period of time, the prognostic value of parameters related to ventricular function has increased; thus, an inadequate blood pressure response was predictive of cardiac events in 60 percent of the studies performed before 1982 and in 86 percent of the studies performed after 1982.

Additional Information Provided by Radionuclide Studies and Echocardiography

Radionuclide techniques can be used in conjunction with exercise testing to provide additional data. Thallium 201 or technetium 99m sestamibi scintigraphy permits detection of transient regional perfusion defects, and radionuclide ventriculography and two-dimensional echocardiography yield information on global and regional wall motion.

Gibson et al. [25] identified the high-risk patient by the presence of multiple thallium defects involving different vascular regions, thallium-201 redistribution, or increased lung uptake by left ventricular dysfunction. The sensitivity and specificity of these findings were superior to those provided by exercise testing alone and by coronary angiography [25]. Other investigations documented a high sensitivity of thallium exercise testing for detecting more extensive coronary artery disease [64, 65].

The exercise ventriculogram also can help identify the patient at high risk. In one study comparing the prognostic value of reversible perfusion defect, time on treadmill, and ejection fraction, the only two independent predictors of prognosis were a peak treadmill workload of 4 METs or less and a decrease of 5 percent or more in the ejection fraction [29]. In another study, the changes in ejection fraction, end-systolic volume, and ratio of systolic blood pressure to end-systolic volume were predictive of subsequent cardiac events [23]. Resting ejection fraction may be more predictive of mortality and the changes during exercise more predictive of subsequent ischemic events [66], although the former can also be influenced by transient left ventricular dysfunction induced by the changing loading conditions, particularly the increased afterload. The sensitivity and specificity of the exercise ventriculogram to detect multivessel disease may be as high as those for thallium perfusion scintigraphy [67]. The specificity of both tests for detecting multivessel disease is reduced in the presence of anterior myocardial infarction [64, 67].

Studies published to date using radionuclide techniques involved only small numbers of patients and used multiple cardiac events as end points. The yield of these tests to evaluate the post–myocardial infarction patient has not yet been determined. They can obviously be advantageous in many clinical circumstances, particularly when the ST segment changes are nonspecific, as with the presence of bundle branch block, left ventricular hypertrophy, Wolff-Parkinson-White syndrome, digitalis effect, and abnormal resting ST segment abnormalities caused by a large anterior Q-wave myocardial infarction. They can also be useful in the presence of chest pain without ST segment changes or when the ST changes are of borderline significance.

The additional information provided by myocardial scintigraphies may not justify their routine use when the exercise test results are completely negative at a high workload or when obvious ischemic ST segment shifts occur at a low workload. In the

Table 34-4
Comparisons of predischarge low-level and symptom-limited exercise tests in 200 myocardial infarction patients*

Test	Low-level test	Symptom-limited test	p value
Exercise duration (sec)	389 ± 125	554 ± 209	.0001
METs	4.2 ± 1.1	5.7 ± 1.8	.0001
Peak HR	108 ± 14	121 ± 20	.0001
Peak systolic BP (mm Hg)	140 ± 25	155 ± 30	.0001
Peak rate-pressure product ($\times 10^{-3}$)	15.2 ± 3.7	18.9 ± 5.6	
ST depression ≥ 1 mm	56 (28)	89 (45)	.0009
ST depression ≥ 2 mm	22 (11)	41 (21)	.0001
Angina	26 (13)	40 (20)	.01
ST depression or angina	66 (33)	105 (53)	.0001
Maximal ST depression (mm)	1.6 ± 0.7	1.8 ± 0.9	NS
Ventricular premature beats	19 (9.5)	33 (17)	<.05

*Values are mean ± standard deviations or number (%) of patients.
BP = blood pressure; HR = heart rate; METs = metabolic equivalents.
Source: From M. Juneau, P. Colles, P. Théroux et al. Symptom-limited versus low level exercise testing before hospital discharge after myocardial infarction. *J. Am. Coll. Cardiol.* 20:927, 1992. With permission.

latter circumstance, they may help localize the site of ischemia and influence the selection of therapy.

Exercise testing coupled with echocardiography also was recently shown to be of prognostic value. This technique is applicable in 85 to 90 percent of post-myocardial infarction patients. Three studies documented the prognostic value of exercise echocardiography to predict coronary events after the occurrence of a noncomplicated myocardial infarction [68–70]. Quiñones et al. [71] recently reported that exercise echocardiography could help identify the stunned versus the necrotic myocardium; the technique could be less sensitive than myocardial scintigraphy.

Exercise Test Protocols

The Naughton protocol is generally selected for the early exercise test performed before hospital discharge and the Bruce protocol for tests performed 2 to 3 weeks later. The workload equivalent calculated in multiples of resting oxygen consumption (METs) is the most useful criterion for comparing results of various tests in the same patient and results from various studies. When the exercise test is performed before hospital discharge, most investigators and clinicians prefer the use of a low-level exercise protocol (5 METs) [8, 30, 34]; symptom-limited exercise testing after myocardial infarction is usually delayed until 3 weeks after discharge [11, 24, 72]. Two recent studies [18, 73], however, showed the feasibility and safety of a predischarge symptom-limited exercise test. In the study from the Montreal Heart Institute [18], the symptom-limited test compared to the low-level exercise test provided a significantly greater stress and was associated with an ischemic response nearly twice as frequently (Table 34-4).

The advantages of the in-hospital test are patient convenience, early detection of high risk, promotion of self-confidence and reassurance for the family, and the potential to institute earlier, more definitive medical or surgical treatment and a rehabilitation program. The late test, however, may provide superior data on overall cardiovascular status and serves as a guideline for more intensive rehabilitation and return to work. Timing of the test is not a critical issue, as both the early and the late tests provide complementary information.

Complications of Post–myocardial Infarction Exercise Testing

Hamm et al. [74] recently reported data compiled from questionnaire responses on 651,949 post–myocardial infarction exercise tests performed in 570 institutions. The overall fatality rate was 0.03 percent (n = 41), 0.04 percent in the 28,052 symptom-limited tests, and 0.03 percent in the 99,695 low-level tests. Cardiac rupture was reported in one symptom-limited and in one low-level test, an incidence that may not be higher than the expected rate at the same period after myocardial infarction, in the absence of an exercise test. When all major fatal complications are grouped together, they represent 0.03 percent for the low-level tests and 0.04 percent for the symptom-limited tests (not significant). The percentage of all nonfatal major complications was 0.07 percent for the low-level tests and 0.15 percent for the symptom-limited tests, a difference of 0.08 percent ($p < .05$).

To reduce complications, careful selection of patients is important and close observation during the test is required so that the test can be stopped when abnormalities are detected.

Selection of Patients

Patients can be selected on the basis of a careful history and physical examination. The two cardiac contraindications to exercise testing are chest pain occurring at rest or during mild exercise and clinical signs of congestive failure, such as pulmonary rales, presence of a third heart sound, and sinus tachycardia. When heart failure is compensated, exercise testing may be performed to assess functional capacity. Some patients are excluded because of other medical conditions, such as chronic obstructive lung disease, peripheral vascular disease, orthopedic conditions, or other severe medical illness. Age per se is not a contraindication. In patients unable to exercise because of a physical condition, alternative methods to unmask ischemia are now available, as will be discussed.

Pharmacologic Stress Testing

Exercise testing with standard electrocardiogram or with an imaging technique (scintigraphy or echocardiography) remains the best method to evaluate post–myocardial infarction patients since it provides important clinical information not provided by pharmacologic testing: maximal functional capacity, maximal heart rate, blood pressure response, and exercise-induced arrhythmias. When patients are unable to exercise, pharmacologic stress testing represents a very useful alternative.

Several studies documented the prognostic value of dipyridamole thallium-201 testing after myocardial infarction. Leppo et al. [75] demonstrated that the redistribution of thallium as observed on scans significantly predicts cardiac events including recurrent infarction and death. These results were subsequently confirmed by Brown et al. [76] and Gimple et al. [77]. However, these studies included a limited number of patients and the coronary events during follow-up were more often recurrent angina than myocardial infarction and cardiac death. More recent studies combined dipyridamole infusion with echocardiography, with some promising results [78–81]. Bolognese et al. [78] reported that dipyridamole-induced dyssynergy was a strong predictor of adverse outcome after myocardial infarction.

Another recently introduced coronary vasodilator is adenosine, which has a very short half-life and is considered to be very safe in coronary patients. Mahmarian et al. [79] reported that adenosine thallium-201 single-photon emission computed tomography (SPECT) can be safely performed after myocardial infarction to assess the extent of coronary disease and determine the risk of in-hospital cardiac events. Long-term follow-up was not available. Further studies are needed to assess the role of this new pharmacologic stress test after myocardial infarction.

Dobutamine is a sympathomimetic agent that causes an increase in heart rate and systolic blood pressure. Because it causes a progressive increase in myocardial oxygen demand, the dobutamine stress test has been referred to as an exercise-simulating test. Atrial pacing had been similarly used for this purpose with positive results [80]. Dobutamine can be coupled with echocardiography [81–83] and myocardial scintigraphy [84, 85]. Dobutamine stress testing has been shown to be safe in coronary patients but experience in post–myocardial infarction patients is limited [81]. Piérard et al. [81] compared dobutamine echocardiography with positron emission tomography in 17 post–myocardial infarction patients treated with thrombolytic therapy. The results indicated that dobutamine echocardiography can accurately identify viable versus nonviable myocardium but no data on prognosis were reported. Because of its physiologic effect, dobutamine coupled with echocardiography, scintigraphy, or standard electrocardiography could comprise a very promising alternative stress test in patients unable to exercise. Coma-Canella et al. [86] performed thallium-201 SPECT studies and radionuclide ventriculography 1 day apart in association with dobutamine in 63 postinfarction patients. They showed that mild to moderate ischemia was compatible with an increase in contractility whereas severe ischemia induced worsening of wall motion.

Further studies are needed to document the prognostic value of the various pharmacologic stress tests in the post–myocardial infarction patient before their routine use can be recommended. Also, the exact pathophysiologic meaning of these tests remains to be investigated more in-depth, particularly the relative contribution to a positive test result of ischemia, left ventricular function, and regional stunning at various times after the infarction.

Exercise Testing and the Patient: Global Approach

All patients recovering from myocardial infarction should be considered for exercise testing. Indeed, the test provides information on prognosis that is not otherwise available [13, 14, 21, 36, 37]. The presence of a cardiac contraindication to the test is already predictive of a poor prognosis [14, 30, 37]. The associated risk varies depending on the severity of the exclusion criteria used, but can be as high as 56 percent.

Good tolerance to exercise without ischemia and with a normal hemodynamic response is associated with a mortality risk of less than 2 percent at 1 year [1, 8, 11, 14, 16, 23, 30, 32]. This point could be the most positive aspect of exercise testing. Indeed, the asymptomatic patient with a low risk would likely not benefit from additional investigation or treatment. On the contrary, this patient is a candidate for a positive rehabilitation program and early return to work [87]. A recent study [88] showed that these low-risk patients can resume occupational work as early as 5 weeks after the infarction occurred. A positive exercise test result, on the other hand, is an indication to further investigation to establish the most appropriate treatment.

Because myocardial ischemia is associated with a high risk of recurrent angina, myocardial infarction, and death, a clear ischemic response is an indication for coronary angiography, often followed by more intensive medical therapy or a revascularization procedure. If myocardial ischemia is suspected but not documented, further investigation should be carried out with radionuclide techniques. This aggressive attitude for the control of ischemia will hopefully reduce further the devastating prognostic impact of this parameter.

Poor tolerance to exercise and an abnormal hemodynamic response should also be more fully investigated to determine whether they are related to ischemia or to left ventricular dysfunction. Echocardiographic and radionuclide studies are then indicated. Depressed left ventricular function with or without clinical congestive heart failure should be managed in light of the recent studies showing improved prognosis with angiotensin-converting enzyme inhibitors [89, 90]. The presence of ventricular premature beats during exercise is also an indication for investigating left ventricular function; beta blockers should then be considered if they are not contraindicated. A recent study also suggested that amiodarone therapy could be useful in these patients [91]. A large multicenter study is now testing the value of amiodarone in the post–myocardial infarction patient with premature ventricular beats on Holter recordings.

Exercise Testing After Myocardial Infarction in the Era of Thrombolysis and Angioplasty

Fibrinolysis and angioplasty are now widely used for the acute management of myocardial infarction. This treatment, particularly when applied within 6 hours after the onset of pain, improves survival [92]. Changes in our scheme of risk stratification and in the relative frequency of the various determinants of prognosis have already been observed. Successful thrombolysis improves left ventricular function and reduces the frequency [93] and severity [94] of ventricular arrhythmias. It also probably results in less-frequent residual ischemia, contrary to earlier thoughts [95, 96]. In a recent study on 202 myocardial infarction patients, the use of a thrombolytic agent compared to no thrombolysis resulted in a longer exercise duration, a higher workload achieved, and less frequent ST depression in both the low-level exercise test and the symptom-limited exercise test (Table 34-5) [18]. Similar data were reported in the Thrombolysis in Myocardial Infarction (TIMI-2) trial [97]. In this randomized

Table 34-5
Influence of thrombolytic therapy on the results of exercise testing[a]

	Low-level test		Symptom-limited test	
	Thrombolysis (n = 113)	No thrombolysis (n = 87)	Thrombolysis (n = 113)	No thrombolysis (n = 87)
Exercise duration (sec)	393 ± 125	385 ± 125	586 ± 204[b]	509 ± 206[b]
METs	4.3 ± 1.1	4.2 ± 1.1	5.9 ± 1.7[b]	5.3 ± 1.7[b]
Peak HR	107 ± 13	108 ± 15	122 ± 19	118 ± 19
% maximal HR	65 ± 8	66 ± 9	74 ± 11	72 ± 11
Peak systolic BP (mm Hg)	136 ± 21[b]	144 ± 26[b]	155 ± 28	154 ± 31
ST depression ≥ 1 mm	23 (20)[b]	33 (38)[b]	40 (35)[c]	49 (56)[c]
Angina	12 (11)	14 (16)	23 (20)	17 (20)

[a]Values are mean ± standard deviations or number (%) of patients. Unless indicated, differences between patients with and those without thrombolytic therapy did not attain statistical significance. Abbreviations as in Table 34-4.
[b]$p = .005$.
[c]$p = .002$.
Source: From M. Juneau, P. Colles, P. Théroux et al. Symptom-limited versus low level exercise testing before hospital discharge after myocardial infarction. *J. Am. Coll. Cardiol.* 20:927, 1992. With permission.

study of 586 patients, the predischarge low-level exercise test induced ST depression in 14 percent of the group treated with early coronary arteriography and if appropriate, angioplasty; 14 percent of the group treated with late arteriography and if appropriate, angioplasty; and 21 percent of the conservative-treatment group (angioplasty only if ischemia is detected) (differences not significant). All patients received recombinant tissue plasminogen activator. Therefore, the early perception that patients treated with thrombolytic therapy will be more unstable and demonstrate more exercise-induced ischemia is not supported by recent data.

Thrombolytic therapy of acute myocardial infarction, with or without coronary angioplasty, does not reduce the value of exercise testing for risk stratification and may indeed enhance it. It certainly is an incitation to perform it earlier in patients with a favorable evolution [98].

The evaluation of the viability of stunned myocardium (viable versus nonviable myocardium) has also gained increasing importance with the advent of thrombolytic therapy and has broadened the indications for the use of exercise testing coupled with imaging techniques (echocardiography and scintigraphy) [99]. Evaluation of myocardial viability has a major clinical significance to determine the prognosis and to select the optimal treatment, particularly surgical or balloon angioplasty. Much remains to be learned in this exciting field of investigation.

References

1. Gunnar, R. M., Bourdillon, P. D. V., Dixon, D. W., et al. Guidelines for the early management of patients with acute myocardial infarction. *J. Am. Coll. Cardiol.* 16:249, 1990.
2. Fortuin, N. J., and Weiss, J. L. Exercise stress testing. *Circulation* 56:699, 1977.
3. Atterhög, J. H., Ekelund, L. G., and Kaijser, L. Electrocardiographic abnormalities during exercise 3 weeks to 18 months after anterior myocardial infarction. *Br. Heart J.* 33:871, 1971.
4. Ericsson, M., Granath, A., Ohlsen, P., et al. Arrhythmias and symptoms during treadmill testing three weeks after myocardial infarction in 100 patients. *Br. Heart J.* 35:787, 1973.
5. Ibsen, H., Kjoller, E., Styperek, J., et al. Routine exercise ECG three weeks after acute myocardial infarction. *Acta Med. Scand.* 198:463, 1975.
6. Granath, A., Södermark, T., Winge, T., et al. Early workload tests for evaluation of long term prognosis of acute myocardial infarction. *Br. Heart J.* 39:758, 1977.
7. Markiewicz, W., Houston, N., and DeBusk, R. Exercise testing soon after myocardial infarction. *Circulation* 56:26, 1977.
8. Théroux, P., Waters, D. D., Halphen, C., et al. Prognostic value of exercise testing soon after myocardial infarction. *N. Engl. J. Med.* 301:341, 1979.
9. Smith, J., Dennis, C., Gassman, A., et al. Exercise testing three weeks after myocardial infarction. *Chest* 75:12, 1979.
10. Sami, M., Kraemer, H., and DeBusk, R. F. The prognostic significance of serial exercise testing after myocardial infarction. *Circulation* 60:1238, 1979.

11. Davidson, D. M., and DeBusk, R. F. Prognostic value of a single exercise test 3 weeks after uncomplicated myocardial infarction. *Circulation* 61:236, 1980.
12. Starling, M. R., Crawford, M. H., Kennedy, G. T., et al. Treadmill exercise tests predischarge and six weeks post-myocardial infarction to detect abnormalities of known prognostic value. *Ann. Intern. Med.* 94:721, 1981.
13. Koppes, G. M., Kruyer, W., Beckmann, C. H., et al. Response to exercise early after uncomplicated acute myocardial infarction in patients receiving no medication: Long-term follow-up. *Am. J. Cardiol.* 46: 764, 1980.
14. Madsen, E. B., Rasmussen, S., and Svendsen, T. L. Multivariate long-term prognosis index from exercise ECG after acute myocardial infarction. *Eur. J. Cardiol.* 11:435, 1980.
15. Schwartz, K. M., Turner, J. D., Sheffield, L. T., et al. Limited exercise testing soon after myocardial infarction. *Ann. Intern. Med.* 94:727, 1981.
16. Lindvall, K., and Kaijser, L. Early exercise tests after uncomplicated acute myocardial infarction before early discharge from hospital. *Acta Med. Scand.* 210: 257, 1981.
17. Velasco, J. A., Tormo, V., Ridocci, F., et al. Early load-limited versus symptom-limited exercise testing: Prognostic value in 200 myocardial infarction patients. *Cardiology* 68(Suppl 2):44, 1981.
18. Juneau, M., Colles, P., Théroux, P., et al. Symptom-limited versus low level exercise testing before hospital discharge after myocardial infarction. *J. Am. Coll. Cardiol.* 20:927, 1992.
19. Fuller, C. M., Raizner, A. E., Verani, M. S., et al. Early post-myocardial infarction treadmill stress testing. An accurate predictor of multivessel coronary artery disease and subsequent cardiac events. *Ann. Intern. Med.* 94:734, 1981.
20. Srinivasan, M., Young, A., Baker, G., et al. The value of postcardiac infarction exercise stress testing: Identification of a group at high risk. *Med. J. Aust.* 2:466, 1981.
21. Saunamäki, K. I., and Andersen, J. D. Early exercise test in the assessment of long-term prognosis after myocardial infarction. *Acta Med. Scand.* 209:185, 1981.
22. Weld, F. M., Chu, K. L., Bigger, J. T., et al. Risk stratification with low level exercise testing 2 weeks after acute myocardial infarction. *Circulation* 64: 306, 1981.
23. Corbett, J. R., Dehmer, G. J., Lewis, S. E., et al. The prognostic value of submaximal exercise testing with radionuclide ventriculography before hospital discharge in patients with recent myocardial infarction. *Circulation* 64:535, 1981.
24. De Feyter, P. J., van Eenige, M. J., Dighton, D. H., et al. Prognostic value of exercise testing, coronary angiography and left ventriculography 6-8 weeks after myocardial infarction. *Circulation* 66:527, 1982.
25. Gibson, R. S., Watson, D. D., Craddock, G. B., et al. Reduction of cardiac events after uncomplicated myocardial infarction: A prospective study comparing predischarge exercise thallium-201 scintigraphy and coronary angiography. *Circulation* 68: 321, 1983.
26. Rapaport, E., and Remedios, P. The high risk patient after recovery from myocardial infarction: Recognition and management. *J. Am. Coll. Cardiol.* 1:391, 1983.
27. Norris, R. M., Barnaby, P. F., Brandt, P. W. T., et al. Prognosis after recovery from first acute myocardial infarction: Determinants of reinfarction and sudden death. *Am. J. Cardiol.* 54:408, 1984.
28. Dwyer, E. M., Jr., McMaster, P., Greenberg, H., et al. Non-fatal cardiac events and recurrent infarction in the year after acute myocardial infarction. *J. Am. Coll. Cardiol.* 4:695, 1984.
29. Hung, J., Goris, M. L., Nash, E., et al. Comparative value of maximal treadmill testing, exercise thallium myocardial perfusion scintigraphy and exercise radionuclide ventriculography for distinguishing high- and low-risk patients soon after myocardial infarction. *Am. J. Cardiol.* 53:1221, 1984.
30. Krone, R. J., Gillespie, J. A., Weld, F. M., et al. Low-level exercise testing after myocardial infarction: Usefulness in enhancing clinical risk stratification. *Circulation* 71:80, 1985.
31. Jespersen, C. M., Kassis, E., Edeling, C. J., et al. The prognostic value of maximal exercise testing soon after first myocardial infarction. *Eur. Heart J.* 6:769, 1985.
32. Fioretti, P., Brower, R. W., Simoons, M. L., et al. Prediction of mortality during the first year after acute myocardial infarction from clinical variables and stress test at hospital discharge. *Am. J. Cardiol.* 55:1313, 1985.
33. Madsen, E. B., Gilpin, E., Ahnvee, S., et al. Prediction of functional capacity and use of exercise testing for predicting risk after acute myocardial infarction. *Am. J. Cardiol.* 56:839, 1985.
34. Waters, D. D., Bosch, X., Bouchard, A., et al. Comparison of clinical variables and variables derived from a limited predischarge exercise test as predictors of early and late mortality after myocardial infarction. *J. Am. Coll. Cardiol.* 5:1, 1985.
35. Handler, C. E. Submaximal predischarge exercise testing after myocardial infarction: Prognostic value and limitations. *Eur. Heart J.* 6:510, 1985.
36. Starling, M. R., Crawford, M. H., Henry, R. L., et al. Prognostic value of electrocardiographic exercise testing and noninvasive assessment of left ventricular ejection fraction soon after acute myocardial infarction. *Am. J. Cardiol.* 57:532, 1986.
37. Fioretti, P., Brower, R. W., Simoons, M. L., et al. Relative value of clinical variables, bicycle ergometry, rest radionuclide ventriculography and 24-hour ambulatory electrocardiographic monitoring at discharge to predict 1 year survival after myocardial infarction. *J. Am. Coll. Cardiol.* 8:40, 1986.
38. Sanz, G., Castaner, A., Betriu, A., et al. Determinants of prognosis in survivors of myocardial infarction:

A prospective clinical angiographic study. *N. Engl. J. Med.* 306:1065, 1982.
39. Multicenter Postinfarction Research Group. Risk stratification and survival after myocardial infarction. *N. Engl. J. Med.* 309:331, 1983.
40. Taylor, G. J., Humphries, J. D., Mellits, E. D., et al. Predictors of clinical course, coronary anatomy and left ventricular function after recovery from acute myocardial infarction. *Circulation* 62:960, 1980.
41. Schulze, R., Strauss, H., and Pitt, B. Sudden death in the year following myocardial infarction. *Am. J. Med.* 62:192, 1977.
42. Mukharji, J., Rude, R. E., Poole, K., et al. Risk factors for sudden death after acute myocardial infarction: Two-year follow-up. *Am. J. Cardiol.* 54: 31, 1984.
43. Bigger, J. T., Fleiss, J. L., Kleiger, R., et al. The relationships among ventricular arrhythmias, left ventricular dysfunction, and mortality in the 2 years after myocardial infarction. *Circulation* 69:250, 1984.
44. Schuster, E. H., and Bulkley, B. H. Early post-infarction angina: Ischemia at a distance and ischemia in the infarct zone. *N. Engl. J. Med.* 305:1101, 1981.
45. Bosch, X., Théroux, P., Waters, D. D., et al. Early postinfarction ischemia: Clinical, angiographic and prognostic significance. *Circulation* 75:988, 1987.
46. Gibson, R. S., Beller, G. A., Gheorghiade, M., et al. The prevalence and clinical significance of residual myocardial ischemia two weeks after uncomplicated non-Q wave infarction: A prospective natural history study. *Circulation* 73:1186, 1986.
47. Théroux, P., Kouz, S., Bosch, X., et al. Clinical and angiographic features of non-Q wave myocardial infarction. *Circulation* 74(Suppl II):303, 1986.
48. Théroux, P. A pathophysiologic basis for the clinical classification and management of unstable angina. *Circulation* 75(Suppl V):103, 1987.
49. Palmieri, S. T., Harrison, D. G., Cobb, F. R., et al. QRS scoring system for assessing left ventricular function after myocardial infarction. *N. Engl. J. Med.* 306:4, 1982.
50. Bosch, X., Moise, A., Roy, D., et al. Clinical and angiographic correlates of ventricular premature beats occurring during an exercise test early after myocardial infarction. *Circulation* 70(Suppl II):422, 1984.
51. Haskell, W. L., and DeBusk, R. Cardiovascular responses to repeated treadmill exercise testing soon after myocardial infarction. *Circulation* 60:1247, 1979.
52. DeBusk, R. F., and Haskell, W. Symptom-limited vs heart-rate-limited exercise testing soon after myocardial infarction. *Circulation* 61:738, 1980.
53. DeBusk, R. F., Houston, M., Haskell, W., et al. Exercise training soon after myocardial infarction. *Am. J. Cardiol.* 44:1223, 1979.
54. Wohl, A. J., Lewis, H. R., Campbell, W., et al. Cardiovascular function during early recovery from acute myocardial infarction. *Circulation* 56:931, 1977.
55. Waters, D. D., Théroux, P., Halphen, C., et al. Clinical predictors of angina following myocardial infarction. *Am. J. Med.* 66:991, 1979.
56. Midwall, J., Ambrose, J., Pichard, A., et al. Angina pectoris before and after myocardial infarction: Angiographic correlations. *Chest* 81:681, 1982.
57. Dillahunt, P. H., II, and Miller, A. B. Early treadmill testing after myocardial infarction: Angiographic and hemodynamic correlations. *Chest* 76:150, 1979.
58. Patterson, R. E., Horowitz, S. F., Eng, C., et al. Can noninvasive exercise test criteria identify patients with left main or 3-vessel coronary disease after a first myocardial infarction? *Am. J. Cardiol.* 51:361, 1983.
59. Benjamin, S. T., MacDonald, P. S., Horowitz, J. D., et al. Usefulness of early exercise testing after non-Q wave myocardial infarction in predicting prognosis. *Am. J. Cardiol.* 57:738, 1986.
60. Haines, D. E., Beller, G. A., Watson, D. D., et al. Exercise-induced ST segment elevation 2 weeks after uncomplicated myocardial infarction: Contributing factors and prognostic significance. *J. Am. Coll. Cardiol.* 9:996, 1987.
61. Stone, P. H., Turi, Z. G., Muller, J. E., et al. Prognostic significance to the treadmill exercise test performance 6 months after myocardial infarction. *J. Am. Coll. Cardiol.* 8:1107, 1986.
62. The Cardiac Arrhythmia Suppression Trial (CAST) Investigators. Preliminary report: Effect of encainide and flecainide on mortality in a randomized trial of arrhythmia suppression after myocardial infarction. *N. Engl. J. Med.* 321:406, 1989.
63. Rouleau, J. L., Moyé, L. A., Pfeffer, M. A., et al. A comparison of management patterns after acute myocardial infarction in Canada and the United States. *N. Engl. J. Med.* 328:779, 1993.
64. Turner, J. D., Schwartz, K. M., Logic, J. R., et al. Detection of residual jeopardized myocardium 3 weeks after myocardial infarction, by exercise testing with thallium-201 myocardial scintigraphy. *Circulation* 61:729, 1980.
65. Rigo, P., Bailey, I. K., Griffith, L. S. C., et al. Stress thallium-201 myocardial scintigraphy for the detection of individual coronary arterial lesions in patients with and without previous myocardial infarctions. *Am. J. Cardiol.* 48:209, 1981.
66. Morris, K. G., Palmeri, S. T., Califf, R. M., et al. Value of radionuclide angiography for predicting specific cardiac events after acute myocardial infarction. *Am. J. Cardiol.* 55:318, 1985.
67. Wasserman, A. G., Katz, R. J., Cleary, P., et al. Non-invasive detection of multivessel disease after myocardial infarction by exercise radionuclide ventriculography. *Am. J. Cardiol.* 50:1242, 1982.
68. Applegate, R. J., Dell'Italia, L. J., and Crawford, M. H. Usefulness of two dimensional echocardiography during low-level exercise testing early after uncomplicated acute myocardial infarction. *Am. J. Cardiol.* 60:10, 1987.
69. Jaarsma, W., Visser, C. A., Funke Kupper, A. J., et al. Usefulness of two dimensional exercise echocardiography shortly after myocardial infarction. *Am. J. Cardiol.* 57:86, 1986.

70. Ryan, T., Armstrong, W. F., O'Donnel, J. A., et al. Risk stratification after acute myocardial infarction by means of exercise two dimensional echocardiography. *Am. Heart J.* 114:1305, 1987.
71. Quiñones, M. A., Verani, M. S., Haichin, R. M., et al. Exercise echocardiography versus ^{201}Tl single-photon emission computed tomography in evaluation of coronary artery disease. *Circulation* 85: 1026, 1992.
72. Saunamäki, K. I., and Anderson, J. D. Prognostic significance of the ST-segment response during exercise test shortly after acute myocardial infarction. Comparison with other exercise variables. *Eur. Heart J.* 4:752, 1983.
73. Jain, A., Myers, H., Sapin, P. M., et al. Superiority and safety of maximal exercise testing early after myocardial infarction. *J. Am. Coll. Cardiol.* 21 (Suppl A):98A, 1993.
74. Hamm, L. F., Crow, R. S., Stull, G. A., et al. Safety and characteristics of exercise testing early after acute myocardial infarction. *Am. J. Cardiol.* 63: 1193, 1989.
75. Leppo, J. A., O' Brien, J., Rothendler, J. A., et al. Dipyridamole-thallium-201 scintigraphy in the prediction of future cardiac events after acute myocardial infarction. *N. Engl. J. Med.* 310:1014, 1984.
76. Brown, K. A., O'Meara, J. O., Chambers, C. E., et al. Ability of dipyridamole-thallium-201 imaging one to four days after acute myocardial infarction to predict in-hospital and late recurrent myocardial ischemic events. *Am. J. Cardiol.* 65:160, 1990.
77. Gimple, L., Hutter, A., Guiney, T., et al. Prognostic utility of predischarge dipyridamole thallium imaging compared to predischarge submaximal exercise electrocardiography and maximal exercise thallium imaging after uncomplicated acute myocardial infarction. *Am. J. Cardiol.* 64:1243, 1989.
78. Bolognese, L., Rossi, L., Sarasso, G., et al. Silent versus symptomatic dipyridamole-induced ischemia after myocardial infarction: Clinical and prognostic significance. *J. Am. Coll. Cardiol.* 19:953, 1992.
79. Mahmarian, J. J., Pratt, C. M., Nishimura, S., et al. Quantitative adenosine ^{201}Tl single-photon emission computed tomography for the early assessment of patients surviving acute myocardial infarction. *Circulation* 87:1197, 1993.
80. Tzivoni, D., Gottlieb, S., Keren, A., et al. Early right atrial pacing after myocardial infarction. I. Comparison with early treadmill testing. *Am. J. Cardiol.* 53:414, 1984.
81. Piérard, L. A., De Landsheere, C. M., Berthe, C., et al. Identification of viable myocardium by echocardiography during dobutamine infusion in patients with myocardial infarction after thrombolytic therapy: Comparison with positron emission tomography. *J. Am. Coll. Cardiol.* 15:1021, 1990.
82. Forster, T., McNeill, A. J., Salustri, A., et al. Simultaneous dobutamine stress echocardiography and technetium-99m isonitrile single-photon emission computed tomography in patients with suspected coronary artery disease. *J. Am. Coll. Cardiol.* 21:1591, 1993.
83. Segar, D. S., Brown, S. E., Sawada, S. G., et al. Dobutamine stress echocardiography: Correlation with coronary lesion severity as determined by quantitative angiography. *J. Am. Coll. Cardiol.* 19:1197, 1992.
84. Pennell, D. J., Underwood, S. R., Swanton, R. H., et al. Dobutamine thallium myocardial perfusion tomography. *J. Am. Coll. Cardiol.* 18:1471, 1991.
85. Marwick, T., Willemart, B., D'Hondt, A. M., et al. Selection of the optimal nonexercise stress for the evaluation of ischemic regional myocardial dysfunction and malperfusion. *Circulation* 87:345, 1993.
86. Coma-Canella, I., del Val Gómez Martínez, M., Rodrigo, F., et al. The dobutamine stress test with thallium-201 single-photon emission computed tomography and radionuclide angiography: Postinfarction study. *J. Am. Coll. Cardiol.* 22:399, 1993.
87. DeBusk, R. F., Blomqvist, C. G., Kouchoukos, N. T., et al. Identification and treatment of low risk patients after acute myocardial infarction and coronary artery bypass graft surgery. *N. Engl. J. Med.* 314:161, 1986.
88. Dennis, C., Houston-Miller, N., Schwartz, R. G., et al. Early return to work after uncomplicated myocardial infarction. *J.A.M.A.* 260:214, 1988.
89. The SOLVD Investigators. Effect of enalapril on mortality and the development of heart failure in asymptomatic patients with reduced left ventricular ejection fractions. *N. Engl. J. Med.* 327:685, 1992.
90. Pfeffer, M. A., Braunwald, E., Moyé, L. A., et al. Effect of captopril on mortality and morbidity in patients with left ventricular dysfunction after myocardial infarction. *N. Engl. J. Med.* 327:669, 1992.
91. Cairns, J. A., Connolly, S. J., Gent, M., et al. Postmyocardial infarction mortality in patients with ventricular premature depolarizations. Canadian Amiodarone Infarction Arrhythmia Trial Pilot Study. *Circulation* 84:550, 1991.
92. GISSI—Gruppo Italiano per lo Studio della Streptochinasi nell'Infarto Miocardico. Effectiveness of intravenous thrombolytic treatment in acute myocardial infarction. *Lancet* 1:397, 1986.
93. Théroux, P., Morissette, D., de Guise, P., et al. Aggressive management of myocardial infarction modifies predischarge risk evaluation. *Circulation* 76 (Suppl II):502:1987.
94. Sager, P., Perlmutter, R., Rosenfeld, L., et al. Thrombolysis decreases sudden death and arrhythmogenic potential after anterior myocardial infarction with aneurysm formation. *Circulation* 76 (Suppl II):261, 1987.
95. Melin, J. A., De Coster, P. M., Renkin, J., et al. Effect of intracoronary thrombolytic therapy on exercise-induced ischemia after acute myocardial infarction. *Am. J. Cardiol.* 56:705, 1985.
96. Schaer, D. H., Ross, A. M., and Wasserman, A. L.

Reinfarction, recurrent angina, and reocclusion after thrombolytic therapy. *Circulation* 76(Suppl II):56, 1987.

97. Rogers, W. J., Baim, D. S., Gore, J. M., et al. Comparison of immediate invasive, delayed invasive, and conservative strategies after tissue-type plasminogen activator. *Circulation* 81:1457, 1990.
98. Topol, E. J., Juni, J. E., O'Neill, W. W., et al. Exercise testing three days after onset of acute myocardial infarction. *Am. J. Cardiol.* 60:958, 1987.
99. Dilsizian, V., and Bonow, R. O. Current diagnostic techniques of assessing myocardial viability in patients with hibernating and stunned myocardium. *Circulation* 87:1, 1993.

35. Rehabilitation Following Acute Myocardial Infarction

Charles A. Dennis

While physicians are more sophisticated than ever in the management of acute myocardial infarction and its complications, individual patients remain ill-equipped to manage the medical and functional aspects of recovery that significantly disrupt their lives for the weeks to months after hospital discharge. Even the uncomplicated patient faces medical restrictions on the most routine of activities such as driving, climbing stairs, lifting, and sexual activity. These restrictions are reinforced by family, friends, and coworkers who generally perceive a poor prognosis and are concerned that physical activity can harm the heart. Because patients have an incomplete understanding of their illness, they fear recurrent cardiac problems. This fear can engender a sense of isolation and loss of control as well as a lack of confidence to resume customary activities.

Rehabilitation after myocardial infarction must address medical, physical, emotional, educational, and perceptual problems. While rehabilitation literally means to restore to a former capacity, cardiac rehabilitation should seek larger goals. The short-term goal is to return patients to their normal physical, emotional, functional, and occupational state as soon as possible. The long-term goals are to optimize physical conditioning, to educate the patient and the family about coronary heart disease, and to slow or reverse the pathophysiologic processes that led to myocardial infarction.

This chapter reviews the pathophysiology of acute myocardial infarction and aspects of treatment that affect physical capacity. The role of risk factors in the progression of coronary disease and its late complications is discussed. The social and psychological impediments to recovery are described. The risks and benefits of rehabilitation after myocardial infarction are presented along with recommendations for rehabilitation services.

Structure of Cardiac Rehabilitation Programs

Cardiac rehabilitation programs are widely available across the United States, but their services are underutilized. It is estimated that only 15 percent of patients recovering from myocardial infarction participate in formal rehabilitation programs [1]. Individual physicians can provide rehabilitation services to patients effectively, but generally do not have the expertise or time to provide the broad-based treatment that is given over a short period by cardiac rehabilitation programs.

Phased Rehabilitation

Cardiac rehabilitation programs are usually centered on physical conditioning with related efforts directed toward risk factor modification, patient education and counseling, and disability assessment. While there is variability between programs, most endorse the concept of phased rehabilitation. Phase I programs are provided in the hospital immediately following myocardial infarction, coronary angioplasty, or coronary surgery. Inpatient programs focus primarily on education, counseling, and progressive ambulation. The patient and family receive fundamental information regarding cardiac disease, symptoms, and risk factors. Counseling concerning the psychological impact of myocardial infarction is often provided. Structured programs of increasing physical activity prepare patients for activities of daily living. A low-level treadmill test before discharge may be provided.

Phases II to IV are outpatient programs distinguished by the time since the acute cardiac event occurred and the type of exercise training provided. Phase II rehabilitation is the first outpatient level and generally begins soon after hospital discharge and lasts 8 to 12 weeks. A symptom-limited treadmill test should be performed at entry to assess physical capacity and screen for high-risk patients requiring further treatment. Supervised exercise, often employing electrocardiographic monitoring, is begun at a low level based on the treadmill test results. Exercise duration and intensity are gradually increased over the 3-month program. Individual and group education regarding risk factor modification is provided. More progressive programs may incorporate systematic risk factor modification, especially smoking cessation, dietary modification, and lipid-lowering drug therapy. Counseling to assist in social and emotional adjustment to myocardial infarction may be performed individually or in groups.

Phase III rehabilitation follows the early reconditioning and allows patients to exercise in a supervised setting with less-intensive monitoring. Patients learn how to self-monitor higher-intensity exercise. In addition, skills in smoking abstinence, dietary modification, and stress management are reinforced. Phase III programs usually last 6 to 12 months but may continue indefinitely. Phase IV rehabilitation refers to unsupervised physical activity. The skills in self-monitoring of exercise and in risk factor modification may be reinforced by periodic visits to the rehabilitation center.

Organization of Programs

Most cardiac rehabilitation programs use a team approach. Whether the program is inpatient, outpatient, or combined, key personnel with specific roles are identified. The two central figures in any program are the medical director and the program director. The medical director is a primary link to the medical community. The medical director is crucial in the intake evaluation of the clinical status of patients, communication with referring physicians, development of the complete rehabilitation program, and maintenance of the quality of the medical aspects of the program. As is true for any form of consultative service, the medical director must ensure that high-quality services are provided to patients without jeopardizing the autonomy of the primary physicians' clinical prerogatives.

The program director is responsible for the organizational, administrative, and operational aspects of the rehabilitation program and is an additional link to the medical and lay community. The program director must be well grounded in all aspects of the rehabilitation process in addition to being skilled in administration and management. The program director must recruit and coordinate the efforts of a highly skilled team. Other members of the multidisciplinary team include nurses, physical therapists, exercise physiologists, exercise leaders, dietitians, vocational counselors, psychologists, a business manager, and clerical help. The size and complexity of the rehabilitation program will dictate the numbers of employees and their time commitments.

The facilities and equipment of a particular program will vary depending on the size of the program and the range of services provided. Inpatient programs have limited equipment for exercise training because of the low volume of patients hospitalized at any particular time and the limited exercise training provided. Outpatient programs necessarily have more elaborate exercise equipment. All programs providing exercise training have emergency resuscitation equipment. Small and large conference rooms meet the needs of group and individual programs for education and counseling.

No two cardiac rehabilitation programs are identical in structure or services provided. Subsequent sections provide guidelines for rehabilitation of patients recovering from myocardial infarction that may be incorporated into individual programs. Five major areas of rehabilitative efforts are discussed: physical conditioning, clinical application of exercise training, secondary prevention, psychological evaluation, and resumption of customary activities, including return to work.

Physical Conditioning

Physical capacity is reduced in virtually all patients who have had an acute myocardial infarction. The degree of physical incapacity is related to several factors: the physical condition of the patient before the infarction occurred, the influence of some standard treatments for myocardial infarction such as bed rest, the extent of myocardial necrosis and residual myocardial ischemia after infarction, medications, age, the presence of other noncardiac medical conditions, and the symptoms experienced by the patient while performing physical activity. Separating these effects can be difficult in the individual patient. However, an understanding of each of these effects is paramount to minimizing the iatrogenic causes of physical impairment and to developing a conditioning program.

Exercise Capacity in Normal Individuals

To understand the mechanisms that influence physical capacity after myocardial infarction, one must understand the determinants of physical capacity in normal individuals. In healthy individuals, the *peak exercise capacity* is a measure of the ability of the cardiovascular system to deliver oxygen to exercising skeletal muscle and the ability of the exercising muscle to extract oxygen from blood. The ability of the cardiovascular system to deliver oxygen is most simply defined as the *cardiac output.* The ability of skeletal muscle to extract oxygen is most simply defined as the *arteriovenous oxygen difference* (a-vO_2 difference). No matter what the physical condition of a healthy individual is, these two factors determine peak exercise capacity. Peak exercise capacity can be increased with exercise training by adaptations in cardiac performance and skeletal muscle oxygen extraction.

Normal Responses to Exercise

Exercise capacity is commonly measured for research purposes using the *maximal oxygen uptake* ($\dot{V}O_2$max). $\dot{V}O_2$max represents the liters of oxygen transported from the lungs and used by skeletal muscle at peak exercise. $\dot{V}O_2$max may be increased by exercise training and decreased by many factors such as physical deconditioning or cardiac illness. Because measurement of $\dot{V}O_2$max is cumbersome, other estimates of exercise capacity are used clinically. The most common clinical measurement of exercise capacity is *multiples of resting oxygen consumption* (METs); 1 MET equals 3.5 ml of oxygen uptake/kg of body weight/min and represents the approximate metabolic cost to stand quietly. Treadmill tests have been calibrated to give approximate MET requirements for each stage, although there is some variability for each patient. MET capacity on treadmill testing generally overestimates the $\dot{V}O_2$max for cardiac patients [2, 3].

The measurement of exercise capacity is complex and includes several factors, which are defined in Table 35-1. $\dot{V}O_2$max is the product of maximal cardiac output and a-vO_2 difference. Cardiac output is the product of heart rate and stroke volume. *Stroke volume* is the product of end-diastolic volume and ejection fraction. a-vO_2 difference is the difference in the concentration of oxygen per liter of blood between arterial and mixed venous (i.e., pulmonary arterial) blood.

In healthy individuals, the heart rate may increase 100 to 200 percent with exercise, making it quantitatively the most important influence on cardiac output. End-diastolic volume increases from 0 to 15 percent and ejection fraction from 10 to 20 percent with exercise. During exercise, skeletal muscle can increase oxygen extraction between 50 and 150 percent, reflected in a widened a-vO_2 difference. The maximal a-vO_2 difference attainable is related to the capillary density and mitochondrial concentration of skeletal muscle [4].

Table 35-1
Formulas and terms used in the calculation of maximal oxygen uptake

Formulas	Terms
$\dot{V}O_2max = CO \times a\text{-}vO_2D$	$\dot{V}O_2$max = maximal oxygen uptake (L of O_2/min)
	CO = cardiac output (L of blood/min)
	a-vO_2D = arteriovenous oxygen difference (L of O_2/L of blood)
$CO = HR \times SV$	HR = heart rate (bpm)
	SV = stroke volume (L of blood/beat)
$SV = EDV \times EF$	EDV = end-diastolic volume (L of blood)
	EF = ejection fraction (%)
$a\text{-}vO_2D = a\text{-}O_2con - vO_2con$	aO_2con = arterial oxygen concentration (L of O_2/L of blood)
	vO_2con = venous oxygen concentration (L of O_2/L of blood)

Adaptations to Exercise Training

Exercise training of healthy individuals causes both cardiac and skeletal muscle adaptations, which increase $\dot{V}O_2$max. The maximal heart rate response to exercise in healthy individuals is roughly related to age and does not change with exercise training. Therefore, other cardiac adaptations must occur to increase cardiac output with exercise above that in the untrained state. Maximal stroke volume increases with exercise training. The change in maximal stroke volume reflects an increase in both end-diastolic volume and ejection fraction. Exercise training also increases capillary density and mitochondrial density in skeletal muscle, causing an increased a-vO_2 difference at maximal exercise [5].

The influence of cardiac and peripheral factors on the exercise capacity of a 50-year-old healthy man in the untrained state and after 4 months of exercise training is shown in Table 35-2. Peak heart rate is unchanged but increases in end-diastolic volume and ejection fraction lead to an increase of 24 percent in cardiac output. Skeletal muscle oxygen extraction is increased, reflected in a widened a-vO_2 difference at peak exercise after training. The combination of cardiac and skeletal muscle adaptations to exercise training results in a 42 percent increase in $\dot{V}O_2$max.

Other cardiac effects of exercise training that are not obvious from examining peak exercise data alone contribute to the increase in $\dot{V}O_2$max. Resting heart rate decreases and a lower heart rate at any given exercise workload is common. This chronotropic adaptation allows increased diastolic filling time and therefore improved ventricular filling and emptying. Blood pressure is usually lowered by chronic exercise training, especially in hypertensive patients. A lower blood pressure at any given workload results in a lower afterload and increased ejection fraction. All of these effects result in an improved cardiac output at higher levels of work and therefore an improved exercise capacity.

Exercise Capacity After Myocardial Infarction

The exercise capacity of individuals recovering from myocardial infarction is influenced by the pathophysiologic effects of the illness and by certain effects of treatment. While the same mechanisms of cardiac output and a-vO_2 difference determine $\dot{V}O_2$max, temporally related changes in chronotropic response, intravascular volume, myocardial perfusion and contractility, and skeletal muscle conditioning all interact to determine peak exercise capacity at any given time. Normal processes of recovery, even in the absence of exercise training, are important contributors to the increases in exercise capacity during the early postinfarction period.

Effects of Bed Rest

While current coronary care emphasizes early mobilization of patients who have had a myocardial infarction, patients still spend significant periods in supine bed rest during hospitalization. Even in healthy individuals, bed rest has a detrimental effect on physical capacity. Several studies demonstrated that 10 to 30 days of bed rest is associated with decrements in $\dot{V}O_2$max of 9 to 30 percent [6–8], with the largest proportion of loss occurring in the first 10 days.

The cause of the decrement in $\dot{V}O_2$max is multifactorial. A prolonged absence of orthostatic stress results in a decreased stroke volume due to hypovolemia [9] and in diminished control of venous ca-

Table 35-2
Adaptations in cardiac and peripheral responses to maximum exercise after 4 months of training in a healthy, 50-year-old man

	Peak exercise values						
	HR (bp/m)	EDV (ml)	EF (%)	SV (ml/b)	CO (L/m)	a-vO_2D (L/L)	$\dot{V}O_2$max (L O_2/min)
Untrained	170	170	60	100	17	0.14	2.4
Trained	170	190	65	124	21	0.16	3.4
Percent change	0	+12	+9	+24	+24	+15	+42

pacitance vessels resulting in a decreased venous return [8]. Blunting of normal postural vasomotor reflexes results in postural tachycardia and hypotension. Losses in skeletal muscle mass of 10 to 15 percent [10] and a shift from aerobic to anaerobic metabolism at moderate levels of exercise [5] also contribute to a diminution of physical capacity. A diminished lung volume and vital capacity and an increased respiratory exchange ratio occur with bed rest, implicating pulmonary mechanisms as well [10].

Vigorous training in the supine position during bed rest fails to prevent the deterioration of upright exercise capacity [11], although as little as 3 hours of daily upright posture significantly decreases the deconditioning effect of bed rest [12]. These effects of bed rest resolve spontaneously after hospitalization. This resolution is related primarily to the resumption of upright posture for prolonged periods. The return to normal dietary habits and the conditioning effects of usual activities such as walking also play a role.

Chronotropic Incompetence

Most postinfarction patients manifest chronotropic incompetence, or the inability to achieve the maximal heart rate response to exercise predicted by age. Maximal heart rate can decrease by as much as 25 percent in the first weeks after myocardial infarction has occurred. While the cause of chronotropic incompetence is unknown, one proposed mechanism relates to a loss of normal vagal reflexes during exercise, which has been demonstrated in an animal model [13].

Because the heart rate response to exercise is quantitatively the most important mechanism for increasing cardiac output, chronotropic incompetence can have a significant effect on $\dot{V}O_2$max. Chronotropic incompetence improves spontaneously over the first 3 to 8 weeks after myocardial infarction has occurred, as shown in serial exercise testing studies [14]. Therefore, even in the absence of formal exercise training, $\dot{V}O_2$max increases during this period.

Left Ventricular Dysfunction

In all patients some degree of left ventricular dysfunction develops after myocardial infarction. While the clinical effects of myocardial necrosis may be obvious by physical examination or noninvasive evaluation of left ventricular function, the effects on exercise performance are variable. A diminished ejection fraction at rest or one that fails to rise normally with exercise might be expected to predict a limited exercise capacity. However, most measures of ventricular performance at rest and with exercise, including left ventricular end-diastolic dimension, velocity of circumferential fiber shortening, systolic time intervals, and ejection fraction, correlate poorly with exercise performance [15].

To determine the major factors influencing exercise capacity in patients with left ventricular dysfunction, Higginbotham et al. [16] compared patients with age-matched sedentary control subjects. Both patients and control subjects had a wide range of exercise capacities with significant overlap. Ejection fractions were significantly lower in patients than control subjects and no overlap was present. In both groups, the major determinants of exercise capacity were the same: the heart rate response to exercise and the a-vO_2 difference at maximum exercise. Chronotropic incompetence was more common in patients than control subjects. In the absence of chronotropic incompetence, the onset of anaerobic metabolism was the major limiting effect [16].

Central and peripheral compensatory mechanisms can improve exercise performance even when severe left ventricular dysfunction is present. These include a preserved chronotropic response to exercise, increasing stroke volume with exercise, decreasing peripheral vascular resistance with exercise, ventricular dilation, increased levels of circulating catecholamines at rest and with exercise, and the ability to tolerate very elevated pulmonary artery wedge pressures [16–19]. Some of these mechanisms can be stimulated by exercise training, while the etiology of others is unclear. The implication of these findings is that the common clinical measures used to evaluate left ventricular function are inadequate to predict exercise capacity and formal exercise testing should be used.

Myocardial Ischemia

Following myocardial infarction, patients may have exercise-induced myocardial ischemia if segments of viable myocardium are served by diseased coronary arteries. Myocardial ischemia can limit exercise tolerance. The first physiologic abnormality caused by myocardial ischemia is a contraction abnormality in the affected segment. If a large segment of myocardium becomes ischemic, filling pressures will increase and ejection fraction and cardiac output will fall. These abnormalities may occur in the absence of angina and patients may be limited by symptoms of dyspnea and fatigue.

Symptoms of angina may also limit exercise performance even in the absence of evidence of exercise-induced left ventricular dysfunction. Because patients perceive angina differently, the same degree of myocardial ischemia may be tolerated by some patients and limit exertion in others. In formal cardiac rehabilitation, patients without evidence of ischemia have a significantly greater training effect than do those with ischemia [20]. Amelioration of symptoms by medical therapy may improve exercise tolerance even in the absence of formal exercise training.

The effect of the normal recovery process on the coronary circulation is unknown. Several investigators [21–24] demonstrated spontaneous improvements in myocardial perfusion as measured by radionuclide techniques. However, these improvements were not reflected in changes in electrocardiographic or symptomatic evidence of myocardial ischemia on serial exercise testing in the absence of treatment [14, 24]. There is some evidence that improvements in ischemic profile reflect the development of new or an opening of preexistent coronary collateral vessels [25]. The double product (peak heart rate × peak systolic blood pressure) is a reasonable measure of myocardial oxygen demand. While exercise capacity may increase spontaneously by the mechanisms described previously, the double product at which ischemia occurs remains relatively constant and reproducible in the absence of medical therapy.

Spontaneous Improvement in Exercise Capacity

The factors discussed previously contribute to spontaneous improvements in exercise capacity in most patients recovering from myocardial infarction. Table 35-3 shows an example of the spontaneous improvement of exercise capacity in a 50-year-old man between 2 and 8 weeks following myocardial infarction in the absence of formal exercise training. Quantitatively, the resolution of chronotropic incompetence is the most important factor. Restoration of intravascular volume and recovery of normal cardiovascular reflexes play a major role in the first several days after hospital discharge. Skeletal muscle reconditioning from the resumption of customary activities contributes to improved physical activity by improving skeletal muscle oxygen extraction, resulting in a widened a-vO_2 difference.

These factors should influence evaluation and treatment after myocardial infarction. Early mobilization and prolonged periods of upright posture should be emphasized during hospitalization, especially in uncomplicated patients. Progressive ambulation in the hospital should precede hospital discharge. The combination of chronotropic incompetence and volume depletion may precipitate a hypotensive response at higher levels of exercise; this physiologic response may be incorrectly interpreted as indicating a poor prognosis, leading to further diagnostic testing and limitation of activity. Physicians performing early exercise testing should plan tests with these considerations in mind.

Table 35-3

Spontaneous improvement in exercise capacity in a 50-year-old man between 2 and 8 weeks after myocardial infarction (MI) in the absence of formal exercise training

	Peak exercise values						
Time since MI	HR (bp/m)	EDV (ml)	EF (%)	SV (ml/b)	CO (L/m)	a-vO_2D (L/L)	$\dot{V}O_2$max (L O_2/min)
2 weeks	140	190	45	86	12	0.14	1.7
8 weeks	170	200	45	90	15	0.16	2.4
Percent change	+21	+5	0	0	+25	+14	+41

Clinical Application of Exercise Training

While spontaneous improvements in exercise capacity occur as a part of the normal postinfarction recovery process, exercise training plays an important role in hastening the return to a normal exercise capacity in uncomplicated patients and improving the exercise capacity and symptomatic state of complicated patients. Exercise testing is the basis for recommendations regarding exercise training.

Exercise Testing

Exercise testing is commonly used to assess prognosis and determine functional capacity in patients recovering from myocardial infarction. Any myocardial infarction patient being considered for an exercise training program should undergo symptom-limited exercise testing. The indications for and the prognostic value of treadmill testing after myocardial infarction are presented in Chapter 34. This section reviews considerations related to using the exercise test for the prescription of physical activity.

The timing of exercise testing relates primarily to the condition of the patients and their suitability for exercise training. Uncomplicated patients without evidence of significant left ventricular dysfunction, myocardial ischemia, or arrhythmias may be tested soon after the myocardial infarction occurred. There is controversy regarding the best timing and type of exercise test to use for prognostication. Exercise testing before hospital discharge is usually performed to a submaximal limit, that is, a target heart rate of 60 percent of predicted maximum or 5 METs. Postdischarge treadmill testing may also use heart rate or workload targets.

The potential limitations of the predischarge, submaximal test for exercise prescription are several. Bed rest–induced volume depletion, chronotropic incompetence, and loss of physical conditioning may transiently limit exercise capacity. Exercising to a predicted heart rate or workload with submaximal testing underestimates physical capacity and results in an inappropriately low-exercise prescription. Delaying treadmill testing until 7 to 14 days after hospital discharge can obviate some of these problems. However, a recent study demonstrated that for low-risk patients, symptom-limited predischarge exercise testing is safe and provides significantly more evidence of myocardial ischemia than does low-level testing [26]. Later testing will give a more realistic evaluation of exercise capacity [14].

With symptom-limited testing, the end points of the exercise test include fatigue, dyspnea, moderate angina or leg cramps, or signs of abnormal blood pressure response or ventricular ectopy (triplets or runs). Symptom-limited treadmill testing should be performed when factors such as volume depletion and chronotropic incompetence will not blunt the exercise capacity or limit the test because of exertional hypotension. Symptom-limited testing may be performed prior to or soon after hospital discharge in uncomplicated patients [26–28], but should be delayed in complicated patients.

Complicated postinfarction patients are not candidates for early symptom-limited exercise testing and therefore are not candidates for early exercise training. Patients with evidence of uncompensated left ventricular dysfunction, such as rales, jugular venous distention, a third heart sound, and peripheral edema are at high risk for cardiac death in the 6 months after the myocardial infarction occurred [29]. After such patients are stabilized with appropriate medical therapy, exercise testing can be performed safely and used as the basis for an exercise training program [30]. Patients with angina at rest or with minimal activity are at high risk for recurrent infarction and death; these patients require more aggressive evaluation and many will undergo coronary bypass surgery or angioplasty [29]. Exercise testing can be used following a revascularization procedure as the basis for an exercise training program.

Other less common complications of myocardial infarction decrease the utility of exercise testing after myocardial infarction. Abnormalities of conduction such as complete heart block or pacemaker-dependent rhythms and high-grade or symptomatic ventricular arrhythmias limit the performance and value of exercise testing. Hemodynamic abnormalities other than left ventricular dysfunction such as ischemic mitral regurgitation can limit exercise performance. Atrial arrhythmias such as atrial fibrillation and flutter can affect both the chronotropic and the ventricular loading responses to exercise. Extensive discussion of each of these problems is beyond the scope of this chapter; management of these problems requires careful coordination between the rehabilitation specialist and the primary cardiologist.

In uncomplicated patients, symptom-limited exercise testing is safe when it is performed 7 to 21 days after the date of infarction [26, 31–33]. This timing for testing is optimal because higher-risk patients with asymptomatic myocardial ischemia are identified soon after myocardial infarction and the problems of chronotropic incompetence and volume depletion are sufficiently resolved to obtain a true measure of physical performance. The exercise test should be performed after cardiac medications have been tapered and withdrawn if possible. Medications can mask significant ischemic and arrhythmic abnormalities during exercise that might require further evaluation and more specific therapy [10, 34]. In addition, some patients treated with prophylactic antianginal and antiarrhythmic medications may show no significant abnormalities if they are tested while not taking medications, and medications may then be discontinued.

In complicated patients, delaying exercise testing for 6 to 8 weeks after the myocardial infarction occurred is appropriate. Complicated patients with left ventricular dysfunction or symptomatic myocardial ischemia do not need early exercise testing for prognostication. These clinical syndromes are sufficient to prompt further diagnostic evaluation and therapy with medications or revascularization procedures [29]. Once stabilized, these patients are candidates for exercise testing to establish an exercise prescription.

In all patients recovering from myocardial infarction, a modified Naughton treadmill protocol is a reasonable choice for exercise testing [35]. A comparison of the Bruce and modified Naughton protocols is shown in Table 35-4. The modified Naughton protocol begins at a lower MET level than the Bruce protocol and progresses at 1-MET increments every 3 minutes. The transition between stages is therefore less dramatic and patients can progress comfortably. Patients ultimately achieve the same peak workload with either protocol, but the longer time of exercise on the modified Naughton protocol can reassure the patients that they are capable of beginning formal exercise training. In addition, patients with significant physical deconditioning or symptoms are not overly stressed in the initial stages of exercise.

Eligibility for Exercise Training

The majority of patients recovering from myocardial infarction will be eligible to undergo exercise training within 3 months after the myocardial infarction occurred. Uncomplicated patients eligible for treadmill testing soon after the occurrence of myocardial infarction can begin exercise training as early as 10 days after hospital discharge. Patients with significant myocardial ischemia, presenting as angina or significant ST segment depression or both at low levels of exercise, are not candidates for exercise training until myocardial ischemia is ameliorated by medical or revascularization therapy. Patients with significant left ventricular dysfunction, manifested by symptoms of exertional dyspnea, physical signs of congestive heart failure, or ejection fractions of less than 30 percent, are not candi-

Table 35-4
Comparison between modified Naughton and Bruce protocols for treadmill exercise testing

Modified Naughton					Bruce				
Stage	Minutes	METs	Speed (mph)	Grade (%)	Stage	Minutes	METs	Speed (mph)	Grade (%)
I	3	3	2.0	3.5					
II	3	4	2.0	7.0					
III	3	5	2.0	10.5	I	3	5	1.7	10
IV	3	6	2.0	14.0					
V	3	7	2.0	17.5	II	3	7	2.5	12
VI	3	8	3.0	12.5					
VII	3	9	3.0	15.0					
VIII	3	10	3.0	17.5	III	3	10	3.4	14

dates for exercise training until their symptoms and signs have been adequately treated.

Other patients are eligible for exercise training with some caveats. Patients with high-grade or symptomatic ventricular arrhythmias should undergo evaluation and treatment as outlined in Chapters 10 and 36. Once high-grade ventricular arrhythmias have been suppressed, developing an exercise prescription using treadmill testing is appropriate. Patients with atrial arrhythmias, especially atrial fibrillation, should receive appropriate therapy to suppress an excessive chronotropic response to exercise before beginning exercise training. Exercise testing is a useful tool in assessing such therapy. Patients with electrocardiographic abnormalities that might obscure evidence of myocardial ischemia on exercise testing, such as left bundle branch block, should undergo exercise testing with radionuclide or echocardiographic imaging to be certain that significant ischemic abnormalities are not present.

Exercise Prescription

The basic principles that apply to exercise training of healthy adults are applicable in a modified form to patients recovering from myocardial infarction. The modifications include changes in type, frequency, intensity, and duration of training sessions; the rate of progression to higher-intensity training; and the level of surveillance of patients. Special considerations are necessary for patients with left ventricular dysfunction, myocardial ischemia, and arrhythmias, both atrial and ventricular.

Basic Principles of Exercise Training

In the healthy adult, the recommendations for achieving and maintaining optimal cardiovascular conditioning are a frequency of training 3 to 5 days per week, a minimum intensity of 60 percent of maximal heart rate, and a duration of 15 to 60 minutes per training session. The intensity and duration of exercise are adjusted to achieve an overall energy expenditure of 300 kcal per session. Kilocalorie expenditure is directly related to duration and intensity; the more intense the exercise, the shorter the duration required to expend 300 kcal [36–40].

Training sessions are commonly divided into four components: warm-up, muscular conditioning, aerobic exercise, and cooldown. The warm-up and cooldown are important aspects of the conditioning program. An adequate warm-up can decrease the incidence of injury, especially muscle and ligament strains. It may also decrease the incidence of exercise-induced angina. The cooldown is equally important in patients with coronary disease. The immediate cessation of aerobic exercise is commonly associated with precipitation of ventricular arrhythmias and with sensations of light-headedness. Ventricular arrhythmias are precipitated by the unopposed cathecholamine stimulation of abnormal myocardium. Light-headedness results from a mismatch between the rapid fall in heart rate and cardiac output with cessation of exercise and the slow return of peripheral vasomotor tone from the intense vasodilation induced by exercise.

The muscular conditioning and aerobic components of exercise have the dual goals of optimizing muscular strength for customary activities and developing cardiac and peripheral training effects. Strength training should emphasize large muscle groups in dynamic exercise with as little an isometric component as possible. Isometric exercises, such as weight lifting or an exercise that requires a strong handgrip component, are associated with significant increases in blood pressure [41]. The size of the muscle group used in strength training is directly related to the increases in blood pressure. Adequate muscular training can be achieved with a well-balanced calisthenics program and the use of light hand weights (3 to 7 lb) either prior to or during aerobic exercise. Dynamic upper extremity exercise, such as arm ergometry or rowing, can provide a conditioning effect and is not associated with the hypertensive response of static exercise [42].

Aerobic conditioning programs commonly use walking, jogging, bicycling, and swimming as the predominant exercise. In the patient recovering from myocardial infarction, swimming is not recommended in the first 3 to 6 months because of potential difficulties in monitoring heart rate and treatment in the event of a cardiac complication. The intensity and duration of the aerobic portion of exercise training are generally thought of as the exercise prescription. Individual prescriptions are developed depending on the timing after myocardial infarction, the presence or absence of symptoms, the degree of left ventricular dysfunction and myocardial ischemia, the level of conditioning, and the presence of other complications such as arrhythmias, conduction abnormalities, and other diseases (e.g., obstructive lung disease, orthopedic abnormalities, and peripheral vascular disease).

The intensity of exercise is most commonly prescribed using heart rate. Heart rate can be monitored using pulse counting at either the radial or the carotid artery. Inexpensive heart rate monitors allow the setting of upper and lower heart rate limits and give an audible signal to patients when the heart rate is out of range. Another method for monitoring exercise intensity is use of the Rate of Perceived Exertion (RPE) scale developed by Borg and Linderholm [43]. The scale originally used numbers between 60 and 200 matched with descriptions such as very light, somewhat hard, and so on. The numbers were estimates of heart rate and correlated well with perceived exertion in healthy men undergoing exercise training. The scale has been simplified (Table 35-5) and now ranges from 6 to 20 with the same descriptions. Using the RPE scale during exercise testing allows the prescription of a heart rate range based on the patient's perception of exertion. Matching the prescribed heart rate to the RPE rating and using the RPE for monitoring exercise can be as reliable as assigning heart rate limits [44].

Inpatient (Phase I) Exercise Training

Inpatient exercise training should prepare patients for customary activities they will undertake at home. Programs for progressive ambulation have been published [38–40] and should serve as general guidelines to gradually increase patient activity. Complete physical reconditioning before hospital discharge is an unrealistic goal for several reasons. The period for reconditioning is short, generally only 3 to 5 days. Other physiologic abnormalities such as volume depletion and chronotropic incompetence are significant impediments to formal exercise training. Exercise testing is not usually performed before progressive ambulation.

Realistic goals for inpatient exercise training include preparation to perform customary activities in the first days to weeks after hospital discharge, evaluation of symptomatic responses to physical activity, instruction in low-level exercise including pulse and symptom monitoring, and determination of the optimal timing of entry into a formal conditioning program. For inpatient and early postdischarge exercise, a heart rate limit of 20 beats per minute above the standing resting heart rate is reasonable. This heart rate limit is recommended because most patients do not perform maximal exercise tests before hospital discharge and the calculation of heart rate targets from predicted maximal heart rates (220 − age) may overestimate peak heart rate responses because of the problem of chronotropic incompetence.

Table 35-5
Borg Scale of Rate of Perceived Exertion

	6
Very, very light	7
	8
Very light	9
	10
Light	11
	12
Somewhat hard	13
	14
Hard	15
	16
Very hard	17
	18
Very, very hard	19
	20

Outpatient (Phase II) Exercise Training

Following the performance of a symptom-limited treadmill test, patients may begin formal exercise training. The time of testing and the exercise prescription depend on the condition of individual patients, as will be discussed. In general, patients with complications of myocardial ischemia, left ventricular dysfunction, or arrhythmias are tested later and exercise at lower levels. The issues of safety and supervision are discussed in later sections.

The exercise prescription is based on the peak heart rate attained on the treadmill test and the symptomatic response. Exercise training is initiated at 60 to 70 percent of the peak treadmill heart rate. Patients should be able to monitor their pulse and understand the concept of a target heart range. Target heart ranges should be given for 10-second counts. For example, if the desired heart rate is 120 beats per minute, dividing by 6 gives a target of 20 for 10 seconds. The usual target rate is then 20 ±1, giving an actual heart rate range of 114 to 126 beats per minute. While the 10-second count range of ± 1 seems narrow, it is easily attained after some practice by patients.

The simplest aerobic exercise to perform and monitor is walking. In the initial exercise session, frequent pulse monitoring should be performed to allow patients to determine the exercise level needed to attain the target heart rate. Some exercise programs begin with a ''30-30'' program [45]. Patients walk for 30 seconds at a speed sufficient to meet their target rate and then slow down for 30 seconds to heart rates below the target rate. This is a valuable technique for demonstrating how heart rate is a good measure of physical activity. As patients progress, the ''30-30'' is shifted to a ''45-15'' program (45 seconds at target, 15 seconds below target) and then to full aerobic periods at the target heart rate. Uncomplicated patients may make this progression in one or two exercise sessions whereas complicated patients may require several sessions.

Significant emphasis should be placed on pulse and symptom monitoring during exercise training because most cardiac complications of exercise occur when patients exceed their target heart rates. Patients should be aware that other factors can influence the heart rate. Elevated body temperature increases the heart rate at any given workload. Factors such as ambient temperature, heavy clothing, and intercurrent febrile illness must be considered. Changes in medical condition can influence the heart rate response. Worsening left ventricular function, development of atrial or ventricular arrhythmias, and changes in drug therapy can all potentially influence the heart rate response to exercise. As chronotropic incompetence resolves, the heart rate response will change. Finally, as physical conditioning occurs, the heart rate will be lower for any given workload.

Uncomplicated Patients

In the uncomplicated patient who does not show significant abnormalities on the treadmill test, target heart rates during early exercise training should be 70 to 85 percent of the peak heart rate achieved during treadmill testing. During the first 7 weeks after the myocardial infarction occurred, the target heart rates should be gradually increased from 70 to 85 percent. At the same time a training effect is occurring, chronotropic incompetence is spontaneously resolving. By the eighth week, most patients can achieve significantly higher peak heart rates during treadmill testing [14]. The target heart rates can then be increased to 85 to 100 percent of the peak heart rate attained on early testing. This target corresponds to 70 to 85 percent of the peak heart rate that would be attained by repeated treadmill testing at 8 weeks after myocardial infarction [14]. Uncomplicated patients performing postinfarction treadmill testing and beginning exercise training later (e.g., 6 to 8 weeks after infarction) do not require this adjustment because chronotropic incompetence has resolved. Further adjustments in exercise prescription should be based on repeated treadmill testing. With the guidelines outlined previously, uncomplicated patients should exercise for 30 to 60 minutes, three to five times weekly. Pulse counting and symptom monitoring are sufficient to monitor the intensity of exercise.

Patients with Myocardial Ischemia

The extent and severity of myocardial ischemia during exercise testing soon after myocardial infarction should guide therapy and modify the exercise prescription. Several studies demonstrated that patients with exercise-induced ischemia after myocardial infarction have higher rates of cardiac death, recurrent infarction, and coronary revascularization in the first 6 to 12 months [29, 32, 46–49]. Patients with more than 0.2 mV of ST segment depression, especially at a low heart rate or workload, have significantly higher event rates [32]. An abnormal blood pressure response [32, 49] or a low exercise tolerance even in the absence of significant ischemic changes on the electrocardiogram [32, 49] also predicts cardiac events.

The best diagnostic and therapeutic approach to patients with exercise-induced myocardial ischemia is unknown. The guidelines for exercise training should be modified depending on the therapy used to treat ischemia. Patients undergoing coronary bypass graft surgery are usually eligible for treadmill testing 4 to 6 weeks after surgery. Treadmill testing should be performed postoperatively even if a preoperative treadmill test was performed. Exercise capacity, ischemic threshold, symptoms, heart rate response, medications, and other parameters affecting exercise training can be modified by surgery and repeat testing is necessary to provide an accurate exercise prescription. The type of exercise postoperative patients perform should be modified initially to avoid stress to the pectoral girdle as the sternum heals. Patients undergoing coronary angioplasty can undergo treadmill testing within 1 week of the procedure and be given an exercise prescription based on the results.

Patients with mild ischemia may receive medical therapy with beta blockers, nitrates, calcium channel blockers, or a combination. All of these agents increase the exercise capacity primarily by decreasing the double product for any given workload [50–54]. Ideally, exercise prescriptions should be based on treadmill testing performed during medical treatment. However, patients will often receive medical therapy because of an ischemic abnormality found on a routine postinfarction treadmill test, and repeat treadmill testing will not be performed. For patients receiving antianginal medications other than beta blockers, it is usually reasonable to provide an exercise prescription without repeating the treadmill test. In such patients, and those with treadmill test–detected ischemia in whom medical therapy is not prescribed, the target heart rate should be set at 5 to 10 beats per minute below the heart rate at which ischemia occurs or to 70 to 85 percent of the peak heart rate, whichever is lower. For patients not performing repeat testing, this prescription may be conservative in comparison to the target rate that might be prescribed if the treadmill test was repeated.

Because beta blockers can have a profound effect on peak heart rate response to exercise, treadmill testing while the patient is on medication is ideal for prescribing exercise training [50, 52]. When repeat testing is not feasible, an exercise prescription at 55 to 70 percent of the peak heart rate attained during treadmill testing while the patient is off medication or 5 to 10 beats per minute below the heart rate at which ischemia is present may be used. This modification of the prescription is commonly used in cardiac rehabilitation programs and is clinically useful. Exercise testing should be repeated at 4 to 6 weeks of exercise training in patients taking beta blockers to ensure that they are receiving a training effect and to determine whether the target heart rates can be increased safely.

The effect on conditioning of patients receiving anti-ischemic therapy is not clear. While some authors suggest that beta blockade attenuates training in angina patients [52], others showed exercise training effects in the presence of beta-blockade therapy [55, 56]. Calcium channel blockers do not appear to attenuate training effects in patients with coronary disease [51, 57]. The majority of studies on the effects of medications on training were performed in mixed populations of patients with coronary disease, rather than only patients recovering from recent myocardial infarction.

Patients with Left Ventricular Dysfunction

Persistent left ventricular dysfunction in the absence of myocardial ischemia occurs in 10 to 15 percent of postinfarction patients. The severity of left ventricular dysfunction and the patient's symptoms are variable. While left ventricular dysfunction is the most powerful predictor of a poor prognosis [29, 32], many patients have few symptoms and a preserved functional capacity. More recent studies showed that survival can be improved with medical therapy, particularly with angiotensin-converting enzyme (ACE) inhibitors [58]. While symptoms and signs of congestive heart failure and measurements of ventricular performance are useful for prognostication, they do not necessarily correlate with exercise capacity as discussed previously.

Unlike uncomplicated patients and those with mild postinfarction ischemia, patients with left ventricular dysfunction should undergo symptom-limited treadmill testing during maximal medical therapy. When revascularization therapy is not an option, exercise testing should be performed when hemodynamics are optimal. Although significantly more physiologic data can be obtained by combined respiratory and cardiac monitoring during an exercise test [30], a standard treadmill test is usually sufficient to develop an exercise prescription.

In addition to determining whether ischemia is present, other specific abnormalities should be searched for during exercise testing in patients with left ventricular dysfunction. The development of mitral regurgitation during exercise testing may reflect either myocardial ischemia with papillary muscle dysfunction or impaired ventricular dynamics. A fall in systolic blood pressure may reflect myocardial ischemia or an inadequate cardiac output response to exercise-induced peripheral vasodilation. Exercise-induced pulmonary congestion may occur due to these and other mechanisms. Exercise prescriptions must be modified in patients with any of these abnormalities.

While patients with significant left ventricular dysfunction are frequently excluded from exercise training because of their high-risk status, there is clear evidence that exercise training can provide beneficial physiologic effects without increased risk [59–62]. Physiologic changes induced by exercise training include decreased peripheral vascular resistance and improved skeletal muscle oxygen extraction. Even in the absence of major central changes, these peripheral influences can improve ventricular function by reducing afterload and increasing the efficiency of skeletal muscle oxygen extraction [63, 64].

The exercise prescription in patients with left ventricular dysfunction uses the same intensity, (i.e., 60 to 85 percent of peak heart rate on the treadmill) but shorter duration initially. The "30-30" program can limit the degree of fatigue experienced by the patient. Patients tolerating interval training can gradually increase the duration of higher-intensity exercise and decrease the duration of lower-intensity exercise. The exercise intensity should be decreased in patients developing any of the hemodynamic abnormalities described previously. Clinically, lowering the prescription by 10 beats per minute below the heart rate at which the abnormality occurs has been suggested [50].

There is evidence that chronic nitrate therapy improves exercise capacity in the long term in patients with left ventricular function, primarily by its effects on the venous circulation [53, 65]. Similarly, long-term improvements in exercise capacity were demonstrated in patients receiving vasodilator therapy alone and in association with exercise training programs [66–69]. Digitalis therapy also improves exercise capacity [70, 71]. Significant changes in medical therapy should prompt repeated exercise testing and prescription.

Patients with Arrhythmias

High-grade ventricular arrhythmias are common when myocardial infarction is complicated by left ventricular dysfunction. Management of left ventricular dysfunction and ventricular arrhythmias is presented in Chapter 36. Once arrhythmias are successfully treated, patients should undergo symptom-limited treadmill testing to develop an exercise prescription.

The postinfarction exercise test may reveal previously unsuspected high-grade ventricular arrhythmias. Ectopy is common in the early recovery phase after exercise because of high levels of unopposed circulating catecholamines. These arrhythmias should not necessarily prompt more aggressive therapy unless they are high grade such as nonsustained ventricular tachycardia. If exercise-induced arrhythmias are high grade, further evaluation and treatment is needed. Exercise testing should be repeated after therapy is instituted.

Even in patients managed with antiarrhythmic drugs, arrhythmias may occur during treadmill testing. Patients who have high-grade ventricular arrhythmias such as triplets or runs during exercise while on medical therapy should be evaluated further. If antiarrhythmic therapy is deemed adequate, the target heart rates for exercise training should be at least 10 beats per minute below the heart rate at which arrhythmias occur.

In some patients, complete suppression of all high-grade ventricular arrhythmia is not possible. In those patients, the benefit of exercise training should be carefully weighed against the risk. If patients are allowed to exercise, electrocardiographic monitoring should be performed during training to assess the reproducibility and prognostic significance of the arrhythmias. The results of monitoring should be used to guide the clinician in further evaluation and therapy as well as the desirability of continued exercise training.

Atrial arrhythmias may be present after myocardial infarction and should be evaluated and treated as outlined in Chapter 11. The most common atrial arrhythmia that influences the exercise prescription is atrial fibrillation. Even when heart rates are well controlled at rest, patients with atrial fibrillation often have an exaggerated chronotropic response to exercise. This response can impair exercise capacity because of the rate-related loss of diastolic filling time and the absence of the atrial component of ventricular filling. If this exaggerated chronotropic response is present during treadmill testing, consideration should be given to beta blockers or verapamil for control of the heart rate and the exercise test should be repeated.

The development of complete heart block after myocardial infarction usually reflects a large amount of myocardial necrosis, especially if the infarction is anterior. Exercise capacity is more often limited by the concomitant left ventricular dysfunction than the heart block. If left ventricular dysfunction is not severe, consideration of placement of a rate-responsive pacemaker should be considered. The exercise prescription should then be based on exercise testing with the pacemaker in place.

Outpatient (Phase III and IV) Exercise Training

After completion of the standard 12-week phase II exercise training program, some patients will want or need further exercise training. Uncomplicated patients desiring prolonged exercise training who have progressed well through phase II training should undergo repeat treadmill testing. If the treadmill test result is normal, patients can be given the option of continued supervised group exercise (phase III) or self-monitored home exercise (phase IV). The prescription is similar to that of phase II, but patients should exercise at an intensity closer to 85 percent of peak treadmill heart rate. The four components of exercise (warm-up, muscular conditioning, aerobic exercise, and cooldown) should be emphasized as should self-monitoring techniques for heart rate response and symptoms.

Complicated patients or those who were severely deconditioned at the beginning of phase II programs may benefit from more prolonged phase III exercise training. These patients should also undergo repeat treadmill testing and a new exercise prescription should be given based on that test. The same caveats described for phase II training of complicated patients are true for phase III training. Complicated patients with stable symptoms may eventually become candidates for unsupervised, self-monitored exercise training. The decision to advance such patients should be made only after careful medical evaluation by the primary physician and the medical director of the rehabilitation program.

Effects of Exercise Training

The physiologic benefits of exercise training after myocardial infarction are well demonstrated. Training studies consistently demonstrate increased peak heart rates, increased functional capacity, decreased heart rates at rest and submaximal exercise, and decreased systolic blood pressure at submaximal exercise [4, 72]. The immediate response to training is a reduced heart rate and systolic blood pressure for a given workload. These changes lower myocardial oxygen demand at any given level of work.

Whether exercise training causes significant improvement in cardiac function after myocardial infarction is controversial. High-intensity exercise and prolonged endurance training were associated with increases in stroke volume, left ventricular ejection fraction, and myocardial perfusion in some studies [22, 73–75]. However, other investigators did not demonstrate significant changes in cardiac performance despite improvements in exercise capacity [24, 59, 62]. While exercise-induced angina and ST segment depression appear at higher workloads after exercise training, they generally occur at a constant double product.

While controversy exists concerning cardiac adaptations to exercise training after myocardial infarction, peripheral adaptations appear in virtually all patients. The primary peripheral adaptations are in the circulation and in skeletal muscle metabolism and include increases in capillary density, skeletal muscle mitochondria, myoglobin content, and oxidative enzymes [61, 64, 76]. These peripheral adaptations lower the double product for a given workload. The workload at which ischemia occurs is therefore increased. Favorable hemodynamic responses such as lower systolic blood pressure can decrease myocardial work in patients with left ventricular dysfunction.

These physiologic changes are usually associated with improvements in symptoms. Patients with angina often have their anginal threshold increased, so they can perform more physical activity without ischemia. The lower mean blood pressure with exercise results in a greater exercise capacity for patients with left ventricular dysfunction. Patients with left ventricular dysfunction often have the greatest symptomatic benefit because their exercise capacity is so low initially.

Whether exercise training decreases cardiac mortality after myocardial infarction is controversial. Postinfarction training studies demonstrated trends toward improved survival in most instances [77–80]. However, design flaws such as an inadequate number of patients or short follow-up time limited results in some studies. In other studies, compliance to exercise training was low and crossovers from the nonexercise to exercise groups occurred. Two meta-analyses evaluated the effects of exercise training and found a reduction in cardiovascular mortality of 20 to 25 percent in patients undergoing exercise training compared to those not training [81, 82].

Other benefits of exercise training are related to secondary prevention and psychosocial outcomes discussed in more detail later in this chapter. Increased caloric expenditure can, with dietary modification, help the patient to achieve ideal body weight. Because energy costs of physical work are proportional to body mass, a loss of fat can reduce the energy requirement of any given activity [40]. Improvements in lipid profiles are associated with exercise training [77, 83]. Reductions in blood pressure occur, especially in hypertensive patients [84]. Psychological benefits include diminished anxiety and depression [85] and improved confidence to undertake physical activity and resume customary activities [86].

Safety of Exercise Training

Ensuring that physical training does not harm the patient is a paramount concern during rehabilitation. The most important factors that ensure safety are patient selection, careful intake evaluation, appropriate prescription, and adequate supervision. The risk of exercise for the individual patient is related primarily to the extent and severity of left ventricular dysfunction, myocardial ischemia, and ventricular arrhythmias. In postinfarction patients without significant abnormalities, the risk of exercise is minimal and rapid progression from supervised to unsupervised exercise is possible. Conversely, in patients with severe manifestations of one or more of these abnormalities, exercise training may be contraindicated or high-level surveillance may be appropriate.

Several clinical and exercise test abnormalities are associated with a higher risk for cardiac events during exercise training. Significant left ventricular dysfunction increases the risk of exercise. It may be manifested by multiple prior infarctions; low ejection fraction as determined by radionuclide, echocardiographic, or angiographic techniques; symptoms of dyspnea at rest or low levels of exercise; low treadmill exercise tolerance; chronotropic incompetence; and abnormal blood pressure response to exercise. Significant myocardial ischemia may be manifested by frequent angina poorly controlled by medical therapy, significant exercise-induced ST segment depression with or without angina, low exercise tolerance, a declining ejection fraction with exercise, and severe anatomic coronary disease at angiography. Significant electrical instability may be manifested as complex atrial and ventricular arrhythmias at rest, high-degree atrioventricular block, and complex ventricular arrhythmias induced by exercise.

If any of these clinical or exercise test abnormalities are present, exercise training should be undertaken with caution after appropriate therapy is begun. The exercise prescription should account for the exercise level at which abnormalities appear. Higher levels of supervision and surveillance should be used in higher-risk patients. Complications of exercise training are directly related to the intensity of exercise. To achieve the desired training effect in higher-risk patients, the intensity can be lowered and the frequency or duration of training sessions increased.

In higher-risk patients, compliance to the exercise prescription is crucial. Exercising above the prescribed intensity may be due to inaccurate monitoring techniques by the patient, a lack of understanding of techniques for monitoring, inadequate frequency of monitoring, or a disregard for the necessity of monitoring. In these circumstances, increased surveillance by the exercise leaders may be required. This surveillance might include electrocardiographic monitoring, either continuous or intermittent; increased frequency of pulse monitoring; the use of electronic heart rate monitors; and increased educational efforts [87].

There is considerable debate among rehabilitation specialists regarding the degree and duration of medical supervision needed for patients undergoing exercise training. Individual programs vary from requiring continuous electrocardiographic monitoring of all patients during early exercise training, to frequent pulse and symptom monitoring by patients and supervising personnel, to home exercise training with patient pulse and symptom monitoring. No single set of guidelines has been established unequivocally as appropriate for all programs. Guidelines suggested by individual investigators [39, 40, 87] and professional organizations [36–38] are consistent in matching the intensity of monitoring with the severity of pathophysiologic manifestations of the individual patient.

On-site supervision with continuous electrocardiographic monitoring is recommended for patients at high risk for cardiac arrest or ventricular fibrillation, such as those with prior cardiac arrest, severe congestive heart failure, exercise-induced ventricular tachycardia, and complex ventricular arrhythmias associated with left ventricular dysfunction. At the other end of the spectrum, very-low-risk patients without left ventricular dysfunction and a peak treadmill capacity of 6 METs or higher without evidence of myocardial ischemia or arrhythmias are recommended for home exercise training with pulse monitoring using an individualized exercise prescription. In the absence of firm guidelines, decisions regarding the degree of medical supervision for exercise need to be made by the responsible physician.

While concerns regarding risks of exercise training are appropriate, supervised exercise training of cardiac patients is associated with a low risk of precipitating cardiac events. A survey of 167 cardiac rehabilitation programs in the mid 1980s evaluated the incidence of major cardiovascular complications over a 4-year period. The level of medical supervision ranged from continuous to limited electrocardiographic monitoring of new patients. The incidence rate per million patient-hours of exercise was 1.3 for fatalities, 3.4 for myocardial infarctions, and 8.9 for resuscitated cardiac arrests. There were no significant differences in these event rates for small compared to large programs or for continuous electrocardiographic monitored compared to intermittent electrocardiographic monitored programs [88].

These rates of major cardiovascular complications are significantly lower than the rates found in a similar study of programs surveyed between 1960 and 1977 [89]. The reasons for improvements in complication rates are speculative. Improved risk stratification, improved medical and revascularization therapies, more rigorous standards in cardiac rehabilitation programs, and increasing awareness of the necessity for monitoring high-risk patients may have contributed to this improved safety record.

Secondary Prevention After Myocardial Infarction

While exercise training is the focus of most rehabilitation programs after the occurrence of myocardial infarction, secondary prevention is at least as important for the long-term health of patients. Secondary prevention measures for patients who have had myocardial infarction commonly include drug therapy for symptoms and prophylaxis of left ventricular dysfunction and myocardial ischemia as discussed in Part VII of this book. Other measures include treatment of conventional risk factors including smoking, lipid abnormalities, hypertension, and type A personality. Smoking cessation has clearly been demonstrated to improve mortality after myocardial infarction. Treatment of elevated plasma lipid levels has not been shown unequivocally to alter outcome after myocardial infarction, but several recent studies showed that coronary atherosclerosis can be positively influenced with lipid management. There is no convincing evidence that treating hypertension alters the outcome after myocardial infarction, although such treatment is customary. Finally, there is controversy regarding the effect of type A personality on prognosis, but some evidence that outcome can be improved with treatment.

Smoking

Risk of Smoking

Cigarette smoking is an established risk factor for the development of angina and myocardial infarction and for the recurrence of myocardial infarction [90, 91]. Survivors of myocardial infarction who continue to smoke have approximately twice the rate of recurrent infarction and cardiac death compared to nonsmokers and patients who quit smoking after the occurrence of a myocardial infarction [91–95]. Smoking cessation was associated with a 61 percent reduction in mortality rate over 6 years in the Framingham Study [95] and a 55 percent reduction in mortality over 13 years in survivors of unstable angina or myocardial infarction [96]. The Norwegian Multi-Center Group Study demonstrated a 45 percent reduction in the reinfarction rate over 17 months after myocardial infarction in patients who quit smoking, compared to those who continued to smoke [93]. The risk for cardiac death and reinfarction appears to decline rapidly in smokers who quit after suffering a myocardial infarction compared to those who continue to smoke. Within 3 years after having a myocardial infarction, exsmokers have approximately the same risk for reinfarction as survivors of myocardial infarction who never smoked [92, 94].

Pathophysiology of Smoking

The pathophysiology underlying the risk for death and reinfarction in smokers is uncertain. Coronary spasm, platelet aggregation, thrombosis [97], and diminished coronary and collateral reserve [98] have been implicated as possible causes. Coronary vascular reserve, the capacity of coronary arteries to dilate and increase blood flow on increased demand, is significantly reduced in smokers compared to nonsmokers. Individuals who smoke more cigarettes have significantly lower coronary vascular reserve than that of those who smoke less [98]. Fibrinogen levels are significantly higher in smokers than nonsmokers and appear to increase the primary risk for myocardial infarction [99]. While the degree of coronary atherosclerosis does not appear to be strongly correlated to smoking habits [100], the risk for myocardial infarction in smokers appears to be strongly correlated with the degree of underlying coronary disease and the plasma level of cholesterol [97]. While some of these data are derived primarily from patients who have not had a previous myocardial infarction, they shed some light on pathophysiologic mechanisms that may be relevant in postinfarction patients.

Factors Influencing Smoking After Myocardial Infarction

The association between smoking and cardiac disease is well known in medical and lay communities. Myocardial infarction is a sufficient impetus to stop smoking in 20 to 60 percent of patients [101]. Several demographic and psychological factors are associated with continued smoking after myocardial infarction. Lower occupational and educational levels, smoking a higher number of cigarettes per day before myocardial infarction occurred, increasing age [101], and higher rates of alcohol consumption [102] are demographic factors associated with continued smoking. Psychological factors such as less negative attitudes regarding smoking, higher anxiety levels, and a lower sense of personal control of life events identify smokers who are less likely to quit after myocardial infarction [101].

Etiology of Tobacco Dependence

Several theories attempt to explain tobacco dependence. No single theory is adequate to explain all aspects of smoking behavior. Smoking is a complex behavior with physiologic, psychological, and sociologic causes. Continued smoking reflects the physiologic dependence on nicotine; abrupt smoking cessation can cause acute craving for cigarettes related to nicotine deprivation [103]. Smoking is also a habit that appears to minimize negative emotions, such as distress, anger, and fear. Smoking may be a coping behavior to transform such negative emotions into a socially acceptable habit [104]. Finally, smoking behavior has sociologic origins related to modeling behavior after others, such as parents or peer groups.

Smoking Abstinence

The significantly higher morbidity and mortality rates of postinfarction patients who continue to smoke is the rationale for including smoking abstinence as a part of comprehensive cardiac rehabilitation. Abstinence from cigarette smoking has two components: smoking cessation and relapse prevention. Smoking abstinence is best achieved through structured programs. However, physicians should not discount their influence on patients who smoke. Patients receiving specific advice to stop smoking from health professionals are more likely to quit and remain abstinent than those who do not receive advice [105, 106]. This is particularly true for individuals who believe that they are at personal risk if they continue smoking [107]. Providing low-cost educational materials available from the American Heart Association, American Lung Association, and the American Cancer Society can reinforce the strong medical advice provided during hospitalization for myocardial infarction.

Smoking Cessation

The majority of smokers will quit smoking at the time of hospitalization for myocardial infarction [106]. For patients unable to quit on their own, a variety of methods for smoking cessation are available. While no one method appears significantly more effective than another, the most effective programs focus on the physiologic dependence on nicotine, the psychological need for a coping mechanism, and aspects of the learned behavior of smoking. Nicotine dependence may be approached using tapering techniques by changing cigarette brands, controlling smoking habits, and substituting nicotine gum. Aversive techniques such as rapid puffing and smoke holding may also be effective.

The availability of nicotine substitutes has improved the cessation and abstinence rates of smoking cessation programs [108–110]. Simple prescription of nicotine substitutes to smokers without a concomitant program to change behavior has not been effective in maintaining long-term smoking abstinence. Nicotine substitutes appear to blunt craving for cigarettes by exposing patients to low levels of nicotine. They are most effective in patients who have a high level of nicotine dependence. Nicotine dependence can be assessed by a variety of scales, one of the more common being the Fagerstrom Nicotine Tolerance Scale [111]. A simple method to assess nicotine dependence is to ask patients how soon they need to smoke after awakening in the morning. Patients needing to smoke within 30 minutes are highly nicotine dependent and will benefit from a nicotine substitute.

Two varieties of nicotine substitutes are available. Nicotine polacrilex was the initial product introduced. A 2-mg dose, the most commonly prescribed amount, gives an average blood nicotine level of 12 ng/ml compared to levels of 35 to 54 ng/ml obtained from cigarette smoking [112]. Nicotine polacrilex is prescribed on an as-needed basis, up to 30 pieces per day. Most patients use 10 pieces per day. Physicians should carefully read the package insert on how to instruct patients in the use of nicotine polacrilex. The medication is frequently misused in ways that make it ineffective. The frequency of use should gradually decrease over a 1- to 3-month period. If smoking cessation has not occurred by 6 months, nicotine polacrilex is most likely being used as a cigarette substitute rather than a cessation aid.

The introduction of nicotine patches has made the use of nicotine substitutes simpler. The most commonly prescribed products are provided in strengths of 21, 14, and 7 mg. The patches release nicotine over a 24-hour period and blood nicotine levels are in the 7 to 25 ng/ml range [113]. Patches must be placed on the trunk or upper arm to be effectively absorbed. In patients without severe angina who weigh more than 110 lb, the usual starting dose is 21 mg/day. The dose is sequentially lowered at 4- to 8-week intervals. The 14-mg dosage is recommended for patients with mild angina or weighing less than 110 lb.

Techniques to eliminate the physiologic dependence on nicotine are most effective when coupled with behavioral counseling such as identifying and avoiding situations in which smoking is likely and substituting behaviors such as exercise. The same behavioral techniques are effective for both smoking cessation and relapse prevention [114].

Relapse Prevention

Once patients stop smoking, relapse prevention becomes the goal of smoking abstinence programs. Education of the patient regarding the effects of continued smoking is the first step in relapse prevention. Informing patients about symptoms associated with smoking abstinence will prepare them for behavior change and allow them to correctly attribute sensations to smoking withdrawal. Intense craving for cigarettes is common and is often behavior specific (e.g., while drinking coffee or alcohol, while talking on the telephone) and situation specific (e.g., at parties, in stressful environments). Irritability, emotionality, anxiety, and inability to concentrate are symptoms of smoking cessation [104]. Physical symptoms such as nausea, headache, increased appetite, and sleep disturbance are common [115, 116].

Teaching patients new ways to deal with situations or behaviors that encourage smoking is the next step in relapse prevention. The majority of smoking is habitual and strongly associated with daily habits, such as following meals, while driving or talking on the telephone, or when drinking alcoholic beverages. Having patients identify and list the circumstances in which they are at high risk of relapse and carry the list wherever they go is useful. Applying self-control strategies to high-risk situations is also helpful. For example, if smoking is associated with the morning coffee break, the patient should switch the time or the activity of the break. If smoking is likely in social situations, role-playing cigarette denial or refusal may be helpful. Substituting healthful behaviors, such as a short walk or a short period of reminding themselves that they and not the cigarettes are in control, are effective strategies to prevent relapse [117]. Enlisting social support from spouses, friends, coworkers, and other participants in a cardiac rehabilitation program may help to reinforce nonsmoking behavior.

Hypercholesterolemia

A large body of basic, clinical, and epidemiologic evidence supports the link between hypercholesterolemia and the development and progression of coronary artery disease. The association between elevated cholesterol levels and the development of coronary disease is well established. Primary prevention trials have demonstrated that lowering low-density-lipoprotein (LDL) cholesterol [118, 119] or raising low levels of high-density-lipoprotein (HDL) cholesterol lowers the risk of coronary events [120], such as myocardial infarction and cardiac death. More recent secondary prevention trials established that aggressive dietary and drug therapy for hypercholesterolemia in patients with established coronary artery disease can slow the progression or even cause regression of coronary atherosclerosis [121–125]. More importantly, there is some evidence that such treatment can decrease the rate of adverse outcomes in a relatively short period of time [125]. This evidence strongly supports the treatment of abnormal cholesterol levels in patients with documented coronary artery disease [126].

Metabolism of Plasma Lipids

The processes of absorption, transport, metabolism, and excretion of the plasma lipids—cholesterol, cholesterol esters, triglycerides, and phospholipids—are complex and well described elsewhere [127]. A comprehensive review of lipid metabolism is beyond the scope of this chapter, but certain concepts are important in the treatment of lipid disorders in patients who have had a myocardial infarction.

Four major families of lipoproteins are defined by density on ultracentrifugation of plasma: chylomicrons, very-low-density lipoprotein (VLDL), LDL, and HDL. The lipoproteins consist of a hydrophilic coat of associated apoproteins and a neutral lipid core. The apoproteins are functionally important as catalysts for some enzymatic reactions and as recognition sites for binding to specific cellular receptors. At a bonding position between the protein surface and neutral core are the polar head groups of unesterified cholesterol and the fatty acyl chains of phospholipids. The density of the lipoproteins is determined by the relative concentrations of the esterified cholesterol and triglycerides in the core. The structure and functions of the major lipoproteins are outlined in Table 35-6.

Chylomicrons are the largest of the lipoproteins and are responsible for the transfer of ingested fats from the intestine into the circulation and to the liver. Lipoprotein lipase, an enzyme in vascular endothelial cells, degrades triglycerides from chylomicrons, leaving remnants that are cleared rapidly by the liver. These cholesterol-rich remnants suppress the de novo synthesis of cholesterol by the liver.

In the liver, VLDL particles are synthesized and released. VLDL particles, which are rich in triglycerides, undergo lipolysis in the circulation by lipoprotein lipase, leaving intermediate lipoproteins

Table 35-6
Structure and function of major classes of lipoproteins

Lipoproteins	Density	Constituents	Function	Comment
Chylomicrons	0.950	Triglyceride	Transport of ingested fat to circulation	Degraded by lipoprotein lipase
VLDL	0.950–1.006	Triglyceride Phospholipid	Transport of endogenous triglyceride and cholesterol	Degraded to LDL by lipoprotein lipase
LDL	1.019–1.063	Esterified cholesterol Triglyceride	Transport of cholesterol to tissues	Uptake by cell-specific receptors
HDL	1.063–1.210	Phospholipid cholesterol	Catabolism of VLDL and transport of cholesterol to liver	Suppresses cholesterol synthesis at HMG-CoA reductase step

VLDL = very-low-density lipoprotein; LDL = low-density lipoprotein; HDL = high-density lipoprotein; HMG = 3-hydroxy-3-methylglutaryl.

that are converted to LDLs, both in the liver and in the peripheral circulation. LDL is the major transport particle for cholesterol, delivering it to both the liver and the peripheral cells, including vascular endothelium. LDL uptake occurs through cell-specific receptors; cholesterol absorption suppresses the de novo synthesis of cholesterol within cells. Elevated LDL cholesterol is the most important lipid abnormality related to risk for the development of coronary disease.

HDL is synthesized by the liver and is partially responsible for the catabolism of VLDL through reactions involving lipoprotein lipase, lecithin-cholesterol acyltransferase (LCAT), and other enzymes that may inhibit the hepatic uptake of cholesterol. HDL is postulated to facilitate cholesterol transport from peripheral tissues to the liver. This process may increase the cholesterol excretion in the form of bile acids and down-regulate the hepatic synthesis of cholesterol by suppression of the rate-limiting step catalyzed by 3-hydroxy-3-methylglutaryl–coenzyme A (HMG-CoA) reductase.

The incorporation of cholesterol into bile acids is an important step in cholesterol metabolism. An enterohepatic recirculation mechanism reclaims cholesterol incorporated into bile acids, thereby conserving a portion of biliary cholesterol. This recirculation phenomenon inhibits the excretion of cholesterol into bile acids, helping to maintain plasma cholesterol levels. Each of the metabolic pathways discussed is of clinical importance because it can be affected by various therapies.

Definition of Hypercholesterolemia

The definition of hypercholesterolemia has been difficult to establish. The mean plasma total cholesterol level for white men over the age of 30 in the Lipid Research Clinics Program prevalence study ranged from 192 to 214 mg/dl and approximated the 50th percentile. The 90th percentile ranged from 239 mg/dl at age 30 to 34 to 262 mg/dl at ages 55 to 59 [128]. Compared to epidemiologic data from other cultures with substantially lower mortality rates from coronary heart disease, cholesterol levels above the 50th to 75th percentile in American men are associated with an increased risk from coronary heart disease. Using these data, the Consensus Conference of the National Institutes of Health defined a moderate-risk and a high-risk category of hypercholesterolemia and recommended therapy for individuals in either category. Their recommendations are primarily based on the absolute level of LDL cholesterol and the presence of either documented coronary heart disease (documented myocardial infarction or ischemia) or two or more risk factors (male gender, family history, cigarette smoking, hypertension, low HDL level, diabetes, peripheral or cerebrovascular disease, or severe obesity) [126].

The moderate-risk category is defined as age-adjusted values of total plasma cholesterol in the 75th to 90th percentiles. The high-risk category is defined as age-adjusted values above the 90th percentile. The moderate-risk category includes large numbers of individuals with elevated cholesterol levels due at least in part to elevated dietary saturated fats and cholesterol. The high-risk category includes most individuals with hereditary forms of hypercholesterolemia [126].

Plasma cholesterol should be determined with a fasting sample and abnormal values confirmed with repeated samples. Secondary causes of hypercholesterolemia, such as diabetes, liver disease, nephrotic syndrome, hypothyroidism, and medications such as beta blockers and thiazide diuretics, should be sought. Fractionation of cholesterol to determine LDL and HDL levels is needed to determine therapy based on the Consensus guidelines [124]. HDL levels below 30 mg/dl appear to be an independent risk factor [129], and might prompt a more aggressive therapy for even moderately elevated levels of total or LDL cholesterol. Screening other family members to search for hereditary forms of hypercholesterolemia is indicated in patients with elevated plasma levels of cholesterol.

Goals of Therapy for Hypercholesterolemia

The goals for therapy for hypercholesterolemia have been defined by the Consensus Conference Report [126]. Primary recommendations are based on levels of LDl and the presence of risk factors. Table 35-7 briefly outlines the recommendations. The target goal for LDL for individuals recovering from myocardial infarction is 130 mg/dl. Patients with LDL levels of 130 to 160 mg/dl should be treated initially with diet alone and then reassessed. Patients with LDL levels above 160 mg/dl should be treated with both diet and drug therapy. There

Table 35-7
National Cholesterol Education Program: Age-adjusted risk categories for total plasma cholesterol suggested by the Consensus Development Conference [126]

Treatment	LDL treatment level (mg/dl)	LDL goal (mg/dl)
Diet only		
Without CHD or risk factors	≥ 160	< 160
With CHD or ≥ 2 risk factors	≥ 130	< 130
Diet and drug		
Without CHD or risk factors	≥ 190	< 160
With CHD or ≥ 2 risk factors	≥ 160	< 130

LDL = low-density lipoprotein; CHD = coronary heart disease.

is controversy surrounding the indications for treatment of low HDL levels. Some experts recommend that patients with HDL levels below 35 mg/dl be treated with a combination of exercise and medications to raise levels [129, 130]. Because of the recent data demonstrating improvements in coronary angiographic assessment of atherosclerosis as well as improved outcomes, an aggressive approach to lowering lipid levels is strongly recommended. Unfortunately, despite the strong evidence of benefit, studies have shown that physicians have not aggressively treated hypercholesterolemia, even in patients hospitalized for coronary angiography [131].

Dietary Treatment of Hypercholesterolemia

In both moderate- and high-risk patients, dietary therapy is the initial step in management. The goals of dietary therapy are to lower total fat, saturated fat, and cholesterol intake and to achieve ideal body weight in patients who are overweight. The dietary modifications suggested by different groups to achieve these goals differ in regard to the manner in which the diet is undertaken. However, most guidelines recommend an initial approach restricting 30 percent of total caloric intake to fats and no more than 300 mg of cholesterol per day (Table 35-8). The total saturated fat intake should be less than 10 percent of total calories. This limitation on total saturated fats will have the greatest

Table 35-8
Recommended daily restrictions on fat as a percentage of total calories and cholesterol in moderate- and high-risk hypercholesterolemic patients

	Total fat	Saturated fat	Cholesterol
Moderate risk	30%	<10%	≤300 mg
High risk	20%	5–10%	100–150 mg

effect on LDL levels. In high-risk groups, progressive restrictions to 20 percent of calories as fats and 100 to 150 mg of cholesterol per day are recommended. Total caloric restriction combined with exercise is important in overweight patients.

Life style changes are among the most difficult for patients to make. However, most patients recovering from myocardial infarction are highly motivated to adopt habits that will reduce their risk of subsequent complications of coronary disease. A major effort by the patient, physician, dietitian, and cardiac rehabilitation specialist is necessary to provide the proper education, motivation, and encouragement needed for dietary modification. The person primarily responsible for buying and preparing food must be actively included in the dietary management.

Drug Therapy for Hypercholesterolemia

For patients failing to achieve the goals for reductions in total and LDL cholesterol levels with dietary measures within 3 months, there are several drugs that can lower cholesterol levels (Table 35-9).

Bile Acid Sequestrants

The bile acid sequestrants cholestyramine and colestipol are nonabsorbable resins which have quaternary amine groups that interact with the acidic moiety of bile acids. Taken orally, they interrupt the normal enterohepatic recirculation of bile acids by binding them so they are excreted in the stool. Enhanced bile acid excretion interrupts the feedback inhibition of bile acid synthesis and increases conversion of cholesterol into bile acids. Lower hepatic cellular cholesterol levels result in increased LDL receptor density on hepatocytes and increased LDL extraction from the bloodstream, causing plasma concentrations of LDL cholesterol to fall.

Table 35-9
Major lipid-lowering drugs, mechanisms of action, and effects on lipid levels

Type	Examples	Mechanism	Effect
Bile acid sequestrants	Cholestyramine Colestipol	Bind bile acids in bowel preventing enterohepatic recirculation of cholesterol	Decreases total cholesterol by 8–25%
Nicotinic acid		Inhibit secretion of VLDL and LDL from the liver	Decreases total cholesterol 15–25% Raises HDL Lowers triglycerides
Fibric acid derivatives	Clofibrate Gemfibrozil	Promote lipolysis of VLDL by activating lipoprotein lipase May increase cholesterol in patients with hypertriglyceridemia	Decreases total cholesterol by 7–15% Raises HDL
Probucol		Unknown, but appears to promote clearance of LDL Has antioxidant effect	Decreases total cholesterol by 15–20% Lowers HDL
HMG-CoA reductase inhibitors	Lovastatin Pravastatin Simvastatin	Inhibits HMG-CoA reductase reaction	Decreases total cholesterol by 18–39% Increases HDL

VLDL = very-low-density lipoprotein; LDL = low-density lipoprotein; HDL = high-density lipoprotein; HMG = 3-hydroxy-3-methylglutaryl.

Small changes in VLDL and triglyceride levels are sometimes noted.

The usual dose for cholestyramine is 16 to 24 gm daily and for colestipol 20 to 25 gm daily in divided doses, mixed with liquid. Treatment is best initiated at half the full dosage and increased gradually over a 1- to 3-week period. The most commonly reported side effects of the resins are gastrointestinal, primarily constipation and heartburn. Other symptoms related to therapy include abdominal pain, diarrhea, bloating, gas, and nausea. Symptoms tend to diminish with prolonged use of the medications and may be ameliorated with antacids and antiflatulents.

In the Coronary Primary Prevention Trial [118, 119], cholestyramine therapy resulted in a mean reduction in total cholesterol of 8.2 percent and in LDL cholesterol of 12 percent. Patients who adhered completely with higher doses of cholestyramine had sustained reductions of 25 and 35 percent, respectively, while poor adherers had little or no change in total and LDL cholesterol levels. Maximum reductions tend to occur early in treatment and cholesterol levels tend to rise with time. This gradual increase in cholesterol probably reflects lower adherence to diet and drug therapy and the effect of aging.

Nicotinic Acid

Nicotinic acid lowers the plasma cholesterol concentration by inhibiting the secretion of both VLDL and LDL from the liver. It also suppresses free fatty acid mobilization from adipose tissue, which suppresses VLDL synthesis. Nicotinic acid also increases HDL levels, probably secondary to decreased VLDL production. Nicotinic acid use was associated with a decrease in the rate of recurrent myocardial infarction in the Coronary Drug Project [123].

The usual dosage for nicotinic acid is 2 to 6 gm/day in three divided doses. Side effects of cutaneous flushing due to capillary dilation and pruritus are common and may result in noncompliance if patients are not counseled to expect them. Flushing generally begins 20 minutes after the dose is taken and lasts 30 to 60 minutes. Gastric irritation is common and can be mitigated by taking the medication with meals. Elevation of hepatic transaminases can occur with the initiation of therapy but is usually transient. Long-acting preparations of nicotinic acid have been reported to cause irreversible hepatic injury. Using a lower dose or avoiding the long-acting preparations has been recommended [132]. Some impairment of carbohydrate tolerance may occur, and is of clinical significance primarily in insulin-dependent diabetics. Uric acid levels may increase with nicotinic acid ingestion and may precipitate gout in some patients. Transient declines in blood pressure may occur and antihypertensive medications may need to be adjusted as doses of nicotine acid are increased.

Intolerance to side effects is a common reason why many patients do not continue nicotinic acid in high doses or for long periods. Side effects can be minimized by several measures. Hot drinks can exacerbate the flushing and patients should be told to avoid them around the time of dosing. Because capillary dilation appears to be prostaglandin mediated, pretreatment with aspirin before dosing is helpful. Tachyphylaxis to flushing and pruritus at any given dose level is common; patients can be counseled to expect the side effects to improve. Beginning at extremely low doses, such as 100 to 250 mg three times daily, and increasing the dose by 250 mg each week will minimize side effects.

In the majority of patients, LDL cholesterol levels will normalize with nicotinic acid alone. In patients with extremely high plasma cholesterol levels, the combination of diet, a bile acid sequestrant, and nicotinic acid can reduce LDL cholesterol levels by as much as 50 percent [127]. Patients receiving nicotinic acid should have pretreatment measurements of plasma glucose, hepatic transaminases, and uric acid in addition to lipid screening. Studies should be repeated after titration to moderate doses and then monitored at 3- to 6-month intervals.

Fibric Acid Derivatives

Two fibric acid derivatives, clofibrate and gemfibrozil, lower cholesterol by lowering VLDL levels. Clofibrate promotes lipolysis of VLDL triglycerides by activating lipoprotein lipase and by reducing hepatic VLDL synthesis. Gemfibrozil also appears to reduce hepatic VLDL synthesis as well as inhibit its secretion. Both drugs reduce triglyceride levels, which is associated with increases in LDL levels in some patients with hypertriglyceridemia.

The usual dose of clofibrate is 1 gm orally twice daily and of gemfibrozil is 600 mg orally twice daily. The most common side effects of clofibrate are nausea, diarrhea, and weight gain. Other important side effects include a rare myositis syndrome, transient hepatic transaminase elevation, and potentiation of the action of warfarin by displacing it from protein-binding sites. A small increase in biliary and gastrointestinal cancers and a failure to decrease cardiac mortality was noted in one primary prevention trial [133]. Gemfibrozil is well tolerated, with the most common side effects being nausea and diarrhea. The fibric acid derivatives should not be given in combination with the HMG-CoA reductase inhibitors because of the significantly increased incidence of myositis with the combination.

The fibric acid derivatives can be expected to lower total cholesterol levels by 7 to 15 percent and triglyceride levels by 30 to 50 percent [127]. Both clofibrate and gemfibrozil raise HDL levels. Because these drugs are less effective than either the bile acid sequestrants or nicotinic acid, they should be considered second-line agents. They are the drugs of choice only in a small group of patients with primary elevations of VLDL.

HMG-CoA Reductase Inhibitors

The HMG-CoA reductase inhibitors are highly effective hypolipidemic agents. The first introduced was lovastatin, an inactive lactone that is hydrolyzed to a beta-hydroxy-acid form after ingestion. This is a principal metabolite of HMG-CoA reductase, which is a key enzyme in the biosynthetic pathway of cholesterol. In pharmacologic doses, lovastatin lowers both total and LDL cholesterol levels by 18 to 39 percent and increases HDL cholesterol levels by 3 to 13 percent by partially blocking the HMG-CoA reductase reaction. The usual dose of lovastatin is 20 to 80 mg orally in single or divided doses daily. Side effects are uncommon and are predominantly gastrointestinal, including constipation, diarrhea, and gas. Persistent elevations of hepatic transaminases are noted in some patients. Some patients develop lenticular opacities seen by slit-lamp examination, but no changes in visual acuity have been noted. Baseline and periodic hepatic transaminase measurements are recommended. Periodic slit-lamp examinations are no longer considered necessary. Many other reductase inhibitors that are now available have minor differences in effect and some potential advantages in dosing.

Probucol

Probucol is a hypolipidemic drug that is not structurally similar to the previously described agents. The mechanism of action is not clear, but it appears to promote the clearance of LDL. Probucol also appears to have important antioxidant effects that may importantly influence subclasses of LDL cholesterol in their atherogenic effect. There is no consistent effect on triglycerides, but HDL levels usually fall [134]. The usual dose of probucol is 500 mg orally twice daily. Side effects are mild, generally consisting of diarrhea, flatulence, and nausea. Lowering of total cholesterol by 15 to 20 percent is reported. The lower efficacy compared to the resins and nicotinic acid and the HDL-lowering effect make probucol a second-line agent, to be used in conjunction with the resins or when first-line agents fail.

Other Medications

Other medications known to lower plasma cholesterol levels include dextrothyroxine, neomycin, and beta-sitosterol. These drugs have a limited role in the majority of patients recovering from myocardial infarction.

HDL Cholesterol

While low HDL cholesterol levels have been associated with higher rates of coronary events in the general population [131], the influence of HDL cholesterol on the outcome of patients recovering from myocardial infarction is unknown. The mechanism of protection is thought to be reverse cholesterol transport [135]. Several factors that may cause HDL levels to be low include sedentary life style, cigarette smoking, obesity, hypertriglyceridemia, some cholesterol-lowering drugs, and other medications including some beta blockers and thiazide diuretics. While exercise training has been shown to increase HDL levels [136], the effects of other interventions are not known. In patients with low HDL cholesterol levels, attention should be directed to factors lowering HDL and exercise should be prescribed as a means of increasing HDL.

Nonpharmacologic Therapy for Hypercholesterolemia

Exercise

The effects of exercise training on plasma lipids is not completely understood. Conflicting reports on the effect of exercise on total cholesterol are probably related to the failure of studies to control for the effects of changes in body weight, diet, and intensity of exercise. In general, low- to moderate-intensity exercise has little influence on total cholesterol [4]. More consistent data demonstrate a beneficial effect of exercise training on HDL levels. Longitudinal training studies consistently demonstrated increases in HDL cholesterol levels at low, moderate, and high durations and intensities of exercise [83, 136]. Coronary patients with low initial HDL levels show the largest increases with training. These changes appear in the HDL_1 subfraction, which has been epidemiologically associated with lower rates of coronary heart disease.

Alcohol

The effect of alcohol consumption on plasma cholesterol levels is not completely understood. Moderate alcohol consumption has been associated with a decreased prevalence of coronary artery disease [137, 138]. This association was initially postulated to be a protective effect of increased HDL concentrations. However, more recent evidence demonstrates that moderate alcohol consumption is associated primarily with increases in the HDL_3 subfraction of cholesterol, which does not appear to have an epidemiologic association with coronary disease [139]. Further study will be required to elucidate the effect of alcohol on cholesterol and coronary heart disease [140].

Fish Oils

The effect of diets rich in fish oils, especially omega-3 fatty acids, on plasma lipid profiles also has been controversial. Recent evidence suggests that fish oils probably reduce VLDL synthesis in the liver or increase the catabolism of VLDL. Through this effect on VLDL metabolism, plasma LDL levels may be decreased [140]. Fish oils may have a role in treating hypercholesterolemic states in which VLDL levels are increased. The influence of dietary fish oils on the development and manifestations of coronary heart disease is unknown [141].

Psychological Evaluation

Psychological Effects of Myocardial Infarction

Even in the absence of underlying psychopathology, myocardial infarction precipitates some degree of psychological dysfunction in all patients. Anxiety is the most common psychological reaction in the acute setting [142], occurring in up to 80 percent of patients. That anxiety is generally focused on fear regarding specific future events: death, disability, isolation, loss of autonomous functioning, physical capacity and sexual activity, and the significance of somatic symptoms. Anger, frustration, and apathy are common reactions to the activity restriction and the dependent role in which patients are placed. These reactions may be translated to frank hostility or agitation.

Most patients can be expected to progress through a predictable sequence of anxiety, denial, depression, and manifestation of chronic personality traits in the acute setting [143]. While some degree of denial is an appropriate coping response to minimize fear, some patients will deny the gravity or presence of illness, which is clearly inappropriate. Such denial is maladaptive and predicts future noncompliance with medical regimens.

As anxiety and denial diminish, the realization of the disease and disability leads to a sense of sadness and loss. The abrupt loss of physical and social power is a marked contrast for most patients who experience myocardial infarction at a time when their social and occupational productivity is high. The depressive reaction may be exacerbated by preexisting depression, other life stresses, and common myths about myocardial infarction, especially those related to a dire prognosis and loss of physical capabilities [144].

During hospitalization and the early weeks after hospital discharge, the profile of psychological disturbance will change. Most patients experience some separation anxiety at the time of transfer from the coronary care unit and again at the time of hospital discharge when they leave an area of support and care and face a situation of self-care. In the early postinfarction period, social support is a critical issue. Social support involves perceptions by the patient that support of a sufficient quantity and quality is available from family and friends after myocardial infarction.

Just as anxiety and depression affect the patient recovering from myocardial infarction, so do they affect the spouse, who generally has less access to psychological support systems than the patient. Common marital conflicts precipitated by myocardial infarction include different perceptions of medical instructions, overprotectiveness for the patient by the spouse, resumption of sexual activities, and return to customary activities [145, 146].

Psychological Evaluation and Treatment After Myocardial Infarction

The majority of adverse psychological effects of myocardial infarction are transient and benign. Physicians and rehabilitation specialists should recognize the usual mood disturbances and loss of confidence experienced by most postinfarction patients. The evaluation and treatment of these mood states vary. While some cardiac rehabilitation programs use standard assessment tools such as the Beck Depression Scale [147] or the Minnesota Multiphasic Personality Inventory (MMPI) [146], others adapt a pragmatic approach of providing nonspecific, supportive therapy to all patients.

These pragmatic approaches include social support, exercise training, and group counseling. These nonspecific interventions are associated with improvements in psychological state although most studies are small and use broad psychological assessment instruments such as the MMPI. There appear to be clear improvements in mood states and activity levels resulting from exercise training programs. Exercise training appears to positively alter patients' perceptions of their physical capabilities, increase their participation in leisure activities, and lower their job-related stress [85].

Physicians and rehabilitation specialists should recognize that significant depression occurs in 5 to 15 percent of patients recovering from myocardial infarction. These patients generally do not respond to the usual, nonspecific approaches. Prompt recognition of depressive symptoms and impaired functional recovery should lead to referral of such patients to an appropriate professional.

Type A Behavior

The psychological response to myocardial infarction may have a significant impact on functional recovery, but has not been shown to significantly affect medical outcomes. An underlying personality trait, type A behavior, may have a significant influence on medical outcomes after myocardial infarction. The type A behavior pattern is an action-emotion complex in which individuals appear to be directed toward achieving more in less time. Individuals with type A personality traits are usually regarded as driven, work oriented, and preoccupied with a sense of time urgency. Anger and hostility are significant components of the type A personality and may be the most important influences on cardiovascular disease. The construct of the type A personality has been developed extensively by the work of Friedman and Rosenman [149].

Effect of Type A Behavior on Prognosis

While type A behavior has been classified as a risk factor for the development of coronary artery disease [150], its relationship to prognosis after myocardial infarction is controversial. The Western Collaborative Group Study (WCGS) demonstrated that patients with prior myocardial infarction or angina were five times more likely to have a recurrent infarction if they were classified as type A rather than type B [151]. This finding was not confirmed by the Aspirin Myocardial Infarction Study (AMIS) [152] or the Multicenter Post-infarction Program (MPIP) [153]: postinfarction patients classified as type A did not suffer more recurrent infarctions or deaths than did those classified as type B.

Data from the Recurrent Coronary Prevention Project (RCPP) [154] challenge the conclusions of the AMIS and MPIP. In the RCPP, type A patients were randomly assigned to participate in either a cardiac education program (control) or a group counseling program designed to reduce the manifestations of type A behavior (treatment). Treatment patients had significant reductions in type A behavior patterns compared to control patients. More importantly, cardiac death and recurrent myocardial infarction rates were reduced in treatment patients compared to control patients. The benefits in morbidity and mortality were seen primarily in patients with less-severe medical complications after myocardial infarction, as indicated by a low Peel Index score [154], a prognostic scale designed to identify high- and low-risk patients.

Treatment of Type A Behavior

Because type A behavior appears to influence the prognosis in patients who have had a myocardial infarction without severe left ventricular dysfunction or myocardial ischemia, treatment of this disorder may be warranted. A treatment approach tested in the RCPP used a focused behavioral counseling intervention to reduce the manifestations of type A behavior. The counseling emphasized three techniques: (1) social modeling to demonstrate desired behavior, (2) encouragement to engage in new behavior, and (3) prompt corrective feedback about performance [155]. This group counseling intervention had a striking effect on recurrent myocardial infarction and cardiac death. The reinfarction rate was 50 percent lower in the intervention group and mortality was reduced by 25 percent over a 4.5-year follow-up period [154].

Resumption of Customary Activities

While health professionals focus on the medical consequences of myocardial infarction, the social consequences are of equal importance to patients. Even the uncomplicated patient faces restrictions on activities that days before were performed as a customary part of daily life. In addition to those restrictions, the patient is surrounded by family, friends, and coworkers who have limited information about the effects of heart disease. Americans harbor many misconceptions about myocardial infarction that are translated into attitudes and actions toward patients recovering from heart attack. The most prevalent misconceptions are the belief in a dire prognosis for cardiac patients and the belief that physical and mental stresses are harmful.

Because of patient and family's limited knowledge and misconceptions about myocardial infarction, patients should receive very specific advice and education in the early phases of recovery. Even seemingly commonsensical knowledge should not be presumed by the health professionals caring for the patient. The spouse or primary caretaker should receive the advice along with the patient for two reasons. First, the retention of information by patients is limited, especially during the hospitalization for myocardial infarction. Second, most disagreements between patient and spouse in the early recovery period are related to perceptions of medical advice given.

Household Activities

In addition to the advice regarding physical activity presented previously, patients should be specifically counseled regarding performance of customary household activities soon after discharge. These activities include climbing stairs, lifting, driving, socializing with visitors, shopping, and walking outdoors. Individual patients may have more specific questions.

A simple approach to providing guidelines for these activities is to treat them as forms of exercise. In the absence of a formal exercise test, limiting patients to a heart rate 20 beats above the standing heart rate is a concrete guideline that the patient can grasp and practice before hospital discharge. After patients are taught how to count their pulse, walking different speeds and climbing stairs can be performed with supervision. The patient will learn very quickly the heart rate response to each activity and will be confident in undertaking such activities at home.

Other activities that may involve more mental than physical stress, such as driving, socializing, and shopping, are best limited until a more formal exercise evaluation is performed. In studies of patients recovering from myocardial infarction who underwent psychological stress testing using standard techniques, the mean resting heart rate rose less than 10 beats per minute and the mean systolic blood pressure rose less than 15 mm Hg with the most stressful intervention. In every case, the hemodynamic response to psychological stress was substantially lower than that to treadmill exercise. In a subset of patients with exercise-induced ST segment depression, none developed ischemic responses to psychological stress testing [156]. These data suggest that the psychological stress of usual social activities is unlikely to precipitate significant cardiovascular abnormalities.

Lifting is often proscribed for 6 to 8 weeks after myocardial infarction. The rationale for this restriction is concern that the marked blood pressure response to static, upper extremity exercise might precipitate cardiac rupture during the 6-week healing phase of myocardial infarction. In an evaluation of 40 men who had a myocardial infarction, static lifting of an average of 36 lb using one arm was associated with a double product of less than 50 percent of that attained by bicycle ergometry [42, 157]. The combination of static lifting and dynamic treadmill walking was not associated with significantly higher double products than walking alone. In both studies, no patient had electrocardiographic evidence of ischemia with static lifting, although 25 percent had ischemic ST segment depression during treadmill testing [157]. These data suggest that lifting of 25 to 50 lb is safe for patients without evidence of severe myocardial ischemia or left ventricular dysfunction. These data also suggest that activities such as carrying moderate loads, such as groceries, should not necessarily be prohibited.

Sexual Activity

Sexual dysfunction is not uncommon following myocardial infarction. The most common sexual problems that occur after myocardial infarction include reduced or absent libido, avoidance of sexual activity even if libido has recovered, impotence, and premature or delayed ejaculation in men. The causes of sexual dysfunction include preexisting conditions, fear of precipitating a cardiac event, depression, and medications, especially beta blockers and diuretics. In addition, the sex partner may believe that sexual activity could precipitate a cardiac event, and therefore avoids sexual activity. Many patients are embarrassed to discuss sexual dysfunction with health professionals and some consider it a natural sequela of myocardial infarction. Therefore, the physician should address issues of sexuality with patients recovering from myocardial infarction and consider the effects of medications on sexual drive.

The hemodynamic response to sexual intercourse has been evaluated in patients recovering from myocardial infarction. The maximal heart rate during sexual intercourse averages 120 beats per minute. In general, this heart rate response approximates maximal heart rates attained in the performance of other customary activities of daily living [158, 159]. The hemodynamic response to sexual activity is far greater with an unfamiliar compared to a familiar partner [160], in unfamiliar settings, and after excessive eating and alcohol consumption.

In patients undergoing exercise testing after myocardial infarction, the hemodynamic response to exercise can be used to gauge the potential cardiac stress of sexual activity. Patients without significant treadmill abnormalities can be advised to resume sexual activity gradually [161]. Masturbation and mutual caressing can be initiated first, followed by progression to sexual intercourse. Cardiac work associated with sexual intercourse can be minimized by adopting relaxed positions such as side-to-side positions rather than top-and-bottom postures that increase the isometric work [162].

Patients should be advised that the development of significant symptoms such as angina, prolonged dyspnea, excessive fatigue, or tachycardia lasting more than 10 minutes after intercourse should be reported to their physician. In sedentary individuals, such symptoms may be the only manifestation of exercise-induced ischemia or left ventricular dysfunction. These symptoms should prompt further evaluation.

Return to Work

The majority of previously employed patients under the age of 60 return to work after they have had a myocardial infarction [163]. However, decisions regarding reemployment are complex. Older patients, especially those with accessible retirement benefits, are less likely to return to work [164]. Patients with lower educational achievement, those with blue-collar jobs, and those unemployed for more than 3 months before the myocardial infarction occurred are significantly less likely to be employed after the infarction [144, 165, 166]. Patients with severe symptoms of angina or congestive heart failure are less likely to return to work. Rehabilitation efforts alone are unlikely to affect these medical, demographic, and social impediments to reemployment after myocardial infarction.

In younger employed patients, the most important consideration is not whether but when they should return to work. Concerns by patients, employers, and physicians that occupational work will precipitate a recurrent cardiac event underlie the current recommendations for a convalescent period of 2 to 4 months before patients return to work. This prolonged convalescence places a significant economic burden on both patients and employers. Patients generally live on more-limited disability income, especially during the later convalescence period, while employers must function without the patients or with less-efficient temporary help.

The two primary issues that must be addressed if earlier reemployment is to be allowed are prognosis and physical capacity. Uncomplicated patients generally have an excellent prognosis and a well-preserved physical capacity. Early, symptom-limited treadmill testing in such patients can confirm these findings [32].

In a study to determine whether the interval between myocardial infarction and return to work could be shortened, Dennis et al. [167] used a predischarge risk stratification model to identify uncomplicated patients [32]. Patients without angina at rest or clinical evidence of congestive heart failure were designated as uncomplicated and comprised 57 percent of all patients and 77 percent of employed patients in four community hospitals. Patients who were uncomplicated and under the age of 60 and, therefore, were most likely to return to work within 6 months comprised 64 percent of all employed patients.

Patients with these criteria were randomized either to receive usual care from their primary physicians or to undergo an occupational work evaluation. The occupational work evaluation consisted of a symptom-limited treadmill test at 3 weeks after the myocardial infarction occurred and specific advice to the patient and primary physician regarding reemployment. The 6 percent of patients demonstrating severe ischemia (e.g., 0.2 mV of ST segment depression at a heart rate less than 135) on the treadmill test were advised to undergo further evaluation with coronary arteriography. The 70 percent of patients without abnormalities on the treadmill test were advised to return to work at 35 days while the 24 percent of patients with mild abnormalities, most commonly 0.1 to 0.2 mV of ST depression or angina at a heart rate greater than 135, were advised to return to work at 42 days, after beginning antianginal medication.

In a 6-month follow-up evaluation, cardiac events were rare. The mortality rate was 1.5 percent and the reinfarction rate was 2 percent in the randomized patients, without differences between the two groups. Events were more common in patients who demonstrated severe ischemia during the treadmill test. All but one event occurred before patients returned to work and no cardiac events occurred while patients were on the job.

At 6 months, 90 percent of patients in both groups were working either full- or part-time. However, patients receiving the occupational work evaluation returned to work at a median of 51 days, compared to 75 days for patients receiving usual care. This 33 percent reduction in the convalescence period resulted in an average of $2102 in increased earned income in the 6 months after myocardial infarction occurred for patients receiving the occupational work evaluation compared to those receiving usual care [168]. A follow-up study to assess the utility of this intervention in community hospitals demonstrated that uncomplicated patients could safely return to work within 37 days after the myocardial infarction occurred [169].

This type of intervention can be employed in outpatient cardiac rehabilitation programs. The intervention may not be sufficient for the evaluation of patients performing heavy manual labor. In the cited study, the average peak treadmill capacity at 3 weeks was 7 METs. This capacity is sufficient for most jobs that are sedentary or involve light physical labor. It may be insufficient for patients performing heavy manual labor. However, only 16 percent of Americans perform manual labor and that percentage declines with age. Patients performing manual labor or those involved with public safety such as police officers, firefighters, and pilots may require more extensive evaluation or prolonged exercise training before they return to work.

References

1. Gattiker, H., Goins, P., and Dennis, C. Cardiac rehabilitation: Current status and future directions. *West. J. Med.* 156:183, 1992.
2. Haskell, W. L., Savin, M., Oldridge, N., and DeBusk, R. Factors influencing estimated oxygen uptake during exercise testing soon after myocardial infarction. *Am. J. Cardiol.* 50:299, 1982.
3. Roberts, J. M., Sullivan, M., Froelicher, V. F., et al. Predicting oxygen uptake from treadmill testing in normal subjects and coronary artery disease patients. *Am. Heart J.* 108:1454, 1984.
4. Franklin, B. A., Wrisley, D., Johnson, S., et al. Chronic adaptations to physical conditioning in cardiac patients. *Clin. Sports Med.* 3:471, 1984.
5. Dehn, M. M., Blomquist, C. G., and Mitchell, J. H. Clinical exercise program. *Clin. Sports Med.* 3:319, 1984.
6. Convertino, V., Hung, J., Goldwater, D., and DeBusk, R. F. Cardiovascular responses to exercise in middle-aged men after 10 days of bedrest. *Circulation* 65:134, 1982.
7. Convertino, V. A., Bisson, R., Bates, R., et al. Effects of anti-orthostatic bedrest on the cardiorespiratory responses to exercise. *Aviat. Space Environ. Med.* 52:251, 1981.
8. Saltin, B., Blomquist, G., Mitchell, J. H., et al. Response to exercise after bedrest and after training. *Circulation* 38(Suppl VII):VII-1, 1968.
9. Fareeduddin, K., and Abelmann, W. H. Impaired orthostatic tolerance after bedrest in patients with acute myocardial infarction. *N. Engl. J. Med.* 280: 345, 1969.
10. Wenger, N. K. Cardiovascular drugs: Effects on exercise testing and exercise training of the coronary patient. *Exerc. Heart Cardiovasc. Clin.* 15:133, 1985.
11. Dittmer, D. K., and Teasell, R. Complications of immobilization and bed rest. Part 1: Musculoskeletal and cardiovascular complications. *Can. Fam. Physician* 39:1428–32, 1435–37, 1993.
12. Greenleaf, J. E., Bernauer, E. M., Ertl, A. C., et al. Isokinetic strength and endurance during 30-day 6 degrees head-down bed rest with isotonic and isokinetic exercise training. *Aviat. Space Environ. Med.* 65:45, 1994.
13. Thoren, P. N. Activation of left ventricular receptors with non-medullated vagal afferent fibers during occlusion of a coronary artery in the cat. *Am. J. Cardiol.* 37:146, 1976.
14. Haskell, W. L., and DeBusk, R. Cardiovascular responses to repeated treadmill exercise testing soon after myocardial infarction. *Circulation* 60:1247, 1979.
15. Franciosa, J. A. Lack of correlation between exercise capacity and indexes of resting left ventricular performance in heart failure. *Am. J. Cardiol.* 47: 33, 1981.
16. Higginbotham, M. B., Morris, K. G., Conn, E. H., et al. Determinants of variable exercise performance among patients with severe left ventricular dysfunction. *Am. J. Cardiol.* 51:52, 1983.
17. Litchfield, R. L., Kerber, R. E., Benge, W., et al. Normal exercise capacity in patients with severe left ventricular dysfunction: Compensatory mechanisms. *Circulation* 66:129, 1982.
18. Wilson, J. R., and Ferraro, N. Exercise tolerance in patients with chronic left heart failure: Relation to oxygen transport and ventilatory abnormalities. *Am. J. Cardiol.* 51:1358, 1983.
19. Jette, M., Heller, R., Landry, F., et al. Randomized 4-week exercise program in patients with impaired left ventricular function. *Circulation* 84:1561, 1991.
20. Ades, P. A., Grunvald, M. H., Weiss, R. M., et al. Usefulness of myocardial ischemia as predictor of training effect in cardiac rehabilitation after myocardial infarction or coronary artery bypass grafting. *Am. J. Cardiol.* 63:1032, 1989.
21. Buda, A. J., Dubbin, J. D., McDonald, I. L., et al. Spontaneous changes in thallium-201 myocardial perfusion imaging after myocardial infarction. *Am. J. Cardiol.* 50:1272, 1978.
22. Froelicher, V. F., Jensen, D., Atwood, E., et al. Cardiac rehabilitation: Evidence for improvement in myocardial perfusion and function. *Arch. Phys. Med. Rehabil.* 61:517, 1980.
23. Franklin, B. A. Introduction: Physiologic adaptations to exercise training in cardiac patients: Contemporary issues and concerns. *Med. Sci. Sports Exerc.* 23:645, 1991.
24. Hung, J., Gordon, E. P., Houston, N., et al. Changes

in rest and exercise myocardial perfusion and left ventricular function 3 to 26 weeks after clinically uncomplicated acute myocardial infarction: Effects of exercise training. *Am. J. Cardiol.* 54:943, 1984.

25. Sasyaama, S., and Fujita, M. Recent insights into coronary collateral circulation. *Circulation* 85:1197, 1992.
26. Juneau, M., Colles, P., Théroux, P., et al. Symptom-limited versus low level exercise testing before hospital discharge after myocardial infarction. *J. Am. Coll. Cardiol.* 20:927, 1992.
27. DeBusk, R. F. Physical conditioning following myocardial infarction. *Adv. Cardiol.* 31:156, 1982.
28. DeBusk, R. F., Houston, N., Haskell, W., et al. Exercise training soon after myocardial infarction. *Am. J. Cardiol.* 44:1223, 1979.
29. Krone, R. J. The role of risk stratification in the early management of a myocardial infarction. *Ann. Intern. Med.* 116:223, 1992.
30. Weber, K. T., and Janicki, J. S. Cardiopulmonary exercise testing for evaluation of chronic cardiac failure. *Am. J. Cardiol.* 55:22A, 1985.
31. DeBusk, R. F., and Haskell, W. L. Symptom-limited vs heart-rate-limited exercise testing soon after myocardial infarction. *Circulation* 61:738, 1980.
32. DeBusk, R. F., Kraemer, H. C., Nash, E., et al. Stepwise risk stratification soon after myocardial infarction. *Am. J. Cardiol.* 52:1161, 1983.
33. Fioretti, P., Brower, R. W., Simoons, M. L., et al. Prediction of mortality during the first year after acute myocardial infarction from clinical variables and stress test at hospital discharge. *Am. J. Cardiol.* 55:1313, 1985.
34. Ho, S. W-C., McComish, M. J., and Taylor, R. R. Effect of beta-adrenergic blockade on the results of exercise testing related to the extent of coronary artery disease. *Am. J. Cardiol.* 55:258, 1985.
35. Naughton, J., Sevelios, G., and Balke, B. Physiological responses of normal and pathological subjects to a modified work capacity test. *J. Sports Med.* 3:201, 1973.
36. American College of Sports Medicine. Position statement on the recommended quantity and quality of exercise for developing and maintaining fitness in healthy adults. *Med. Sci. Sports* 10:vii, 1978.
37. Erb, B., Fletcher, J. F., and Sheffield, T. L. Standards for cardiovascular exercise treatment programs. *Circulation* 59:1084A, 1979.
38. *American Association of Cardiovascular and Pulmonary Rehabilitation: Guidelines for Cardiac Rehabilitation Programs* (1st ed.). Champaign, IL: Human Kinetics, 1991.
39. Pollock, M. L., and Pells, A. E., III. Exercise prescription for the cardiac patient: An update. *Clin. Sports Med.* 3:425, 1984.
40. Shephard, R. J. Exercise regimens after myocardial infarction: Rationale and results. *Exerc. Heart Cardiovasc. Clin.* 15:145, 1985.
41. Bezucha, G. R., Lenser, M. L., Hanson, P. G., et al. Comparison of hemodynamic responses to static and dynamic exercise. *J. Appl. Physiol.* 53:1589, 1982.
42. DeBusk, R., Pitts, W., Haskell, W., and Houston, N. Comparison of cardiovascular responses to static-dynamic effort and dynamic effort alone in patients with chronic ischemic heart disease. *Circulation* 59:977, 1979.
43. Borg, G., and Linderholm, H. Exercise performance and perceived exertion in patients with coronary insufficiency, arterial hypertension and vasoregulatory asthenia. *Acta Med. Scand.* 187:17, 1970.
44. Juneau, M., Rogers, F., deSantos, V., et al. Comparison of the effectiveness of self-monitored home-based moderate-intensity exercise training in middle-aged men and women. *Am. J. Cardiol.* 60:66, 1987.
45. Fry, G., and Berra, K. *YMCArdiac Therapy.* Chicago: National Council of the Young Men's Christian Associations, 1981.
46. Koppes, G. M., Kruyer, W., Beckman, C. H., and Jones, F. G. Response to exercise early after uncomplicated acute myocardial infarction in patients receiving no medication: Long-term follow-up. *Am. J. Cardiol.* 46:764, 1980.
47. Miller, D. H., and Borer, J. S. Exercise testing early after myocardial infarction: Risks and benefits. *Am. J. Med.* 72:427, 1982.
48. Weiner, D. A. Predischarge exercise testing after myocardial infarction: Prognostic and therapeutic features. *Exerc. Heart Cardiovasc. Clin.* 15:95, 1985.
49. Waters, D. D., Bosch, X., Bouchard, A., et al. Comparison of clinical variables and variables derived from a limited predischarge exercise test as predictors of early and late mortality after myocardial infarction. *J. Am. Coll. Cardiol.* 5:1, 1985.
50. Williams, R. S., Miller, H., and Koisch, F. P. Guidelines for unsupervised exercise in patients with ischemic heart disease. *J. Cardiac Rehabil.* 1:213, 1981.
51. Hossack, K. F., and Bruce, R. A. Improved exercise performance of persons with stable angina pectoris receiving diltiazem. *Am. J. Cardiol.* 47:95, 1981.
52. Hossack, K. F., Bruce, R. A., and Clark, L. J. Influence of propranolol on exercise prescription of training heart rates. *Cardiology* 65:47, 1980.
53. Leier, C. V., Huss, P., Magonen, B. D., et al. Improved exercise capacity and differing arterial and venous tolerance during chronic isosorbide dinitrate therapy for congestive heart failure. *Circulation* 67:817, 1983.
54. Malborg, R., Isaaccson, S., and Kallivroussis, G. The effects of beta blockade and/or physical training in patients with angina pectoris. *Curr. Ther. Res.* 16:171, 1974.
55. Gordon, N. F., Kruger, P. E., Hons, B. A., et al. Improved exercise ventilatory responses after training in coronary heart disease during long-term beta-adrenergic blockade. *Am. J. Cardiol.* 51:755, 1983.
56. Pratt, C. M., Welton, D. E., Squires, W. G., et al. Demonstration of training effect during chronic

beta-adrenergic blockade in patients with coronary artery disease. *Circulation* 64:1125, 1981.

57. Koiwaya, Y., Nakamura, M., Mitsutake, A., et al. Increased exercise tolerance after oral diltiazem, a calcium antagonist, in angina pectoris. *Am. Heart J.* 101:143, 1981.
58. Feldman, A. M. Can we alter survival in patients with congestive heart failure? *J.A.M.A.* 267:956, 1992.
59. Cobb, F. R., Williams, P. S., McEwan, P., et al. Effects of exercise training on ventricular function in patients with recent myocardial infarction. *Circulation* 66:100, 1982.
60. Conn, E., Williams, R. S., and Wallace, A. G. Exercise responses before and after conditioning in patients with severely depressed left ventricular function. *Am. J. Cardiol.* 49:296, 1982.
61. Coats, A. J., Adamopoulos, S., Radaelli, A., et al. Controlled trial of physical training in chronic heart failure. Exercise performance, hemodynamics, ventilation and autonomic function. *Circulation* 85:2119, 1992.
62. Verani, M. S., Hartung, G. H., Hoepfel-Harris, J., et al. Effects of exercise training on left ventricular performance and myocardial perfusion in patients with coronary artery disease. *Am. J. Cardiol.* 47: 797, 1981.
63. Sullivan, M. J., and Cobb, F. R. The anaerobic threshold in chronic heart failure. Relation to blood lactate, ventilatory basis, reproducibility and response to exercise training. *Circulation* 81(Suppl 1):II47, 1990.
64. Ogawa, T., Vyden, J., Rose, H. B., et al. Peripheral circulatory changes after physical conditioning in coronary artery disease patients. *J. Cardiac Rehabil.* 1:269, 1981.
65. Cohn, J. N. Mechanisms of action and efficacy of nitrates in heart failure. *Am. J. Cardiol.* 70:88B, 1992.
66. Awan, N. A., Miller, R. R., DeMaria, A. N., et al. Efficacy of ambulatory systemic vasodilator therapy with oral prazosin in chronic refractory heart failure. *Circulation* 56:346, 1977.
67. Francis, G. S., and Rucinska, E. J. Long-term effects of a once-a-day versus twice-a-day regimen of enalapril for congestive heart failure. *Am. J. Cardiol.* 63:17D, 1989.
68. Cohn, J. N., Johnson, G., Ziexche, S., et al. A comparison of enalapril with hydralazine-isosorbide dinitrate in the treatment of chronic congestive heart failure. *N. Engl. J. Med.* 325:303, 1991.
69. Goldsmith, S. R., Franciosa, J. A., and Cohn, J. N. Contrasting acute and chronic effects of nitrates on exercise capacity in heart failure. *Am. J. Cardiol.* 43:404, 1979.
70. Kulick, D. L., and Rahimtoola, S. H. Current role of digitalis therapy in patients with congestive heart failure. *J.A.M.A.* 266:2995, 1991.
71. Sullivan, M., Atwood, J. E., Myers, J., et al. Increased exercise capacity after digoxin administration in patients with heart failure. *J. Am. Coll. Cardiol.* 13:1138, 1989.
72. DeBusk, R. F. Physical conditioning following myocardial infarction. *Adv. Cardiol.* 31:156, 1982.
73. Jensen, D., Atwood, J. E., Froelicher, V., et al. Improvement in ventricular function during exercise studied with radionuclide ventriculography after cardiac rehabilitation. *Am. J. Cardiol.* 46:770, 1980.
74. Williams, R. S., McGinnis, R. D., Cobb, F. C., and Califf, R. C. Enhanced left ventricular ejection fraction during exercise in subjects with coronary artery disease following physical conditioning (Abstract). *Circulation* 68(Suppl III):377, 1983.
75. Paterson, D. H., Shepard, R. J., Cunningham, D., et al. Effects of physical training upon cardiovascular function following myocardial infarction. *J. Appl. Physiol.* 47:487, 1979.
76. Buchwalsky, R. Hemodynamics before and after physical endurance training in patients with myocardial infarction under various physical and psychomotor stress tests. *Clin. Cardiol.* 5:332, 1982.
77. Shaw, L. W. Effects of a prescribed supervised exercise program on mortality and cardiovascular morbidity in patients after a myocardial infarction. *Am. J. Cardiol.* 48:39, 1981.
78. Naughton, J. Contributions of exercise clinical trials to cardiac rehabilitation. *Clin. Sports Med.* 3:545, 1984.
79. Rechnitzer, P. A., Cunningham, D. A., Andrew, G. M., et al. Relation of exercise to the recurrence rate of myocardial infarction in men: Ontario exercise-heart collaborative study. *Am. J. Cardiol.* 51:65, 1983.
80. Shaw, L. W. Effects of a prescribed supervised exercise program on mortality and cardiovascular morbidity in patients after a myocardial infarction: The National Exercise and Heart Disease Project. *Am. J. Cardiol.* 48:39, 1981.
81. Oldridge, N. B., Guyatt, G. H., Fisher, M. E., et al. Cardiac rehabilitation after myocardial infarction. Combined experience of randomized clinical trials. *J.A.M.A.* 260:945, 1988.
82. O'Connor, G. T., Buring, J. E., Yusuf, S., et al. An overview of randomized trials of rehabilitation with exercise after myocardial infarction. *Circulation* 80: 234, 1989.
83. Heath, G. W., Ehsani, A. A., Hagberg, J. M., et al. Exercise training improves lipoprotein lipid profiles in patients with coronary artery disease. *Am. Heart J.* 105:889, 1983.
84. Boyer, J. L., and Cash, F. W. Exercise therapy in hypertensive men. *J.A.M.A.* 211:1668, 1970.
85. Gentry, W. D., and Stewart, M. A. Psychologic effects of exercise training in coronary-prone individuals and in patients with symptomatic coronary heart disease. *Exerc. Heart Cardiovasc. Clin.* 15:255, 1985.
86. Ewart, C. K., Stewart, K. J., Gillilan, R. E., et al. Usefulness of self-efficacy in predicting overexer-

tion during programmed exercise in coronary artery disease. *Am. J. Cardiol.* 57:557, 1986.

87. Haskell, W. L. Safety of outpatient cardiac exercise programs. *Clin. Sports Med.* 3:455, 1984.
88. Van Camp, S. P., and Peterson, R. A. Cardiovascular complications of outpatient cardiac rehabilitation programs. *J.A.M.A.* 256:1160, 1986.
89. Haskell, W. L. Cardiovascular complications during exercise training of cardiac patients. *Circulation* 57:920, 1978.
90. The Pooling Project Research Group. Relationship of blood pressure, serum cholesterol, smoking habit, relative weight and ECG abnormalities to incidence of major coronary events: Final report of the Pooling Project. *J. Chronic Dis.* 31:201, 1978.
91. Gordon, T., Kannel, W. B., and McGee, D. Death and coronary attacks in men giving up cigarette smoking: A report from the Framingham Study. *Lancet* 2:1345, 1974.
92. Dobson, A. J., Alexander, H. M., Heller, R. F., et al. How soon after quitting smoking does risk of heart attack decline? *J. Clin. Epidemiol.* 44:1247, 1991.
93. Ronnevik, P. K., Gundersen, T., and Abrahamsen, A. M. Effect of smoking habits and timolol treatment on mortality and reinfarction in patients surviving acute myocardial infarction. *Br. Heart J.* 54:134, 1985.
94. Rosenberg, L., Kaufman, D. W., Helmrich, S. P., and Shapiro, S. The risk of myocardial infarction after quitting smoking in men under 55 years of age. *N. Engl. J. Med.* 313:1511, 1985.
95. Sparrow, D., Dawber, T. R., and Colton, T. The influence of cigarette smoking on prognosis after a first myocardial infarction: A report from the Framingham Study. *J. Chronic Dis.* 31:425, 1978.
96. Daly, L. E., Mulcahy, R., Graham, I. M., and Hickey, N. Long-term effect on mortality of stopping smoking after unstable angina and myocardial infarction. *B.M.J.* 287:324, 1983.
97. Hartz, A. J., Barboriak, P. N., Anderson, A. J., et al. Smoking, coronary artery occlusion and nonfatal myocardial infarction. *J.A.M.A.* 246:851, 1981.
98. Klein, L. W., Pichard, A. D., Holt, J., et al. Effects of tobacco smoking on the coronary circulation. *J. Am. Coll. Cardiol.* 1:421, 1983.
99. Wilhelmsen, L., Svardsudd, K., Korsan-Bengfsen, K., et al. Fibrinogen as a risk factor for stroke and myocardial infarction. *N. Engl. J. Med.* 311:501, 1984.
100. Vliestra, R. E., Kronmal, R. A., Frye, R. L., et al. Factors affecting the extent and severity of coronary artery disease in patients enrolled in the CASS. *Arteriosclerosis* 2:208, 1982.
101. Ockene, J. K., Hosmer, D., Rippe, J., et al. Factors affecting cigarette smoking status in patients with ischemic heart disease. *J. Chronic Dis.* 38:985, 1985.
102. Taylor, C. B., Houston-Miller, N., Killen, J. D., et al. Smoking cessation after acute myocardial infarction: Effects of a nurse-managed intervention. *Ann. Intern. Med.* 113:118, 1990.
103. Sachs, D. P. L. Cigarette smoking: Health effects and cessation strategies. *Clin. Geriatr. Med.* 2:337, 1986.
104. Benfari, R. C., Ockene, J. K., and McIntyre, K. M. Control of cigarette smoking from a psychological perspective. *Annu. Rev. Public Health* 3:101, 1982.
105. Cohen, S. J., Stookey, G. K., Katz, B. P., et al. Encouraging primary care physicians to help smokers quit. A randomized, controlled trial. *Ann. Intern. Med.* 110:648, 1989.
106. Rigotti, N. A., Singer, D. E., Mulley, A. G., et al. Smoking cessation following admission to the coronary care unit. *J. Gen. Intern. Med.* 6:305, 1991.
107. Weinblatt, E., Shapiro, S., and Frank, C. W. Changes in personal characteristics of men over five years following first diagnosis of coronary heart disease. *Am. J. Public Health* 61:831, 1971.
108. Lee, E. W., and D'Alonzo, G. E. Cigarette smoking, nicotine addiction and its pharmacologic treatment. *Arch. Intern. Med.* 153:34, 1993.
109. Hjalmarson, A. I. Effect of nicotine chewing gum in smoking cessation: A randomized, placebo-control double-blind study. *J.A.M.A.* 252:2835, 1984.
110. Fiore, M. C., Jorenby, D. E., Baker, T. B., et al. Tobacco dependence and the nicotine patch. Clinical guidelines for effective use. *J.A.M.A.* 268:2687, 1992.
111. Benowitz, N. L. Cigarette smoking and nicotine addiction. *Med. Clin. North Am.* 76:415, 1992.
112. McNabb, M. E., Ebert, R. V., and McCusker, K. Plasma nicotine levels produced by chewing nicotine gum. *J.A.M.A.* 248:865, 1982.
113. Gorsline, J., Gupta, S. K., Dye, D., et al. Nicotine dose relationships for nicotine transdermal system at steady state. *Pharmacol. Res.* 8(Suppl 299):S-299, 1991.
114. Miller, G. H., Golish, J. A., and Cox, C. E. A physician's guide to smoking cessation. *J. Fam. Pract.* 34:759, 1992.
115. Carney, R. M., and Goldberg, A. P. Weight gain after cessation of cigarette smoking. *N. Engl. J. Med.* 310:614, 1984.
116. Soldatos, C. R., Kales, J. D., Sharf, M. B., et al. Cigarette smoking associated with sleep difficulty. *Science* 207:551, 1980.
117. Marlatt, G. A., and Parks, G. A. Self-management of addictive behaviors. In P. Karoly and F. H. Kanfer (eds.), *Self-Management and Behavior Change.* New York: Pergamon, 1982.
118. Lipid Research Clinics Program. The Lipid Research Clinics Coronary Primary Prevention Trial results: I. Reduction in incidence of coronary heart disease. *J.A.M.A.* 251:351, 1984.
119. Lipid Research Clinics Program. The Lipid Research Clinics Coronary Primary Prevention Trial results: II. The relationship of reduction in incidence of coronary heart disease to cholesterol lowering. *J.A.M.A.* 251:365, 1984.
120. Miller, N. E. Pharmacotherapy of disorders of plasma

lipoprotein metabolism. *Am. J. Cardiol.* 66:16A, 1990.

121. Brensike, J. F., Levy, R. I., Kelsey, S. F., et al. Effects of therapy with cholestyramine on progression of coronary atherosclerosis: Results of the NHLBI type II coronary intervention study. *Circulation* 69:313, 1984.
122. Artzenius, A. C., Krombout, D., Barth, J. D., et al. Diet, lipoproteins and progression of coronary atherosclerosis. The Leiden intervention trial. *N. Engl. J. Med.* 312:805, 1985.
123. Coronary Drug Project Research Group. Natural history of myocardial infarction in a coronary drug project: Long-term prognostic importance of serum lipid levels. *Am. J. Cardiol.* 41:489, 1978.
124. Leren, P. The effect of plasma cholesterol lowering diet in male survivors of myocardial infarction. *Acta Med. Scand. Suppl.* 466:142, 1966.
125. Brown, G., Albers, J. J., Fisher, L. D., et al. Regression of coronary artery disease as a result of intensive lipid-lowering therapy with high levels of apolipoprotein B. *N. Engl. J. Med.* 323:1337, 1990.
126. National Cholesterol Education Program. Report of the Expert Panel on Population Strategies for Blood Cholesterol Reduction: Executive summary. National Heart, Lung and Blood Institute, National Institutes of Health. *Arch. Intern. Med.* 151:1071, 1991.
127. Gotto, A. M., Jr., Jones, P. H., and Scott, L. W. The diagnosis and management of hyperlipidemia. *Dis. Mon.* 32:247, 1986.
128. The Lipid Research Clinics Program Epidemiology Committee. Plasma lipid distributions in selected North American populations: The Lipid Research Clinics Program prevalence study. *Circulation* 60: 427, 1979.
129. Rifkind, B. M. High density lipoprotein cholesterol and coronary artery disease: Survey of the evidence. *Am. J. Cardiol.* 66:3A, 1990.
130. Grundy, S. M., Goodman, D. W., Rifkind, B. M., et al. The place of HDL in cholesterol management. A perspective from the National Cholesterol Education Program. *Arch. Intern. Med.* 149:505, 1989.
131. Ginsburg, G. S., Safran, C., and Pasternak, R. C. Frequency of low serum high-density lipoprotein cholesterol levels in hospitalized patients with "desirable" total cholesterol levels. *Am. J. Cardiol.* 68:187, 1991.
132. Henkin, Y., Oberman, A., Hurst, D. C., et al. Niacin revisited: Clinical observations on an important but underutilized drug. *Am. J. Med.* 91:239, 1991.
133. Committee of Principal Investigators. WHO Cooperative Trial on primary prevention of ischemic heart disease using clofibrate to lower serum cholesterol: Mortality follow-up. *Lancet* 23:379, 1980.
134. Walldiu, G., Regnstrom, J., Nilsson, J., et al. The role of lipids and antioxidative factors for development of atherosclerosis. The Probucol Quantitative Regression Swedish Trial (PQRST). *Am. J. Cardiol.* 71:15B, 1993.
135. Gwynne, J. T. High density lipoprotein cholesterol levels as a marker of reverse cholesterol transport. *Am. J. Cardiol.* 64:10G, 1989.
136. Hartung, G. H., Squires, W. G., and Gotto, A. M. Effect of exercise training on plasma high density, lipoprotein cholesterol and coronary disease patients. *Am. Heart J.* 101:181, 1981.
137. Klatsky, A. L., Friedman, G. D., and Sieglaub, A. B. Alcohol consumption before myocardial infarction: Results from the Kaiser Permanente epidemiologic study of myocardial infarction. *Ann. Intern. Med.* 81:294, 1974.
138. Dyer, A. R., Stamler, J., Paul, O., et al. Alcohol consumption and seventeen year mortality in the Chicago Western Electric Company Study. *Prev. Med.* 9:78, 1980.
139. Haskell, W. L., Camargo, C., Jr., Williams, P. T., et al. The effect of cessation and resumption of moderate alcohol intake on serum high-density-lipoprotein subfractions: A controlled study. *N. Engl. J. Med.* 310:805, 1984.
140. Steinberg, D., Pearson, T. A., and Kuller, L. H. Alcohol and atherosclerosis. *Ann. Intern. Med.* 114: 967, 1991.
141. Israel, D. H., and Gorlin, R. Fish oils in the prevention of atherosclerosis. *J. Am. Coll. Cardiol.* 19:174, 1992.
142. Hackett, T. P., Cassem, N. H., and Wishnie, H. A. The coronary care unit: An appraisal of its psychological hazards. *N. Engl. J. Med.* 279:1365, 1968.
143. Tesar, G. E., and Hackett, T. P. Psychiatric management of the hospitalized cardiac patient. In D. S. Krantz and J. A. Blumenthal (eds.), *Behavioral Assessment and Management of Cardiovascular Disorders.* Sarasota, FL: Professional Resource Exchange, 1987.
144. Garrity, T. F. Vocational adjustment after first myocardial infarction; comparative assessment of several variables suggested in the literature. *Soc. Sci. Med.* 7:705, 1973.
145. Wishnie, H. A., Hackett, T. P., and Cassem, N. H. Psychological hazards of convalescence following myocardial infarction. *J.A.M.A.* 215:1292, 1971.
146. Wiklund, I., Sanne, H., Vedin, A., and Wilhelmsson, C. Psychosocial outcome one year after a first myocardial infarction. *J. Psychosom. Res.* 28:309, 1984.
147. Beck, A. T., Ward, C. H., Mendelson, M., et al. An inventory for measuring depression. *Arch. Gen. Psychiatry* 4:561, 1961.
148. Hathaway, S. R., and McKinley, J. C. *The Minnesota Multiphasic Personality Inventory Manual.* Minneapolis: University of Minnesota Press, 1943.
149. Friedman, M., and Rosenman, R. *Type A Behavior and Your Heart.* New York: Knopf, 1974.
150. The Review Panel on Coronary-Prone Behavior and Coronary Heart Disease. Coronary-prone behavior and coronary heart disease: A critical review. *Circulation* 63:1199, 1981.
151. Jenkins, C. D., Zyzanski, S. J., and Rosenman, R. H. Risk of new myocardial infarction in middle-

aged men with manifest coronary heart disease. *Circulation* 53:342, 1976.

152. Shekelle, R. B., Gale, M., and Norusis, M. (for the Aspirin Myocardial Infarction Study Research Group). Type A score (Jenkins Activity Survey) and risk of recurrent coronary heart disease in the Aspirin Myocardial Infarction Study. *Am. J. Cardiol.* 56:221, 1985.
153. Case, R. B., Heller, S. S., Case, N. B., Moss, A. J., and the Multicenter Post-infarction Research Group. Type A behavior and survival after acute myocardial infarction. *N. Engl. J. Med.* 312:737, 1985.
154. Friedman, M., Thoresen, C. E., Gill, J. J., et al. Alteration of type A behavior and its effect on cardiac recurrences in post myocardial infarction patients: Summary results of the Recurrent Coronary Prevention Project. *Am. Heart J.* 112:653, 1986.
155. Thoresen, C. Treatment of type A behavior. In D. S. Krantz and J. A. Blumenthal (eds.), *Behavioral Assessment and Management of Cardiovascular Disorders.* Sarasota, FL: Professional Resource Exchange, 1987.
156. DeBusk, R. F., Taylor, C. B., and Agras, W. S. Comparison of treadmill exercise testing and psychologic stress testing soon after myocardial infarction. *Am. J. Cardiol.* 43:907, 1979.
157. DeBusk, R. F., Valdez, R., Houston, N., and Haskell, W. Cardiovascular responses to dynamic and static effort soon after myocardial infarction: Application to occupational work assessment. *Circulation* 58:368, 1978.
158. Hellerstein, H., and Friedman, E. J. Sexual activity in the post-coronary patient. *Med. Aspects Human Sex.* March:70, 1969.
159. Jackson, S. Sexual intercourse and angina pectoris. *B.M.J.* 2:16, 1978.
160. Massie, R. E., Rapp, J., and Whelton, R. Sudden death during coitus: Fact or fiction. *Med. Aspects Human Sex.* March:22, 1969.
161. Tardif, G. S. Sexual activity after a myocardial infarction. *Arch. Phys. Med. Rehabil.* 70:763, 1989.
162. Cooper, A. J. Myocardial infarction and advice on sexual activity. *Practitioner* 229:575, 1985.
163. Wenger, N. K., Hellerstein, H. K., Blackburn, H., and Castranova, S. J. Physician management and the practice of patients with uncomplicated myocardial infarction: Changes in the past decade. *Circulation* 65:421, 1982.
164. Shapiro, S., Weinblatt, E., and Frank, C. W. Return to work after first myocardial infarction. *Arch. Environ. Health* 24:17, 1972.
165. Kjoller, E. Resumption of work after acute myocardial infarction. *Acta Med. Scand.* 199:379, 1976.
166. Weinblatt, E., Shapiro, S., Frank, C. W., and Sager, R. V. Return to work and work status following first myocardial infarction. *Am. J. Public Health* 56:169, 1966.
167. Dennis, C. A., Houston-Miller, N., Schwartz, R. G., et al. Early return to work after uncomplicated myocardial infarction: Results of a randomized trial. *J.A.M.A.* 260:214, 1988.
168. Picard, M. H., Dennis, C. A., Schwartz, R. G., et al. Cost-benefit analysis of early return to work after uncomplicated acute myocardial infarction. *Am. J. Cardiol.* 63:1308, 1989.
169. Pilote, L., Thomas, R. J., Dennis, C., et al. Return to work after uncomplicated myocardial infarction: A randomized clinical trial of practice guidelines in a community setting. *Ann. Intern. Med.* 117:383, 1992.

36. Coronary Artery Bypass Surgery in Patients with Recent Myocardial Infarction

Vibhu R. Kshettry and R. Morton Bolman III

Coronary artery disease and its sequelae continue to be the leading cause of death in the Western world. The relationship between coronary artery occlusion and myocardial infarction was established by Malmsten and Düben of Sweden in 1859 [1]. Since then, our understanding of the subtle pathophysiologic changes of myocardial infarction has progressed greatly. Few areas in medicine have witnessed as radical a change in the past decade as has the management of acute myocardial infarction.

Myocardial infarction involves segmental myocardial injury produced by sudden occlusion of a major coronary artery. This occlusion is caused, in most instances, by an intravascular thrombosis superimposed at the site of a preexisting atheromatous plaque. The rationale for the reperfusion of infarcting myocardium derives from experimental studies performed to salvage ischemic but viable myocardium by reestablishing blood flow and limiting myocardial loss [2, 3]. In the early postinfarction period, not only the infarcted myocardium but also adjacent viable muscle perform suboptimally due to a loss of contractile function.

However, the process of myocardial infarction is not necessarily instantaneous and complete, but evolves over several hours [4]. This provides a window of opportunity for partially or completely reversing the ischemic insult [5, 6]. Reperfusion after 6 hours or more increases the myocardial damage mediated by hemorrhage into the infarct and results in the "no-reflow" phenomenon [7, 8]. These considerations have led to interventions after the occurrence of a acute myocardial infarction to establish early reperfusion with thrombolytics, angioplasty, and surgery. The evolution of the application of coronary artery bypass surgery in these patients is discussed in this chapter. In addition, a number of mechanical complications that also require surgical intervention, such as ventricular free wall or septal rupture, acute mitral insufficiency, and ventricular aneurysm, can occur after myocardial infarction; discussions regarding these complications are presented elsewhere in this text.

Acute Myocardial Infarction

Acute myocardial infarction has traditionally been associated with a mortality of 10 to 15 percent in the first year. More than a third of the deaths occur in the first 6 weeks, and half in the first 3 months [9]. Thus, early surgery seemed logical to correct underlying coronary artery stenoses causing ischemia or to avoid a catastrophe later. The goals of early surgical revascularization are to restore blood flow, limit myocardial damage, and offer long-term protection from subsequent ischemia. Since the evolving necrosis occurs rapidly, surgery should be performed within 6 hours after the onset of chest pain. Unfortunately, the initial experience in the early 1970s with such surgery was disappointing, with high morbidity and mortality [10, 11].

The early 1980s saw a resurgence of interest in early revascularization. DeWood et al. [12] reviewed 701 patients who underwent surgery an average of 6 hours after the onset of chest pain. Their operative mortality was 5.2 percent for patients with transmural infarction and 3 percent for those with nontransmural infarction. At follow-up of 10 years, the late mortality rate was 12.5 percent for patients with transmural infarction and 6.5 percent for those with nontransmural infarction. While these results were encouraging, certain subsets of patients had higher mortality rates. The in-hospital mortality rate was 2.3 percent for patients with transmural infarction and one-vessel disease but increased to 4.4 percent for those with two-vessel and 9 percent for those with three-vessel coronary artery disease. In addition, the timing of surgery relative to the onset of chest pain appeared to affect the surgical outcome for patients with transmural infarction. If the operation took place within 6 hours after onset, there was a 4 percent early and 8 percent total mortality rate; if it took place after 6 hours, surgery was associated with an 8 percent early and 21 percent total mortality rate.

Phillips et al. [13] reported a similar experience with 339 patients with evolving myocardial infarction, 181 of whom were selected for bypass surgery (160 primarily, 21 after intracoronary thrombolysis failed) from 1 to 36 hours after the onset of chest pain. The overall mortality rate was 4.4 percent. However, patients undergoing surgery as primary therapy had a mortality rate of 1.2 percent (2/160), whereas patients undergoing surgery after intracoronary thrombolysis failed had a mortality rate of 29 percent (6/21). Phillips et al. [14] updated this experience in 1986: Of 738 patients with evolving myocardial infarction, 261 underwent surgical reperfusion; the overall mortality rate was 5.7 percent. In addition to low mortality rates, these studies reported improvement in ventricular function after successful revascularization. For patients whose operation takes place within 4 hours after the onset of chest pain, infarct size (as estimated by thallium scrintigraphy) can be limited [15].

Many years have passed since these two reports (12, 13) were published. Although the surgical results were impressive, these studies have been validly criticized. They were neither randomized nor prospective studies. They were flawed by patient selection bias, especially by the inclusion of low-risk patients: 80 percent had one- or two-vessel coronary artery disease (50 percent one-vessel, 30 percent two-vessel disease) [14, 15]. True surgical emergencies were either not included or comprised a minority of patients. Patients with multivessel disease undergoing percutaneous transluminal coronary angioplasty (PTCA) were excluded. Furthermore, the indications for surgical intervention in many patients were not signs of profound ischemia (e.g., intractable chest pain or shock). Emergency surgery was performed for patients with angiographic evidence of multiple-vessel disease.

Many recent studies attempted to clarify the role of emergency revascularization for patients with acute myocardial infarction [16–19]. Like the earlier studies in the 1980s, the recent ones also were nonrandomized, but their conclusions more accurately predict current results. These studies included patients with persistent ischemia refractory to aggressive medical therapy with intravenous nitroglycerin, and patients who first underwent thrombolytic therapy or PTCA. Operative mortality rates ranged from 10 to 15 percent. Important risk factors that increased mortality included left main coronary artery disease, reoperation, left ventricular dysfunction, and cardiogenic shock. Long-term results were not different from results for patients who underwent surgery for a remote infarction [20].

Current management of acute myocardial infarction includes thrombolytic therapy followed by, if necessary, coronary angiography to delineate coronary anatomy and to guide further therapy. PTCA and coronary bypass surgery both play a role in treating persistent ischemia. PTCA is clearly a good option for one- or two-vessel disease, whereas surgery is a better alternative when the site, extent, and characteristics of the offending coronary lesions make PTCA unsuitable or hazardous. When opting for surgery, one must take into account the availability of resources for providing surgical care to an acutely ill patient, so that reperfusion occurs within a reasonable time frame.

Emergency Surgery After Thrombolytic Therapy or Failed PTCA

For most patients, thrombolytic therapy is the front line of treatment of acute evolving myocardial infarction. Results of early surgery after thrombolytic therapy have been reported by many institutions. In a review of 13 reports between 1979 and 1986, comprising 1514 patients, Akins [21] reported that about a third of patients who receive thrombolytic therapy require surgery 1 hour to 2 weeks later. The mortality rate ranged from 0 to 16.7 percent, with an average of 4.1 percent. These rates seem acceptable, considering the clinically urgent situation. Postoperative bleeding complications and thus the use of blood products are increased in these patients.

Since its introduction in 1978, PTCA has emerged as a major tool in the armamentarium for treating coronary artery disease [22]. Initially it was restricted to select patients. However, as interventional cardiologists have gained more experience and as equipment has become more sophisticated, use of PTCA has expanded. Yet 3 to 8 percent of patients undergoing PTCA will still require emergency coronary bypass surgery for complications resulting in acute myocardial infarction [23]. Of 9360 patients who underwent PTCA at various institutions between 1979 and 1986, 491 (5.2 percent) required surgery, according to Akins's review [21]. The average mortality rate was 5.3 percent (range, 0 to 11.3 percent). In addition, a third of the patients had a myocardial infarction, and a fourth required an intra-aortic balloon pump.

Similarly, Parsonnet et al. [24] reviewed 15 series. Of 15,802 patients undergoing PTCA, 902 required emergency surgery. The average mortality rate was 5.9 percent (range, 0 to 24 percent). Barner et al. [25] reviewed 701 patients undergoing PTCA between 1982 and 1988. The average mortality rate was 3.6 percent (range, 0 to 7.7 percent). In contrast, a comparable group of patients undergoing elective surgery would have an operative mortality rate of less than 2 percent.

These series clearly point to increased complication rates for patients undergoing emergency bypass after thrombolytic therapy or PTCA failure. Repeated attempts at PTCA should be avoided. Ischemic insult should not be prolonged. Intra-aortic balloon pump support is recommended in patients with persistent ischemia. Emergency bypass with complete surgical revascularization is the preferred therapy.

Postinfarction Angina

In the early era of coronary artery bypass graft surgery, operative morbidity and mortality rates were believed to be too high for the procedure to be done within 2 to 4 weeks after a myocardial infarction occurred. In 1974 Dawson et al. [26] described 1700 patients who underwent coronary artery bypass surgery. The operative mortality rate was twice as high for patients undergoing revascularization within 30 days after infarction (14.5 percent) as for those who had had an infarction in the remote past (6.9 percent), and three to four times higher than that for patients with no previous infarction. Furthermore, patients who underwent surgery within the first 7 days after the occurrence of an acute infarction had a sixfold higher risk of early death, compared with patients undergoing surgery between days 31 and 60. Dawson et al. recommended deferring surgery for 30 days after acute myocardial infarction occurred, if possible. However, this recommendation was altered in the early 1980s, with further understanding of the pathophysiology of myocardial infarction and advances in myocardial protection techniques during cardiac surgery [27, 28].

The rationale for early surgical revascularization for patients with persistent or recurrent angina pectoris after an acute myocardial infarction has occurred derives from high rates of reinfarction and cardiac-related mortality, and the need for subsequent interventional therapy for patients who initially receive medical therapy [29, 30]. Persistent angina pectoris developing after myocardial infarction signifies viable, but persistently ischemic myocardium, either in the area of infarction (in the so-called border zone) or in some area remote from the infarction that is supplied by a severely stenosed artery [31, 32]. Reperfusion should be performed with surgery or PTCA, within hours to days after the onset of chest pain to salvage viable myocardium. Overall, coronary bypass surgery is now relatively safe to perform within 30 days after acute myocardial infarction for hemodynamically stable patients with preserved left ventricular function.

Recent studies examined variables that predict operative mortality and morbidity for patients undergoing coronary artery bypass early after a myocardial infarction has occurred [33–36]. Stuart et al. [33] looked at 226 patients who underwent bypass within 30 days after acute myocardial infarction between 1982 and 1986. The operative mortality rate was 5.3 percent. Significant independent predictors of perioperative mortality, by univariate and multivariate analyses, included transmural and anterior myocardial infarction and the need for preoperative intra-aortic balloon pumping for angina or congestive heart failure. Kennedy et al. [34] reported on 793 patients who underwent bypass within 30 days after acute myocardial infarction between 1982 and 1987. The overall mortality rate was 5.7 percent. However, subgroup mortality rates varied: For patients who underwent bypass 1 day after the myocardial infarction occurred, the rate was 9.9 percent; 2 to 7 days, 8.2 percent; and 8 to 30 days, 2.4 percent. The mortality rate for patients undergoing elective bypass surgery without a prior acute myocardial infarction was 1.9 percent. Kennedy et al. [34] also identified risk factors for increased morbidity and mortality, such as age over 70 years, emergency surgery, reoperations, congestive heart failure, and Q-wave myocardial infarction. Similarly, Kouchoukos et al. [35] reported on 240 patients who underwent bypass within 30 days after acute myocardial infarction for persistent or recurrent ischemia between 1985 to 1987. Significant independent predictors of increased mortality were left main coronary artery disease, female sex, and left ventricular dysfunction.

In summary, patients with postinfarction angina should undergo revascularization and their individual risk factors assessed (Table 35-1). Relief of angina occurs with a frequency equal to that for patients who underwent bypass more than 30 days after the infarction occurred. The long-term survival rate does not differ from that for patients who had an elective bypass. However, postoperative mortality and morbidity are higher, especially when surgery is done within 24 to 48 hours after the infarction occurred.

Cardiogenic Shock

Cardiogenic shock represents the failure of the myocardium to maintain a level of cardiac output necessary for adequate organ perfusion. Acute transmural myocardial infarction is followed in 10 to 15 percent of patients by cardiogenic shock, which in turn carries a high risk of mortality [37]. Considerable judgment is required to treat this difficult group of patients. Prompt inotropic support and intra-aortic balloon counterpulsation may help stabilize the patient. Numerous therapeutic interventions can now reduce infarct size with varying degrees of effectiveness, yet the mortality rate for patients without surgery remains in the 90 percent range [38]. However, timely revascularization in selected patients may reduce the mortality.

Patients should undergo urgent coronary angiography as they are being stabilized. Angiography is invaluable: Half of the patients undergoing catheterization become surgical candidates. Patients with proximal coronary stenosis with good-quality by-

Table 36-1
Mortality and risk assessment of patients undergoing CABG after recent MI

Authors	Year	No. of patients	Overall mortality rate	Significant predictors of perioperative mortality
Stuart et al. [33]	1988	226	5.3%	Transmural and anterior MI Preoperative IABP
Kennedy et al. [34]	1989	793	5.7%	Age > 70 yr Emergency surgery Reoperation Congestive heart failure Q-wave MI
Kouchoukos et al. [35]	1989	240	3.3%	Left main coronary artery disease Female sex Left ventricular dysfunction
Floten et al. [20]	1989	832	4.1%	Surgery within 24 hr of MI
Gardner et al. [36]	1989	300	5%	Ejection fraction Anterior and transmural MI Use of IABP
Edwards et al. [17]	1990	117	14.5%	Previous MI Hypertension Cardiopulmonary resuscitation Reoperation

MI = myocardial infarction; IABP = intra-aortic balloon pump; CABG = coronary artery bypass grafting.

passable distal vessels are considered for surgery. Early surgery in this group of patients results in a survival rate of at least 50 percent. If revascularization is done within 12 to 16 hours after the onset of symptoms, the survival rate can approach 75 to 80 percent [39].

Ventricular Assist Devices and Cardiac Transplantation

This review of coronary artery bypass surgery for patients with recent myocardial infarction would be incomplete without mentioning ventricular assist devices and cardiac transplantation. Obviously, these are reserved for patients who otherwise have no chance of survival. Ventricular assist devices (VADs) are best used in patients with reversible myocardial insufficiency. According to the VAD registry, 965 patients received a VAD between 1985 to 1990, for postcardiotomy cardiogenic shock. However, less than half of these patients could be weaned from circulatory assistance and only a fourth could be discharged from the hospital [40]. A total of 32 received a VAD as a bridge to cardiac transplantation, 20 (62.5 percent) of whom were discharged from the hospital. Such intervention is to be considered only in centers with experience and resources. Obviously a therapy of last resort, cardiac transplantation is severely limited by the shortage of donor organs.

Current management of patients with recent myocardial infarction entails a well-planned approach to achieve early restoration of blood flow to the myocardium, to limit myocardial damage and preserve ventricular function, and to improve the patient's quality of life. In recent years, many refinements in preoperative and postoperative care, anesthetic management, and myocardial preservation techniques during cardiac surgery have contributed to reduction in morbidity and mortality following coronary artery bypass surgery in patients with recent myocardial infarction. However, patient selection, clinical judgement, and understanding of various therapeutic options are paramount. Patients with three-vessel coronary artery disease with persistent postinfarction angina, cardiogenic shock, and mechanical lesions following myocardial infarction are better served with surgery. A close communication between cardiology and cardiac surgery teams is essential and will expedite care of this group of patients.

References

1. Haeser, K. *The Illustrated History of Surgery.* Gothenburg, Sweden: AB Nordbok, 1988. P. 256.
2. Reimer, K. A., Lowe, J. E., Rasmussen, M. M., and Jennings, R. B. The wave-front phenomenon of ischemic cell death. 1. Myocardial infarct size versus duration of coronary occlusion in dogs. *Circulation* 56:786, 1977.
3. Lavallee, M., Cox, D., Patrick, T. A., and Vatner, S. F. Salvage of myocardial function by coronary artery reperfusion 1, 2, and 3 hours after occlusion in conscious dogs. *Circ. Res.* 53:235, 1983.
4. DeWood, M. A., Spores, J., Notske, R., et al. Prevalence of total coronary occlusion during early hours of transmural myocardial infarction. *N. Engl. J. Med.* 303:897, 1980.
5. Maroko, P. R., Libby, P., Ginks, W. R., et al. Coronary artery perfusion, I. Early effects on local myocardial function and extent of myocardial necrosis. *J. Clin. Invest.* 51:2710, 1972.
6. Costantino, C., Corday, E., and Tsu-Wang, L. Revascularization after 3 hours of coronary artery occlusion: Effects of regional cardiac metabolic function and infarct size. *Am. J. Cardiol.* 36:368, 1975.
7. Bresnahan, G. F., Roberts, R., Shell, W. E., et al. Deleterious effects due to hemorrhage after myocardial reperfusion. *Am. J. Cardiol.* 33:82, 1974.
8. Kloner, R. A., Ganote, C. E., and Jennings, R. B. "No-reflow" phenomenon after temporary coronary occlusion in the dog. *J. Clin. Invest.* 54:1496, 1974.
9. Gazes, P. C., Kitchell, J. R., and Meltzer, L. E. Cooperative study: Death rate among 795 patients in first year after myocardial infarction. *J.A.M.A.* 197:906, 1966.
10. Dawson, J. T., Hall, R. J., Hallman, G. L., and Cooley, D. A. Mortality in patients undergoing coronary artery bypass surgery after myocardial infarction. *Am. J. Cardiol.* 33:483, 1974.
11. Berg, R., Jr., Kendall, R. W., Duvoisin, G. E., et al. Acute myocardial infarction: A surgical emergency. *J. Thorac. Cardiovasc. Surg.* 70:432, 1975.
12. DeWood, M. A., Spores, J., Berg, R. J. R., et al. Acute myocardial infarction. A decade of experience with surgical reperfusion in 701 patients. *Circulation* 68(Suppl II):118, 1983.
13. Phillips, S. J., Kongtahworn, C., Skinner, J. R., and Zeff, R. M. Emergency coronary artery reperfusion. A choice of therapy for evolving myocardial infarction. Results in 339 patients. *J. Thorac. Cardiovasc. Surg.* 86:679, 1983.
14. Phillips, S. J., Zeff, R. H., Skinner, J. R., et al. Reperfusion protocol and results in 738 patients with

evolving myocardial infarction. *Ann. Thorac. Surg.* 41:119, 1986.
15. Venhaecke, J., Flameng, W., Sergent, P., et al. Emergency bypass surgery: Late effects on size of infarction and ventricular function. *Circulation* 71:179, 1985.
16. Spencer, F. C. Emergency coronary artery bypass for acute infarction: An improved clinical experiment. *Circulation* 68:17, 1983.
17. Edwards, F. H., Bellamy, R. F., Burge, J. R., et al. True emergency coronary artery bypass surgery. *Ann. Thorac. Surg.* 49:603, 1990.
18. Fremes, S. E., Goldman, B. S., Weisel, R. D., et al. Recent preoperative myocardial infarction increases the risk of surgery for unstable angina. *J. Cardiac Surg.* 6:2, 1991.
19. Lichtenstein, S. V., Abel, J. G., and Salerno, T. A. Warm heart surgery and results of operation for recent myocardial infarction. *Ann. Thorac. Surg.* 52: 455, 1991.
20. Floten, H. S., Amad, A., Swanson, J. S., et al. Long-term survival after postinfarction bypass operation: Early versus late operation. *Ann. Thorac. Surg.* 48:757, 1989.
21. Akins, C. W. Early surgical revascularization following thrombolytic therapy or PTCA failure. In: A. Baue, A. Geha, G. L. Hammond, et al. (eds.), *Glenn's Thoracic and Cardiovascular Surgery.* East Norwalk, CT: Appleton & Lange, 1991. Pp. 1263–1270.
22. Grüntzig, A. R., Senning, A., and Seigenthaler, W. E. Nonoperative dilation of coronary artery stenosis: Percutaneous transluminal coronary angioplasty. *N. Engl. J. Med.* 301:61, 1979.
23. Lazar, H. L., and Hann, C. K. Determinants of myocardial infarction following emergency coronary artery bypass for failed PTCA. *Ann. Thorac. Surg.* 44:646, 1987.
24. Parsonnet, V., Fisch, D., Gielchinsk, I., et al. Emergency operation after failed angioplasty. *J. Thorac. Cardiovasc. Surg.* 96:198, 1988.
25. Barner, H. B., Lea, J. W., IV, Naunheim, K. S., et al. Emergency coronary bypass not associated with preoperative cardiogenic shock in failed angioplasty, after thrombolysis and for acute myocardial infarction. *Circulation* 79:152, 1989.
26. Dawson, J. T., Hell, R. T., Hallmann, G., et al. Mortality in patients undergoing coronary artery bypass surgery after myocardial infarction. *Am. J. Cardiol.* 33:483, 1974.
27. Jones, E. L., Waites, T. F., Craver, J. M., et al. Coronary bypass for relief of persistent pain following acute myocardial infarction. *Ann. Thorac. Surg.* 32:33, 1981.
28. Fudge, T. L., Harrington, O. B., Crosby, V. G., et al. Coronary artery bypass after recent myocardial infarction. *Arch. Surg.* 117:1418, 1982.
29. Gibson, R. S., Beller, G. A., Gheorghiade, M., et al. The prevalence and clinical significance of residual myocardial ischemia 2 weeks after uncomplicated non-Q-wave infarction. A prospective natural history study. *Circulation* 71:1186, 1986.
30. Bosch, X., Theroux, P., Waters, D. D., et al. Early postinfarction ischemia: Clinical, angiographic and prognostic significance. *Circulation* 75:988, 1987.
31. Hearse, D. J., and Yellon, D. M. The "border zone" in evolving myocardial infarction. Controversy or confusion? *Am. J. Cardiol.* 74:1321, 1981.
32. Schuster, E. H., and Bulkeley, B. H. Ischemia at a distance after myocardial infarction: A cause of early postinfarction angina. *Circulation* 62:509, 1980.
33. Stuart, R. S., Baumgartner, W. A., Soule, L., et al. Predictors of perioperative mortality in patients with unstable postinfarction angina. *Circulation* 78(Suppl I):163, 1988.
34. Kennedy, W. J., Ivey, T. D., Misbach, G., et al. Coronary artery bypass graft surgery early after acute myocardial infarction. *Circulation* 79(Suppl I):73, 1989.
35. Kouchoukos, N. T., Murphy, S., Philpott, T., et al. Coronary artery bypass grafting for postinfarction angina pectoris. *Circulation* 79(Suppl 1):1-68, 1989.
36. Gardner, T. J., Stuart, S., Greene, E. S., et al. The risk of coronary bypass surgery for patients with postinfarction angina. *Circulation* 79(Suppl 1):1-79, 1989.
37. Scheidt, S., Wilner, G., Mueller, H., et al. Intraaortic balloon counterpulsation in cardiogenic shock. Report of cooperative trial. *N. Engl. J. Med.* 288:979, 1973.
38. Dunkman, W. B., Leinbach, R. C., Buckley, M. J., et al. Clinical and hemodynamic results of intraaortic balloon pumping and surgery for cardiogenic shock. *Circulation* 46:465, 1972.
39. Moran, J. M., and Singh, A. K. Cardiogenic shock. In H. C. Grillo, G. W. Austen, W. E. Wilkins, et al. (eds.), *Current Therapy in Cardiothoracic Surgery.* Philadelphia: Decker, 1989. P. 432.
40. Pae, W. E., Miller, C. A., Matthews, Y., et al. Ventricular assist devices for postcardiotomy cardiogenic shock. A combined registry experience. *J. Thorac Cardiovasc. Surg.* 104:541, 1992.

37. Programmed Electrical Stimulation After Acute Myocardial Infarction

David A. Rawling and Jay W. Mason

The role of electrophysiologic studies in determining prognosis and guiding therapy in patients who have had a myocardial infarction is undergoing evaluation and evolution. At the present time electrophysiologic studies are used in four situations: (1) to evaluate the need for temporary prophylactic pacing in patients with acute bifascicular block, (2) to evaluate the need for a permanent pacemaker in patients who develop or have progression of conduction disturbances during their myocardial infarction, (3) to evaluate and guide therapy in patients developing sustained ventricular tachycardia or having a cardiac arrest during the postinfarct period (i.e., not occurring during the initial period of the myocardial infarction), and (4) to assess the patient's risk of sudden death after infarction so that those at highest risk can be selected for intervention to reduce their high sudden death risk.

Assessing the Need for Temporary Prophylactic Pacing for Acute Bundle Branch Block

Limited data are available regarding temporary prophylactic pacing for acute bundle branch block. Lie et al. [1] studied 50 consecutive patients with a new right bundle branch block, with or without hemiblock, complicating an acute anteroseptal myocardial infarction. His bundle recordings were made in 35 of these patients at the time of appearance of bundle branch block. Ten patients had only right bundle branch block. Only one had a prolonged HV interval (defined as an HV $\geq$ 60 msec), and none went on to develop complete heart block. Ten of 25 patients with bifascicular block had a normal HV interval; only one of these developed complete heart block. Eleven of 15 patients with bifascicular block and prolonged HV interval developed complete heart block. Thus 11 of 12 patients who developed complete heart block had a prolonged HV interval. Lie et al. concluded that His bundle recording was useful in patients with a *new* right bundle branch block and hemiblock that occurs during the first 24 hours of acute anteroseptal myocardial infarction as patients in this group with prolonged HV intervals are at high risk for development of complete heart block and should have a temporary pacemaker placed.

Two important limitations of the above-described study must be noted: First, Lie et al. specifically excluded patients without anteroseptal infarction; and, second, they excluded patients with left bundle branch block. Thus their results are based on a highly selected group of patients. Also, although the authors thought that 10 of 14 patients who developed complete heart block benefited from temporary pacing (by prevention of Stokes-Adams attacks), all 14 died in a hospital. Thus an overall benefit of HV interval measurement on in-hospital mortality has not been demonstrated.

Lichstein et al. [2, 3] reported two studies in which the HV interval was measured in patients who developed new bifascicular block as a result of an acute myocardial infarction. Measurements were made at the time of temporary pacemaker insertion, which was placed as soon as an electrocardiographic (ECG) pattern of bifascicular block developed. In the initial report of 15 patients [2], 4 had normal and 11 had prolonged HV intervals (defined as an HV interval of $\geq$ 55 msec). None of the 4 patients with normal HV intervals developed complete heart block, and only 1 of 11 patients with prolonged HV intervals developed complete heart block. This patient died suddenly 6 weeks later (2 weeks after permanent pacemaker implant).

Lichstein et al. [3] later extended the series to 28 patients. None of the 5 patients with normal HV intervals developed complete heart block, and just 4 (17 percent) of 23 patients with prolonged HV intervals developed complete heart block. Thus in this less selected patient population, Lichstein et al. found a prolonged HV interval to be less useful. Also, all patients in their study who developed complete heart block died, with an average postinfarct survival time of 3 weeks.

In summary, although electrophysiologic studies appear to be useful for identifying those within specific subsets of patients with acute infarction who will develop complete heart block, the overall mortality rate in this group is sufficiently high that the therapeutic value of HV interval measurement is reduced.

Assessing the Need for Permanent Pacemaker After Myocardial Infarction

Although several groups of investigators have suggested that patients who develop conduction disturbances or advanced degrees of atrioventricular (AV) block during an acute myocardial infarction require permanent pacing [4–8], the Birmingham pacer trial [9] suggested it was not the case. Given these conflicting opinions, it would be useful to have an objective means to determine which patients need permanent pacemaker placement. In 1973 Lichstein et al. [2] used electrophysiologic studies to assess long-term prognosis in patients who developed conduction abnormalities in association with acute infarction. Patients who developed a new bifascicular block had an HV interval measured at the time of temporary pacemaker insertion. In an initial study of 15 patients, Lichstein et al. [2] found that 3 of 4 patients with normal HV intervals (HV < 55 msec) who survived their infarction remained alive at follow-up, whereas 3 of 6 patients with prolonged HV intervals who survived the acute infarct died early during follow-up. Later the study was extended to 28 patients [3]. Now 4 of 5 patients with normal HV intervals survived the acute infarct and remained alive (3 weeks to 22 months' follow-up), whereas only 8 of 23 patients with prolonged HV intervals remained alive at an average of 9.2 months' follow-up. Thus all patients who survived an acute infarct and had a normal HV interval were alive at follow-up, whereas only 53 percent of those with a prolonged HV interval survived. However, of 7 "late" deaths in those with prolonged HV intervals, only 2 were sudden, and 1 of these patients had a permanent pacemaker.

Harper et al. [10] studied 72 patients with AV or bundle branch block associated with acute infarction. They divided the patients into three groups: Group 1 consisted of 32 patients with AV block of more than first degree but with no intraventricular conduction defect (i.e., the QRS duration was normal). Group 2 consisted of 18 patients with either complete right or left bundle branch block, with or without hemiblock. Patients with both acute and chronic bundle branch block were included. Group 3 consisted of 22 patients with complete bundle branch block (right or left) *plus* an acute episode of any degree of AV block.

Harper et al. found that 30 of 32 patients in group 1 had normal HV intervals, including 7 of 9 in complete heart block at the time of study. Only 5 of these 32 patients died, 4 in a hospital. One-half of the group 2 patients had prolonged HV intervals; none died in a hospital, and there were two late deaths. Seventeen group 3 patients had distal His block; 3 also had a prolonged AH interval. Of 14 with distal His block alone, 10 died in a hospital. Also 12 of the group 3 patients progressed to second- or third-degree AV block; 9 of them died in a hospital despite having a temporary pacemaker in place. Harper et al. concluded that His bundle recording added little in determining the site of the AV block.

The authors repeated His bundle recordings in 19 patients 10 to 14 days after the infarction occurred. They found that only 2 group 3 patients showed a more than 10-msec change in HV interval over the intervening period.

Pagnoni et al. [11] studied 59 patients at the time they developed a new conduction disturbance (except Mobitz II or third-degree AV block) during an acute infarction. Fourteen patients (24 percent) had a prolonged HV interval (> 55 msec). Although the mortality rate was higher in these patients than in those with a normal HV interval (50 versus 13 percent), those with a prolonged HV interval had greater cardiac dysfunction. Only 1 patient (with an HV interval of 90 msec) progressed to complete heart block. During follow-up there were only three sudden deaths, one of a patient with a normal HV interval. Thus in this study and that of Lichstein et al. [3] there were only 4 of 78 patients in whom a permanent pacemaker might have influenced outcome.

The Birmingham trial [9] approached the issue differently. Fifty patients with a new, but persistent, conduction defect after an acute myocardial infarction were randomized either to receive a permanent pacemaker (23 patients) or to a control group. Patients with left bundle branch block were excluded. HV intervals were measured at the time of randomization. Throughout the follow-up period, up to 5 years, there was no difference in survival between the paced and unpaced groups. Furthermore, no conduction disorder progression was observed, and no significant differences were found in the average HV interval in the two groups. Thus the HV interval did not appear predictive of outcome, but few patients in the study had HV intervals of more than 70 msec, which has been found to identify patients at higher risk by some authors [12, 13].

How does the HV interval change over time after an acute myocardial infarction? Lichstein et al. [3] repeated HV measurements in ten patients an average of 18 days after the first measurement. The HV interval decreased an average of 2 msec between the two recordings. Only one patient had a "significant" (10-msec) increase in HV interval. Harper et al. [10] found only 2 of 19 patients to have a more than 10-msec HV interval increase at 10 to 14 days. Pagnoni et al. [11] remeasured the HV interval in 48 surviving patients an average of 7.2 months after infarction and found no significant change. Overall, the available data, though somewhat limited, suggest that the HV interval remains relatively constant during the first few weeks to months after myocardial infarction.

In summary, although a prolonged HV interval in association with a new conduction disturbance occurring during an acute myocardial infarction is associated with a poor prognosis, at present there is insufficient information to determine that HV interval measurement can be used to decide the need for permanent pacemaker placement. Only a large, prospective study can resolve this issue. Such a study should be patterned after the Birmingham trial [9] and should include both early and late measurement of HV interval. Also, those patients receiving pacemakers should receive units with rate hysteresis in which the lower rate is set low (e.g., 40 beats per minute); the units should provide a count of pacing events. In contrast to the Birmingham trial, however, patients with new left bundle branch block should be included.

Studies in Patients with Ventricular Tachycardia or Ventricular Fibrillation After Myocardial Infarction

Although most ventricular tachyarrhythmia episodes occur within the first 48 hours of acute myocardial infarction, some patients, usually those with extensive, complicated infarction [14–16], develop recurrent, sustained ventricular tachyarrhythmias after the first 2 days of infarction. The prognosis of these patients is grim. They have a 1-year mortality rate of 50 to 80 percent [14–20]. Because these patients are at high risk, several approaches have been tried to reduce the risk. In a retrospective study, Wald et al. [15] performed coronary artery bypass grafting or aneurysmectomy (or both) in 16 of 25 patients who developed medically intractable ventricular tachyarrhythmias an average of 5 weeks after a large anterior infarction occurred. The survival rate in the surgically treated group was 62 percent, whereas all 9 medically treated patients died either in a hospital or within 2 months of hospital discharge. Although Wald et al. concluded that surgery improved survival, their results appear seriously flawed, as surgery was actually offered to *all* patients. Therefore the medically treated group was *not* randomly selected, but was selected by either patient or physician choice, often because of a projected high operative mortality rate.

In another retrospective study Marchlinski et al. [20] used electrophysiologic studies to guide therapy in 40 patients with sustained ventricular tachyarrhythmias early after infarction. Thirty-three patients with inducible ventricular tachyarrhythmias were tried on several "standard" antiarrhythmic agents; if they failed, mexiletine or amiodarone (occasionally with another drug) was tried. If all drugs failed, the patient was referred for surgical management. Patients ultimately received a variety of therapies, including electrophysiologically guided antiarrhythmic therapy (7 patients), amiodarone (8 patients), clinically guided antiarrhythmic therapy (3 patients), and guided endocardial resection (11 patients). Also, 1 patient had a "non-directed" aneurysmectomy, and 3 patients were discharged without testing of their discharge drug. Finally, 2 of 7 patients in whom tachyarrythmias were not inducible at baseline electrophysiology study received no therapy, 3 received procainamide, and 2 had surgery (aneurysmectomy and "guided" endocardial resection).

During 20 months' mean follow-up, one-half of these patients died, 11 suddenly. As subgroup analyses failed to show superior results for any treatment, Marchlinski et al. [20] concluded that prognosis was poor in these patients regardless of therapy. A problem with this interpretation, however, is that patient number in each subgroup was small.

As reported in a subsequent abstract [21] these investigators divided 85 patients into two treatment groups: electrophysiologically guided medical therapy or surgical management. Patients with one or two clinical episodes of ventricular tachycardia prior to their baseline electrophysiology study (group A) were compared with those who had three or more episodes (group B). No difference in rates of survival (78 percent medical, 67 percent surgical) or ventricular tachycardia recurrence/sudden death (22 percent medical, 0 percent surgical) was found between the two treatment modalities in group A patients, but an improvement in ventricular tachycardia recurrence/sudden death rate was seen in surgically treated group B patients (59 percent medical, 22 percent surgical). Thus medical or surgical therapy appeared to work well for patients with less ventricular tachycardia, but surgery was better for those with frequent arrhythmias. However, with the variety of medical therapy probably used, the significance of these findings is questionable.

Finally, DiMarco et al. [16] reported 53 patients who developed sustained ventricular tachyarrhythmias within 2 months of myocardial infarction. Thirty-four patients were considered clinically stable after their initial event and underwent electrophysiology study. Twenty of 29 patients who had ventricular tachyarrhythmias inducible were discharged on antiarrhythmic therapy (14 on amiodarone). Nine underwent elective cardiac surgery because of limiting angina or heart failure and had intraoperative mapping and arrhythmia focus ablation also attempted. In 4 patients tachyarrhythmias were not inducible and the patients did not receive any antiarrhythmic therapy.

Nineteen patients were considered clinically unstable after their initial event. Three of them died from cardiac arrest; the other 16 underwent emergency cardiac surgery, which included aneurysmectomy, attempted arrhythmia focus ablation, and bypass surgery in 12. There were four operative deaths. Only 13 patients (52 percent) were considered successfully mapped, and 5 of them required long-term antiarrhythmic therapy. Nevertheless, 19 of the 21 surviving surgically treated patients were alive at 17.9 months' average follow-up. In the medically treated group, 21 of the 24 patients were alive at 15 months' average follow-up. DiMarco et al. concluded that an aggressive medical and surgical approach offered the best chance of survival for these patients.

In summary, electrophysiologic studies have been used in patients with sustained ventricular tachyarrhythmias "early" after myocardial infarction to guide antiarrhythmic or surgical therapy. However, as all reported series were retrospective and used a variety of therapies, it is difficult to determine how much the electrophysiology studies contributed to improving patient survival. Regardless of the mode of therapy, however, the long-term prognosis for these patients appears poor.

Assessing the Risk of Sudden Death After Myocardial Infarction

Sustained ventricular tachyarrhythmias are a major cause of mortality in patients who survive an acute myocardial infarction [22, 23]. As a result, numerous investigators have tried to identify specific risk factors for sudden death [24–41]. Two factors that have been found to provide the greatest prognostic information are (1) left ventricular function and (2) the presence of frequent or complex ventricular arrhythmias, or both [23, 25–27, 29–37, 39–43].

Once these prognostic factors were identified, investigators began to look for ways to improve patient survival. In patients with poor left ventricular function, inotropes, vasodilators, calcium channel blockers, and even beta blockers [44] were tried. In patients with frequent or complex ventricular ectopy, or both, several trials of prophylactic antiarrhythmic therapy were carried out. To date, however, the overall results of these antiarrhythmic trials have been disappointing [45–47, 120].

Several reasons have been proposed to explain the failure of these trials to show benefit: (1) The choice of antiarrhythmic drugs was suboptimal. Two studies used phenytoin and two trials used aprindine. (2) The trials were too small. Only two trials included more than 350 patients. (3) In most studies a fixed drug dose was used. Drug levels therefore varied from subtherapeutic to toxic. (4) In most trials no effort was made to document arrhythmia suppression with the drug. (5) Adverse effects were common and led to withdrawal of a significant portion of patients on active drug. (6) Finally, patient selection was poor as ''high-risk'' patients were not selectively enrolled.

Because of the problems with these studies, investigators have been trying to improve antiarrhythmic trial design [48] and find other ways to better identify high-risk patients so that future antiarrhythmic drug trials can be better focused. One method currently being explored is electrophysiologic study. The hypothesis is that patients with inducible ventricular arrhythmias are more prone to clinical ventricular tachyarrhythmias and that antiarrhythmic drug therapy will improve survival.

Tables 37-1 and 37-2 highlight the studies published to date. Studies have appeared as full manuscripts (Table 37-1) or as abstracts (Table 37-2). Nine of 17 full manuscript studies have been said to show that electrophysiologic studies provide useful prognostic information; 2 of 5 studies reported in abstract form reached similar conclusions. Thus one-half of the published studies support electrophysiologic testing, and one-half do not. How can we explain this difference?

We have found six study features that strongly influence the study's results: (1) the time after the acute infarct when the patients were studied, (2) the stimulation protocol used, (3) the endpoint for a positive study, (4) the length of follow-up, (5) the number of ''events'' that occurred, and (6) any treatment modalities patients received that could alter their inherent risk of developing an ''event.'' When we compare the studies in Tables 37-1 and 37-2, the most striking finding is the *lack* of uniformity in study design or method, with the four most consistent studies [49–51, 121] coming from the same group of investigators.

How might the above-mentioned features influence the results of the studies? First, let us consider the time after infarct when patients were studied. As summarized in Table 37-3, the time after infarction when the patients were studied ranged from 5 days to more than a year, although most were studied during the first 4 weeks. This factor is important, as several studies [52–58, 124] showed that there is variable concordance between electrophysiologic findings ''early'' and ''late'' after myocardial infarction. Kuck et al. [56] studied 18 patients 5 and 24 days after an infarct and found 2 patients with inducible sustained ventricular tachycardia at day 5, but in 9 patients sustained ventricular tachycardia was inducible at day 24. Also, Aonuma et al. [55] studied 19 patients at three time periods after infarction. A positive study was defined as one in which six or more repetitive ventricular responses were induced. Fifty-three percent of the patients had a positive study 2 to 3 weeks after the infarction occurred, 37 percent were positive at 4 to 6 weeks, and 21 percent were positive at 12 to 14 weeks. Furthermore, 80, 85, and 100 percent of patients had sustained ventricular tachycardia induced at the respective intervals. Aonuma et al. [55] concluded that electrophysiologic study results were time dependent. Roy et al. [57], however, found a 76 percent concordance in 21 patients studied an average of 12 days and 8 months after infarction. A group of 150 patients were initially studied; in 21, arrhythmias were inducible (2 had ventricular fibrillation, 8 had sustained ventricular tachycardia, and 11 had nonsustained ventricular tachycardia). During the repeat study, six of the ten patients with sustained tachyarrhythmias initially still had a sustained tachycardia, two had nonsustained ventricular tachycardia, and in two, arrhythmias were not inducible. Eleven patients had nonsustained arrhythmias at the first study; 1 now had ventricular fibrillation, 7 had nonsustained ventricular tachycardia, and in 3, arrhythmias were not inducible. Because 16 pa-

Table 37-1
Electrophysiologic studies (published as articles)

Parameter	Greene et al. [73]	Hamer et al. [74]	Richards et al.[a] [49 (100, 101)]	Marchlinski et al. [75, 102]	Kowey et al. [103]	Somberg et al. [61, 63]	Santarelli et al. [104 (105)]	Waspe et al. [95]	Denniss et al. [50]
No. of pts. studied	48[b]	70[c]	165	46	57[d]	29[e]	50	50[g]	175
No. eligible	?	?	304	?	?	47[e]	119	~250[g]	339
Av. time post-MI pts. studied	24 days	11 days (median)	10 days	22 days	12 mo	10–20 days	25 days	16 days	1–4 wk
Age (av.)	51	59	54	57	56	?	53	65	55
S_1–S_1	AP (700)	SR, AP (600,500) VP (500,400)	VP (600)	SR, VP (600,400)	VP (< sinus, 500)	VP (500)	VP (600,460)	SR, VP (600,425)	VP (600)
No. of extrastimuli	1	1–2	1–2	1–2	1–3	1–4	1–2	1–3[h]	1–2
Sites stimulated	RVA, RVOT	RVA, RVOT	RVA, RVOT	RVA	RVA	RVA, RVOT	RVA, RVOT	RVA, RVOT	RVA, RVOT
Current strength	2 × DT	2 V, 4–10 V	2 × DT, 20 mA	2 × DT	2 × DT	2 × DT	2 mA, 10 mA	4 × DT	2 × DT, 20 mA
P.W. (msec)	0.9	2	2	1	2	2	2	1	2
Reproducible?	NS	Yes	NS	NS	Yes	NS	NS	NS	NS
Endpoint for positive study	≥2 RVRs	≥2 RVRs; > 5 RVRs gave better discrimination	>10 sec VT/VF	≥ 2 RVRs	≥ 5 RVRs	≥ 10 beats VT	≥ 10 RVRs	≥ 8 RVRs	> 10 sec VT/VF
RVRs	19			13					
NSVT		12	–	5	13	10	13	6	–
Sust. VT		8	–	5	5	18	10	11	–
VF		0	–	0	0	0	0	0	–
Pos. study	19	20	38	23	18	28	23	17	38
LVEF (av.)	48%	–	55%	44%	49%	37%	45%	44%	52%
Follow-up (mo)	12 (av.)	12 (av.)	8 (av.)	18 (av.)	None	12.5 (av.)	11.2 (av.)	22.8 (av.)	12 (minimum)
a.a.	?	26 pts. (37%)	8%	15%	?	96%[f]	24%	14 (28%)[i]	8 (5%)
β-Block	?	"Some"	20%	39%	51%	17%	16%	13 (26%)	48 (27%)
CABG or PTCA	?	5 pts. (7%)	13%	9%	?	?	14%	9 (18%)	27 (15%)
+ pts. - SD	8	4	9	4		0	0	6	10
+ pts. - VT	7	0	4	0		1	3	1	–
– pts. - SD	4	1/17 full study. 4/33 limited studies	1	2		0	0	0	8
– pts. - VT	0		2	0		0	0	0	–
EPS worthwhile	Yes	Yes	Yes	No	?	Yes	Not sure	Yes	Yes

MI = myocardial infarction; AP = atrial paced rhythm; SR = sinus rhythm; VP = ventricular paced rhythm; RVA = right ventricular apex; RVOT = right ventricular outflow tract; LV = left ventricle; P.W. = pulse width; DT = diastolic threshold; NS = not studied; RVRs = repetitive ventricular responses; VT = ventricular tachycardia; VF = ventricular fibrillation; NSVT = nonsustained ventricular tachycardia; LVEF = left ventricular ejection fraction; a.a. = antiarrhythmia therapy; CABG = coronary artery bypass graft; PTCA = percutaneous transluminal coronary angioplasty; + pts. = positive study; – pts. = negative study; SD = sudden death; EPS = electrophysiologic study, VB = ventricular burst pacing.

[a]Large patient overlap between this study and that of Denniss et al. [50].

[b]Patients had ventricular arrhythmias after first 24 hr in coronary care unit.

[c]Patients had mechanical or electrical complications of their acute MI.

[d]17 Patients had VF with acute MI.

[e]On preentry Holter, 15% had cardiac arrest, 62% had symptomatic ventricular arrhythmias, 15% had asymptomatic ventricular arrhythmias.

[f]Lorcainide in 67%; all but two had EP-guided therapy.

Parameter	Roy et al. [94 (106, 107)]	Bhandari et al. [64, 125 (108)]	Breithardt et al. [96, 97 (109–111)]	Denniss et al. [51 (112, 113)]	McComb et al. [87]	Cripps et al. [126]	Iesaka et al. [127]	Richards et al. [121]	Nogami et al. [124]
No. of pts. studied	150	75	132	403	92[l]	75	133	313	32
No. eligible	320	164	379	495	92	209	180	457	44
Av. time post-MI pts. studied	12 days	11 days	22 days	12 days	12 days	21 days	1.8 mo	7–10 days	19 and 36 days
Age (av.)	52	53	56	52	52	55	57	<71 yr	61
S_1–S_1	VP (600,400)	VP (500,400)	SR, VP (500,430, 370,330)	VP (600)	SR, VP (600,500, 400)	SR, VP (600,500, 430)	VP (600,400)	Protocol 1: VP (600) Protocol 2:	VP (600,400)
No. of extrastimuli	1–2	1–3, VB	1–2	1–2	SR 1–3; VP 1–2	1–3	1–3	P1: 1–2 P2: 1–5	1–3
Sites stimulated	RVA, RVOT	RVA, RVOT, LV apex	RVA	RVA, RVOT	RVA	RVA	RVA, RVOT	P1: RVA, RVOT P2: ?	RVA, RVOT
Current strength	2 × DT	2 × DT	2 × DT	2 × DT, 20 mA	2.5 mA	2 × DT	?	P1: 2 × DT, 20 mA P2: 2 × DT	2 × DT
P.W. (msec)	1.5	2	1.8	2	2	2	?	?	1.0
Reproducible?	No	No	NS	No	NSVT only	NSVT only	NS	NS	"Not checked"
Endpoint for positive study	≥ 6 RVRs	Sust. VT/VF	≥ 4 RVRs	> 10 sec VT/VF	≥ 5 RVRs	Sust. mono. VT	Sust. mono. VT	> 10 sec VT/VF	Sust. VT
RvRs	85	5	27	–	–	44	?	?	Day 19: ? Day 36: ?
NSVT	17	6	6	–	12	23	21	?	2 16
Sust. VT	16	19	28	80	20	8	25	27	12 8
VF	2	14		56	–	14	11	132	8 8
Pos. study	35	33	61	136	32	8	25	27	12 8
LVEF (av.)	46%	48%	–	35% (meas. in those with + EPS)	50%	<40% in 85%	51%	?	41%
Follow-up (mo)	10 (av.)	18 (av.)	15 (av.)	12	30	16 mo	21	Min. 1 yr, median 2.0 yr	21 mo
a.a.	5 (3%)	10 (13%)[j]	26 (20%)	63 (16%)[m]	32 (35%)[n]	0	0		
β-Block	66 (44%)	7 (9%)	44 (33%)[k]	126 (31%)	35 (38%)	?	?	136 (43%)	9 (28%)
CABG or PTCA	21 (14%)	11 (15%)	22 (17%)	66 (16%)	?	9	?	?	1
+ pts. - SD	1	3	1	0.90 (1-yr actuarial survival)	0	1	70% 1-yr	15.2 times	Day 19: 4/12
+ pts. - VT	1	2	9		1	5	Event free	Risk for electrical event	Day 36: 5/8
− pts. - SD	1	1	3	0.96 (1-yr actuarial survival)	1	0	98% 1-yr		Day 19: 1/20
− pts. - VT	1	1	0		0	0	Event free	with + EPS	Day 36: 0/24
EPS worthwhile	No	No	Probably	Yes	Cannot say	Not cost-effective	Yes	Yes	

[g]All had complicated MI (new conduction disturbance and/or ventricular tachyarrhythmias and/or congestive heart failure).
[h]Varied during study (10-1, 10-2, 30-3).
[i]Some EP-guided therapy; more positive patients got treated.
[j]Given to patients with positive EPS for first 3–6 mo.
[k]Most with positive EPS.
[l]All received thrombolytic therapy for their acute MI.
[m]Mostly given to patients with positive EPS.
[n]Given to patients with positive EPS.

Table 37-2
Electrophysiologic studies (published as abstracts)

Parameter	Gonzales et al. [114]	Pumphrey et al. [86]	Korn et al. [62]	Bhandari et al. [83]	Iesaka et al. [115]
No. pts. studied	84	70	38	75	133
No. eligible	?	?	?	?	?
Time post-MI studied	6–8 wk	≤ 4 wk	7–10 days	14 days av.	1.8 mo av.
Age	32–70				
S_1–S_2		SR, VP (600,500)	2 C.L.		
No. extrastimuli	1–2	1–2	1–4, VB	1–3	1–3
Sites stim.	RVA		RVA, RVOT	RVA, RVOT, LV	RVA, RVOT
Current strength	2 × DT		5 mA		
Pulse width			2		
Reproducibility	NS	NS	NS	NS	NS
Endpoint for positive study	≥ 6 RVRs	≥ 4 RVRs	NSVT or sust. VT	Sust. VT/VF	
RVRs	29				21
NSVT	} 19		} 33		36
Sust. VT				19	
VF				14	
+ Study	19	16		33	57
LVEF (av.)		48%			
Follow-up (mo)	20	3 mo (minimum)	12.3	16	20
Other therapy					
a.a.		9 pts.[a]			
β-Blocker			About 75%		
CABG					
+ pts. - SD	0	2[b]			8
+ pts. - VT	0			} 5	1
− pts. - SD	4		} 4 S.D.		
− pts. - VT	0			} 2	
EPS of value	No	?	No	Yes	Yes

[a]Given to patients with positive EPS.
[b]Both on sotalol.
See Table 37-1 for key to abbreviations.

Table 37-3
Time after infarct: Influence on studies

Ref.	No. of pts.	Time after MI studied	Endpoint	No. of pts. with pos. study	% Pos. studies	Av. follow-up (mo)	Pts. with VT/SD No.	Pts. with VT/SD %
73	48	24 days	≥ 2 RVRs	19	40	12	19	40
74	70	11 days	≥ 2 RVRs	20	29*	12	9	13
49	165	10 days	≥10 sec VT/VF	38	23	8	16	10
75	46	22 days	≤ 2 RVRs	23	50	18	6	13
103	57	12 mo	≥ 5 RVRs	18	32			
61, 63	29	10–20 days	≥10 betas VT	28	97*	12.5	1	3
104	50	25 days	≥10 RVRs	23	46	11.2	3	6
95	50	16 days	≥ 8 RVRs	17	34*	22.8	7	14
50	175	1–4 wk	>10 sec VT/VF	38	22	Min. 12	10	6
94	150	12 days	≥ 6 RVRs	35	23	10	4	3
64	45	14 days	Sust. VT/VF	20	44	10	3	7
96, 97	132	22 days	≥ 4 RVRs	61	46	15	13	10
51	403	12 days	>10 sec VT/VF	136	34	12	34	9
87	92	12 days	≥ 5 RVRs	32	35*	30	2	2
114	84	6–8 wk	≥ 6 RVRs	19	23	20	4	5
86	70	≤4 wk	≥ 4 RVRs	16	23	Min. 3	2	3
62	38	7–10 days	?	33	87	12.3	4	11
83	75	14 days	Sust. VT/VF	33	44	16	7	9
115	133	1.8 mo	?	57	43	20	9	7
81	72	3–4 wk	Sust. VT/VF	53	74			
54	70	3–4 wk	≥ 6 RVRs	33	47	10.3	3	4
56	18	5 days	Sust. VT/VF	2	11	24	0	0
55	19	2–3 wk	≥ 6 RVRs	10	53			
84	84	5–10 days	Sust. VT/VF	18	21*			
82	36	26 days	Sust. VT/VF	25	69*	14	1	3
58	62	15 days	Sust. VT/VF	26	42	19	5	8
116	84	4 wk	≥ 6 RVRs	25	30			
117	33	<6 wk	?	9	27	12	2	6
85	111	2–52 wk	Sust. VT/VF	92	83	12	2	2
126	7 5	21 days	Sust. MVT	8	11	16	6	8
127	133	1.8 mo	Sust. MVT	25	19	21		
121	313	7–10 days	>10 sec VT/VF	27	9	Median 24		
124	32	19+36 days	Sust. VT	12/8	38/25	21	5	16
Total (or mean)	3054	32.3		1027	34	15.8	177	7.7

*Selected patients studied.
See Table 37-1 for key to abbreviations.

tients with inducible tachyarrhythmias at the first study had tachyarrhythmias induced at the second study, Roy et al. calculated the concordance to be 76 percent, although only 60 percent of patients with sustained ventricular arrhythmias and 64 percent of patients with nonsustained ventricular arrhythmias had the same type of arrhythmia induced at the second study.

Bhandari et al. [58, 123] reported on two series examining the reproducibility of induced arrhythmias in postinfarction patients. In the first [58], they studied 27 patients an average of 15 and 150 days after an acute myocardial infarction occurred. Of the 17 patients with inducible sustained arrhythmias at the first study, only 8 (47 percent) had a sustained tachyarrhythmia induced at the follow-up study. In the second series, Bhandari et al. [123] performed programmed stimulation on 56 patients on 2 consecutive days an average of 12 days after an acute myocardial infarction occurred. No patient had a history of documented or suspected sustained ventricular tachycardia or fibrillation occurring more than 48 hours after their infarct. Of the 21 patients with a sustained arrhythmia induced at the initial study, 16 (76 percent) had a sustained arrhythmia induced at the follow-up study. Of the 35 patients without a sustained arrhythmia inducible at the initial study, 31 (89 percent) also did not have a sustained arrhythmia induced on the follow-up study.

Finally, Nogami et al. [124] studied 32 patients 19 and 36 days after an acute myocardial infarction occurred. At the "early study" (day 19), sustained monomorphic ventricular tachycardia was induced in 12 patients; sustained polymorphic ventricular tachycardia in 1; nonsustained arrhythmias, in 2; and 10 patients had no arrhythmia induced. At the "late study" (day 36), only 8 patients had sustained monomorphic ventricular tachycardia induced; 5 of these patients had sustained monomorphic ventricular tachycardia induced at the early study.

These studies show that induction of ventricular tachyarrhythmias changes over time after infarction. This finding should not be surprising as other investigators have reported *day-to-day* changes in ventricular tachyarrhythmia induction [59, 60]. However, for postinfarction studies, the time after an infarction at which ventricular tachyarrhythmia inducibility stabilizes or the time at which specificity peaks remains largely unknown. As mentioned already, Nogami et al. [124] studied 32 patients 19 and 36 days after an acute myocardial infarction occurred. During the follow-up period (average 21 months) there were five arrhythmic events (sustained ventricular tachycardia or sudden death). Nogami et al. found the inducibility of sustained monomorphic ventricular tachycardia at the late study to have both a higher sensitivity and a higher specificity than at the early study (sensitivity, 100 versus 80 percent; specificity, 89 versus 70 percent). These authors concluded that studying patients at more than 4 weeks after a myocardial infarction occurred increased both the sensitivity and the specificity of electrophysiologic studies, and reduced the incidence of nondiagnostic responses. As shown in Table 37-3, however, very few of the published studies waited this long after infarction to begin testing.

The second feature to examine is the stimulation protocol used. Except for studies done by the same investigators, none of the protocols were the same. The basic drive varied from sinus rhythm to an atrial paced rhythm to ventricular paced rhythms; pacing cycle lengths also varied. One to two extrasystoles were used in most studies, but two groups used up to four extrastimuli [61–63] and two groups used ventricular burst pacing [62, 64]. In studies in which four extrastimuli were used, the percentage of positive studies was high (97 and 87 percent), raising the question of the specificity of the induction protocol, as several groups of investigators showed that specificity decreases as the number of extrastimuli is increased, especially above two extrastimuli [65–69].

Other stimulation protocol variations included the number of pacing sites used; most groups used two, but a few used only one, and Bhandari et al. [64] performed left ventricular stimulation. Stimulation current strength also varied. Most groups used current strengths of twice diastolic threshold, but some used current strengths of 10 to 20 mA. This point is a concern, as several studies questioned the sensitivity and specificity of using higher stimulus current strengths [69–72]. Finally, even pulse width varied among studies.

Richards et al. [121] tested the predictive ability of two different stimulation protocols. One protocol used up to two premature stimuli at two right ventricular sites; it also used a 20-mA stimulus intensity. (This protocol was used in their previously published studies [49–51].) The other protocol used up to five premature stimuli, each repeated three times, in an attempt to identify an optimal protocol for programmed stimulation after a myocardial infarction. Richards et al. found that maximal sensitivity and positive predictive accuracy were achieved when three extrastimuli were introduced at twice diastolic threshold.

The third feature to examine is the endpoint for a positive study, as it can profoundly influence the sensitivity and specificity of results. Again, significant variability was present (see Table 37-3). In three studies [73–75] induction of two repetitive ventricular responses was classified as a positive result. Although it may have increased study sensitivity, several other reports raised serious questions about the specificity of using so few repetitive ventricular responses [76–80]. In most studies a minimum of five repetitive ventricular responses had to be induced for a positive result. Several studies, however, required that a sustained ventricular tachyarrhythmia be induced for a positive result [53, 56, 58, 64, 81–85, 124, 126, 127]. Thus it is not surprising that reported ventricular tachyarrhythmia induction varied from 9 to 97 percent.

Only four groups reported testing arrhythmia induction reproducibility. Reproducibility was not tested in four studies, and in the rest it could not be determined.

The fourth feature to examine is the length of follow-up. Related to this point is the fifth feature, the number of events that occurred during follow-up. As the cumulative probability of a patient having an event increases with time, the longer the follow-up, the greater the number of events that should occur. This point is important because should no events occur (as in one study [56]), the study does not provide meaningful information. Table 37-3 shows that follow-up varied from a "minimum of 3 months" [86] to a 30-month average follow-up [87]. Because patients are at greatest risk of sudden death during the first 6 to 12 months after infarction [23, 88, 89], a well-designed study should have a minimum of 12 months' follow-up. As can be seen from Table 37-3, however, only 17 of the 33 studies had follow-up times of more than 12 months.

Given the variable follow-up periods, and the recruitment of specific patient groups in some studies, it is not surprising that the incidence of ventricular tachycardia or sudden death was variable (from 0 [56] to 40 percent [73]). This point is a concern because if the event rate is "too low," the power of the study to show that electrophysiologic testing has predictive value is low (a type II error).

The final factor is other therapies that might have altered the subject's risk of having an event and thus biased the outcome of the study. Three such therapeutic interventions and the percentage of patients receiving them are listed in Tables 37-1 and 37-2. The interventions are (1) use of antiarrhythmics, (2) use of beta blockers, and (3) coronary artery bypass surgery or angioplasty. The last is probably least important. Although there are data suggesting bypass surgery can decrease recurrence in patients who have had ventricular tachycardia or a cardiac arrest [90, 91], this effect appears to be uncertain and poorly defined [90–93]; for angioplasty no data are available. Nevertheless, these interventions could alter mortality and, depending on study endpoint, alter the study's conclusions. In the studies cited, 3 to 18 percent of patients underwent bypass surgery or angioplasty during follow-up.

In contrast to bypass surgery or angioplasty, antiarrhythmic therapy certainly could alter patient outcome, particularly if the results of the electrophysiology study were used to select those who would receive antiarrhythmic therapy. In the listed studies 3 percent [94] to 96 percent [61, 63] of the patients were given antiarrhythmic agents. Although most patients received antiarrhythmics without the results of the electrophysiology study influencing their use, in six studies [51, 61, 63, 64, 86, 87, 95] antiarrhythmics were preferentially given to patients with positive results. For example, Somberg et al. [61, 63] treated all (except one) patients with positive electrophysiology studies. Most were given lorcainide, with therapy guided by electrophysiology testing. McComb et al. [87] placed all 32 patients with positive electrophysiology studies on antiarrhythmic therapy using electrophysiologic testing to determine drug efficacy. Finally, Denniss et al. [51, 122] entered 96 of 136 patients with a positive electrophysiology study into a randomized trial; 49 of the 96 patients received quinidine, disopyramide, or mexiletine at dosages that achieved "therapeutic" serum levels. Denniss et al. [68, 122] found that antiarrhythmic therapy did *not* reduce subsequent events, perhaps

Table 37-4
Several studies using alternate techniques to determine risk after infarction

Ref.	No. of pts.	Test and criteria	Percent				Notes
			Sens.	Spec.	PPV	NPV	
31	430	HM; VT	30	92	38	88	
118	430	HM; ≥ 1 PVC/hr	75	56	23	93	
		HM; ≥ 10 PVC/hr	48	78	27	90	
		HM; ≥ 100 PVC/hr	13	94	26	86	
35	766	HM; ≥ 30 PVC/hr	18	90	19	92	a
		HM; VT	24	90	23	91	
		RNV; EF < 30%	42	88	30	92	
36	533	HM + RNV					
		EF > 40%, < 10 PVCs/hr	17	39	2	89	b
		EF < 40%, ≥ 10 PVCs/hr	24	93	18	96	
41	1640	HM: > 0 PVCs/24 hr	92	16			c
		≥ 10 PCVs/hr	25	88			
		Pairs or VT	34	81			
		Multiform PVCs	62	69			
		≥10 PVCs/hr or pairs or VT or multiform	67	61			
33	1739	HM; R-on-T or pairs or VT or multiform or bigeminy	56	74	5	99	d
34	139	HM + RNV; complex PVCs, age, EF <50%, anterior MI	85	79			
28	55	QT_c > 440 msec on 12-lead	57	81	76	65	e
39	750	RNV or cath					
		EF < 30%	20				
		EF < 40%	57				
		EF < 45%	77				
		RNV or cath + HM: EF <45% + PVCs ≥ Lown grade 2	41				
98	165	SAECG; late potential and/or long QRS	92	62			
		RNV or cath; EF < 40%	92	75			
		HM; Lown grade 3–5 PVCs	73	67			
43	200	SAECG; late potential only	93	65			
		SAECG; late potential and/or long QRS	50	90	28		
		SAECG + HM: abn. SAECG and complex PVCs	65	89			
		SAECG + RNV or cath; abn. SAECG and EF < 40%	80	89			
119	138	SAECG; late potentials occurring 350–500 msec after QRS	79	80			
99	102	SAECG; late potentials and/or long-duration low-amp. signals and/or long QRS	87	63	29	96	
		RNV; EF < 40%	80	54	24	94	
		HM; ≥ 10 PVCs/hr and/or couplets and/or NSVT	80	42	23	91	
		SAECG + RNV; abn. SAECG + EF < 40%	100	59	36	100	
		SAECG + HM; abn. SAECG + high-grade ectopy (as above)	100	45	35	100	
		HM + RNV; high-grade ectopy + EF < 40%	92	44	37	94	
		Abn. SAECG + high-grade ectopy + EF < 40%	100	53	50	100	
62	58	EPS; VT	80	28			
73	48	EPS; ≥ 2 RVRs	79	86	79	86	
		HM; Lown grade 4B–5	54	88			
74	70	EPS; ≥ 2 RVRs	44	74	20	90	
49	165	EPS; > 10 sec VT/VF	81	83	65	91	
75	46	EPS; ≥ 4 RVRs	17	82	13	86	b
		EPS; ≥ 2 RVRs	67	55	19	91	
		HM; Lown grade 3–4	50	58	16	88	
		RNV or cath or 2-D echo; EF < 40%	83	70	31	96	
		RNV or cath or 2-D echo; presence of LV aneurysm	83	78	38	97	

Table 37-4 (continued)

Ref.	No. of pts.	Test and criteria	Percent Sens.	Spec.	PPV	NPV	Notes
		EPS + HM; ≥ 4 RVRs and Lown grade 3–4	17	83	13	87	
		EPS + EF deter.; ≥4 RVRs + EF < 40%	17	98	50	89	
		HM + EF deter.; Lown grade 3–4 + EF < 40%	33	87	29	89	
104	50	EPS; ≥ 10 RVRs	100	57	13	100	
95	50	EPS; > 7 RVRs	100	57			
		RNV or cath; EF < 40%	100	52			
		RNV or cath; LV aneurysm	50	68			
		HM; Lown grade 4B	33	79			
		Patients receiving antiarrhythmic drug	50	75			
		Patients receiving CABG	17	82			
		Patients not treated	17	70			
50	228	EPS; > 10 sec VT/VF	56	82	26	94	
		ETT; ≥ 2 mm ST segment depression or elevation	58	70	11	96	
		EPS + ETT; both positive	88	65	13	99	
94	150	EPS; ≥ 6 RVRs	50	77	6	98	
64	45	EPS; sust. VT/VF	67	57	10	96	
96,97	132	EPS; ≥ 4 RVRs	77	57	16	96	
		SAECG; presence of late potential	77	59	17	96	
		EPS + SAECG; ≥ 4 RVRs + late potential	62	77	23	95	
51	403	EPS; > 10 sec VT/VF	57	83			
		SAECG; presence of delayed potentials	65	77			
		EPS + SAECG; > 10 sec VT/VF *and* late potentials	39	92			
		EPS + SAECG; > 10 sec VT/VF *or* late potentials	83	68			
		EPS; >10 sec VT/VF, 2 × DT current *only*	30	91			
87	92	EPS; ≥ 5 RVRs	50	66	3	98	f
121	361	EPS; > 10 sec VT	58	95	30	98	
		RNV; ≤ 40%	71	74	11	98	
		SAECG; vent. activation ≥ 120 msec	57	82	17	97	
		HM; > 60 PVCs/hr, couplets, NSVT, R-on-T	82	40	6	98	
		Left ventricular aneurysm	13	93	7	96	
126	75	Killip class > II	50	97	60		
		Cardiogenic shock, pulm. edema, persistent sinus tachycardia, elevated blood urea nitrogen	83	68	19		
		EF < 40% (RNV or cath)	67	76	22		
		SAECG; long QRS and late potentials	83	78	25		
		HM; PVCs > 10/hr	67	85	31		
		EP; NSVT	33	67	8		
		EP; SMVT	100	97	75		
127	133	EP; SMVT	82	87	36	98	
		Cath EF < 40%	55	87	27	95	
		EPS + EF	36	97	50	94	
		EPS or EF	100	75	28	100	
Range			13–100	16–98	2–79	65–100	

HM = Holter monitoring; VT = ventricular tachycardia; PVC = premature ventricular contractions; RNV = radionuclide ventriculography; EF = ejection fraction; SAECG = signal-averaged electrocardiography; VF = ventricular fibrillation; RVRs = repetitive ventricular responses; EPS = electrophysiologic study; NSVT = nonsustained ventricular tachycardia; CABG = coronary artery bypass graft; ETT = exercise treadmill test.

[a]Figured for 2-yr follow-up.

[b]Figured for 13-mo follow-up.

[c]For sudden death only.

[d]One hour of monitoring; figured for 5-yr follow-up.

[e]Figured for 10-yr follow-up.

[f]Patients had received thrombolytic therapy.

because the antiarrhythmics suppressed inducible ventricular arrhythmias in only 31 percent of treated patients. Thus several studies were possibly influenced by patients receiving antiarrhythmic agents, and six studies were definitely tainted as antiarrhythmic agents were selectively given to those with positive electrophysiology studies.

Arguments similar to those just mentioned can be made regarding the use of beta blockers. Beta blocker use varied from 0 percent to almost 80 percent, with an average of about one-third of patients in most studies receiving a beta blocker. Also, in one study [96, 97] beta blockers were preferentially given to patients with a positive electrophysiology result. Again, as with antiarrhythmic drugs, the substantial use of beta blockers may have had an important impact on the results of these studies.

Table 37-3 reviews selected aspects of the studies. The percentage of positive electrophysiology studies varied from 9 percent [121] to 97 percent [61, 63], with an average of 34 percent of patients having a positive study. None to 40 percent of patients had a major arrhythmic event during follow-up; the overall average was 7.7 percent during a 15.8-month average follow-up period. The wide percentage range of positive studies suggests that selection of certain patients for study inclusion and the variability in stimulation protocols, as well as the variable definitions of a positive result, significantly influenced the incidence of study positivity. On the other hand, the widely variable incidence of follow-up events suggests that administration of antiarrhythmics and beta blockers may have influenced this figure.

The above-mentioned considerations suggest that the prognostic usefulness of electrophysiologic testing soon after infarction has occurred remains to be established. Perhaps other trials, such as the Multicenter Automatic Defibrillator Implantation Trial (MADIT) [128], will help clarify the situation. In the MADIT, patients with poor left ventricular function, nonsustained ventricular tachycardia, and a prior myocardial infarction (at least 1 month after infarction) undergo electrophysiologic testing. If a sustained arrhythmia is induced (with specific caveats) and this arrhythmia is not suppressed by intravenous procainamide, the patient is randomized to receive either "conventional" (antiarrhythmic) therapy or an AICD. The primary objective of the trial is to determine whether implantation of an AICD in high-risk patients will reduce the overall mortality rate. Since the time after infarction when the patient enters the study is dichotomized (< 6 months and > 6 months), the ability of electrophysiologic testing to define a high-risk group of patients early after infarction may be able to be assessed.

Because electrophysiologic testing is both invasive and expensive, there has been ongoing concern regarding its cost-effectiveness in evaluating prognosis in postinfarction patients [123, 126, 129]. Table 37-4 provides an overview of several studies that used other techniques to determine risk after infarction. What is clear in the table is that we are much better at predicting that an event *will not occur* (negative predictive value) than we are at predicting its occurrence (positive predictive value). It produces a problem in antiarrhythmic therapy, as several patients must be treated to prevent an event in one.

Holter monitoring seems to be the least useful of the other techniques that have been used. Otherwise, there seems to be little difference in the overall usefulness of ejection fraction, presence of late potentials as measured by the signal-averaged ECG, and ventricular tachyarrhythmia induction by electrophysiology testing. For example, in the study by Kuchar et al. [98] information derived from the signal-averaged ECG and measurement of ejection fraction gave similar results, whereas Holter monitoring did less well. In contrast, in the study of Gomes et al. [99] information derived from the signal-averaged ECG did best, whereas measurement of ejection fraction and Holter monitoring indexes gave less predictive information.

Studies involving electrophysiologic testing do not show clear superiority for the technique. In the study of Marchlinski et al. [75] the presence of a left ventricular aneurysm gave the best predictive information, followed by ejection fraction. Holter monitoring did less well, and electrophysiologic testing was only marginally useful. In the study of Waspe et al. [95] both electrophysiologic testing and ejection fraction provided highly sensitive results, and Holter monitoring did poorly. Two studies compared electrophysiologic testing with the signal-averaged ECG. Breithardt et al. [96, 97] found that electrophysiologic testing and the signal-averaged ECG provided almost identical prognostic information. In the large study of Denniss et al. [51] the signal-averaged ECG again closely matched electrophysiologic testing for predictive ability. However, if the electrophysiologic results were based on using a stimulus strength of two times diastolic threshold, rather than the results with 20-mA stimulation, electrophysiologic testing did much worse.

In summary, the case for using electrophysiologic testing to help determine prognosis after infarction is weak. The reasons are as follows: First, studies to date give conflicting information about the usefulness of the technique, although part of it may be due to methodologic differences. Second, prognostic information similar to that obtained from electrophysiologic testing is available from other less invasive and less expensive techniques. Finally, when the results of electrophysiologic testing were used to identify patients needing antiarrhythmic therapy, treatment did not substantially improve survival. To determine the prognostic usefulness of electrophysiologic testing after myocardial infarction, a large, prospective study is required in which other tests thought to provide prognostic information are performed on each patient: Holter monitoring, signal-averaged ECG, radionuclide measurement of ejection fraction, and an exercise test. These tests should all be done 2 to 4 weeks after infarction. Test results should *not* alter therapy. The electrophysiologic testing protocol *must* be standardized; whether to use a high stimulus current could be a major issue. Finally, at least a 12-month follow-up is needed. Such a study should allow determination of the most cost-effective and accurate way to determine prognosis in patients after a myocardial infarction.

References

1. Lie, K. I., Wellens, H. J., Schuilenburg, R. M., et al. Factors influencing prognosis of bundle branch block complicating acute antero-septal infarction: The value of His bundle recordings. *Circulation* 50:935, 1974.
2. Lichstein, E., Gupta, P. K., Chadda, K. D., et al. Findings of prognostic value in patients with incomplete bilateral bundle branch block complicating acute myocardial infarction. *Am. J. Cardiol.* 32:913, 1973.
3. Lichstein, E., Gupta, P. K., and Chadda, K. D. Long-term survival of patients with incomplete bundle-branch block complicating acute myocardial infarction. *Br. Heart J.* 83:924, 1975.
4. Atkins, J. M., Leshin, S. J., Blomqvist, G., and Mullins, C. B. Ventricular conduction blocks and sudden death in acute myocardial infarction: Potential indications for pacing. *N. Engl. J. Med.* 288: 281, 1973.
5. Waugh, R. A., Wagner, G. S., Haney, T. L., et al. Immediate and remote prognostic significance of fascicular block during acute myocardial infarction. *Circulation* 47:765, 1973.
6. Ritter, W. S., Atkins, J. M., Blomqvist, C. G., and Mullins, C. B. Permanent pacing in patients with transient trifascicular block during acute myocardial infarction. *Am. J. Cardiol.* 38:205, 1976.
7. Hindman, M. C., Wagner, G. S., Jaro, M., et al. The clinical significance of bundle branch block complicating acute myocardial infarction. 1. Clinical characteristics, hospital mortality, and one-year follow-up. *Circulation* 58:679, 1978.
8. Hindman, M. C., Wagner, G. S., Jaro, M., et al. The clinical significance of bundle branch block complicating acute myocardial infarction. 2. *Circulation* 58:689, 1978.
9. Watson, R. D. S., Glover, D. R., Page, A. J. F., et al. The Birmingham trial of permanent pacing in patients with intraventricular conduction disorders after acute myocardial infarction. *Am. Heart J.* 108: 496, 1984.
10. Harper, R., Hunt, D., Vohra, J., et al. His bundle electrogram in patients with acute myocardial infarction complicated by atrioventricular or intraventricular conduction disturbances. *Br. Heart J.* 37:705, 1975.
11. Pagnoni, F., Finzi, A., Valentini, R., et al. Long-term prognostic significance and electrophysiological evolution of intraventricular conduction disturbances complicating acute myocardial infarction. *PACE* 9:91, 1986.
12. Scheinman, M. M., Peters, R. W., Sauve, M. J., et al. Value of the H-Q interval in patients with bundle branch block and the role of prophylactic permanent pacing. *Am. J. Cardiol.* 50:1316, 1982.
13. Scheinman, M. M., Peters, R. W., Morady, F., et al. Electrophysiologic studies in patients with bundle branch block. *PACE* 6:1157, 1983.
14. Lie, K. I., Liem, K. L., Schuilenburg, R. M., et al. Early identification of patients developing late in-hospital ventricular fibrillation after discharge from the Coronary Care Unit: A 5 1/2 year retrospective and prospective study of 1,897 patients. *Am. J. Cardiol.* 41:674, 1978.
15. Wald, R. W., Waxman, M. B., Corey, P. N., et al. Management of intractable ventricular tachyarrhythmias after myocardial infarction. *Am. J. Cardiol.* 44:329, 1979.
16. DiMarco, J. P., Lerman, B. B., Kron, K. L., and Sellers, T. D. Sustained ventricular tachyarrhythmias within 2 months of acute myocardial infarction: Results of medical and surgical therapy in patients resuscitated from the initial episode. *J. Am. Coll. Cardiol.* 6:759, 1985.

17. Wilson, C., and Adgey, A. A. J. Survival of patients with late ventricular fibrillation after acute myocardial infarction. *Lancet* 2:124, 1974.
18. Goldberg, R., Szklo, M., Tonascia, J., and Kennedy, H. L. Length of time between hospital admission and ventricular fibrillation or cardiac arrest: Complicating acute myocardial infarction: Effect on prognosis. *Johns Hopkins Med. J.* 145:187, 1979.
19. Wellens, H. J. J., Bar, F. W., Vanagt, E. J., and Brugada, P. Medical treatment of ventricular tachycardia: Considerations in the selection of patients for surgical treatment. *Am. J. Cardiol.* 49:186, 1982.
20. Marchlinski, F. E., Waxman, H. L., Buxton, A. D., and Josephson, M. E. Sustained ventricular tachyarrhythmias during the early postinfarction period: Electrophysiologic findings and prognosis for survival. *J. Am. Coll. Cardiol.* 2:240, 1983.
21. Kleiman, R. G., Marchlinski, F. E., Buxton, A. E., and Josephson, M. E. Ventricular tachycardia early after infarct (Abstract). *Circulation* 74(Suppl II): 11, 1986.
22. Horowitz, L. N., and Morganroth, J. Can we prevent sudden cardiac death? *Am. J. Cardiol.* 50:535, 1982.
23. Rosenthal, M. E., Oseran, D. S., Gang, E., and Peter, T. Sudden cardiac death following acute myocardial infarction. *Am. Heart J.* 109:865, 1985.
24. Kotler, M. N., Tabatznik, B., Mower, M. M., and Tominaga, S. Prognostic significance of ventricular ectopic beats with respect to sudden death in the late postinfarction period. *Circulation* 47:959, 1973.
25. Ruberman, W., Weinblatt, E., Goldberg, J. D., et al. Ventricular premature beats and mortality after myocardial infarction. *N. Engl. J. Med.* 297:750, 1977.
26. Schulze, R. A., Strauss, H. W., and Pitt, B. Sudden death in the year following myocardial infarction: Relation to ventricular premature contractions in the late hospital phase and left ventricular ejection fraction. *Am. J. Med.* 62:192, 1977.
27. Anderson, K. P., DeCamilla, J., and Moss, A. J. Clinical significance of ventricular tachycardia (3 beats or longer) detected during ambulatory monitoring after myocardial infarction. *Circulation* 57: 890, 1978.
28. Schwartz, P. J., and Wolf S. QT interval prolongation as predictor of sudden death in patients with myocardial infarction. *Circulation* 57:1074, 1978.
29. Hammermeister, K. E., DeRouen, T. A., and Dodge, H. T. Variables predictive of survival in patients with coronary artery disease. *Circulation* 59:421, 1979.
30. Moss, A. J., Davis, H. T., DeCamilla, J., and Bayer, L. W. Ventricular ectopic beats and their relation to sudden and nonsudden cardiac death after myocardial infarction. *Circulation* 60:998, 1979.
31. Bigger, J. T., Weld, F. M., and Rolnitzky, L. M. Prevalence, characteristics and significance of ventricular tachycardia (three or more complexes) detected with ambulatory electrocardiographic recording in the late hospital phase of acute myocardial infarction. *Am. J. Cardiol.* 48:815, 1981.
32. Ruberman, W., Weinblatt, E., Frank, C. W., et al. Repeated 1 hour electrocardiographic monitoring of survivors of myocardial infarction at 6 month intervals: Arrhythmia detection and relation to prognosis. *Am. J. Cardiol.* 47:1197, 1981.
33. Ruberman, W., Weinblatt, E., Goldberg, J. D., et al. Ventricular premature complexes and sudden death after myocardial infarction. *Circulation* 64:297, 1981.
34. Rapaport, E., and Remedios, P. The high risk patient and recovery from myocardial infarction: Recognition and management. *J. Am. Coll. Cardiol.* 1:391, 1983.
35. Bigger, J. T., Fleiss, J. L., Kleiger, R., et al. The relationships among ventricular arrhythmias, left ventricular dysfunction, and mortality in the 2 years after myocardial infarction. *Circulation* 69:250, 1984.
36. Mukharji, J., Rude, R. E., Poole, W. K., et al. Risk factors for sudden death after acute myocardial infarction: Two-year follow-up. *Am. J. Cardiol.* 54:3 1, 1984.
37. Olson, H. G., Lyons, K. P., Troop, P., et al. Prognostic implications of complicated ventricular arrhythmias early after hospital discharge in acute myocardial infarction: A serial ambulatory electrocardiography study. *Am. Heart J.* 108:1221, 1984.
38. Luria, M. H., Debanne, S. M., and Osman, M. I. Long-term follow-up after recovery from acute myocardial infarction: Observations on survival, ventricular arrhythmias, and sudden death. *Arch. Intern. Med.* 145:1592, 1985.
39. Ahnve, S., Gilpin, E., Henning, H., et al. Limitations and advantages of the ejection fraction for defining high risk after acute myocardial infarction. *Am. J. Cardiol.* 58:872, 1986.
40. Bigger, J. T., Fleiss, J. L., Rolnitzky, L. M., et al. Prevalence, characteristics and significance of ventricular tachycardia detected by 24-hour continuous electrocardiographic recordings in the late hospital phase of acute myocardial infarction. *Am. J. Cardiol.* 58:1151, 1986.
41. Kostis, J. B., Byington, R., Friedman, L. M., et al. Prognostic significance of ventricular ectopic activity in survivors of acute myocardial infarction. *J. Am. Coll. Cardiol.* 10:231, 1987.
42. Moss, A. J., DeCamilla, J., Mietlowski, W., et al. Prognostic grading and significance of ventricular premature beats after recovery from myocardial infarction. *Circulation* 51/52(Suppl III):204, 1975.
43. Kuchar, D. L., Thorburn, C. W., and Sammel, N. L. Prediction of serious arrhythmic events after myocardial infarction: Signal-averaged ECG, Holter monitoring and radionuclide ventriculography. *J. Am. Coll. Cardiol.* 10:531, 1987.
44. Furberg, C. D., and Yusuf, S. Effect of drug therapy on survival in chronic congestive heart failure. *Am. J. Cardiol.* 62:41A, 1988.
45. Furberg, C. D. Effect of antiarrhythmic drugs on mortality after myocardial infarction. *Am. J. Cardiol.* 52:32C, 1983.
46. IMPACT Research Group. International mexilitine

and placebo antiarrhythmic coronary trial. I. Report on arrhythmia and other findings. *J. Am. Coll. Cardiol.* 4:1148, 1984.
47. Gottlieb, S. H., Achuff, S. C., Mellits, E. D., et al. Prophylactic antiarrhythmic therapy of high-risk survivors of myocardial infarction: Lower mortality at 1 month but not at 1 year. *Circulation* 75:792, 1987.
48. Cardiac Arrhythmia Pilot Study Investigators. Effects of encainide, flecainide, imipramine, and moricizine on ventricular arrhythmias during the year after acute myocardial infarction: The CAPS. *Am. J. Cardiol.* 61:501, 1988.
49. Richards, D. A., Cody, D. V., Denniss, A. R., et al. Ventricular electrical instability: A predictor of death after myocardial infarction. *Am. J. Cardiol.* 51:75, 1983.
50. Denniss, A. R., Baaijens, H., Cody, D. V., et al. Value of programmed stimulation and exercise testing in predicting one-year mortality after acute myocardial infarction. *Am. J. Cardiol.* 56:213, 1985.
51. Denniss, A. R., Richards, D. A., Cody, D. V., et al. Prognostic significance of ventricular tachycardia and fibrillation induced at programmed stimulation and delayed potentials detected on the signal-averaged electrocardiograms of survivors of acute myocardial infarction. *Circulation* 74:731, 1986.
52. Bhandari, A., Rose, J., Au, P., and Rahimtoola, S. H. Long-term reproducibility of the stimulus induced ventricular arrhythmia during pre-hospital discharge phase of acute myocardial infarction (Abstract). *Circulation* 72(Suppl III):360, 1985.
53. Costard, A., Schluter, M., and Geiger, M. Inducibility of ventricular arrhythmias after acute myocardial infarction: Influence of time on stimulation results and prognostic significance (Abstract). *Circulation* 72(Suppl III):477, 1985.
54. Klein, H., Trappe, H. J., Hartwig, C. A., et al. Repeated programmed stimulation within the first year after myocardial infarction (Abstract). *Circulation* 72(Suppl III): 359, 1985.
55. Aonuma, K., Iesaka, Y., Ri, K., et al. Time dependent response to ventricular programmed stimulation in post acute myocardial infarction patients (Abstract). *Circulation* 74(Suppl II):189, 1986.
56. Kuck, K. H., Costard, A., Schluter, M., and Kunze, K. P. Significance of timing programmed electrical stimulation after acute myocardial infarction. *J. Am. Coll. Cardiol.* 8:1279, 1986.
57. Roy, D., Marchand, E., Theroux, P., et al. Long-term reproducibility and significance of provokable ventricular arrhythmias after myocardial infarction. *J. Am. Coll. Cardiol.* 8:32, 1986.
58. Bhandari, A. K., Au, P. K., Rose, J. S., et al. Decline in inducibility of sustained ventricular tachycardia from two to twenty weeks after acute myocardial infarction. *Am. J. Cardiol.* 59:284, 1987.
59. McPherson, C. A., Rosenfeld, L. E., and Batsford, W. P. Day-to-day reproducibility of responses to right ventricular programmed electrical stimulation: Implications for serial drug testing. *Am. J. Cardiol.* 55:689, 1985.
60. Lombardi, F., Stein, J., Podrid, P. J., et al. Daily reproducibility of electrophysiologic test results in malignant ventricular arrhythmias. *Am. J. Cardiol.* 57:96, 1986.
61. Somberg, J. C., Butler, B., Torres, V., et al. Lorcainide therapy for the high-risk patient post myocardial infarction. *Am. J. Cardiol.* 54:34B, 1984.
62. Korn, J., Li, C., Broudy, D., et al. Lack of prognostic value of programmed electrical stimulation in patients with recent myocardial infarction or unstable angina (Abstract). *J. Am. Coll. Cardiol.* 5:471, 1985.
63. Somberg, J. C., Butler, B., Torres, V., et al. Therapy for late post infarction ventricular tachycardia. *Angiology* 36:181, 1985.
64. Bhandari, A. K., Rose, J. S., Kotlewski, A., et al. Frequency and significance of induced sustained ventricular tachycardia or fibrillation two weeks after acute myocardial infarction. *Am. J. Cardiol.* 56:737, 1985.
65. Mann, D. E., Luck, J. C., Griffin, J. C., et al. Induction of clinical ventricular tachycardia using programmed stimulation: Value of third and fourth extrastimuli. *Am. J. Cardiol.* 52:501, 1983.
66. Brugada, P., Green, M., Abdollah, H., and Wellens, H. J. J. Significance of ventricular arrhythmias initiated by programmed stimulation: The importance of the type of ventricular arrhythmia induced and the number of premature stimuli required. *Circulation* 69:87, 1984.
67. Buxton, A. E., Waxman, H. L., Marchlinski, F. E., et al. Role of triple extrastimuli during electrophysiologic study of patients with documented sustained ventricular tachyarrhythmias. *Circulation* 69:532, 1984.
68. Denniss, A. R., Ross, D. L., Cody, D. V., et al. Randomized trial of antiarrhythmic drugs in patients with inducible ventricular tachyarrhythmias after recent myocardial infarction (Abstract). *Circulation* 74(Suppl II):213, 1986.
69. Herre, J. M., Mann, D. E., Luck, J. C., et al. Effect of increased current, multiple pacing sites and number of extrastimuli on induction of ventricular tachycardia. *Am. J. Cardiol.* 57:102, 1986.
70. Morady, F., DiCarlo, L. A., Liem, L. B., et al. Effects of high stimulation current on the induction of ventricular tachycardia. *Am. J. Cardiol.* 56:73, 1985.
71. Kennedy, E. E., Rosenfeld, L. E., McPherson, C. A., et al. Mechanisms and relevance of arrhythmias induced by high-current programmed ventricular stimulation. *Am. J. Cardiol.* 57:598, 1986.
72. Weissberg, P. L., Broughton, A., Harper, R. W., et al. Induction of ventricular arrhythmias by programmed ventricular stimulation: A prospective study on the effects of stimulation current on arrhythmia induction. *Br. Heart J.* 58:489, 1987.
73. Greene, H. L., Reid, P. R., and Schaeffer, A. H. The repetitive ventricular response in man: A pre-

dictor of sudden death. *N. Engl. J. Med.* 299: 729, 1978.

74. Hamer, A., Vohra, J., Hunt, D., and Sloman, G. Prediction of sudden death by electrophysiologic studies in high risk patients surviving acute myocardial infarction. *Am. J. Cardiol.* 50:223, 1982.
75. Marchlinski, F. E., Buxton, A. D., Waxman, H. L., and Josephson, M. E. Identifying patients at risk of sudden death after myocardial infarction: Value of the response to programmed stimulation, degree of ventricular ectopic activity and severity of left ventricular dysfunction. *Am. J. Cardiol.* 52:1190, 1983.
76. Mason, J. W. Repetitive beating after single ventricular extrastimuli: Incidence and prognostic significance in patients with recurrent ventricular tachycardia. *Am. J. Cardiol.* 45:1126, 1980.
77. Akhtar, M. The clinical significance of the repetitive ventricular response (Editorial). *Circulation* 63:773, 1981.
78. Ruskin, J. N., DiMarco, J. P., and Garan, H. Repetitive responses to single ventricular extrastimuli in patients with serious ventricular arrhythmias: Incidence and clinical significance. *Circulation* 63:767, 1981.
79. Horowitz, L. N., and Morganroth, J. Can we prevent sudden cardiac death? *Am. J. Cardiol.* 50:535, 1982.
80. Roy, D., Brugada, P., Bar, F. W. H. M., and Wellens, H. J. J. Repetitive responses to ventricular extrastimuli: Incidence and significance in patients without organic heart disease. *Eur. Heart J.* 4:79, 1983.
81. Brugada, P., Waldecker, B., Kersschot, Y., et al. Ventricular arrhythmias initiated by programmed stimulation in four groups of patients with healed myocardial infarction. *J. Am. Coll. Cardiol.* 8:1035, 1986.
82. Kersschot, I. E., Brugada, P., Ramentol, M., et al. Effects of early reperfusion in acute myocardial infarction on arrhythmias induced by programmed stimulation: A prospective, randomized study. *J. Am. Coll. Cardiol.* 7:1234, 1986.
83. Bhandari, A., Hong, R., Au, P., et al. Prognostic significance of programmed ventricular stimulation in patients at "low-risk" two weeks after acute myocardial infarction (Abstract). *J. Am. Coll. Cardiol.* 9:107A, 1987.
84. Grigg, L. E., Chan, W., Hamer, A., et al. Correlation between electrophysiological studies. Holter recordings, and signal-averaged ECGs in the postinfarction period (Abstract). *Circulation* 76(Suppl IV):32, 1987.
85. Zehender, M., Brugada, P., Geibel, A., et al. Programmed electrical stimulation in healed myocardial infarction using a standardized ventricular stimulation protocol. *Am. J. Cardiol.* 59:578, 1987.
86. Pumphrey, C. W., Skehan, J. D., and Rothman, M. T. Responses to ventricular extrastimuli following myocardial infarction are independent of ventricular function and can be modified by therapy (Abstract). *Circulation* 70(Suppl II): 401, 1984.
87. McComb, J. M., Gold, H. K., Leinbach, R. C., et al. Electrically induced ventricular arrhythmias in acute myocardial infarction treated with thrombolytic agents. *Am. J. Cardiol.* 62:186, 1988.
88. Moss, A. J., DeCamilla, J., Chilton, J., and Davis, H. T. The chronology and suddenness of cardiac death after myocardial infarction. *Ann. N.Y. Acad. Sci.* 382:465, 1982.
89. Moss, A. J., DeCamilla, J., and Davis, H. Cardiac death in the first 6 months after myocardial infarction: Potential for mortality reduction in the early posthospital period. *Am. J. Cardiol.* 39:816, 1977.
90. Anderson, K. P., and Mason, J. W. Surgical management of ventricular tachyarrhythmias. *Clin. Cardiol.* 6:415, 1983.
91. Garan, H., Ruskin, J. N., DiMarco, J. P., et al. Electrophysiologic studies before and after myocardial revascularization in patients with life-threatening ventricular arrhythmias. *Am. J. Cardiol.* 51:519, 1983.
92. Horowitz, L. N., Harken, A. H., Josephson, M. E., and Kastor, J. A. Surgical treatment of ventricular arrhythmias in coronary artery disease. *Ann. Intern. Med.* 95:88, 1981.
93. Boineau, J. P., and Cox, J. L. Rationale for a direct surgical approach to control ventricular arrhythmias. *Am. J. Cardiol.* 49:381, 1982.
94. Roy, D., Marchand, E., Theroux, P., et al. Programmed ventricular stimulation in survivors of an acute myocardial infarction. *Circulation* 72:487, 1985.
95. Waspe, L. E., Seinfeld, D., Ferrick, A., et al. Prediction of sudden death and spontaneous ventricular tachycardia in survivors of complicated myocardial infarction: Value of the response to programmed stimulation using a maximum of three ventricular extrastimuli. *J. Am. Coll. Cardiol.* 5:1292, 1985.
96. Breithardt, G., Borggrefe, M., and Haerten, K. Role of programmed ventricular stimulation and noninvasive recording of ventricular late potentials for identification of patients at risk of ventricular tachyarrhythmias after acute myocardial infarction. In *Cardiac Electrophysiology and Arrhythmias.* Orlando: Grune & Stratton, 1985. Pp. 553–561.
97. Breithardt, G., Borggrefe, M., and Haerten, K. Ventricular late potentials and inducible ventricular tachyarrhythmias as a marker for ventricular tachycardia and myocardial infarction. *Eur. Heart J.* 7 (Suppl A):127, 1986.
98. Kuchar, D. L., Thorburn, C. W., and Sammel, N. L. Late potentials detected after myocardial infarction: Natural history and prognostic significance. *Circulation* 74:1280, 1986.
99. Gomes, J. A., Winters, S. L., Stewart, D., et al. A new noninvasive index to predict sustained ventricular tachycardia and sudden death in the first year after myocardial infarction: Based on signal-aver-

aged electrocardiogram, radionuclide ejection fraction and Holter monitoring. *J. Am. Coll. Cardiol.* 10:349, 1987.

100. Richards, D. A., Cody, D. V., Denniss, A. R., et al. Ventricular electrical instability during the first year following myocardial infarction (Abstract). *Am. J. Cardiol.* 49:929, 1982.
101. Holley, L. K., Denniss, A. R., Cody, D. V., et al. Comparison of clinical significance of programmed stimulation induced ventricular tachycardia and fibrillation in survivors of acute myocardial infarction (Abstract). *PACE* 6:73, 1983.
102. Marchlinski, F. E., Waxman, H. L., Buxton, A. D., and Josephson, M. E. Predictive value of programmed stimulation in determining electrical instability after myocardial infarction (Abstract). *PACE* 6:73, 1983.
103. Kowey, P. R., Friehling, T., Meister, S. G., and Engel, T. R. Late induction of tachycardia in patients with ventricular fibrillation associated with acute myocardial infarction. *J. Am. Coll. Cardiol.* 3:690, 1984.
104. Santarelli, P., Bellocci, F., Loperfido, F., et al. Ventricular arrhythmia induced by programmed ventricular stimulation after acute myocardial infarction. *Am. J. Cardiol.* 55:391, 1985.
105. Santarelli, P., Bellocci, F., Loperfido, F., et al. Ventricular electrical instability in acute myocardial infarction: Clinical, angiographic and electrophysiologic correlations (Abstract). *Circulation* 68(Suppl III):108, 1983.
106. Marchand, E., Roy, D., Theroux, P., et al. Induction of ventricular arrhythmias after myocardial infarction: Relation to other determinants of prognosis (Abstract). *Circulation* 70(Suppl II):19, 1984.
107. Roy, D., Marchand, E., Theroux, P., et al. Reproducibility and significance of ventricular arrhythmias induced after an acute myocardial infarction (Abstract). *Circulation* 70(Suppl II): 18, 1984.
108. Bhandari, A., Rose, F., Kotlewski, A., et al. Programmed ventricular stimulation two weeks after acute myocardial infarction (Abstract). *J. Am. Coll. Cardiol.* 5:471, 1985.
109. Haerten, K., Borggrefe, M., and Breithardt, G. Repetitive ventricular response and late potentials in patients early after myocardial infarction (Abstract). *Circulation* 68(Suppl III):174, 1983.
110. Breithardt, G., Borggrefe, M., and Haerten, K. Programmed ventricular stimulation and recording of late potentials for risk stratification after myocardial infarction (Abstract). *Circulation* 70(Suppl II):19, 1984.
111. Borggrefe, M., Haerten, K., and Breithardt, G. Electrophysiological characteristics of stimulus-induced ventricular tachycardia after myocardial infarction (Abstract). *J. Am. Coll. Cardiol.* 5:471, 1985.
112. Denniss, A. R., Richards, D. A., Cody, D. V., et al. Comparable prognostic significance of delayed potentials and inducible ventricular tachycardia after myocardial infarction (Abstract). *Circulation* 72(Suppl III):359, 1985.
113. Denniss, A. R., Ross, D. L., Cody, D. V., et al. Randomized trial of antiarrhythmic drugs in patients with inducible ventricular tachyarrhythmias after recent myocardial infarction. (Abstract). *Circulation* 74(Suppl II):213, 1986.
114. Gonzalez, R., Arriagada, D., Corbalan, R., et al. Programmed electrical stimulation of the heart does not help to identify patients at high risk post myocardial infarction (Abstract). *Circulation* 70(Suppl II):19, 1984.
115. Iesaka, Y., Anuma, K., Nogami, A., et al. Prognostic significance of induced ventricular tachycardia, Holter monitor grade and ejection fraction in recent myocardial infarction patients (Abstract). *Circulation* 76(Suppl IV):33, 1987.
116. Treese, N., Pop, T., Erbel, R., et al. Outcome of primary coronary recanalization and arrhythmia profile in survivors of acute myocardial infarction. *Int. J. Cardiol.* 15:19, 1987.
117. Moses, J. W., Tamari, I., Friedman, C., et al. Arrhythmogenic effects of procainamide in high risk patients after myocardial infarction (Abstract). *Clin. Res.* 32:678A, 1984.
118. Bigger, J. T., Weld, F. M., and Rolnitzky, L. M. Which postinfarction ventricular arrhythmias should be treated? *Am. Heart J.* 103:660, 1982.
119. Potratz, J., Mentzel, H., Djonlagic, H., and Diederich, K. The significance of late potentials in the acute and chronic infarction period (Abstract). *Circulation* 74(Suppl II):470, 1986.
120. Hine, L. K., Laird, N. M., Hewitt, P., et al. Meta-analysis of empirical long-term antiarrhythmic therapy after myocardial infarction. *J.A.M.A.* 262:3037, 1989.
121. Richards, D. A., Byth, K., Ross, D. L., et al. What is the best predictor of spontaneous ventricular tachycardia and sudden death after myocardial infarction? *Circulation* 83:1090, 1991.
122. Denniss, A. R., Ross, D. L., Cody, D. V., et al. Randomized trial of antiarrhythmic drugs in patients with inducible ventricular tachyarrhythmias after recent myocardial infarction (Abstract). *Circulation* 74(Suppl II):213, 1986.
123. Bhandari, A. K., Hong, R., Kulick, D., et al. Day to day reproducibility of electrically inducible ventricular arrhythmias in survivors of acute myocardial infarction. *J. Am. Coll. Cardiol.* 15:1075, 1990.
124. Nogami, A., Aonuma, K., Takahashi, A., et al. Usefulness of early versus late programmed ventricular stimulation in acute myocardial infarction. *Am. J. Cardiol.* 68:13, 1991.
125. Bhandari, A. K., Hong, R., Kotlewski, A., et al. Prognostic significance of programmed ventricular stimulation in survivors of acute myocardial infarction. *Br. Heart J.* 61:410, 1989.
126. Cripps, T., Bennett, E. D., Camm, A. J., et al. Inducibility of sustained monomorphic ventricular tachycardia as a prognostic indicator in survivors

of recent myocardial infarction: A prospective evaluation in relation to other prognostic variables. *J. Am. Coll. Cardiol.* 14:289, 1989.

127. Iesaka, Y., Nogami, A., Aonuma, K., et al. Prognostic significance of sustained monomorphic ventricular tachycardia induced by programmed ventricular stimulation using up to triple extrastimuli in survivors of acute myocardial infarction. *Am. J. Cardiol.* 65:1057, 1990.
128. MADIT Executive Committee. Multicenter Automatic Defibrillator Implantation Trial (MADIT): Design and clinical protocol. *PACE* 14:920, 1991.
129. Goldman, L. Electrophysiological testing after myocardial infarction. A paradigm for assessing the incremental value of a diagnostic test. *Circulation* 83:1090, 1991.

38. Prognosis of Acute Myocardial Infarction

Hartmut Henning

Since 1968 there has been a decline in the mortality from cardiovascular disease and especially coronary artery disease. These declining mortality trends have been confirmed over the subsequent two decades and have been observed in all age groups, in both sexes, and in the major race groups [1, 2]. Data indicate that there has been a more than 25 percent decrease in the overall age-adjusted death rate from coronary heart disease. The causes for this impressive decline in the death rates from coronary artery disease are not unique to the North American continent but are seen as well in other countries including Australia, South America, Europe, and Japan. It remains uncertain whether the decline in coronary artery disease death rates is the result of a decreased incidence of acute myocardial infarction (AMI) and sudden death or the result of changes in survival in patients with coronary heart disease [3]. Other causes for the decline in coronary heart disease mortality include the development of acute coronary care, noninvasive diagnostic methods for early detection of myocardial infarction, new treatment modalities with drugs as well as coronary artery bypass graft surgery, and lastly the identification and modification of specific cardiovascular risk factors.

The decrease in the incidence rates of coronary artery disease and the associated decrease in mortality could be attributed to changes in the prevalence and severity of the major coronary risk factors. However, with an unchanged incidence in coronary heart disease and an associated decline in coronary heart disease death, the progressive decrease in mortality could be related to effects from secondary preventive efforts. It appears that both primary prevention through life style changes and improved treatment regimens have played a role in the decline in mortality in patients with AMI.

With the introduction of prehospital care and greater access and use of emergency medical services, the out-of-hospital death rate in patients with AMI has been reduced. Prior to the development of the coronary care unit (CCU), early mortality after AMI had been approximated at 30 percent. Treatment in the CCU has reduced in-hospital mortality to 10 to 18 percent [4–18]. A further reduction in early mortality to approximately 12 percent has been accomplished with the use of anti-ischemic therapy early in the course of AMI. An approximately 8 percent further reduction in early and late mortality has been observed in acute infarct patients who undergo thrombolysis and invasive reperfusion therapy [19, 20]. However, mortality following discharge from hospital after recovery from AMI remains high, with an approximately 10 percent mortality within the first year after myocardial infarction. Most of these deaths occur within the first 6 months after discharge, owing to sudden death, recurrent myocardial infarction, and congestive heart failure [4–6]. A large proportion of cardiac deaths within the first 6 months are due to sudden arrhythmic death. The death rates decline during the second half of the first year after myocardial infarction, further decline to 5 percent during the second year, and subsequently approach 3 to 4 percent annual mortality in the years thereafter [4, 7] (Fig. 38-1).

Prognostic Variables

The short-term and long-term survival after AMI depends on certain patient characteristics that signify independent risk for morbidity and mortality early and late after AMI. The reported variables that predict high risk after AMI have varied largely because of differences in study design that examined historical and objective information [4–13].

Studies on prognostication and stratification of postinfarction patients have used different patient selection criteria, commonly introducing an age limit to 60 or 65 years or restriction to a specific population criterion that may include the capability

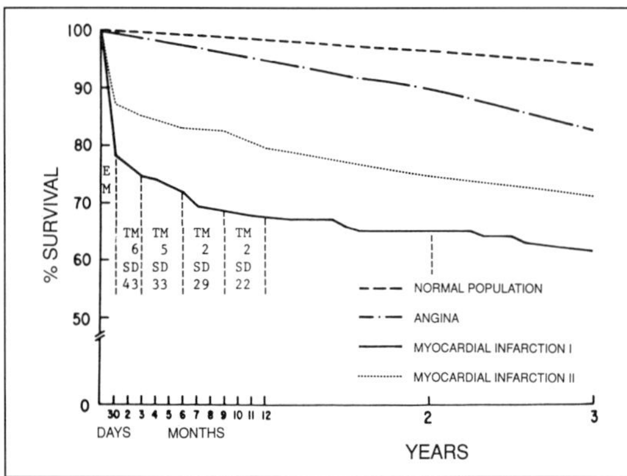

Fig. 38-1
Actuarial survival curves for patients with myocardial infarction. The solid line depicts the survival of 1420 patients with acute myocardial infarction (I) studied between 1979 and 1984 and the dotted line, the survival of 1266 patients (II) followed between 1987 and 1992. The survival rates of an age- and sex-matched normal population (*dashed line*) and patients with angina pectoris (*dashed/dotted line*) are shown for comparison. The survival rates in the normal population and angina population were significantly higher at 1, 2, and 3 years [7]. EM = early (30-day) mortality; TM = total mortality (percent) for time interval; SD = sudden death (percent of total mortality) for time intervals during the first year after acute myocardial infarction.

of early postinfarction exercise testing [21] or the availability of rest and exercise perfusion imaging [22]. The eligibility for predischarge exercise stress testing has been shown to define an already lower-risk group, as these patients are free of complications that may indicate poor prognosis, such as postinfarction angina, congestive heart failure, or complex ventricular arrhythmias during the postinfarction period. Thus in one study the 1-year mortality rate for patients who did not undergo exercise testing was 14 percent compared to only a 5 percent mortality rate for patients who were able to undergo exercise testing [21].

Another factor that may influence the variables and the importance of these variables for prediction of mortality and survival is the era in which the study has been carried out. During the 1950s characteristics from the history and the electrocardiographic, radiographic, and laboratory examinations were available; during the 1970s more objective parameters were included to define high risk and low risk after myocardial infarction with hemodynamic measurements, accurate assessment of the extent of ischemia by myocardial perfusion imaging, and estimation of left ventricular function by radionuclide angiography or contrast ventriculography. The development of quantitative techniques to accurately determine the extent of continuing myocardial ischemia, the severity of ventricular arrhythmias, and impairment of left ventricular function has provided a better definition of high-risk patients and established risk stratification schemes for patients after myocardial infarction. Similarly, early and late mortality after AMI may have been altered by the changing treatment modalities that have become available through the past decades. These have included prophylactic aspirin [23] and beta blockers [24–26], early coronary artery bypass graft surgery [27, 28], and more recently thrombolytic therapy [19, 20]. Such treatment during the acute phase, convalescent phase, and postdischarge period has been shown to improve subsequent morbidity and mortality and is to be taken into account when natural history and outcome are examined in postinfarction patients.

Prognostic variables may vary in terms of their significance of predicting death and survival depending on the timing of the start of the follow-up period after acute infarction. Variables examined at the time of admission with AMI may be a significant predictor for in-hospital mortality but may not predict 1-year or long-term mortality [7]. The mortality rates are highest during the first two 3-month intervals after hospital discharge, and therefore studies showing lower mortality rates may be the result of late enrollment rather than specific therapy. Studies following patients 2 to 10 years after AMI showed that most deaths occur within the first several months and differing mechanisms of mortality have been implied [4, 7–13]. Beyond the first year after acute infarction, the mortality rate stays relatively constant at about 3 to 5 percent a year, and from there on it may not differ from mortality rates reported for chronic stable angina pectoris [7]. Certain variables obtained at the time of admission or hospital discharge may be predictive of short-term mortality within 1 month after AMI but not beyond this time. Objective patient characteristics obtained at the time of discharge similarly may predict outcome during the first year after AMI but not during the subsequent long-term follow-up period. Complications of recurrent angina pectoris, recurrent myocardial infarction, or need for coronary artery bypass graft surgery are predictive from data obtained at the time of hospital discharge but not from data obtained at the time of admission with AMI [18, 29–38].

The difference in the identification of risk variables after myocardial infarction has also been attributed to the method of statistical analysis applied to the data obtained during the early and late phases after myocardial infarction. More sophisticated statistical techniques have been utilized for risk factor assessment following AMI. Multivariate analytic techniques can define the significant factors that identify death and survivors with high accuracy and correctly classify death in a studied infarct population [7, 39–45]. These methods determine the importance and independence of predictor variables and have been validated in subsequent test populations. The recognition of the similarity of basic characteristics in infarct populations in different institutions and different countries and mortality trends during the time periods after infarction as well as validation of prognostication schemes have provided a means of reliably identifying high-risk and low-risk patients for decision-making on treatment.

Early Mortality After Acute Myocardial Infarction

Early mortality rates after AMI have shown a wide variability for the early prognosis following AMI. Table 38-1 shows the in-hospital mortality rates from selected studies ranging from 12 to 41 percent. Studies on mortality and risk stratification often included different periods after the onset of acute symptoms, including the first day after admission [43] and the hospital period [39], intervals ranging from 2 to 20 days; in other studies early mortality was defined as a death within 30 days after AMI [7]. These defined intervals are the result of an observed mortality pattern in the study population. Early mortality rates and in-hospital mortality during the 1950s and 1960s were high (approximately 28 percent). An improving short-term prognosis has been observed in study populations of different intervals in the same institution showing an early mortality rate of 29 percent in 1967 compared with mortality of 22.4 percent in patients hospitalized in 1971 [50]. In later studies during the 1970s and 1980s, the in-hospital mortality ranged from 9 to 21 percent [7, 17, 18, 49].

Goldberg et al. [51] found a decreasing in-hospital and long-term mortality rate over consecutive study periods in the Worcester Heart Attack Study. The age-adjusted in-hospital mortality rate declined by 32 percent over the 10-year period between 1975 (22.2 percent) and 1984 (15.1 percent). A decline of 37 percent was seen in the patients with first myocardial infarction, and a decline of 26 percent was reported for patients with recurrent AMI between 1975 and 1984. Similarly, declining mortality rates may be related to changes in the extent and severity of AMI. In some studies, an increase in non-Q-wave myocardial infarction, which has a low early mortality as compared with Q-wave infarction, was observed [52, 53]. A decrease in the

Table 38-1
Studies on early mortality after acute myocardial infarction

First author	Study period	Population size	Early mortality rate (%)
Juergens [8]	1935–1951	279	15.8
Honey [9]	1940–1954	543	32.2
Zukel [46]	1943–1944	1090	17.0
Hughes [47]	1953–1960	445	32.8
Pell [10]	1956–1961	1331	30.0
Day [14]	1962–1964	126	15.9
Mosbech [48]	1963	1094	41.0
Norris [11]	1966–1967	757	26.0
Peterson [16]	1966–1969	6955	29.5
Henning [7]	1969–1973	221	21.0
	1973–1976	150	18.0
Gillum [18]	1970	3842	16.7
	1980	3736	11.9
Wolffenbuttel [49]	1977	132	12.1

extent of myocardial damage in the acute infarction phase as determined by peak creatinine phosphokinase levels also was observed when study periods of 1975, 1978, and 1981 were compared. It appears that in-hospital mortality rates from AMI have declined over time from 24 percent in 1970 to 18 percent in 1977 and 14 percent in 1984.

Long-Term Survival After Acute Myocardial Infarction

The long-term survival rates in patients with AMI discharged from hospital are shown in Table 38-2, demonstrating the highest risk for death within the first year. The 1-year mortality rate for discharged patients varies between 10 and 15 percent, with subsequent annual mortality rates between 4 and 6 percent. Longitudinal studies of cardiac mortality after myocardial infarction found an exponential fall in mortality for the 6- and 8-month periods after myocardial infarction [4, 57]. In a study of a population of 2290 patients from three geographically different populations, colleagues and I observed that 50 percent of all deaths during the first year had occurred by day 19 and 70 percent of all deaths by day 100 [4] (Fig. 38-2). The cardiac mortality between day 2 and 3 weeks was 11.4 percent and for the remainder of the year 10.5 percent. We found that separate exponential curves best delineate the survival distributions up to 3 weeks and for the remainder of the first year after myocardial infarction.

Several studies examined the changes of long-term mortality in hospital survivors of AMI to assess improvement over time in the long-term prognosis of AMI [17, 50, 54, 58]. Studies on hospital survivors of AMI failed to observe an improvement in the long-term survival over time, with no differences between first or recurrent myocardial infarction [17, 50]. However, after introduction of thrombolytic agents, both short-term and long-term survival rates appear to be improved [19, 20], but these therapeutic advances require further documentation of changes in the long-term survival patterns.

Risk factor assessment and prognostication begin at the time of admission with AMI. Data from the patient's history, physical examination, electrocardiogram, chest radiograph, and laboratory examinations, including serum enzyme determinations, are available. During the patient's stay in the CCU, further clinical information becomes available. Clinical data obtained during the patient's stay in the CCU and from the hospital predischarge evaluation by special studies such as exercise testing, radionuclide left ventriculography, 24-hour ambulatory electrocardiographic recording, and coronary angiography are available to derive prognostic information.

Prognostic Indicators for Mortality and Survival

Certain patient characteristics indicate an increased risk for cardiac death and sudden cardiac death

Table 38-2
Long-term survival rates after acute myocardial infarction

			Survival rates at follow-up points				
First author	Study period	Population size	1 yr	2 yr	3 yr	5 yr	10 yr
Juergens [8]	1935–1951	224			68.8	55.4	29.2
		1030				59.0	39.0
Beard [55]	1950–1952	427				69.0	44.0
Pell [10]	1956–1961	932	90.5	86.8	81.8	74.0	
Kjoller [33]	1966–1969	644	84.9		67.0		
Goldberg [50]	1966–1967	334	85.0	79.0		64.0	
Martin [56]	1970–1971	666	87.7	80.0	73.6	60.8	
Luria [36]	1970–1973	143		76.9		60.1	
Henning [7]	1969–1973	224	68.5		61.0		

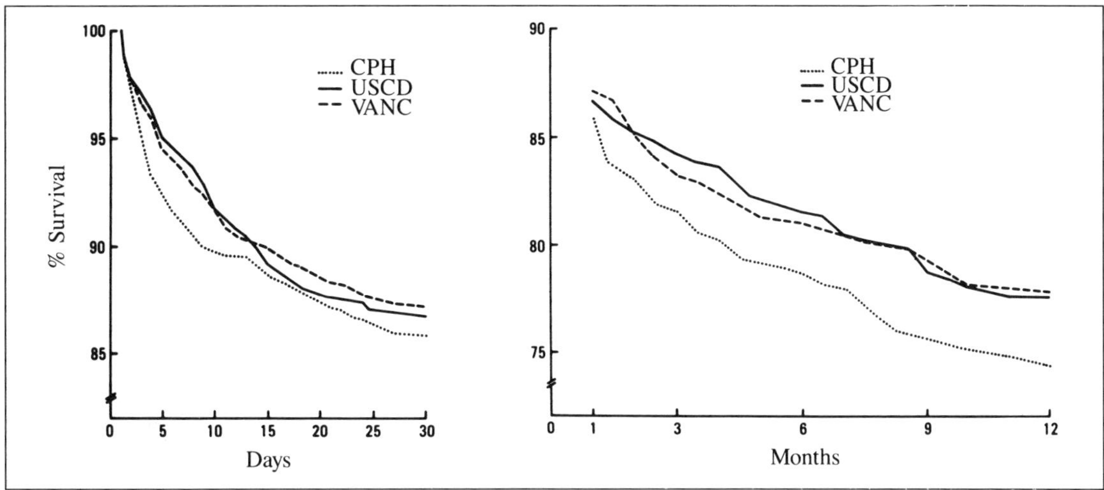

Fig. 38-2
Survival curves for patients with acute myocardial infarction from three institutions. *Left.* Percent of patients alive at the end of day 1 after admission with acute myocardial infarction through day 30. *Right.* Percent survival from the end of 1 month through 12 months. The curves are extensions of those in the left panel on a different time scale. CPH = Copenhagen, Denmark; UCSD = University of California (San Diego); VANC = Vancouver, British Columbia, Canada.

during the in-hospital phase and postdischarge phase after AMI. The major risk indicators are related to the reduction in left ventricular performance, ongoing myocardial ischemia, and ventricular arrhythmias after AMI. Many investigations during the past decades have identified many simple independent risk factors for mortality and morbidity. There have been multiple studies on the relation of prognosis to historical and clinical factors prior to the availability of invasive hemodynamic monitoring and techniques of left ventricular function measurement. The historical factors such as advanced age, female sex, previous myocardial infarction, previous congestive heart failure, previous angina, and chronic obstructive pulmonary disease are associated with a twofold or more mortality compared with infarct patients without the abnormal variable [4, 7–9, 11, 59–61]. The clinical factors and results of the standard laboratory examinations are often an indirect indication of the extent of myocardial damage and the resulting impairment of myocardial function. Data from the physical examination include heart rate, systolic blood pressure, respiratory rate, temperature, ventricular third heart sound gallop rhythm, bilateral pulmonary rales, and peripheral edema; and these abnormalities contribute to early and late outcome after AMI [4, 7, 9–11, 29, 42, 62, 63]. The initial chest radiograph provides information on cardiac enlargement and the presence and severity of congestive heart failure [64]. Composites of clinical findings relate to left ventricular function and severity of congestive heart failure as devised by Killip and Kimball [65]. Twenty to 30 percent of patients present on admission to the CCU without signs of left ventricular congestive heart failure and have a low 1-month mortality; 40 to 60 percent of patients on admission exhibit mild to moderate left ventricular failure, which carries a twofold mortality (approximately 15 percent) compared with patients who do not show signs of left ventricular failure [7, 65]. A fivefold early mortality is associated with the presence of pulmonary edema and a tenfold early mortality with the presence of cardiogenic shock at the time of admission [7]. Congestive heart failure in patients with AMI was identified in most prognostication studies as the most important clinical variable [7, 8, 11, 43, 66, 67], even in the presence of quantitative indicators of mechanical or ischemic dysfunction. Clinical and radiologic abnormalities of congestive heart failure have been heavily weighed in composite prognostic schemes [11, 60].

Thus the clinical prognostic indexes of Peel and Norris [60, 61] selected congestive heart failure as the most important variable. The Multicenter Postinfarction Research Group reported four independent risk predictors of mortality that ranked the presence of bilateral pulmonary rales above left ventricular ejection fraction (LVEF), ventricular ectopic depolarization activity, and advanced New York Heart Association (NYHA) functional class before infarction [67].

Other historical and demographic factors are associated with a poor prognosis and have included the female gender [68], a history of diabetes mellitus [69], and prior angina pectoris [70]. Diabetes mellitus affects the risk after an AMI for both early and late mortality [69]. The in-hospital mortality rate among diabetic patients has been reported to be 30 percent compared with less than 20 percent for nondiabetic patients. Similarly, the 1-year mortality rate after hospital discharge is increased at 20 to 30 percent compared with 8 to 15 percent in nondiabetic patients. The exact mechanism contributing to increased early and late mortality in diabetic patients remains unclear but may possibly be related to more extensive myocardial infarctions, more previous infarctions, and the greater prevalence of heart failure in diabetic infarct patients. Isolated elevation of systolic blood pressure and combined systolic and diastolic hypertension appear to have prognostic indication [71]. Studies on the influence of obesity on early and late prognosis after AMI showed that obese patients with a body mass index over 30 kg/cm^2 have a similar mortality rate of 13 percent when compared with a 14 percent hospital mortality rate in normal-weight patients [72]. Obese patients over age 65 showed a mortality rate of 30 percent compared with 17 percent in patients over 65 years old with normal weight. Excessive early mortality was strongly influenced by obesity in older patients, but the obesity appears to have no significant influence on 1-year outcome or on early prognosis in patients younger than age 65.

Laboratory data such as white blood cell count, blood urea nitrogen, serum creatinine, uric acid, and serum enzyme levels (creatine kinase [CK], aspartate aminotransferase [AST], lactate dehydrogenase [LDH]) have been reported as independent risk predictors for early and late mortality [73]. The electrocardiogram demonstrates multiple indicators of poor prognosis [73–75]. There is a greater mortality after anterior wall infarction than after inferior infarction even when corrected for infarct size [76, 77]. Further prognostic information can be derived from the QRS duration, the QT interval, the QRS score of electrocardiographic infarct size, ST segment changes, conduction defects, atrial and ventricular arrhythmias, and sinus tachycardia. Early and late prognosis is worsened by the persistence of advanced heart block, new bifascicular or trifascicular block, and preexisting left bundle branch block. The persistence of ischemic ST segment depression on serial electrocardiograms and ischemic ST segment abnormalities found on ECG leads other than leads with new Q waves is associated with a higher subsequent mortality and reinfarction rate compared with patients without persisting ischemic ST abnormality [75]. Similarly, patients with ischemic ST abnormalities developing with recurrent angina early after myocardial infarction distant from the acute infarct have a worse prognosis than those with angina associated with ischemia in the infarct zone.

The electrocardiogram may be diagnostic of a prior myocardial infarction in the absence of a diagnostic history of infarction. Although the incidence of an unrecognized myocardial infarction is not known, the long-term prognosis after a "silent" infarction is similar to that for hospitalized diagnosed infarction [78]. There appears to be a lesser incidence of angina pectoris after silent myocardial infarction. Prognostic importance has been attributed to silent ischemia after previously unrecognized myocardial infarction, which also is associated with a high incidence of congestive heart failure. Estimation of the extent of myocardial damage by serial CK values relates to anatomic infarct size and to the impairment of left ventricular function. In previous studies, CK areas of over 40 IU/L/hr and elevated plasma CK levels over 2000 IU have been associated with poor prognosis and high incidence of left ventricular failure [7]. Large defects on thallium 201 perfusion scintigrams [79] and large infarcts on technetium 99m scintigrams [80] are associated with increased mortality and recurrent cardiac events. The extent of transmural infarct involvement is characterized by electrocardiographic Q-wave development in contrast to the subendocardial, nontransmural, or non-Q-wave infarction. Despite the poor correlation between the electrocardiographic definitions of transmural or subendocardial infarction and the pathologic myocardial findings, marked similarities between the two types of infarction have been found [53, 81]. Many investigations showed that acute mortality in patients with non-Q-wave infarcts is significantly lower than that in patients with Q-wave infarcts [82–84]. Non-Q-wave myocardial infarction has a variable incidence of 16 to 36 percent in infarct populations. Non-Q-wave infarction is more common in patients with previous coronary artery bypass graft surgery, with an incidence as high as 60 percent in postsurgery patients [85]. Patients with non-Q-wave infarction tend to have smaller infarctions [86]. It is supported by lower CK levels, a lower incidence of heart failure, and a lower average Killip class as well as a mean higher ejection fraction compared with Q-wave infarct patients [85]. Non-Q-wave infarct patients have less commonly total occlusions of the infarct-related coronary artery but may have more than 60 percent critical stenotic lesions in two or three coronary arteries and a higher incidence of left main coronary artery disease [87]. Patients with non-Q-wave infarctions tend to have subtotal but severe stenosis of the infarct-related artery and a high incidence of recurrent angina early after infarction or after hospital discharge; 20 percent of patients develop acute Q-wave infarction within 3 months after the onset of a non-Q-wave infarct [81]. Hutter et al. [84] reported a high recurrence rate of 21 percent at 9 months after initial infarction and 57 percent when patients were followed up to 54 months. Increased complications are found in patients with non-Q-wave infarcts that show large perfusion abnormalities within the infarct zone on thallium 201 perfusion scintigrams [88]. Patients studied in a 30-month follow-up period had a reinfarction rate of 18 percent in non-Q-wave and 6 percent in Q-wave infarction. Eighty-eight percent of recurrent infarctions in non-Q-wave infarction patients related to the previous area of infarct compared with only 20 percent in patients with Q-wave infarctions.

Comparable late mortality rates have been found in patients with both types of infarction [83, 84, 88]. In a collaborative study we studied early and late mortality rates in 277 patients with non-Q-wave infarction and compared these with the rates for 959 patients with Q-wave infarction [53]. One-year cumulative survival rates for patients with Q-wave and non-Q-wave infarcts were nearly identical when patients with infarct extensions were excluded. The hospital mortality in patients with infarct extension was 15 percent in those with Q-wave infarcts, whereas 43 percent in those with non-Q-wave infarcts died. During the follow-up period, there was a significantly higher incidence of 24 percent of infarct extension in the nonsurvivors than the 6 percent incidence in the survivors. For patients with infarct extension, the 1-year survival rate of 66 percent in patients with Q-wave infarction was higher than 35 percent in patients with non-Q-wave infarction. Extension of infarction was a strong predictor of a 1-year mortality in patients with non-Q-wave infarctions. Thus non-Q-wave infarctions are considered relatively unstable situations with a low early mortality rate but a higher risk of infarct extension and later infarction with a high late mortality rate. The recognition of this entity and the associated coronary artery findings provide the basis for early coronary arteriography in this patient group.

Hemodynamic measurements obtained by bedside pulmonary artery catheter monitoring during the acute phase and complications of myocardial infarction have provided quantitative parameters to further define early and late prognosis after AMI. Hemodynamic indices reflect the severity of congestive heart failure and inotropic dysfunction of the left and right ventricles and correlate to early and late mortality after AMI. An elevated left ventricular filling pressure, decreased cardiac output, cardiac index, increased arteriovenous oxygen difference, decreased stroke volume index, and left ventricular stroke work index signify poor early prognosis after AMI [7, 49, 89, 90]. Hemodynamic measurements can be abnormal in the absence of clinical manifestations of pump failure [91]. The presence of acute pulmonary edema that may be associated with normal ejection fraction can further identify patients at high risk of early death after AMI [7, 92]. We found that abnormal invasive measurements yielded a fivefold mortality when left ventricular filling pressure was over 20 mm Hg, cardiac index was less than 2 L/min/m^2, stroke volume index was less than 25 ml/beat/m^2, and arteriovenous oxygen difference was more than 5.6 ml/dl [7]. Hemodynamic measurements improve the predictive accuracy of early death and survival, compared to historical and clinical data. When discriminant function analysis was used for the development of a prognostication scheme, the factors from the history, physical examination, and noninvasive assessment correctly classified 73 percent of the deaths. The inclusion of hemodynamic data improved the correct classification of early death to 97 percent. Also, in this study, during a follow-up period of 26 months late mortality was increased twofold in patients with a left ventricular filling pressure over 20 mm Hg. Only the two other indicators of cardiac enlargement and previous myocardial infarction signified a twofold higher late mortality after 30 days and after hospital discharge [7]. The accurate identification of high-risk patients by hemodynamic data was demonstrated in patients with cardiogenic shock [89]. Accurate prediction of in-hospital mortality is improved by admission hemodynamic measurements with the added information on left ventricular failure from the initial chest radiograph and the Peel index [93].

Late Postinfarct Evaluation of Prognosis

During the late postinfarct period, the risk of subsequent cardiac death is the result of recurrent myocardial ischemia, complex or frequent ventricular ectopic activity, and left ventricular dysfunction [42, 67, 94]. It is suggested that the impairment of left ventricular function is the most important indicator for 1-year and 2-year cardiac mortality after myocardial infarction [67, 95]. Depressed LVEF is often associated with persistent sinus tachycardia, a third heart sound, palpable left ventricular dyssynergy, bibasilar rales, and a murmur of papillary muscle dysfunction after AMI [96]. Significant correlations between both Killip and NYHA classes for congestive heart failure with ejection fraction have been reported [67]. An abnormal chest radiograph after myocardial infarction may predict the presence of depressed LVEF in more than 50 percent of patients [97]. Dewhurst and Muir [98] reported the relation between rest ejection fraction and infarct location on the discharge electrocardiogram. Patients exhibiting Q waves in the anterior or lateral leads or in both the anterior and inferior leads had the most severely depressed ejection fractions. The same authors reported a significant association between depressed ejection fraction and peak CK after both anterior and inferior infarction. A study on survivors of AMI indicated that abnormal rest or exercise ejection fraction was related to a history of previous infarction, cardiomegaly, functional class for congestive heart failure at the time of discharge, infarct location, and Killip class, whereas depressed ejection fraction did not correlate to significant exercise-induced ST segment depression [99].

It has been suggested that impaired left ventricular performance is related to complex ventricular arrhythmias with ejection fractions of less than 40 percent [95]. Similarly, patients identified with high-grade ventricular arrhythmias after acute infarction have lower rest and exercise ejection fractions [93, 100].

The LVEF within the first 24 hours after admission relates to short-term mortality [91]. Ejection fraction stabilizes within the subsequent 24 to 48 hours [101], and ejection fraction measured during the later hospital stay relates to postdischarge mortality over the subsequent 2 years [67, 94]. Various separation points in the measurement of rest ejection fraction have been reported to best predict in-hospital and postdischarge mortality [102, 103]. Patients with acute infarction and resting ejection fraction of less than 30 percent showed an early mortality of 55 percent [103], and an ejection fraction of less than 40 percent at the time of discharge was associated with a 30 percent 1-year mortality [67, 95]. We found that a separation point of 45 percent can provide optimal sensitivity and specificity for cardiac death up to 1 year [92]. Significant differences in mortality are found in patients with abnormal ejection fractions of less than 52 percent (24 percent 1-year mortality) compared with patients with normal values (10 percent 1-year mortality). In our study, an LVEF of less than 45 percent classified 62 percent of deaths correctly and 64 percent of the survivors who had an ejection fraction over 45 percent. Only 19 percent of patients who died within the first year had an LVEF of less than 30 percent, but 90 percent of survivors had an LVEF over 30 percent.

The 1-year cardiac mortality progressively increases as the ejection fraction decreases below 40 percent, and an LVEF of less than 30 percent carries a fivefold increase in the risk of dying during the first year after infarction [67] (Fig. 38-3). Studies on the role of ejection fraction combined with other prognostic parameters suggest that rest ejection

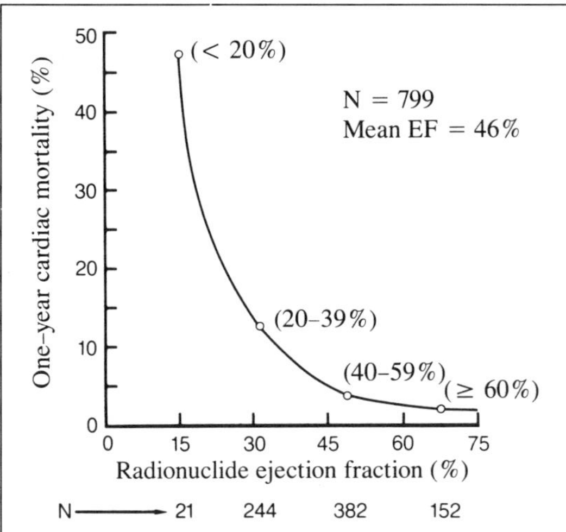

Fig. 38-3
One-year cardiac mortality as a function of left ventricular ejection fraction (EF) during the first year following hospital discharge after acute myocardial infarction. Mortality increases greatly as the ejection fraction before hospital discharge falls below 40 percent. (From The Multicenter Postinfarction Research Group: Risk stratification and survival after myocardial infarction. *N. Engl. J. Med.* 309:331, 1983. With permission.)

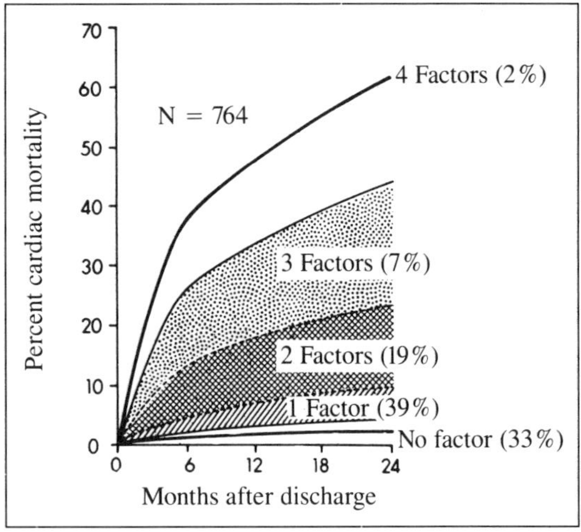

Fig. 38-4
Mortality curves and zones of risk according to the increasing number of risk factors. The risk factors included New York Heart Association (NYHA) functional classes II to IV before hospital admission, pulmonary rates, occurrence of 10 or more premature ventricular contractions per hour, and a left ventricular ejection fraction below 40 percent. The risk zones indicate the spectrum of relative risk for single factors and the range of multiple risks for combinations of two, three, and four factors. The numbers in parentheses indicate the proportions of the population with the specified number of risk factors. (From The Multicenter Postinfarction Research Group: Risk stratification and survival after myocardial infarction. *N. Engl. J. Med.* 309:331, 1983. With permission.)

fraction is the most important predictor of mortality after hospital discharge [93, 102].

The Multicenter Postinfarction Research Group reported progressive increases in 1-year mortality in patients with ejection fractions less than 40 percent [67]. Four risk factors were independent predictors of mortality: an ejection fraction below 40 percent, evidence of congestive heart failure with bilateral extensive pulmonary rales in the CCU, ventricular ectopy of 10 beats or more per hour, and advanced NYHA functional class before infarction. These factors were analyzed in a logistic regression analysis for mortality, and the most important independent prognostic factors were pulmonary rales and LVEF. An increasing number of these risk factors are associated with an increasing mortality, the lowest-risk group without any prognostic factors having a less than 3 percent 2-year mortality rate, and the highest-risk group with all four factors having a 60 percent 2-year mortality rate (Fig. 38-4). The combination of pulmonary rales and ejection fraction of less than 40 percent identified patients with a 2-year mortality rate of 38.1 percent, whereas the mortality rate in the remaining patient group was only 8.9 percent, and the combination of pulmonary rales and a history of previous infarction indicated a high mortality rate of 39.4 percent within 2 years.

In the Multicenter Investigation of the Limitation of Infarct Size (MILIS), ejection fraction was examined with 15 other variables for prognostic importance in a Cox regression analysis [94]. LVEF of less than 40 percent ranked as the second most important indicator after ventricular premature beats of more than 10 per hour, followed by the use of digitalis at discharge and a history of previous infarction.

The presence or absence of clinical or radiographic heart failure gives further prognostic information in patients with normal or depressed LVEF [92]. In our multicenter study of 972 patients with AMI, the effect of the presence or absence of in-hospital heart failure on late mortality was studied in three groups divided according to LVEF; group I had an LVEF of 40 percent or less; group II, 41 to 50 percent; and group III, 51 percent or more. In group I patients with clinical signs of left ventricular failure, 1-year mortality rate after hospital discharge was 26 percent, significantly higher than the 19 percent rate in group II and the 8 percent rate in group III. In the absence of left ventricular failure, mortality rates were significantly lower at 12, 6, and 3 percent, respectively. The 1-year mortality rates were markedly increased for patients who had radiographic signs of congestive heart failure during the CCU period at 36, 24, and 14 percent in groups I, II, and III, respectively, and markedly lower at 13, 9, and 3 percent when no radiographic heart failure was seen. Moderate or severe depression of LVEF in the absence of clinical or radiographic heart failure predicted an increased 1-year mortality compared with patients with a normal LVEF but at much lower mortality levels than when heart failure was present. Patients with a normal ejection fraction without heart failure had a 1-year mortality rate of 3 percent, which increased to 8 or 14 percent when clinical or radiologic signs of left ventricular failure were present.

Comparative Prognostic Value of Ejection Fraction with Other Clinical and Laboratory Parameters

Other studies compared the prognostic value of radionuclide ejection fraction with other clinical and laboratory parameters [98, 104, 105] and suggested that LVEF is a more potent predictor of subsequent mortality and events than those available from history, physical examination, electrocardiogram, and other noninvasive examinations. Similarly, the LVEF was also ranked higher than other clinical variables or the prognostic indices of Peel and Norris [106].

Exercise-induced ST segment abnormalities have been shown not to be as potent predictors of subsequent cardiac events as the radionuclide angiographic variables. Submaximal exercise testing variables such as maximal heart rate, blood pressure, workload, angina, ST segment changes, and arrhythmias were found to be less significantly related to subsequent events than the radionuclide angiographic variables [104, 105].

Thallium 201 myocardial imaging has been used prognostically in survivors of AMI [22]. Prognostic information from the rest and exercise radionuclide ventriculogram was compared to thallium 201 myocardial perfusion scintigraphy [107]. The results of thallium imaging were significantly related to subsequent combined events, but radionuclide angiographic variables were superior to thallium scintigraphic variables for predicting cardiac events in postinfarction patients.

The prognostic value of exercise radionuclide angiography parameters has been examined [106]. Exercise ejection fraction and the change in ejection fraction were predictive of major cardiac events, which included cardiac death and recurrent myocardial infarction. Rest ejection fraction, left ventricular wall motion score, and left ventricular end-systolic volume index also had a significant association with subsequent events. The peak LVEF during exercise was the most important variable in determining the highest-risk groups if ventricular ejection fraction at rest was less than 40 percent. The change in the LVEF with exercise distinguished best the patients with minor cardiac events of angina pectoris and congestive heart failure rather than identifying patients with subsequent major events and cardiac death.

Cardiac Arrhythmias

Certain cardiac arrhythmias during the acute phase of myocardial infarction and the late postinfarct phase have been associated with an increased in-hospital and short-term mortality [108–113]. Supraventricular tachyarrhythmias including atrial fibrillation and sinus tachycardia, ventricular fibrillation, and complete atrioventricular block were associated with a more than twofold early mortality, and multivariate analyses identified sinus tachycardia, ventricular fibrillation, and complete atrioventricular block as independent predictors for poor early prognosis [7, 114]. Early prognosis with increased in-hospital mortality or 40-day mortality after acute infarction is affected by the occurrence of supraventricular tachycardia, atrial fibrillation, sinus bradycardia, atrioventricular block, ventricular premature beats, ventricular tachycardia, and ventricular fibrillation [114]. Also, the new occurrence of left bundle branch block, bifascicular block, and trifascicular conduction block was associated with increased early mortality.

Ventricular arrhythmias occurring during the acute phase of myocardial infarction have been established as important predictors of subsequent mortality. Investigations documented the prognostic value of ventricular arrhythmias that occur before discharge and are associated with an increased risk of cardiac and sudden death after hospital discharge [108, 109, 111, 112, 115]. Sudden cardiac death after hospital discharge is attributed to ventricular fibrillation and accounts for a large proportion of cardiac deaths within the first year after myocardial infarction. We observed an incidence of 45 percent sudden arrhythmic death among all cardiac patients who died during the first 2 months after hospital discharge after myocardial infarction, with a subsequent decreasing incidence of 33, 29, and 22 percent sudden death for the following 3-month intervals during the first year after myocardial infarction. Frequent and complex ventricular premature beats documented by ambulatory electrocardiographic recordings or telemetry and exercise testing with electrocardiographic monitoring were related to prognosis, with improved prediction of subsequent mortality in association with either impaired left ventricular function or myocardial ischemia [67, 110, 113].

Thus 1-hour electrocardiographic recordings in postinfarction patients showed that ventricular premature beats in combination with congestive heart failure carried a sevenfold risk of sudden death compared to patients without both findings [115]. Residual ventricular ectopic activity after AMI has a more adverse impact on prognosis in the presence of myocardial dysfunction [110]. In a follow-up study of 81 patients, all the patients who died suddenly had complex ventricular arrhythmias and a LVEF of less than 40 percent by radionuclide ventriculography [110]. Taylor et al. [103] documented that complex ventricular arrhythmias during the late hospital phase and after discharge are associated with multivessel coronary artery disease, left ventricular dysfunction, and sudden death. This study defined complex ventricular arrhythmias as multiform ventricular premature beats, bigeminy, or runs of ventricular beats recorded with a 24-hour Holter monitor 10 to 24 days after AMI. In this study, 60 percent of patients had complex ventricular arrhythmias at some time during the 1-year follow-up period, and their common presence resulted in a low predictive value for morbidity and mortality.

Controversy exists concerning whether complex ventricular arrhythmias have prognostic value independent of other major risk indicators. Similarly, a uniform definition of "complex" ventricular arrhythmias and the frequency indicative of poor prognosis remain undefined. The Multicenter Postinfarction Research Group established that 10 ventricular premature beats per hour indicates an increased risk for subsequent mortality [67]. In this study, 866 patients underwent 24-hour Holter monitoring and determination of the resting radionuclide ventricular ejection fraction; 1-year and 2-year mortality rates were independently related to ventricular ectopy of 10 or more depolarizations per hour but, more importantly, to the ejection fraction of less than 40 percent and the occurrence of advanced left ventricular failure with the presence of extensive pulmonary rales and a history of previous congestive heart failure. A progressive increase in 1-year cardiac mortality was observed as the frequency of ventricular ectopic depolarizations rose above 1 per hour and the ejection fraction fell below 40 percent. However, ejection fraction had a considerably stronger effect on mortality than did ectopic depolarizations. The same group reported from another study that an ejection fraction of less than 30 percent was significantly more important for the prediction of total cardiac mortality than ventricular ectopic beats of more than 3 per hour, with a 50 percent mortality rate for patients with both risks compared to 6 percent of patients without these findings [95]. Similarly, patients with low ejection fractions (< 40 percent) and frequent depolarizations (> 10/hr) had a 3.8-fold increased risk of cardiac death compared with the patient without these risk indicators.

The MILIS identified in 533 patients ventricular ectopic activity of more than 10 per hour as the most important type of ventricular arrhythmia and strongest predictor for subsequent sudden death [94]. LVEF of less than 40 percent was identified as the next important predictor among many historical and clinical variables. The occurrence of both ventricular premature beats of more than 10 per hour and a reduced LVEF of less than 40 percent identified a group of postinfarction patients with a sudden death rate of 18 percent during an 18-month follow-up period compared to only 2 percent for the patients without these findings. Thus the additive risk for sudden death among the group of patients with ventricular premature beats of more than 10 per hour was five times that of the group with neither frequent ventricular beats nor left ventricular dysfunction. The additive risk for sudden death was 11 times greater in the group with both left ventricular dysfunction and frequent premature ventricular beats. Patients with good left ventricular function have a relatively low mortality, even in the presence of a high frequency of ventricular ectopic beats. The MILIS study identified ventricular premature beat frequency of more than 10 per hour as the most important ventricular arrhythmia, to a lesser degree complex features of premature ventricular contractions (PVCs) including couplets, R on T phenomenon, runs, and multiform ventricular premature beats, which were also predictive of sudden death.

An association between silent myocardial ischemia after myocardial infarction and arrhythmias has been suggested [116, 117]. Patients with myocardial infarction and ventricular fibrillation had exercise-induced painless myocardial ischemia. Malignant ventricular arrhythmias in patients with prior myocardial infarction were inducible by programmed ventricular stimulation in the presence of ischemia and were not inducible in the absence of ischemia.

Early ventricular fibrillation after AMI is associated with an increased in-hospital mortality rate [118]. In one study [118] we observed a 7 percent incidence of ventricular fibrillation within 48 hours of hospital admission, which carried a 25 percent hospital mortality compared with 13 percent in patients without early ventricular fibrillation. The common causes of death in these patients were congestive heart failure and cardiogenic shock. Multivariate analysis identified ventricular fibrillation as an independent prognostic factor for the in-hospital mortality. The 1-year mortality rate after hospital discharge was not significantly greater in patients with than in those without early ventricular fibrillation (15 percent and 11 percent, respectively), even in the subgroup of patients with anterior myocardial infarction.

In another study, we investigated the relation of complex ventricular arrhythmias including multiform PVCs, couplets, and ventricular tachycardia to infarct location [119]. Sixty-two percent of patients with non-Q-wave infarcts who did not survive 1 year had complex PVCs compared with 32 percent of survivors. No differences were seen in the Q-wave group. In patients with complex PVCs, survival was higher (92 percent) in patients with Q-wave infarction compared to those with non-Q-wave infarction (76 percent). For the Q-wave infarct group, survival was similar in patients with and those without complex ectopic activity, and the incidence of complex ectopic activity was similar in patients with LVEF above and those with LVEF below 45 percent. Complex PVCs were independent of ejection fraction in patients with non-Q-wave infarction but closely associated with ejection fraction in patients with Q-wave infarction. The presence of complex PVCs at the time of hospital discharge appears to be an important predictor of 1-year mortality in patients with non-Q-wave infarction.

Exercise Testing

Exercise stress testing soon after recovery from an uncomplicated myocardial infarction has been shown to be a safe and useful technique that aids in patient management and prognostic assessment. The predischarge submaximal or symptom-limited exercise test is useful for the detection of myocardial ischemia and arrhythmias in patients without clinical features apparent during the early hospital stay after acute infarction [120–122]. Furthermore, maximal stress testing performed 4 to 6 weeks after the hospital stay may identify a large number of patients with residual myocardial ischemia [123].

Studies have shown that 30 to 40 percent of postinfarction patients demonstrate ischemic electrocardiographic abnormalities during early treadmill exercise testing that relate to the extent of coronary artery disease in the risk area of recent infarction and other sites adjacent or remote from the recent infarct [124, 125]. Even in uncomplicated patients after myocardial infarction who do not exhibit symptoms of residual or recurrent ischemia, exercise testing has identified those with multiple-vessel coronary artery disease. Further methods used to identify residual myocardial ischemia include exercise myocardial imaging with thallium

201, exercise radionuclide angiography, and exercise two-dimensional echocardiography.

Most clinical studies indicate that the ST segment depression or the development of angina during electrocardiographic exercise testing prior to hospital discharge relates to mortality and subsequent reinfarction or unstable angina [120–122, 126]. Other exercise test variables that predict subsequent cardiac events after infarction are the development of angina pectoris [120–122], complex ventricular arrhythmias [120, 127], the heart rate response [128], the blood pressure response [121–129], and the rate-pressure product at the time of chest pain or ST depression [129]. In patients unable to increase their systolic blood pressure by at least 10 mm Hg or in whom the systolic blood pressure decreases by 20 mm Hg during continued exercise, a high incidence of severe three-vessel or left main coronary artery disease with a high associated cardiac mortality is found [120, 123]. In such patients, a symptom-limited treadmill exercise test demonstrates myocardial ischemia better than a heart-rate-limited exercise test [123]. Most studies identified the exercise functional capacity to be of predictive value for subsequent mortality as determined by the duration of exercise [129, 130], the early termination of exercise, the maximum accomplished workload in watts [131], and the total cardiac capacity expressed in multiples of resting oxygen consumption (METs) [121, 127]. The more important prognostic indicators from exercise testing largely reflect impaired left ventricular function. Cardiac mortality is high in patients who achieve 4 METs or less of exercise [132]. Patients achieving 4 METs or less had a cardiac event rate of 18 percent with cardiac death or new myocardial infarction within 1 year, compared with a 2 percent cardiac event rate in patients with a more than 4 METs exercise capacity. A good functional capacity over 4 METs was predicted from age and ST segment abnormalities at rest. Among the 60 percent of patients who were predicted to have good functional capacity of more than 4 METs, only 15 percent had poor functional capacity at the time of exercise testing. Multivariate analysis identified only functional capacity but not ST depression as a predictor of subsequent death. An important indicator of poor prognosis is the inability to perform an exercise test [132, 133]. Similarly, patients selected for exercise testing have a more favorable prognosis than those who are not tested. Reasons for the inability to perform an exercise test include age, poor general medical condition, severe peripheral vascular disease, congestive heart failure, and markedly impaired left ventricular function. The inability to perform an exercise test was identified as the strongest predictor of outcome in a study that examined variables with clinical factors and LVEF [131].

ST segment depression of 1 mm or more during exercise testing has been related to subsequent mortality [120–122, 127]. Studies reported a significantly higher mortality rate (4 to 25 percent) for patients with ST depression in contrast to a low mortality rate (0 to 7 percent) for patients without exercise-induced ST depression. Waters et al. [134] investigated 225 patients with a predischarge exercise test to 5 METs or 70 percent of maximum predicted heart rate, and only exercise-induced ST segment abnormality and the failure to increase the systolic blood pressure by 10 mm Hg predicted mortality during the first year after myocardial infarction. Cardiac mortality during the follow-up period after the first year could no longer be predicted by ST segment abnormalities, but exercise-induced ventricular arrhythmias and a history of previous myocardial infarction predicted mortality beyond the first year. Other investigators ascribed a high risk to the development of angina during exercise testing in association with ST segment depression [123]. Patients who manifest angina with exercise-induced ST depression were shown to have an 88 percent prevalence of multivessel coronary artery disease with increased subsequent mortality. In the presence of more marked ST depression of 2 mm or more at peak heart rates of less than 135 per minute, a high-risk group with a 10 percent mortality is identified, compared to a 1.3 percent mortality rate in patients without these exercise test abnormalities.

Exercise-induced asymptomatic myocardial ischemia has been identified as an important predictor of poor prognosis [135]. In one study [135], 63 percent of patients who underwent low-level exercise treadmill testing early after myocardial infarction had a positive exercise test without angina. The group with anginal chest pain and the group without exercise angina had similar extents of coronary artery disease and LVEF. Silent myocardial ischemia recorded as intermittent ST depression on ambulatory electrocardiographic recording was associated with an increased risk of cardiac events during the postinfarction period [136].

Exercise Test Variables and Other Prognostic Variables

The importance of variables from exercise testing has been investigated for the prediction of mortality and other cardiac events [137, 138]. Different multivariate methods ranked exercise duration highest for prediction of death, with lesser importance for the heart rate-pressure product, exercise-induced ventricular arrhythmias, heart rate, and female gender; ST segment depression was not selected as a significant predictor of subsequent death [127].

Madsen et al. [114] examined prognosis from both clinical and exercise test variables and ranked heart failure over exercise-induced ventricular ectopic activity and exercise duration. For the endpoints of death and nonfatal new myocardial infarction, exercise duration was most important compared with exercise-induced arrhythmias, female gender, age, and atrioventricular block. In this study, clinical variables alone provided the highest correct prediction of death.

Patients who are able to exercise after myocardial infarction are at a lower risk for subsequent death. The Multicenter Postinfarction Research Group study found a 7.5 percent 1-year mortality rate in the total study population, but the mortality rate was low, at 5 percent, in patients who were able to perform a low-level exercise tolerance test, compared to 17 percent in patients who were unable to exercise [67]. The same study group identified a subgroup of exercised postinfarction patients who had no evidence of congestive heart failure on chest radiograph with an only 1 percent 1-year cardiac mortality rate.

DeBusk et al. [126] studied postinfarction patients to develop a risk stratification scheme. A high-risk group with an 80 percent mortality or recurrent infarction rate during the subsequent 6 months was identified by the presence of a history of previous infarction or angina and recurrent angina in the CCU. Of the remaining patients, the ineligibility for exercise testing further identified a risk group with a 6.4 percent event rate. Of the patients who performed an exercise test, those with a positive finding of 2 mm or more of ST segment depression had a high event rate compared with those with a negative exercise test, indicating the value of exercise testing for defining high- and low-risk subgroups after myocardial infarction.

Thallium Scintigraphy

Myocardial thallium 201 imaging in conjunction with exercise testing enhances sensitivity and specificity for detection of ischemia in patients with functionally important multivessel coronary artery disease [139]. In patients with negative exercise tests, scintigraphic evidence of residual myocardial ischemia, either within the infarct zone or in myocardial regions remote from the site of infarction, is common. Patients with demonstrated ischemia on thallium 201 testing were found to have a significantly greater mortality, a higher incidence of reinfarction during long-term follow-up, and a higher risk of experiencing subsequent cardiac events compared with patients without scintigraphic evidence of residual ischemia [22, 140]. The prognostic value of thallium perfusion imaging was similarly demonstrated in postinfarction patients with painless ST segment depression during predischarge exercise testing and in patients who exhibited false-positive electrocardiographic responses after recent myocardial infarction [141].

Exercise scintigraphy detects significant disease in the anterior descending coronary artery, right coronary artery, and the circumflex coronary artery with a sensitivity of 91, 87, and 63 percent, respectively [139]. The presence of thallium 201 perfusion abnormalities in multiple different vascular distributions allows identification of multivessel and left main coronary artery disease after myocardial infarction.

Gibson et al. [22] compared the results of submaximal exercise testing, thallium 201 scintigraphy, and coronary angiography prior to hospital discharge after myocardial infarction for identification of patients at high risk, as defined by defects in more than one vascular region, redistribution within or remote from the infarct zone, or abnormal lung uptake [22]. Thallium scintigraphy was more sensitive (95 percent) than either treadmill exercise testing or coronary angiography for identifying nonfatal recurrent myocardial infarction and rehospitalization with class 3 and class 4 angina during a follow-up period of 15 months. Exercise electrocardiographic studies identified only 50 percent of patients with either cardiac death or recurrent infarction. In contrast, the total cardiac event rate was 6 percent and the cardiac mortality rate was 2 percent in patients with normal perfusion or single persistent defects in the infarct zone. All patients who died from cardiac causes during the follow-up period had underlying multiple-vessel disease, and 90 percent of them had one or more high-risk scintigraphic findings. Of patients with single-vessel disease and subsequent cardiac events, 92 percent demonstrated redistribution within the infarct region. However, for the prediction of death, multivessel disease by coronary angiography was a stronger predictor than exercise thallium scintigraphy. Hung et al. [140] reported that the magnitude of exercise-induced thallium 201 defects and the extent of redistribution during symptom-limited exercise testing 3 weeks after infarction were strongly predictive of subsequent events. In a study of 117 men followed over 12 months, variables from exercise thallium scintigraphy, maximal exercise electrocardiographic testing, and radionuclide angiography were examined by regression analysis together with the clinical data [140]. A decreased exercise capacity and an inability to raise ejection fraction by 5 percent with exercise predicted cardiac death, nonfatal recurrent infarction, and ventricular fibrillation better than did thallium scintigraphic abnormalities.

Thallium 201 exercise scintigraphy following myocardial infarction may identify 50 percent of postinfarction patients with multivessel disease. Twenty-eight percent of these patients with multiple perfusion defects on exercise scintigrams 3 months after myocardial infarction had a subsequent cardiac event, compared to 6 percent of patients with a monovessel disease pattern on scintigrams [142].

The relative prognostic value of rest thallium 201 imaging, radionuclide ventriculography, and 24-hour ambulatory electrocardiographic monitoring was studied for the prediction of 1-year mortality after AMI [143]. High-risk patients were identified by an abnormal thallium perfusion score, LVEF of less than 40 percent, and complex ventricular arrhythmias (three or more consecutive PCVs, paired PCVs, or more than 10 PVCs in 1 hour) and were important predictors of survival by univariate Cox survival analysis. The thallium perfusion score, however, was the only important predictor by multivariate analysis, and the predictive power of the thallium perfusion score was comparable to that of combined ejection fraction and ambulatory electrocardiographic monitoring. Conversely, patients with a small, persistent thallium 201 defect in a single region and without increased lung uptake appear at very low risk for a future cardiac event and mortality and are candidates for early hospital discharge and rehabilitation.

Two-Dimensional Echocardiography

Two-dimensional echocardiography at rest and during exercise is useful in the diagnosis of coronary artery disease, left ventricular function, and wall motion abnormalities [144–148]. Two-dimensional echocardiography was shown to be comparable to radionuclide ventriculography for the quantitation of LVEF and left ventricular wall motion abnormalities in anterior infarction, with superior detection of wall motion abnormalities of the inferoposterior wall [149, 150]. Among 93 patients studied with two-dimensional echocardiography and radionuclide ventriculography, high- and low-risk patients were identified by LVEF and left ventricular wall motion indices by both techniques [150]. In repeated studies, 10 days after myocardial infarction in 81 survivors, risk groups with similar 1-year mortality rates by either technique were defined.

Two-dimensional echocardiography within 12 hours after admission with AMI was performed to assess the location and extent of contraction abnormalities [151]. Patients with a high abnormal wall motion score were at high risk of subsequent cardiac death, left ventricular failure, and malignant ventricular arrhythmias during the hospital stay. Of the 27 patients with a high-risk echocardiographic wall motion score at 12 hours after infarction, 24 (89 percent) had one or more cardiac events compared to an 18 percent event rate in the low-risk group with a low abnormal wall motion score. Patients with a high abnormal wall motion score had a 37 percent in-hospital mortality rate, and patients with a lesser extent of wall motion abnormalities only a 6 percent mortality rate.

Ryan et al. [152] examined the value of prognostic information from exercise two-dimensional echocardiography compared to treadmill exercise testing in patients recovering from AMI. During a 10-month follow-up period, 80 percent of patients who had exercise-induced echocardiographic wall motion abnormalities had subsequent cardiac events—cardiac death, readmission with unstable angina, recurrent myocardial infarction, or coronary artery bypass graft surgery. Treadmill exercise tests were positive in only 55 percent of patients with subsequent events. No cardiac deaths occurred in patients with negative exercise echocardiograms, and there was a significant decrease in the event-free survival rate in patients without exercise-induced wall motion abnormalities compared to those with new abnormalities. Exercise echocardiography was more sensitive and specific than treadmill exercise testing for the prediction of subsequent cardiac events after AMI.

Cardiac Catheterization, Coronary Angiography

Cardiac catheterization can be safely performed early after AMI to identify subgroups of patients with variable extent and severity of coronary artery disease and the related prognosis [153–156]. Coronary artery bypass surgery improves survival in certain subgroups with narrowing of the left main coronary artery and in patients with three-vessel coronary artery disease and left ventricular dysfunction. Approximately 10 percent of patients recovering from an AMI have critical stenosis of the left main coronary artery, and 30 to 40 percent have three-vessel disease. Thus a substantial proportion of patients who survive an AMI may be recommended for coronary artery bypass surgery based on the coronary arteriographic findings after infarction.

Clinical features of patients with multivessel disease include advanced age [155], postinfarction angina [155, 157], complex arrhythmias during 24-hour electrocardiographic monitoring [156], ventricular tachycardia and ventricular fibrillation in the CCU [158], congestive heart failure, pulmonary edema, or shock [158]. One study identified weight, systolic blood pressure, serum cholesterol, and infarct location as common features in patients with three-vessel disease [157]. Other historical information of previous myocardial infarction [158, 159], history of angina [157, 158] or changing angina prior to infarction [153], family history of coronary artery disease [157], and history of hypertension [103] were related to the extent of coronary artery disease. Left ventricular function was inversely related to the number of involved arteries [158]. More extensive coronary disease is commonly found in the presence of increased left ventricular end-diastolic pressure, increased end-diastolic volume, and reduced stroke work index [160]. Multivariate statistical techniques have been applied to identify patients with multivessel disease. These variables included the occurrence of postinfarction angina, a family history of coronary disease, a high serum cholesterol level [157], anterior ST and T-wave abnormalities, and a positive treadmill exercise test after myocardial infarction [161].

The results from coronary angiography were examined using multivariate analysis to determine subsequent cardiac events and mortality. In a study of 179 survivors of AMI who underwent coronary angiography and left ventriculography within 8 weeks after infarction, the prevalence of multivessel disease was high (79 percent) in the symptomatic patients [130]. Three-vessel disease or an ejection fraction of less than 30 percent identified a subgroup of patients with a high mortality rate (22 percent) during an average 20-month follow-up period, but recurrent myocardial infarction was best predicted from exercise test variables. Another study examined prognosis in relation to the location and severity of coronary artery stenosis defined by a coronary artery jeopardy score [162]. Patients with the highest jeopardy score had a 56 percent 5-year survival rate and those with low jeopardy scores a 95 percent survival rate. However, the LVEF was more closely related to prognosis than the coronary artery jeopardy score, and only the maximal percent stenosis in the left anterior descending artery added prognostic information to the jeopardy score.

Sanz et al. [45] investigated predictors for late mortality in 259 consecutive patients who underwent coronary arteriography after myocardial infarction. An ejection fraction of 50 percent or less, the number of diseased vessels, and the occurrence of congestive heart failure in the CCU were the only independent predictors of survival. Survival was lowest in patients with ejection fractions between 21 and 49 percent, and the proportion with three-vessel disease was high in this group, who stand to benefit the most from coronary artery bypass surgery.

The severity of coronary artery disease and the degree of left ventricular dysfunction have been useful for prognostication and risk stratification up to 5 years after AMI [163]. In this study one-half of the patients had three-vessel disease, and only 7 percent had an LVEF of less than 30 percent. Of multiple clinical and angiographic variables, combined right and left anterior descending coronary artery stenosis, ejection fraction, and the presence of myocardial risk segments were significant predictors of subsequent cardiac death, nonfatal reinfarction, or coronary artery bypass surgery over the 5-year follow-up period. These angiographic variables added significant information for prognosis and prediction of cardiac events to the clinical variables over the entire 5-year period after myocardial infarction.

One study identified left ventricular end-systolic volume as a stronger indicator of survival than either ejection fraction or the number of coronary occlusions after myocardial infarction [164]. LVEF, however, can be assessed by noninvasive techniques, which may further reduce the indications for cardiac catheterization as a means for risk stratification.

Programmed Electrical Stimulation

Although the prognostic importance of complex ventricular arrhythmias during the in-hospital and postdischarge phase after AMI has been documented, the role of programmed electrical stimulation (PES) is uncertain. Provoked ventricular tachyarrhythmias may identify patients with late sudden death and poor prognosis after AMI [165–169]. Patients who develop sustained ventricular tachycardia or ventricular fibrillation spontaneously during the early recovery period after infarction have an increased in-hospital mortality. Electrical instability produced by PES has been related to subsequent sudden death after myocardial infarction, and associated myocardial ischemia may be a requirement for the induction of ventricular tachycardia in patients with coronary artery disease who have survived a "sudden death" event [170]. Patients with AMI who sustained ventricular tachycardia in a hospital or were resuscitated from ventricular fibrillation had more frequently inducible ventricular tachycardia with a lesser number of premature stimuli required. Forty percent of patients with PES-inducible ventricular tachycardia had also documented spontaneous early ventricular tachycardia or fibrillation after infarction. In contrast, nonsustained ventricular tachyarrhythmia was more frequently induced in patients without earlier ventricular arrhythmias or with nonsustained ventricular tachycardia. The temporal evolution of inducible sustained ventricular arrhythmias after myocardial infarction was studied in clinically stable patients early and late after myocardial infarction [171]. During the initial programmed ventricular stimulation at an average of 2 weeks after myocardial infarction, sustained ventricular tachycardia or ventricular fibrillation was inducible in most of the patients but was reproduced at an average of 5 months later in only 47 percent of patients. A decrease in late inducibility of the sustained ventricular arrhythmias was greater for patients in whom arrhythmias were induced during initial programmed ventricular stimulation by triple extrastimuli and burst pacing than for those in whom arrhythmias were induced by double extrastimuli; but it appeared to be unrelated to other clinical, hemodynamic, or angiographic variables. Only 7 percent of patients with initially inducible ventricular arrhythmias died during a 1-year follow-up period, and all patients in the noninducible group were surviving. Higher mortality rates were reported, with 32 percent incidence of sudden death in patients with inducible ventricular tachycardia or fibrillation [167], but sudden death rates of 14 percent were reported for nonresponders during 1-year follow-up periods. One study suggested that ventricular arrhythmias induced early after myocardial infarction can be reproduced late in these survivors of acute infarction, but the persistent electrical instability is not a predictor of the risk of sudden death during the first year after myocardial infarction [172]. Denniss et al. [173] compared the relative prognostic significance of ventricular tachycardia and fibrillation inducible by PES within 1 month after AMI in a prospective study of 403 survivors of transmural myocardial infarction and found that 20 percent of the patients had inducible ventricular tachycardia and 14 percent had inducible ventricular fibrillation. For the patients with inducible ventricular tachycardia, the 1-year probability of survival was significantly lower than the respective probability for patients without inducible arrhythmias, and the probability of remaining incident free of cardiac death or nonfatal arrhythmia was significantly lower than in the group with no inducible arrhythmias.

The prognostic significance of programmed ventricular stimulation and its usefulness in relation to other forms of invasive and noninvasive testing were investigated in 150 survivors of myocardial infarction, with inducibility of ventricular arrhythmias in 23 percent of these patients [174]. No significant differences existed between patients with and those without inducible ventricular tachyarrhythmias in relation to spontaneous ventricular arrhythmias during the acute and recovery phases after infarction, inducible ischemia or arrhythmias on predischarge treadmill exercise testing, severity of coronary artery disease on angiography, or degree of left ventricular dysfunction. A higher incidence of inferior infarction was observed in patients with inducible ventricular tachycardia. Patients with and those without inducible ventricular arrhythmias had a similar occurrence of sudden death, cardiac death, and ventricular tachyarrhythmias during the subsequent year. In this population, a low LVEF, presence of a left ventricular aneurysm, and exercise-induced PVCs were predictors of subsequent death and spontaneous ventricular tachycardia, whereas PES-induced ventricular tachycardia in the patients recovering from infarction could not identify a group at high risk for subsequent sudden cardiac death.

The combined use of PES and the exercise test allows definition of high- and low-risk groups after infarction [169]. In one study [169], patients with inducible ventricular arrhythmias had a higher mortality rate than those without inducible arrhythmias (26 versus 6 percent). Patients with an exercise-induced ST segment change of 2 mm or more had a higher (11 percent) mortality rate than did those with ST changes of less than 2 mm (4 percent). Of patients who had both tests, 62 percent had no inducible arrhythmia and an ST change of less than 2 mm; only 1 percent died during the first year. Of the patients with inducible ventricular arrhythmias and/or ST segment depression of 2 mm or more, 13 percent died within 1 year. Programmed stimulation and exercise testing together predicted death within the first year and identified a large group of patients with a low mortality rate.

The contribution of PES to risk assessment in patients after myocardial infarction was compared to that of clinical variables, information from exercise testing, and 24-hour ambulatory electrocardiographic recording and radionuclide ejection fraction [175]. In 19 (23 percent) of the 84 patients, ventricular tachycardia of more than six repetitive beats was produced, but none of these patients died during an average 20 months of follow-up, whereas 9 percent in the group without inducible arrhythmias died. In the patients with inducible ventricular tachycardia, complex ventricular ectopy and ventricular tachycardia were commonly detected on ambulatory electrocardiographic recording. No relation was found between the response to PES and the abnormalities of exercise testing and radionuclide ejection fraction. All but 1 of the patients who died had an LVEF under 40 percent, and 4 of the 6 patients had ventricular tachycardia on ambulatory electrocardiographic recording. PES at 6 weeks after myocardial infarction appears not to contribute to identification of high-risk patients after myocardial infarction; high-risk patients were more accurately characterized by ventricular function, exercise testing, and complex ventricular arrhythmias on ambulatory electrocardiographic recording.

The identification of high-risk patients with inducible ventricular arrhythmias during the postinfarction period may, however, define a group at high risk for arrhythmic death in whom control of ventricular arrhythmias by medical and surgical therapy may improve long-term mortality and form the basis for a population for controlled randomized antiarrhythmic therapy trials.

Prognostic Indices

Multiple risk factors were investigated by univariate analyses and found to be important prognostic indicators of mortality and survival after AMI [7, 9, 39, 43, 57, 59, 60, 61, 63, 176]. These univariately significant indicators for prognosis may be selected at different times during and after hospitalization and may differ in their significance, although the importance and independence of such variables cannot be assessed by simple statistical methods [4, 7, 73, 177]. In simple prognostication and stratification schemes, principles of prognostic risk factor selection are used to classify a patient into a high-risk or a low-risk group. Such prognostic schemes utilize the frequency of risk factors from historical, standard laboratory, and clinical data, which may provide an indirect measure of the extent of myocardial damage and the resulting impairment of cardiac performance [114, 178]. Prognostic information from the physical examination has included heart rate, systolic blood pressure, respiration rate, temperature, shock, S_3 gallop rhythm, pulmonary rales, and peripheral edema [179]. Cardiomegaly and severity of pulmonary congestion on the chest radiograph and laboratory data (including leukocyte count and blood urea nitrogen, serum creatinine, cholesterol, and serum enzyme levels) have been related to outcome. Prognostic information from the electrocardiogram includes the site of infarction, QRS duration, QT interval, ST segment abnormalities, conduction blocks, atrial and ventricular arrhythmias, and sinus tachycardia [179]. The hemodynamic measurements of compromised left ventricular function during AMI more accurately distinguish death and survivors by such indices as left ventricular filling pressure, stroke volume index, left ventricular stroke work index, cardiac output, cardiac index, arteriovenous oxygen difference, and LVEF [7, 89, 90].

First prognostic indices were devised by assigning weights to the various factors observed during the first 24 hours after admission [59]. Schnur's pathologic index rating system [59] used 19 historical and clinical variables, some of which were graded according to the severity of the finding. This prognostic scoring system was applied to 230 patients surviving the first 24 hours after hospitalization and allowed distinction of five patient groups. The long-term mortality in the lowest group was 8 percent and for the highest patient group 95 percent.

Peel et al. [60] developed a prognostic index in 1962 based on assigned weights from the clinical impressions of their relative prognostic importance. Their index assigned numerical values to six factors—age, sex, previous history, shock, heart failure, and the electrocardiogram and rhythm disturbances during the first 24 hours after admission—to obtain a patient's prognostic score. The index was applied to 628 patients with five score ranges that produced patient groups with 30-day mortality rates from 2.5 to 88.5 percent. An accurate prediction of early death was obtained only in patients with very high scores, but precise prediction of death and survival was not possible in patients with lower scores. The Peel index was tested by other investigators and used as a single variable within other multivariate prognostic schemes [39, 93].

The construction of more precise prognostic indices was facilitated by the development of multivariate statistical methodologies and the use of computers, including multiple objective and quantitative indicators, and considering the relative importance and interdependency of risk variables to a final prognostic function. Hughes et al. [47] attempted to predict hospital mortality in a retrospective study of 445 patients from three hospitals using 20 historical, admission, and early postadmission variables in a linear discriminant function analysis. From the variables of age, white blood cell count, temperature, systolic blood pressure, presence of conduction defects, pulmonary infarction, congestive heart failure, and shock, 97 percent of the survivors and 80 percent of the deaths were correctly classified. Lemlish et al. [180] applied multiple linear regression to 368 patients to develop a ranking system of several important factors for 30-day mortality or survival. The relative importance of prognostic indicators was identified by the ranking order of blood pressure, history of a previous myocardial infarction, age, temperature, and duration of elevated temperature. McHugh and Swan [93] used multiple linear regression in 42 patients predicting in-hospital mortality by a weighted combination of mixed venous oxygen saturation, chest radiographic determination of left ventricular failure, and the Peel index as an individual variable. Shubin et al. [89] predicted outcome for 20 shock patients by discriminant analysis from stroke volume index and diastolic arterial pressure measured serially over the first 80 hours after admission, with a 94 percent predictive accuracy.

Norris et al. [11] presented in 1970 a method using discriminant function analysis that had selected indicators from historical and admission data for the prediction of in-hospital and 3-year mortality. Univariately significant factors were further quantitated and discriminant weights computed for index scores that divided patients into six groups, each with increasing mortality. Prognostic indicators for in-hospital outcome included age, location of infarct, admission systolic blood pressure, heart size, and the presence of congestive heart failure from the chest radiograph and the history of infarction or angina. Prognostic indicators for late outcome were only age, heart size and congestive failure on the chest radiograph, and previous infarction or angina. The Norris and Peel indices were tested by other investigators on various infarct populations [181, 182].

Studies of late outcome after myocardial infarction utilized historical and clinical variables from the time of admission, from the early hospital course and prior to the time of discharge from the CCU [43, 57, 61], or the entire hospital course [13, 36, 41, 57, 178]. The only prognostic variables consistently identified during the later in-hospital period were pulmonary congestion on the chest radiograph [43, 178, 183] and certain ventricular arrhythmias [13, 36, 39, 41, 43, 57, 61, 112]. However, data from the first 24 to 48 hours after the onset of myocardial infarction may allow risk prediction from 6 to 36 months after acute infarction [43, 57, 61]. In one study, linear regression selected from 42 factors from the history and the first 48 hours after admission the ten variables of age, female gender, diabetes, previous angina, blood pressure, clinical and radiographic left ventricular failure, high LDH level, high blood urea nitrogen, and high leukocyte count [43]. The prognostic score from these variables correctly classified 90 percent of the patients at 1 month and 86 percent at 6 months, allowing early in-hospital identification of patients with risk of late death.

In a study from our group, data from the history and the first 24 hours of hospitalization predicted 1-year death and survival; they predicted equally well as the data from the entire hospital course [57]. Discriminant function analysis identified in 818 patients discharged from the hospital five important factors from the 24-hour data: maximal level of blood urea nitrogen, previous myocardial infarction, age, displaced left ventricular apex on physical examination, and sinus bradycardia. When data from the entire hospital stay were included, extension of infarction and maximal heart rate in the CCU were also selected. Examining variables including discharge parameters, the presence of S_3 gallop, and abnormal apex were important for prediction of 1-year mortality. LVEF and the presence of complex ventricular arrhythmias during a 24-hour ambulatory electrocardiographic recording were independent predictors of 6-month and 1-year mortality, but correct classification of 58 percent of the deaths and 79 percent of the survivors from clinical data alone was not further improved by more than 2 percent with the inclusion of ejection fraction and ambulatory electrocardiographic monitoring.

Studies on risk factor identification, high-risk prediction, and stratification used different infarct populations and different analytic methodologies. The commonly employed multivariate schemes provide similar precise prognostic evaluation with applicability to test populations in the same or a different institution [7, 13, 36, 37, 184]. A reliable risk identification scheme requires validation before its generalization to other populations. These problems were investigated in one of our studies that used four separate multivariate methodologies for predicting death and survival at 30 days after myocardial infarction [185]. Predictive schemes were constructed using stepwise discriminant analysis, logistic regression, recursive partitioning, and a nearest neighbor procedure. The four methods were then used on a second population, and the reliability of a risk identification scheme within each population was assessed by a cross-validation procedure. Subsequently, each scheme constructed from the data of one population was tested on the data from the other. One study population had 295 patients who were admitted to the University of California (San Diego) Medical Center (UCSD) and the other 407 patients admitted to the Vancouver General Hospital (VGH) in British Columbia [185]. Similar predictors showed the same trends and patterns of significance for both populations. Population differences indicated that the VGH population was older but had a lower incidence of predictive factors of previous myocardial infarction, history of chronic obstructive lung disease, S_3 gallop on admission, rales above the scapula on admission, third-degree atrioventricular block, and anterior infarct location. Maximum heart rate within the first 24 hours and admission heart rate were higher for the UCSD population, whereas respiration rate was higher for the VGH population.

Using stepwise discriminant analysis, logistic regression, and recursive partitioning, we identified the relative importance of each of the candidate predictor variables included in the analyses for both populations. Only one predictor (maximum heart rate during the first 24 hours after admission) played a role in all six analyses. Four other variables were identified in five of the six analyses and included age, third-degree atrioventricular block, pulmonary congestion on chest radiograph, and minimum systolic blood pressure during the first 24 hours after admission. Age and pulmonary congestion on chest radiograph had a high rank in each of the analyses, whereas the importance of the other two factors varied. Variables that were highly significant for one population but not for the other, such as history of congestive heart failure, tended to enter the analysis for that population only and not the other.

Cross-Validation Within Populations

The three methodologies cross-validated performed better on the complete UCSD data (a reduction in error risk of close to 50 percent) than on the complete data from VGH (a reduction in error risk of about 30 percent). For both populations, recursive partitioning produced the lowest error risk and correctly classified 72 percent of early deaths and 85 percent of survivors within the UCSD population and 85 percent of early deaths but only 65 percent of survivors within the VGH population [185]. When patients with some missing data for UCSD were included, the error risk increased. However, for the VGH population only a minor increase in the error risk was observed, indicating that some missing data are tolerable but that too much decreases the performance for the method of recursive partitioning.

Between-Population Classification

When the risk prediction schemes for VGH were used to predict for UCSD, the error risks for the three methods were lower than those when UCSD data were used to predict for VGH. This finding represented a reduction in error risk by 40, 44, 11, and 11 percent for UCSD and by 20, 30, 11, and 3 percent for VGH, similar to the reduction in error risk achieved by cross-validation within each population.

Another study from our institution examined four methodologies for predicting short-term outcome after acute infarction using risk factor selection, discriminant function analysis, recursive partitioning, and Cox multivariate analysis [186]. Similar correct classification rates were obtained in the four multivariate schemes providing equally precise prognostic evaluation. Thus the choice of methodology for prognostication is often based on other considerations, such as ease of use as in the method of recursive partitioning, or the ability to accurately assess individual risk as provided in the Cox models.

Madsen et al. [73] compared linear discriminant analysis, Cox regression, and recursive partitioning for prediction of short-term (36-day) and long-term (1-year) mortality using two independent populations. Each scheme performed similarly for prediction of short-term mortality, with a 90 percent correct classification rate of deaths in the base sample and an 87 percent correct classification rate in a test population by discriminant analysis, and 89 percent for the other two methods. For 1-year mortality, recursive partitioning performed better than the two other methods on the test population using congestive heart failure in the CCU as the first discriminant variable.

Validation Studies of Risk Prediction Schemes

Previously developed risk prediction schemes showed good performance in risk identification in the population used to develop such schemes rather than in an independent test population. The need for validation was first developed by Peel et al. [60], who used a cohort of patients admitted to their center from 1958 to 1961 to assess and amend the weightings for each risk factor in their original prognostic index. The factors and their weights were introduced into that prognostic index based on general clinical impressions of their importance for prognosis at 4 weeks. The scheme was then applied to additional earlier cohorts comprised of patients who were admitted from 1946 to 1950 and those admitted from 1951 to 1957. Both the percentages of patients falling in the four prognostic categories established from the index and the mortality for each prognostic group varied, however, by as much as 100 percent among the three cohorts. Other studies applied the Peel index to their own population groups [93, 181]. The validation studies used small patient samples. The high Peel scores predictive of death were associated with error rates of up to 37 percent for survivors and 21 percent for deaths; similar error rates were seen for the base population used to construct the index, with a 31 percent error rate for survivors and 18 percent for deaths.

The Norris index for in-hospital mortality, developed by discriminant function analysis, was tested in other institutions [181, 184]. In the original population of 757 patients, high index scores predictive of death had a 30 percent error rate for deaths and 40 percent for survivors [11, 187]. Error rates in subsequent test populations were lower than those in the original population, ranging from 12 to 22 percent for survivors and 4 to 19 percent for deaths.

Previous studies attempted to validate the prognostic indices in groups of patients from another institution or new populations from the same institution [8, 13, 36, 75, 178, 184]. Some studies carry low prediction error rates for survivors and others low prediction rates for deaths at the relative cost for misclassification of either deaths or survivors (Table 38-3). The prediction schemes developed by linear discriminant function analysis were associated with overall error rates within 6 percent of those derived from their base population. Habib et al. [182] compared the Norris index developed by discriminant function analysis with the Chapman index [188] developed by multiple regression in a small independent population. They found 88.3 percent total correct classification for the Chapman index and 77.7 percent for the Norris index. However, Rotmensch et al. [181] found a lesser performance for the Norris index, with only 38.6 percent correct classification. This study also tested the Peel index, with higher total correct classification but with very low correct classification of the deaths (15 percent).

Moss et al. [178] applied their two prognostic stratification schemes for a 4-month mortality that was developed on a 1973 cohort to patients studied during 1974. Only one of the schemes performed satisfactorily on the 1974 population, as the mortalities for the low- and high-risk groups were not statistically different using the other scheme.

The application of prognostic stratification techniques developed by Moss et al. showed high error rates when applied to populations of other institutions [11, 183]. The identified prognostic predictors (20 or more PVCs/hr, history of angina with moderate activity or at rest, and hypotension or heart failure in the CCU) were applied by Bigger et al. [183], without differences in mortality rates when compared to patients in their population without these predictors. The lack of cross-validation of a

Table 38-3
Validation results for risk stratification schemes

First author	Period	Method	No. of pts.[a]	No. of survivors[a]	No. of deaths[a]
Chapelle [184]	14 days	LDF	B 159 (.18)	142 (.18)	17 (.18)
			T 201 (.16)	176 (.15)	25 (.24)
Henning [7]	30 days	LDF	B 177 (.07)	143 (.03)	33 (.27)
			T 150 (.12)	123 (.04)	27 (.48)
Evans [66]	3 mo	LDF	B 298 (.29)	249 (.33)	49 (.04)
			T 437 (.35)	362 (.44)	95 (.04)
Moss [178]	4 mo	PS	B 269 (.13)	258 (.12)	11 (.36)
			T 234 (.16)	223 (.14)	11 (.55)
Helmers [13]	1 yr	AID	B 308 (.24)	255 (.21)	53 (.38)
			T 163 (.21)	141 (.20)	22 (.32)
Luria [36]	2 yr	LDF	B 137 (.17)	110 (.06)	27 (.59)
			T 105 (.14)	91 (.08)	22 (.57)

LDF = linear discriminant function analysis; PS = prognostic stratification; AID = automatic interaction detection; B = base sample; T = test sample.
[a]Numbers in parentheses are the percent error (percent of the group incorrectly classified).

prediction scheme in this study was attributed to the discrepancy of the two patient populations with respect to age, mortality at 4 months, cardiac status, and urban versus suburban locale.

In a much larger study involving the placebo group of 2789 patients in the Coronary Drug Project, it was observed that even though very different variables proved important within each of two geographically separated subpopulations, acceptable performance for 3-year mortality was achieved when this scheme was applied to the other population and subsequently to a third group of patients from clinics not part of the Coronary Drug Project [41]. Our studies indicated that cross-population testing of various prediction schemes produces acceptable classification results for deaths and survivors when applied to new populations, with total correct classification ranging from 50 to 68 percent [185, 186].

Low-Risk Identification

The goal of risk stratification and prognostication after AMI is to include a scheme that allows stratification of the individual patient into high-risk or low-risk status. A low-risk status implies a less than 2 percent risk of cardiac death during the first year after myocardial infarction and a reduced probability of recurrent infarction and rehospitalization for new-onset angina [66, 189–191]. Postinfarction patients identified as having low-risk status would be candidates for early discharge and early resumption of normal physical activities and reemployment.

There has been a decreasing trend in median hospitalization time for patients with uncomplicated myocardial infarction, from a 21-day average hospital stay in 1970 to 14 days in 1979 [192]. A number of studies showed that discharge even earlier than days 5 to 9 after acute infarction is feasible for selected patients, with apparently small increase in risk [66, 189, 193, 194]. In a controlled study of 268 patients, which comprised 70 percent of the total studied population randomized to be discharged on day 9 or day 16 after admission with acute infarction, no significant differences during a 6 weeks' follow-up were reported for death, chest pain, congestive heart failure, arrhythmias, or readmission [66]. The same authors developed a prognostic index by discriminant function analysis in 298 patients that allocated 56 percent of the total infarct population to a risk group that carried a 3-month mortality rate of 1.2 percent, in contrast to a high-risk group that had a 36 percent mortality rate and represented 43.6 percent of their study population [189]. The low-risk identification required the absence of certain risk variables: electrocardiographic ST segment elevation of more than 2 mm, more than 40 ventricular ectopic beats per hour, the presence of R on T ventricular ectopic beats, persistent sinus tachycardia, blood urea nitrogen concentration over 12 mmol/L, signs of congestive heart failure on chest radiograph, and age. In a smaller study, 67 patients (42 percent of the study population) without serious complications from day 1 to day 4 were randomized to be discharged 1 week after admission in the absence of ventricular tachycardia or fibrillation, advanced-degree heart block, pulmonary edema, cardiogenic shock, sinus tachycardia, hypotension, rapid atrial arrhythmias, or extension of infarction [195]. No complications or death occurred in either of these small groups of patients during a 6-month follow-up period. These studies used insufficient sample sizes to detect an event rate that is significantly greater than the 4 to 6 percent event rate during the first year after myocardial infarction expected in the low-risk patients.

Other uncontrolled studies defined low-risk criteria for the selection of patients for early discharge resulting in low event rates of 0 to 2.7 percent during the early postdischarge period of 2 to 6 months [190, 191]. Madsen et al. [189], in a retrospective study of 1140 patients with AMI, used a daily risk assessment scheme on a Cox regression analysis that assigned the patient to a low risk of events of death, cardiac arrest, or cardiogenic shock with a projected incidence of less than 2 percent. Of the study population, 47 percent of patients fulfilled early discharge criteria but were kept in a hospital until day 18 after admission. Only one death and a 2 percent event rate occurred in this group during a 30-day observation period. The same institution prospectively discharged 67 percent of 169 consecutive patients who survived day 5, and only 1.7 percent unexpected deaths occurred between 12 and 24 days after discharge. For low-risk identification most investigators used a set of exclusion criteria that included infarct extension, persistent chest pain, signs of congestive heart failure, hypotension or cardiogenic shock, or severe arrhythmias (ventricular tachycardia, ventricular fibrillation, supraventricular tachycardia, atrial fibrillation, atrioventricular block, nodal rhythm, or frequent or complex ventricular ectopic beats). Other studies also identified elderly patients and those with a history of previous myocardial infarction not suitable for early discharge [66, 196].

Our previous studies identified a group of patients at low risk of cardiac endpoints between days 9 and 90 after acute infarction [4, 73]. Patients with complications from days 1 to 8 that would preclude early discharge were excluded when death, persistent pain beyond the first day after admission, extension of infarct, ventricular tachycardia or fibrillation, cardiac arrest, second- or third-degree heart block, or congestive heart failure occurred. Linear discriminant analysis identified a group comprising 25 percent of the total population with a 2.3 percent mortality rate between days 9 and 90, as well as a 4.6 percent combined death and complication rate during this period. The events in the low-risk group included one patient with extension of infarction on day 9, recurrent infarction on days 42 and 45, and one sudden death 23 days after discharge. In this identified low-risk group, younger age, a lower incidence of previous congestive heart failure, hypertension, family history, complex Holter arrhythmias, and higher ejection fractions were noted.

Exercise testing [120–123] and exercise thallium 201 scintigraphy testing [139, 141, 142] were shown to identify low-risk patients after myocardial infarction with annual mortality rates of less than 2 percent. Similarly, we identified a low-risk group among patients with a first myocardial infarction [197]. Patients with a first myocardial infarction at age less than 50 years with an LVEF over 40 percent and those patients between 51 and 70 years with an LVEF over 50 percent had only a 1.2 percent cardiac mortality rate within the first year. In this study, ejection fraction as the only predischarge test identified a sizable low-risk group of patients with a first myocardial infarction that comprised 47 percent of individuals with a first myocardial infarction. Studies on low-risk identification in patients undergoing coronary reperfusion therapy by thrombolysis, angioplasty, or both defined low risk in the absence of angina, congestive heart failure, ventricular arrhythmias, and provocable ischemia on exercise testing; and they discharged these patients 3 days after admission without fatal events occurring during the 6-month follow-up period, with a substantial reduction in hospital costs [198].

Further studies on low-risk identification and its applicability for early discharge are required to provide general implications for low-risk stratification after myocardial infarction and to provide a safe selection procedure for the early discharge of patients after AMI.

Prognostic Changes by Therapeutic Interventions During and After Acute Myocardial Infarction

AMI remains the most common cause of death in all Western industrialized countries. In recent years unadjusted rates of mortality from myocardial infarction have been decreasing, similar to rates of mortality due to all other causes. However, the proportion of deaths caused by AMI has not changed, accounting for 37 percent of all deaths in the United States for which a cause could be identified in 1950, for 39 percent in 1960, 1970, and 1980, and for 36 percent in 1986 [199]. A decline of in-hospital mortality from AMI was observed during the past 20 years [51, 200], although this favorable trend in improved mortality could not be demonstrated in compared mortality rates between 1973 to 1979 [201], 1974 to 1981 [202], and 1970 to 1985 [203]. The changes in early death rates after AMI before the thrombolytic era were often attributed to a single major therapeutic intervention or to differences in study populations [204, 205]. The observed decline in the incidence of ventricular fibrillation [206] and cardiogenic shock [207], which signify important predictors of early cardiac death, may have also resulted in a decrease in early and in-hospital mortality from AMI.

In the past 10 years, the hospital mortality rates from AMI have been reduced from approximately 20 percent to nearly 10 percent with the use of thrombolytic and other pharmacologic and interventional treatment methods [208, 209]. In our institution, the early mortality rate in the prethrombolytic era between 1984 and 1987 was 11.0 percent and not different from the 12.4 percent mortality rate between 1987 and 1992 when 30 percent of

Table 38-4
Mortality after thrombolytic therapy

Trial	Patients	Agent, dose	Time (hr)	Follow-up	Mortality: Therapy (%)	Mortality: Control (%)	Mortality: Risk reduction (%)	Mortality: Odds reduction (%)	p
Intravenous SK vs placebo									
Yusuf [208]	5284	SK			15.4	19.2	20	24	<.001
Intravenous SK vs placebo									
GISSI [210]	11,806	SK 1.5 MU, 1 hr	< 12	Hospital	10.7	13.0	18	20	.0002
ISAM [219]	1741	SK 1.5 MU, 1 hr	< 6	21 days	6.3	7.1	11	12	NS
White [211]	219	SK 1.5 MU, 1 hr	< 4	30 days	3.7	12.5	70	73	.016
Western Washington [220]	368	SK 1.5 MU, 1 hr	< 6	14 days	6.3	9.6	34	37	.23
ISIS-2 [212]	17,187	SK 1.5 MU, 1 hr	< 24	5 wk	9.3	12.0	23	25	<.0001
EMERAS [221]	3568	SK 1.5 MU, 1 hr	6–24	5 wk	11.2	11.8	6		NS
Intravenous APSAC vs placebo									
AIMS [214]	1258	APSAC 30 U	< 6	30 days	6.4	12.1		50.5	.0006
Intravenous rt-PA vs placebo									
ASSET [216, 217]	5011	rt-PA 100 mg, 3 hr	< 5	1 mo	7.2	9.8	26	28	.001
European Coop. [222]	129	rt-PA 0.75 mg/kg, 1.5 hr	< 6	Hospital	1.6	6.2			NS
National Heart Australia [223]	144	rt-PA 100 mg, 3 hr	< 4	Hospital	9.6	4.2			NS
European Coop. [218]	721	rt-PA 100 mg, 3 hr; ASA 250 mg, heparin 5000 U	< 5	14 days	2.8	5.7	51		NS
Intracoronary SK vs control									
Yusuf [208]	944	SK			12.5	14.7	15	18	NS
Western Washington [224]	250	SK 286,000 U	Mean 4 hr	30 days	3.7	11.2	71	71	.02
Dutch [225]	533	SK ic first 302 patients, then iv followed by ic next 231 patients	< 4 hr	14 days	5.2	9.8	46	51	.05

APSAC = anisoylated plasminogen streptokinase activator complex; ASA = acetylsalicylic acid; ic = intracoronary; iv = intravenous; NS = not significant; rt-PA = recombinant tissue-type plasminogen activator; sc = subcutaneous; SK = streptokinase.

the patients with AMI received early thrombolytic therapy. Similarly, 1-year mortality rates of 8.6 and 8.9 percent, respectively, were unchanged in the thrombolytic period. The 30-day and 1-year mortality rates of 5.4 and 2.2 percent, respectively, in the patients receiving early thrombolytic therapy, were significantly lower ($p < .001$) than the early mortality rate of 14.8 percent and 1-year mortality rate of 9.4 percent for patients who did not receive thrombolytic treatment.

Thrombolytic Therapy

Since 1986 there has been increasing evidence for the reduction of early and late mortality by streptokinase, anisoylated plasminogen streptokinase activator complex (APSAC), and recombinant tissue-type plasminogen activator (rt-PA) for patients treated intravenously early after the onset of AMI [208]. An overview [208] (Table 38-4) of 24 randomized trials of intravenous thrombolytic therapy in 5284 patients with AMI showed a significantly lower early mortality rate of 15.4 percent in the treatment group compared to a 19.2 percent mortality rate in the control group, resulting in a significant odds reduction of 24 percent. Table 38-4 reviews the mortality trials of thrombolytic therapy, which differed in the type and dose of the thrombolytic agent, patient selection and time of administration in relation to the onset of infarction, and the concurrent therapies.

An overview of results of randomized clinical trials of thrombolytic therapy utilizing intravenous streptokinase estimated a significant 24 percent mortality reduction and an increased benefit on mortality by early administration of the thrombolytic agent within 6 hours after the onset of infarct symptoms [208]. The large-scale trials conducted since 1986 demonstrated mortality reduction by intravenous streptokinase [210–212]. The Gruppo Italiano per lo Studio della Streptokinase nell infarcto Miocardico (GISSI) study [210] enrolled 11,806 patients in 176 coronary care units in Italy and randomized them to receive streptokinase or conventional therapy. In both groups, 21 percent of patients received intravenous heparin and/or oral anticoagulants and antiplatelet therapy was used in 14 percent of patients. The GISSI study demonstrated a reduction in hospital mortality from 13 to 10.7 percent, a significant 18 percent risk reduction (Fig. 38-5). The Second International Study of Infarct Survival (ISIS-2) [212] randomized 17,187 patients in 417 hospitals in Europe, Australia, New Zealand, the United States, and Canada, with placebo control, to receive intravenous streptokinase, acetylsalicylic acid (ASA), both, or neither in a factorial design. A significant 5-week vascular mortality reduction from 12.0 to 9.2 percent was demonstrated, signifying a 23 percent risk reduction by streptokinase compared with no streptokinase. The combined use of streptokinase and ASA compared with no streptokinase or ASA showed a significant 39 percent risk reduction and decreased the 5-week mortality rate from 13.2 to 8 percent. This significant reduction in the risk of early death was also seen in patients who did not receive routine anticoagulation therapy, and the magnitude in reduction of mortality was similar among patients who did and those who did not receive anticoagulants. White et al. [211] showed a significant 72 percent risk reduction and reduced 30-day mortality rate by streptokinase, from 12.5 to 3.7 percent. An overview of the thrombolytic trials with intravenous streptokinase demonstrated a significant average odds reduction of 23 percent with the use of streptokinase within 24 hours and a further significant average odds reduction of 27 percent when streptokinase was administered within 6 hours after the onset of infarct symptoms.

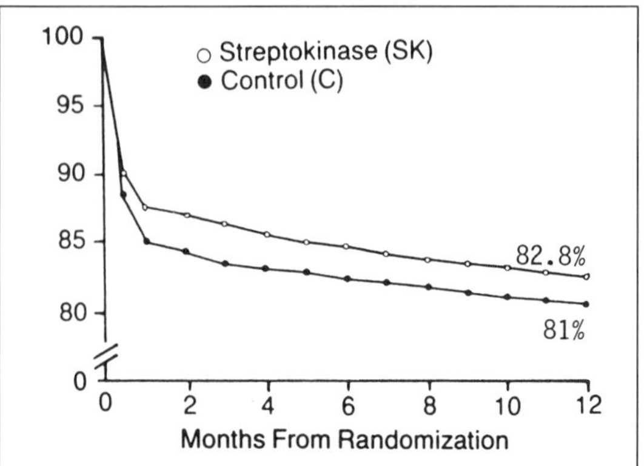

Fig. 38-5
Cumulative percent survival in the GISSI trial. The 1-year survival rate of 82.8 percent in the 5851 patients with acute myocardial infarction treated with streptokinase was significantly higher than the 81 percent in the 5846 control patients. A significant improvement in 21-day survival was also demonstrated in the streptokinase-treated patients.

Tables 38-4 and 38-5 review other thrombolytic agents and their effect on early and late mortality.

The APSAC Intervention Mortality Study (AIMS) [213, 214] randomized 1258 patients to receive 30 U of APSAC or placebo within 6 hours after AMI. The 30-day mortality rate was significantly reduced from 12.1 to 6.4 percent, which represented a 50.5 percent odds reduction of mortality. Combining data from previous trials of APSAC on a total of about 2000 patients suggested a significant 50 percent reduction in mortality [215].

The Anglo-Scandinavian Study of Early Thrombolysis (ASSET) [216, 217] in 1988 examined the effect of intravenous rt-PA on 1-month mortality. In this study, 5011 patients were randomized to receive intravenous rt-PA or placebo; all patients received intravenous heparin for 24 hours, but no aspirin was given. The 1-month mortality rate was reduced by rt-PA to 7.2 percent from 9.8 percent, a 26 percent risk reduction. The European Cooperative trial [218] compared rt-PA with placebo to examine the effects of rt-PA on left ventricular function, infarct size, and morbidity in 722 patients randomized to receive rt-PA; all patients received heparin and 250 mg of aspirin. There was an insignificant decrease in mortality rate to 3.7 percent with rt-PA from 6.8 percent with placebo. The overview of rt-PA trials shows a significant 29 percent pooled odds reduction of mortality.

Comparison of Thrombolytic Agents and Their Effect on Mortality and Survival

The earlier trials on thrombolytic therapy showed conclusive evidence on the reduction of risk of death after AMI by the available thrombolytic agents streptokinase, APSAC, and rt-PA, without any distinct advantage of any thrombolytic agent on relative efficacies and side effect profiles. This resulted in comparative trials because of the apparent effect sizes observed in different trials potentially influenced by differences in patient selection, timing of treatment, and concurrent interventions.

The comparisons of thrombolytic agents, doses and routes of administration, and their effects on mortality and risk reduction are reviewed in Table 38-5. In the GISSI-2 trial [228, 229], 20,891 patients with AMI were randomized within 6 hours of symptom onset, to compare the benefits and risks of streptokinase and tissue plasminogen activator (t-PA). Patients were also randomly allocated to receive heparin (12,500 U subcutaneously twice daily starting within 12 hours of thrombolysis) or usual therapy. All patients were given aspirin, 325 mg daily for 30 days; intravenous atenolol followed by oral atenolol was administered to 45 percent of the patients. No significant differences were observed in 35-day mortality rates between t-PA and streptokinase (9.6 compared with 9.2 percent) or between heparin and no heparin (9.3 compared with 9.4 percent). No significant differences were observed among groups regarding major cardiac complications. The long-term follow-up of patients in GISSI-2 showed no significant changes in the differences for survival between t-PA and streptokinase.

The Third International Study of Infarct Survival (ISIS-3) [234] was a randomized trial directly comparing the effectiveness of three thrombolytic agents—streptokinase, standard-dose t-PA, and APSAC—in reducing mortality and the additive effects of heparin to a thrombolytic ASA regimen. The 41,299 patients admitted within 24 hours after onset of suspected AMI were randomly assigned to receive streptokinase, t-PA, or APSAC. All patients received aspirin, 162 mg daily, and were further randomly assigned to receive heparin (12,500 U subcutaneously twice daily for 7 days starting 4 hours after randomization) or not to receive heparin. The vascular mortality rates at 35 days were 10.3 percent for the t-PA group, 10.6 percent for the streptokinase group, and 10.5 percent for the APSAC group, without differences in mortality rates among the three thrombolytic treatment groups. Similarly, in the subset of patients randomized within 6 hours after the onset of symptoms, no difference in mortality was seen among the three thrombolytic treatment groups. No difference in mortality existed among the heparin-treated patients (10.3 percent) and the patients not treated with heparin (10.6 percent). The rates for major in-hospital clinical events including cardiogenic shock, heart failure requiring treatment, ventricular fibrillation, and cardiac rupture were also identical. A small but significant deficit of in-hospital reinfarctions was observed in the t-PA treatment group. In data-derived subgroup analysis in patients from ISIS-3 who received intravenous heparin as a protocol deviation, no differential mortality effect was found when one agent was compared with another: the 35-day mortality rates were 10 percent for t-PA with heparin treatment compared with 10.7 percent without heparin treatment, 10.5 percent for strepto-

Table 38-5
Mortality after thrombolytic therapy: comparisons of thrombolytic agents

Trial	Patients	Agent, dose	Time (hr)	Follow-up	Mortality: Therapy (%)	Mortality: Control (%)	Mortality: Risk reduction (%)	Mortality: Odds reduction (%)	p
Intravenous SK vs intravenous APSAC									
Anderson [226]			< 4	Hospital	SK: 7.1	APSAC: 5.9			.61
Intravenous SK vs intravenous rt-PA									
TIMI-I [227]	290	rt-PA 80 mg, 3 hr or SK 1.5 MU, 1 hr	< 7	21 days	SK: 5	rt-PA: 4			.61
European Coop. [222]	129	rt-PA 0.75 mg/kg, 1.5 hr or SK 1.5 MU, 1 hr	< 6	Hospital	SK: 4.6	rt-PA: 4.7			NS
White [211]	270	rt-PA 100 mg, 3 hr vs SK 1.5 MU, 0.5 hr, heparin at 30 min → 48 hr ASA/DIP	< 3	30 days	7.4	3.7			NS
GISSI-2 [228]	12,490	rt-PA 100 mg, 3 hr vs SK 1.5 MU, 0.5–1.0 hr	< 6	Hospital	SK: 8.6	rt-PA: 9.0			NS
International Study Group [229]	20,891	rt-PA 100 mg, 3 hr vs SK 1.5 MU, 0.5–1 hr	< 6	Hospital	8.5	8.9			NS
Intravenous SK vs intravenous scuPA									
PRIMI [230]	401	SK 1.5 MU, 1 hr scuPA 80 mg 1 hr + heparin bolus at 3 hr then infusion → oral	< 4	Hospital	SK: 4.9	scuPA: 3.5			NS

Intravenous APSAC vs intravenous rt-PA									
Bassand [231]	183	APSAC 30 U, rt-PA 100 mg, 3 hr	< 4	3 wk	APSAC: 5.5	rt-PA: 7.5			NS
TAPS [232]	435	APSAC 30 U, rt-PA 100 mg, 1.5 hr + heparin	< 6	Hospital	8.1	2.4	70		.0095
Intravenous rt-PA vs intravenous UK									
GAUS [233]	245	rt-PA 70 mg single, 1.5 hr vs UK 3 MU, 1.5 hr + heparin → oral	< 6	Hospital	t-PA: 4.8	UK: 4.1			NS
Intravenous SK vs APSAC vs intravenous rt-PA									
ISIS-3 [234]	46,091	SK 1.5 MU 1 hr, APSAC 30 U, 3 to 5 min, immediate ASA, random sc heparin	< 24	35 days	SK: 10.5	APSAC: 10.6	rt-PA: 10.3		NS
Intravenous SK vs SK/rt-PA vs rt-PA									
GUSTO [235]	41,021	SK 1.5 MU 1 hr + heparin sc or iv, or SK 1.5 MU 1 hr + rt-PA 1.0 mg/kg 1 hr + heparin, or rt-PA 1.25 mg/kg 1.5 hr + heparin	< 6	30 days	SK-sc heparin: 7.2	SK-iv heparin: 7.4	SK/rt-PA: 7.0; rt-PA: 6.3	14	.001 (accel. rt-PA vs SK)

APSAC = anisoylated plasminogen streptokinase activator complex; ASA = acetylsalicylic acid; DIP = dipyridamole; iv = intravenous; MI = myocardial infarction; NS = not significant; rt-PA = recombinant tissue-type plasminogen activator; sc = subcutaneous; scuPA = single-chain urokinase-type plasminogen activator; SK = streptokinase; UK = urokinase.

kinase with heparin and 10.6 percent without heparin, and 10.5 percent with APSAC and heparin and 10.6 percent without heparin. However, the stroke rate among patients receiving intravenous heparin was twice that among patients treated with subcutaneous heparin, regardless of whether they were receiving streptokinase, t-PA, or APSAC. An overview of the GISSI-2 and ISIS-3 data indicated a 35-day mortality rate of 10 percent associated with both t-PA and streptokinase. An overview of the heparin effect for the two trials showed mortality rates of 10 percent with heparin and 10.2 percent with no heparin. During the 7-day heparin treatment period, the mortality rate of 6.8 percent with heparin was significantly lower than the 7.3 percent rate without heparin. It has been suggested that the GISSI-2 and ISIS-3 studies had an insufficiently vigorous heparin regimen for a maximum benefit from t-PA or streptokinase. It appears that full-dose intravenous heparin treatment may have a beneficial effect in sustaining infarct vessel patency among patients treated with t-PA. The rt-PA–APSAC Patency Study (TAPS) group [232] randomized 435 patients within 6 hours after the onset of symptoms to receive ''front-loaded'' t-PA or APSAC, and all patients received an initial bolus injection of 5000 U of heparin and intravenous infusion started after 90 minutes in the t-PA group and after 6 hours in the APSAC group with continued anticoagulation during the hospital stay. A significantly lower in-hospital death rate of 2.4 percent was observed in the t-PA group compared to 8.1 percent for the APSAC group.

The multinational Global Utilization of Streptokinase and Tissue Plasminogen Activator for Occluded Arteries (GUSTO) trial [235] examined the relation of a specific thrombolytic regimen for rapid and sustained infarct vessel recanalization and improved survival after AMI. The GUSTO study evaluated two new ''accelerated'' t-PA regimens and compared them with streptokinase given with either intravenous or subcutaneous heparin. Within 6 hours after the onset of AMI, the 41,021 patients were randomly assigned to receive one of the following four treatments: accelerated-dose rt-PA combined with intravenous heparin, accelerated-dose rt-PA combined with streptokinase and intravenous heparin, standard-dose streptokinase combined with intravenous heparin, and standard-dose streptokinase combined with subcutaneous heparin. All patients also received 160 mg of aspirin. The 30-day mortality rates were 6.3 percent for rt-PA (intravenous heparin), 7 percent for rt-PA with streptokinase (intravenous heparin), 7.2 percent for streptokinase (subcutaneous heparin), and 7.4 percent for streptokinase (intravenous heparin). The accelerated-dose rt-PA plus intravenous heparin had a 0.9 percent mortality advantage over standard-dose streptokinase plus subcutaneous heparin, although a higher stroke rate was associated with rt-PA, a 1.55 percent incidence compared with 1.22 percent in the streptokinase group. The small absolute reduction of 0.7 percent in the combined rate of death and nonfatal stroke was statistically significant. This finding was restricted to patients treated within 4 hours after the onset of symptoms. In the GUSTO trial, the median time to treatment was 2.8 hours, but most patients with AMI in the United States and Canada come to the hospital more than 4 hours after the onset of symptoms. Among the patients treated in the GUSTO study who were admitted more than 4 hours after the onset of symptoms, no thrombolytic regimen indicated an advantage in terms of mortality, a finding consistent with the ISIS-3 and GISSI-2 results. The standard-dose streptokinase plus intravenous heparin had no advantage in terms of combined mortality and nonfatal stroke rates when compared with standard-dose streptokinase plus subcutaneous heparin (8.2 compared with 7.9 percent). The accelerated-dose rt-PA combined with streptokinase and intravenous heparin had no beneficial effect when compared with standard doses of streptokinase plus subcutaneous heparin (7.9 percent for both groups). In this study the patients treated with accelerated-dose rt-PA were significantly more likely to have emergency coronary artery bypass graft surgery than were patients treated with streptokinase (9.5 compared with 8.5 percent), despite somewhat lower rates of congestive heart failure, pulmonary edema, and cardiogenic shock in patients receiving accelerated-dose rt-PA than in those receiving streptokinase. The benefit of accelerated-dose rt-PA for improved survival appeared to be restricted to US patients in the GUSTO trial. In the GUSTO trial, 7803 patients were studied outside the United States. In this group, the lowest mortality rate was seen in patients receiving the regimen of accelerated-dose rt-PA plus streptokinase. No difference was found in the mortality benefit from accelerated-dose rt-PA plus intravenous heparin when compared with standard-dose streptokinase plus subcutaneous heparin, suggesting the possibility of inadvertently introduced bias by the open-label design of the study.

Intracoronary Thrombolytic Therapy

Intracoronary thrombolytic trials [236, 237] were carried out to study mortality, coronary artery patency, and left ventricular function and are reviewed in Table 38-6. The Western Washington trial [224, 237] randomized 250 patients to receive intracoronary streptokinase or conventional therapy after coronary angiography, at a mean of 4.5 hours after the onset of acute infarct symptoms. The 30-day mortality rate for patients who received a mean of 286,000 U of streptokinase was 3.7 percent, significantly lower than the 11.2 percent rate in the control group and a 67 percent reduction. An improved 1-year survival rate was observed in patients with an infarct in an anterior location after early intracoronary streptokinase treatment. The Dutch trial [236] of intracoronary streptokinase randomized 533 patients within 4 hours after acute infarction to receive conventional therapy or rapid recanalization of the occluded coronary artery. In the first 136 patients, 250,000 U of intracoronary streptokinase was used and in the subsequent 117 patients intravenous streptokinase was given and followed by intracoronary streptokinase if persisting occlusion was observed at the time of cardiac catheterization. The 2-week mortality was significantly reduced from 9.8 to 5.2 percent following intracoronary streptokinase treatment and similarly showed a significantly improved 1-year mortality rate. The comparison of intravenous APSAC and intracoronary streptokinase administered within 6 hours after the onset of symptoms did not reveal significant differences in hospital mortality [239]. Because intracoronary thrombolytic therapy requires urgent cardiac catheterization, it is rarely used today as a strategy for treatment of AMI.

Mortality Reduction in Subgroups of Patients

Large-scale randomized and placebo-controlled thrombolytic trials have accumulated large patient numbers and subsets for comparison of effectiveness of thrombolytic therapy in defined risk groups. Immediate risk stratification at the time of presentation with AMI may identify patients who would be expected to have a poor prognosis without reperfusion and in whom reperfusion may provide improved survival and preservation of left ventricular function. Risk indicators of poor early prognosis at the time of admission with myocardial infarction include advanced age, previous myocardial infarction, hypotension with a systolic blood pressure less than 100 mm Hg, heart rate greater than 100 beats per minute, the presence of atrial fibrillation, Killip class III or IV, and anterior ST segment elevation on the initial electrocardiogram. Both the benefit and the risk of therapy may depend on patient subgroups (i.e., a potential greater absolute mortality reduction could be experienced after thrombolytic therapy in advanced age), while a greater risk of hemorrhage and stroke with associated increased mortality could result from the same treatment.

Age

The effect of age on mortality was examined in the recent thrombolytic trials [210, 216, 228]. A consistent deleterious effect of advancing age on mortality in both treatment and control groups was found. An approximately 2.4 times increased mortality was observed in older patients. Most studies [212, 213, 216] demonstrated a significant reduction in mortality with treatment of patients over 70 years old. Pooled data indicate that thrombolytic treatment in the elderly results in two additional lives saved per 100 patients treated when compared with younger patients receiving thrombolytic therapy.

Gender

The thrombolytic trials demonstrating improved short-term mortality had a similar favorable influence in both males and females; however, in the GISSI-1 trial [210], the overall mortality in the placebo group was twofold in females (22.6 percent) compared with males (10.6 percent). Other studies [212, 213, 216] revealed a consistent 1.5 to 2 times increase in mortality in females (10.9 to 22.6 percent) versus males (9.4 to 12.0 percent). The overall benefit of thrombolytic therapy is estimated to save two lives per 1000 patients; an additional 1.5 to 2 female lives versus male lives would be saved.

Table 38-6
Total mortality at 6 to 12 months of follow-up after thrombolytic therapy

Trial	Patients	Agent, dose	Follow-up	Mortality: Therapy (%)	Mortality: Placebo (%)	Mortality: Risk reduction (%)	Mortality: Odds reduction (%)	*p*
Intravenous SK vs placebo								
GISSI [210]	11,806	SK	1 yr	17.2	19	9.5	11	.008
ISAM [238]	1741	SK	7 mo	10.9	11.1	1.8	2	NS
ISIS-2 [212]	17,187	SK	1 yr	13	16.3	20	23	.0001
Intracoronary SK vs placebo								
Dutch [236]	533	SK iv/ic	1 yr	9	16	44	52	.01
	533	ic SK	3 yr	13	21			
			5 yr	19	29	39		
Intracoronary SK vs conventional								
Western Washington [237]	250	SK	1 yr	8.2	14.7	44	52	.10 (unadjusted); .03 (adjusted for LV function and MI location)
Intravenous APSAC								
AIMS [214]	1258	APSAC	1 yr	11.1	17.8	42.7		.0007
Intravenous rt-PA								
ASSET [217]	5013	rt-PA	6 mo	10.4	13.1	21		.0026
			12 mo	13.2	15.1	12.6		
Intravenous SK vs intravenous rt-PA				SK	rt-PA			
TIMI-I [227]	290	SK vs rt-PA	6 mo	9.5	7.7			NS
			12 mo	11.6	10.5			NS

APSAC = anisoylated plasminogen streptokinase activator complex; ic = intracoronary; iv = intravenous; LV = left ventricular; MI = myocardial infarction; NS = not significant; rt-PA = recombinant tissue-type plasminogen activator; sk = streptokinase.

Previous Myocardial Infarction

The beneficial effect on the reduction in mortality in patients with a previous myocardial infarction has been variable [210, 212, 213]. In the GISSI-1 trial, placebo patients with a previous infarction had a higher mortality rate (16.5 percent) compared with those without a previous myocardial infarction (12.3 percent). No treatment effect could be demonstrated in patients with a previous myocardial infarction. Both the ISIS-2 [212] and AIMS study [214] showed a benefit for survival from thrombolytic therapy in patients with a previous myocardial infarction. In the high-risk group of patients with prior myocardial infarction, thrombolytic therapy leads to the saving of at least two lives per 100 patients treated.

Time to Treatment

The interval after the onset of acute symptoms during which treatment is beneficial for reduction in mortality extends over the first 12 hours after the onset of infarction [212, 228]. A pooled analysis of large trials demonstrated that treatment within 6 hours significantly reduced mortality by 26 percent and that later treatment between 6 and 24 hours results in a lesser reduction of mortality by 17 percent [208, 219]. In the GISSI-1 study [210], the largest effect on mortality was observed with early treatment of the 0- to 1-hour treatment group. This marked benefit of mortality reduction during this very early time window was not confirmed in the ISIS-2 trial [212]. The ISIS-2 study included large numbers of patients after 6 hours and observed a significant mortality reduction even when treatment was started between 6 and 24 hours. A benefit for the reduction in vascular mortality was observed for treatment between 5 and 12 hours and between 13 and 24 hours. The AIMS trial [213] and Anglo-Scandinavian Study of Early Thrombolysis (ASSET) [216] did not show any difference in the treatment effect between 0 and 3 hours as opposed to 3 to 5 hours. The Late Assessment of Thrombolytic Efficacy (LATE) study [240] randomized patients with AMI presenting 6 to 24 hours after the onset of symptoms to receive rt-PA and aspirin or aspirin alone. The results showed a significant 14 percent relative reduction in mortality rate from 10.3 to 8.8 percent, and the analysis of patients presenting 6 to 12 hours after symptom onset showed a significant 27 percent mortality reduction from 11.9 to 8.7 percent. The patients presenting between 12 and 24 hours after symptom onset experienced no benefit on survival. Therefore, the relative risk reduction and significance of the mortality reduction are more marked in patients receiving thrombolytic treatment between 0 and 6 hours, somewhat less in patients treated at 7 to 12 hours, and uncertain for the patients treated between 13 and 24 hours. The primary indication for thrombolytic therapy between 12 and 24 hours after myocardial infarction has been the persistence of pain or ischemia.

Hemodynamic Status on Admission

The hemodynamic status and clinical class on admission determine early and late mortality after myocardial infarction and the therapeutic effect on reduced mortality by early thrombolytic treatment. The GISSI-1 trial [210] showed a twofold to threefold rise in the mortality rate according to the Killip class on admission. Placebo-treated patients in class I had a 7.3 percent early mortality rate; class II, 19.9 percent; class III, 39 percent; and class IV, 70.1 percent. Beneficial treatment effects of streptokinase were observed in Killip class I and II patients, there was a trend for such improvement in Killip class III patients, and no benefit was evident in patients in Killip class IV.

Infarct Location and Electrocardiographic Abnormalities

In recent randomized and placebo-controlled thrombolytic trials [210, 212, 213, 216], patients with anterior ST elevation and infarct location had high mortality rates of 7.5 to 20.6 percent when they were untreated, and patients with inferior ST elevation and infarct location had mortality rates from 7.2 to 10.2 percent. While some studies suggested that only patients with anterior myocardial infarction were likely to benefit from thrombolytic therapy in terms of mortality reduction [210], other studies [208, 212] demonstrated a reduction in mortality among patients with inferior myocardial infarction, patients with undefined or multiple sites of myocardial infarction, and patients with previous myocardial infarction. The ISIS-2 trial [212] demonstrated that the beneficial effect in patients with anterior myocardial infarction results in an expected four lives per 100 saved with thrombolytic therapy. A recent pooled analysis [241] indicated benefits of two per 100 lives saved in patients with an inferior infarction. In the GUSTO trial [235], both patients with anterior and those with inferior myocardial infarctions derived a mortality benefit from accelerated-dose rt-PA as compared with streptokinase, although the benefit in those with anterior infarctions was greater, with a mortality rate of 8.6 versus 10.5 percent, compared with 4.7 versus 5.3 percent, respectively, for patients with an inferior infarction. Patients with left bundle branch block showed a marked benefit from treatment in the ISIS-2 trial [212]. The 27.7 percent mortality rate in the control group was significantly higher than the 14.1 percent rate in the treated group. Such mortality benefit for patients with left bundle branch block was not demonstrated in the GISSI-1 trial. Similarly, no benefit was evident in patients presenting with ST depression or normal electrocardiograms.

Mortality and Patency of the Infarct-Related Artery

Thrombolytic therapy can lead to recanalization and reperfusion of the infarct-related artery. Early reperfusion results in preservation of the myocardium and improved left ventricular function. It is generally believed that improvement in left ventricular function after reperfusion is the major mechanism by which survival is improved, left ventricular function and ejection fraction being the strongest independent predictors of survival. Several placebo-controlled trials demonstrated improved ejection fraction and reduced mortality [242, 243]. Other studies demonstrated significant improvement in left ventricular function without a significant reduction in deaths, but an associated consistent trend for improved survival [223, 232]. A Dutch study [225] of patients treated within 2 hours after the onset of symptoms revealed a benefit for improvement in survival, recovery of left ventricular function, and salvage of myocardium. It appears that early patency of the infarct artery results in better left ventricular function and lower morbidity and mortality [244], improvements in ejection fraction and regional wall motion, and decreases in the enzyme index of infarct size [219]. There are sufficient data to support the relationship between thrombolysis-induced myocardial preservation and a reduction in mortality; however, there are also data suggesting that late therapy, beyond the time when substantial myocardial salvage is probable, may improve survival [210, 212, 219], although by comparison with early initiated thrombolytic therapy, a lesser benefit is observed.

Variable early patency rates after thrombolytic therapy have been reported in 44 to 78 percent of patients treated with streptokinase and higher patency rates of 60 to 91 percent following rt-PA treatment. The GUSTO trial [235, 245] examined the speed of restoration of patency of the infarct artery and its effect on improvement in survival after AMI. In 2431 patients who were randomly assigned to receive one of the four thrombolytic treatment strategies, coronary arteriography was randomly assigned to be performed 90 minutes, 180 minutes, 24 hours, or 5 to 7 days after the initiation of thrombolytic therapy. The patency of the infarct-related artery was highest at 90 minutes in the group given accelerated-dose rt-PA and heparin. The 81 percent patency rate was significantly higher than the 54 percent rate in the group receiving streptokinase and subcutaneous heparin, the 60 percent patency rate after streptokinase and intravenous heparin treatment, and the 73 percent patency rate in the group receiving combined rt-PA and streptokinase therapy. A TIMI grade 2 or 3 flow in the infarct artery was achieved at 90 minutes in 54 percent of patients given rt-PA and heparin but in less than 40 percent of patients in the three other treatment groups. By 180 minutes the patency differences disappeared, and patency was essentially the same in all four treatment groups. There was a relationship between left ventricular function and coronary artery patency status across all groups. Ejection fraction was better among patients demonstrating TIMI grade 3 flow at 90 minutes and at 5 to 7 days when compared with those who demonstrated TIMI grade 2 flow. Left ventricular function was best in the group given rt-PA with heparin and in patients with normal flow in the infarct-related artery, irrespective of treatment group. The infarct artery patency status at 90 minutes related to 30-day mortality: the 4.4 percent mortality rate in patients with normal coronary flow at 90 minutes was significantly lower than the 8.9 percent mortality rate in patients with no flow in the infarct artery. This suggests that the mechanism of more rapid and complete restoration of coronary flow in the infarct-related artery results in improved ventricular performance and lower mortality and the more significant reduction of mortality with the use of accelerated rt-PA therapy. This is the rationale for preferring t-PA in young patients who present very early with a presumed anterior myocardial infarction.

A recent study examined the patency of the infarct-related artery and left ventricular function and its relation to mortality after Q-wave myocardial infarction [246]. In this study of Q-wave myocardial infarction from single-vessel coronary artery disease, only the infarct artery patency and end-systolic volume index were independently related to survival. Long-term survival was significantly higher in patients who had patent infarct-related arteries and TIMI grade 2 to 3 flow than in patients with grade 0 or 1 flow. The importance of patency of the infarct-related artery for short-term and long-term mortality was demonstrated in patients with cardiogenic shock complicating AMI [247]. Identified predictors of in-hospital death were patency of the infarct-related artery, patient age, and lowest cardiac index. The 33 percent mortality rate in patients with patent infarct-related arteries was significantly lower than the 75 percent rate in those with closed arteries. Patients who survived cardiogenic shock to hospital discharge had a 1-year mortality rate of 18 percent and postdischarge mortality was independently predicted by patency of the infarct-related artery, age, and ejection fraction.

It appears that the fibrin-specific fibrinolytic agents rt-PA and single-chain urokinase plasminogen activator are more effective in achieving early infarct artery patency than the nonselective agents streptokinase, urokinase, and APSAC [222, 227, 230, 232, 248]. Generally a higher early patency or recanalization rate is achieved with rt-PA rather than streptokinase; however, patency rates at 24 hours and at discharge are similar with all thrombolytic agents. Front-loaded doses of rt-PA administered over 90 minutes resulted in early patency rates of 80 to 90 percent, potentially enhancing myocardial preservation and survival, when compared with previously employed 3- to 6-hour regimens [232, 249]. Reocclusion results in poor left ventricular function and a mortality rate similar to that in patients who do not achieve any patency [250]. A combination of a clot-selective agent with a nonselective thrombolytic agent may reduce the rate of reocclusion [251, 252] but this was not confirmed in the combined rt-PA–streptokinase treatment arm in the GUSTO study. No difference in improvement of LVEF following treatment with the different thrombolytic agents has been demonstrated [248, 253].

Use of intravenous heparin with rt-PA improves infarct artery patency [254]. Early patency appears to be reduced when heparin is not administered with rt-PA. In a recent study [255] a higher late patency rate was found in patients who were given heparin and this difference was greater in those who had an activated partial thromboplastin time in a therapeutic range as compared with those in whom this parameter was in a subtherapeutic range. In the GISSI-2 [228] and ISIS-2 [212] trials, randomized treatment with heparin was delayed by 4 to 12 hours and heparin was administered subcutaneously. Heparin treatment did not result in any added benefit of survival. The GUSTO trial [245] established a correlation between infarct artery patency and the degree of anticoagulation with intravenous heparin. The treatment with accelerated-dose rt-PA together with intravenous heparin resulted in a higher infarct artery patency rate and lower mortality rate than when streptokinase was given with either intravenous or subcutaneous heparin. Treatment with intravenous or subcutaneous heparin was not associated with a difference in mortality for the patients in the GUSTO trial who received streptokinase, although higher early rates of infarct artery patency were observed in the streptokinase-treated patients who also received intravenous heparin.

Adjunctive Medical Therapy for Thrombolysis

Adjunctive therapy with thrombolysis aims at achieving maximal myocardial preservation and achieving and maintaining coronary artery patency and potential improvement in survival. Management strategies and medical modalities initiated during and following the acute phase of myocardial infarction aim at secondary prevention and reduction of long-term morbidity and mortality. Large trials of adjunctive and postlytic treatment regimens have been evaluated for the additional benefit over thrombolytic therapy alone and for the added benefit on infarct size reduction of promoting and maintaining patency of the infarct-related artery and improvement in left ventricular function and mortality. Thus, antithrombotic treatment potentiates the efficacy of the thrombolytic agent by decreasing the time to reperfusion and preventing reocclusion of the infarct artery.

Aspirin

Aspirin is an antithrombotic agent that reduces mortality following AMI. The ISIS-2 pilot study showed that the early administration of aspirin at a dose of 160 mg/day resulted in a significant 21 percent reduction in mortality compared with a control group. In addition, there was a significant 44 percent reduction in nonfatal myocardial infarction. The ISIS-2 trial [212] demonstrated the additional benefit of aspirin for AMI treated with thrombolytic therapy. The beneficial effects of streptokinase and aspirin appear to be largely independent of each other and their combined benefits appear additive. In this trial, 7187 patients presenting within 24 hours of symptoms were randomly selected for treatment with intravenous streptokinase, 160 mg of oral aspirin daily for 30 days, both, or neither. With aspirin alone there was a significant decrease in mortality from 13.2 to 10.7 percent, which was similar to the mortality reduction with streptokinase alone (13.2 to 10.4 percent). A further reduction in mortality to 8 percent was observed with the combined use of aspirin and streptokinase. The reduction in mortality appeared more marked when treatment with streptokinase and aspirin was initiated within 6 hours after the onset of symptoms, but the relative benefit of aspirin did not differ with a time interval from onset of symptoms to treatment initiation. The benefit from aspirin appeared to be related to the reduction of reinfarction. The 1.8 percent reinfarction rate in the combined-treatment group was significantly lower than the 3.8 percent rate in patients treated with streptokinase alone and the 2.9 percent incidence of reinfarction in the placebo group. The combination of streptokinase and aspirin, like aspirin alone, was associated with a reduction in strokes (0.6 percent in the combined-treatment group, 0.6 percent in the aspirin group, and 1.1 percent in the placebo group).

Heparin

The effect of the addition of heparin to thrombolytic therapy (streptokinase) was investigated in the SCATI trial [256], which randomly assigned patients to receive within 24 hours after the onset of acute symptoms intravenous heparin (2000-U bolus) and subcutaneous heparin (12,500 U twice daily) or no anticoagulation. Patients admitted within 6 hours after the onset of symptoms received intravenous streptokinase, but no aspirin. In the patients treated with streptokinase, the 4.5 percent mortality rate in the heparin group was significantly lower than the 8.8 percent rate in patients not receiving heparin. No significant differences in the rates of recurrent ischemia or nonfatal reinfarction were observed. Thus, heparin appears beneficial for patients treated with streptokinase during the acute phase of infarction.

In the ISIS-2 trial [212] patients receiving intravenous heparin had a reduction in mortality rate from 13.1 to 6.4 percent and patients with subcutaneous heparin from 13.5 to 7.6 percent as compared with a reduction from 12.9 to 9.6 percent in patients not receiving heparin. The GISSI-2 [228] and ISIS-3 [234] studied the usefulness of subcutaneous heparin in patients receiving rt-PA and streptokinase. Heparin was initiated 12 hours after thrombolysis in the GISSI-2 trial and 4 hours afterward in the ISIS-3 trial. No significant effect on mortality was demonstrated. The anticoagulation therapy with heparin in these trials may have been inadequate because of the subcutaneous use of heparin resulting in subtherapeutic anticoagulation for 1 to 2 days after acute infarction. The GUSTO trial [235] did not demonstrate any differences in 24-hour and 30-day mortality with intravenous or subcutaneous heparin when used with streptokinase. In the streptokinase-treated patients, intravenous heparin was commenced immediately and continued to at least 48 hours and subcutaneous heparin was initiated 4 hours after initiation of streptokinase treatment and repeated every 12 hours for 7 days. The 30-day mortality rates were 7.4 percent with intravenous heparin and 7.2 percent with subcutaneous heparin. Higher coronary artery patency rates and a significantly lower mortality rate of 6.3 percent were demonstrated when accelerated-dose rt-PA was given with intravenous heparin than when streptokinase was given with intravenous (7.4 percent mortality) or subcutaneous heparin (7.2 percent).

The heparin-induced enhancement of the efficacy of rt-PA for the reperfusion of the infarct-related artery was demonstrated in several angiographic studies [255, 257, 258]. The TAPS trial [232] compared rt-PA with APSAC, with concomitant heparin treatment with each thrombolytic agent using 5000 U intravenously and an intravenous heparin infusion started after 1 hour in the rt-PA group and after 6 hours in the APSAC group and continued through hospitalization. The coronary artery patency rate at 90 minutes was 84.4 percent in rt-PA–treated patients, significantly higher than the 70.3 percent in the APSAC-treated group. Despite a higher reocclusion rate in the rt-PA–treated patients and a significantly higher patency rate at 48 hours with APSAC (93.4 versus 84.9 percent), the in-hospital mortality rate of 2.4 percent in the rt-PA treatment group was significantly lower than the 8.1 percent rate in the APSAC treatment group. In the GUSTO angiographic trial [245], the patency rate of the infarct-related artery was highest at 90 minutes in the group treated with accelerated-dose rt-PA (81 percent) that also received intravenous heparin with a bolus of 5000 U followed by continuous infusion of 1000 U/hr, compared with a significantly lower patency rate of 54 to 60 percent in the streptokinase-treated groups that received either subcutaneous or intravenous heparin and in the group given combination therapy with intravenous heparin. Patency of the infarct-related artery and normal flow at 90 minutes was highest in the group given rt-PA and heparin and associated with a significantly lower 30-day mortality rate of 6.3 percent as compared with 7.0 to 7.4 percent mortality rates for patients treated with streptokinase or combined thrombolytic agents. Further, the mortality rate was lowest (at 4.4 percent) in patients with normal coronary flow at 90 minutes when compared to patients with no flow (8.9 percent), supporting the relation of rapid and complete recovery of coronary flow through the infarct-related artery and associated decreased mortality.

Nitroglycerin and Nitrates

A meta-analysis of seven previous trials [259] of intravenous nitroglycerin administered within 24 hours after the onset of infarction suggested a significant reduction in mortality rates from 20.5 percent in 425 control patients to 12.0 percent in 406 treated patients. The largest single trial in the prethrombolytic era examined the nitroglycerin effect on mortality in 310 patients receiving intravenous nitroglycerin within 12 hours after the onset of acute symptoms to obtain a mean blood pressure reduction of 10 percent and continued for 40 hours [260]. Intravenous nitroglycerin reduced in-hospital mortality rates from 26 to 14 percent and 1-year mortality rates from 31 to 21 percent with a favorable effect on reinfarction. These benefits appeared greater in patients with anterior myocardial infarction. The addition of nitroglycerin to thrombolysis appears to provide earlier and better improvement in left ventricular function, when combined nitroglycerin and streptokinase were compared with streptokinase alone and placebo [261]. In a $2 \times 2 \times 2$ factorial design, the ISIS-4 trial [262] randomized patients within 24 hours after the onset of symptoms of suspected AMI to receive oral isosorbide mononitrate or placebo for 1 month, oral captopril or placebo for 1 month, and intravenous magnesium sulfate for 24 hours, in addition to streptokinase therapy and antiplatelet therapy. Oral isosorbide mononitrate was initiated early with 30 mg and the dose was repeated 12 hours later followed by 60 mg daily. The preliminary data presented did not indicate any difference in 35-day mortality and 6-month survival rates in the isosorbide mononitrate–treated patients compared with the placebo group. In this study, intravenous magnesium sulfate administration over 24 hours did not result in any improved mortality, although meta-analysis of magnesium treatment in AMI patients suggested a significant reduction in mortality [263, 264].

The GISSI-3 study was a randomized trial designed to evaluate the efficacy of lisinopril, nitrates, and their combination on survival and left ventricular function in patients with AMI, 72 percent of whom received thrombolytic therapy. In the 2×2 factorial design, lisinopril alone, nitrates alone, combined therapy, and no trial therapy were evaluated. Patients randomized to receive nitroglycerin therapy received a 24-hour nitroglycerin infusion followed by 10 mg of transdermal nitroglycerin daily for 6 weeks. The 6.5 percent 6-week mortality rate was not different from the 6.9 percent rate in the control group. These studies did not demonstrate any gain in short-term mortality by nitroglycerin as adjunctive treatment to thrombolysis. Nevertheless, intravenous nitroglycerin continues to be widely used in the treatment of AMI.

Beta Blockers

Clinical trials carried out in the prethrombolytic era showed that treatment with beta blockers within 12 hours after the acute onset of myocardial infarction may reduce myocardial damage, the risk of reinfarction, ventricular fibrillation, and cardiac rupture as mechanisms for reduction of early and late mortality. A review of pooled data from 27 randomized trials totaling about 27,000 patients [265–267] documented a favorable effect on the rate of reinfarction and cardiac arrest. Treatment reduced mortality significantly by 13 percent in the first week. The more marked mortality reduction in the first 2 days suggested that maximum benefit is likely to be obtained by initiation of very early treatment. Similarly, the rates of nonfatal reinfarction and nonfatal cardiac arrests in hospital were significantly reduced by 19 and 16 percent, respectively. In the ISIS-1 trial [266], vascular mortality was reduced by 15 percent during the 7 days of treatment. Mortality rates were 3.9 percent in the beta-blocker treatment group and 4.6 percent in the control group.

The TIMI-II B trial [268] examined the beneficial effect of beta blockers as adjunctive treatment to thrombolysis with rt-PA. Patients assigned to the beta-blocker treatment group received 15 mg of intravenous metoprolol followed by oral metoprolol or oral metoprolol started on day 6. Hospital mortality and left ventricular function were not different between the group treated earlier and the group treated later. Rates of nonfatal reinfarction and recurrent ischemic episodes were significantly lower in the group with early initiation of beta-blocker treatment.

Calcium Channel Blockers

Pooled data from randomized trials of calcium channel blockers in patients with AMI could not demonstrate a reduction in mortality or morbidity. A 10 percent increase in mortality was observed in patients receiving calcium channel blockers [209]. In a randomized study of 171 patients with threatened or acute myocardial infarction, no benefit was observed with nifedipine in terms of the incidence of infarction, infarct size, and mortality [269]. The 2-week mortality rate was insignificantly higher in the nifedipine-treated patients compared with the placebo group. Similarly, the Norwegian Nifedipine Multicenter Trial [270] in patients given nifedipine within 12 hours after the acute onset of symptoms failed to show a beneficial effect on mortality or infarct size. A trial of diltiazem in patients with non-Q-wave myocardial infarction observed a significant reduction in early recurrence of infarction, but no effect on 2-week mortality [271]. The use of calcium channel blockers as adjunctive treatment to thrombolysis was investigated only in a few studies. In a randomized double-blind study of nifedipine or placebo during streptokinase treatment and coronary angioplasty, nifedipine treatment resulted in an insignificantly higher mortality rate (13 versus 8 percent) and more frequent reocclusion after thrombolysis [272]. Routine use of calcium channel blockers cannot be recommended for treatment of AMI.

Angiotensin-Converting Enzyme Inhibitors

Experimental data have shown that angiotensin-converting enzyme (ACE) inhibitors may reduce the size of the infarct zone, the extent of contraction abnormality, and resulting infarct expansion [273]. These factors and adaptive changes of left ventricular remodeling ultimately determine left ventricular function after myocardial infarction, the most important determinant of short- and long-term prognosis. Captopril was shown to reduce left ventricular dilatation and subsequent mortality in rats [274]. The Survival and Ventricular Enlargement (SAVE) trial [275] randomized 2231 asymptomatic patients with a LVEF of less than 40 percent to receive captopril (25 mg three times daily during the in-hospital treatment and subsequently 50 mg three times daily) or placebo within 3 to 16 days after infarction. One-third of the patients had received thrombolytic therapy. After an average follow-up period of 42 months, a deterioration of 9 percent or more in ejection fraction had occurred in 16 percent of the surviving patients in the placebo group as compared with 13 percent of captopril-treated patients. Patients receiving captopril treatment were 37 percent less likely to develop overt congestive heart failure and had a significant 25 percent lower relative risk in reinfarction and a 22 percent relative risk reduction of hospitalization for congestive heart failure. During the mean follow-up period of 42 months, mortality of 20 percent was significantly lower in the captopril group as compared to 25 percent in the placebo group, resulting in a significant risk reduction of 19 percent with active treatment (Fig. 38-6). The vast majority of deaths were due to cardiovascular causes, which were reduced by 21 percent with captopril. Similarly, captopril treatment resulted in a 36 percent

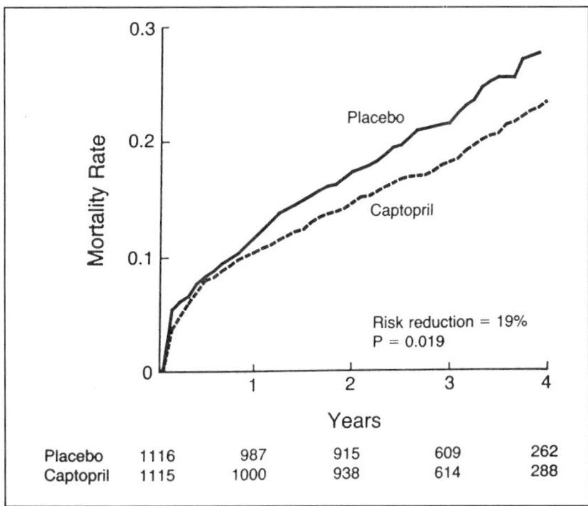

Fig. 38-6
Cumulative mortality for 1115 patients treated with captopril after acute myocardial infarction and 1116 patients with placebo in the Survival and Ventricular Enlargement (SAVE) trial. The number of patients at risk at the beginning of each year is shown at the bottom. During an average follow-up of 42 months, total mortality was 20.4 percent in the captopril group and 24.6 percent in the placebo group, indicating a significant 19 percent reduction in the risk of death.

reduction in mortality from progressive heart failure.

The Cooperative New Scandinavian Enalapril Survival Study (CONSENSUS II) trial [276] could not demonstrate any benefit on survival with the use of the ACE inhibitor enalapril. The multicenter trial enrolled 6090 patients with AMI within 24 hours after the onset of symptoms. The treatment regimen included 1 mg of enalapril given intravenously over 2 hours followed by 2.5 mg of oral enalapril 6 hours later; the dose was increased to 20 mg daily by the fifth day. At 6-month follow-up, the mortality rate was 10.2 percent in the enalapril-treated group, not different from the 9.4 percent mortality rate in the placebo group. Patients 70 years and older tended to have a higher mortality when given enalapril. It has been suggested that a beneficial effect on mortality could not be apparent in a 6-month follow-up period since significant mortality reduction in the SAVE trial became apparent at approximately 1 year of follow-up.

The Studies of Left Ventricular Dysfunction (SOLVD) trial [277] studied the effect of enalapril on mortality, development of heart failure, and hospitalization for heart failure in patients with ejection fractions of 35 percent or less and who were not receiving drug treatment for congestive heart failure. Of the 4228 patients, 80 percent had sustained myocardial infarction and were treated with enalapril (20 mg daily) or placebo. During an average follow-up of 3 years, mortality was 14.8 percent in the enalapril group and 15.8 percent in the placebo group. This risk reduction was not significant. However, there was a significant risk reduction of 29 percent of the combined endpoints of death or development of congestive heart failure and similarly, a significant 20 percent risk reduction for death or hospitalization for congestive heart failure; thus, enalapril significantly lowers the incidence of heart failure and tends to reduce cardiovascular mortality.

The beneficial effect of an ACE inhibitor in conjunction with thrombolytic therapy was also analyzed in the CONSENSUS II trial; 56 percent of the patients had received thrombolytic therapy [276]. In these patients, mortality was not different in the enalapril-treated group compared with the placebo group (7.8 and 7 percent, respectively); however, the trial had insufficient power to evaluate a benefit of early ACE inhibitor therapy.

Recently presented results of the ISIS-4 trial suggest a beneficial effect of an ACE inhibitor added to thrombolytic therapy. There were 58,000 patients randomly allocated in a $2 \times 2 \times 2$ factorial design to receive captopril at 6.25 mg for the initial dose, 12.5 mg 2 hours later, 25 mg 12 hours later, and then 50 mg twice daily, or placebo; oral isosorbide mononitrate or placebo; and intravenous magnesium sulfate for 24 hours. Patients received streptokinase and aspirin. The 30-day mortality rate of 6.8 percent was lower in the captopril-treated patients after thrombolysis as compared with the 7.3 percent mortality rate in the control group. A significantly improved 6-month survival rate was observed in the captopril-treated patients. The GISSI-3 study examined the effect of 6 weeks of treatment with the ACE inhibitor lisinopril on 6-week and 6-month mortality in 19,394 patients with AMI. Patients were randomized within 24 hours after the onset of symptoms to receive oral lisinopril at 10 mg daily or open control, and 72 percent of the randomized population received thrombolytic therapy. The lisinopril-treated group had a significantly lower mortality rate of 6.3 percent compared with 7.1 percent rate in the control group. Lisinopril also significantly reduced left ventricular damage identified by an LVEF of 35 percent or less or by 45 percent or more myocardial segment involvement measured by two-dimensional echocardiography. These two large randomized trials demonstrated a beneficial effect of ACE inhibitors as adjunct to thrombolytic therapy on 35- to 40-day and 6-month mortality after myocardial infarction.

Coronary Angioplasty

Coronary angioplasty after thrombolytic therapy attempts to open 20 percent of coronary occlusions that have not been opened with thrombolytic treatment, reduce ischemia and allow earlier and better recovery of left ventricular function, and potentially reduce the risk of reocclusion and mortality. Studies that examined the routine delayed angioplasty after thrombolysis showed that such strategy does not improve left ventricular function or subsequent mortality. The routine intervention of immediate angioplasty [268, 278–281] over a general approach made on a clinical basis has no advantage. Studies of the use of early elective [278, 279, 282] and elective conservative [268, 280] angioplasty showed a trend to higher mortality and an increased need for coronary artery bypass graft surgery. Routine angioplasty has not produced lower reinfarction rates. In the TIMI-II B trial [268] patients were randomly assigned to an invasive strategy following thrombolytic treatment with rt-PA and 60 percent underwent percutaneous transluminal coronary angioplasty (PTCA). The patients receiving the invasive approach had a trend to higher rates of reinfarction and death in 42 days and a higher rate of coronary artery bypass graft surgery. Ejection fraction at 6 weeks was not different between invasive and conservative groups, but the invasive group had a lower incidence of positive exercise tests at hospital discharge. At 1 year of follow-up there were no differences in mortality rates (invasive 6.9 percent, conservative 7.4 percent) or rates of reinfarction (invasive 9.4 percent, conservative 9.8 percent) between the two treatment strategies. In the SWIFT trial [280], 43 percent of the patients underwent coronary angioplasty and 15 percent coronary bypass surgery following thrombolytic therapy with anistreplase. In the conventional group, 5 percent required revascularization during hospital admission. The mortality rates at 12 months were 5.8 percent in the delayed elective intervention group, and 5.0 percent in the conventional treatment group. There was no difference in the rate of death or recurrent infarction within 12 months, which occurred in 19.1 percent of the intervention group and 16.6 percent of the conventional treatment group. No improvement in ejection fraction could be demonstrated in the intervened group at 3 months and at 1 year. These studies indicate that a strategy of routine deferred angioplasty following thrombolytic therapy has no benefit on mortality, reinfarction, or left ventricular function compared with conventional medical therapy.

Direct angioplasty without prior thrombolytic therapy was evaluated in randomized trials comparing angioplasty alone with thrombolytic therapy alone [283–285]. Immediate PTCA compared with rt-PA therapy in patients with AMI reduced the combined rate for occurrence of nonfatal reinfarction and death from 12 to 5.1 percent. Similarly, reinfarction or death was significantly reduced at 6 months in patients who had direct PTCA [283]. No difference in ejection fraction was observed in the rt-PA and PTCA groups at 6 weeks. A comparison of immediate coronary angioplasty with intravenous streptokinase treatment showed a significantly lower rate of reinfarction and unstable angina in the group with direct PTCA [284]. A higher patency rate of the infarct-related artery and higher ejection fraction were observed in the patients treated with immediate angioplasty after AMI. Another randomized trial of direct coronary angioplasty versus intravenous streptokinase [286] did not demonstrate any difference in 48-hour infarct-related artery patency or LVEF. The mortality rate of 6 percent with direct coronary angioplasty did not differ significantly from the 2 percent mortality rate in the streptokinase-treated group. These studies support the direct approach in patients who have contraindications to thrombolytic therapy and when an intervention laboratory is available. Similarly, patients in cardiogenic shock may benefit from early direct angioplasty [287].

Secondary Prevention and Improved Survival

The use of beta blockers, anticoagulants, antiplatelet agents, and ACE inhibitors can prevent recurrent events and improve survival after myocardial infarction but no benefit on mortality by nitroglycerin and nitrates, calcium channel blockers, and antiarrhythmic agents has been demonstrated. The effects of medical management on mortality, survival, and reinfarction after an acute infarction were reviewed in previous chapters of this publication.

Beta blockers can provide effective secondary prophylaxis after myocardial infarction [265–267]. An overview of the available randomized trials indicates that both early and delayed treatment with beta blockers significantly reduces mortality by 22 percent [265]. This benefit is apparent in both high- and low-risk groups. Analysis of the long-term effect on mortality after 7 days in trials in which therapy was started within a day of the onset of AMI showed a similar risk reduction of 23 percent and was applicable to various subgroups of risk such as age, sex, infarct location, risk category, and presence or absence of ventricular arrhythmia on Holter monitoring. Similarly, significant risk reduction by 19 percent for nonfatal reinfarction and a 32 percent reduction in sudden death were achieved with beta blockers. The early use of intravenous beta blockers after AMI and continuation of oral treatment within the first 2 years after infarction are indicated for improving survival.

Oral anticoagulation treatment may reduce mortality after myocardial infarction. An overview of randomized trials of anticoagulant treatment after myocardial infarction suggested a significant mortality reduction by 22 percent in patients who received anticoagulants [288]. The use of antiplatelet treatment after AMI yielded a decreased risk of vascular death by 13 percent, which appears to be evident beyond the first year of follow-up after acute infarction [289]. Similarly, ASA treatment produces a 42 percent reduction in nonfatal reinfarction and a 31 percent reduction in nonfatal stroke during 2 years of follow-up. There is no evidence that the addition of dipyridamole or sulfinpyrazone increases the benefit obtained with aspirin alone. Comparison of different doses of aspirin suggest that 160 mg daily, 300 to 325 mg daily, and 900 to 1500 mg daily provide similar benefit.

ACE inhibitors improve the short-term and long-term survival rate in patients with symptomatic heart failure and reduced left ventricular function [276, 277, 290]. Captopril lessens progressive left ventricular dilatation in AMI patients with an ejection fraction less than 45 percent when such treatment is initiated 1 week after the infarction occurred or later [291, 292]. Earlier treatment within 48 hours after AMI may result in a greater benefit in the prevention of left ventricular dilatation [293], although enalapril did not produce a mortality benefit over the first 6 months after acute AMI when treatment was started within 24 hours after AMI occurred [276]. ACE inhibitors appear to reduce mortality by 19 percent, and significantly reduce the incidence of reinfarction and readmission for congestive heart failure after myocardial infarction.

The role of coronary angioplasty and coronary bypass surgery following AMI with and without thrombolysis and other adjunctive treatment and their effect on short-term and long-term survival is reviewed in an earlier chapter.

References

1. Stern, M. P. The recent decline in ischemic heart disease mortality. *Ann. Intern. Med.* 91:630, 1979.
2. Thom, T. J., and Kannel, W. B. Downward trend in cardiovascular mortality. *Annu. Rev. Med.* 32:427, 1981.
3. Havlik, R. K., and Feinleib, M. *Proceedings of the Conferences on the Decline in Coronary Heart Disease Mortality.* NIH Publication 79:1610. U.S. Department of Health, Education and Welfare, 1979.
4. Gilpin, E. A., Koziol, J. A., Madsen, E. B., et al. Periods of differing mortality distribution during the first year after acute myocardial infarction. *Am. J. Cardiol.* 52:240, 1983.
5. Helmers, C., Lundman, R., Maasing, R., and Wester, P. O. Mortality pattern among initial survivors of acute myocardial infarction using a life table technique. *Acta Med. Scand.* 200:469, 1976.
6. Carlisle, R., and Lewis, A. F. Survival curves applied to acute myocardial infarction. *Am. Heart J.* 94:807, 1977.
7. Henning, H., Gilpin, E., Covell, J. W., et al. Prognosis after acute myocardial infarction: A multivariate analysis of mortality and survival. *Circulation* 59: 1124, 1979.
8. Juergens, J. L., Edwards, J. E., and Achor, R. W. Prognosis of patients surviving first clinically diagnosed myocardial infarction. *Arch. Intern. Med.* 105:444, 1960.
9. Honey, G. E., and Truelove, S. C. Prognostic factors in myocardial infarction. *Lancet* 1:1155, 1957.
10. Pell, S., and D'Alonzo, C. A. Immediate mortality and five year survival of employed men with a first myocardial infarction. *N. Engl. J. Med.* 270:915, 1964.
11. Norris, R. M., Caughey, D. E., Deeming, L. W., et al. Coronary prognostic index for predicting sur-

vival after recovery from acute myocardial infarction. *Lancet* 2:485, 1970.
12. Norris, R. M., Caughey, D. E., and Deeming, L. W. Prognosis following acute myocardial infarction. *N. Z. Med. J.* 77:12, 1973.
13. Helmers, C. Short and long-term prognostic indices in acute myocardial infarction: A study of 606 patients initially treated in a CCU. *Acta Med. Scand. Suppl.* 555, 1973.
14. Day, H. W. Effectiveness of an intensive coronary care area. *Am. J. Cardiol.* 15:51, 1965.
15. Goble, A. J., Sloman, G., and Robinson, J. S. Mortality reduction in a coronary care unit. *B.M.J.* 1: 1005, 1966.
16. Peterson, D. R., Thompson, D. J., and Chinn, N. Ischemic heart disease prognosis: A community-wide assessment (1966–1969). *J.A.M.A.* 219:1423, 1972.
17. Elveback, L. K., Connolly, D. C., and Kurland, L. T. Coronary heart disease in residents of Rochester, Minnesota. II. Mortality, incidence and survivorship 1950–1975. *Mayo Clin. Proc.* 56:665, 1981.
18. Gillum, R. F., Folsom, A., and Luepker, R. V. Sudden death and acute myocardial infarction in a metropolitan area, 1970–1980: The Minnesota Heart Survey. *N. Engl. J. Med.* 309:1353, 1983.
19. Gruppo Italiano per lo Studio della Streptokinase nell Infarcto Miocardico (GISSI). Effectiveness of intravenous thrombolytic treatment in acute myocardial infarction. *Lancet* 1:397, 1986.
20. ISIS Steering Committee. Intravenous streptokinase given within 0–4 hours of onset of myocardial infarction reduced mortality in ISIS-2. *Lancet* 1:502, 1987.
21. Krone, R. J., Gillespie, J. A., Weld, F. M., et al. Low-level exercise testing after myocardial infarction: Usefulness in enhancing clinical risk stratification. *Circulation* 71:80, 1985.
22. Gibson, R. S., Watson, D. D., Craddock, G. B., et al. Prediction of cardiac events after uncomplicated myocardial infarction: A prospective study comparing predischarge exercise thallium-201 scintigraphy and coronary angiography. *Circulation* 68:321, 1983.
23. Elwood, P. C. Aspirin in the prevention of myocardial infarction: Current status. *Drugs* 28:1, 1984.
24. Norwegian Multicenter Study Group: Timolol-induced reduction in mortality and reinfarction in patients surviving acute myocardial infarction. *N. Engl. J. Med.* 302:801, 1981.
25. Herlitz, J., Elmfeldt, D., Holmberg, S., et al. Goteborg metoprolol trial: Mortality and causes of death. *Am. J. Cardiol.* 53:9D, 1984.
26. Beta-Blocker Heart Attack Study Group. The Beta-Blocker Heart Attack Trial. *J.A.M.A.* 246:2073, 1981.
27. CASS Principal Investigators and Their Associates. Coronary Artery Surgery Study (CASS): A randomized trial of coronary artery bypass surgery: Survival data. *Circulation* 68:939, 1983.
28. CASS Principal Investigators and Their Associates. Myocardial infarction and mortality in the Coronary Artery Surgery Study (CASS) randomized trial. *N. Engl. J. Med.* 310:750, 1984.
29. Moss, A. J., DeCamilla, J., Davis, H., and Bayer, L. The early posthospital phase of myocardial infarction. *Circulation* 54:58, 1976.
30. Kannel, W. B., Sortic, P., and McNamara, P. M. Prognosis after initial myocardial infarction: The Framingham Study. *Am. J. Cardiol.* 44:53, 1979.
31. Vedin, J. A., Wilhelmsson, C., Elmfeldt, D., et al. Sudden death: Identification of high risk groups. *Am. Heart J.* 86:124, 1973.
32. Jelinek, V. M., McDonald, I. G., Ryan, W. F., et al. Assessment of cardiac risk 10 days after uncomplicated myocardial infarction. *B.M.J.* 284:227, 1982.
33. Kjoller, E., Mortensen, L. S., Larsen, S., et al. Long term prognosis after acute myocardial infarction. *Dan. Med. Bull.* 26:199, 1979.
34. Lofmark, R. Clinical features in patients with recurrent myocardial infarction. *Acta Med. Scand.* 206: 367, 1979.
35. Kentala, E., Pyorala, K., Heikkila, J., et al. Factors related to long-term prognosis following acute myocardial infarction: Importance of left ventricular function. *Scand. J. Rehabil. Med.* 7:118, 1975.
36. Luria, M. H., Knoke, J. D., Margolis, R. M., et al. Acute myocardial infarction prognosis after recovery. *Ann. Intern. Med.* 85:561, 1976.
37. Vedin, A., Wilhelmsen, L., Wedel, H., et al. Prediction of cardiovascular deaths and nonfatal reinfarctions after myocardial infarction. *Acta Med. Scand.* 201:309, 1977.
38. Davis, H. T., DeCamilla, J., Bayer, L. W., and Moss, A. J. Survivorship patterns in the posthospital phase of myocardial infarction. *Circulation* 60:1252, 1979.
39. Moss, A. J., DeCamilla, J., Engstrom, F., et al. The posthospital phase of myocardial infarction: Identification of patients with increased mortality risk. *Circulation* 49:460, 1974.
40. Bay, K. S., Lee, S. J. K., Flathman, D. P., and Roll, J. W. Application of step-wise discriminant analysis and Bayesian classification procedure in determining prognosis of acute myocardial infarction. *Can. Med. Assoc. J.* 115:887, 1976.
41. Coronary Drug Project Research Group. Factors influencing long-term prognosis after recovery from myocardial infarction—three year findings of the coronary drug project. *J. Chronic Dis.* 27:267, 1974.
42. Helmers, C. Assessment of 3-year prognosis in survivors of acute myocardial infarction. *Br. Heart J.* 37:593, 1975.
43. Beaune, J., Touboul, P., Boissel, J. P., and Belhaye, J. P. Quantitative assessment of myocardial infarction prognosis to 1 and 6 months from clinical data. *Eur. J. Cardiol.* 8:629, 1978.
44. Ruberman, W., Weinblatt, E., Goldberg, J. D., et al. Ventricular premature beats and mortality after myocardial infarction. *N. Engl. J. Med.* 297:750, 1977.

45. Sanz, G., Castaner, A., Betriu, A., et al. Determinants of prognosis in survivors of myocardial infarction. *N. Engl. J. Med.* 306:106, 1982.
46. Zukel, W. J., Cohen, B. M., and Mattingly, T. W. Survival following first diagnosis of coronary heart disease. *Am. Heart J.* 78:159, 1969.
47. Hughes, W. I., Kalbfleisch, J. M., Brandt, E. N., and Costiloe, J. P. Myocardial infarction prognosis by discriminant analysis. *Arch. Intern. Med.* 3:120, 1963.
48. Mosbech, J., and Dreyer, K. Coronary occlusion in Denmark: Morbidity and mortality. *Acta Med. Scand.* 180:429, 1966.
49. Wolffenbuttel, B. H. R., Verdouw, P. D., and Hugenholtz, P. G. Immediate and two year prognosis after acute myocardial infarction: Prediction from noninvasive as well as invasive parameters in the same individuals. *Eur. Heart J.* 2:375, 1981.
50. Goldberg, R., Szklo, M., and Tonascia, J. Time trends in prognosis of patients with myocardial infarction: A population-based study. *Johns Hopkins Med. J.* 144:73, 1979.
51. Goldberg, R. J., Gore, J. M., and Alpert, J. S. Recent changes in attack and survival rates of acute myocardial infarction (1975 through 1981): The Worcester Heart Attack Study. *J.A.M.A.* 255:2774, 1986.
52. Goldberg, R. J., Gore, J. M., and Alpert, J. S. Non-Q wave myocardial infarction: Recent changes in occurrence and prognosis—a community-wide perspective. *Am. Heart J.* 113:273, 1987.
53. Maisel, A. S., Ahnve, S., Gilpin, E., et al. Prognosis after extension of myocardial infarct: The role of Q-wave or non-Q-wave infarction. *Circulation* 71: 211, 1985.
54. Kjoller, E. The long-term prognosis after acute myocardial infarction. *Dan. Med. Bull.* 22:202, 1971.
55. Beard, O. W., Hipp, H. R., Robins, M., et al. Initial myocardial infarction among veterans: Ten-year survival. *Am. Heart J.* 73:317, 1967.
56. Martin, C. A., Thompson, P. L., Armstrong, B. K., et al. Long-term prognosis after recovery from myocardial infarction: A nine year follow-up of the Perth Coronary Register. *Circulation* 68:961, 1983.
57. Madsen, E. B., Gilpin, E., Henning, H., et al. Prediction of late mortality after myocardial infarction from variables measured at different times during hospitalization. *Am. J. Cardiol.* 53:47, 1984.
58. Weinblatt, E., Goldberg, J. D., Ruberman, W., et al. Mortality after first myocardial infarction: Search for a secular trend. *J.A.M.A.* 247:1576, 1982.
59. Schnur, S. Mortality rates in acute myocardial infarction. II. A proposed method for measuring quantitatively severity of illness on admission to the hospital. *Ann. Intern. Med.* 39:1018, 1953.
60. Peel, A. A. F., Semple, T., Wang, I., et al. A coronary prognostic index for grading the severity of infarction. *Br. Heart J.* 24:745, 1962.
61. Norris, R. M., Caughey, D. E., Mercer, C. J., et al. Coronary prognostic index for predicting survival after recovery from acute myocardial infarction. *Lancet* 2:485, 1970.
62. Rosenbaum, F. F., and Levine, F. A. Prognostic value of various clinical and electrocardiographic features of acute myocardial infarction. *Arch. Intern. Med.* 68:913, 1941.
63. Cole, D. R., Singian, E. B., and Katz, L. N. The long-term prognosis following myocardial infarction and some factors which affect it. *Circulation* 9:321, 1954.
64. Battler, A., Karliner, J. S., Higgins, C. B., et al. The initial chest x-ray in acute myocardial infarction: Prediction of early and late mortality and survival. *Circulation* 61:1004, 1980.
65. Killip, T., and Kimball, J. I. Treatment of myocardial infarction in a coronary care unit: A two-year experience with 250 patients. *Am. J. Cardiol.* 20:457, 1967.
66. Evans, A. E., Boyle, D. Mc. C., Barber, J. M., et al. Safe selection of coronary patients for early discharge. *Eur. Heart J.* 2:395, 1981.
67. Multicenter Postinfarction Research Group. Risk stratification and survival after myocardial infarction. *N. Engl. J. Med.* 309:331, 1983.
68. Toller, G. H., Stone, P. H., Muller, J. E., et al. Effects of gender and race on prognosis after myocardial infarction: Adverse prognosis for women, particularly black women. *J. Am. Coll. Cardiol.* 9:473, 1987.
69. Smith, J. W., Marcus, F. I., Serokman, H., et al. Prognosis of patients with diabetes mellitus after acute myocardial infarction. *Am. J. Cardiol.* 54:718, 1984.
70. Merrilees, M. A., Scott, P. J., and Norris, H. M. Prognosis after myocardial infarction: Results of 15-year follow-up. *B.M.J.* 288:356, 1984.
71. Coronary Drug Project Research Group. Blood pressure in survivors of myocardial infarction. *J. Am. Coll. Cardiol.* 4:134, 1984.
72. Hoit, B. D., Gilpin, E. A., Maisel, A. S., et al. Influence of obesity on morbidity and mortality after acute myocardial infarction. *Am. Heart J.* 114:1334, 1987.
73. Madsen, E. B., Gilpin, E., and Henning, H. Short-term prognosis in acute myocardial infarction: Evaluation of different prediction methods. *Am. Heart J.* 107:1241, 1984.
74. Coronary Drug Project Research Group. The prognostic importance of the electrocardiogram after myocardial infarction: Experience in the coronary drug project. *Ann. Intern. Med.* 77:677, 1972.
75. Schuster, E. H., and Bulkley, B. H. Early post-infarction angina: Ischemia at a distance and ischemia in the infarct zone. *N. Engl. J. Med.* 35:1101, 1981.
76. Maisel, A. S., Gilpin, E., Hoit, B., et al. Survival after hospital discharge in matched populations with inferior or anterior myocardial infarction. *J. Am. Coll. Cardiol.* 6:731, 1985.
77. Hands, M. E., Lloyd, B. L., Robinson, J. S., et al.

Prognostic significance of electrocardiographic site of infarction after correction for enzymatic size of infarction. *Circulation* 73:885, 1986.
78. Kannel, W. B., and Abbott, R. D. Incidence and prognosis of unrecognized myocardial infarction. *N. Engl. J. Med.* 311:1144, 1984.
79. Becker, L. C., Silverman, K. J., Bulkley, B. H., et al. Comparison of early thallium-201 scintigraphy and gated blood pool imaging for predicting mortality in patients with acute myocardial infarction. *Circulation* 67:1272, 1983.
80. Holman, B. L., Chisholm, B. J., and Braunwald, E. The prognostic implications of acute myocardial infarct scintigraphy with 99m Tc-pyrophosphate. *Circulation* 57:320, 1978.
81. Madias, J. E., Chahine, R. A., Gorlin, R., and Blacklow, D. J. A comparison of transmural and nontransmural myocardial infarction. *Circulation* 49:498, 1974.
82. Rigo, P., Murray, M., Taylor, D. R., et al. Hemodynamic and prognostic findings in patient with transmural and nontransmural infarction. *Circulation* 51:1064, 1975.
83. Szklo, M., Goldberg, R., and Kennedy, H. L. Survival of patients with transmural infarction: A population-based study. *Am. J. Cardiol.* 42:648, 1978.
84. Hutter, A. M., DeSanctis, R. W., Flynn, T., and Yeatman, L. A. Nontransmural myocardial infarction: A comparison of hospital and late clinical course of patients with that of matched patients with transmural anterior and transmural inferior myocardial infarction. *Am. J. Cardiol.* 48:595, 1981.
85. Waters, D. D., Pelletier, G. B., and Hache, M. Myocardial infarction in patients with previous coronary artery bypass surgery. *J. Am. Coll. Cardiol.* 3:909, 1984.
86. Nicholson, M. R., Boubin, G. S., Bernstein, L., et al. Prognosis after an initial non-Q-wave myocardial infarction related to coronary arterial anatomy. *Am. J. Cardiol.* 52:462, 1983.
87. Theroux, P., Kouz, S., and Bosch, X. Clinical and angiographic features of non-Q and Q wave myocardial infarction. *Circulation* 74(Suppl II):303, 1986.
88. Gibson, R. S., Beller, G. A., Gheoghiade, M., et al. The prevalence and clinical significance of residual myocardial ischemia 2 weeks after uncomplicated non-Q wave infarction: A prospective natural history study. *Circulation* 73:1186, 1986.
89. Shubin, H., Afifi, A. A., Rand, W. M., and Weil, M. H. Objective index of hemodynamic status for quantification of severity and prognosis of shock complicating myocardial infarction. *Cardiovasc. Res.* 4:329, 1968.
90. Verdouw, P. D., Hagemeijer, F., van Dorp, W. G., et al. Short-term survival after acute myocardial infarction predicted by hemodynamic parameters. *Circulation* 52:413, 1975.
91. Battler, A., Slutsky, R., Karliner, J., et al. Left ventricular ejection fraction and first-third ejection fraction early after acute myocardial infarction: Predictive value for mortality and survival. *Am. J. Cardiol.* 45:797, 1980.
92. Nicod, P., Gilpin, E., Dittrich, H., et al. Influence on prognosis and morbidity of left ventricular ejection fraction with and without signs of left ventricular failure after acute myocardial infarction. *Am. J. Cardiol.* 61:1165, 1988.
93. McHugh, T. J., and Swan, H. J. C. Prognostic indicators in acute myocardial infarction. *Geriatrics* 26:72, 1971.
94. Mukharji, J., Rude, R. E., Poole, W. K., et al. Risk factors for sudden death after acute myocardial infarction: Two-year follow-up. *Am. J. Cardiol.* 54:31, 1984.
95. Bigger, J. T., Fleiss, J. L., Kleiger, R., et al. The relationships among ventricular dysfunction, and mortality in the 2 years after myocardial infarction. *Circulation* 69:250, 1984.
96. Ahvne, S., Gilpin, E., Henning, H., et al. Limitations and advantages of the ejection fraction for defining high risk after acute myocardial infarction. *Am. J. Cardiol.* 58:872, 1986.
97. Madsen, E. B., Gilpin, E., Slutsky, R. A., et al. Usefulness of the chest x-ray for predicting abnormal left ventricular function after acute myocardial infarction. *Am. Heart J.* 108:1431, 1984.
98. Dewhurst, N. G., and Muir, A. L. Comparative prognostic value of radionuclide ventriculography at rest and during exercise in 100 patients after first myocardial infarction. *Br. Heart J.* 49:111, 1983.
99. Morris, K. G., Palmeri, S. T., Califf, R. M., et al. Value of radionuclide angiography for predicting specific cardiac events after acute myocardial infarction. *Am. J. Cardiol.* 55:318, 1985.
100. Kuchar, D. L., Throburn, C. W., and Neville, L. S. Prediction of serious arrhythmic events after myocardial infarction: Signal averaged electrocardiogram, Holter monitoring and radionuclide ventriculography. *J. Am. Coll. Cardiol.* 9:531, 1987.
101. Schelbert, H. R., Henning, H., Ashburn, W. L., et al. Serial measurements of left ventricular ejection fraction by radionuclide angiography early and late after myocardial infarction. *Am. J. Cardiol.* 38:407, 1976.
102. Greenberg, H., McMaster, P., Dwyer, E. M., et al. Left ventricular dysfunction after acute myocardial infarction: Results of a prospective multicenter study. *J. Am. Coll. Cardiol.* 4:867, 1984.
103. Taylor, G. J., Humphries, J. O., Mellits, E. D., et al. Predictors of clinical course, coronary anatomy and left ventricular function after recovery from acute myocardial infarction. *Circulation* 62:960, 1980.
104. Corbett, J. K., Dehmer, G. J., Lewis, S. E., et al. The prognostic value of submaximal exercise testing with radionuclide ventriculography before hospital discharge in patients with recent myocardial infarction. *Circulation* 64:535, 1981.
105. Corbett, J. R., Nicod, P., and Lewis, S. E. Prognostic value of submaximal exercise radionuclide ventric-

ulography after myocardial infarction. *Am. J. Cardiol.* 52:82A, 1983.

106. Morris, K. G., Califf, R. M., and Palmeri, S. T. Independent prognostic value to rest and exercise radionuclide angiography 3 and 8 weeks after infarction. *Circulation* 68:111, 1983.
107. Hung, J., Goris, M. L., Nash, E., et al. Comparative value of maximal treadmill testing, exercise thallium myocardial perfusion scintigraphy and exercise radionuclide ventriculography for distinguishing high- and low-risk patients soon after myocardial infarction. *Am. J. Cardiol.* 53:1221, 1984.
108. Moss, A. J., David, H. T., DeCamilla, J., and Bayer, L. W. Ventricular ectopic beats and their relation to sudden and nonsudden cardiac death after myocardial infarction. *Circulation* 60:998, 1979.
109. Ruberman, W., Weinblatt, E., Goldberg, J. D., et al. Ventricular premature beats and mortality after myocardial infarction. *N. Engl. J. Med.* 297:750, 1977.
110. Schultze, R. A., Strauss, H. W., and Pitt, B. Sudden death in the year following myocardial infarction: Relation to ventricular premature contractions in the late hospital phase and left ventricular ejection fraction. *Am. J. Med.* 62:192, 1977.
111. Lown, B., and Wolf, M. Approaches to sudden death from coronary heart disease. *Circulation* 44: 130, 1971.
112. Vismara, L. A., Amsterdam, E. A., and Mason, D. T. Relationship of ventricular arrhythmias in the late hospital phase of acute myocardial infarction to sudden death after hospital discharge. *Am. J. Med.* 59:6, 1975.
113. Lesch, M., and Kehoe, R. F. Predictability of sudden cardiac death: A partially fulfilled promise. *N. Engl. J. Med.* 310:255, 1984.
114. Madsen, B., Svendsen, L. T., and Rasmussen, S. Multivariate long-term prognostic index from exercise ECG after acute myocardial infarction. *Eur. J. Cardiol.* 11:435, 1980.
115. Coronary Drug Project Research Group. Factors influencing long-term prognosis after recovery from myocardial infarction: Three-year findings of the Coronary Drug Project. *J. Chronic Dis.* 27:267, 1974.
116. Sharma, B., Asinger, R., Francis, G. S., et al. Demonstrations of exercise-induced painless myocardial ischemia in survivors of out-of-hospital ventricular fibrillation. *Am. J. Cardiol.* 59:740, 1987.
117. Morady, F., DiCarlo, L. A., Krol, R. B., et al. Role of myocardial ischemia during programmed stimulation in survivors of cardiac arrest with coronary artery disease. *J. Am. Coll. Cardiol.* 9:1004, 1987.
118. Nicod, P., Gilpin, E., Dittrich, H., et al. Late clinical outcome in patients with early ventricular fibrillation after myocardial infarction. *J. Am. Coll. Cardiol.* 11:464, 1988.
119. Maisel, A. S., Scott, N., Gilpin, E., et al. Complex ventricular arrhythmias in patients with Q wave versus non-Q wave myocardial infarction. *Circulation* 72:963, 1985.
120. Theroux, P., Water, D. D., Halphen, C., et al. Prognostic value of exercise testing soon after myocardial infarction. *N. Engl. J. Med.* 301:341, 1979.
121. Davidson, D. M., and DeBusk, R. F. Prognostic value of a single exercise test 3 weeks after uncomplicated myocardial infarction. *Circulation* 61:236, 1980.
122. Starling, M. R., Crawford, M. H., Kennedy, G. T., and O'Rourke, R. A. Exercise testing early after MI: Predictive value for subsequent unstable angina and death. *Am. J. Cardiol.* 46:909, 1980.
123. Starling, M. R., Crawford, M. H., Kennedy, D. T., and O'Rourke, R. A. Treadmill exercise tests predischarge and six weeks post-myocardial infarction to detect abnormalities of known prognostic value. *Ann. Intern. Med.* 94:721, 1981.
124. Akhras, F., Upward, J., Keates, J., and Jackson, G. Early exercise testing and elective coronary artery bypass surgery after uncomplicated myocardial infarction: Effect on morbidity and mortality. *Br. Heart J.* 52:413, 1984.
125. Akhras, F., Upward, J., Stott, R., and Jackson, G. Early exercise testing and coronary angiography and uncomplicated myocardial infarction. *B.M.J.* 284:1293, 1982.
126. DeBusk, R. F., Kraemer, H. C., and Nash, E. Stepwise risk stratification soon after acute myocardial infarction. *Am. J. Cardiol.* 52:1161, 1983.
127. Weld, F. M., Chu, K. L., Bigger, J. T., and Rolnitzky, L. M. Risk stratification with low-level exercise testing 2 weeks after acute myocardial infarction. *Circulation* 64:306, 1981.
128. Jennings, K., Reid, D. S., Hawkins, T., and Julian, D. J. Role of exercise testing early after myocardial infarction in identifying candidates for coronary surgery. *B.M.J.* 288:185, 1984.
129. Birk Madsen, E., and Gilpin, E. Prognostic value of exercise test variables after myocardial infarction. *J. Cardiac Rehabil.* 3:481, 1983.
130. DeFeyter, P. J., van Eenige, M. J., Dighton, D. H., et al. Prognostic value of exercise testing, coronary angiography and left ventriculography 6–8 weeks after myocardial infarction. *Circulation* 66:527, 1982.
131. Fioretti, P., Brower, R. W., Simoons, M. L., et al. Prediction of mortality in hospital survivors of myocardial infarction: Comparison of predischarge exercise testing and radionuclide ventriculography at rest. *Br. Heart J.* 52:292, 1984.
132. Birk Madsen, E., Gilpin, E., Ahnve, S., et al. Prediction of functional capacity and use of exercise testing for predicting risk after acute myocardial infarction. *Am. J. Cardiol.* 56:839, 1985.
133. Deckers, W., Fioretti, P., Brower, R. W., et al. Ineligibility for predischarge exercise testing after myocardial infarction in the elderly: Implications for prognosis. *Eur. Heart J.* 5(Suppl E):97, 1984.
134. Waters, D. D., Bosch, X., Bourchard, A., et al. Comparison of clinical variables and variables de-

rived from a limited predischarge exercise test as predictors of early and late mortality after myocardial infarction. *J. Am. Coll. Cardiol.* 5:1, 1985.
135. Ouyang, P., Shapiro, E. P., Chandra, N. C., et al. An angiographic and functional comparison of patients with silent and symptomatic treadmill ischemia early after myocardial infarction. *Am. J. Cardiol.* 59:730, 1987.
136. Gottlieb, S. H., Gerstenblith, G., Achuff, S. C., et al. Ischemic ST segment changes by ambulatory Holter predict one year mortality in high risk post-infarct patients (Abstract). *Circulation* 74(Suppl II): 58, 1986.
137. Jelinek, V. M., McDonald, I. G., Ryan, W. F., et al. Assessment of cardiac risk 10 days after uncomplicated myocardial infarction. *B.M.J.* 284:227, 1982.
138. Sami, M., Kraemer, H., and DeBusk, R. F. The prognostic significance of serial exercise testing after myocardial infarction. *Circulation* 60:1238, 1979.
139. Gibson, R. S., Taylor, G. J., and Watson, D. D. Predicting the extent and location of coronary disease during the early post-infarction period by quantitative thallium-201 scintigraphy. *Am. J. Cardiol.* 47:1010, 1981.
140. Hung, J., Goris, M. L., Nash, E., et al. Comparative value of maximal treadmill testing, exercise thallium myocardial perfusion scintigraphy and exercise radionuclide ventriculography for distinguishing high- and low-risk patients soon after acute myocardial infarction. *Am. J. Cardiol.* 53:1221, 1984.
141. Gibson, R. S., Beller, G. A., and Kaiser, D. L. Prevalence and clinical significance of painless ST segment depression during early postinfarction exercise testing. *Circulation* 75(Suppl 2):36, 1987.
142. Smeets, J. P., Rigo, P., and Legrand, V. Prognostic value of thallium-201 stress myocardial scintigraphy with exercise ECG after myocardial infarction. *Cardiology* 68:67, 1981.
143. Hakki, A. H., Nestico, P. F., Heo, J., et al. Relative prognostic value of rest thallium-201 imaging, radionuclide ventriculography and 24 hour ambulatory electrocardiographic monitoring after acute myocardial infarction. *J. Am. Coll. Cardiol.* 10(1): 25, 1987.
144. Heger, J. J., Weyman, A. E., Wann, L. S., et al. Cross-sectional echocardiographic analysis of the extent of left ventricular asynergy in acute myocardial infarction. *Circulation* 60:531, 1987.
145. Gibson, R. S., Bishop, H. L., Stamm, R. B., et al. Value of early two dimensional echocardiography in patients with acute myocardial infarction. *Am. J. Cardiol.* 49:1110, 1982.
146. Horowitz, R. S., and Morganroth, J. Immediate detection of early high-risk patients with acute myocardial infarction using two-dimensional echocardiographic evaluation of left ventricular regional wall motion abnormalities. *Am. Heart J.* 103:814, 1982.
147. Horowitz, R. S., Morganroth, J., Parrotto, C., et al. Immediate diagnosis of acute myocardial infarction by two-dimensional echocardiography. *Circulation* 65:323, 1982.
148. Morganroth, J., Chin, C. C., David, D., et al. Exercise cross-sectional echocardiographic diagnosis of coronary artery disease. *Am. J. Cardiol.* 47:20, 1981.
149. Crawford, M. H., Amon, K. W., and Vance, W. S. Exercise 2-dimensional echocardiography: Quantitation of left ventricular performance in patients with severe angina pectoris. *Am. J. Cardiol.* 51:1, 1983.
150. Van Reet, R. E., Quinones, M. A., Poliner, L. R., et al. Comparison of two-dimensional echocardiography with gated radionuclide ventriculography in the evaluation of global and regional left ventricular function in acute myocardial infarction. *J. Am. Coll. Cardiol.* 3:243, 1984.
151. Nishimura, R. A., Tajik, A. J., Shub, C., et al. Role of two-dimensional echocardiography in the predication of in-hospital complications after acute myocardial infarction. *J. Am. Coll. Cardiol.* 4:1080, 1984.
152. Ryan, T., Armstrong, W. F., O'Donnell, J. A., and Feigenbaum, H. Risk stratification after acute myocardial infarction by means of exercise two-dimensional echocardiography. *Am. Heart J.* 114:1305, 1987.
153. Madigan, N. P., Rutherford, B. D., and Frye, R. L. The clinical course, early prognosis and coronary anatomy of subendocardial infarction. *Am. J. Med.* 60:634, 1976.
154. Califf, R. A., Burks, J. M., Behar, V. S., et al. Relationships among ventricular arrhythmias, coronary artery disease and angiographic and electrocardiographic indicators of myocardial fibrosis. *Circulation* 57:725, 1978.
155. Chaitman, B. R., Waters, D. D., Corbara, F., and Bourassa, M. G. Prediction of multivessel disease after inferior myocardial infarction. *Circulation* 57: 1085, 1978.
156. Bertrand, M. E., Lefebvre, J. M., Laisne, C. L., et al. Coronary arteriography in acute transmural myocardial infarction. *Am. Heart J.* 97:61, 1979.
157. Vanhaecke, J., Piessens, J., Willems, J. L., and DeGeest, H. Coronary arterial lesions in young men who survived a first myocardial infarction: Clinical and electrocardiographic predictors of multivessel disease. *Am. J. Cardiol.* 47:810, 1981.
158. Roubin, G. S., Harris, P. J., Bernstein, L., and Kelly, D. T. Coronary anatomy and prognosis after myocardial infarction in patients 60 years of age and younger. *Circulation* 67:743, 1983.
159. Turner, J. D., Rogers, W. J., Mantle, J. A., et al. Coronary angiography soon after myocardial infarction. *Chest* 77:58, 1980.
160. Betriu, A., Castaner, A., Sanz, G. A., et al. Angiographic findings 1 month after myocardial infarction: A prospective study of 259 survivors. *Circulation* 65:1099, 1982.
161. Veenbrink, T. W. G., van der Werf, T., Westerhof, P. W., et al. Is there an indication for coronary

angiography in patients under 60 years of age with no or minimal angina pectoris after a first myocardial infarction? *Br. Heart J.* 53:30, 1985.

162. Califf, R. M., Phillips, H. R., Hindman, M. C., et al. Prognostic value of a coronary artery jeopardy score. *J. Am. Coll. Cardiol.* 5:1055, 1985.
163. Schulman, S. P., Achuff, S. C., Griffith, L. S., et al. Prognostic cardiac catheterization variables in survivors of acute myocardial infarction: A five year prospective study. *J. Am. Coll. Cardiol.* 11: 1164, 1988.
164. White, H. D., Norris, R. M., Brown, M. A., et al. Left ventricular end-systolic volume as the major determinant of survival after recovery from myocardial infarction. *Circulation* 76:44, 1987.
165. Waspe, L. E., Seinfeld, D., Ferrick, A., et al. Prediction of sudden death and spontaneous ventricular tachycardia in survivors of complicated myocardial infarction: Value of response to programmed stimulation using a maximum of three ventricular extrastimuli. *J. Am. Coll. Cardiol.* 5:1292, 1985.
166. Hammer, A., Vohra, J., Hunt, D., and Sloman, G. Prediction of sudden death by electrophysiologic studies in high risk patients surviving acute myocardial infarction. *Am. J. Cardiol.* 50:223, 1982.
167. Richards, D. A., Cody, D. V., Denniss, A. R., et al. Ventricular electrical instability: A predictor of death after myocardial infarction. *Am. J. Cardiol.* 51:75, 1983.
168. Marchlinski, F. E., Buxton, A. E., Waxman, H. L., and Josephson, M. E. Identifying patients at risk of sudden death after myocardial infarction: Value of the response to programmed stimulation, degree of ventricular ectopic activity and severity of left ventricular dysfunction. *Am. J. Cardiol.* 52:1190, 1983.
169. Denniss, A. R., Baaijens, H., Cody, D. V., et al. Value of programmed stimulation and exercise testing in predicting one-year mortality after acute myocardial infarction. *Am. J. Cardiol.* 56:213, 1985.
170. Morady, F., DiCarlo, L. A., Krol, R. B., et al. Role of myocardial ischemia during programmed stimulation in survivors of cardiac arrest with coronary artery disease. *J. Am. Coll. Cardiol.* 9:1004, 1987.
171. Bhandari, A. K., Au, P. K., Rose, J. S., et al. Decline in inducibility of sustained ventricular tachycardia from two to twenty weeks after acute myocardial infarction. *Am. J. Cardiol.* 59:284, 1987.
172. Roy, D., Marchand, L., Theroux, P., et al. Long-term reproduction and significance of provokable ventricular arrhythmias after myocardial infarction. *J. Am. Coll. Cardiol.* 8:32, 1986.
173. Denniss, A. R., Richards, D. A., Cody, D. V., et al. Prognostic significance of ventricular tachycardia and fibrillation induced at programmed stimulation and delayed potentials detected on the signal-averaged electrocardiograms of survivors of acute myocardial infarction. *Circulation* 74:731, 1986.
174. Roy, D., Marchand, E., Theroux, P., et al. Programmed ventricular stimulation in survivors of an acute myocardial infarction. *Circulation* 72:487, 1985.
175. Gonzalez, R., Arriagada, D., Corbalan, R., et al. Role of programmed electrical stimulation of the heart in risk stratification post-myocardial infarction. *PACE* 11:283, 1988.
176. Rapaport, E., and Remedios, P. The high risk patient after recovery from myocardial infarction: Recognition and management. *J. Am. Coll. Cardiol.* 1: 391, 1983.
177. Madsen, E. B., Gilpin, E., and Henning, H. Evaluation of prognosis one year after myocardial infarction. *J. Am. Coll. Cardiol.* 1:985, 1983.
178. Moss, A. J., Decamilla, J., Davis, H., and Bayer, L. The early posthospital phase of myocardial infarction. *Circulation* 54:58, 1976.
179. Gilpin, E. A., Karliner, J. S., and Ross, J., Jr. Risk assessment after acute myocardial infarction. In J. S. Karliner and G. Gregoratos (eds.), *Coronary Care.* New York: Churchill-Livingstone, 1980. P. 1040.
180. Lemlish, A., Covo, G., and Ziffer, J. Multivariate analysis of prognostic factors in myocardial infarction. In K. Enslein (ed.), *Data Acquisition and Processing in Biology and Medicine. Proceedings* (Vol. 3):Rochester Conference on Data Acquisition and Processing in Biology and Medicine. New York: Macmillan, 1963. P. 65.
181. Rotmensch, H. H., Terdiman, R., Cheffer, M., et al. Dynamic prognostic profile for acute myocardial infarction. *Chest* 76:663, 1979.
182. Habib, T., Taylor, D. J. E., and Dalton, R. Comparison of two coronary prognostic indices. *Postgrad. Med. J.* 55:255, 1979.
183. Bigger, J. T., Heller, C. A., Wengler, T. L., and Weld, F. M. Risk stratification after acute myocardial infarction. *Am. J. Cardiol.* 42:202, 1978.
184. Chapelle, J. P., Albert, A., Smeets, J. P., et al. Early assessment of risk in patient with acute myocardial infarction. *Eur. Heart J.* 2:187, 1981.
185. Gilpin, E., Olshen, R., Henning H., and Ross, J., Jr. Risk prediction after acute myocardial infarction: Comparison of three multivariate methodologies. *Cardiology* 70:73, 1983.
186. Olshen, R. A., Gilpin, E. A., Henning, H., et al. Twelve month prognosis following myocardial infarction: Classification trees, logistic regression, and stepwise linear discrimination. In L. M. LeCam and R. A. Olshen (eds.), *The Proceedings of the Berkeley Conference in Honor of Jerzy Neyman and Jack Kiefer* (Vol. 1). Monterey, CA: Wadsworth Advanced Books and Software, 1985. P. 245.
187. Norris, R. M., Brandt, P. W. T., Caughey, D. E., et al. A new coronary prognostic index. *Lancet* 1: 224, 1969.
188. Chapman, B. L., and Gray, C. H. Prognostic index for myocardial infarction treated in a coronary care unit. *Br. Heart J.* 35:135, 1973.
189. Madsen, E. B., Hougaard, P., Gilpin, E., and Pedersen, A. The length of hospitalization after acute

myocardial infarction determined by risk calculation. *Circulation* 68:9, 1983.
190. Chaturvedi, N. C., Walsh, M. J., Evans, A., et al. Selection of patients for early discharge after acute myocardial infarction. *Br. Heart J.* 36:533, 1974.
191. Lindvall, K., Erhardt, L. R., Lundman, T., et al. Early mobilization and discharge of patients with acute myocardial infarction. *Acta Med. Scand.* 206: 169, 1979.
192. Wenger, N. K., Hellerstein, H. K., Blackburn, H., and Castranova, S. J. Physician practice in the management of patients with uncomplicated myocardial infarction: Changes in the past decade. *Circulation* 65:421, 1982.
193. Hutter, A. M., Jr., Sidel, V. W., Shine, K. L., and DeSanctis, R. W. Early hospital discharge after myocardial infarction. *N. Engl. J. Med.* 288:1141, 1973.
194. Hayes, M. J., Morris, G. K., and Hampton, J. R. Comparison of mobilization after two and nine days in uncomplicated myocardial infarction. *B.M.J.* 3: 10, 1974.
195. McNeer, J. F., Wagner, G. S., Ginsburg, P. B., et al. Hospital discharge one week after acute myocardial infarction. *N. Engl. J. Med.* 298:229, 1978.
196. Birk Madsen, E. Time of discharge for patients with acute myocardial infarction. *Cardiovasc. Rev. Rep.* 4:1301, 1983.
197. Ahnve, S., Gilpin, E., Dittrich, H., et al. First myocardial infarction: Age and ejection fraction identify a low risk group. *Am. Heart J.* 116:925, 1988.
198. Topol, E. J., Burek, K., O'Neill, W. W., et al. A randomized controlled trial of hospital discharge three days after myocardial infarction in the era of reperfusion. *N. Engl. J. Med.* 318:1083, 1988.
199. Sutherland, J. E., Perksy, V. W., and Brody, J. A. Proportionate mortality trends: 1950 through 1986. *J.A.M.A.* 264:3178, 1990.
200. De Vreede, J. J. M., Gorgels, A. P. M., Verstraaten, G. M. P., et al. Did prognosis after acute myocardial infarction change during the past 30 years? A meta-analysis. *J. Am. Coll. Cardiol.* 18:698, 1991.
201. Goldman, L., Cook, F., Hashimoto, B., et al. Evidence that hospital care for acute myocardial infarction has not contributed to the decline in coronary mortality between 1973–1974 and 1978–1979. *Circulation* 65:936, 1982.
202. Stewart, A., Beaglehole, R., Fraser, G. E., et al. Trends in survival after myocardial infarction in New Zealand, 1974–81. *Lancet* 2:444, 1984.
203. McGovern, P. G., Folsom, A. R., Sprafka, J. M., et al. Trends in survival of hospitalized myocardial infarction patients between 1970 and 1985. *Circulation* 85:172, 1992.
204. Klein, H. H., Hengstenberg, C., Peuckert, M., et al. Comparison of death rates from acute myocardial infarction in a single hospital in two different periods (1977–1978 versus 1988–1989). *Am. J. Cardiol.* 71:518, 1993.
205. Dellborg, M., Eriksson, P., Riha, M., et al. Declining hospital mortality in acute myocardial infarction. *Circulation* 84(Suppl II):334, 1991.
206. Antman, E. M., and Berlin, J. A. Declining incidence of ventricular fibrillation in myocardial infarction. *Circulation* 86:764, 1992.
207. Goldberg, R. J., Gore, J. M., Alpert, J. S., et al. Cardiogenic shock after acute myocardial infarction. Incidence and mortality from a community-wide perspective, 1975 to 1988. *N. Engl. J. Med.* 325:1117, 1991.
208. Yusuf, S., Collins, R., Peto, R., et al. Intravenous and intracoronary fibrinolytic therapy in acute myocardial infarction: Overview of results on mortality, reinfarction and side-effects from 33 randomized controlled trials. *Eur. Heart J.* 6:556, 1985.
209. Yusuf, S., Wittes, J., and Friedman, L. Overview of results of randomized clinical trials in heart disease. I. Treatments following myocardial infarction. *J.A.M.A.* 260:2088, 1988.
210. Gruppo Italiano per lo Studio della Streptokinase nell Infarcto Miocardico (GISSI). Effectiveness of intravenous thrombolytic treatment in acute myocardial infarction. *Lancet* 1:397, 1986.
211. White, H. D., Norris, R. M., Brown, M. A., et al. Effect of intravenous streptokinase on left ventricular function and early survival after acute myocardial infarction. *N. Engl. J. Med.* 317:850, 1987.
212. ISIS-2 (Second International Study of Infarct Survival) Collaborative Group. Randomized trial of intravenous streptokinase, oral aspirin, both or neither among 17,187 cases of suspected acute myocardial infarction. *Lancet* 2:349, 1988.
213. AIMS Trial Study Group. Effect of intravenous APSAC on mortality after acute myocardial infarction: Preliminary report of a placebo-controlled clinical trial. *Lancet* 1:545, 1988.
214. AIMS Trial Study Group. Long-term effects of intravenous anistreplase in acute myocardial infarction: Final report of the AIMS study. *Lancet* 335:427, 1990.
215. Monk, J. P., and Hoel, R. C. Anisoylated plasminogen streptokinase activator complex (APSAC): A review of the mechanism of action, clinical pharmacology and therapeutic use in acute myocardial infarction. *Drugs* 34:25, 1987.
216. Wilcox, R. G., Van der Lippe, G., and Olsson, C. G. Trial of tissue plasminogen activator for mortality reduction in acute myocardial infarction. Anglo-Scandinavian Study of Early Thrombolysis (ASSET). *Lancet* 2:525, 1988.
217. Wilcox, R. G., von der Lippe, G., Olsson, C. G., et al. Effects of alteplase in acute myocardial infarction: 6-months results from the ASSET study. *Lancet* 335:1175, 1990.
218. Van der Werf, F., and Arnold, A. E. R. Intravenous tissue plasminogen activator and size of infarct, left ventricular function, and survival in acute myocardial infarction. *B.M.J.* 287:1374, 1988.
219. The ISAM Study Group. A prospective trial of intravenous streptokinase in acute myocardial in-

farction (ISAM): Mortality, morbidity and infarct size at 21 days. *N. Engl. J. Med.* 314:1465, 1986.
220. Kennedy, J. W., Martin, G. V., Davis, K. B., et al. The Western Washington intravenous streptokinase in acute myocardial infarction randomized trial. *Circulation* 77:345, 1988.
221. EMERAS (Estudio Multicentrico Estreptokinasa Republicas de America del Sur) Collaborative Group. Randomized trial of late thrombolysis in patients with suspected acute myocardial infarction. *Lancet* 342:767, 1993.
222. Verstraete, M., Bernard, R., Bory, M., et al. Randomized trial of intravenous recombinant tissue-type plasminogen activator versus intravenous streptokinase in acute myocardial infarction: Report from the European Cooperative Study Group for recombinant tissue-type plasminogen activator. *Lancet* 1:842, 1985.
223. National Heart Foundation of Australia Coronary Thrombolysis Group. Coronary thrombolysis and myocardial salvage by tissue plasminogen activator given up to 4 hours after onset of myocardial infarction. *Lancet* 1:203, 1988.
224. Kennedy, J. W., Ritchie, J. L., Davis, K. B., et al. Western Washington randomized trial of intracoronary streptokinase in acute myocardial infarction. *N. Engl. J. Med.* 304:1477, 1983.
225. Simoons, M. L., Serruys, P. W., Brand, M., et al. Improved survival after early thrombolysis in acute myocardial infarction: A randomized trial by Interuniversity Cardiology Institute in the Netherlands. *Lancet* 2:578, 1985.
226. Anderson, J. L., Sorensen, S. G., Moreno, F. L., et al. Multicenter patency trial of intravenous anistreplase compared with streptokinase in acute myocardial infarction. *Circulation* 83:126, 1991.
227. Chesebro, J. H., Knatterud, G., Roberts, R., et al. Thrombolysis in Myocardial Infarction (TIMI) trial, phase I: A comparison between intravenous tissue plasminogen activator and intravenous streptokinase. *Circulation* 76:142, 1987.
228. Gruppo Italiano per lo Studio della Sopravvivenza nell Infarcto Miocardico. GISSI-2: A factorial randomized trial of alteplase and heparin versus no heparin among 12,490 patients with acute myocardial infarction. *Lancet* 336:65, 1990.
229. The International Study Group. In-hospital mortality and clinical course of 20,891 patients with suspected acute myocardial infarction randomized between alteplase and streptokinase with or without heparin. *Lancet* 336:71, 1990.
230. PRIMI Trial Study Group. Randomized double-blind trial of recombinant pro-urokinase against streptokinase in acute myocardial infarction. *Lancet* 1:863, 1989.
231. Bassand, J.-P., Cassagnes, J., Machecourt, J., et al. Comparative effects of APSAC and rt-PA on infarct size and left ventricular function in acute myocardial infarction. A multicenter randomized study. *Circulation* 84:1107, 1991.
232. Neuhaus, K. L., Von Essen, R., Tebbe, U., et al. Improved thrombolysis in acute myocardial infarction with front-loaded administration of alteplase: Results of the rt-PA–APSAC Patency Study (TAPS). *J. Am. Coll. Cardiol.* 19:885, 1992.
233. Neuhaus, K.-L., Tebbe, U., Gottwik, M., et al. Intravenous recombinant tissue plasminogen activator (rt-PA) and urokinase in acute myocardial infarction: Results of the German Activator Urokinase Study (GAUS). *J. Am. Coll. Cardiol.* 12:581, 1988.
234. ISIS-3 Collaborative Group. ISIS-3: A randomized comparison of streptokinase vs tissue plasminogen activator vs anistreplase and of aspirin plus heparin vs aspirin alone among 41,299 cases of suspected acute myocardial infarction. *Lancet* 339:753, 1992.
235. The GUSTO (The Global Utilization of Streptokinase and Tissue Plasminogen Activator for Occluded Arteries) Investigators. An international randomized trial comparing four thrombolytic strategies for acute myocardial infarction. *N. Engl. J. Med.* 329:673, 1993.
236. Simoons, M. L., Vos, J., Tijssen, J. G. P., et al. Long-term benefit of early thrombolytic therapy in patients with acute myocardial infarction: 5 year follow-up of a trial conducted by the Interuniversity Cardiology Institute of the Netherlands. *J. Am. Coll. Cardiol.* 14:1609, 1989.
237. Kennedy, J. W., Martin, G. V., Davis, K. B., et al. Western Washington randomized trial of intracoronary streptokinase in acute myocardial infarction (a 12-month follow-up report). *N. Engl. J. Med.* 312:1073, 1985.
238. Schroder, F., Neuhaus, K. I., Leizorovicz, A., et al. Trial of intravenous streptokinase in acute myocardial infarction. Long-term mortality and morbidity. *J. Am. Coll. Cardiol.* 9:197, 1987.
239. Anderson, J. F., Rothburd, R. L., Hackworthy, R. A., et al. Multicenter reperfusion trial of intravenous anisoylated plasminogen activator complex (APSAC) in acute myocardial infarction: Controlled comparison with intracoronary streptokinase. *J. Am. Coll. Cardiol.* 11:1153, 1988.
240. Wilcox, R. G., and the LATE Study Group. Late Assessment of Thrombolytic Efficacy (LATE) study: Alteplase 6–24 hours after onset of acute myocardial infarction. *Lancet* 342:759, 1993.
241. Grines, C. L., and DeMaria, A. N. Optimal utilization of thrombolytic therapy for acute myocardial infarction: Concepts and controversies. *J. Am. Coll. Cardiol.* 16:223, 1990.
242. Simoons, M. L., Serruys, P. W., van den Brand, M., et al. Early thrombolysis in acute myocardial infarction: Limitation of infarct size and improved survival. *J. Am. Coll. Cardiol.* 7:717, 1986.
243. Van de Werf, F., and Arnold, A. E. R. Intravenous tissue plasminogen activator and size of infarct, left ventricular function and survival in acute myocardial infarction. *B.M.J.* 297:1374, 1988.
244. Barbash, G. I., Roth, A., Hod, H., et al. Rapid resolution of ST elevation and prediction of clinical

outcome in patients undergoing thrombolysis with alteplase (recombinant tissue-type plasminogen activator): Results of the Israeli Study of Early Intervention in Myocardial Infarction. *Br. Heart J.* 64: 241, 1990.

245. The GUSTO Angiographic Investigators. The effects of tissue plasminogen activator, streptokinase, or both on coronary-artery patency, ventricular function and survival after acute myocardial infarction. *N. Engl. J. Med.* 329:1615, 1993.
246. Galvani, M., Ottani, F., Ferrini, D., et al. Patency of the infarct-related artery and left ventricular function as the major determinants of survival after Q-wave acute myocardial infarction. *Am. J. Cardiol.* 71:1, 1993.
247. Bengtson, J. R., Kaplan, A. J., Pieper, K. S., et al. Prognosis in cardiogenic shock after acute myocardial infarction in the interventional era. *J. Am. Coll. Cardiol.* 20:1482, 1992.
248. Magnani, B. Plasminogen Activator Italian Multicenter Study (PAIMS). Comparison of intravenous recombinant single-chain human tissue-type plasminogen activator (rt-PA) with intravenous streptokinase in acute myocardial infarction. *J. Am. Coll. Cardiol.* 13:19, 1989.
249. Neuhaus, K. L., Feuerer, W., Jeep-Tebbe, S., et al. Improved thrombolysis with a modified dose regimen of recombinant tissue-type plasminogen activator. *J. Am. Coll. Cardiol.* 14:1566, 1989.
250. Ohman, E. M., Califf, R. M., Topol, E. J., et al., and the TAMI Study Group. Characteristics and importance of reocclusion following successful reperfusion therapy in acute myocardial infarction. *Circulation* 82:781, 1990.
251. Califf, R. M., Topol, E. J., Stack, R. S., et al. Evaluation of combination thrombolytic therapy and timing of cardiac catheterization in acute myocardial infarction. *Circulation* 83:1543, 1991.
252. Grines, C. L., Nissen, S. E., Booth, D. C., et al., and the Kentucky Acute Myocardial Infarction Trial (KAMIT) Group. A prospective, randomized trial comparing combination half-dose tissue-type plasminogen activator and streptokinase with full-dose tissue-type plasminogen activator. *Circulation* 84: 540, 1991.
253. Anderson, J. L., Becker, L. C., Sorensen, S. G., et al. Anistreplase versus alteplase in acute myocardial infarction: Comparative effects on left ventricular function, morbidity and 1-day coronary artery patency. *J. Am. Coll. Cardiol.* 20:753, 1992.
254. Bleich, S. D., Nichols, T. C., Schumacher, R. R., et al. Effect of heparin on coronary arterial patency after thrombolysis with tissue plasminogen activator in acute myocardial infarction. *Am. J. Cardiol.* 66:1412, 1990.
255. The European Cooperative Study Group (ECSG). The effect of early intravenous heparin on coronary patency, infarct size and bleeding complications after alteplase thrombolysis: Results of a randomized double-blind European Cooperative Study Group Trial. *Br. Heart J.* 67:122, 1992.
256. The SCATI Group. Randomized controlled trial of subcutaneous calcium-heparin in acute myocardial infarction. *Lancet* 2:182, 1989.
257. Topol, E. J., George, B. S., Kereiakes, D. J., et al. A randomized controlled trial of intravenous tissue plasminogen activator and early intravenous heparin in acute myocardial infarction. *Circulation* 79: 281, 1989.
258. Hsia, J., Hamilton, W. P., Kleiman, N., et al. A comparison between heparin and low-dose aspirin as adjunctive therapy with tissue plasminogen activator for acute myocardial infarction. *N. Engl. J. Med.* 323:1433, 1990.
259. Yusuf, S., Collins, R., MacMahon, S., et al. Effects of intravenous nitrates on mortality in acute myocardial infarction: An overview of the randomized trials. *Lancet* 1:1088, 1988.
260. Jugdutt, B. I., and Warnica, J. W. Intravenous nitroglycerin therapy to limit myocardial infarct size, expansion and complications. Effects of timing, dosage and infarct location. *Circulation* 78:906, 1988.
261. Jugdutt, B. I., Tymchak, W. J., and Burton, J. R. Preservation of left ventricular geometry and function after late reperfusion and intravenous nitroglycerin in acute transmural myocardial infarction (Abstract). *Circulation* 84(Suppl II):11524, 1991.
262. ISIS-4. Randomized study of oral isosorbide mononitrate in over 50,000 patients with suspected acute myocardial infarction. *Circulation* 88:I-394, 1993.
263. Teo, K. T., Yusuf, S., Collins, R., et al. Effects of intravenous magnesium in suspected acute myocardial infarction. *B.M.J.* 303:1499, 1991.
264. Horner, S. M. Efficacy of intravenous magnesium in acute myocardial infarction in reducing arrhythmias and mortality. *Circulation* 86:774, 1992.
265. Yusuf, S., Peto, R., Lewis, J., et al. Beta-blockage during and after myocardial infarction: An overview of the randomized trials. *Prog. Cardiovasc. Dis.* 27:335, 1985.
266. ISIS-1 (First International Study of Infarct Survival) Collaborative Group. Randomized trial of intravenous atenolol among 16,027 cases of suspected acute myocardial infarction: ISIS-1. *Lancet* 2:57, 1985.
267. The MIAMI Trial Research Group. Metoprolol in Acute Myocardial Infarction (MIAMI). A randomized placebo-controlled intervention trial. *Eur. Heart J.* 6:199, 1985.
268. The TIMI Study Group. Comparison of invasive and conservative strategies after treatment with intravenous tissue plasminogen activator in acute myocardial infarction: Results of the Thrombolysis in Myocardial Infarction (TIMI) phase II trial. *N. Engl. J. Med.* 320:618, 1989.
269. Muller, J. E., Morrison, J., Stone, P. H., et al. Nifedipine therapy for patients with threatened and acute myocardial infarction: A randomized double-blind, placebo-controlled comparison. *Circulation* 69:740, 1984.
270. Sirnes, P. A., Overskeid, K., Pedersen, T. R., et al.

Evolution of infarct size during the early use of nifedipine in patients with acute myocardial infarction: The Norwegian Nifedipine Multicenter Trial. *Circulation* 70:638, 1984.
271. Gibson, R. S., Boden, W. E., Theroux, P., et al. Diltiazem and reinfarction in patients with non-Q wave myocardial infarction. *N. Engl. J. Med.* 315:423, 1986.
272. Erbel, R., Pop, T., Meinertz, T., et al. Combination of calcium channel blocker and thrombolytic therapy in acute myocardial infarction. *Am. Heart J.* 115:529, 1988.
273. Pfeffer, J. M., Pfeffer, M. A., and Braunwald, E. Influence of chronic captopril therapy on the infarcted left ventricle of the rat. *Circ. Res.* 57:84, 1985.
274. Pfeffer, M. A., Pfeffer, J. M., Steinberg, C., et al. Survival after an experimental myocardial infarction: Beneficial effects on long-term therapy with captopril. *Circulation* 72:406, 1985.
275. Pfeffer, M. A., Braunwald, E., Moye, L. A., et al. Effect of captopril on mortality and morbidity in patients with left ventricular dysfunction after myocardial infarction. *N. Engl. J. Med.* 327:669, 1992.
276. Swedberg, K., Held, P., Kjekshus, J., et al. Effects on the early administration of enalapril on mortality in patients with acute myocardial infarction. Results of the Cooperative New Scandinavian Enalapril Survival Study II (CONSENSUS II). *N. Engl. J. Med.* 327:678, 1992.
277. The SOLVD Investigators. Effect of enalapril on survival in patients with reduced left ventricular ejection fractions and congestive heart failure. *N. Engl. J. Med.* 325:293, 1991.
278. Topol, E. J., Califf, R. M., George, B. S., et al., and the Thrombolysis and Angioplasty in Myocardial Infarction Study Group. A randomized trial of immediate versus delayed elective angioplasty after intravenous tissue plasminogen activator in acute myocardial infarction. *N. Engl. J. Med.* 317:581, 1987.
279. Simoons, M. L., Betriu, A., Col, J., et al. Thrombolysis with tissue plasminogen activator in acute myocardial infarction: No additional benefit from immediate percutaneous coronary angioplasty. *Lancet* 1:197, 1988.
280. SWIFT Trial Study Group. SWIFT trial of delayed elective intervention v conservative treatment after thrombolysis with anistreplase in acute myocardial infarction. *B.M.J.* 302:555, 1991.
281. The TIMI Research Group. Immediate vs delayed catheterization and angioplasty following thrombolytic therapy for acute myocardial infarction. TIMI II A results. *J.A.M.A.* 260:2849, 1988.
282. Erbel, R., Pop, T., Diefenbach, C., et al. Long-term results of thrombolytic therapy with and without percutaneous transluminal coronary angioplasty. *J. Am. Coll. Cardiol.* 14:276, 1989.
283. Grines, C. L., Browne, K. F., Marco, J., et al. A comparison of immediate angioplasty with thrombolytic therapy for acute myocardial infarction. *N. Engl. J. Med.* 328:673, 1993.
284. Zijlstra, F., deBoer, M. J., Hvorntje, J. C. A., et al. A comparison of immediate angioplasty with intravenous streptokinase in acute myocardial infarction. *N. Engl. J. Med.* 328:680, 1993.
285. Gibbons, R. J., Holmes, D. R., Reeder, G. S., et al. Immediate angioplasty compared with the administration of a thrombolytic agent followed by conservative treatment for myocardial infarction. *N. Engl. J. Med.* 328:685, 1993.
286. Ribeiro, E. E., Silva, L. A., Carneiro, R., et al. Randomized trial of direct coronary angioplasty versus intravenous streptokinase in acute myocardial infarction. *J. Am. Coll. Cardiol.* 22:376, 1993.
287. O'Neill, W. W., Timmis, G. C., Bourdillon, P. D., et al. A prospective randomized clinical trial of intracoronary streptokinase versus coronary angioplasty for acute myocardial infarction. *N. Engl. J. Med.* 314:812, 1986.
288. Chalmers, T. G., Matta, R. J., Smith, H., Jr., et al. Evidence favoring the use of anticoagulants in the hospital phase of acute myocardial infarction. *N. Engl. J. Med.* 297:1091, 1977.
289. Antiplatelet Trialists' Collaboration. Secondary prevention of vascular disease by prolonged antiplatelet treatment. *B.M.J.* 296:320, 1988.
290. Cohn, J. N., Archibald, D. G., Ziesche, S., et al. Effect of vasodilator therapy on mortality in chronic congestive heart failure. Results of a Veterans Administration Cooperative Study. *N. Engl. J. Med.* 314:1547, 1986.
291. Sharpe, D. N., Murphy, J., Smith, H., et al. Treatment of patients with symptomless left ventricular dysfunction after myocardial infarction. *Lancet* 1: 255, 1988.
292. Pfeffer, M. A., Lamas, G. A., Vaughan, D. E., et al. Effect of captopril on progressive ventricular dilatation after acute myocardial infarction. *N. Engl. J. Med.* 319:80, 1988.
293. Sharpe, N., Smith, H., Murphy, J., et al. Early prevention of left ventricular dysfunction following myocardial infarction with angiotensin converting enzyme inhibition. *Lancet* 337:872, 1991.

39. Overall Risk Stratification and Management Strategies for Patients with Acute Myocardial Infarction

Andrew A. Wolff and Joel S. Karliner

Myocardial oxygen demand in excess of supply is the basic pathophysiologic derangement underlying myocardial ischemia, which, when unrelieved, progresses to myocardial infarction (MI). The latter implies myocardial cell death and subsequent necrosis and is, as such, irreversible. It is the goal of the clinician to interrupt ischemia in progress (thus limiting infarction) and to prevent its recurrence. A logical therapeutic strategy is to increase oxygen supply while decreasing demand.

Initial Management

Acutely, the first step in this effort is to provide supplemental inspired oxygen to the patient. Three factors can act, singly or in combination, to reduce the supply of oxygen-rich coronary arterial blood to an area of myocardium: (1) fixed obstruction of the vascular lumen due to atheroma; (2) dynamic reduction of the vessel diameter due to increases in coronary vascular smooth muscle tone (i.e., "coronary spasm"); and (3) intracoronary thrombus formation, usually in an area of fixed obstruction and often with accompanying coronary spasm. Thus subsequent acute and chronic interventions are directed toward reducing the influence of these three factors in decreasing coronary blood flow while striving whenever possible to diminish the myocardial demand for oxygen.

In the most acute setting, little can be done to effect a reduction in the degree of fixed stenosis underlying an episode of myocardial ischemia. Coronary artery bypass surgery (CABG) and percutaneous transluminal coronary angioplasty (PTCA) are the only proved therapies directed toward rectifying the problems caused by fixed atherosclerotic lesions; although they may benefit selected patients when they can be expeditiously initiated and undertaken by experienced personnel, the expense of maintaining such sophisticated teams on a 24-hour basis is far too great to consider these procedures routinely in first-line management of acute myocardial ischemia and myocardial infarction (AMI). On the other hand, the definitive nature of CABG has rendered the best results in the long-term management of coronary artery disease in certain subsets of patients [1–3]. Similarly, because PTCA is clearly effective in directly reducing the stenosis underlying ischemia or infarction, the improvement in the systolic motion of jeopardized myocardium offered by this technique may eventually be translated into gains in long-term survival [4].

Several drugs act to reduce coronary arterial tone, thereby increasing coronary flow. Nitrates, administered sublingually or intravenously, represent the mainstay of therapy for acute myocardial ischemia; in their topical and orally active preparations, nitrates are similarly the cornerstone of prophylaxis against recurrent attacks of ischemia. Nitrates cause vascular smooth muscle relaxation by activating the cytosolic enzyme guanylate cyclase, thereby increasing intracellular levels of 5′-cyclic guanosine monophosphate (cGMP). In turn, increased levels of this cyclic nucleotide activate the enzyme protein kinase G, which promotes smooth muscle relaxation both directly, via effects on the contractile apparatus, and indirectly, by reducing the intracellular free calcium ion concentration [5]. In addition to directly relaxing the vascular smooth muscle of the coronary conductance vessel, nitrates exert a similar effect on the systemic capacitance venules and resistance arterioles. The action on the capacitance venules allows some degree of systemic venous pooling, which reduces venous return to the heart, effecting decreases in ventricular end-diastolic volume and pressure, reflected as a reduction in myocardial preload. Similarly, the arteriolar effects of nitrates are translated into a decline in myocardial afterload. Because myocardial preload and afterload are major determinants of myocardial stroke work, which is in turn a major determinant of myocardial oxygen consumption, nitrates act not only to increase myocardial oxygen supply but to decrease myocardial oxygen demands as well.

Calcium channel blockers, such as nifedipine, diltiazem, and verapamil, offer all the beneficial vascular actions of nitrates but act via a separate mechanism; thus their effect, when used in combination with nitrates, is additive. Whereas the effects of nitrates on guanylate cyclase in smooth muscle are limited to this tissue, calcium channel blockers act to reduce the influx of calcium ion across the cell membranes of both smooth muscle cells and cardiac myocytes. The subsequent reduction of intracellular free calcium ion causes a parallel decrease in the resting tension of vascular smooth muscle cells. Secondarily, these agents also decrease intracellular calcium stores available for efflux from the sarcoplasmic reticulum during depolarization of cardiac myocytes; thus cardiac contractility is reduced. This direct negative inotropic effect of calcium channel blockers, which can be titrated to therapeutic benefit, decreases myocardial oxygen consumption, thereby favorably altering the myocardial oxygen supply-demand ratio; however, calcium channel blockers have the potential for precipitating congestive heart failure (CHF). These drugs also exhibit significantly longer half-lives (3 to 6 hours) than sublingual, intravenous (IV), or topical preparations of nitrates (about 5 minutes). This longer half-life represents a disadvantage in the management of an acutely ill patient, where rapid fluctuations in the clinical situation may necessitate equally rapid adjustments in therapy. Alternatively, the longer half-life constitutes an advantage in prophylaxis against recurrent ischemia in the stable patient [6]. Studies of verapamil and nifedipine in AMI have shown these agents not to be beneficial but, in fact, to be deleterious in some high-risk patients [7]. Long-term studies of diltiazem have demonstrated a harmful effect in patients with depressed left ventricular (LV) function. Hence, this class of drugs should be used extremely cautiously in patients with MI [8].

Morphine sulfate, injected intravenously, is used primarily for the relief of anginal pain due to myocardial ischemia. Although this pain relief is largely the result of the central nervous system effects of the drug on pain perception, morphine also reduces systemic venous tone, with the attendant beneficial effect on preload described above for nitrates and calcium channel blockers. There is also a modest dilatory effect on the coronary vessels. Perhaps most importantly, the direct pain relief and sedation offered by morphine are often advantageous; pain and anxiety, nearly universal in conscious patients during the acute stages of MI, contribute to elevations in heart rate and blood pressure, which in turn increase myocardial oxygen demands [9].

Beta blockers competitively antagonize the coupling of beta-adrenergic agonists, such as epinephrine and norepinephrine, with their specific cell-surface receptors. Consequently, the ability of beta agonists to activate cellular adenylate cyclase via their receptors is reduced by beta blockade, resulting in a decrease in intracellular levels of the "second messenger" compound, 5′-cyclic adenosine monophosphate (cAMP). In cardiac myocytes, decreased intracellular levels of cAMP in turn decrease the number of calcium channels available for calcium influx, thereby lowering intracellular calcium ion concentrations, with attendant decreases in heart rate and myocardial contractility; thus myocardial oxygen demand is reduced. In contrast, the effect of cAMP on calcium influx does not occur in vascular smooth muscle; in fact, much like cGMP, cAMP acts to decrease vascular smooth muscle tone by activating protein kinase A, which has effects similar to those of protein kinase G [5]. As a result, beta blockers, by reducing intracellular levels of cAMP in coronary vascular smooth muscle, actually function to increase coronary tone and thus decrease myocardial oxygen supply. Fortunately, the beneficial effects of beta blockers on myocardial oxygen demand outweigh their deleterious effects on oxygen supply, and their net effect on the balance between the two is favorable.

Beta blockers are used primarily to prevent recurrent ischemia in patients with coronary artery disease; however, there are two additional uses specific to the treatment of MI. Acutely, the IV administration of metoprolol or atenolol has been associated with a modest reduction (about 13 percent) in in-hospital mortality [10, 11]. This reduction in mortality appears to be greater (30 to 50 percent) in older patients with previous MI, angina, CHF, hypertension, or diabetes [12]; nonetheless, early IV beta blockade as an approach to the management of AMI has not gained widespread acceptance among clinicians. In contrast, therapy with a variety of beta blockers, begun prior to discharge and continued for at least 1 year thereafter, is frequently prescribed. This treatment has been associated with mean 21 and 24 percent reductions in subsequent mortality and nonfatal reinfarction, respectively, during the first postinfarction year. The effect on mortality is due largely to the prevention of sudden cardiac death [13]. A short-acting beta blocker, esmolol, may also be useful in reducing heart rate and blood pressure, two major determinants of myocardial oxygen demand, in patients presenting with tachycardia and hypertension.

Elimination of intracoronary thrombus represents an established approach to early treatment of AMI; prevention of thrombus reformation actually represents the renaissance of an old concept. Studies have shown that the earlier coronary angiography is performed during AMI, the higher the prevalence of intracoronary thrombus [14]. Thus, the involvement of thrombus in most AMIs has been widely acknowledged. Accordingly, the development of thrombolytic agents represented a milestone in the treatment of AMI. The bacterial enzyme streptokinase (SK) binds with circulating plasminogen to form a complex that accelerates the cleavage of unbound plasminogen to its active form, plasmin. Plasmin, in turn, degrades both fibrin and fibrinogen; thus, it dissolves formed thrombus but also precipitates a systemic fibrinolytic state predisposing to hemorrhage. Recombinant tissue plasminogen activator (rt-PA) is more specific for fibrin, because it cleaves only plasminogen in proximity to fibrin. When administered within several hours of the onset of ischemic symptoms (preferably less than 3 to 4 hours and ideally less than 1 to 2 hours), both agents can effect reperfusion of an infarct-related coronary artery with essentially equal efficiency: approximately 80 percent with intracoronary administration, and about 65 to 70 percent when given intravenously [15]. By either route, the incidence of successful thrombolysis decreases with time from the onset of symptoms, as do the beneficial effects of thrombolysis on left ventricular ejection fraction (LVEF) and mortality. In general, the greatest salvage of life and ventricular function occurs when these agents are given as early as possible (even less than 1 hour) after the onset of symptoms [16, 17]. A recent large trial has suggested a small advantage of rt-PA over SK, but at the expense of a small increase in stroke rate [18].

Although its more specific mechanism suggests that rt-PA should be associated with fewer bleeding complications than SK, to date this suggestion has not been verified in clinical trials [18, 19]. It is probably because once successful reperfusion has been accomplished with either agent, systemic anticoagulation must be instituted to prevent early reocclusion of the infarct-related artery. Unfortunately, heparin also increases the rate of hemorrhagic complications associated with thrombolytic therapy [15]; therefore it is usually discontinued within the first several days of reperfusion, once treatment with an antiplatelet agent, usually aspirin, has been instituted to prevent reocclusion.

With these therapeutic principles in mind, strategies for the initial management of patients with AMI can be outlined. When an anterior AMI (or any first MI) can be confidently diagnosed in any patient without contraindications to the use of a thrombolytic agent, the agent should be given intravenously without delay. How this principle can be best implemented is currently a matter of some clinical controversy. For example, if emergency medical personnel begin IV thrombolysis in the field, improvement in survival and myocardial salvage might be expected because of shorter elapsed time from the onset of symptoms to the initiation of therapy. It is possible, however, that this benefit would be offset by an increase in serious hemorrhagic complications due to inappropriate administration of the drugs.

While ongoing trials attempt to resolve such issues, there is no doubt that IV thrombolysis should be instituted in the emergency department after an initial evaluation by a physician has determined such therapy to be appropriate for the patient. In general, thrombolysis is indicated for a patient under the age of 75 years who is seen within 6 hours of the onset of ischemic symptoms, whose electrocardiogram (ECG) displays ST segment elevation, who has no history of stroke or recent trauma (including external chest compression during cardiopulmonary resuscitation that has resulted in significant sternocostal damage), and who is not actively bleeding. Successful reperfusion is recognized clinically by relief of chest pain with resolution of ST segment elevation; "reperfusion arrhythmias," typically accelerated idioventricular complexes, may occur at this time [20]. These arrhythmias are rarely associated with hemodynamic compromise but should be monitored because of their occasional degeneration to ventricular tachycardia and fibrillation.

As the decision whether to administer thrombolysis is made, other therapeutic interventions against ischemia can begin. All of the drugs described above can be given concurrently with thrombolytic agents, although extra caution should be exercised when using those that predispose to hypotension, because thrombolytic agents, particularly SK, are also known to lower the blood pressure in some patients. Sublingual nitrates are usually the agents of first choice: They can be administered even before IV access is available, act rapidly, and have beneficial effects on both myocardial oxygen supply and demand, without the price of negative inotropy. Based on the results of the Second International Study of Infarct Survival (ISIS-2) trial [17], chewable aspirin, 325 mg, is recommended acutely, followed by a 325-mg enteric-coated tablet given orally each day. When anginal pain persists, morphine may be added, and IV nitrate therapy can be augmented while blood pressure is monitored. When a hyperdynamic state is believed to contribute to ongoing ischemia, the use of the rapidly acting beta blocker esmolol, which can be given intravenously and has an extremely short half-life, should be considered. Supplemental oxygen should be given to all patients. A prophylactic bolus and infusion of lidocaine is no longer recommended, particularly where facilities for resuscitation are available [7]. Noncardiac factors that may complicate treatment of ischemia by increasing myocardial oxygen demands (e.g., systemic arterial hypertension, even of modest degree, or fever causing tachycardia) should receive prompt attention. The goal is a hemodynamically stable patient without ischemic symptoms. Intravenous magnesium also appears to be beneficial, although its mechanism of action is unknown [21].

Risk Stratification and Management Strategies for Surviving Patients

Events during the initial hospitalization most accurately predict the subsequent course of patients with AMI. Patients who survive their first MI without recurrent chest pain, CHF, or significant late arrhythmias enjoy a good prognosis, suffering less than 3 percent mortality during the first 2 years after infarction. Unfortunately, each of these complications increases the likelihood of future cardiovascular morbidity and mortality [22, 23]. Data from noninvasive and, where warranted, invasive testing help to further refine the prognosis and aid in the management of each of these groups.

Infarct localization by ECG at admission is of great value in initial risk stratification. When compared with patients with inferior infarctions, patients with anterior infarction experience increases in both in-hospital (12 percent versus 3 percent) and long-term mortality (27 percent versus 11 percent at 2.5 years). This poorer outcome with anterior infarction persists, even when adjustments are made for infarct size [24]. The prognostic value of the ECG type of infarction (i.e., Q wave versus non-Q wave) continues to be debated. Some studies have found patients with non-Q-wave infarctions to sustain a more benign in-hospital course but to suffer a higher rate of recurrent infarction and mortality after discharge. Such data are consistent with the hypothesis that non-Q-wave infarctions represent "incomplete" infarctions, with substantial viable myocardium remaining at risk in the distribution of the infarcted vessel [25, 26], and they have been used to support an aggressive management strategy for patients with non-Q-wave infarction, including routine predischarge coronary angiography with, when appropriate, subsequent revascularization. Although the non-Q-wave pattern clearly reflects a smaller infarction (assessed by changes in plasma creatine kinase-MB (MB-CK) activity) attended by fewer in-hospital complications, other studies have found no differences in survival or reinfarction rates after discharge between patients with Q-wave and those with non-Q-wave infarctions [24]. However, these two patterns of infarction are not useful for determining whether an infarction is "transmural" or "nontransmural"; the use of these terms to denote, respectively, Q-wave and non-Q-wave infarctions is inaccurate and should be abandoned [27]. In addition, diltiazem treatment of patients surviving non-Q-wave infarctions is associated with a reduction in the rate of reinfarction during the first 14 days after the acute event [6]; this benefit has not been shown to extend to survivors of Q-wave infarctions, or to survivors with reduced LV function [8].

Management of any patient surviving MI, whether complicated or not, must include an aggressive program of overall cardiovascular risk reduction. Smokers must be encouraged to quit and obese patients advised to lose weight. When present, hypertension and diabetes should be controlled. Total serum cholesterol should be measured and fractionated into high (HDL) and low density (LDL) components. If abnormalities are found, they should be treated with dietary restrictions and, when necessary, drug therapy. In this regard, it is important to remember that any acute intercurrent illness, including MI, can abruptly lower serum cholesterol; therefore a normal serum cholesterol level during the initial hospitalization does not rule out clinically significant hypercholesterolemia. Such patients should have their cholesterol and HDL and LDL levels rechecked at a follow-up visit 4 to 6 weeks after discharge.

In addition to these major cardiovascular risk factors, nearly any acute medical illness harbors the potential for aggravating the consequences of coronary artery disease by increasing metabolic rates and, subsequently, the demand on the heart. Obviously, the clinician optimizes the general medical condition of any patient, but particular care must be taken to ensure that the sinus tachycardia, low-grade fever, and mild leukocytosis observed frequently during the first days after MI do not serve to mask, for instance, an underlying infection or concomitant hyperthyroidism.

The administration of low doses of aspirin has been shown in controlled studies to reduce the reinfarction and cardiovascular death rates in patients after MI [28–30]. Its use is associated with few complications, probably because the effective dose appears to be low and administration need not be frequent (as little as 300 mg every day has been beneficial in some studies). Furthermore, enteric-coated preparations can be used with similar benefit. Theoretical concerns that higher doses might prove to be less beneficial (or even deleterious) due to inhibition of synthesis of the vasodilator prostacyclin, in addition to inhibition of synthesis of the potent vasoconstrictor thromboxane A_2, have not been borne out by clinical investigation [31]. In view of this safety and efficacy, all patients who survive MI should be treated on admission with chewable aspirin, then placed indefinitely on a dose of at least 300 mg of aspirin per day, excluding only those patients with active peptic ulcer disease, a documented history of true aspirin hypersensitivity, or demonstrated gastrointestinal intolerance of 300 mg per day. Often the latter can be overcome by using an enteric-coated preparation.

The reductions in mortality and reinfarction attendant to beta-antagonist treatment of survivors of AMI have been noted above. Propranolol or timolol probably should be given to most survivors of AMI who can tolerate this therapy without symptomatic bradycardia or CHF. A reduced LVEF is not itself a contraindication to beta-blocker therapy if symptomatic CHF is absent; indeed, these patients may benefit most from the protective effects of beta blockade. Treatment should be continued for at least 1 year; however, benefit has not been shown to extend beyond 2 years after infarction. In fact, the adverse effects of most beta-adrenergic antagonists on serum lipid profiles argue against indefinite therapy with these agents.

The management strategies outlined below refer only to patients who have not undergone reperfusion with a thrombolytic agent, either because such an agent was not administered, or because thrombolytic therapy was unsuccessful in restoring flow through the involved coronary artery. Strategies for management of the successfully reperfused patient continue to evolve. Early coronary angiography in these individuals has demonstrated a substantial incidence of high-grade residual stenosis of successfully reperfused infarct vessels [4] with an appreciable rate of reocclusion/reinfarction in the absence of anticoagulation [1]. These observations support the emerging consensus that patients successfully reperfused with thrombolytic agents should remain anticoagulated until they undergo coronary angiography, anticipating the performance of PTCA on the infarct-related vessel, if the anatomy of the culprit lesion is amenable to this procedure. Although this intervention should occur prior to hospital discharge, there appears to be no advantage to urgent angiography/angioplasty, as results are equally good when these procedures are delayed until several days after the AMI, so long as the patient remains adequately anticoagulated during this interval [32]. Some have advocated routine risk stratification (see below) after thrombolysis, since routine PTCA appears to confer no additional advantage on survival [33]. If catheterization is performed, PTCA may be found to be an unfeasible management strategy. The anatomy of the infarct-related stenosis may be unfavorable or the coexistence of multiple critical stenoses may mandate CABG. If surgical revascularization is elected, full anticoagulation with heparin should be continued until 4 hours before surgery in order to prevent rethrombosis. To date, trials of numerous agents prescribed to prevent restenosis after PTCA have been disappointing, and the restenosis rate remains at 30 to 50 percent.

Uncomplicated Myocardial Infarction

Patients with an uncomplicated MI include those without recurrent angina or malignant ventricular arrhythmias detected beyond 48 hours after admission to the coronary care unit (CCU) and without clinical evidence of CHF at any time during their hospital course. Clinical experience indicates that mild to moderate chest discomfort frequently persists for some hours after relief of the acute pain that prompted the patient to seek medical attention. This symptom usually does not evoke complaints from the patient but, rather, is elicited by questioning a patient who appears to be resting comfortably. Such discomfort may originate from the irreversibly damaged myocardium as it undergoes necrosis; it generally does not last beyond the first hospital day, is not associated with new ECG changes, and is not of particular significance. Such discomfort must be distinguished from a recurrence of angina after initial stabilization of the patient, which indicates that further viable myocardium is at risk of infarction and constitutes a complication of the original MI. Obviously, when doubt exists regarding the etiology of a patient's chest discomfort after MI, recurrent angina must be presumed until proved otherwise. Finally, hemodynamically significant ventricular tachycardia or ventricular fibrillation during the first 48 hours after AMI does not constitute a complication of the MI for purposes of risk stratification. Although the occurrence of this dysrhythmia is associated with a doubling of in-hospital mortality (largely due to severe pump failure), it does not affect the long-term prognosis of patients who survive to hospital discharge [34, 35].

Because of their favorable prognosis (approximately 1 to 2 percent mortality per year [22]), patients surviving an uncomplicated first MI require little in the way of routine testing before discharge from the hospital; however, because the single objectively quantifiable variable that best predicts reduced survival after AMI is depressed LV function [22, 36] and because LV function can be accurately measured noninvasively at a relatively low cost, some quantification of this parameter is recommended for all patients surviving AMI prior to hospital discharge. In patients with an LVEF greater than 0.40, 1-year mortality is 5 percent or less; however, mortality increases sharply as the LVEF falls below 0.40 [22] (Fig. 39-1). In addition to aiding in prognosis, this measurement provides baseline data for comparison during follow-up evaluation.

The most common methods employed in the noninvasive quantitation of LV function are echocardiography and (RVG); the choice of techniques may be reasonably based on their relative availability or cost at a given institution. RVG offers greater

Fig. 39-1
Relation between the predischarge radionuclide ejection fraction and 1-year cardiac mortality after myocardial infarction. (From A. J. Moss for The Multicenter Postinfarction Research Group. *New Engl. J. Med.* 309:331, 1983. With permission.)

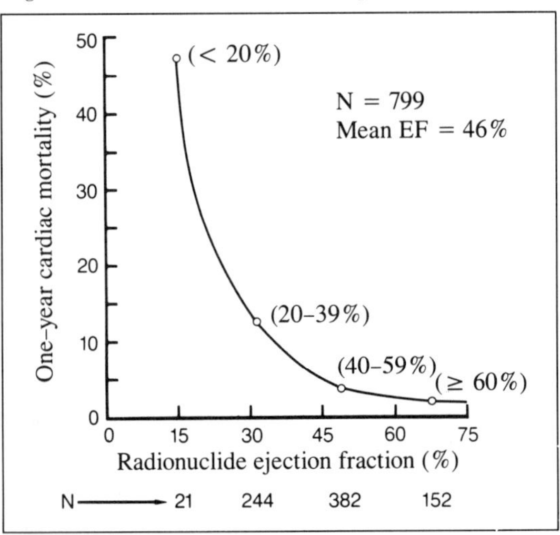

accuracy and reproducibility than echocardiography in measuring the EF but is perhaps less sensitive in identifying regional wall motion abnormalities (especially smaller ones) and cannot assess the structure or function of the cardiac valves, as can echocardiography, particularly when Doppler techniques are used. Thus if the clinician expects the predischarge evaluation to disclose some impairment of LV function and anticipates future serial evaluations to discover whether improvement occurs with time or adjustments in therapy, RVG may be the better choice. If, on the other hand, normal LV function is likely, echocardiography offers a wider screen for the unanticipated structural abnormality (e.g., significant LV hypertrophy) and is clearly preferable if any valvular pathology is suspected.

Once adequate global LV function (EF $\geqslant$ 0.40) has been documented in the patient with an uncomplicated MI, predischarge submaximal exercise testing is of limited use. Only a few such patients would be found to have severe myocardial ischemia induced by a low level of exercise and would indeed be at high risk for subsequent cardiovascular morbidity and mortality; however, these patients would also be identified by a symptom-limited exercise test at 4 to 6 weeks postinfarction. The risk to this subgroup of interval cardiovascular death or reinfarction associated with delaying the exercise test is well under 1 percent [37].

Later symptom-limited exercise testing identifies those additional patients at risk for recurrent cardiovascular events that the predischarge test would have missed and provides useful information about the functional status of the patient that the submaximal test cannot. It then allows the clinician to prescribe exercise for patients without an early positive result. Therefore, a single symptom-limited exercise test, performed 4 to 6 weeks after discharge, constitutes the most effective management of patients with an uncomplicated MI and adequate global LV function who have remained angina-free to that time, as well as those who have developed since discharge class I or class II angina that has responded well to medical therapy.

This strategy is also appropriate for patients surviving an uncomplicated MI who unexpectedly are found to have an EF below 0.40 despite the absence of clinically apparent CHF at any time during their hospitalization; however, such patients are clearly at increased risk for subsequent cardiovascular morbidity and mortality, and a substantially larger percentage of them could be expected to have a positive result during a predischarge exercise test compared with patients with a similar hospital course but with adequate LV function. Therefore, predischarge exercise testing of patients surviving a clinically uncomplicated MI, but with a reduced EF, should provide early identification of those among this group most likely to benefit from CABG (those with three-vessel disease and, by definition of this group, depressed LV function, in addition to those with left main coronary artery disease [1, 2]). Patients with reduced LV function and a positive submaximal exercise test before discharge should undergo early coronary angiography.

Exercise testing should be performed while the patient has optimal medical therapy, as the issue is not if the patient has coronary disease but, rather, whether medical therapy (if any) allows the patient to tolerate successfully the burden of coronary disease. There is little useful information to be gained from exercise testing a patient on a medical regimen he or she cannot maintain because of unacceptable side effects. If at any time the patient's angina cannot be adequately controlled by well tolerated medicines, referral for coronary angiography is indicated.

Many post-MI patients have abnormal resting ECGs; the addition of stress and rest thallium 201 imaging to the exercise test helps to determine how much, if any, myocardium remains jeopardized in these patients, because the exercise ECGs of these patients may be of little use in this regard. In fact, because the severity and extent of reversible perfusion defects detected by exercise thallium 201 scintigraphy are themselves of prognostic value [38, 39], it is appropriate to routinely perform the 6-week postdischarge exercise test with thallium 201 imaging in all patients. In patients unable to exercise, scintigraphy may be performed using pharmacologic interventions (dipyridamole, adenosine).

In general, interpretation of the exercise data must be individualized. The patient's desired life style must be considered in concert with such predictors of future cardiovascular morbidity and mortality as objectively measured exercise tolerance and the size and number of myocardial areas made ischemic during exercise. Clearly, large, widespread areas of myocardial ischemia warrant referral for coronary angiography; however, one or two ischemic areas of small or moderate size might reasonably prompt continued medical therapy in an elderly patient who achieves a workload significantly in excess of the demands placed on the individual's heart during usual daily activities. Alternatively, if a single, small area of ischemia, associated with limiting angina at a relatively low workload, persists during repeated tests despite an escalation to maximal medical therapy in an otherwise healthy patient wishing to return to a program of regular strenuous physical activity, invasive evaluation with an eye toward revascularization becomes indicated.

With these considerations in mind, one of the three management options presents itself to the clinician after the 6-week postdischarge, symptom-limited exercise test in the uncomplicated MI patient with adequate global LV function. If the patient performs well, with good exercise tolerance for age, and exhibits little or no evidence of exercise-induced myocardial ischemia, the risk of subsequent cardiovascular morbidity and mortality is low [40], and the patient may be followed on the current regimen. Repeat exercise testing every 6 months for 1 year and yearly thereafter is adequate follow-up for patients who remain asymptomatic. In contrast, patients with markedly poor exercise tolerance, with ECG or scintigraphic evidence suggesting proximal stenosis of the left anterior descending coronary artery, or with large or numerous exercise-induced ischemic defects by thallium 201 scintigraphy should be referred for coronary angiography and, if possible, subsequent revascularization (PTCA or CABG).

The third option, increasing medical therapy followed by repeat exercise testing, should be used sparingly and be reserved for three types of patients in this group: (1) those on a minimal to moderate medical regimen who experience early limiting angina from a demonstrably small area of ischemia (particularly inferior ischemia) without evidence of LV dysfunction during the exercise test (i.e., normal blood pressure response to exercise); (2) patients who develop a small to moderate-sized ischemic area in a single coronary distribution but only at a workload clearly in excess of the usual daily activity and again without evidence of LV dysfunction during the test; (3) patients who are poor surgical candidates for a noncardiac reason. Particularly in the group with adequate global LV function, it is prudent to err on the side of catheterization. First, the risk of the procedure itself is low. Second, documentation of surgical disease, where mortality is clearly reduced by surgical revascularization—generally accepted to include significant left main coronary artery disease and severe proximal triple-vessel disease with LVEF less than 0.50—could be life-saving. Third, CABG, if indicated, is of comparatively low risk in patients with preserved LV function.

There is little rationale for routine ambulatory ECG monitoring of patients surviving an uncomplicated AMI with adequate global LV function. Only about 10 percent of these patients are found to have frequent ventricular ectopy, defined as a mean of ten or more ventricular premature contractions (VPCs) per hour during 24 hours of ambulatory monitoring [36]. The prognostic value of this finding in the setting of adequate ventricular function is uncertain. In the Multicenter Investigation of the Limitation of Infarct Size (MILIS) study [36], this small subgroup sustained a disturbingly high 18 percent mortality by 1.5 years postinfarction. Other data, however, indicate only 10 percent mortality at 22 months for all patients with ten or more VPCs per hour [22], suggesting that the subgroup with adequate LV function would enjoy an even better prognosis. In a more recent study, no patient with an EF of more than 0.40 and ten or more VPCs per hour died during a year of follow-up, despite a median frequency of more than 100 VPCs per hour in that group [41]. Beyond this information, there is no evidence that attempts to suppress these ventricular arrhythmias with drug therapy alter subsequent mortality. Indeed, the proarrhythmic effects of agents that suppress VPCs may lead to excess mortality in such patients [42]. Accordingly, drug or device therapy should be reserved for patients who have symptomatic tachyarrhythmias or who have been resuscitated from sudden death unassociated with the AMI. Thus, routine ambulatory ECG monitoring of patients surviving an uncomplicated AMI with adequate LV function appears to be a low-yield procedure, identifying few patients at an uncertain (but likely low) degree of risk, for whom no proved therapy exists.

Myocardial Infarction Complicated by Congestive Heart Failure

As demonstrated by Killip and Kimball in 1967 [43], the occurrence of increasingly severe CHF soon after MI is associated with a parallel increase in hospital mortality. Similarly, late mortality is increased in survivors of MI complicated by CHF [22]. These clinical observations reflect the direct relation between the extent of ischemic myocardial dysfunction causing pump failure and the extent and severity of the underlying coronary disease. Although the occurrence of severe CHF or cardiogenic shock at any point during the course of AMI indicates the presence of widespread coronary disease, all the ischemically dysfunctional myocardium does not necessarily progress irreversibly to infarction and permanent damage [44]. Observations of spontaneous improvement in LV function after CHF due to AMI gave rise to the concept of *stunned myocardium.* This term refers to myocardium unable to support normal electromechanical cardiac events but capable of an eventual full recovery given restitution and maintenance of an adequate blood supply [45]. Advances in thrombolytic therapy have improved the salvage of such ischemic myocardium jeopardized during the initial clinical presentation, as reflected by improvement in regional LV function [46] and in both early and late mortality in patients treated with these agents [16, 17, 47].

Thus, the first question to be answered in the management of the patient whose MI is complicated by CHF is whether pump failure is a consequence of active, ongoing ischemia or a sequel to some other irreversible cause, such as a previous, completed ischemic event. Accordingly, the clinical strategy is, first, to relieve any ischemia contributing to the pump failure; second, to prevent recurrent ischemia; and finally, to provide inotropic support, where necessary, without reaggravating the imbalance between oxygen supply and demand that always underlies myocardial ischemia. In any of these situations, supplemental oxygen should be administered. If the presence of suggestive chest pain, ECG changes, or other clinical data indicate an AMI, thrombolytic therapy, if not contraindicated, must be instituted as early as possible to maximize its beneficial effects on impaired LV function.

If the clinical situation is more compatible with active ischemia than with infarction, or when thrombolytic therapy is not an option, aggressive therapy with nitrates is indicated. By dilating coronary conductance vessels, as well as peripheral arterioles and venules, nitrates favorably alter the myocardial oxygen supply-demand ratio by decreasing preload and afterload while increasing coronary blood flow. In addition to improving ventricular dysfunction by relieving ischemia, the preload reduction itself reduces pulmonary congestion. Beta-adrenergic antagonists and calcium channel blockers, though not absolutely contraindicated in this setting, must be used cautiously in order to avoid exacerbating CHF by their negative inotropic effects. Beta-adrenergic antagonists are useful when inappropriate tachycardia is thought to underlie the ischemia and CHF; calcium channel blockers can be added to nitrates when hypertension or coronary spasm believed to be aggravating the clinical syndrome does not respond satisfactorily to aggressive nitrate treatment.

As treatment of active ischemia progresses, specific therapy for CHF can be instituted. Gentle diuresis is appropriate. If an inotropic agent is required, IV dobutamine or amrinone offer better inotropic support for the same degree of tachycardia compared with dopamine or epinephrine, because dobutamine and amrinone increase myocardial oxygen demands less. Dobutamine or amrinone are thus the agents of choice when the possibility of inducing recurrent myocardial ischemia with an inotropic drug is a concern. Small amounts of dopamine (''renal dose'') may be used in conjunction with other inotropic agents to augment renal blood flow. The therapeutic response to these drugs is best evaluated, and thus most easily titrated, when serial measurements of cardiac output and pulmonary artery pressures are readily available. In view of this point and because patients in CHF due to AMI can deteriorate abruptly, the clinician should be very cautious about placing a pulmonary artery catheter into these patients. Afterload reduction with nitroprusside is beneficial when the calculated systemic vascular resistance is elevated.

Noninvasive assessment of LV function should be performed as early as is practical to provide a baseline for serial evaluations. Spontaneous improvement in the function of stunned myocardium is most rapid within the first days after the ischemic event and is usually complete within 1 week [40]. As improvement occurs, the patient can be weaned from IV inotropic agents and vasodilators and switched to oral digoxin, diuretics, and, when necessary, vasodilators. The combination of preload reduction with nitrates and afterload reduction with hydralazine improves mortality in patients with CHF from a variety of causes, including coronary artery disease and previous MI [48]. Treatment with the angiotensin-converting enzyme inhibitor enalapril confers a similar benefit on these patients [49]. Salt restriction should always accompany drug treatment of CHF. Recent data indicate that patients with reduced LV function after MI respond favorably to captopril [50]. Administration of this agent within 3 to 16 days after infarction, with a target dose of 50 mg tid, resulted in a highly significant reduction in cardiovascular morbidity and mortality [50].

Because serious CHF in the setting of AMI usually indicates the presence of widespread, hemodynamically significant coronary artery stenoses, its occurrence represents a probable indication for coronary angiography. The exceptions to this recommendation are patients with an LVEF remaining below 0.30, despite optimal medical therapy, by 6 weeks postinfarction; by this time, further recovery of stunned myocardium is no longer likely [45]. In this subgroup, the risk of CABG is greatest and usually (but not always) outweighs the potential benefits [23]. Continued medical therapy, directed to prevention of ischemia and optimal management of CHF, is appropriate.

In other patients who survive an MI complicated by Killip class III or IV CHF with subsequent improvement in the signs and symptoms of CHF, the incidence of left main or proximal three-vessel coronary artery disease with significant viable but jeopardized myocardium is high [44]. CABG has been shown to decrease mortality in patients with these coronary lesions [1, 2]. In the absence of other contraindications to major thoracic surgery, these patients have an acceptable surgical risk and often display an increase in LVEF after coronary revascularization. Therefore, they should undergo coronary angiography followed by CABG when the latter is appropriate.

In order to minimize risk to patients with CHF during an AMI, it is preferable, whenever possible, to delay surgery until at least 2 weeks after the acute event in order to stabilize the patient medically and await maximal spontaneous recovery of ventricular function; indeed, surgical mortality is probably further decreased when more than 6 weeks elapse after AMI. In some patients, however, pump failure, which can lead to overt cardiogenic shock, is clearly due to recurrent ischemia that cannot be successfully managed by aggressive medical therapy. Definition of the coronary anatomy in anticipation of revascularization offers the only hope for myocardial salvage and must proceed, in the absence of other contraindications, to surgery. In such cases, placement of an intra-aortic balloon pump often can enhance the treatment of both CHF and underlying ischemia by reducing the impedance to ejection during systole and increasing the coronary perfusion pressure during diastole. The balloon pump frequently stabilizes the condition of a critically ill patient, allowing cardiac catheterization to be performed safely, and maintains adequate perfusion of the heart and other vital organs until a definitive myocardial revascularization procedure can be performed. If, after intra-aortic balloon pumping, a patient remains in a tenuous hemodynamic state and is thus a poor surgical candidate, judicious PTCA of the most easily approached lesion, although not providing complete revascularization, may allow sufficient improvement to enable the patient to tolerate surgery. Such a strategy should be reserved for patients who would die, despite balloon pumping, without an emergency revascularization procedure.

Finally, many patients whose infarction is complicated only by mild CHF leave the hospital with no congestive signs or symptoms on their medical regimen at that time. Management options at that point are similar to those described earlier for patients who have sustained an uncomplicated MI based on the predischarge resting EF. As noted above, therapy with captopril, which reduces excessive dilation (remodeling) in surviving myocardium appears to be routinely indicated in such patients [50]. Whether long-acting angiotensin-converting enzyme inhibitors will confer similar benefit remains to be determined [51, 52].

The prevalence of malignant ventricular arrhythmias detected by ambulatory ECG monitoring is known to be significantly increased among patients left with symptomatic CHF after an AMI. Because frequent VPCs (≥10 per hour) documented beyond 48 hours after an AMI pose an independent risk for cardiovascular death [22, 36], routine ambulatory ECG monitoring of postinfarction patients with CHF should be considered. By 6 weeks after discharge, according to the management strategies discussed above, these patients have undergone either treadmill exercise testing or cardiac catheterization, depending on the severity of the CHF that complicated their MI. If the results of either of these investigations have not suggested the need for further studies or revascularization, it is reasonable to perform ambulatory ECG monitoring at that time. Otherwise, it is preferable to wait until after revascularization has been completed or the need for it has been excluded.

Once malignant ventricular arrhythmias have been identified in patients with reduced LV function, and treatment of CHF or recurrent ischemia has been optimized with all appropriate pharmacologic and invasive measures, their management should probably involve either electrophysiologic testing with programmed electrical stimulation or treatment with an agent such as amiodarone. The problem of postinfarction ventricular arrhythmias is addressed in a separate section of this chapter.

Myocardial Infarction Complicated by Recurrent Ischemia

In general, the problem of recurrent myocardial ischemia can be equated with recurrent angina pectoris; of course, the possibility of anginal equivalents as clinical signs of recurrent ischemia must be borne in mind. For example, dyspnea or lightheadedness may be due to LV dysfunction as a result of recurrent ischemia, even in the absence of typical angina pectoris. The clinician must also remember that the character of a patient's angina sometimes changes after an AMI, as myocardium that had previously contributed to symptoms has died and is therefore no longer a source of ischemia. The pharmacologic management of an individual attack of postinfarction angina is no different from that already outlined for the initial ischemic event or for ischemia underlying CHF. As always, the general strategy is to improve myocardial oxygen supply while decreasing the demand.

Patients experiencing ischemic symptoms soon after an AMI clearly have additional myocardium at risk for reinfarction. Because the 6-month postinfarction mortality exceeds 50 percent in such patients [53], they should undergo coronary angiography prior to discharge from the hospital. Knowledge of the coronary anatomy allows rational management of these patients. Patients with single-vessel coronary artery disease have a good prognosis following an AMI [54]. In one study, none of 97 such patients died during a mean follow-up period of more than 3 years, and only six sustained a recurrent nonfatal infarction. Those patients who displayed thallium redistribution during exercise scintigraphy had a higher incidence of nonfatal infarction and readmission with unstable angina [53]; this subgroup may benefit from prophylactic PTCA, whereas medical management is sufficient for the others. At the other end of the spectrum, patients with postinfarction angina found at coronary angiography to have significant left main or three-vessel coronary artery disease clearly require CABG. When two-vessel coronary disease is found in patients with early postinfarction angina, management may be aided by the location of ECG changes associated with the postinfarction ischemic events. The 6-month mortality of patients with ischemic changes observed in a distribution different from the ECG location of the index infarction ("ischemia at a distance") is three times greater than that of patients whose early postinfarction angina is associated with ECG changes limited to the leads involved by the original infarction [53]; a revascularization procedure (surgery or angioplasty), chosen on the basis of the individual's specific coronary anatomy, is a reasonable strategy. Prognostic information from exercise thallium scintigraphy can also be useful when deciding between medical therapy and a revascularization procedure in patients with two-vessel disease, as the number and severity of reversible defects predict subsequent cardiac events and survival [38, 39]. Finally, guidance comes from the VA Cooperative Study Group; in addition to the well known angiographic criteria for the identification of patients benefiting from CABG with prolonged survival, this study also clinically defined a group that enjoyed an enhanced survival after CABG without regard to the angiographically defined coronary anatomy. The latter group included patients with at least two of the following: (1) resting ST depression, (2) a history of MI, or (3) a history of hypertension [1].

Myocardial Infarction Complicated by Complex Ventricular Arrhythmias

The results of several large studies of postinfarction patients leave little doubt that an average of ten or more VPCs per hour (documented over 24 hours of ambulatory ECG monitoring performed more than 48 hours after the infarction) is associated with an increased risk of overall cardiac mortality [22] and sudden death [36]. Unfortunately, what impact these associations should have on the care of postinfarction patients is far less clear.

First, frequent and complex ventricular ectopy is so common after MI that its predictive value for morbidity is relatively low [55]. Second, whereas such ectopy is not limited to patients with LV dysfunction, it is heavily concentrated among them [56] (Fig. 39-2); the prognosis of these patients is influenced far more prominently by their degree of LV dysfunction than by their ventricular dysrhythmias [22]. Conversely, in patients with LVEFs of more than 0.40, mortality is low despite frequent VPCs; in one study, the 1-year mortality of postinfarction patients with an EF of 0.40 or more and a median VPC frequency of more than 100 per hour was 0 percent [41]. Most distressing is the fact that antiarrhythmic therapy of these postinfarction ventricular arrhythmias has never been shown to reduce the incidence of either sudden death or overall cardiac mortality. An early report that electrophysiologic testing of survivors of AMI could predict subsequent ventricular tachycardia and sudden death [57] raised hope that this technique would allow effective, directed prophylaxis against these fatal sequelae; however, the results of later investigations have not been as encouraging [58, 59]. This therapeutic nihilism can be tempered somewhat by observations of the efficacy of invasive electrophysiologic studies for guiding therapy of recurrent ventricular tachycardia and out-of-hospital cardiac arrest in patients without recent MI [60, 61]. Moreover, the results of the Cardiac Arrhythmia Suppression Trial (CAST), indicating that agents efficacious in the suppression of PVCs are also the most proarrhythmic [42], throw serious doubt on the routine use of antiarrhythmic agents for the suppression of PVCs after MI.

In the absence of direct scientific evidence to support any recommendations for the evaluation and treatment of myocardial electrical instability after AMI, the following suggestions appear to constitute a rational approach to the problem (Fig. 39-3):

1. Routine ambulatory ECG monitoring of survivors of AMI with LVEF of more than 0.40 is not necessary.
2. Patients with sustained or symptomatic ventricu-

Fig. 39-2
A. Distribution of ventricular ectopic activity (VEA; noncomplex versus complex) among patients with ejection fractions ≤ 0.40 versus ≥ 0.40. Complex VEA is rare in the group with the higher ejection fraction. *B.* Distribution of ejection fractions (≤ 0.40 versus ≥ 0.40) in patients with noncomplex versus complex ventricular ectopic activity. An ejection fraction ≥ 0.40 is rare in the group with complex ventricular ectopic activity. (Adapted from the data of R. A. Schultze et al. *Am. J. Med.* 62:192, 1977 by N. Goldschlager. *Cardiology* (Vol. 2.). Philadelphia: Lippincott, 1987. With permission.)

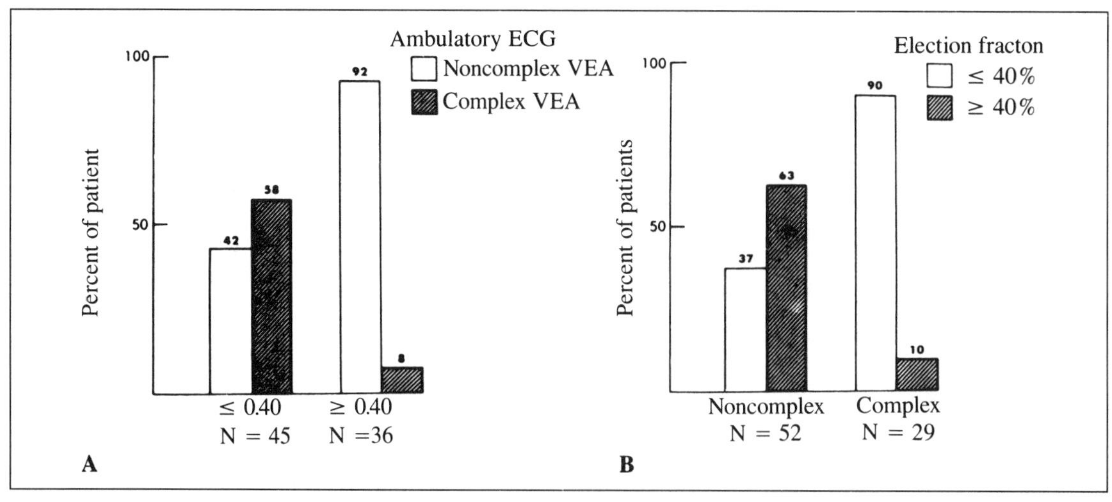

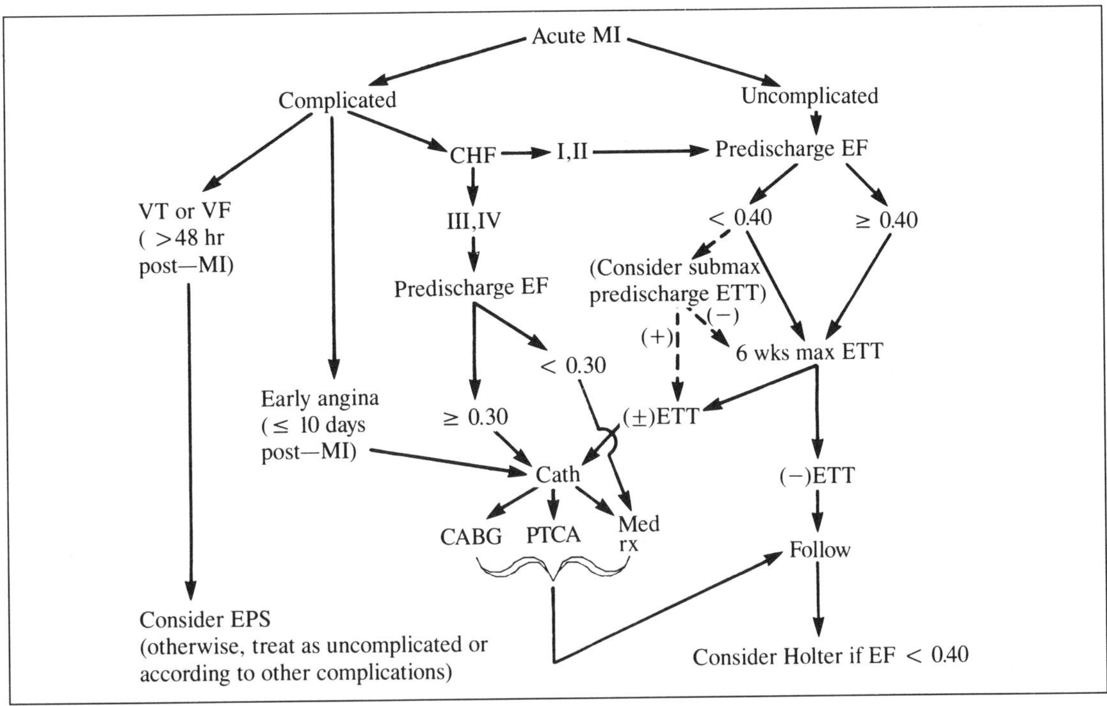

Fig. 39-3
Management strategies for patients surviving acute myocardial infarction. MI = myocardial infarction; CHF = congestive heart failure; I,II = Killip class I or II; III,IV = Killip class III or IV; EF = ejection fraction; VT = ventricular tachycardia; VF = ventricular fibrillation; ETT = exercise tolerance test; cath = cardiac catheterization and coronary angiography; CABG = coronary artery bypass grafting; PTCA = percutaneous transluminal coronary angioplasty; med rx = medical therapy; EPS = electrophysiologic study.

lar tachycardia discovered by any means more than 48 hours after AMI should be considered for programmed electrical stimulation in an attempt to direct therapy. Alternatively, such patients may be placed on amiodarone, or considered for treatment with a newer antiarrhythmic drug with beta-blocking properties such as sotalol.

3. If survivors of AMI with an LVEF of less than 0.40 are to undergo ambulatory ECG monitoring, it should be with the intention of referring them for programmed electrical stimulation if runs of ventricular tachycardia are recorded. The documentation of frequent or complex ventricular ectopy during ambulatory ECG monitoring of these patients is likely, but it does not necessarily constitute an indication for antiarrhythmic therapy. If antiarrhythmic therapy is undertaken for the treatment of frequent ventricular ectopy, it should be with the understanding that there is no evidence that such treatment impacts favorably on survival; indeed, follow-up monitoring should be performed to determine that the drug chosen does not exert a proarrhythmic effect on the patient's ventricular ectopy.

References

1. Veterans Administration Coronary Artery Bypass Surgery Cooperative Study Group. Eleven-year survival in the Veterans Administration randomized trial of coronary bypass surgery for stable angina. *N. Engl. J. Med.* 311:1333, 1984.
2. Passamani, E., Davis, K. B., Gillespie, M. J., et al. A randomized trial of coronary artery bypass surgery. *N. Engl. J. Med.* 312:1665, 1985.
3. Vigilante, G. J., Weintraub, W. S., Klein, L. W., et al. Improved survival with coronary bypass surgery in patients with three vessel coronary disease and

abnormal left ventricular function. *Am. J. Med.* 82: 697, 1987.

4. O'Neill, W., Timmis, G. C., Bourdillon, P. D., et al. A prospective randomized clinical trial of intracoronary streptokinase versus coronary angioplasty for acute myocardial infarction. *N. Engl. J. Med.* 314: 812, 1986.
5. Sasaguri, T., Itoh, T., Hirata, M., et al. Regulation of coronary artery tone in relation to the activation of signal transductors that regulate calcium homeostasis. *J. Am. Coll. Cardiol.* 9:1167, 1987.
6. Gibson, R. S., Boden, W. E., Theroux, P., et al. Diltiazem and reinfarction in patients with non-Q-wave myocardial infarction. *N. Engl. J. Med.* 315: 423, 1986.
7. Yusuf, S., Sleight, P., Held, P., et al. Routine medical management of acute myocardial infarction. Lessons from overview of recent randomized controlled trials. *Circulation* 82(Suppl II):II-117, 1990.
8. The Multicenter Diltiazem Postinfarction Trial Research Group. The effect of diltiazem on mortality and reinfarction after myocardial infarction. *N. Engl. J. Med.* 319:385, 1988.
9. Ryan, W. F., Henning, H., and Karliner, J. S. Effects of morphine on left ventricular dimensions and function in patients with previous myocardial infarction. *Clin. Cardiol.* 2:417, 1979.
10. MIAMI Trial Research Group. Metoprolol in acute myocardial infarction (MIAMI): A randomised placebo-controlled international trial. *Eur. Heart J.* 6: 199, 1985.
11. ISIS-1 (First International Study of Infarct Survival) Collaborative Group. Randomized trial of intravenous atenolol among 16,207 cases of suspected acute myocardial infarction: ISIS-1. *Lancet* 2:60, 1986.
12. Hjalmarson, A. International beta-blocker review in acute and postmyocardial infarction. *Am. J. Cardiol.* 61:26B, 1988.
13. Yusuf, S., Peto, R., Lewis, J., et al. Beta blockade during and after myocardial infarction: An overview of the randomized trials. *Prog. Cardiovasc. Dis.* 27: 335, 1985.
14. DeWood, M. A., Spores, J., Notske, R., et al. Prevalence of total coronary occlusion during the early hours of transmural myocardial infarction. *N. Engl. J. Med.* 303:897, 1980.
15. Sherry, S. Recombinant tissue plasminogen activator (rt-PA): Is it the thrombolytic agent of choice for an evolving acute myocardial infarction? *Am. J. Cardiol.* 59:984, 1987.
16. Gruppo Italiano per lo Studio della Streptochinasi nell'Infarto Miocardico (GISSI). Long-term effects of intravenous thrombolysis in acute myocardial infarction: Final report of the GISSI study. *Lancet* 2:871, 1987.
17. ISIS-2 (Second International Study of Infarct Survival) Collaborative Group. Intravenous streptokinase given within 0–4 hours of onset of myocardial infarction reduced mortality in ISIS-2. *Lancet* 1:502, 1987.
18. The GUSTO Investigators. An international randomized trial comparing four thrombolytic strategies for acute myocardial infarction. *N. Engl. J. Med.* 329: 673, 1993.
19. ISIS-3: Third International Study of Infarct Survival Collaborative Group. ISIS-3: A randomised comparison of streptokinase vs tissue plasminogen activator vs anistreplase and of aspirin plus heparin vs aspirin alone among 41,299 cases of suspected acute myocardial infarction. *Lancet* 339:753, 1992.
20. Gorgels, A. P. M., Vos, M. A., Letsch, I. S., et al. Usefulness of the accelerated idioventricular rhythm as a marker for myocardial necrosis and reperfusion during thrombolytic therapy in acute myocardial infarction. *Am. J. Cardiol.* 61:231, 1988.
21. Yusuf, S., Teo, K., and Woods, K. Intravenous magnesium in acute myocardial infarction. An effective, safe, simple, and inexpensive intervention. *Circulation* 87:2043, 1993.
22. Multicenter Postinfarction Research Group. Risk stratification and survival after myocardial infarction. *N. Engl. J. Med.* 309:331, 1983.
23. DeBusk, R. F., Blomqvist, G., Kouchoukos, N. T., et al. Identification and treatment of low-risk patients after acute myocardial infarction and coronary-artery bypass graft surgery. *N. Engl. J. Med.* 314:161, 1986.
24. Stone, P. H., Raabe, D. S., Jaffe, A. S., et al. Prognostic significance of location and type of myocardial infarction: Independent adverse outcome associated with anterior location. *J. Am. Coll. Cardiol.* 11:453, 1988.
25. Krone, R. J., Friedman, E., Thanavaro, S., et al. Long-term prognosis after first Q-wave (transmural) or non-Q-wave (nontransmural) myocardial infarction: Analysis of 593 patients. *Am. J. Cardiol.* 52: 234, 1983.
26. Gibson, R. S., Beller, G. A., Gheorghiade, M., et al. The prevalence and clinical significance of residual myocardial ischemia 2 weeks after uncomplicated non-Q-wave infarction: A prospective natural history study. *Circulation* 73:1186, 1986.
27. Phibbs, B. "Transmural" versus "subendocardial" myocardial infarction: An electrocardiographic myth. *J. Am. Coll. Cardiol.* 1:561, 1983.
28. Elwood, P. C., Cochrane, A. L., Burr, M. L., et al. A randomized controlled trial of acetyl salicyclic acid in the secondary prevention of mortality from myocardial infarction. *B.M.J.* 1:436, 1974.
29. Aspirin Myocardial Infarction Study Research Group. A randomized, controlled trial of aspirin in persons recovered from myocardial infarction. *J.A.M.A.* 243: 661, 1980.
30. Canner, P. L. Aspirin in coronary heart disease. *Isr. J. Med. Sci.* 19:413, 1983.
31. Marcus, A. J. Aspirin as an antithrombotic medication. *N. Engl. J. Med.* 309:1515, 1983.
32. Topol, E. J., Califf, R. M., George, B. S., et al. A randomized trial of immediate versus delayed elective angioplasty after intravenous tissue plasminogen activator in acute myocardial infarction. *N. Engl. J. Med.* 317:581, 1987.
33. Ellis, S. G., Mooney, M. R., George, B. S., et al.

Randomized trial of late elective angioplasty versus conservative management for patients with residual stenoses after thrombolytic treatment of myocardial infarction. *Circulation* 86:1400, 1992.
34. Volpi, A., Maggioni, A., Franzosi, M. G., et al. In-hospital prognosis of patients with acute myocardial infarction complicated by primary ventricular fibrillation. *N. Engl. J. Med.* 317:257, 1987.
35. Nicod, P., Gilpin, E., Dittrich, H., et al. Late clinical outcome in patients with early ventricular fibrillation after myocardial infarction. *J. Am. Coll. Cardiol.* 11:464, 1988.
36. Mukharji, J., Rude, R. E., Poole, K., et al. Risk factors for sudden death after acute myocardial infarction: Two-year follow-up. *Am. J. Cardiol.* 54:31, 1984.
37. DeBusk, R. F., and Dennis, C. A. "Submaximal" predischarge exercise testing after acute myocardial infarction: Who needs it? *Am. J. Cardiol.* 55:499, 1985.
38. Smeets, J. P., Rigo, P., Legrand, V., et al. Prognostic value of thallium-201 stress myocardial scintigraphy with exercise ECG after myocardial infarction. *Cardiology* 68:67, 1981.
39. Gibson, R. S., Watson, D. D., Craddock, G. B., et al. Prediction of cardiac events after uncomplicated myocardial infarction: A prospective study comparing predischarge exercise thallium-201 scintigraphy and coronary angiography. *Circulation* 68:321, 1983.
40. De Feyter, P. J., van Eenige, M. J., Dighton, D. H., et al. Prognostic value of exercise testing, coronary angiography and left ventriculography 6–8 weeks after myocardial infarction. *Circulation* 66:527, 1983.
41. Gottlieb, S. H., Ouyang, P., and Gottlieb, S. O. Death after acute myocardial infarction: Interrelation between left ventricular dysfunction, arrhythmias and ischemia. *Am. J. Cardiol.* 61:7B, 1988.
42. Cardiac Arrhythmia Suppression Trial (CAST) Investigators. Preliminary report: Effect of encainide and flecainide on mortality in a randomized trial of arrhythmia suppression after myocardial infarction. *N. Engl. J. Med.* 321:406, 1989.
43. Killip, T., and Kimball, J. T. Treatment of myocardial infarction in a coronary care unit: A two-year experience with 250 patients. *Am. J. Cardiol.* 20:457, 1967.
44. Warnowicz, M. A., Parker, H., and Cheitlin, M. D. Prognosis of patients with acute pulmonary edema and normal ejection fraction after acute myocardial infarction. *Circulation* 67:330, 1983.
45. Braunwald, E., and Kloner, R. A. The stunned myocardium: Prolonged, postischemic ventricular dysfunction. *Circulation* 66:1146, 1982.
46. Stack, R. S., Phillips, H. R., Grierson, D. S., et al. Functional improvement of jeopardized myocardium following intracoronary streptokinase infusion in acute myocardial infarction. *J. Clin. Invest.* 72:84, 1983.
47. Mathey, D. G., Schofer, J., Sheehan, F. H., et al. Improved survival up to four years after early coronary thrombolysis. *Am. J. Cardiol.* 61:524, 1988.
48. Cohn, J. N., Archibald, D. G., Ziesche, S., et al. Effect of vasodilator therapy on mortality in chronic congestive heart failure: Results of a Veterans Administration cooperative study. *N. Engl. J. Med.* 314:1547, 1986.
49. CONSENSUS Trial Study Group. Effects of enalapril on mortality in severe congestive heart failure: Results of the cooperative north Scandinavian enalapril survival study. *N. Engl. J. Med.* 316:1429, 1987.
50. Pfeffer, M. A., Braunwald, E., Moye, L. E., et al. Effect of captopril on mortality and morbidity in patients with left ventricular dysfunction after myocardial infarction. *N. Engl. J. Med.* 3217:669, 1992.
51. Yusuf, S., Pepine, C. J., Garces, C., et al. Effect of enalapril on myocardial infarction and unstable angina in patients with low ejection fractions. *Lancet* 340:1173, 1992.
52. Swedberg, K., Held, P., Kjekhus, J., et al. Effect of the early administration of enalapril on mortality in patients with acute myocardial infarction. *N. Engl. J. Med.* 340:1173, 1992.
53. Schuster, E. H., and Bulkley, B. H. Early post-infarction angina: Ischemia at a distance and ischemia in the infarct zone. *N. Engl. J. Med.* 305:1101, 1981.
54. Wilson, W. W., Gibson, R. S., Nygaard, T. W., et al. Acute myocardial infarction associated with single vessel coronary artery disease: An analysis of clinical outcome and the prognostic importance of vessel patency and residual ischemic myocardium. *J. Am. Coll. Cardiol.* 11:223, 1988.
55. Taylor, G. J., Humphries, J. O., Mellits, E. D., et al. Predictors of clinical course, coronary anatomy and ventricular function after recovery from acute myocardial infarction. *Circulation* 62:960, 1980.
56. Schulze, R. A., Strauss, H. W., and Pitt, B. Sudden death in the year following myocardial infarction: Relation to ventricular premature contractions in the late hospital phase and left ventricular ejection fraction. *Am. J. Med.* 62:192, 1977.
57. Greene, H. L., Reid, P. R., and Schaeffer, A. H. The repetitive ventricular response in man: A predictor of sudden death. *N. Engl. J. Med.* 299:729, 1978.
58. Richards, D. A., Cody, D. V., Denniss, A. R., et al. Ventricular electrical instability: A predictor of death after myocardial infarction. *Am. J. Cardiol.* 51:75, 1983.
59. Marchlinski, F. E., Buxton, A. E., Waxman, H. L., et al. Identifying patients at risk of sudden death after myocardial infarction: Value of the response to programmed stimulation, degree of ventricular ectopic activity and severity of left ventricular dysfunction. *Am. J. Cardiol.* 52:1190, 1983.
60. Mason, J. W., and Winkle, R. A. Electrode-catheter arrhythmia induction in the selection and assessment of antiarrhythmic drug therapy for recurrent ventricular tachycardia. *Circulation* 58:971, 1978.
61. Wilber, D. J., Garan, H., Finkelstein, D., et al. Out-of-hospital cardiac arrest: Use of electrophysiologic testing in the prediction of long-term outcome. *N. Engl. J. Med.* 318:19, 1988.

IX. Administrative Decisions in the Coronary Care Unit

40. Administration of the Extended Coronary Care Unit

Galen S. Wagner, Bradi L. Bartrug, Wanda M. Bride, and Robert M. Califf

During the past 35 years, patients with symptoms suggestive of acute myocardial infarction (AMI) have been admitted into a specialized nursing area called a Coronary Care Unit (CCU). Recently, coronary care has been extended to include pre- and posthospital periods. It may begin with either general practioners [1] or paramedics [2] at the location where the patient's symptoms occur, and extend through cardiac rehabilitation programs [3]. The prehospital initiation of specialized coronary care has been required for optimal benefit from intravenous (IV) thrombolytic agents [4]; its posthospital extension has been indicated by the feasibility of early hospital discharge [5] and the efficacy of rehabilitative interventions in returning the individual to a functioning life style [6]. Coordination of pre-, intra-, and posthospital coronary care requires extensive personal and electronic communication, and this, in turn, requires an extended CCU Administrative Team.

Since the documentation of the effectiveness of direct coronary angioplasty [7], which is available only in some communities, patients are commonly emergently transported by helicopter soon after symptom onset [8]. This requires efficient communication between two geographically separated coronary care systems, and further extension of the CCU Administrative Team.

Attainment of optimal coronary care may be confounded by absence from hospital emergency facilities of the patient's primary physician and any cardiovascular specialist. Instead, there may be an emergency physician specialized in providing a wide range of patient care, but not familiar with the history of the individual patient or the intricacies of the rapidly changing approaches to delivery of thrombolytic therapy [9]. The CCU Administrative Team must meet the challenge of developing an electronic communication system that provides the insight of the patient's primary physician and the expertise of the cardiologist when they are most needed to assist the emergency physician in providing appropriate coronary care for the patient.

The CCU Administrative Team

To accomplish its extended responsibilities, the CCU Administrative Team should include, in addition to the Medical Director and Nurse Manager of the CCU itself, the leaders of all of the areas into which the CCU extends:

- Emergency Department
- Emergency Medical Services
- Helicopter Transport
- Catheterization Laboratory
- Rehabilitation Program
- Electronic Communications
- Computerized Databank
- Medical Center Administration

This team should develop guidelines for the function of multiple extensions of the CCU, guidelines that the team continues to evolve during regular meetings.

The Prehospital CCU Extension

The clinical test that is most useful in coronary care, the electrocardiogram (ECG), is commonly recorded by a computerized system and interpreted by automated diagnostic algorithms. A method is currently being developed to include automated prognostic algorithms, at the time of patient presentation, to indicate the potential cost/benefit of thrombolytic therapy [10]. The technology has been developed for transmission of an ECG from the paramedics at the scene to the hospital emergency department. Its use has decreased the time to administration of intravenous thrombolytic therapy from 57 minutes in the Myocardial Infarction Triage and Intervention—Phase I (MITI-I) feasibility study [11] to 20 minutes during the MITI randomized trial [2].

The technology has also been developed for electronic archiving of previous ECG recordings, and these can provide valuable comparison with the patient's recording at the time of presentation with acute symptoms. The patient's primary physician and cardiologist must be able to immediately access, via a small portable computer, both the patient's baseline ECG from the archives and the AMI ECG from the paramedics. Ideally, for easy access, this computer would be incorporated into the physician's electronic paging device.

The emergency physician functions as coordinator of the input from paramedics at the scene and from the patient's primary physician and cardiologist. This group can develop the plan for initiation of the posthospital phase of acute coronary care during the time the patient is in transit to the hospital. A brief checklist of the required patient data was developed in the MITI study and this can be carried on a laminated card by the paramedics. This list includes the potential contraindications for IV thrombolytic therapy [11].

Routine patient access to the prehospital extension of the CCU requires efficient functioning of the Administrative Team. This group, at a referral medical center, should help to develop similar teams in surrounding communities. If there is a Helicopter Transport System, an Interventional Catheterization Laboratory, or both, the director(s) of these facilities should be included in the CCU Administrative Team. Since electronic communications equipment has been developed only recently, representatives from the manufacturers should be included in the discussions. Site visits to communities with model extended coronary care systems in operation are necessary to minimize errors in design and integration of the multiple components.

The In-Hospital CCU Extension

Because of the specialized nature of coronary care with use of thrombolytic agents, the patient's primary physician may be excluded. This is even more likely when the patient has been transported outside his or her local community. The primary physician should be kept informed of the patient's day to day condition and have input into clinical decisions. With the exception of required emergency interventions, the cost/benefit of coronary care can be positively influenced by maintenance of the primary doctor-patient relation. Consideration of both past and future medical, personal, and social situations may alter decisions about the management of such matters as comorbid conditions, anticoagulation, aggressiveness of prophylactic interventions, and initiation or discontinuation of life-support systems.

The CCU Administrative Team should provide access for the patient's primary physician via an electronic communication system. Presently, the fax and telephone are the only components commonly available. The primary physician should be integrated into the daily CCU rounds for the patient. This would require two-way video and audio communication from the patient's bedside via personal computer, modem, and telephone. The primary physician could then directly review the patient's tests, such as ECGs, echocardiograms, serum enzyme levels, and angiograms. When possible, final non-emergency decisions should be made by consultation between the patient's primary physician and the coronary care specialist.

Several pilot programs instituted in some areas of the United States are currently exploring advanced telemedicine systems. At this time, these systems create a continuous link with the patient's primary care physician, the consulting cardiologist, the care nurse and the patient via a communication network. Although the network is still in the embryonic stage of development, it allows transmission of medical records, images (x-ray), and diagnostic tests (cath, ECHO) to and from a PC terminal via modem. Voice transmission capability, currently in the refinement stage, will allow the primary care physician to play a more active role in the decision making process, especially during rounds at the referral CCU.

The Posthospital CCU Extension

The bedside electronic communication system can be used to plan the most effective transfer of the patient from the CCU to a local medical community or outpatient facility. The time required for dedicated coronary care inside or outside the local community should be kept to a minimum. During the 1970s, prior to the advent of thrombolytic therapy, serious complications rarely made their first appearance after the fourth day [5]. Currently, with infarct size limited by early and effective thrombolytic therapy [1, 2], there should be less risk of serious complications, with the possible exception of infarct extension. It has been considered likely that the incidence of extension might be increased by initial limitation of the infarct size, but to date there has been no documentation that this occurs. Before the patient's discharge from the CCU, the primary and consultant physicians can use the electronic communication system to determine the anticoagulation regimen for maintaining patency of the patient's infarct-related artery.

In preparation for the patient's transition to the posthospital phase of coronary care, it is important to determine the patient's prognosis and functioning capacity [12]. Persistent ischemic symptoms at rest, or occurrence of either symptoms or signs of ischemia during stress testing, suggest the need for examination of the coronary artery anatomy to determine the feasibility of revascularization. Stress testing has also been demonstrated to be useful in developing realistic expectations about the capacity of patients to return to their usual activities following an AMI [13]. Consultation among the primary physician, coronary care specialists, and cardiac rehabilitation specialists is necessary to determine the optimal time and method for the patient's stress testing.

If the data from each patient's history and extended CCU experience are entered into a computerized databank for comparison with all previous patients, the patient's immediate and long-term prognosis can be assessed. The Duke Cardiovascular Databank was developed as an extension of the Duke CCU as early as 1969 [14, 15]. The longitudinal study in Framingham, Massachusetts, has demonstrated the ability of such a system to characterize all patients receiving coronary care within a particular community [16]. At the time of the patient's transfer from the CCU to the posthospital extension and at discharge from the cardiac rehabilitation program, reports generated from the cardiovascular data bank can serve as a communication link to all members of the extended CCU Administrative Team and to the patient's primary physician.

References

1. Rawles, J. Halving of mortality at 1 year by domiciliary thrombolysis in the Grampian Region Early Anistreplase Trial (GREAT). *J. Am. Coll. Cardiol.* 23: 1, 1994.
2. Weaver, W. D., Cequeira, M., Hallstrom, A. P., et al. Prehospital-initiated vs hospital-initiated thrombolytic therapy. The Myocardial Infarction Triage and Intervention Trial. *J.A.M.A.* 270:1211, 1993.
3. Wenger, N. K., Hellerstein, H. K., Blackburn, H., et al. Physician practice in the management of patients with uncomplicated myocardial infarction: Changes in the past decade. *Circulation* 65:421, 1982.
4. Gruppo Italiano per lo Studio della Streptochinase nell'Infarcto Miocardio (GISSI). Effectiveness of intravenous thrombolytic treatment in acute myocardial infarction. *Lancet* 1:397, 1986.
5. McNeer, J. F., Wallace, A. G., Wagner, G. S., et al. The course of acute myocardial infarction. Feasibility of early discharge of the uncomplicated patient. *Circulation* 51:410, 1975.
6. Miller, N. H., Haskell, W. L., Berra, K., et al. Home versus group exercise training for increasing functional capacity after myocardial infarction. *Circulation* 70:645, 1984.
7. Grines, C. L., Browne, K. F., Marco, J., et al. A Comparison of Immediate Angioplasty with Thrombolytic Therapy for Acute Myocardial Infarction. *N. Engl. J. Med.* 328:673, 1993.
8. LaPlante, G., and Gaffney, T. M. Helicopter transport of the patient receiving thrombolytic therapy. *J. Emerg. Nurs.* 15:196, 1989.
9. Eisenberg, M. S., and Smith, M. The farmer and the cowman should be friends: Emergency physicians and cardiologists must work together to ensure rapid initiation of thrombolytic therapy. *Ann. Emerg. Med.* 17:6, 1988.
10. Selker, H. P., Griffith, J. L., Beshansky, J. R., et al. A thrombolytic predictive instrument for acute myocardial infarction. *Circulation* 86:1, 1992.
11. Weaver, W. D., Eisenberg, M. S., Martin, J. S., et al. Myocardial Infarction Triage and Intervention Project—Phase I: Patient characteristics and feasibil-

ity of prehospital initiation of thrombolytic therapy. *J. Am. Coll. Cardiol.* 15:925, 1990.
12. DeBusk, R. F., Blomqvist, C. G., Kouchoukos, N. T., et al. Identification and treatment of low-risk patients after acute myocardial infarction and coronary-artery bypass graft surgery. *N. Engl. J. Med.* 314:161, 1986.
13. Ewart, C. K., Taylor, C. B., Reese, L. B., et al. The effects of early post-myocardial infarction exercise testing on self-perception and subsequent physical activity. *Am. J. Cardiol.* 51:1076, 1983.
14. Rosati, R. A., Simon, S. B., Ripperton, L. A., et al. Medical interactive data system: Prognostic stratification of patients with acute myocardial infarction. Reprint from Proceedings of the San Diego Biomedical Symposium. 10:179, 1971.
15. Rosati, R. A., McNeer, J. F., Starmer, C. F., et al. A new information system for medical practice. *Arch. Intern. Med.* 135:1017, 1975.
16. Jones, M. G., Anderson, K. M., Wilson, P. W. F., et al. Prognostic use of a QRS scoring system after hospital discharge for initial acute myocardial infarction in the Framingham cohort. *Am. J. Cardiol.* 66:546, 1990.

41. Ethical and Legal Dilemmas in the Coronary Care Unit

John J. Paris and Frank E. Reardon

The high-technology medicine available in today's coronary care unit (CCU) not only provides near miraculous benefits for some patients, it also creates new and troublesome ethical and legal dilemmas for patients and practitioners. Standards for access to and discharge from the CCU, the question of withdrawal of nutrition and fluids, Do Not Resuscitate (DNR) orders, determination of death, advanced directives, decision-making capacity, and substantive and procedural guidelines for termination of treatment in incomptetent patients are among the problems. These issues are discussed in this chapter.

In one of the first and most significant studies of the public policy implications of intensive care delivery, Knaus and colleagues [1] at George Washington University Medical Center identified two principal roles for intensive care: "life support of organ system failure in critically ill patients or close monitoring of stable noncritically ill patients in case the need for life support suddenly occurs." From their study they determined there is little evidence that the widespread use of such services has resulted in improved survival or quality of life for a substantial portion of the patients presently admitted to such intensive care units (ICU). In fact, they concluded that approximately 25 percent of the total ICU therapy is used for patients who either have little need for unique ICU services or are too acutely and chronically ill to benefit from them.

Their study confirmed the findings of others who have examined the indications and outcomes of intensive care medicine [2–5], pointing to the need for more vigorous standards for ICU admission and discharge. Such an attempt was made at Memorial Sloan-Kettering Cancer Center, where early it was recognized that many of the patients admitted to the ICU were surviving acute episodes only to die shortly thereafter from underlying cancer. Rather than subject these patients (and their families) to the trauma of spending their final days in an ICU, the medical staff adopted a policy of formally classifying all hospital patients according to the underlying prognosis of their disease. As Turnbull and associates reported [6], those patients whose short-term prognosis was poor and for whom no definitive therapy existed were not considered candidates for transfer to the ICU regardless of the acute problems that might develop.

To limit the inappropriate institution of other invasive lifesaving therapy, similar classifications were developed for patients suffering from advanced cystic fibrosis [7], severe burns [8], and nontraumatic coma [9]. In addition, work began on establishing quantitative predictive models such as the Acute Physiology and Chronic Health Evaluation (APACHE) scale developed by Knaus and colleagues as an objective measure of the severity of illness of ICU patients [10]. By design, however, the APACHE I and II scales [11] are more appropriate for predicting outcomes for populations of ICU patients, rather than for individuals. That task, at least in the initial stages, remains notoriously uncertain [12] and varied [13].

Knaus' [14] recent data indicated that of 571 acutely ill ventilated patients admitted to the ICUs of 12 hospitals, 48 percent could be identified on admission to be at a 75 percent or greater risk of hospital death; by day 4 of ICU treatment, estimates for hospital mortality increased to 97 percent. Of those predicted to die, a single 56-year-old patient who had severe long-standing multiple organ system failure with an episode of septic shock survived. Such survivals, even though extremely rare, led to a reluctance by clinicians to withdraw or withhold intensive care from those apparently too ill to benefit [15].

To overcome the statistical character of the predictive index, Chung [16] proposed the development of a dynamic rather than a static model, one that would identify individual patients who would not survive the course of their illness. Although it remains impossible to predict which acutely ill ICU patients will survive, Chung established that focusing on changes in homeostasis allows the observer to identify accurately that subset of ICU patients who are not likely to survive. With his predictive index, 40 percent of nonsurvivors can be identified.

The remarkable growth of the hospice movement from only one program in 1974 to over 1600 programs today [17] is another phenomenon in the attempt to limit inappropriate care of the critically ill. Many of these programs, however, are still in the fledgling stage and are available to only a small fraction of the nation's terminally ill patients. Most critically and terminally ill patients continue to be cared for in institutions in which aggressive intervention and treatment of acute episodes is the norm.

There are many reasons for the general practice of maximal response to crises in the seriously ill patient. Several of them have been identified by Angell [18]: (1) the current fee-for-service reimbursement schedule, which rewards physicians preferentially for performing tests and procedures; (2) the ever-present spectre of malpractice; and (3) the American propensity to believe that every problem has a solution, often a technical one. This last factor leads to the familiar request of patients and families to "do everything possible," which is all too often translated into what Thurow [19] perceptively characterized as using every experimental technique on the outside chance that one of the procedures just might work.

This process, which Fuchs labeled "the technological imperative" [20], when combined with other forces now operative in our society, has produced a health care system in crisis. The cost of care has risen beyond our ability, or at least our willingness, to pay for it. Among the measures to control and limit the rising costs and thereby curb the demands for rationing of health care, Angell [18] suggested that we re-examine the proposition that in health care, as in other commodities, more is better. She insisted that, far from being beneficial, much of the medical care now provided in this country is unnecessary, that much medical care is of no demonstrated value to those who receive it, and that some is positively harmful. She cited among unnecessary items the aggressive treatment of terminally ill patients for whom treatment other than palliative care is no longer appropriate.

In an essay, Moore [21] condemned "desperate measures for desperately ill patients desperately hopeless from the outset." Moore's insight is more readily adopted by European than American physicians. European physicians understand that the ICU is designed for patients with acute reversible diseases and those at risk for developing complications, for example, after extensive surgery. As a result, the physicians have "a policy of admitting only those patients who have a reasonable chance of recovery to a meaningful life and deny ICU admissions to terminally ill patients" [22]. ICU use is confined to those who are expected to recover from acute episodes; it is not used as a high-tech hospice.

As Ramsey [23] noted, it is imperative to distinguish between treatments that will benefit the patient and those that are useless and false remedies. For the patient who has truly entered the dying process, comfort and company, not further and futile attempts at treatment, are appropriate care. Ramsey's comment forces us into the difficult but nonetheless important distinction of medical ethics, a distinction whose origin can be traced back to the earliest formulations of the Hippocratic Corpus. There we find the antidote to the notion that the physician's duty is to do everything possible to prolong life. As Admundsen's [24] historical analysis established,

> The treatise entitled *The Art* in the Hippocratic Corpus defines medicine as having three roles: doing away with the sufferings of the sick, lessening the violence of their diseases, and refusing to treat those who are overmastered by their diseases, realizing that in such cases medicine is powerless.

The best contemporary restatement of the standards for appropriate care of the sick is found in the report of the President's Commission for the Study of Ethical Problems in Medicine and Biomedical and Behavioral Research [25]. That report, which was formulated by ethicists, physicians, lawyers, theologians, and academics, had enormous impact on hospital policies, regulatory directives, court opinions, and the direction of medicine. Many of the topics in the report responded to the concerns, fears, and worries of physicians, nurses, and patients, particularly those in the highly sophisticated setting of an ICU. The Commission approached its task primarily from the perspective of ethics, the traditions of medicine, and issue of human choice. Only secondarily did the Commission turn to the narrower and, necessarily, more limited perspective of law for its contributions to the development of standards and formation of public policy. The result is a balanced, sensitive, humane, and strikingly sensible approach to complex, difficult ethical dilemmas, an approach that is helpful to practitioners and patients alike.

Several of the issues reviewed by the Commission are of particular interest to those involved with intensive care medicine: Do Not Resuscitate (DNR) orders, brain death, living wills, and decision-making for the incompetent patient.

Guidelines for Resuscitation Decisions

Current American Medical Association Guidelines

After nearly a decade of turmoil concerning DNR orders, the Ethical and Judicial Council of the American Medical Association issued a policy statement designed to provide guidance for physicians and hospitals on that topic [26]. Lo indicates [27] that the Council's guidance is ambiguous, somewhat convoluted, and certain to evoke hostility from some physicians. The ambiguity and confusion is engendered in part by the Council's efforts to find a compromise between those who support complete patient autonomy [28] and those who insist that physician determination of potential effectiveness [29] should govern whether to attempt cardiopulmonary resuscitation (CPR).

In its search for a middle course, the Council rejected Blackhall's proposal that futility be defined as survival to discharge [30]. Instead, the Council defined futility as that which cannot restore heartbeat or, if it can, fails to achieve the expressed goals of the informed patient or the patient's family. The Council's approach thus sided with those who favor patient or family determination on whether to attempt CPR.

The outer reaches of that approach are found in a New York statute enacted on the recommendation of the New York State Task Force on Life and the Law [31] that requires physicians to obtain the informed consent of a competent patient or the family of a decisionally incapable patient before they may legally write a DNR order. The only exception for direct involvement of a competent patient is the assessment by the attending physician plus a second independent physician that the patient would suffer "immediate and severe" harm from the discussion, i.e., the very posing of the question would prove so threatening to the patient as to trigger an immediate cardiac arrest or would prove so unsettling to a patient with severe paranoia, depression, or suicidal tendencies that it might drive the patient to self-inflicted harm.

When asked at a medical meeting if this policy meant that a physician would be required to undertake what was believed to be a futile attempt at cardio-resuscitation if requested to do so by a competent patient (or presumably by the family of a decisionally incapable terminally ill patient), the New York Health Commissioner, Dr. David Axelrod, replied: "There is a right to CPR so I think the patient has to get it." "But," he continued, "that's pretty rare. How often does that happen?" The response from the assembled physicians: "Often." "Everyday." "All the time." [32].

Historical Development of DNR Orders

In formulating CPR or DNR policies, ethics committees and the hospitals they serve are aware of these conflicting views and the sometimes unreasonable expectations and demands of dying patients and their families. Nurses, physicians, and families regularly find themselves at odds over the topic; yet until recently, the subject was left unaddressed and unresolved. A help in designing policies as well as understanding the context for the AMA guidelines can be found in the historical background of the present debate.

With the development of resuscitation techniques in the 1960s came the need for reflection and guidance on their effectiveness and appropriate usage. These were first provided in the 1974 American Medical Association's *Report on Standards for Cardiopulmonary Resuscitation* [33] that set standards and initiated a massive and highly effective CPR training program. The report declared that

> The purpose of cardiopulmonary resuscitation is the prevention of sudden, unexpected death. Cardiopulmonary resuscitation is not indicated in certain situations, such as in cases of terminal irreversible illness where death

is not unexpected or where prolonged cardiac arrest dictates the futility of resuscitation efforts. Resuscitation in these circumstances may represent a positive violation of an individual's right to die with dignity.

That thoughtful and carefully formulated statement was all but forgotten as paramedics, nurses, and physicians trained in the new lifesaving techniques respond to "code blues" with "crash carts" and portable defibrillators like firemen answering an alarm. In the words of Dr. Mitchell Rabkin, President of Boston's Beth Israel Hospital, "When the bell rings, you run!"

Such a response pattern soon led to attempted resuscitations for virtually all in-hospital deaths, regardless of a patient's medical history and prognosis. As Lampton and Winship reported, "Many medical staffs adopted universal, hospital-wide policies stating that CPR would be instituted on all patients experiencing sudden and unexpected cardiopulmonary arrest" [34]. They observed that "ultimately, it appears that many persons view CPR as a mandatory activity for all patients dying in a hospital." In an insightful and humane essay, Steven Spenser [35] noted that tendency has evolved into a fixed policy of attempting to overcome the death of all patients unless the physician has written a specific "no-code" order. Consequently, physicians find themselves in the position of having to write a negative, inhibiting order to protect terminally ill patients from unwanted and unwarranted intrusions into their dying.

A further complication in this litigation-conscious era is that physicians are now looking to the courts and the legal profession for guidance and protection on the proper treatment of the dying patient. They are also asking families to share the burden of responsibility for such decisions to a degree that Spenser observed would have been unthinkable a few years ago.

How this predicament evolved, and possible resolutions to it, were the subject of a 2-year study by the 1983 President's Commission. Dr. Rabkin provided the most complete explanation to the Commission. Rabkin testified that before this institution's well known 1976 "Orders Not to Resuscitate" directive [36] was in effect, "a significant percentage of patients who died received cardiopulmonary resuscitation upon their *quietus* even though it was acknowledged that the resuscitation efforts for many would be useless. In his words, "The emergency code was called, and all of the troops—cardiologists, anesthetists, nurses, respiratory therapists, and others—responded in full."

The folly of that policy was epitomized for Rabkin when he encountered a nurse weeping in the corridor outside her patient's room. The patient, an octogenarian with widespread terminal cancer, had just stopped breathing, and a staff member had called the code. A horde of professionals was applying intravenous medication and electrical current to stimulate the heart, and the anesthetist was ventilating the patient through an endotracheal tube just inserted—all to no avail, of course. "Why can't they just let him die in peace?" wept the nurse. The answer was straightforward and hinted at in the 1976 Beth Israel directive [36]:

Both as a standard of medical care and a statement of philosophy, it is the general policy of hospitals to act affirmatively to preserve the life of all patients, including persons who suffer from irreversibly terminal illness. It is essential that all hospital staff understand this policy and act accordingly.

That pro-life policy, good in itself, was so rigidly interpreted that a DNR order could be entered only after (1) it was determined that the patient was irreversibly and irreparably ill and death was imminent (within 2 weeks); (2) an ad hoc committee of senior physicians and nurses concurred in that evaluation; and (3) the informed choice of the competent patient (or the family of an incompetent patient) was given. If, in the judgment of the responsible physician, the patient would be unable to cope psychologically with the consent stipulation, no order could be written. Here a misplaced emphasis on patient autonomy and informed consent pressured the dying patient into the trauma of a code versus no-code choice as a final discretionary decision.

Several years' experience with those stringent stipulations and the increasing realization that these ill-considered resuscitation efforts in no way represented an affirmative act to preserve life led the medical staff to rewrite the DNR policy. In addition to the hospital's own experiences, a Massachusetts appellate court had ruled that DNR decision-making should rest with the physician acting in accordance with the standards of good medical practice and the wishes of the patient or the patient's family [37].

That ruling led numerous Massachusetts hospitals to establish formal DNR policies or to reconsider existing procedures. The 1981 Beth Israel Hospital guidelines omitted the attempt to define the candidates for DNR orders; they left that determination to the judgment of the attending physician. The 1981 policy specified the process by which such possibilities were to be considered and orders written. It also eliminated the need for a bureaucratic ad hoc committee and substituted the notification of the chief of service that such an order had been given.

Then, in a dramatic shift from the previous emphasis on individual autonomy and informed consent, the new guidelines stated that

> If, in the opinion of the attending physician, the competent patient might be harmed by a full discussion of whether resuscitation would be appropriate in the event of an arrest, the competent patient should be spared the discussion; therefore, if the physician and the Chief of Service deem a DNR order appropriate and the family members are in agreement that the discussion might harm the patient and the resuscitation is not appropriate, a DNR order may be entered by the physician [38].

This policy, which recognized the difference between an automaton and an autonomous patient, conformed to Spenser's [35] insight that explanations of DNR orders to dying patients "are thoughtless to the point of being cruel except for the extremely unlikely case where the patient himself inquires."

Rabkin [36] reported that the new Beth Israel policy allowed more open discussion among caregivers on the appropriateness of orders not to resuscitate a given patient. Concomitantly, slow codes and partial codes [39] (e.g., "Walk, don't run," "Page but don't stat page," and "Do not intubate if a code is called") declined. Not only did partial orders such as these place unwarranted burdens on the hospital staff, but they were, in Goldenring's [40] explicit phrasing, "an ethical fraud." Under Beth Israel's 1981 guidelines a code was called and answered as a well-considered affirmative act to benefit the patient. As such, when a code was issued, the staff responded knowing that they were not deliberately imposing a final, useless indignity on the end of life.

In its 1983 report, the President's Commission [25] devoted an entire chapter to resuscitation decisions for hospitalized patients. The Commission noted that, among the general hospital population, in which virtually all deaths were attended by resuscitation efforts, only 3 percent of the attempts were successful. Further, 1 in 20 patients who survived resuscitation sustained severe brain damage, and about 1 in 4 had some serious and permanent injury. Consequently, the Commission concluded that the reflex resuscitation efforts attempted in hospitals were frequently a misguided adventure that injured the patient and violated personal control over his or her life.

In response, the Commission called for a reevaluation of resuscitation practices by hospitals, health care providers, and especially treatment areas (e.g., ICUs and cardiac care units) where many patients are at risk for cardiac arrest and where CPR frequently is attempted automatically without appropriate deliberation.

In the advanced technical setting of today's acute-care hospital, the physician-patient-family relationship has been expanded to include health teams, rotating residents, triple shifts of nurses, and many other allied health professionals. Decisions that were once commonly agreed upon and easily effected directly by the physician now involve a large, diverse, and frequently unknown cadre of caregivers. Hence, the emerging need for explicit policies and guidelines for procedures, including those for resuscitate–DNR orders.

Prior deliberation in such cases (1) enables the patient's rights and decisions regarding self-determination to be respected, (2) guarantees that medical interventions serve the patient's best interest, (3) allows adequate evaluation of resource allocation and equity considerations, and (4) reduces nurse-physician-family misunderstandings on resuscitation practices. To protect both the patient and caregivers, hospital policies should require appropriate communication with the patient (or the family) about the resuscitation decision. If a DNR order is deemed appropriate, the order should be written in the patient's chart, along with its rationale and supporting documentation.

There is an ongoing dispute over the extent to which the competent patient should or must be involved in the decision to write a DNR order [41]. Clearly, if the patient expresses an explicit desire for or against resuscitation, and the patient's comprehension of the medical situation is not questionable, that decision should be honored. The difficulty arises from the fact that most seriously ill patients have not directly expressed any opinion on the subject. Further, many of these patients are unwilling to make a decision [42].

How, then, should the decision-making process be approached? In its original 1976 directive, and its recent 1991 update, Beth Israel Hospital followed the standard adopted by the Commission: the focus is on patient autonomy and informed consent, which means that patients must make their preferences known. The New York Task Force on Life and the Law went even further in its recommendation (since adopted as law in New York state), that competent patients must provide informed consent for a DNR order unless, in the physician's judgment, the very seeking of the consent would lead to immediate cardiac arrest or suicide. The impact of this mandate and its potentially negative effect on decision makers is not lessened by a footnoted qualification that "other care-giving professionals, religious advisors, or family members are in a good or better position to discuss the issue and convey the information (as is the attending physician)" [25].

Although Miles and coworkers [43] rightly placed the question of resuscitation within the context of the patient's total medical care and prognosis, their insistence on a frank but not overly technical discussion of resuscitation with the patient might well exacerbate the patient's plight. Among the nontechnical factors they believed the patient should understand was that "resuscitation may be followed by the need for life support including intratracheal tube, tracheotomy, respiratory ventilator assistance, arterial lines and monitoring, and continuous intravenous medication, all for an indeterminate period."

Such an approach to CPR decision-making might have been modified had it been compared with the 1974 and 1980 standards for CPR issued by the National Conference of the American Heart Association and with Siegler's [44] reminder that "the principal ethical grounds for making a decision not to resuscitate a patient should be the sound medical judgment that the patient's death from the primary disease is imminent and that further treatment for the primary disease is futile."

The Issue of Futility

The futility of attempting CPR in certain cases is documented in a study by Bedell and colleagues [45] that reveals a 98 to 100 percent mortality rate in patients with metastatic disease, acute strokes, sepsis, renal failure, and pneumonia. The same statistics apply to those for whom resuscitation took longer than 30 minutes. The physician, aware of the outcome data and the futility of intervention in such cases, has a professional obligation to provide care consonant with medical reality. In such cases, Blackhall believed, "the issue of patient autonomy is irrelevant" [30]. When that issue arose, he believed that the physician should write DNR orders on the chart with the following type of documentation: "This patient has a condition for which CPR has been shown not to be effective. In case of cardiopulmonary arrest, CPR should not be performed."

Tomlinson and Brody [46] distinguished three rationales for DNR orders: no medical benefit, poor quality of life after CPR, and poor quality of life before CPR. They adopted Blackhall's position that "physicians have no obligation to provide, and patients and families no right to demand, medical treatment that is of no demonstrable benefit." In such cases, they, too, believed that the patient, or family's desire for CPR was irrelevant, the decision was entirely within the physician's technical expertise, and that the physician's duty was to communicate with the family to explain that the patient's physical condition was such that no intervention could reverse the dying process and, hence, none would be attempted. They believed the most physicians should do when CPR is believed futile was to communicate that information to the patient or family so that the decision the physician has made will be understood. If the present or anticipated quality of life of the patient was such that the patient did not desire CPR, then the patient's values or desires were of import. In such cases, the patient's personal values, not the physician's preferences would prevail.

Murphy [47] and colleagues applied similar thinking to the issue of resuscitation in the elderly. Their data showed resuscitation of elderly patients was successful in only 3.8 percent of cases, never successful for cardiac arrests that were unwitnessed or occurred outside the hospital, and were also unsuccessful in witnessed hospital events in elderly patients with nonventricular arrhythmias.

Similar outcomes were found by Applebaum and colleagues [125] with regard to CPR initiated in elderly nursing home patients, by Gray [126] for out-of-hospital resuscitation efforts in which heartbeat had not been restored in the field, by Blackhall [127] for acutely sick patients in county hospitals, and by McIntyre [128] and (independently) by Landry [129] and colleagues for chronically ill patients in intensive care units.

The same was true for cardiac arrests in the first 72 hours of life in very low birthweight babies. In a study by Lantos and colleagues [48] at the University of Chicago, none of 38 babies who received CPR in the first 3 days of life survived. They concluded that, in such instances, CPR was an "innovative" or "nonvalidated" therapy. As such, it need not be provided or, if offered, should be presented to the family as an experimental procedure.

One additional insight into DNR practice is found in the study by Wachter and others [49] regarding the discrepancy in the use of DNR orders by disease. Despite similar prognoses by clinicians, physicians, according to Wachter, are far more willing to write DNR orders for patients with lung cancer and acquired immunodeficiency syndrome (AIDS) than for those with equally untreatable cirrhosis or severe congestive heart failure. In Wachter's study, 52 percent of terminally ill AIDS patients and 47 percent of those with lung cancer had DNR orders, but only 16 percent of patients with cirrhosis and 4 percent of those with congestive heart failure and coronary artery disease received a DNR order. The differences persisted even after the results had been adjusted for severity of illness and similarity of prognosis.

These studies suggest that the focus on the process of patient involvement rather than on the purpose and restricted effectiveness of CPR is a misplaced emphasis, one that will not affect the outcome of resuscitation efforts appreciably. The concern with patient autonomy and consent distracts and distorts the attention and actions of patients, families, and caregivers. For most dying patients, the issue is purely a technical assessment: given the patient's physiologic status, the data indicate CPR will be futile.

Policy Decisions Regarding DNR Orders

Present hospital policies of instituting "full codes" on all patients for whom a DNR order is not written may be inappropriate. In cases in which the responding team has no knowledge of the patient, it is imperative to institute a full code. But in many situations, the responding residents are fully aware of the terminal status of the patient and the reluctance of the family or the attending physician to authorize a DNR order. The response team must then participate in a charade or an exercise in futility. Neither is good medicine.

In response to such situations, the Tufts-New England Medical Center Hospitals adopted the following policy [50]. If there is no written DNR order (1) It is the responsibility of the nursing staff to call a "Code 99" and to initiate CPR. (2) It is the responsibility of all appropriate staff and hospital personnel to respond as quickly as possible to the Code 99. (3) It is the responsibility of the physician(s) responding to the Code 99 to determine what efforts are medically appropriate to treat the patient who has cardiac arrest; this responsibility includes continuing, or discontinuing, CPR when, in the judgment of the physician(s), aggressive treatment is medically inappropriate.

The American Heart Association's (AHA) 1992 *Guidelines on Cardiopulmonary Resuscitation and Emerging Cardiac Care* [51] also take this position. In addition to withholding CPR when there is a "No-CPR order" (AHA guidelines use that phrase for DNR), the AHA guidelines state that resuscitation efforts "should be withheld . . . when, in the judgment of the physician, such efforts cannot restore or sustain cardiopulmonary function; or when widely accepted scientific data indicate that there is no likelihood of survival."

Beth Israel Hospital's 1991 guidelines for Withholding, Withdrawing or Limiting Life-Sustaining Treatment [52], which adopted as hospital policy the fact that in some cases CPR will not work, were the first in the nation to incorporate the outcome data of multiple studies done on the efficacy of CPR. These guidelines recognized that in certain classes of identifiable patients, CPR is not effective and therefore would not be offered to patients or families. Beth Israel's guidelines make a critical distinction between a DNR order that is based on the patient's or surrogate's choice as to whether or not to attempt resuscitation in the event of a cardiac arrest and a situation in which a CPR Not Indicated order is appropriate. The latter occurs when "a *medical evaluation* of the patient has led to the conclusion that resuscitation efforts would be futile—such efforts would not be expected to restore cardiac or respiratory function or the patient is dying and resuscitative efforts will not benefit the patient." In such situations, Beth Israel's policy followed Blackhall's admonition that patient or (more likely) surrogate authorization is "irrelevant." Consent to withhold CPR is neither sought nor required in such instances since to provide it would be both medically futile and "an unwarranted abuse of the patient."

Beth Israel's policy adopted Tomlinson and Brody's advice that the physician should inform the family that nothing more could be done in the way of resuscitative efforts to apprise them of the situation, not to seek their permission or their approbation. Beth Israel's policy stated "There is no option which benefits the patient; the patient must therefore be allowed to expire in peace."

It is important to keep in mind Ingelfinger's admonition that "a physician who merely spreads an array of vendibles in front of the patient (or family) and then says, 'Go ahead and choose, it's your life,' is guilty of shirking his duty, if not malpractice" [53]. The physician certainly should explain the patient's condition to the family and the realistic options available. However, Ingelfinger reminds us that it is the physician's responsibility to recommend a specific course of action instead of merely asking the family to choose among courses. In addition, the physician is not asking the family to substitute its judgment for that of the patient, but is, rather, asking them to reflect the patient's own value choice as close as humanly possible.

A frustrating situation may arise if, in the physician's judgment, there is no further treatment that can benefit the irreversibly dying patient, yet the family, through ignorance, misunderstanding, fear, or guilt demands that "everything possible" be done. Conversely, the problem may be insistence by the family on a No-CPR order for a patient whom the physician believes has a good opportunity of recovery. In these situations, an intrainstitutional consultation or ethics committee should assess the case. Perhaps a simple airing of the issues or the benefit of consultation will dispel the disagreement. Sometimes a change of physician may be in order. Alternatively, the review committee may decide to petition a court to appoint a legal guardian to protect the patient's interests.

Another problem that frequently arises in major hospital settings is the elderly dying patient who has outlived all family and friends. Rather than unreflectively resuscitating all such patients or overusing the complex and somewhat costly role of legal guardian, decisions against resuscitation might continue to be made as they customarily have been—by the attending physician with the concurrence of a disinterested physician, staff consensus, or an institutionally designated patient advocate. These decisions are well within the scope of common medical practice and should not be elevated to the role of moral dilemma or judicial problem. Decisions that are more complex or uncertain might, of course, demand more formal institutional review or legal guardianship. Here, as in almost all of its recommendations, the President's Commission of 1983 was firm in its stance that rarely, if ever, is decision-making about life-sustaining care improved by resort to courts.

In fact, with regard to these questions the only court ever to address itself directly to the issue of DNR orders ruled that "the question (DNR) is not one for judicial decision, but one for the attending physician, in keeping with the highest traditions of his profession." It was, in the court's words, "a question peculiarly within the competence of the medical profession of what measures are appropriate to ease the imminent passing of an irreversibly, terminally ill patient in light of the patient's history and condition and the wishes of [the patient's] family" [37].

The possibility that the highly invasive, costly, and often violent resuscitation procedures available in acute-care settings might not be appropriate to a particular patient should be considered as a positive and prospective part of the delivery of high-quality medical care. Such decisions should not be made arbitrarily, hastily, or casually, nor should they depend on the personal fears or predilections of the individual physician. Rather, they should reflect a careful consideration of the particular patient's medical condition, prognosis, and values.

Further, the writing of a DNR order does not diminish the physician's continuing responsibility to provide active medical care to the patient. As the Minnesota Medical Society's guidelines make clear: "DNR orders are compatible with maximal therapeutic care. The patient may be receiving vigorous support in all other therapeutic modalities and yet justifiably be considered a proper subject for the DNR order" [54].

The Issue of Brain Death

Despite the opposition of radical right-to-life forces and of a small but influential group of Orthodox Jews [55–57] who share the belief that only destruction of the brain can be entertained as a possible definition of death, there seems to be little doubt as to what the medically accepted standards are for brain death. The *Guidelines for the Determination of Death,* a document summarizing accepted medical practices of the time, was published in 1981 [58].

Signed by the nation's leading authorities in neurology, neurosurgery, critical care, and legal medicine, the document represented "a consensus that is truly a remarkable achievement, [one] of which the medical profession can be proud" [59]. That document endorsed the Uniform Determination of Death Act. To date, some 38 states, excluding such major medical areas as Massachusetts. New York, and Minnesota, have adopted statutes regarding brain death.

One remaining moral dilemma that some physicians continue to perceive is the need for family permission to remove a respirator from brain-dead patients. A classic statement of that problem was seen in the case of a 13-year-old girl who was brain dead as the result of encephalitis [130]. The physicians approached her parents, informed them of the girl's diagnosis, told them that her condition was hopeless, and recommended the removal of the life-support system. The parents opted for continued treatment in the hope of a "miracle." The hospital, fearful of opposing the parents' wishes and unwilling to face the adverse publicity of a court proceeding to override the parents' decision, kept the child in the pediatric ICU until several months later, when she "succumbed" to cardiac failure.

Not only is there no need to ask family permission to remove a respirator, to ask is highly inappropriate; it gives a purported choice when, in fact, none exists. Furthermore, to ask, as happened with the encephalitis victim, opens the family to unnecessary feelings of ambivalence, anxiety, and guilt—feelings that may result in moral paralysis or a steadfast denial of death. Those emotions, in turn, may result in a decision to continue medical intervention in the hope of a miracle. An approach more attuned to the reality of the situation would have been to inform the encephalitis victim's family of her condition: "She is dead. The motions you see in her body are only the result of air being forced into her lungs by the ventilator."

As William Curran, Professor of Legal Medicine at Harvard Medical School and member of the original Harvard ad hoc committee on brain death [60], repeatedly emphasized, the determination of brain death is a technical medical issue, one that does not involve patient consent or family approval. Once the medical staff has made a well-informed determination of brain death, the patient is dead. The only moral issue remaining is the proper disposition of the corpse.

After allowing the family time to adjust, the physician should inquire about the family's willingness to donate the patient's organs. If the response is negative, the physician should present the family with the available options: "You may go in and see [the patient] before we remove the respirator or you may choose to wait until after it has been removed."

The physician should avoid using the phrase "brain dead." Dead is dead. Modification of the reality of death may lead to confusion and false hopes on the part of both health care providers and families. As the study by Younger and colleagues [61] revealed, physicians and other health care professionals involved in determining brain death and seeking organ procurement have confused and self-contradictory understandings of the concept. Only 38 percent of those surveyed could correctly identify and apply the criterion for brain death. If, as was proved, some of the professionals' explanations of brain death suggested they really believed the patient was alive, 40 percent of them rejected any brain-oriented concept of death whatsoever, and the majority (58 percent) did not use a coherent concept of death consistently, it is clear that the term conveys ambiguity and confusion about its meaning and implications.

Informing the family that the patient who meets the criterion for brain death is "dead" avoids creating the sense that the family is being asked to sign a "death warrant" and saves them from the possible guilt of thinking they did not do everything available to save the patient's life.

Pitts used an alternative approach [62]. Following the Harvard ad hoc directive that the decision and the responsibility for declaring death and turning off the respirator belongs to the physician, Pitts recommended informing the family that clinical evidence suggests the patient is brain dead and that several tests, including one for apnea, will be done to confirm that diagnosis. The family is asked whether it wants to see the patient before the tests are done. After the family has gone, the tests, the last of which is for apnea, are performed. In that controlled situation, after the respirator has been removed, if the patient is unable to breathe, death is pronounced. The physician then informs the family that the evidence was correct: the patient is dead. There is no question of removing a respirator; none is in use.

The Issue of Advance Directives

A problem in the CCU more common than brain death is what to do for the critically ill patient who is unable to make personal preferences known because of physical condition, age, or medication. The well-documented legal history of informed consent makes clear that the primary responsibility of caregivers is to ascertain as much as possible what the individual, if competent, would choose [63, 64]. The decision should reflect as closely as possible the patient's preferences, choices, and values.

That decision can be made by learning the patient's values and discovering what the patient would have done for others in similar situations. The clearest and most convincing evidence is the individual's direct testimony on the extent and duration of medical treatment. Ideally, the attending physician explores and learns this over the course of the illness. Unfortunately, such conversations are rare.

What leads to a breakdown in communication in an area as vital as life and death decisions? The limited empirical studies of the topic indicate a widespread belief on the part of both patients and physicians that the other party has the responsibility to initiate the conversation. A study by La Puma showed that physicians and providers view advance directives as a responsibility of the patient rather than a responsibility of a professional or institution [65]. Further support for that finding comes from a national study of hospitals with policies on advance directives. The study showed only 4 percent of hospital personnel asked their patients whether they had advance directives; 96 percent of the institutions assumed that patients who had such directives would inform the hospital [66].

Patients have just the opposite expectation. Emanuel's study of advanced directives revealed that the most frequently cited barrier to their use was patients' expectation that the physician would take the initiative in raising the topic [67]. The study found that although 93 percent of outpatients and 89 percent of the general public who were surveyed wanted a document specifying future care, only 7 percent had one and only 5 percent had ever had a discussion on the topic with their physicians.

The Patient Self-Determination Act of 1990 (PSDA) [68], which Congress passed as part of the Omnibus Budget Reconciliation Act, was designed, in part, to break this stalemate. The law, which took effect on December 1, 1991, requires all hospitals, nursing facilities, hospices, home health care services and health maintenance organizations that receive Medicare or Medicaid to inform their adult patients on admission or enrollment of their right to make decisions regarding their medical care and of their right under applicable state law to write a living will or durable power of attorney. The PSDA also requires as a condition for Medicare or Medicaid funding that these institutions do the following:

1. Document in the patient's medical record whether the individual has executed an advance directive.
2. Follow the directives in compliance with state laws.
3. Educate both their own staffs and the general community concerning advanced directives.

The PSDA did not create new rights or privileges for patients. It granted no new rights to citizens. The PSDA merely required health care providers to inform patients of their existing rights to refuse unwanted medical treatment. The United States Supreme Court noted in its 1990 *Cruzan* opinion that the common law right to refuse treatment is constitutionally protected as part of our fundamental "liberty interests" [69]. An earlier Supreme Court had stated, "No right is held more sacred, or is more carefully guarded by the common law, than the right of every individual to the possession and control of his person, free from all restraint or interference of others, unless by clear and unquestionable authority of law" [70].

The medical implications of a person's right of autonomy were first articulated in 1914 by Justice Benjamin Cardozo, then of the New York Court of Appeals, when he wrote in his landmark Schloendorff opinion: "Every human being of adult years and sound mind has a right to determine what shall be done with his own body; and a surgeon who performs an operation without his patient's consent commits an assault, for which he is liable in damages" [71]. Schloendorff's opinion, which forms the basis for the doctrine of informed consent, made clear, as the *Cruzan* case was to reiterate 75 years later, that the competent patient has a right to decline all medical interventions including those that might prolong life.

Difficulties arise when the question of patient autonomy is applied to noncompetent patients. How does one determine what medical treatment, if any, the unconscious Karen Ann Quinlan [72] or Nancy Cruzan would want? The problem is exacerbated by technological advances that have increased medicine's ability to preserve and prolong life. Procedures that once were only dreams have become reality—artificial means to replace failed lungs, hearts, and kidneys are now commonplace. However, sophisticated techniques can be abused; the very means used to preserve life may transform it into a sublethal extension of monitoring machines and sustaining apparatus.

A solution to the problem of protecting the rights and dignity of the incompetent patient was proposed in 1969 by Louis Kutner, who described a document, which he termed a "living will," in which a competent adult could put in writing directions for future medical care to be used by the health care provider should the individual become incapacitated and unable to communicate his or her wishes [73].

By 1993, 41 states and the District of Columbia had enacted living will statutes. Though differing widely in detail, all the statutes grant immunity to physicians and health care providers who follow the patient's expressed wishes [74]. George Annas noted that most of the statutes suffer from four major shortcomings: (1) they are applicable only to those who are terminally ill; (2) they limit the types of treatment that can be refused to artificial or extraordinary therapies; (3) they make no provisions for the person to designate another person to make the decision on his or her behalf and set criteria for such decisions; and (4) they do not provide for a penalty in the event that health care providers fail to honor these documents [75].

The American Medical Association's Committee on Medico-Legal Problems also evaluated these statements and found significant drawbacks [76]. First, and most important, no matter how carefully crafted, no legislation provides guidance for unanticipated circumstances. If drafted in language general enough to cover a broad range of circumstances, the law seems too vague, too abstract, or too ambiguous to apply to specific situations. Ambiguity and the need for physicians to make decisions based on an interpretation of a document, rather than on a discussion with someone acting on behalf of the patient, can result in decisions contrary to what a patient would want. For example, Tom Wirth, a New York City man with AIDS, signed a living will stating that should he become incapable of making his own decisions and should his condition be "irreversible," he would not want "extraordinary" measures taken to extend his life. When Mr. Wirth developed a brain infection from toxoplasmosis, his physician, over the strenuous objections of Mr. Wirth's companion, continued to treat Mr. Wirth because, in the physician's judgment, "toxoplasmosis is potentially reversible." The court upheld the physician's position [77]. Despite intensive treatment, Mr. Wirth eventually succumbed to the infection. The appointment of the companion as health care proxy would have obviated the difficulties found in Mr. Wirth's blunt, unnuanced, written statement. The appointment of an identifiable person, especially one who knows the patient and the patient's values, assures that the decision will be clinically situated, attuned to changing conditions, and in the hands of someone whom the patient knows and whose judgment the patient trusts.

The static nature of a living will has led to proposals to replace what one commentator labeled "a bloodless document" with a flesh-and-blood person who could speak for the patient [78]. This can be done effectively by assigning a durable power of attorney to a designated person who will speak for an individual should that individual become incapacitated. The terminology used for the document that identifies the surrogate, proxy, or agent (the terms are used interchangeably in the literature)—the "durable power of attorney"—is confusing and misleading. The instrument, though developed from probate law, has nothing to do with lawyers. One does not need a lawyer to draft a durable power of attorney, and the proxy or agent named therein need not be an attorney.

Any competent adult can write a statement naming any other competent adult—spouse, parent, child, sibling, companion, friend—as his or her proxy for health care decisions. To prevent potential abuses or conflicts of interest, it is best that, except for relatives, direct health care providers not be named as agents. (Many statutes, in fact, exclude such providers from being named as health care proxies.) Once designated in a written, witnessed document, the proxy has the same health care decision-making power the patient would have had were he or she able to make decisions.

The actual statement need not be complex, nor need it be drafted by an attorney. One can simply

Fig. 41-1
Bok's "Directions for My Care."

I wish to live a full and long life, but not at all costs. If my death is near and cannot be avoided, and if I have lost the ability to interact with others and have no reasonable chance of regaining this ability, or if my suffering is intense and irreversible, I do not want to have my life prolonged. I would then ask not to be subjected to surgery or resuscitation. Nor would I then wish to have life support from mechanical ventilators, intensive care services, or other life-prolonging procedures, including the administration of antibiotics, blood products, or artificially provided nutrition and fluids. I would wish, rather, to have care which gives comfort and support, which facilitates my interaction with others to the extent that this is possible, and which brings peace.

In order to carry out these instructions and to interpret them, I authorize ____________________ to accept, plan, and refuse treatment on my behalf in cooperation with my attending physicians and health personnel. This person knows how I value the experience of living, weigh incompetence, suffering and dying. Should it be impossible to reach this person, I authorize ____________________ to make such choices for me. I have discussed these desires concerning terminal care with them, and I trust their judgment on my behalf. In addition, I have discussed with them the following specific instructions regarding my care:

Signature ____________________

Address ____________________

Date ____________________

Name of proxy ____________________

Address of proxy ____________________

Telephone number of proxy ____________________

Name of substitute ____________________

Address of substitute ____________________

Telephone number of substitute ____________________

Date ____________________

Witnessed ____________________

Signed ____________________

and by ____________________

write in plain prose what he or she wants done in such circumstances. If the person wishes a prewritten form, the best and most readily available is Bok's "Directions for My Care" [79] (see Fig. 41-1).

Patients with Inadequate Capacity for Decision-Making

Although it is relatively easy to make medical decisions for patients who have provided clear directives for their care, the overwhelming majority of patients with impaired decision-making capacity have not done so. These patients present several dilemmas to health care providers. The first of these dilemmas is how to determine that the patient has become too incapacitated to be a competent decision-maker. Many physicians' initial impulse is to call for psychiatric consultation or seek a court order to declare the patient incompetent [80]. In most cases, neither approach is appropriate. As the 1983 President's Commission emphatically noted, "'Decision making incapacity' is not a medical or a psychiatric diagnostic category; it rests on a judgment of the type an informed layperson might make—that the patient lacks sufficient ability to understand a situation and to make a choice in light of that understanding" [25]. More specifically, the physician wants to ascertain that the patient understands his or her condition, the treatment options (including nontreatment), the consequences of each option, and is able to make a reasoned choice among them. However, this choice need not be what the physician would consider reasonable, rational, or medically appropriate; the patient's decision need only reflect a reasoned choice among the options. As the Massachusetts Appeals Court stated in *Lane v Candura*—a case involving an admittedly confused 78-year-old woman's refusal to have her gangrenous leg amputated—what must be determined is whether the "areas of forgetfulness and confusion cause or relate in any way to impairment of her ability to understand that in rejecting the treatment she is, in effect, choosing death over life" [81].

Once it has been determined that the patient lacks adequate decision-making capacity, the need arises for a surrogate or proxy. Generally, the surrogate should be a family member or a friend who knows the patient's interests and values—and can address them directly. Even if the patient had never made any specific statements on treatment decisions, the proxy might legitimately be able to infer from the patient's known values and beliefs what he or she would want in such a situation and thereby preserve the subjective and idiosyncratic values of the individual. In the event that no prior discussion of the issues has occurred and the surrogate is unable to assess what the incompetent individual would have chosen, the proxy must use a "best interests" test that examines the patient's welfare and well-being. The President's Commission spelled out several factors that should be considered in such a determination, factors that the California Court of Appeals in the *Barber v Superior Court* case [82] adopted as normative: "relief of suffering, the preservation or restoration of functioning; the quality as well as the extent of life sustained . . . and the impact of a decision on the incapacitated patient's loved ones." The caveat is that the "quality of life and impact on family should be viewed exclusively from the perspective of the patient."

One attempt to ensure that the process produces an objective, disinterested, and publicly accountable decision is to take the issue to court [83–86]. That route, however, is costly, cumbersome, traumatic, and uncertain. The personal predilections of judges, the highly diverse formulations of the law, and the fact that judges are poorly equipped for, and not fond of, handling such issues makes that route fraught with potential peril for patients, physicians, hospitals, and society [87, 88]. Furthermore, even court approbation does not protect a hospital and physicians from explosive societal repercussions. This is illustrated by the Bloomington, Indiana *Baby Doe* case, in which a family physician's decision not to treat a Down's syndrome infant with an esophageal fistula was approved by three courts, including the Indiana Supreme Court. Those repercussions, in the form of highly restrictive and counterproductive original Baby Doe regulations with their hot line, anonymous tipsters, and "flying Doe squads," proved a better way than inflexible bureaucratic regulations is needed to resolve these problems [89].

The Decision-Making Process

Whatever the process, good decision-making on behalf of incompetent patients must consider three factors: the physician, the patient, and the community. Although the era of the paternalistic physician and the passive patient has passed [90], the physician continues to have a primary role and responsibility. The physician must make the diagnosis, provide the prognosis, and, after forming a professional judgment on the range of options, make a recommendation. Here, once again, we are reminded of Ingelfinger's admonition [53] that a physician who merely presents options to an uncounseled patient and expects a decision is guilty of, at least, shirking duties and, at most, malpractice.

Given the physician's recommendation, the patient or proxy must address the subjective values that determine whether the proposal offers proportionate benefit. Here the entire range of factors, such as cost, burden, pain, anticipated outcome, dislocation, family structure, and personal plans comes into play. The patient or the person acting on behalf of the patient must plumb these and make a choice.

Although the combination of patient-family choice is generally final, a third factor—society—must be considered. With the change in attitude from the strong paternalism of ''the doctor knows best'' to the elevation of autonomy into a near absolute, individuals sometimes forget that their actions and decisions have implications for, and impact on, others. Consequently, society, for the protection of individuals and the common good, places constraints and limits, both positive and negative, on individual rights [91]. Several examples of these constraints have emerged as ethical problems in health care delivery. For example, as seen in the Johns Hopkins case [92] and the Bloomington Baby Doe dispute, many persons believe that parents should have the right to deny lifesaving corrective surgery to a Down's syndrome infant because a retarded child would prove a burden on the family [93, 94]. However, a strong consensus has emerged in our society that such an infant may not be denied the necessary surgery simply because of its mental handicap [95, 96]. Likewise, though parents may have a right to decline blood transfusions based on religious convictions, a consensus believes they have no right to impose those beliefs on their immature minor children [97].

An example of the restriction on one's right to positive claims is the denial of a family request to have a rapidly deteriorating critically ill patient remain in or be moved to the ICU to satisfy the demand that ''everything possible be done'' [98–101]. Use of the ICU must rest on the medical staff's professional assessment of the usefulness of the ICU to the patient and the comparative merit of others' claims for that scarce resource [102]. To hold otherwise transforms the physician from a professional charged with making informed and sometimes difficult judgments into one who simply strives to fulfill family demands.

Perhaps the most succinct statement of the physician's professional role is found in a discussion on termination of treatment decisions in the Vatican's 1980 Declaration on Euthanasia [103]:

> For such a decision to be made, account will have to be taken of the wishes of the patient and the patient's family, as also of the advice of the doctors who are especially competent in the matter. The latter may in particular judge that the investment in instruments and personnel is disproportionate to the results foreseen; they may also judge that the techniques applied impose on the patient strain or suffering out of proportion with the benefits which he or she may gain from such techniques.

Here, an institution highly protective of the sanctity of life indicated not only that there are limits to the burdens an individual must undergo to preserve life, but that there are limits that can and ought to be set by physicians concerning what may legitimately be offered to, or demanded for, such patients.

Responsibility for the Decision

Judgments concerning burden and benefit to the patient are value judgments, moral choices. They are judgments in which, all things considered, the continuance of life is either called for or is not worthwhile to the patient. Such judgments are the onerous prerogative of those who are primarily responsible for the welfare of the incompetent patient—the family or other surrogate. When a surrogate exercises this prerogative in a way that is questionably no longer in the best interests of the patient, such as allowing a patient with a good prognosis to go untreated, society has the duty to intervene. That intervention can take many forms, such as legislation, criminal prosecution, or neglect hearings. The purpose of such proceedings is to guarantee that the primary decision-maker acts responsibly in a manner that should be able to sustain public scrutiny. Public accountability and review, which guarantees that the values of the society are respected and adhered to, can be invoked short of judicial intervention.

One approach to achieving this goal is found in the President's Commission report [25]. In the opinion of the Commission, "routine judicial oversight [of medical decision-making] is neither necessary or appropriate." A court's remoteness from a clinical situation and subsequent inability to keep pace with ongoing fluctuations in a patient's condition, particularly in an intensive care setting, are strong arguments in support of the Commission's view. The Commission favored having the surrogate's decision in difficult cases reviewed by an in-place, broadly based, multidisciplinary hospital bioethics committee familiar with both the medical setting and the community's standards. That consultative body, which would have the ongoing charge of establishing standards of treatment and issuing guidelines for the medical institution, should provide a framework for impartial but sensitive review of hard choices [104–106] and guarantee that the interests of the patient were being considered without the formality and intensely adversarial character of a court proceeding. If, after all this, irreconcilable disagreement still persisted, the President's Commission recommended referral to the court for the appointment of a legal guardian who would be empowered to evaluate the options and make a decision "in the best interest" of the patient. The decision would be subject to judicial scrutiny as a last resort.

Such an approach ensures that the decision-maker has received the most reliable information available, that the decision is within the range of acceptable options, and that those uncomfortable with it have had an opportunity to discuss their reservations with a concerned and disinterested representative of the public. It also insulates the choices from the glare of publicity, the distortion of public posturing, and the costly and tangled involvement of court proceedings.

The implementation of bioethics committees as mediators was greatly enhanced in January 1984, when the Department of Health and Human Services, in response to the criticism of its revised, proposed Infant Doe Regulations [107] adopted the suggestion of the American Academy of Pediatrics [108] that the resolution of treatment-issue decisions for seriously ill newborns should be made in each hospital by a multidisciplinary Infant Care Review Committee [95]. Institutionally based, clinically sensitive, multidisciplinary bodies can educate physicians, staff, and patients on difficult ethical issues. These bodies can also establish institutional policies and guidelines on treatment decisions, and they have proved valuable for consultation on new or particularly difficult cases. Such benefits have led to the widespread use of institution-based bodies for discussing ethics [109–113].

Legal Guidelines

The procedural aspects of good decision-making assure that patient autonomy, physician responsibility, and societal values are considered, but they do not produce the decision or guarantee its character. Further, the range of ethically acceptable options, the complexity of individual cases, and the variable situation of institutions and specific patients precludes prepackaged solutions to ethical dilemmas.

Nonetheless, there are some agreed-upon norms and guidelines that are helpful in resolving difficult ethical questions. The most practical and readily available source for the clinician is Jonsen's *Clinical Ethics* [114], a short text in which an ethicist, a physician, and an attorney set out some of the more agreed-on principles and illustrate them with brief case studies. However, the best summary of ethical norms is found not in discursive philosophical texts but in major court opinions issued since the *Quinlan* case [72]. Four of these, *Superintendent of Belchertown State School v Saikewicz* [115], *Barber v Superior Court* [82], *In the matter of Claire Conroy* [116], and the *Cruzan* case [69] illustrate the emerging consensus of law and ethics on appropriate care for an incompetent, terminally ill, or irreversibly comatose patient.

In *Saikewicz,* the Massachusetts Supreme Judicial Court ruled that the court could determine whether a 67-year-old, profoundly retarded (I.Q. of 10), institutionalized man with acute myelogenous leukemia would, if competent, opt for nontreatment. The argument was that the administration of chemotherapy, which for the nonretarded patient might be endured in the hope of a remission, would inexplicably change the character of Joseph Saikewicz's life from a peaceful routine into a bewildering nightmare of pain, fear, and physical restraint. As such, it would surely constitute extraordinary treatment. If the patient had no obligation to undergo such treatment, neither had the physician any moral obligation to provide it nor the judge to order it.

In forming this opinion, the Massachusetts Supreme Judicial Court gave judicial support to the distinction between ordinary and extraordinary means: "We should not use *extraordinary* means of prolonging life or its semblance when, after careful consideration . . . it becomes apparent that there is no hope of recovery for the patient" [117]. Further, the court concurred with *Quinlan* in adopting the thesis of both Ramsey [23] and Kubler-Ross [118] that the distinction between "curing the ill and comforting and easing the dying" can be and ought to be elucidated. The court accepted the thesis that physicians ought not to treat the hopeless and the dying as though they are curable. In the court's view, physicians should recognize that the dying need comfort more than treatment. These positions, buttressed by recent developments in the law on informed consent and respect for the right of privacy, were the basis for the court's authorization of the withholding of chemotherapy for Saikewicz. However, the court reversed the thesis that the value of life is lessened or cheapened by a decision to refuse treatment. It ruled that the value of life is diminished by the failure to allow a competent human being the right of choice and the right of privacy, that is, the right to be left alone.

The more difficult problem was the attribution of these rights to the incompetent. There are those who argue strenuously that the state must always provide treatment for the incompetent or risk devaluing their dignity and worth. The Massachusetts Supreme Judicial Court rejected that proposition and, in a precedent-shattering contribution to the developing trend in the law, ruled that "the principles of equality and respect for all individuals require that a choice exist for incompetents as well as competents. To do otherwise would be to treat wards of the state as a person of lesser status or dignity than others" [115].

Having recognized the right of an incompetent to refuse life-prolonging treatment, the Massachusetts court faced the task of framing an adequate rationale to explain how that right may be exercised in a case of first impression. It yoked the long-standing legal doctrine of substituted judgment with a Rawlsian reconstruction of the mental world of a "rational" incompetent. Substituted judgment, a doctrine first articulated in English law over 150 years ago, deals with the authorization of gifts from the estate of incompetents [119]. The English court reasoned this could be done by "donning the mental mantle of the incompetent," that is, what one might reasonably conclude the individual would do if he or she could understand the situation.

That theory of respect for the integrity and autonomy of all persons found renewed vigor in John Rawls's highly influential *A Theory of Justice* [120], in which he wrote that maintaining the integrity of the person means that we act towards him "as we have reason to believe he would choose for himself if he were capable of reasoning and deciding rationally." This does not mean that one can impute preferences that the patient never held. But, as is true in the case of Saikewicz where no preferences had been made, the task is to ask how the patient would act if he or she could perceive the present situation.

Applying the substituted judgment theory to Saikewicz, the Massachusetts Supreme Judicial Court concluded that the probate court, the guardian *ad litem,* the physicians, and the staff operated in the best interests of Joseph Saikewicz (i.e., they chose what appeared to be the least detrimental available alternative). That choice, they argued, is what Saikewicz would have chosen if he were capable of doing so.

The California Court of Appeals in the *Barber* case refined and developed the ethical standards found in *Saikewicz.* Reflecting on the moral propriety of the physicians who honored the family request to remove the intravenous feeding tube from the irreversibly comatose Clarence Herbert, the California court confronted a host of medical-ethical questions: Is the physician bound by the Hippocratic oath to do everything possible to save life? When, if ever, is it appropriate to stop treatment? What is the difference between killing or letting die, acts of omission or commission, withholding or withdrawing treatment? How does one distinguish ordinary from extraordinary means? Is not use of an intravenous tube ordinary? Who decides for the incompetent patient? Must there be a legal guardian? Is a court order necessary?

In the course of its 25-page opinion, the California Court of Appeals addressed all of these issues. In doing so, it adopted as normative nearly all of the recommendations on what constitutes appropriate care of the terminally ill or irreversibly comatose patient that were proposed in the 1983 President's Commission report. For the first time, a court equated the stopping of intravenous feeding with the removal of a respirator or any other medical intervention [121–123]. Each intervention, it declared, is a medical treatment and is to be used only if it benefits the patient. If the intervention merely sustains biologic function, it is not a treatment but a useless and futile gesture, one which the physician need not continue. As the court phrased it, "there is no duty to continue [life-sustaining machinery] once it has become futile in the opinion of qualified medical personnel" [82]. The court discarded the traditional "ordinary–extraordinary" language in favor of the increasingly common usage of "proportionate–disproportionate" and "benefit–burden" to the patient. That approach shifted the emphasis from the technique used to the condition of the patient. In the court's words:

> Thus, even if a proposed course of treatment might be extremely painful or intrusive, it would still be proportionate treatment if the prognosis was for complete cure or significant improvement in the patient's condition. On the other hand, a treatment course which is only minimally painful or intrusive may nonetheless be considered disproportionate to the potential benefits if the prognosis is virtually hopeless for any significant improvement in condition.

Finally, bringing to completion a trend in the law that was first articulated in *Quinlan,* the court noted that in the case of incompetents, the surrogate, if unable to ascertain the patient's actual choices, should be guided by the patient's best interests. These, as previously noted, included factors such as relief from suffering, the preservation or restoration of functioning, the quality and the extent of the life sustained, and the impact of the decision on the family. The court held that, without evidence of malevolence, the family was the proper surrogate for the incompetent patient, and that there was no need for the surrogate to seek prior judicial approval before a decision to withdraw treatment could be made. Such judicial involvement, the court concluded, was not only unnecessary, but might be unwise.

The New Jersey Supreme Court in *In the Matter of Claire Conroy* [116] further refined the standards articulated in the Barber case on the withholding or withdrawing of medical treatments, including nutrition and fluids, from incompetent seriously ill patients who, even with treatment, will probably die within 1 year. After observing that there was no doubt that if competent, an individual in Miss Conroy's condition would have the right to have a nasogastric tube withdrawn, the New Jersey Supreme Court declared the same right should be accorded to the incompetent. It then articulated three tests to guide the substitute decision-maker. The first—"subjective standard"—was to apply if the patient had previously communicated his or her wishes by a written living will, an oral directive, or a durable power of attorney. The other two tests—labeled "limited-objective" and "purely objective"—were best interests tests to be used when there had been no prior directives from the patient. The New Jersey court avoided the idea that it could discern the mind-set of an incompetent patient, and did not take the position of the New York Court of Appeals in the O'Connor decision [86] that precluded any cessation of treatment for persons who had never expressed their desires about life-sustaining treatment.

The New Jersey court's limited objective test allowed the termination of treatment for someone in Claire Conroy's situation if there were some trustworthy evidence, such as life style, attitudes, or values that indicated the patient would not want treatment or feeding continued because "it would involve too heavy a burden of unavoidable pain and suffering." In the absence of reliable evidence, or indeed, of any evidence, treatment could be withheld or withdrawn if the purely objective test was satisfied. Under this standard "the net burdens of the patient's life with treatment" would "clearly and markedly outweigh the benefits derived from life," for example, if the patient were suffering from such severe pain that the administration of life-sustaining treatment or feeding would be inhumane. The New Jersey court cautioned that it expressly denied authority under this third test to remove life support from any patient (1) on a quality-of-life basis other than extreme pain, or (2) on the ground that the patient's value to society was negligible.

In a commentary on this case, Curran [124] observed that the importance of this decision "on the medical obligation to the dying cannot be overstated." For the first time in American jurisprudence, a state supreme court had approved the removal of nutrition and hydration as well as other forms of life support and had reinforced the legitimacy of allowing surrogates, in good faith and without a conflict of interest, to determine that the patient's best interests would not be served by prolonging a painful, hopeless existence.

The broad sweep of the Conroy decision reflects one state's approach to treatment decisions for incompetent patients. As the United States Supreme Court's 1990 opinion in *Cruzan v Director Missouri Department of Health* makes clear, individual states can set their own evidentiary standards with regard to treatment decisions for incompetent patients. In its first ruling on the right to die, the Court stated that although a competent person would have a constitutionally protected right to refuse potentially lifesaving medical treatment including artificially provided nutrition and hydration, the United States Constitution does not prohibit a state from requiring clear and convincing evidence of an incompetent patient's prior wishes with regard to withdrawal of life-sustaining treatment before such treatment can be terminated.

Since such evidence was found to be lacking in the case of Nancy Cruzan, the United States Supreme Court upheld the ruling of the Missouri Supreme Court that no surrogate, including her parents, could make the decision to terminate her medical treatment. Since the Cruzans could not meet the evidentiary standard set by Missouri, Nancy Cruzan was to continue to receive artificially provided nutrition and fluids at the state facility where she had been cared for in a persistent vegetative state for eight years. However, the Supreme Court's opinion ought not be interpreted too broadly. The ruling did not consign all incompetent patients who had not made their treatment preferences known to a regimen of unlimited treatment. The ruling said only that there was no constitutional prohibition forbidding states from setting procedural guidelines and evidentiary standards for surrogate decision makers. The Supreme Court itself set no standards nor did it require states to establish specific guidelines to control proxy medical decision making.

The Supreme Court's opinion in *Cruzan* provided several positive outcomes for the complex area of law and medicine. It recognized "the principle that a competent person has a constitutionally protected liberty interest in refusing unwanted medical treatment." It also resolved the debate over whether artificially provided nutrition and fluids are medical treatments. Further, it concluded that these treatments should be assessed and evaluated on the same standard as any other medical intervention—on the basis of the patient's subjective assessment of benefits and burdens.

The opinion also gave legal recognition to advance directives. It indicated that the prior expressed wishes of an incompetent patient are to be accorded the same constitutional protection given to the competent patient's wishes. That assures that even in the absence of specific statutes recognizing their status, written advance directives (living wills) are to be honored as explicit instructions of the patient. Justice O'Connor's concurrence signaled that a majority of the Cruzan Court also gave the same constitutional status to the decisions of a designated proxy or health care agent and that a competent individual could be assured the same protection to his or her directions by signing a durable power of attorney.

In addition, the Court recognized that incompetent persons have and retain constitutional rights with regard to refusing medical treatment. Although all of the Justices agreed that a state can establish procedural safeguards to protect the rights of incompetent persons, they were divided on the level of evidence a state may require to indicate what the incompetent person would want. A majority found that Missouri's requirement of clear and convincing evidence of the patient's expressed wishes with regard to the withdrawal of life-sustaining medical treatment did not violate the constitutional rights of the patient.

Practical Implications for Physicians and Hospitals

The Supreme Court's opinion in the Cruzan case did not impose any new standards on the practice of medicine. It recognized that states may establish procedural guidelines for treatment decisions for incompetent patients, and it upheld Missouri's right to demand clear and convincing evidence of the patient's expressed wishes before treatment can be terminated. States are free to set their own standards. New York, like Missouri, requires clear and convincing evidence. Massachusetts uses substituted judgment. Other states, including California, that have addressed the issue of withholding or withdrawing medical treatment from incompetent patients have allowed caring families or close friends to determine the best interest of the patient. Most states have never addressed the question of medical treatment for incompetents. The traditional practice of physician-family assessment of physical findings and known values or best interest are used to determine what should be done. Nothing in the Supreme Court's *Cruzan* opinion changes the way those decisions are to be made. In all states—except Missouri and New York—physicians may, at the direction of a caring family, legally withhold or withdraw life-sustaining medical treatments including artificially provided nutrition and fluids from a terminally ill or irreversibly comatose patient.

The high-technology medicine available today not only provides near miraculous benefits for some patients, but also creates challenging and troublesome ethical and legal dilemmas for patients, families, and practitioners. Fortunately, the process of moral reflection and analysis necessary to meet these challenges has begun. The task now is to continue to reflect so that we come to understand, as others since the time of Hippocrates have tried to understand, the appropriate duties and limits of medicine.

References

1. Knaus, W., Draper, E., and Wagner, D. P. The use of intensive care: New research initiatives and their implications for national health policy. *Milbank Mem. Fund. Q.* 61:561, 1983.
2. Schroeder, S. A., Showstack, J. A., and Roberts, H. E. Frequency and clinical description of high-cost patients in 17 acute-care hospitals. *N. Engl. J. Med.* 300:1306, 1979.
3. Thibault, G. E., Mulley, A. G., and Barnett, G. O. Medical intensive care: Indications, interventions, and outcome. *N. Engl. J. Med.* 302:938, 1980.
4. Zook, C. J., and Moore, F. D. High-cost users of medical care. *N. Engl. J. Med.* 302:996, 1980.
5. Teres, D., Brown, R. B., and Lemeshow, S. Predicting mortality of intensive care patients: The importance of coma. *Crit. Care Med.* 10:65, 1982.
6. Turnbull, A. D., Goldiner, P., Silverman, D., et al. The role of an intensive care unit in a cancer center. *Cancer* 37:82, 1976.
7. Davis, P. B., and di Sant'Angnese, P. A. Assisted ventilation for patients with cystic fibrosis. *J.A.M.A.* 239:1851, 1978.
8. Imbus, S. H., and Zawacki, B. E. Autonomy for burned patients when survival is unprecedented. *N. Engl. J. Med.* 297:308, 1977.
9. Levy, D. E., Bates, D., Cardonna, J. J., et al. Prognosis in non-traumatic coma. *Ann. Intern. Med.* 94:293, 1981.
10. Knaus, W. A., Zimmerman, J. E., Wagner, D. P., et al. APACHE—acute physiology and chronic health evaluation: A physiologically based classification system. *Crit. Care Med.* 9:591, 1981.
11. Knaus, W. A., Draper, E. A., Wagner, D. P., et al. APACHE II: A severity of disease classification system. *Crit. Care Med.* 13:818, 1985.
12. Rodman, G. H., Etlint, T., Civetta, J. M., et al. How accurate is clinical judgment? *Crit. Care Med.* 6:127, 1978.
13. Pearlman, R. A., Inui, T. S., and Carter, W. B. Variability in physician bioethical decision-making: A case study of euthanasia. *Ann. Intern. Med.* 97:420, 1982.
14. Knaus, W. A. Prognosis with mechanical ventilation: The influence of disease, severity of disease, age, and chronic health status on survival from an acute illness. *Am. Rev. Respir. Dis.* 140:S8, 1989.
15. Intensive Care Audit (Editorial). *Lancet* 1:1, 1985.
16. Chung, R. W. Individual outcome prediction models for intensive care patients. *Lancet* ii:143, 1989.
17. Seale, C. F. What happens in hospice: A review of research evidence. *Soc. Sci. Med.* 28:551, 1989.
18. Angell, M. Cost containment and the physician *J.A.M.A.* 254:1203, 1985.
19. Thurow, L. Medicine versus economics. *N. Engl. J. Med.* 313:611, 1985.
20. Fuchs, V. R. Who shall live? In Fuchs, V. R. (ed.) *Health, Economics and Social Choice.* New York: Basic Books, 1974.
21. Moore, F. D. The desperate case: CARE (costs, applicability, research, ethics). *J.A.M.A.* 261:1483, 1989.
22. Vincent, J. L., Parquier, J. N., Preiser, J. C., et al. Terminal events in the intensive care unit: Review of 258 fatal cases in one year. *Crit. Care Med.* 17:530, 1989.
23. Ramsey, P. *The Patient as Person.* New Haven: Yale University Press, 1970.
24. Admundsen, D. The physician's obligation to prolong life: A medical duty without classical roots. *Hastings Cent. Rep.* 8:23, 1978.
25. President's Commission for the Study of Ethical Problems in Medicine and Biomedical and Behavioral Research. *Deciding to Forego Life-Sustaining Treatment.* Washington, D.C.: U.S. Government Printing Office, 1983.
26. Council on Ethical and Judicial Affairs, American Medical Association. Guidelines for the appropriate use of do-not-resuscitate orders. *J.A.M.A.* 265:1868, 1991.
27. Lo, B. Unanswered questions about DNR orders. *J.A.M.A.* 265:1874, 1991.
28. Wolfe, S. M. Near death—In the moment of decision. *N. Engl. J. Med.* 322:208, 1990. Decision

making in "near death" (Correspondence). *N. Engl. J. Med.* 322:1604, 1990.

29. Hachler, J. C., and Hiller, F. C. Family consent to orders not to resuscitate: Reconsidering hospital policy. *J.A.M.A.* 264:1281, 1990.
30. Blackhall, L. Must we always use CPR? *N. Engl. J. Med.* 317:1281, 1987.
31. The New York State Task Force on Life and the Law. *Do Not Resuscitate Orders: The Proposed Legislation and Report.* New York: New York State Task Force, 1986.
32. Rosenthal, E. New rules for saving the dying are being misused, doctors say. *New York Times,* Oct. 4, 1990. P. B20
33. National Conference Steering Committee: Standards for cardiopulmonary resuscitation (CPR) and emergency cardiac care (ECC). *J.A.M.A.* 227:837, 864, 1974.
34. Lampton, L. M., and Winship, D. H. The no-code blue issue: Missouri is not Massachusetts. *Mo. Med.* 76:259, 1979.
35. Spenser, S. S. Code or no code: A non-legal opinion. *N. Engl. J. Med.* 300:138, 1979.
36. Rabkin, M. T., Gillerman, G., and Rice, N. R. Orders not to resuscitate. *N. Engl. J. Med.* 295:364, 1976.
37. *Dinnerstein,* 380 NE2d, 134, 135 (Mass App 1978).
38. *Guidelines: Orders not to resuscitate.* Boston: Beth Israel Hospital, March 5, 1981.
39. Fowler, M. D. Slow code, partial code, limited code. *Heart Lung* 18:533, 1989.
40. Goldenring, J. Code or no code decisions (Correspondence). *N. Engl. J. Med.* 300:1058, 1979.
41. Hashimoto, D. M. A structural analysis of the physician-patient relationship in no-code decision making. *Yale Law J.* 93:362, 1983.
42. Schade, G. S., and Muslin, H. Do not resuscitate discussions with patients. *J. Med. Ethics* 15:186, 1989.
43. Miles, S. H., Cranford, R., and Schulty, A. L. The do-not resuscitate order in a teaching hospital. *Ann. Intern. Med.* 96:660, 1982.
44. Siegler, M. Does everything include CPR? *Hastings Cent. Rep.* 12:28, 1982.
45. Bedell, S. E., Delbanco, T. L., Cook, E. F., et al. Survival after cardiopulmonary resuscitation in the hospital. *N. Engl. J. Med.* 309:569, 1983.
46. Tomlinson, T., and Brody, H. Ethics and communication in do-not-resuscitate orders. *N. Engl. J. Med.* 318:43, 1988.
47. Murphy, D. J., Murray, A. M., Robinson, B. E., et al. Outcomes of cardiopulmonary resuscitation in the elderly. *Ann. Intern. Med.* 111:119, 1989.
48. Lantos, J. D., Miles, S. H., Silverstein, M. D., et al. Survival after cardiopulmonary resuscitation in babies of very low birthweight: Is CPR futile therapy? *N. Engl. J. Med.* 318:91, 1988.
49. Wachter, R. M., Luce, J. M., Hearst, N. H., et al. Decisions about resuscitation: Inequities among patients with different diseases but similar prognoses. *Ann. Intern. Med.* 111:525, 1989.
50. Grossman, J. H. *Do not resuscitate (DNR) orders-revised.* Boston: New England Medical Center Hospitals, September, 1989.
51. The Emergency Cardiac Care Committee of the American Heart Association. Guidelines on cardiopulmonary resuscitation and emergency cardiac care: Ethical considerations in resuscitation. *J.A.M.A.* 268:2282, 1992.
52. *Guidelines for Withholding, Withdrawing or Limiting Life-Sustaining Treatment Including Resuscitation.* Boston: Beth Israel Hospital, 1991.
53. Ingelfinger, F. Arrogance. *N. Engl. J. Med.* 303: 1507, 1980.
54. Minnesota Medical Association. Do Not Resuscitate (DNR) Guidelines. In President's Commission for the Study of Ethical Problems in Medicine and Biomedical and Behavioral Research, *Deciding to Forego Life-Sustaining Treatment.* Washington, D.C.: U.S. Government Printing Office, 1983. P. 499.
55. Committee for Pro-Life Activities. *Definition of death legislation* (Resource paper). Washington, D.C., National Conference of Catholic Bishops, April, 1983.
56. Byrne, P. A., O'Reilly, S., Quay, P. M. Brain death: An opposing viewpoint. *J.A.M.A.* 242:1985, 1979.
57. Rosner, F., and Bleich, J. D. *Jewish Bioethics.* New York: Hebrew Publishing, 1979.
58. Guidelines for the determination of death. *J.A.M.A.* 246:2184, 1981.
59. Barclay, W. R. Guidelines for the determination of death (Editorial). *J.A.M.A.* 246:2194, 1981.
60. Harvard Medical School ad hoc Committee to Examine the Definition of Brain Death. A definition of irreversible coma. *J.A.M.A.* 205:337, 1968.
61. Younger, S. J., Landefeldt, C. S., and Coulton, C. J. "Brain death" and organ retrieval: A cross-sectional survey of knowledge and concepts among health professionals. *J.A.M.A.* 261:2205, 1989.
62. Pitts, L. H. Maintenance of a cadaver donor for multiple organ procurement. Presented at National Institutes of Health Conference. Washington, D.C.: Jan. 21, 1984.
63. Katz, J. *The Silent World of Doctor and Patient.* New York: Free Press, 1984.
64. Applebaum, P. S., Lidz, C. W., and Meisel, A. *Informed Consent: Legal Theory and Clinical Practice.* New York: Oxford University Press, 1987.
65. La Puma, J., Orentlicher, D., and Moss, R. J. Advanced directives on admission: Clinical implications and analysis of the Patient Self-Determination Act of 1990. *J.A.M.A.* 66:402, 1991.
66. Finucane, T. E., Schumway, J. M., Powers, R. L., et al. Planning with elderly patients for contingencies of severe illness. *J. Intern. Med.* 3:322, 1988.
67. Emanuel, L. L., Barry, M. J., Stockle, J. D., et al. Advanced directives for medical care—a case for greater use. *N. Engl. J. Med.* 324:889, 1991.
68. 42 U.S.C. §1395 cc(a)(1) et seq. (as amended Nov. 1990).

69. *Cruzan v Director Missouri Dept. of Health.* 110 S. Ct. 2841, 1990.
70. *Union Pacific R. Co. v Bostford.* 141 U.S. 250, 1891.
71. *Schloendorff v Society of New York Hospitals.* 211 N.Y. 125, 105 NE 92, 1914.
72. In re Quinlan, 70 N.J. 10, 355 A.2d 647(1976).
73. Kutner, L. Due process of euthanasia: The living will a proposal. *Ind. Law J.* 44:539, 1969.
74. Silverman, H. J., Vinicky, J. K., and Gasner, M. R. Advance directives: Implications for critical care. *Crit. Care Med.* 20:1029, 1992.
75. Annas, G. The health care proxy and the living will. *N. Engl. J. Med.* 324:1210, 1991.
76. Report of the Board of Trustees of the American Medical Association. *Living Wills, Durable Powers of Attorney, and Durable Powers of Attorney for Health Care.* Chicago: American Medical Association, 1989.
77. Rosenthal, E. Filling the gap where a living will won't do. *New York Times,* Jan. 17, 1991. P. B9.
78. Alper, P. R. A living will is a bloodless document. *Wall Street Journal,* January 11, 1991, P. 15.
79. Bok, S. Directions for my care. *N. Engl. J. Med.* 295:367, 1976.
80. Perk, M., and Shelp, E. E. Psychiatric consultation making moral dilemmas in medicine. *N. Engl. J. Med.* 307:618, 1982.
81. *Lane v Candura,* 6 Mass 377, 576 NE2d 1232 (1978).
82. *Barber v Superior Court,* 195 Cal 484 (1983).
83. Baron, C. H. Medical paternalism and the rule of law: A reply to Dr. Relman. *Am. J. Law Med.* 4:337, 1979.
84. Rhoden, N. Litigating life and death. *Harvard Law Rev.* 102:375, 1988.
85. Johnson, S. H. From medicalization to legalization to politicization: O'Connor, Cruzan and refusal of treatment in the 1980s. *Conn. Law Rev.* 21:685, 1989.
86. Gindes, D. Judicial postponement of death recognition: The tragic case of Mary O'Connor. *Am. J. Law Med.* 15:301, 1989.
87. Paris, J. J. Court intervention and the diminution of patients' rights: The case of Brother Joseph Fox. *N. Engl. J. Med.* 303:876, 1980.
88. Rothenberg, L. S. The empty search for an imprimatur, or Delphic oracles are in short supply. *Law Med. Health Care* 20:115, 1982.
89. Committee on the Legal and Ethical Aspects of Health Care for Children. Comments and recommendations on the "Infant Doe" proposed regulations. *Law Med. Health Care* 11:203, 1983.
90. Collins, J. Should doctors tell the truth? *Harpers* 155:320, 1927.
91. Callahan, D. Shattuck lecture: Contemporary biomedical ethics. *N. Engl. J. Med.* 302:1228, 1980.
92. Gustafson, J. Mongolism, parental desires and the right to life. *Perspect. Biol. Med.* 524:429, 1973.
93. Shaw, A., Randolph, J. G., and Manard, B. Ethical issues in pediatric surgery: A national survey of pediatricians and pediatric surgeons. *Pediatrics* 60: 588, 1977.
94. Todres, I. D., Krane, D., Howell, M. C., et al. Pediatricians' attitudes affecting decision making in defective newborns. *Pediatrics* 60:197, 1977.
95. Department of Health and Human Services. Nondiscrimination on the basis of handicap: Procedures and guidelines relating to health care for handicapped infants. *Fed. Register* 49:1622, 1984.
96. Kopelman, L. M., Irons, T. G., and Kopelman, A. E. Neonatologists judge the "Baby Doe" regulations. *N. Engl. J. Med.* 318:677, 1988.
97. *In re E. G.,* Ill. S. Ct., slip op., Nov. 13, 1989.
98. Callahan, D. Allocating health care resources. *Hastings Cent. Rep.* 18:14, 1988.
99. Regan, M. Health care rationing: A problem in ethics and policy. *J. Health Polit. Pol. Law* 14:627, 1989.
100. Callahan, D. *What Kind of a Life: The Limits of Medical Progress.* New York: Simon & Schuster, 1990.
101. Zussman, R. *Intensive Care, Medical Ethics and the Medical Profession.* Chicago: University of Chicago, 1992.
102. Schwartz, W. B., and Aaron, H. J. Rationing health care: Lessons from Britain. *N. Engl. J. Med.* 310: 52, 1983.
103. Sacred congregation for the doctrine of the faith: Declaration on euthanasia. Vatican City, 1980. In President's Commission for the Study of Ethical Problems in Medicine and Biomedical and Behavioral Research, *Deciding to Forego Life-Sustaining Treatment.* Washington, D.C.: U.S. Government Printing Office, 1983. Pp. 300-307.
104. Ruark, J. E., Raffin, T. A., and the Stanford University Medical Center Committee on Ethics. Initiating and withdrawing life support. *N. Engl. J. Med.* 318: 25, 1988.
105. Smedira, N., Evans, B. H., Grais, L. S., et al. Withholding and withdrawal of life-support from the critically ill. *N. Engl. J. Med.* 322:309, 1990.
106. Luce, J. Ethical principles in critical care. *J.A.M.A.* 263:696, 1990.
107. Department of Health and Human Services. Nondiscrimination on the basis of handicap. *Fed. Register* 48:846, 1983.
108. Committee on Bioethics, American Academy of Pediatrics. Treatment of critically ill newborns. *Pediatrics* 72:556, 1983.
109. Cranford, R. E., and Doudera, A. E. (eds.). *Institutional Ethics Committees and Health Care Decision Making.* Ann Arbor: Health Administration Press, 1984.
110. Ross, J. W., Bayley, C., Michael, V., et al. *Handbook for Hospital Ethics Committees.* Chicago: American Hospital Publishing, 1986.
111. Brennan, T. A. Ethics committees and decisions to limit care. *J.A.M.A.* 260:803, 1988.
112. Wolf, S. M. Toward a theory of process. *Law Med. Health Care* 20(4):278, 1992.
113. Cohen, C. B. Avoiding "cloudcuckooland" in eth-

ics committee case review. *Law Med. Health Care* 20(4):294, 1992.
114. Jonsen, A. R., Siegler, M., and Winslade, W. J. *Clinical Ethics.* New York: Macmillan, 1982.
115. *Superintendent of Belchertown State School v Saikewicz,* 370 NE2d 417, 1977.
116. *In the matter of Claire Conroy,* 486 A2d 1209 NJ, 1985.
117. Paris, J. J. Withholding of life-supporting treatment from the mentally incompetent. *Linacre Q.* 8:237, 1978.
118. Kubler-Ross, E. *On Death and Dying.* New York: Macmillan, 1969.
119. *Ex parte Whitebread in re Hinde,* a lunatic. *English Rep.* 35:878, 1816.
120. Rawls, J. *A Theory of Justice.* Cambridge: Harvard University Press, 1971.
121. Lynn, J., and Childress, J. F. Must patients always be given food and water? *Hastings Cent. Rep.* 13: 17, 1983.
122. Paris, J. J., and Fletcher, A. B. Infant Doe regulations and the absolute requirement to use nourishment and fluids for the dying infant. *Law Med. Health Care* 11:210, 1984.
123. Paris, J. J., and Reardon, F. E. Court responses to withholding or withdrawing artificial nutrition and fluids. *J.A.M.A.* 253:2243, 1985.
124. Curran, W. J. Defining appropriate medical care: Providing nutrients and hydration for the dying. *N. Engl. J. Med.* 313:940, 1985.
125. Applebaum, G. E., King, J. E., and Finucane, T. E. The outcome of CPR initiated in nursing homes. *J. Am. Geriatr. Soc.* 38:197, 1990.
126. Gray, W. A. Prehospital resuscitation: The good, the bad and the futile. *J.A.M.A.* 270:1471, 1993.
127. Blackhall, L. J., Ziogas, A., and Azen, S. P. Low survival rate after cardiopulmonary resuscitation in a county hospital. *Arch. Intern. Med.* 152:2045, 1992.
128. McIntyre, K. M. Cardiopulmonary resuscitation in chronically ill patients in the intensive care unit. *Arch. Intern. Med.* 152:2181, 1992.
129. Landry, F. J., Parker, J. M., and Phillips, Y. Y. Outcomes of cardiopulmonary resuscitation in the intensive care setting. *Arch. Intern. Med.* 152:2305, 1992.
130. Thompson, R. State says hospital can decide girl's fate. *Sarasota (Florida) Herald Tribune.* Feb. 26, 1994. P. 1A.

Index

Index